Y0-DKL-352

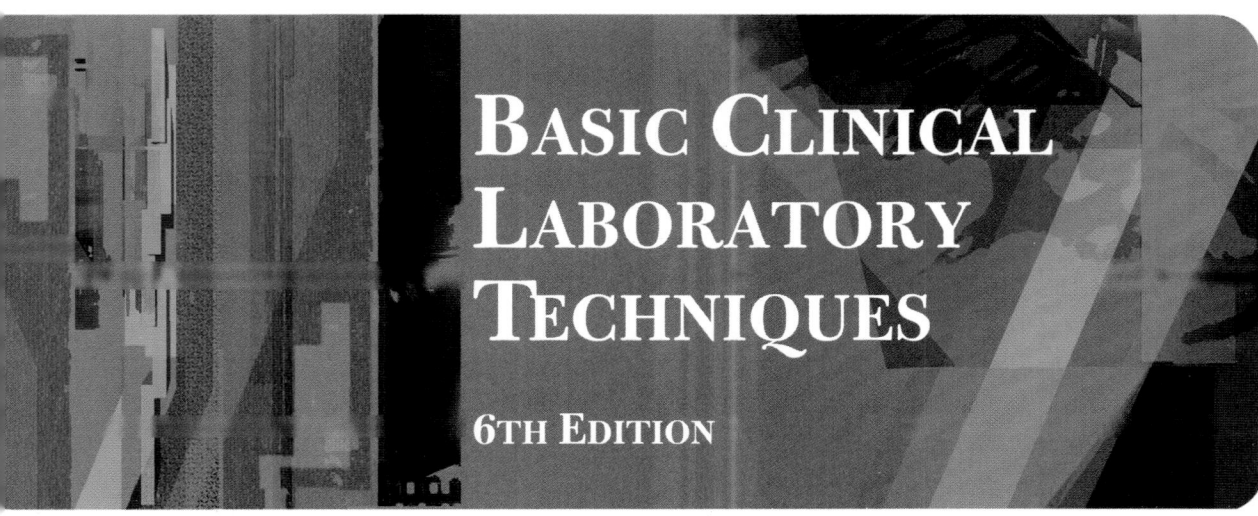

BASIC CLINICAL LABORATORY TECHNIQUES

6TH EDITION

BASIC CLINICAL LABORATORY TECHNIQUES

6TH EDITION

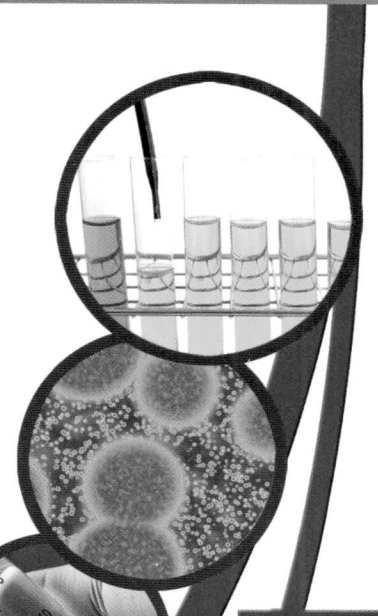

BARBARA H. ESTRIDGE, BS, MT (ASCP)

ANNA P. REYNOLDS, MS, BS, MT (ASCP)

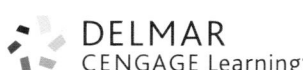

DELMAR
CENGAGE Learning·

Australia • Brazil • Japan • Korea • Mexico • Singapore • Spain • United Kingdom • United States

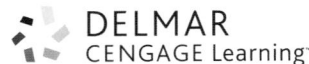
DELMAR
CENGAGE Learning

Basic Clinical Laboratory Techniques, Sixth Edition
Barbara H. Estridge and Anna P. Reynolds

Vice President, Editorial: Dave Garza

Director of Learning Solutions: Matthew Kane

Associate Acquisitions Editor: Tom Stover

Managing Editor: Marah Bellegarde

Product Manager: Natalie Pashoukos

Editorial Assistant: Anthony Souza

Vice President, Marketing: Jennifer Baker

Marketing Director: Wendy Mapstone

Senior Marketing Manager: Nancy Bradshaw

Production Manager: Andrew Crouth

Content Project Manager: Thomas Heffernan

Senior Art Director: David Arsenault

© 2012, 2008, 2000 Delmar, Cengage Learning

ALL RIGHTS RESERVED. No part of this work covered by the copyright herein may be reproduced, transmitted, stored, or used in any form or by any means graphic, electronic, or mechanical, including but not limited to photocopying, recording, scanning, digitizing, taping, Web distribution, information networks, or information storage and retrieval systems, except as permitted under Section 107 or 108 of the 1976 United States Copyright Act, without the prior written permission of the publisher.

For product information and technology assistance, contact us at
Cengage Learning Customer & Sales Support, 1-800-354-9706

For permission to use material from this text or product,
submit all requests online at **www.cengage.com/permissions**.
Further permissions questions can be e-mailed to
permissionrequest@cengage.com

Library of Congress Control Number: 2011938571

ISBN-13: 978-1-1111-3836-3

ISBN-10: 1-1111-3836-2

Delmar
5 Maxwell Drive
Clifton Park, NY 12065-2919
USA

Cengage Learning is a leading provider of customized learning solutions with office locations around the globe, including Singapore, the United Kingdom, Australia, Mexico, Brazil, and Japan. Locate your local office at:
international.cengage.com/region

Cengage Learning products are represented in Canada by Nelson Education, Ltd.

To learn more about Delmar, visit **www.cengage.com/delmar**

Purchase any of our products at your local college store or at our preferred online store **www.cengagebrain.com**

Notice to the Reader
Publisher does not warrant or guarantee any of the products described herein or perform any independent analysis in connection with any of the product information contained herein. Publisher does not assume, and expressly disclaims, any obligation to obtain and include information other than that provided to it by the manufacturer. The reader is expressly warned to consider and adopt all safety precautions that might be indicated by the activities described herein and to avoid all potential hazards. By following the instructions contained herein, the reader willingly assumes all risks in connection with such instructions. The publisher makes no representations or warranties of any kind, including but not limited to, the warranties of fitness for particular purpose or merchantability, nor are any such representations implied with respect to the material set forth herein, and the publisher takes no responsibility with respect to such material. The publisher shall not be liable for any special, consequential, or exemplary damages resulting, in whole or part, from the readers' use of, or reliance upon, this material.

Printed in the United States of America
3 4 5 6 14

DEDICATION

To our instructors for their guidance, our students for inspiration, our families for their encouragement and patience, and especially to our husbands, Ron and George, for the unconditional support they have provided through the years

CONTENTS

UNIT 6
Basic Clinical Chemistry ● 597

UNIT 7
Basic Clinical Microbiology ● 689

UNIT 8
Basic Parasitology ● 815

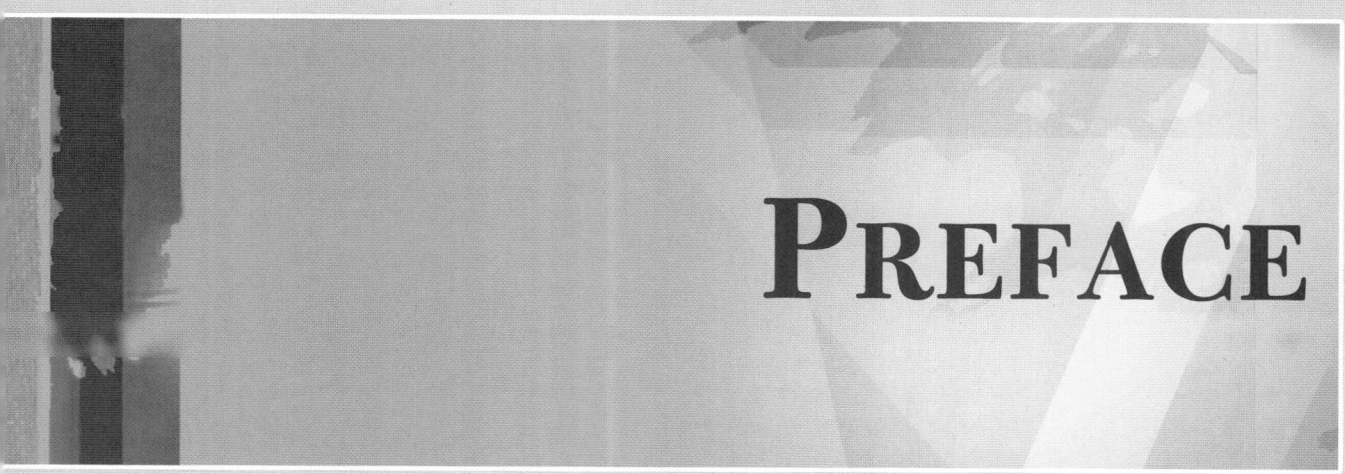

PREFACE

Basic Clinical Laboratory Techniques, 6th edition, is a performance-based text for use in allied health programs at postsecondary levels. The text is appropriate for medical laboratory technician and medical assistant programs, as well as for introductory survey courses or orientation classes in medical or clinical laboratory science. This text is also useful as a reference for personnel who perform CLIA-waived tests in point-of-care (POC) settings or physician office laboratories (POLs).

   Almost 30 years have passed since the first publication of this text, and these years have brought many advances in the field of medical laboratory science. Although this text includes only the most basic procedures, the principles, skills, and techniques presented continue to be core to understanding the more sophisticated technologies used in the clinical laboratory.

TEXT ORGANIZATION

Basic Clinical Laboratory Techniques, 6th edition, presents fundamentals of techniques used throughout the discipline of clinical laboratory science as well as an introduction to current technologies and instrumentation. The text is organized into eight units, encompassing the major departments in the clinical laboratory:

- The Clinical Laboratory
- Basic Hematology
- Basic Hemostasis
- Basic Immunology and Immunohematology
- Urinalysis
- Basic Clinical Chemistry
- Basic Clinical Microbiology
- Basic Parasitology

Unit Organization

The Unit Overview at the beginning of each unit provides a snapshot of the information contained in the unit as well as a list of references, readings, resources and web sites pertinent to that unit. Each unit is divided into several lessons.

   UNIT 1—The Clinical Laboratory, is an introduction to the field of clinical laboratory science. Information about changing trends in clinical laboratories and credentialing for laboratory personnel is included. Emphasis is placed on safe work practices such as Standard Precautions, hand hygiene techniques, use of antiseptics and disinfectants, and prevention of healthcare-associated infections (HAIs). In addition, Unit 1 presents other general knowledge used in all laboratory departments, including:

- Quality assessment policies and procedures
- Medical terminology
- Use of the metric system
- Use of general laboratory equipment
- Preparation of reagents
- Use of the clinical microscope
- Capillary and venipuncture blood collection techniques

   UNIT 2—Basic Hematology, contains introductory information about blood and hemopoiesis, the formation of blood cells. Lessons in the unit explain basic hematology principles and include procedures for hemoglobin, hematocrit, blood cell counts, white blood cell differential count, reticulocyte count, erythrocyte sedimentation rate, as well as information about hematology automation. Two lessons on blood cell morphology provide guidelines for identifying normal and abnormal blood cells.

   UNIT 3—Basic Hemostasis, explains principles of hemostasis and coagulation, discusses diseases and disorders affecting blood coagulation, and presents procedures for several coagulation tests.

UNIT 4—Basic Immunology and Immunohematology, introduces the student to the broad field of immunology. This includes immunity, antigen-antibody reactions, and types of immunological tests. Three lessons describing immunological tests introduce the student to principles used in immunology testing. Unit 4 also includes three lessons about the field of immunohematology, also called blood banking. Procedures for ABO and Rh typing are given.

UNIT 5—Urinalysis, includes an overview of the anatomy and function of the urinary system including formation of urine, urine collection methods, and procedures for performing the physical, chemical and microscopic examinations that make up the routine urinalysis.

UNIT 6—Basic Clinical Chemistry, introduces the student to the field of clinical chemistry and the many types of chemistry tests available. Lessons in the unit provide the student an opportunity to perform tests such as glucose measurement, cholesterol measurement, and the test for fecal occult blood, as well as to use various chemistry instruments.

UNIT 7—Basic Clinical Microbiology, introduces the student to four subgroups of microbiology: bacteriology, parasitology, virology and mycology. The lessons in the unit focus on procedures commonly performed in a bacteriology laboratory. Basic culture techniques are presented as well as the procedures for performing throat culture, urine culture and colony count, bacterial identification, susceptibility testing, and tests for sexually transmitted diseases (STDs). Also included is information on preventing transmission of infections in healthcare settings and information about emerging infectious diseases and biological threat agents.

UNIT 8—Basic Parasitology, is an introduction to the field of parasitology and the procedures used to identify parasitic infections. Several parasitic diseases are discussed.

Lesson Organization

Each lesson covers a specific topic or test procedure. In general, each lesson contains:

- List of learning objectives
- Glossary of important or new terms with definitions—each term is highlighted and defined when it first occurs in a lesson
- Introductory material, including principle and rationale of the procedure or test
- Safety information and reminders
- Quality assessment information and reminders
- Basic theoretical and technical information
- Current topics for enrichment
- Case studies and critical thinking questions
- Summary
- Review questions
- Suggested student activities, including web-based activities
- Student Performance Guides: Step-by-step guides to performing specific procedures, including worksheets when appropriate

NEW TO THE SIXTH EDITION

All lessons have been updated to reflect current technology and accepted practice at the time of writing. New student activities, web activities, worksheets, case studies, current topics, and critical thinking problems have been added. Other changes include:

- Numerous new tables and figures
- Expanded discussions on healthcare-associated infections, hand hygiene, and antiseptics and disinfectants
- General laboratory equipment and labware combined into one lesson
- Explanation of venipuncture procedure using winged collection sets
- Emphasis on CLSI order of draw
- Explanation of new CLSI designations for types of laboratory reagent water
- New photomicrographs of blood cells
- Explanations of two new commercial systems for manual cell counts
- New lesson on manual and automated D-dimer tests
- New lesson on coagulation instrumentation
- Comparisons of coagulation tests that use plasma with whole blood coagulation tests
- Expanded discussions on instrumentation and technologies such as nephelometry, turbidimetry, and flow cytometry.
- Two new lessons on specimen collection and processing, one in clinical chemistry and one in bacteriology
- Discussion of the H1N1 influenza pandemic of 2009–2010
- Expanded discussions on types of media for bacterial identification and antibiotic susceptibility testing
- Several new and updated current topics including
  - ○ *Clostridium difficile*
  - ○ Methicillin-resistant *Staphylococcus aureus* (MRSA)
  - ○ Healthcare-associated infections
  - ○ Infections caused by free living amebae such as *Naegleria*
  - ○ Chagas disease

Graphic icons are used throughout the test to call attention to safety, quality assessment, critical timing, critical temperatures, student activities, and use of math skills:

 Biological hazard: Use Standard Precautions

 Chemical hazard: Follow chemical safety rules

 Physical hazard: Follow safety precautions to protect from fire, electrical shock, or other physical hazards

 Critical timing: Pay careful attention to timing

 Critical temperature: Observe temperature requirements

Quality Assessment: Follow quality assessment policies and techniques

 Math: Use basic math skills

 Web-based activity: Use Internet to explore additional learning opportunities

 Critical thinking: Apply principles from the lesson(s) to make a decision or solve a problem

INSTRUCTOR RESOURCES

An Instructor Resources CD accompanying the sixth edition of *Basic Clinical Laboratory Techniques* contains:

- Instructor's Manual, including
  - ○ Lesson plans
  - ○ Answers to review questions
  - ○ Answers to case studies and critical thinking problems
  - ○ Answers to worksheets (when applicable)
- ExamView test bank with more than 1700 questions
- More than 800 PowerPoint Slides
- Student Performance Guides, Worksheets and Report Forms
- Resources such as references, pertinent web sites, and a list of healthcare-related agencies, societies, and organizations that are relevant to medical laboratory science
- A Laboratory Supply and Equipment List is provided for instructor use and shows the methods, instruments, and test supplies suggested for teaching the lessons

The *Instructor's Manual* contains the unit overviews and lists of objectives for each unit, as well as lesson plans for each lesson. Each lesson plan includes lesson objectives, glossary terms with definitions, list of teaching aids and resources, lesson content outline, student learning activities, web activities, and answers to case studies, critical thinking problems, review questions, and worksheets (when possible). It is not possible to provide answers to web activities, student performance guide activities, report forms or several of the worksheets because the students' results will vary depending on the samples provided to them and the resources available in their laboratories.

The test bank contains more than 1,700 questions (and answers) in multiple choice, matching, fill-in-the-blank (completion), problem, and true/false formats. The test bank is in ExamView software, and allows the instructor to mix and match questions to customize a printable test form, as well as to modify questions or add their own questions to the test bank. Also included are more than 800 PowerPoint slides to assist with classroom presentations, and downloadable, printable versions of the Student Performance Guides, Worksheets, and Report Forms.

- Instructor Resources CD (ISBN: 978-1-1111-3838-7)

ADDITIONAL STUDENT RESOURCES

To access additional course materials including CourseMate, please visit www.cengagebrain.com. At the CengageBrain.com home page, search for the ISBN of your title (from the back cover of your book) using the search box at the top of the page. This will take you to the product page where these resources can be found.

CourseMate

The CourseMate that accompanies *Basic Clinical Laboratory Techniques, Sixth Edition* helps you make the grade.

CourseMate includes:

- An interactive eBook, with highlighting, note taking and search capabilities
- Interactive learning tools including:
  - ○ Quizzes
  - ○ Flashcards
  - ○ PowerPoint slides
  - ○ Glossary
  - ○ and more!

CourseMate

- Printed Access Card (ISBN: 978-1-1337-3232-7)
- Instant Access Code (ISBN: 978-1-1337-3231-0)

ACKNOWLEDGMENTS

We are indebted to our many editors, colleagues, friends, and family members who have provided technical advice, encouragement, and support throughout this project. Since the first edition of this book came to life approximately 30 years ago, this list has continued to grow.

In particular, we would like to thank our Delmar, Cengage Learning editorial and production staff for their guidance and assistance with this edition: Natalie Pashoukos, Product Manager, Sherry Dickinson, Senior Acquisitions Editor, and Tom Stover, Associate Acquisitions Editor. We also wish to thank those individuals who reviewed the manuscript and offered valuable feedback and suggestions:

Angela R. Bell, M.S., MT(ASCP) SM, DLM
Associate Professor and MLT Program Director
Tidewater Community College
Virginia Beach, Virginia

Mary Elizabeth Browder, M. Ed.
Associate Professor
Raymond Walters College|UC Blue Ash
Cincinnati, Ohio

Patricia A. Chappell, M.A. B.S. MT (ASCP)
Allied Health Coordinator
Camden County College
Blackwood, New Jersey

Ernest Dale Hall, MA Ed. MT(ASCP)
Clinical Coordinator and Instructor MLT/PBT
Southwestern Community College
Sylva, North Carolina

Karen Golemboski, Ph.D., MT(ASCP)
Associate Professor, Medical Laboratory Science
Bellarmine University
Louisville, Kentucky

Additionally, we would like to thank the following companies and individuals for providing images, image processing, or access to enhance this edition:

Abbott Laboratories, Abbott Park, IL

Alpha Scientific, Malvern, PA

Bayer Healthcare Diagnostic Division, Norwood, MA

Beckman Coulter, Fullerton, CA

Becton Dickinson and Co., Franklin Lakes, NJ

Bio/Data Corporation, Horsham, PA

BioMedical Polymers, Gardner, MA

bioMérieux, Durham, NC

Biosite, Inc., San Diego, CA

BioTek Instruments, Inc., Winooski, VT

Brevis Corporation, Salt Lake City, UT

Bridgman, R., Hybridoma Facility, Auburn University, AL

Centers for Disease Control and Prevention, Atlanta, GA

Estridge, A., Warner Studios, Los Angeles, CA

HemoCue Inc., Lake Forest, CA

Hycor Biomedical Inc., Garden Grove, CA

ITC, Edison, NJ

Metrika Inc., Sunnyvale, CA

Mitchell Plastics, Inc., Norton, OH.

Nova Biomedical, Waltham, MA

Quidel Corporation, San Diego, CA

Remel, Inc., Lenexa, KS

Roche Diagnostics Corp., Indianapolis, IN

Scientific Device Lab, Des Plaines, IL

Smith's Medical ASD, Inc., Keene, NH

StatSpin, Inc., Norwood, NJ

Sundermann, C. A., Auburn University, AL

Sysmex America, Inc., Mundelein, IL

West, K. M., Medical and Laboratory Technology Program, Auburn University, AL

NOTE TO THE READER

Clinical laboratory science is a rapidly changing field. Instruments and test methods are constantly being improved, modified, and updated. We have performed extensive research to ensure that the information in this work is complete, accurate, and up-to-date. However, because of the possibility of human error and the time lapse between writing and publication, no guarantee can be given that the information contained herein is accurate in every respect by the time this text is published. The authors, publishers, and all other parties involved in this work disclaim all responsibility for errors and/or omissions in this work. Students, instructors, and others who use this work are encouraged to consult other appropriate sources to confirm information. It is especially important to follow established safety guidelines, to always read and follow the operating manuals for the particular instrument being used, and to consult the instructions and package inserts that accompany the reagents and test kits being used. Questions, comments, or suggestions can be made to the authors by contacting the publisher.

Barbara H. Estridge, BS, MT (ASCP)
Anna P. Reynolds, MS, BS, MT (ASCP)

HOW TO USE THIS BOOK

Basic Clinical Laboratory Techniques, 6th edition, is organized into eight units, each containing several lessons that all follow the same format. Each lesson contains learning objectives listing the key points you will learn or procedures you will master, a glossary of new terms, lesson content, review questions, student activities, and, in most cases, a student performance guide or worksheet. In the lesson content, the subject is introduced, the procedure is explained, safety and quality issues are emphasized, and the lesson is summarized. In addition, most lessons include case studies, critical thinking problems, and current topics. These features are described below.

OBJECTIVES

Review the objectives at the beginning of each lesson to understand the overall purpose and salient points to be learned in the lesson.

GLOSSARY

The glossary contains terms that might be new and that are critical to understanding the lesson material. Look for the glossary words in **bold** font the first time they are used and defined in a lesson.

LESSON CONTENT

Introduction. The introduction gives a brief overview of the lesson and leads into the principle and performance of a procedure.

Principle and Procedure. Lessons covering a particular test procedure describe the procedure principle and explain how to perform the test. Reference ranges, test interpretation, and clinical significance of the tests are given.

Icons. Look for icons throughout the text and in the Student Performance Guides. The icons are to remind you of procedures or situations that require extra attention to safety, quality assessment, timing, temperature considerations, math skills, critical thinking, or procedural details.

  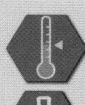 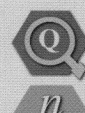 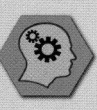

Quality Assessment. Quality Assessment (QA) information reminds you of the importance of following the specified procedure when performing tests. The QA sections emphasize specimen collection and processing, correct analytical technique, instrument maintenance, and use of control materials to achieve reliable test results.

Case Studies and Critical Thinking Problems. Case studies and critical thinking problems present problem-solving situations such as might be encountered in daily laboratory work. These give you a chance to apply your knowledge to a practical situation.

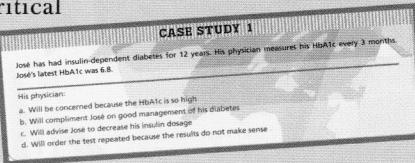

xv

Current Topics. Current Topics are scattered throughout the text. They offer more in-depth information about topics of current interest in medical laboratory science, such as stem cells, diabetes, leukemia, and drug-resistant strains of bacteria.

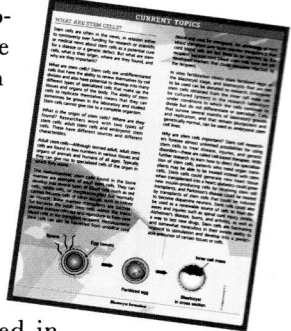

Safety Precautions. Safety Precautions are included in each lesson to call attention to biological, chemical, or physical hazards that might be present when performing the procedure described in the lesson.

Reminders. Procedural reminders and safety reminders at the end of the lessons reinforce important quality and safety issues to remember before beginning a laboratory procedure.

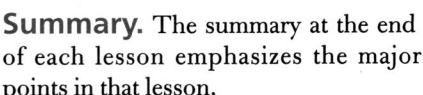

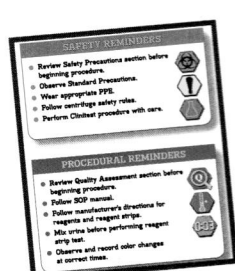

Summary. The summary at the end of each lesson emphasizes the major points in that lesson.

REVIEW QUESTIONS

Review questions are provided to test your understanding of the lesson. If you are unable to answer some of the questions after studying the lesson, the material should be reviewed.

STUDENT ACTIVITIES AND WEB ACTIVITIES

Student activities help you practice skills and expand knowledge. Through various web activities you learn to use reliable web sites to find valuable, up-to-date information from a variety of online resources.

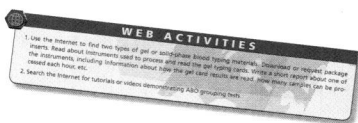

STUDENT PERFORMANCE GUIDES

Student Performance Guides contain step-by-step instructions for laboratory procedures. Icons are included to remind of safety and other considerations that must be kept in mind while performing the procedure. A list of materials you will need to perform the procedure is also included. The Guides provide a chance to practice most procedures until you are proficient enough to have the instructor evaluate your performance.

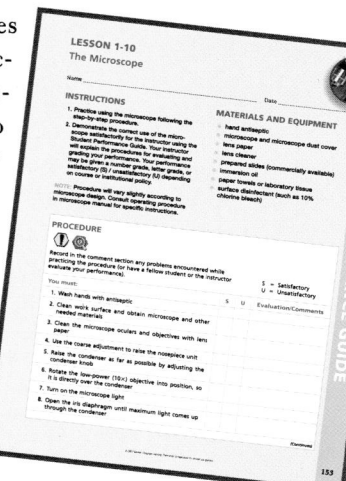

UNIT 1

The Clinical Laboratory

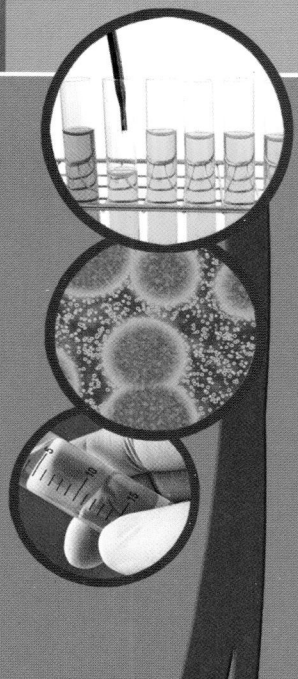

UNIT OBJECTIVES

After studying this unit, the student will:

- Discuss the regulation, organization, and function of the clinical laboratory.
- Discuss the qualifications, job functions, and ethical responsibilities of clinical laboratory personnel.
- Identify and define selected abbreviations and acronyms commonly used in the clinical laboratory.
- Identify, define, and use prefixes, suffixes, and stems in selected medical terms.
- Discuss and implement laboratory safety rules that must be followed to guard against chemical, physical, and biological hazards.
- Identify common types of labware and demonstrate their correct uses.
- Discuss and demonstrate safe use of general laboratory equipment.
- Use the metric system to perform measurements and calculations.
- Use laboratory math to prepare simple laboratory reagents.
- Discuss the importance and use of quality assessment programs in the clinical laboratory.
- Use the compound bright-field microscope.
- Perform a capillary puncture.
- Perform a venipuncture.

The clinical laboratory is a place where blood, body fluids, and other biological specimens are tested, analyzed, or evaluated. The observations can be qualitative or quantitative. The tests can be performed manually or using automated analyzers. Precise measurements are made, and the results are calculated and interpreted. Because of this, laboratory workers must have the skills necessary to perform a variety of tasks.

Unit 1 is an introduction to the laboratory environment as a workplace and to the profession of clinical laboratory science, also called medical laboratory science. Key concepts and procedures laboratory professionals need to know to work in the laboratory are described in the introductory unit.

The regulation, organization, and function of the clinical laboratory are addressed in Lesson 1-1. Qualifications and job functions of laboratory personnel are reviewed in Lesson 1-2.

As an introduction to the structure of medical terms, Lesson 1-3 gives basic information about medical terminology and abbreviations and acronyms used in the laboratory. As other units are studied, additional vocabulary terms will be introduced and defined.

Two lessons on laboratory safety (Lessons 1-4 and 1-5) are included in Unit 1 because workers must understand and follow all safety procedures and practices before any laboratory exercises can be performed. Every worker in the clinical laboratory must be thoroughly aware of potential hazards in the workplace and must perform tasks in a manner that keeps them, coworkers, and patients safe.

The correct and safe use of general laboratory equipment such as centrifuges, pH meters, autoclaves, and laboratory balances is described in Lesson 1-6. Also explained is the care, use, and cleaning of frequently used labware such as beakers, cylinders, test tubes, and flask.

Because laboratory analyses use metric units, a brief introduction to the metric system is given in Lesson 1-7. Knowledge of the metric system is required for exercises in other units.

Basic laboratory math, methods of reagent preparation, and the correct use of pipets are explained in Lesson 1-8.

Principles, methods, and procedures for ensuring the reliability and accuracy of laboratory analyses are presented in Lesson 1-9. These quality assessment principles are included in Unit 1 because they must be integrated into all aspects of laboratory operations, from employee training and evaluation to specimen collection and processing, specimen analysis, and interpretation and reporting of results.

The proper care and use of the microscope is included in Unit 1 (Lesson 1-10) because knowledge of its use is required for lessons in the microbiology, hematology, urinalysis, and parasitology units. Lessons 1-11 and 1-12 introduce techniques for collecting capillary and venous blood.

Unit 1 is an introduction to the techniques, rules, and skills needed to perform the exercises in Units 2 through 8. Unit 1 can also be used alone as an introduction to the profession of clinical laboratory science. After Unit 1 has been completed, the remaining units can be studied in order of the instructor's preference depending on available time, laboratory space, and equipment.

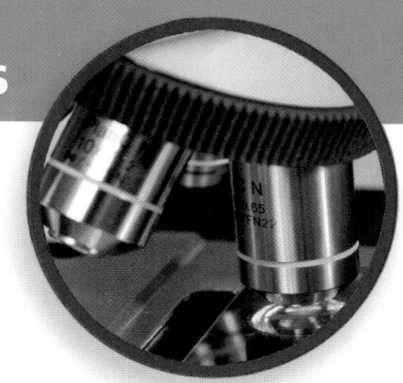

General—Clinical Laboratory Science

Baker, F. J., et al. (2001). *Baker & Silverton's introduction to medical laboratory technology*. (7th ed.). Oxford, UK: Oxford University Press.

Burtis, C. A., et al. (Eds.). (2005). *Tietz textbook of clinical chemistry and molecular diagnostics*. (4th ed.). Philadelphia: W. B. Saunders Company.

Clinical Laboratory Improvement Amendments of 1988. (1992). In *Federal Register, 57*(40): 7001–7288.

Karni, K. (2002). *Opportunities in clinical laboratory science*. Lincolnwood, IL: VGM Career Books, McGraw-Hill.

Laposata, M. (1992). *SI unit conversion guide*. Boston: NEJM Books.

Lindh, W. Q., et al. (2009). *Delmar's comprehensive medical assisting*. (4th ed.). Clifton Park, NY: Delmar Cengage Learning.

McPherson, R.A. & Pincus, M.R. (Eds.) (2007). *Clinical diagnosis & management by laboratory methods*. (21st ed.). Philadelphia: Saunders Elsevier.

Simmers, L. (2004). *Diversified health occupations*. (6th ed.). Clifton Park, NY: Thomson Delmar Learning.

Turgeon, M. L. (2006). *Linné and Ringsrud's clinical laboratory sciences: The basics and routine techniques*. (5th ed.). St. Louis: Mosby

Westgard, J. O. (2002). *Basic QC practices*. (2nd ed.). Washington, DC: AACC Press.

Medical Terminology

Chabner, D. (Ed.). (2005). *The language of medicine*. (7th ed.). Philadelphia: W. B. Saunders Company.

Dennerll, J. T. (2006). *Medical terminology made easy*. (4th ed.). Clifton Park, NY: Delmar Cengage Learning.

Dorland, W. A. N. (Ed.). (2011). *Dorland's illustrated medical dictionary*. (32nd ed.). Philadelphia: W. B. Saunders Company.

Ehrlich, A. & Schroeder, C. L. (2003). *Medical terminology for health professions*. (4th ed.). Clifton Park, NY: Thomson Learning.

Sormunen, C. (2009). *Terminology for health professionals*. (6th ed.). Clifton Park, NY: Delmar Cengage Learning.

Venes, D. (Ed.). (2009). *Taber's cyclopedic medical dictionary*. (21st ed.). Philadelphia: F. A. Davis Company.

Phlebotomy

Hoeltke, L. B. (2006). *The complete textbook of phlebotomy*. (3rd ed.). Clifton Park, NY: Thomson Delmar Learning.

Kalanick, K. (2004). *Phlebotomy technician specialist*. Clifton Park, NY: Thomson Delmar Learning.

Turgeon, M. L. (2011). *Clinical hematology theory & procedures*. (5th ed.). Hagerstown, MD: Lippincott Williams & Wilkins.

Safety

American Hospital Association, Division of Quality Resources. (1992). OSHA's final bloodborne pathogens standard: A special briefing.

Centers for Disease Control and Prevention. (1987). Recommendations for prevention of HIV transmission in healthcare settings. *Morbidity and Mortality Weekly Report, 36*(Suppl. 25):3S–18S.

Centers for Disease Control and Prevention. (2002). Guidelines for hand hygiene in health care settings. *Morbidity and Mortality Weekly Report, 51*(No. RR-16):1–45.

Centers for Disease Control and Prevention and National Institutes of Health. (2005). *Biosafety in microbiological and biomedical laboratories*. (5th ed.). Washington, D.C.: U.S. Government Printing Office. Available free online at www.cdc.gov/biosafety/publications/bmbl5/index.htm

Joint Advisory Notice; Department of Labor/Department of Health and Human Services; HBV/HIV. (1982). In *Federal Register, 52*(210):41818–41823.

Longtin, Y., et al. (2011). Videos in Clinical Medicine: Hand Hygiene. N Engl J Med 2011:364;e24. March 31, 2011. http://www.nejm.org/doi/full/10.1056/NEJMvcm0903599

March 2006, brochure #6. DHHS: CMS/CDC. Clinical Laboratory Improvement Amendments (CLIA): How to Obtain a Certificate of Waiver.

Occupational Safety and Health Administration. Occupational exposure to bloodborne pathogens, final rule, labor. In *Federal Register, 56*(235): Rules and regulations. Often referred to as 29 CFR Part 1910.0130.

Occupational Safety and Health Administration. (1987). Hazard communication, labor. In *Federal Register, 52*(163): 31852–31886.

Occupational Safety and Health Administration. (1999). How to prevent needlestick injuries: Answers to some important questions. (Publication 3161). Washington, D.C.: U.S. Department of Labor.

OSHA Publications. Safety pamphlets. Available online at www.osha.gov.

Safety Alert Network. OSHA-compliant safety training programs. Available online at www.safetyalert.com.

Safety sense: A laboratory guide. (2001). Cold Spring Harbor, NY: Cold Spring Harbor Laboratory Press.

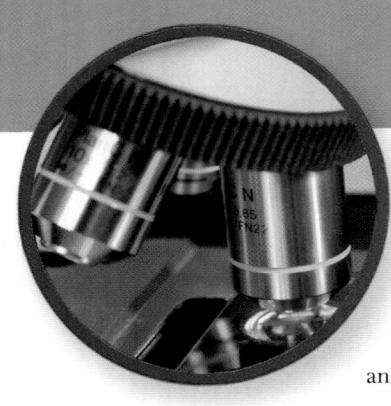

Web Sites of Interest

Association for Professionals in Infection Control and Epidemiology, www.apic.org

Centers for Disease Control and Prevention, www.cdc.gov

Center for Phlebotomy Education, www.phlebotomy.com

Clinical Laboratory Improvement Amendments, www.cma.gov/clia/

Federal Drug Administration, www.fda.gov

National Institute for Occupational Safety and Health, www.cdc.gov/NIOSH

National Institutes of Health, www.nih.gov

Occupational Safety and Health Administration, www.osha.gov

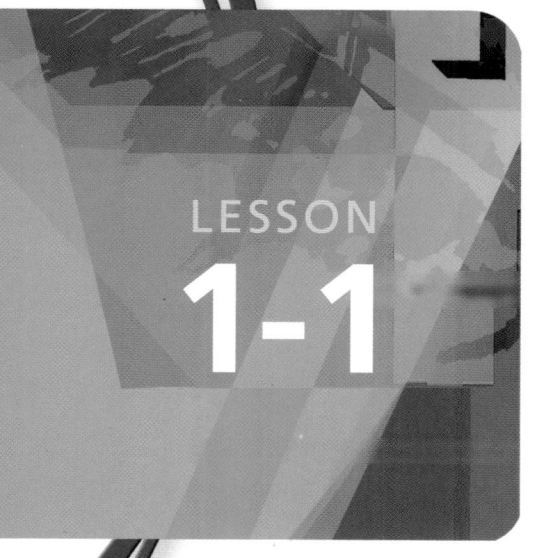

LESSON 1-1

Introduction to the Clinical Laboratory

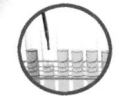

LESSON OBJECTIVES

After studying this lesson, the student will:

⊙ Explain the function of a medical or clinical laboratory.

⊙ Discuss the organization of a typical hospital clinical laboratory.

⊙ Describe the functions of the different levels of laboratory personnel.

⊙ List the major departments of a typical clinical laboratory and name a test that would be performed in each department.

⊙ List three examples of nonhospital clinical laboratories and describe the function of each.

⊙ Explain how clinical laboratories are regulated.

⊙ Explain the relationships between Centers for Medicare and Medicaid Services (CMS), Clinical Laboratory Improvement Amendments of 1988 (CLIA '88), and clinical laboratories.

⊙ Discuss benefits of point-of-care (POC) testing.

⊙ Explain how the Health Insurance Portability and Accountability Act (HIPAA) affects the laboratory and laboratory workers.

⊙ Discuss the use and value of electronic health records (EHRs).

⊙ Describe the purpose and scope of quality assessment programs in the clinical laboratory.

⊙ Explain the reason for proficiency testing.

⊙ Explain the purpose of laboratory accreditation.

⊙ Define the glossary terms.

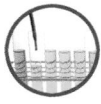

GLOSSARY

accessioning / the process by which specimens are logged in, labeled, and assigned a specimen identification code

accreditation / a voluntary process in which an independent agency grants recognition to institutions or programs that meet or exceed established standards of quality

American Association of Blood Banks (AABB) / international association that sets blood bank standards, accredits blood banks, and promotes high standards of performance in the practice of transfusion medicine

anticoagulant / a chemical or substance that prevents blood coagulation

bacteriology / the study of bacteria

blood bank / clinical laboratory department where blood components are tested and stored until needed for transfusion; immunohematology department; transfusion services; also the refrigerated unit used for storing blood components

(continues)

Centers for Disease Control and Prevention (CDC) / central laboratory for the national public health system

Centers for Medicare and Medicaid Services (CMS) / the agency within the Department of Health and Human Services (DHHS) responsible for implementing CLIA '88

Clinical and Laboratory Standards Institute (CLSI) / an international, nonprofit organization that establishes guidelines and standards of best current practice for clinical laboratories; formerly National Committee for Clinical Laboratory Standards (NCCLS)

clinical chemistry / the laboratory section that uses chemical principles to analyze blood and other body fluids

Clinical Laboratory Improvement Amendments of 1988 (CLIA '88) / a federal act that specifies minimum performance standards for clinical laboratories

coagulation / the process of forming a fibrin clot

College of American Pathologists (CAP) / organization that offers accreditation to clinical laboratories

COLA / agency that offers accreditation to physician office laboratories, hospitals, clinics, and other healthcare facilities; formerly the Commission on Office Laboratory Accreditation

Department of Health and Human Services (DHHS) / the governmental agency that oversees public healthcare matters; also called HHS

electronic health record (EHR) / comprehensive, portable electronic patient health record

electronic medical record (EMR) / a digital form of a patient chart created in a physician's office or a hospital where a patient received treatment

epidemiology / the study of the factors that cause disease and determine disease frequency and distribution

Food and Drug Administration (FDA) / the division of the Department of Health and Human Services (DHHS) responsible for protecting the public health by ensuring the safety and efficacy of foods, drugs, biological products, medical devices, and cosmetics

Health Care Financing Administration (HCFA) / see Centers for Medicare and Medicaid Services (CMS)

hematology / the study of blood and the blood-forming tissues

HIPAA / Health Insurance Portability and Accountability Act of 1996

immunohematology / the study of the human blood groups; in the clinical laboratory, often called blood banking or transfusion services

immunology / the branch of medicine encompassing the study of immune processes and immunity

Joint Commission (JC) / an independent agency that accredits hospitals and large healthcare facilities; formerly known as the Joint Commission on Accreditation of Healthcare Organizations (JCAHO)

Laboratory Response Network (LRN) / a nationwide network of public and private laboratories coordinated by the Centers for Disease Control and Prevention (CDC) with the ability for rapid response to threats to public health

microbiology / the branch of biology dealing with microbes

mycology / the study of fungi

National Committee for Clinical Laboratory Standards (NCCLS) / see Clinical and Laboratory Standards Institute (CLSI)

pathologist / a physician specially trained in the nature and cause of disease

phlebotomist / a healthcare worker trained in blood collection

physician office laboratory (POL) / small medical laboratory located within a physician office, group practice, or clinic

plasma / the liquid portion of blood in which the blood cells are suspended; the straw-colored liquid remaining after blood cells are removed from anticoagulated blood

point-of-care testing (POCT) / testing outside the traditional laboratory setting; also called bedside testing, off-site testing, near-patient testing or alternative-site testing

proficiency testing (PT) / a program in which a laboratory's accuracy in performing analyses is evaluated at regular intervals and compared to the performance of similar laboratories

Provider-Performed Microscopy Procedure (PPMP) / a certificate category under CLIA '88 that permits a laboratory to perform waived tests and also permits specified practitioners to perform on-site microscopy procedures

quality assessment (QA) / in the laboratory, a program that monitors the total testing process with the aim of providing the highest-quality patient care

reference laboratory / an independent regional laboratory that offers routine and specialized testing services to hospitals and physicians

serology / the study of antigens and antibodies in serum using immunological methods; laboratory testing based on the immunological properties of serum

serum / the liquid obtained from blood that has been allowed to clot

standard operating procedure (SOP) / established procedure to be followed for a given operation or in a given situation with the purpose of ensuring that a procedure is always carried out correctly and in the same manner

virology / the study of viruses

waived test / a category of test defined under CLIA '88 as being simple to perform and having an insignificant risk for error

INTRODUCTION

Laboratories that perform chemical and microscopic tests on blood, other body fluids, and tissues are called *clinical* or *medical laboratories*. These laboratories play a major role in patient care and are found in a variety of settings, both government and private. A clinical laboratory can be in a large institution, offer sophisticated services, and employ many highly trained workers who interact daily with patients and other allied health personnel in the institution. Clinical laboratories can also be small, with only one or two employees.

Today clinical laboratories as well as other healthcare delivery systems face a variety of challenges. These include coping with rapidly rising costs, maintaining quality personnel, keeping up with advancing technologies, and complying with increased governmental regulations. These issues must be addressed without sacrificing the quality of patient care. This lesson describes the types of clinical laboratories and their organization, function, and regulation.

REGULATION OF CLINICAL LABORATORIES

All clinical laboratories that perform tests on human specimens (except for research laboratories) are regulated by both federal and state agencies. The **Clinical Laboratory Improvement Amendments of 1988 (CLIA '88)**, a revision of the Clinical Laboratory Improvement Act of 1967, specifies minimum performance standards for all clinical laboratories. The objective of CLIA '88 is to improve and ensure the quality of laboratory testing. Even though CLIA was passed in 1988, the amendments have been continually revised, updated, clarified, refined, and strengthened.

The Division of Laboratory Services, under the **Centers for Medicare and Medicaid Services** (**CMS**, www.cms.gov/clia/) has the responsibility for implementing CLIA '88. All clinical sites that perform laboratory tests on humans must register and obtain a certificate from the CMS to be legally allowed to operate. Under CLIA '88, laboratories are classified as performing:

- Waived tests
- Tests of moderate and high complexity
- **Provider-performed microscopy procedures (PPMP)**

The classifications are based on the difficulty or complexity of the test procedures and the level of training required to accurately perform the tests. Laboratory personnel standards differ for each of these categories. The more complex the test, the more highly trained the testing personnel must be. Each laboratory must obtain a certificate stating its classification.

States can enact their own regulations regarding the operation of laboratories. However, state standards must be at least as stringent as federal regulations and must not violate or counteract federal regulations.

TYPES OF CLINICAL LABORATORIES

Clinical laboratories can be placed into two groups: hospital laboratories and nonhospital laboratories. Although most people think of hospitals when they think of clinical laboratories, laboratories can also be in clinics, group practices, physician offices, nursing homes, veterinary offices, government agencies, industry settings, and military installations. Some clinical laboratories, such as regional reference laboratories, are independent from medical facilities that provide direct patient care.

In December 2010, the **Department of Health and Human Services (DHHS)**, Centers for Medicare and Medicaid Services (CMS), formerly known as the **Health Care Financing Administration (HCFA)**, listed more than 221,000 private and commercial laboratories as providing services to humans in the United States. This number does not include laboratories limited to research or veterinary laboratories.

Table 1-1 lists the numbers of CMS-registered clinical laboratories by type of facility. From the pie chart shown in Figure 1-1, it can be seen that more than half of the registered laboratories are in physician office laboratories (POLs). Although far more laboratories are in the POL category than in any other category, hospital and reference laboratories perform the overwhelming majority of laboratory tests. CMS data show that more than 60% of registered laboratories perform only waived tests. However, these account for only about 10% of the total test volume.

Hospital Laboratories

Clinical laboratories are found in private hospitals, university teaching hospitals, and government-operated institutions such as military hospitals and veterans' hospitals. The clinical laboratory is one of many hospital departments (Figure 1-2). The level of

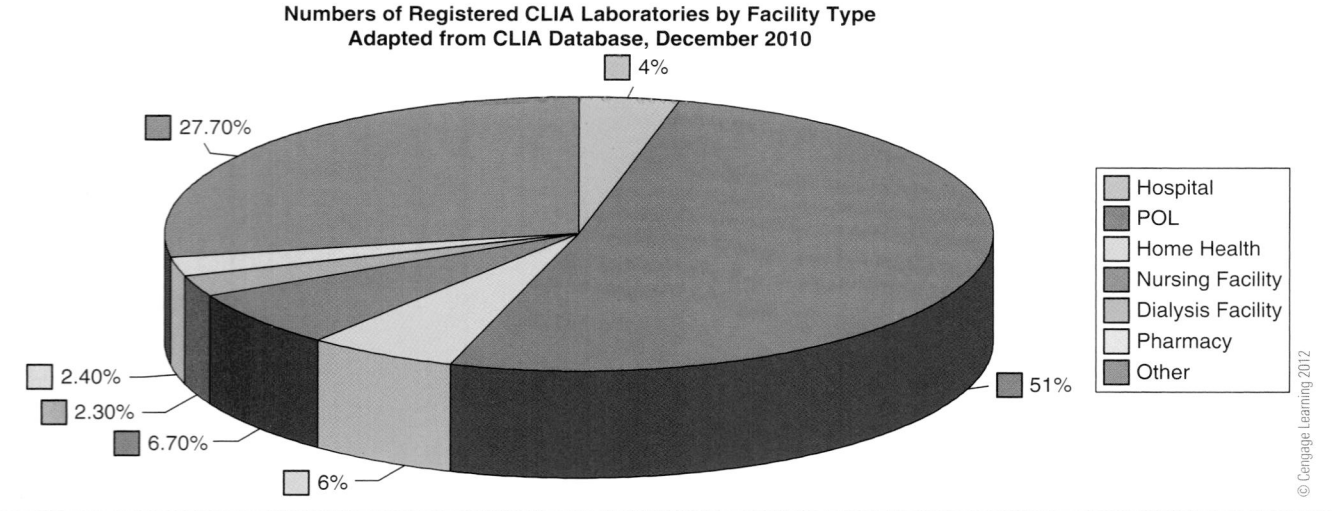

Numbers of Registered CLIA Laboratories by Facility Type
Adapted from CLIA Database, December 2010

- Hospital
- POL
- Home Health
- Nursing Facility
- Dialysis Facility
- Pharmacy
- Other

4%
27.70%
2.40%
2.30%
6.70%
6%
51%

© Cengage Learning 2012

FIGURE 1-1 Pie chart showing registered CLIA laboratories by facility type (Adapted from CMS, CLIA database, December 2010)

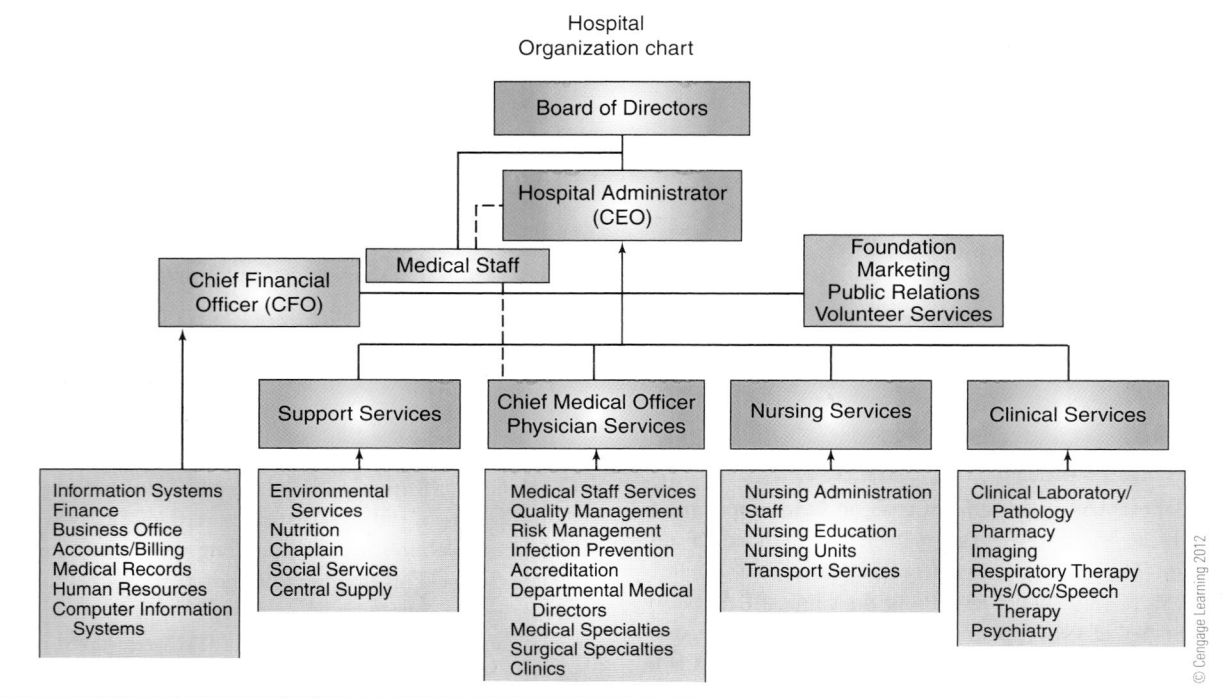

Hospital
Organization chart

Board of Directors

Hospital Administrator
(CEO)

Chief Financial
Officer (CFO)

Medical Staff

Foundation
Marketing
Public Relations
Volunteer Services

Support Services

Chief Medical Officer
Physician Services

Nursing Services

Clinical Services

Information Systems
Finance
Business Office
Accounts/Billing
Medical Records
Human Resources
Computer Information
Systems

Environmental
Services
Nutrition
Chaplain
Social Services
Central Supply

Medical Staff Services
Quality Management
Risk Management
Infection Prevention
Accreditation
Departmental Medical
Directors
Medical Specialties
Surgical Specialties
Clinics

Nursing Administration
Staff
Nursing Education
Nursing Units
Transport Services

Clinical Laboratory/
Pathology
Pharmacy
Imaging
Respiratory Therapy
Phys/Occ/Speech
Therapy
Psychiatry

© Cengage Learning 2012

FIGURE 1-2 Example of a hospital organizational chart

services available from a hospital laboratory is usually determined by the size of the hospital. A laboratory in a small hospital (fewer than 100 beds) performs primarily routine test procedures; complicated or infrequently requested tests are sent to reference laboratories.

In a clinical laboratory in a medium-size hospital (up to 300 beds), routine tests as well as many more complicated test procedures are performed. Only the most recently developed tests, infrequently requested tests, or tests with high levels of complexity or requiring special instrumentation need to be sent to reference laboratories. Clinical laboratories in large hospitals

(more than 300 beds) handle large volumes of work and perform complex tests (Figure 1-3).

Nonhospital Clinical Laboratories

Nonhospital clinical laboratories can be publicly (government) or privately operated. They provide a variety of services and employment for many skilled workers. In the United States in 2010, the majority of registered clinical laboratories were in nonhospital settings (Table 1-1).

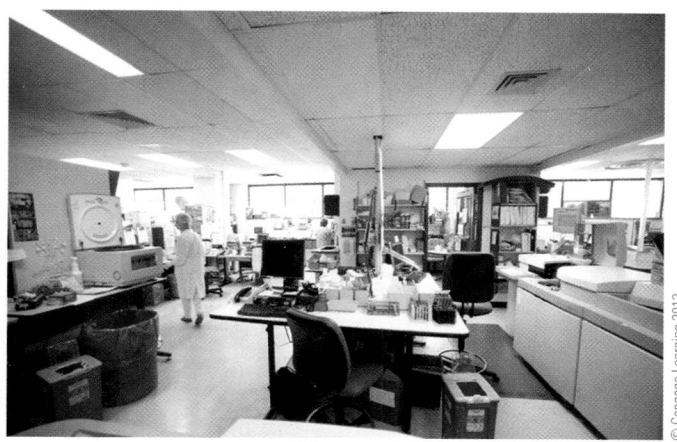

© Cengage Learning 2012

FIGURE 1-3 A clinical laboratory in a large hospital

Physician Office Laboratories

Physician office laboratories (POLs) are laboratories in a physician's office or physicians' group practice. In 2010, more than half of all CMS-registered clinical laboratories were classified as POLs. The increased availability of rapid-test kits and small, easy-to-operate analyzers has broadened the scope of testing in the POL. Several laboratory tests, such as hemoglobin, hematocrit, urine reagent strip, urine pregnancy test, blood glucose, and occult blood, are classified as **waived tests** (Table 1-2) and can be performed in the POL by multiskilled personnel such as medical assistants. As defined by CLIA, waived tests are simple laboratory tests and procedures that "have an insignificant risk of an erroneous result." The **Food and Drug Administration (FDA)** determines which tests meet the criteria of being simple and with low risk for error. The FDA currently lists over 100 analytes for which waived tests are available.

Reference Laboratories

Reference laboratories are usually privately owned, regional laboratories that do high-volume testing and offer a wide variety of tests. Large hospitals use reference laboratories primarily to perform complex or infrequently ordered tests. Small hospitals or physicians' offices use their services for a wide range of tests. Reference laboratories provide courier service to transport specimens from the collection site to the testing laboratory.

Government Laboratories: Federal

The central laboratory for the national public health system is the **Centers for Disease Control and Prevention (CDC)** in Atlanta, Georgia. This agency provides consulting services to state public health laboratories and to individual physicians in unique cases. The CDC provides educational materials and safety guidelines for workers in a variety of healthcare areas, as well as for the general public.

Epidemiology is another important function of the CDC. Data are gathered concerning the origin, distribution, and occurrence of various diseases, and outbreaks are investigated to

determine the causes. This function of the CDC has gained much public attention because of its role in investigating emerging infectious diseases and multidrug resistant microbes that have appeared worldwide in recent years.

The CDC also coordinates the **Laboratory Response Network (LRN)**. This laboratory network was established to ensure that state and private laboratories are equipped to respond effectively to threats to public health, such as biological or chemical bioterrorism events, emerging infectious diseases, or natural disasters.

TABLE 1-1. Numbers and types of CLIA-registered clinical laboratories performing tests on humans, December 2010. (Source: Adapted from Division of Laboratory Services, CMS/CLIA Database)

TYPE OF LABORATORY	NUMBER
Ambulance	3687
Ambulatory surgical center	5051
Community clinic	6376
Comprehensive outpatient rehabilitation facility	313
Ancillary testing site in healthcare facility	2849
Renal dialysis facility	5044
Health fair	616
Health maintenance organization	672
Home health agency	13,433
Hospice	2378
Hospital	8731
Independent	5357
Industrial	1820
Insurance	55
Intermediate care/mentally handicapped	1195
Mobile laboratory	1592
Pharmacy	5412
School/student health facility	2049
Skilled nursing facility/nursing facility	14,831
Physician office	113,124
Other practitioner	3209
Tissue bank/repository	69
Blood bank	457
Rural health clinic	1570
Federally qualified health center	1109
Assisted living facility	987
Prison	210
Public health laboratory	526
Other	19,071
Total	**221,793**

TABLE 1-2. Examples of analytes* for which there are CLIA waived tests (as published by FDA, 2010)

Hemoglobin by copper sulfate

Hemoglobin by single instrument with direct readout

Blood glucose by meters cleared for home use

Glycated hemoglobin (HbA1c)

Fecal occult blood

Lyme disease antibodies

HIV antibodies

Spun hematocrit

Ovulation tests by color comparison

Urine pregnancy tests by visual color comparison

Urine qualitative dipstick tests

Microalbumin

Rapid strep test from throat swab

Erythrocyte sedimentation rate

Immunoassay for *Helicobacter pylori*

Prothrombin time

Fructosamine

Cholesterol; high-density lipoprotein (HDL) and low-density lipoprotein (LDL) cholesterol

Infectious mononucleosis antibodies

* This list contains only a few of the more than 100 analytes for which waived tests are available. A complete up-to-date list can be found on the FDA web site, www.fda.gov

TABLE 1-3. Types of certificates issued under CLIA '88 and the activity(ies) each certificate permits

CERTIFICATE	ACTIVITY PERMITTED
Certificate of Waiver (COW)	Permits a laboratory to perform only CLIA-waived tests
Certificate of Registration	Permits the laboratory to conduct moderate- or high-complexity laboratory testing (or both) until the laboratory is determined by survey to be in compliance with CLIA regulations
Certificate of Compliance (COC)	Issued to a laboratory operating under a certificate of registration after an inspection finds the laboratory to be in compliance with all applicable CLIA regulations
Certificate of Accreditation (COA)	Issued to a laboratory that has been accredited by a CMS-approved accrediting organization and allows moderate- and high-complexity testing
Certificate for PPMP	Allows a physician, mid-level practitioner, or dentist to perform only select permitted microscopy procedures but no other tests of complexity; this certificate also permits the laboratory to perform waived tests

Government Laboratories: State

Each U.S. state and territory has a clinical laboratory operated (usually) by the state's department of public health. These state laboratories provide testing and consulting services to hospitals, physicians, and clinics within the state.

Services available from state laboratories vary from state to state. In general, state laboratories perform tests mandated by state regulations, for example, premarital blood tests and phenylketonuria (PKU) testing of newborns. State laboratories also offer tests not routinely available in other laboratories such as culture of fungi, viruses, and mycobacteria (which include the pathogens causing tuberculosis); tests for parasites; confirmatory tests for reportable infectious diseases such as HIV infection; and some environmental testing. Special-case specimens to be sent to the CDC for testing are usually sent via state public health laboratories.

CLIA CERTIFICATE CATEGORIES

The five CLIA certificate categories are (1) Certificate of Waiver, (2) Certificate for PPMP, (3) Registration Certificate, (4) Certificate of Compliance, and (5) Certificate of

Accreditation. Table 1-3 explains conditions under which each certificate would be issued.

Under CLIA '88, laboratories with a certificate of waiver can only perform waived tests, tests determined to be simple, to have insignificant risk for error, and to pose no harm or risk to patient if the test is performed incorrectly. Many of the tests in this category began as tests that could be performed at home, such as glucose testing, or home pregnancy tests. (Examples of some analytes for which there are waived tests are listed in Table 1-2.) Because of advances in technology, the number and types of waived tests have increased, and the number of laboratories performing waived tests has grown tremendously since CLIA '88 implementation.

Laboratories with a PPMP certificate perform microscopy-based tests during the course of a patient visit on specimens that are not easily transportable. Examples of PPMP include urine microscopic examination and wet mounts.

Most POLs perform only waived tests; others perform more complex (nonwaived) tests. Most hospital laboratories perform moderate- to high-complexity tests. Laboratories performing moderate- to high-complexity tests must have a certificate of registration, compliance, or accreditation. These laboratories must also adhere to mandated personnel guidelines, comprehensive recordkeeping, and quality assessment programs; participate in proficiency testing programs; and be subject to government inspections.

ORGANIZATION OF THE HOSPITAL LABORATORY

The organization schemes of most hospital laboratories follow a general outline (Figure 1-4) that can vary slightly depending on the size of the laboratory. In recent years, some laboratories have changed department and personnel titles to reflect the terminology used in the CLIA '88 rules. Table 1-4 lists personnel titles as stated in CLIA '88 and gives the commonly used equivalent titles. The personnel qualifications for each category are specified in the Clinical Laboratory Improvement Amendments of 1988, Final Rule (*Federal Register*, Vol. 7, No. 40, February 28, 1992).

Clinical Laboratory Personnel

Laboratory Director

The director of the hospital laboratory has customarily been a **pathologist**, a physician specially trained in the nature and cause of disease. Hospital pathologists usually oversee two branches of pathology, anatomical pathology and clinical pathology. The anatomical pathology department includes cytology, histology, and autopsy services. The clinical laboratory department can also be called clinical pathology or clinical laboratory services.

Under CLIA '88, persons other than pathologists can qualify to be clinical laboratory director. The type of CMS certificate held by the laboratory determines the qualifications for a director. In general, the laboratory director must be licensed by the state in which the laboratory operates; hold the degree of doctor of medicine, doctor of osteopathy, or an earned doctorate in a related

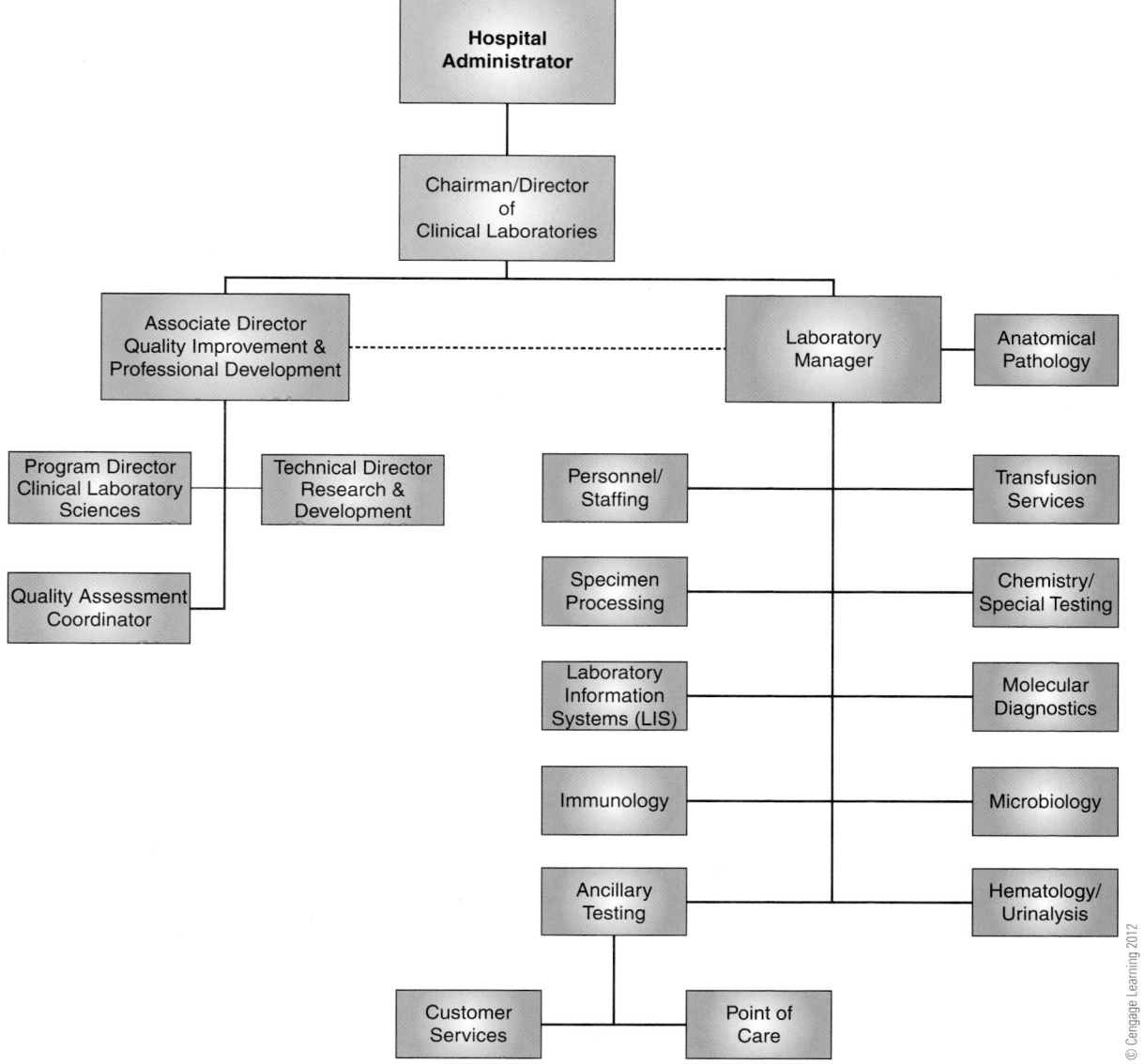

© Cengage Learning 2012

FIGURE 1-4 Organizational chart of a typical hospital laboratory

TABLE 1-4. Titles of clinical laboratory personnel as listed in CLIA '88 Final Rule and commonly used equivalent titles

CLIA '88 JOB TITLE	EQUIVALENT JOB TITLE
Laboratory director	Laboratory director (usually a pathologist)
Technical supervisor	Laboratory manager
	Chief technologist
Clinical consultant	Consultant
Technical consultant or general supervisor	Department head
	Section head
	Section supervisor
	Technical specialist
Testing personnel	Medical technologist
	Medical laboratory scientist
	Clinical laboratory scientist
	Medical laboratory technician
	Clinical laboratory technician
	Laboratory assistant

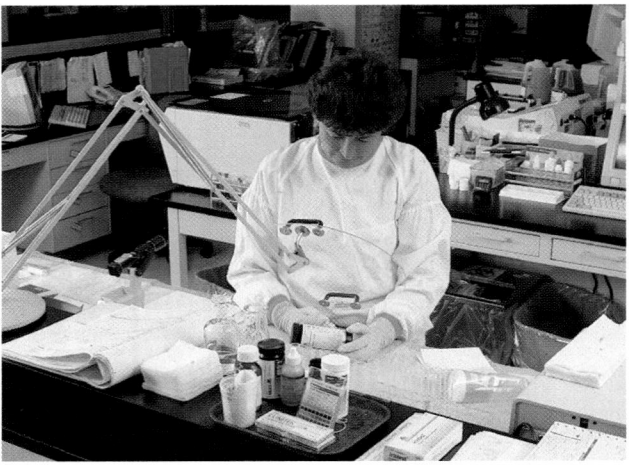

© Cengage Learning 2012

FIGURE 1-5 A clinical laboratory professional at work

clinical field; hold certification from an appropriate body; and have supervisory and clinical laboratory experience. The laboratory director has ultimate responsibility for all laboratory operations.

Small hospitals might not have a full-time pathologist on staff or on-site. Depending on the qualifications of the laboratory director, laboratories in these hospitals can be required to contract with certified individuals to serve as *clinical consultants* and *technical consultants*. These consultants assist the laboratory director in matters of test appropriateness and interpretation or in technical matters relating to test methods.

Technical Supervisor and Laboratory Manager

Directly under the laboratory director's authority is the technical supervisor or laboratory manager (Figure 1-4). This is someone educated in the clinical laboratory sciences with additional business or management training or experience.

The technical supervisor (laboratory manager) is responsible for the day-to-day operation of the laboratory. The technical supervisor is also responsible for setting personnel standards, establishing training and evaluation procedures, establishing appropriate quality assessment programs, observing and documenting employee performance and competence, and making sure that all regulatory mandates are followed.

The technical supervisor is responsible for making available to all personnel an up-to-date procedure manual containing detailed instructions for every procedure performed in the laboratory. This is called the **standard operating procedure (SOP)** manual. The **Clinical and Laboratory Standards Institute (CLSI)** develops standards of current best practice for clinical laboratory procedures. Laboratory procedure manuals must follow CLSI standards, and the manual must be reviewed

and updated at specified intervals. (CLSI was formerly known as the **National Committee for Clinical Laboratory Standards**, or **NCCLS**, until their name change in 2005.)

General Supervisor and Department Head

Each department has a general supervisor or department head responsible for the quality of work performed in the department, training employees, and evaluating employee performance. General supervisors report to the technical supervisor.

Testing Personnel

Testing personnel perform the laboratory analyses (Figure 1-5). These include medical technologists, medical laboratory scientists, clinical laboratory scientists, medical laboratory technicians, and clinical laboratory technicians. Nonlaboratory personnel such as medical assistants and nursing staff often perform tests in POLs and point-of-care testing or testing in other settings outside the laboratory proper. Clinical laboratory personnel qualifications are discussed in Lesson 1-2, The Clinical Laboratory Professional.

Departments of the Clinical Laboratory

The number of departments in clinical laboratories varies. Clinical chemistry, hematology, microbiology, blood bank, and support services (phlebotomy and specimen processing) usually operate as departments or sections, each with its own department head or general supervisor (Figure 1-4). The subdivisions within each department differ from one laboratory to another. Large laboratories often have separate departments for urinalysis, coagulation, immunology, and parasitology.

Hematology

Most **hematology** tests involve studying the cellular components of blood. Hematology procedures can be qualitative or quantitative. The *quantitative* procedures include counts of the various blood components, such as the number of leukocytes (white blood cells), erythrocytes (red blood cells), or platelets; hemoglobin and hematocrit tests are commonly performed and can aid in diagnosis of anemia. These tests can be performed manually but are usually performed on a cell counter or hematology analyzer. Many analyzers are capable of performing several hematological procedures simultaneously.

In *qualitative* procedures, blood components are observed for qualities such as cell size, shape, and maturity. Using a microscope, a laboratory worker can view a blood smear to determine the types of leukocytes present; estimate the size, shape, and hemoglobin content of erythrocytes; or estimate the number of platelets. Cell abnormalities, including immature leukocytes or erythrocytes, are noted during microscopic examination of the blood smear.

In large laboratories, complicated tests such as special stains to classify leukemic cells might be performed in a hematology section called *special hematology*. Some tests in special hematology are performed manually.

Coagulation. Coagulation tests are used to diagnose and monitor patients who have defects in their blood-clotting mechanism or are being treated with **anticoagulants**, drugs that prevent blood coagulation. Coagulation tests can be performed in the hematology department or, in large laboratories, in a separate department. Automated coagulation testing systems, which were once used primarily in larger laboratories, are now available in small, easy-to-use models that allow even small POLs to have the capability of performing some coagulation procedures. **Plasma**, the liquid portion of anticoagulated blood, is the specimen used for most coagulation studies.

Urinalysis. Like coagulation, urinalysis can be a separate department in a large laboratory or a subdivision of another department, usually hematology or chemistry. In the urinalysis department, physical, chemical, and microscopic examinations of urine specimens are performed. These tests can be performed manually or using automated methods.

Clinical Chemistry

In the **clinical chemistry** department, test procedures can be performed on plasma, serum, urine, and other body fluids such as spinal fluid and joint fluid. **Serum** is the liquid part of blood remaining after a clot has formed. Serum is obtained by collecting blood without anticoagulant, allowing it to clot, and centrifuging it to separate blood cells from the serum. Many chemistry analyzers can perform assays using plasma; this eliminates the time delay required for blood to clot if serum is used.

Clinical chemistry is the largest department in most laboratories. Procedures performed in the clinical chemistry department include blood glucose, cholesterol, assays of heart and liver enzymes, and electrolytes (chloride, bicarbonate, potassium, and sodium). Common subdepartments in clinical chemistry are *special chemistry* and *toxicology*. Procedures such as electrophoresis and measurement of hormone levels are performed in special chemistry. In toxicology, blood or urine can be analyzed to determine the drug involved in an overdose or blood levels of prescribed drugs.

The types of chemistry analyzers have increased rapidly in the last several years (see Lessons 6-3 and 6-4). Many of these analyzers provide a wide range of test procedures yet are relatively simple to operate. Thus, it is possible for even the smallest laboratory to perform some routine chemistry tests.

Immunology

Immunology can be a separate department or, in small laboratories, a part of another department such as blood bank or microbiology. In the past, this department was called **serology** because serum was the specimen most often used in the tests. In the immunology department, many tests are based on antigen-antibody methods. Among tests performed in this section are those for pregnancy, arthritis, and autoimmune diseases. Tests for infectious mononucleosis, HIV infection, influenza, hepatitis, sexually transmitted diseases, and other infectious diseases are also performed using immunological methods.

Blood Bank/Transfusion Services

The **blood bank** department is also called **immunohematology** or transfusion services. Procedures performed in this department are critical to patient well-being. If a transfusion is required, the patient's ABO group and Rh type are determined by blood bank technologists. Before blood is transfused, stored components of donor blood are tested for compatibility with patient blood. The blood bank department might also have the capability to collect special blood donations or process donated blood into specialized components. The blood bank is the only area of the clinical laboratory for which there are no waived tests.

Microbiology

The **microbiology** department is responsible for culturing and identifying microorganisms.

Bacteriology. **Bacteriology** procedures make up the majority of the work in microbiology. Bacteria can be isolated from specimens such as sputum, wounds, blood, urine, or other body fluids by inoculating the specimen to culture media. Organisms that grow in the culture are identified, and susceptibility tests are performed to determine the most effective antibiotic treatment. This is done by exposing the bacterial culture to different antibiotics and observing their effect on the organism's growth. Automated systems that can detect growth of an organism, identify an organism, and determine its antibiotic susceptibility are widely used in bacteriology.

Virology and Mycology. Procedures involving **virology**, the study of viruses, and **mycology**, the study of fungi, are usually performed in the microbiology department. Often specimens for virology and mycology are sent to a **reference laboratory** for culture and identification. Because cultures of pathogenic fungi as well as mycobacteria must be handled with special care, specimens suspected of containing these organisms are usually inoculated to media and then sent to a reference laboratory for identification.

Parasitology. In parasitology, usually a part of the microbiology department, patient specimens are examined for parasites. Fecal samples are examined microscopically for evidence of intestinal parasites such as intestinal ameba, tapeworms, or hookworms. Immunological tests are performed to detect parasite antigens in fecal samples. Tests for blood parasites, such as the malarial parasite, are usually performed in the hematology department.

Laboratory Support Services

Laboratory tests begin with the laboratory request form, which must be completed before the test is performed. This can be a written request (Figure 1-6) or a computer-generated request. After the request is received, the laboratory will begin the test process—collecting the specimen; performing the test; and interpreting, recording, reporting, and charting results.

FIGURE 1-6 Example of a laboratory request form

The form shown includes the following sections and elements:

MID AMERICA CLINICAL LABORATORIES

STAT ☐

BILL TO:
☐ DOCTORSOFFICE
☐ INSURANCE
☐ PATIENT

PATIENT INFORMATION - PLEASE PRINT
PATIENT NAME (LAST)
(FIRST)
BIRTH DATE (MM/DD/YYYY)   SEX   PATIENT SOCIAL SECURITY #
OFFICE/PATIENT ID#   PATIENT PHONE #
PRINT NAME OF INSURED/RESPONSIBLE PARTY (LAST, FIRST, MIDDLE) - IF OTHER THAN PATIENT
PATIENT ADDRESS (OR INSURED/RESPONSIBLE PARTY)   APT. #
CITY   STATE   ZIP

REFERRED BY

DATE COLLECTED   TIME   AM PM   TOTAL VOL/HRS.   ML   HR   ☐ Fasting

REQUIRED - COPY OF BOTH FRONT AND BACK OF INSURANCE CARD. IF NOT AVAILABLE COMPLETE BELOW SECTION
RELATIONSHIP TO INSURED: ☐ SELF   ☐ SPOUSE   ☐ DEPENDENT

U.P.I.N. REFERRING PHYSICIAN AND FULL NAME

INSURANCE PRIMARY/SECONDARY
INSURANCE CO. NAME
MEMBER / INSURED ID#   GROUP REQUIRED
INSURANCE ADDRESS
CITY   STATE   ZIP
INSURED EMPLOYER NAME REQUIRED
INSURED SOCIAL SECURITY # (if not patient)   INSURED BIRTH DATE (MM/DD/YYYY)

ICD9 DIAGNOSIS CODE(S) FOR TESTS ORDERED (MUST BE PROVIDED)

☐ Call Results to: (   )   ☐ Fax Results to: (   )
Send Duplicate Report to:
MACL Client # OR NAME: _____
ADDRESS: _____
CITY: _____ STATE: ____ ZIP: _____

Medicare Limited Coverage Tests
@ = May not be covered for the reported diagnosis.
F = Has prescribed frequency rules for coverage.
& = A test or service performed with research/experimental kit.
B = Has both diagnosis and frequency-related coverage limitations

PANELS

Code	Panel	
34392	ELECTROLYTE PANEL: (Na, K, Cl, CO2)	S
10165	BASIC METABOLIC PANEL: (Na, K, Cl, CO2, Glu, BUN, Creat, Ca)	S
10256	HEPATIC FUNCTION PANEL: (Alb, DBili,TBili, AlkP, AST, ALT, TP)	1-S
10306 @	ACUTE HEPATITIS PANEL: (Hep. B Core AB IgM, Hep. B Surface AG*, Hep. C AB*, Hep. A AB IgM)	S
20210	OBSTETRIC PANEL: (CBC with Dif, Hep. B Surface AG, RPR*, Rubella IgG, ABO & Rh, Antibody Screen*)	P,R,L,S
7573 @	IRON STUDIES: (Iron, TIBC, UIBC, %Sat.)	S
7600 B	LIPID PANEL: (TChol, Trig, HDL, calc LDL)	S
10231	COMP METABOLIC PANEL: (Na, K, Cl, CO2, Glu, BUN, Creat, Ca. TP, Alb, TBili, AlkP, AST, ALT)	S
10314	RENAL PANEL: (Alb, Ca, CO2, Cl, Creat, Glu, Phos, K, Na, BUN)	S

INDIVIDUAL TESTS

Code	Test	
7788	ABO GROUP & RH TYPE	P
223	ALBUMIN	S
234	ALKALINE PHOSPHATASE	S
823	ALT (SGPT)	S
243	AMYLASE	S
795	ANTIBODY SCN* REFLEX	P
249	ANTINUCLEAR AB (ANA)*	S
265	ASO, QUANT	S
822	AST, (SGOT)	S

Code	Test	
285	BILIRUBIN, DIRECT	1-S
287	BILIRUBIN, TOTAL	1-S
4420	C-REACTIVE PROTEIN	S
29256 @	CA125	S
303	CALCIUM	S
310	CARBON DIOXIDE (CO2)	S
1759 @	CBC w/Plt & Indices	L
6399	CBC w/Plt, Indices and Diff	L
978 B	CEA	S
330	CHLORIDE (CL)	S
334 B	CHOLESTEROL, TOTAL	S
374 @	CK, TOTAL	S
375	CREATININE	S
418 @	DIGOXIN	R
457 @	FERRITIN	S
466	FOLIC ACID	S
470	FSH	S
483 B	GLUCOSE	S
484 B	GLUCOSE, FASTING	S
8477	GLUCOSE, GESTATION SCREEN	S
29407 @	H PYLORI IgG AB QL	S
8435	HCG, QUAL SERUM	S
8396 B	HCG, QUANT SERUM	S
608 B	HDL	S
509	HEMATOCRIT	L
510 @	HEMOGLOBIN	L
7998 @	HEMOGLOBIN AND HEMATOCRIT	L
496 B	HEMOGLOBIN A1C	L
512	HEP A AB IgM	S
4848	HEP B Core AB IgM	S

Code	Test	
498	HEP B SURFACE AG* REFLEX	S
8472	HEP C AB* REFLEX	S
6449 B	HIV SCREEN * REFLEX	S
	CONSENT ON FILE	
571 @	IRON	S
593	LDH	S
599	LEAD (BLOOD)	1
615	LH	S
622 @	MAGNESIUM	S
654	MONO SCREEN	S
718	PHOSPHORUS	S
723 @	PLATELET COUNT	L
733	POTASSIUM (K)	S
754	PROTEIN, TOTAL	S
5363 B	PSA DIAGNOSTIC	S
10157 F	PSA MEDICARE SCREEN	S
8847 B	PT WITH INR	1-B
763 @	PTT, ACTIVATED	1-B
4418	RHEUMATOID FACTOR	S
36126	RPR* REFLEX	S
802	RUBELLA IgG	S
5780	RUBELLA, IgG PRE-MARITAL	S
836	SODIUM (Na)	S
809	SED RATE	L
867 B	T-4, (THYROXINE)	S
866 B	T-4, FREE	S
873	TESTOSTERONE	S
896 B	TRIGLYCERIDES	S
899 B	TSH	S
294	UREA NITROGEN (BUN)	S

Code	Test	
905	URIC ACID	S
7909	URINALYSIS, *REFLEX	X
5463	URINALYSIS, COMPLETE	X
6448	URINALYSIS, Dipstick Only	X
8563	URINALYSIS, Microscopic	X
927	VITAMIN B12	S
937 @	WBC	S

MICROBIOLOGY
ADDITIONAL CHARGE FOR ID AND SUSCEPTIBILITIES
SOURCE:

Code	Test
389	Culture, Blood
4550	Culture, Aerobic
4469	Culture, Anaerobic Reflex
4446	Culture, Aerobic/Anaerobic (includes gram stain)
4558	Culture, Genital (Bacterial)
4485	Culture, Gp. A Strep (Throat)
5617	Culture, Gp. B Strep (Vag/Rect)
2692	Culture, Fungus
395 @	Culture, Herpes Rapid
6649	Culture, Routine Urine
8756	Culture, Stool
8502	C difficile Toxin A Screen
8501	DNA Probe, Chlamydia
6919	DNA Probe, GC
497	Chlamydia & GC DNA probe
681	Gram Stain
	Parasite Exam (O&P)

(*) Indicates additional reflex testing will be performed if indicated

COLLECTION COMMENTS
R = Red Top Tube
L = Lavender Top
B = Lt. Blue Top
P = Pink Tube
S = Serum Separator Tube
1 = Consult Service Manual
CY = Ur. Preservative Tube

STANDING ORDERS
Begin Date: _____ End Date: _____
FREQUENCY: _____
☐ ORIGINATING ORDER   ☐ RECURRENT ORDER

CODE	ADDITIONAL TESTS	CODE	ADDITIONAL TESTS	
				TOTAL TESTS ORDERED

COMMENTS, CLINICAL INFORMATION:

Physician Signature

For any patient of any payor (including Medicare and Medicaid) that has a medical necessity requirement, you should only order those tests which are medically necessary for the diagnosis and treatment of the patient.

© Cengage Learning 2012

Most hospital laboratories have a separate department responsible for collecting and processing specimens. This department is called by a variety of names such as support services, phlebotomy, or specimen collection and processing. **Phlebotomists** are the specially trained laboratory personnel who collect the blood specimens; sometimes this responsibility is shared by nursing personnel.

In small laboratories, specimens are usually taken directly to the appropriate laboratory department. Many hospitals have pneumatic delivery systems that provide rapid delivery of specimens to the laboratory from the patient room, nursing station, outpatient clinic, surgery, emergency room, or intensive care unit.

In larger laboratories, specimens are delivered to a central **accessioning** area where they are processed, logged into the computer using the barcodes on their labels (Figure 1-7), and given a *specimen identification code* before being distributed to the departments for testing. High-volume laboratories use robotic specimen processing systems, automated systems that perform many of the manipulations usually performed by laboratory personnel. Actions that can be automated include accessioning; sorting according to test ordered and preparation required; centrifugation; decapping, labeling, and aliquoting specimens; and transporting to testing instruments or storage. Robotic systems increase efficiency, improve specimen integrity, reduce errors, and contribute to personnel safety by reducing exposure to the specimen.

Laboratory Information Systems

Large laboratories have integrated laboratory information systems (LIS) that improve efficiency and reduce errors. In hospitals, the LIS can be linked into the institution-wide computer system. Computerization in the laboratory and hospital has reduced errors in specimen identification and tracking. Specimens are labeled with preprinted bar-coded labels that match bar-coded test requisitions and patient identification bracelets. Data can be entered directly into the computer system using bar-code scanners. Even small laboratories usually have a system for preprinting bar-coded specimen labels with patient data. Advantages of laboratory information systems include:

- Elimination of charting errors
- Improved efficiency
- Automatic identification of abnormal or unusual test results
- Matching of patient specimens to test results
- Prevention of unauthorized testing and reporting

Point-of-Care Testing

Rapid advancements in technology make possible rapid changes in all aspects of health care. One of the major changes in the clinical laboratory has been the implementation and increased use of **point-of-care testing (POCT)**. POCT brings the laboratory test to the patient rather than obtaining a specimen from the patient and transporting it to the laboratory for testing. This makes laboratory test results available more rapidly, providing improved patient care.

POCT is commonly used in settings such as clinics, health maintenance organizations (HMOs), nursing homes, home health care, physician offices, emergency departments, intensive care units, and surgery suites. POCT is also referred to as bedside testing, near-patient testing, off-site testing, or alternative-site testing.

The evolution of small, simple-to-use analyzers that provide rapid results has led to widespread POCT implementation. Handheld portable analyzers can measure substances such as hemoglobin, glucose, cholesterol, and electrolytes, and results can be directly uploaded to the central LIS. Most POC analyzers require only a drop of blood, usually obtained by fingerstick. The majority of nonhospital POCT tests are CLIA-waived.

The emergence and growth of POCT has created the opportunity for more collaboration between the laboratory and other members of the healthcare team. Although nonlaboratory personnel from the nursing service, surgery, or emergency department teams can perform the tests, the laboratory is usually responsible for selecting instrumentation, training personnel, developing procedure manuals, and monitoring quality assessment procedures and instrument maintenance.

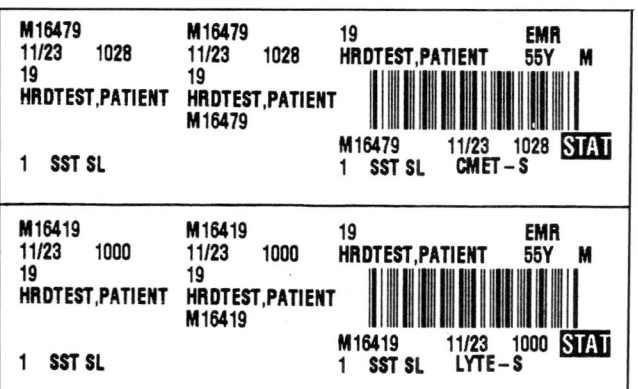

© Cengage Learning 2012

FIGURE 1-7 Use of bar codes and patient identification numbers allows computer accessioning and reduces pre-analytical errors

QUALITY ASSESSMENT IN THE LABORATORY

For many years, clinical laboratories have had programs in place to monitor the quality of laboratory results. These program requirements expanded under CLIA '88 and associated legislation. All laboratories now must have comprehensive programs to evaluate, monitor, and improve overall laboratory performance. These programs have evolved through many changes, beginning as quality control (QC), progressing to quality assurance and broader programs such as total quality management (TQM) and continuous quality improvement (CQI). The name recommended by CMS is **quality assessment (QA)**, part of a comprehensive quality system (QS). In this text the symbol is used to emphasize quality assessment considerations in a method or activity.

CURRENT TOPICS

ELECTRONIC HEALTH RECORDS (EHRs)

Information technology (IT) is an integral part of all facets of our lives, so it is not surprising that health information is going "electronic." One section of the 1996 HIPAA (the Administrative Simplification provisions) requires that national standards for sharing electronic health information be established, with special attention to ensuring the privacy and security of personal health data. The overall intent of the provisions is to improve patient care and healthcare efficiency and reduce healthcare costs.

Electronic Medical Records vs. Electronic Health Records: What is the difference?

Many physicians and hospitals have been using electronic medical records (EMRs) for years. An EMR is a digital form of a patient chart created in a physician's office or a hospital where a patient received treatment (Figure 1-8). Hospital EMRs allow physicians, surgeons, and specialists to easily monitor test results and changes in a patient's condition while they are hospitalized. However, the hospital electronic record does not follow patients when they are discharged and return to the care of their personal physician. The EMR remains in the hospital or medical practice where the record originated. Physicians on a hospital's medical staff can have remote access to view a patient's hospital records, but the records remain hospital property and responsibility. If a patient requires a copy of their medical record, or a specialist requires information from a primary care physician, the medical record will still have to be printed to be shared.

Patient care and the efficiency of healthcare delivery can be improved by making it possible to easily share health information. Unlike EMRs, electronic health records (EHRs) are comprehensive digital records that give a broad view of a patient's health. EHRs contain information compiled from all physicians and facilities involved in a patient's care over time.

Benefits of EHRs

EHRs are designed to be constantly updated, portable, and accessible by all who provide patient care, and also by the patient. An EHR can travel with the patient, allowing electronic sharing of patient medical information with specialists, laboratories, and other healthcare providers, whether in the same practice or across the country.

The use of EHRs instead of paper records to store health information is expected to:

- Allow better coordination of patient care, especially in emergency, life-threatening situations
- Improve follow-up care after hospitalization
- Maintain comprehensive up-to-date information about a patient's health in one file
- Provide a secure way to share patient information over the Internet
- Motivate patients to comply with health recommendations, because they will be able to access their own records and follow their progress
- Reduce medical errors
- Aid in more rapid diagnoses
- Prevent duplicate testing because records are instantly updated
- Reduce costs and storage space required to maintain paper records

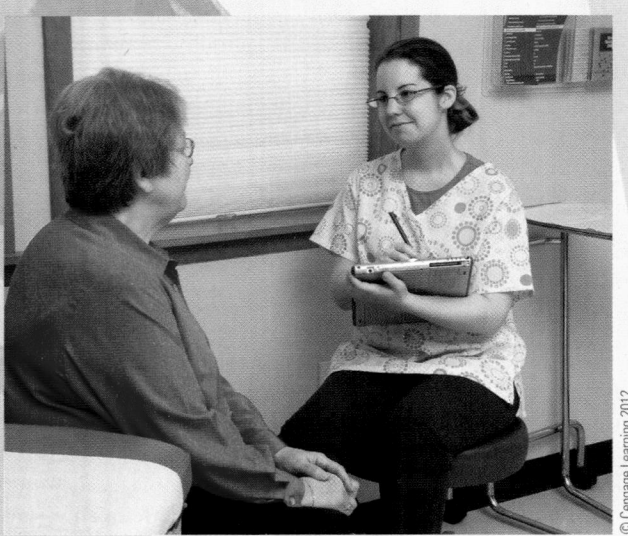

© Cengage Learning 2012

FIGURE 1-8 Using an electronic notepad to record patient medical history allows an electronic medical record to be created in a physician's office

(continues)

CURRENT TOPICS (Continued)

- Simplify compilation of records from multiple sources
- Lower healthcare costs by increasing efficiency and reducing paperwork

EHR Concerns

Several hurdles must be overcome before the use of EHRs is accepted by the general public and implemented nationwide.

- Systems must be developed that ensure adequate patient confidentiality; privacy and security standards must be stringent
- Format(s) must be designed that allow easy exchange between different electronic record systems
- EHR authenticity must be maintained and records must be unalterable
- A standard way of representing imaging test results must be implemented

- Methods of preventing unauthorized access and documenting access must be put in place

It is estimated that during one hospitalization approximately 150 employees (physicians, nursing and laboratory staff, business office staff, etc.) could be able to access a portion of a patient's hospital medical record. When insurance providers and other ancillary services are included, the number of people with access can reach the thousands.

In the United States, health records are considered protected health information and management is addressed under the HIPAA as well as local laws. The creator of a health record (usually a medical practice or a healthcare facility) is the owner and custodian of the physical record and has responsibility for patient records, whether in paper or electronic form. Under HIPAA, the patient has a right to view original records and to obtain copies. The ability to securely share comprehensive, up-to-date patient health records should enhance patient-centered health care and ultimately benefit the patient.

The QA programs are incorporated into each department's procedure manual and day-to-day operation. Usually one person in a supervisory position, such as the assistant laboratory manager, is responsible for implementing the QA programs throughout the laboratory and documenting the results. Every aspect of a test procedure, from ordering the test and collecting the specimen to reporting of results, falls under the QA umbrella. QA responsibilities can also include managing POCT or off-site and satellite laboratory testing; evaluating personnel, training, and providing continuing education; updating procedure manuals; monitoring compliance with regulatory agencies; keeping records; documenting equipment maintenance, calibration, and repairs; and participating in proficiency testing programs.

All institutions receiving Medicare or Medicaid funds are required to develop and maintain a QA program. The intent of this requirement is to improve health care, focusing on patient safety and ways to reduce medical errors. Lesson 1-9 describes in detail how QA is used in the clinical laboratory.

Proficiency Testing

Laboratories performing moderate- or high-complexity testing are required by CLIA '88 to participate in an approved **proficiency testing (PT)** program. Participation in these programs is a part of a laboratory's QA program. PT programs send

"unknown" samples to laboratories at regular intervals. The laboratory performs specific tests on the unknowns and reports the results to the PT agency, which evaluates the results for accuracy and for the laboratory's performance compared to those of other laboratories in the program.

Participation in a PT program is an important part of a laboratory's QA program and allows the laboratory to have confidence in testing methods and identify deficient areas. The PT agency provides documentation of performance for accrediting and regulatory agencies.

Accreditation

Accreditation is a voluntary process by which an independent agency grants recognition to institutions or programs that meet or exceed established standards of quality. Most healthcare institutions seek accreditation because it enhances the institution's reputation and gives the public a way to assess the institution's quality of care.

An institution desiring accreditation invites the accrediting agency to inspect its facility to determine if established standards are being met. Several agencies accredit hospitals, departments within hospitals, and clinical laboratories. Examples of accrediting agencies include the **Joint Commission (JC), College of American Pathologists (CAP), American Association of Blood Banks (AABB),** and **COLA** (Appendix D).

TABLE 1-5. Accrediting agencies with deeming authority under CLIA '88

ACCREDITING AGENCY	ENTITIES ELIGIBLE FOR ACCREDITATION
Joint Commission (JC)	Hospitals
College of American Pathologists (CAP)	Clinical laboratories
American Association of Blood Banks (AABB)	Blood bank departments
American Society for Histocompatibility and Immunogenetics (ASHI)	Laboratories performing histocompatibility testing and testing for genetic studies, transplantation, and blood transfusion
American Osteopathic Association (AOA)	Osteopathic healthcare facilities
COLA	Hospital laboratories, POLs and other smaller laboratories

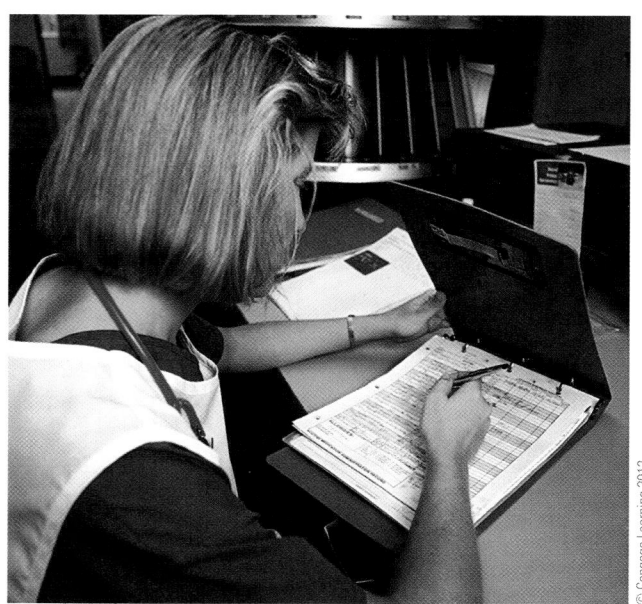

© Cengage Learning 2012

FIGURE 1-9 A patient's right to privacy must be maintained when accessing patient records

In order for a healthcare organization to participate in and receive payment from Medicare or Medicaid programs, it must obtain the appropriate certification as set forth in federal regulations. Institutions desiring certification are required to be inspected by an agency on behalf of CMS, usually a state agency. If an independent accrediting organization, such as the JC or AABB, has and enforces standards that meet or exceed CMS requirements, CMS can grant that accrediting organization *deeming authority* (Table 1-5). This means that accreditation by these agencies is recognized and accepted by CMS as meeting all government standards under CLIA '88. Each institution or laboratory accredited by the deeming authority would have *deemed status* and would not be subject to CMS's routine inspection and certification process.

Accreditation is voluntary; seeking deemed status through accreditation is also voluntary. However, organizations not seeking accreditation are still subject to CMS inspection in order to be able to receive Medicare and Medicaid funds. All inspections are unannounced, whether performed by a state agency or an independent deeming authority.

PRIVACY ISSUES

In 1996, Congress passed the **Health Insurance Portability and Accountability Act (HIPAA)**. From this act, a privacy rule was issued, providing federal protections for personal health information and guaranteeing a patient's right to privacy. This was a response to the potential for loss of privacy created by the increased use and availability of electronic patient records as computers came into wider use in healthcare recordkeeping. The privacy rule requires healthcare facilities to use all necessary measures and procedures to ensure that patient information remains private and confidential. At the same time, the rule permits disclosure of

information that is needed for patient care. All healthcare agencies must now inform patients of their privacy rights, and patients must give written permission for health information to be shared, even with family members. (See Current Topics section in this lesson for more information on electronic health records.)

Much communication in laboratories and healthcare institutions is facilitated by computers. Most laboratories have a central computer information system through which tests are requested and test results are reported and entered into a database. Use of computers in health care contributes to efficiency and improved patient care. However, it also presents the opportunity for violation of patient privacy, whether intentional or unintentional. Computers storing patient information must be password protected so that only authorized persons can access information. The use of specimen identification codes, instead of patient names, helps protect patient privacy.

Computer monitors and printers receiving or printing laboratory results should be positioned so that the monitor or document is not visible to visitors, other patients, or unauthorized employees. Personnel accessing patient charts must do so in a protected area so that patient information is not visible to the public (Figure 1-9).

It must be emphasized to employees that all patient information must remain private and confidential and must be shared only with authorized persons to facilitate and improve patient care.

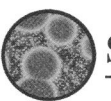 **SUMMARY**

Clinical laboratories are found in both hospital and nonhospital settings. Laboratories must meet specific qualifications to gain government permission to operate. They are regulated by CLIA '88, which contains standards and regulations designed to protect patients,

CRITICAL THINKING

Timothy is a medical assistant working in a small POL. His laboratory operates under a certificate of waiver. The physician requests a microscopic examination of urine for patient Mary Smith. During Timothy's medical assistant training, he learned to perform microscopic examination of urine, classified by CLIA as a moderate complexity test.

1. What is the appropriate action for Timothy to take?
   a. Tell the physician that it is not possible to have the test performed.
   b. Send the specimen to a laboratory approved for performing moderate- to high-complexity testing.
   c. Perform the test and report the results to the physician.
2. Explain your answer.

laboratory personnel, other healthcare workers, and society as a whole. The aims are to ensure that laboratory tests are performed in a manner that ensures reliable results and that laboratory employees work in a safe, healthy environment.

Laboratory personnel must adhere to HIPAA guidelines that guarantee protection of patient privacy. The development of portable EHRs will also require special attention to securing personal medical data.

The clinical laboratory is a dynamic workplace and an important partner on the healthcare team. As rapid changes continue in medical technology and healthcare delivery systems, laboratories must be able to adjust to future trends. The increase in POCT and use of automated specimen processing are two examples of current laboratory trends.

The organization of a clinical laboratory is determined by the laboratory size, types and number of tests performed, and personnel qualifications. Hospital laboratories usually are organized into several departments, such as hematology, chemistry, microbiology, and blood bank. Each department is responsible for performing specific tests in its area and maintaining a QA program.

The clinical laboratory has a role in fostering good channels of communication in the laboratory and also between the laboratory and physicians, other departments in the hospital, and other healthcare providers. By educating healthcare partners about clinical laboratory medicine, such as appropriateness of tests and interpreting and understanding laboratory test results, the best interest of the patient is served.

REVIEW QUESTIONS

1. What is the function of a clinical laboratory?
2. Draw an organizational chart of a typical hospital laboratory.
3. Name five major departments found in a hospital laboratory.
4. Name two procedures performed in the hematology department.
5. Name two tests performed in the chemistry department.
6. How does the HIPAA affect workers in the laboratory?
7. Name three benefits of electronic health records.
8. List three locations of clinical laboratory facilities other than in hospitals.
9. Explain the job functions of the laboratory director, technical supervisor, and department head or general supervisor.
10. Who is responsible for creating the laboratory's SOP manual?
11. What is contained in the SOP manual?
12. What is the purpose of CLIA '88?
13. What federal agency is responsible for implementing CLIA '88?
14. What are waived tests?
15. List the five certificates issued under CLIA '88, and state the activities each certificate permits.
16. What is the advantage of proficiency testing?
17. How do laboratories become accredited?
18. Define accessioning, accreditation, American Association of Blood Banks (AABB) anticoagulant, bacteriology, blood bank, Centers for Disease Control and Prevention (CDC), Centers for Medicare and Medicaid Services (CMS), Clinical and Laboratory Standards Institute (CLSI), clinical chemistry, Clinical Laboratory Improvement Amendments of 1988 (CLIA '88), coagulation, College of American Pathologists (CAP), COLA, Department of Health and Human Services (DHHS), electronic health record (EHRzz), electronic

medical record (EMR), epidemiology, Food and Drug Administration (FDA), Health Care Financing Administration (HCFA), hematology, HIPAA, immunohematology, immunology, Joint Commission (JC), Laboratory Response Network (LRN), microbiology, mycology, National Committee for Clinical Laboratory Standards (NCCLS), parasitology, pathologist, phlebotomist, physician office laboratory (POL), plasma, point-of-care testing (POCT), proficiency testing, Provider-Performed Microscopy Procedure (PPMP), quality assessment, reference laboratory, serology, serum, standard operating procedure (SOP), virology, and waived test.

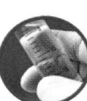

STUDENT ACTIVITIES

1. Complete the written examination on this lesson.

2. Interview an employee of a clinical laboratory and report on your interview. Inquire about the laboratory's organization, the types of tests performed, how specimens are received and how results are recorded and delivered to physicians. Obtain various laboratory test report forms and note the types of tests performed in each department.

3. Tour a hospital laboratory or reference laboratory in your area.

4. Visit a POL and find out the types of tests performed there.

WEB ACTIVITIES

1. Select five analytes from Table 1-2. Find information about the analytes from the CMS or FDA web site. List two brands of test kits that qualify as waived for each of the five analytes.

2. Find web sites of three clinical laboratories. Note the types of information provided on each web site. Look for organizational charts for the laboratories and compare them with what you have learned in this lesson about how laboratories are organized.

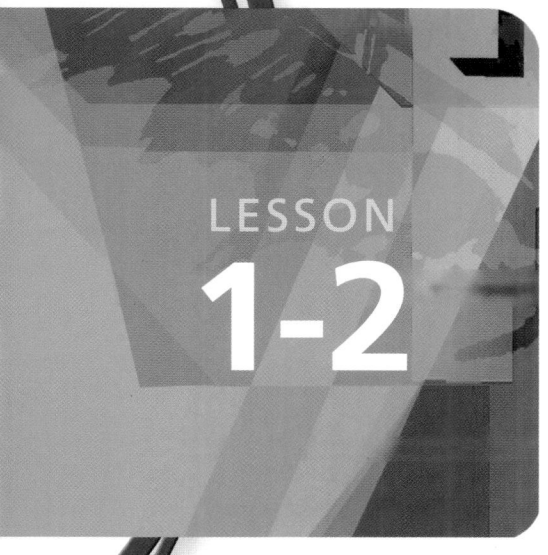

The Clinical Laboratory Professional

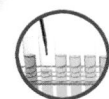

LESSON OBJECTIVES

After studying this lesson, the student will:

- ⊙ Give a brief history of medical technology.
- ⊙ List five personal qualities that are desirable in a clinical laboratory professional.
- ⊙ Describe the educational requirements for medical laboratory scientists and technicians.
- ⊙ Explain the functions of accrediting agencies and credentialing agencies.
- ⊙ Discuss the relationship between the laboratory professional and the patient.
- ⊙ Explain the laboratory professional's responsibility in relation to patient privacy.
- ⊙ Explain the purpose and benefits of professional societies.
- ⊙ Discuss the importance of ethical conduct by laboratory professionals.
- ⊙ Name five areas of employment for clinical laboratory professionals other than in hospital laboratories.
- ⊙ Define the glossary terms.

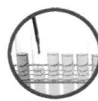

GLOSSARY

American Association of Medical Assistants (AAMA) / professional society and credentialing agency for medical assistants

American Medical Technologists (AMT) / professional society and credentialing agency for several categories of medical laboratory personnel

American Society for Clinical Laboratory Science (ASCLS) / professional society for clinical/medical laboratory personnel

American Society for Clinical Pathology (ASCP) / professional society for clinical/medical laboratory personnel and allied health personnel

American Society of Phlebotomy Technicians (ASPT) / professional society and credentialing agency for phlebotomists, as well as credentialing agency for specialty areas such as point-of-care technician

ASCP Board of Certification (ASCP BOC) / a separate body within the ASCP organizational structure, formed in 2009 by merging NCA with the ASCP BOR and providing certification for medical laboratory personnel

clinical laboratory science / the health profession concerned with performing laboratory analyses used in diagnosing and treating disease, as well as in maintaining good health; synonymous with medical laboratory science and medical (laboratory) technology

(continues)

clinical laboratory scientist (CLS) / the NCA term for a professional who has a baccalaureate degree from an accredited college or university, has completed clinical training in an accredited clinical/medical laboratory science program, and has passed a national certifying examination; also called medical laboratory scientist (MLS) or medical technologist (MT)

clinical laboratory technician (CLT) / the NCA term for a professional who has completed a minimum of 2 years of specific training in an accredited clinical/medical laboratory technician program and has passed a national certifying examination; also called medical laboratory technician (MLT)

Commission on Accreditation of Allied Health Education Programs (CAAHEP) / agency that accredits educational programs for allied health personnel; formerly CAHEA

ethics / a system of conduct or behavior; rules of professional conduct

Health Insurance Portability and Accountability Act (HIPAA) / 1996 act of Congress, a part of which guarantees protection of privacy of an individual's health information

medical laboratory science / the health profession concerned with performing laboratory analyses used in diagnosing and treating disease, as well as in maintaining good health; synonymous with clinical laboratory science and medical (laboratory) technology

medical laboratory scientist (MLS) / a professional who has a baccalaureate degree from an accredited college or university, has completed clinical training in an accredited medical laboratory science program, and has passed a national certifying examination; synonymous with medical technologist (MT) or NCA certified clinical laboratory scientist (CLS)

medical laboratory technician (MLT) / a professional who has completed a minimum of 2 years of specific training in an accredited medical laboratory technician program and has passed a national certifying examination; synonymous with NCA certified clinical laboratory technician (CLT)

medical technologist (MT) / a term gradually being replaced but referring to the professions of medical laboratory scientist (MLS) or clinical laboratory scientist (CLS)

medical technology / synonymous for clinical laboratory science and medical laboratory science

National Accrediting Agency for Clinical Laboratory Sciences (NAACLS) / agency that accredits educational programs for clinical laboratory personnel

National Credentialing Agency for Laboratory Personnel (NCA) / a credentialing agency for clinical laboratory personnel that merged with the ASCP Board of Registry (BOR) in 2009 to form the ASCP Board of Certification (BOC)

National Phlebotomy Association (NPA) / professional society and credentialing agency for phlebotomists

INTRODUCTION

Clinical laboratory science, medical laboratory science, and **medical technology** are all terms used to refer to the health profession concerned with performing laboratory analyses. These analyses are performed by trained, skilled laboratory personnel. Information gained from the analyses is used in diagnosing and treating disease, as well as in preventive care.

What do these clinical laboratory personnel do? They work as medical detectives. They use microscopes to observe changes in cells and use special stains to identify microorganisms. They test blood to find compatible blood for transfusions. They culture organisms and determine which antibiotics are most effective against microbes. They measure substances such as glucose and cholesterol in the blood. They operate complex analytical instruments. They use standards and controls to ensure reliable results. They work under pressure with speed, accuracy, and precision. They adhere to high ethical standards.

This lesson examines the role the laboratory professional plays in today's healthcare settings. Personal and educational qualifications required, job responsibilities, employment opportunities, ethics, and professionalism are all discussed.

HISTORY OF MEDICAL TECHNOLOGY

The origins of medical technology can be traced back several centuries. Papyrus writings dating before 1000 B.C. record descriptions of intestinal parasites, an early example of parasitology. Before medieval times, Hindu doctors performed crude urinalyses when they observed that some urine had a sweet taste and attracted ants. With the invention of the microscope in the seventeenth century, the study of biological specimens progressed from simple visual examination to microscopic examination.

Early Medical Laboratories

The first medical laboratories in the United States appeared in the late nineteenth century and were primitive by today's standards. Some consisted of only a table and a microscope.

They were staffed mostly by doctors who had a special interest in "laboratory medicine." The 1900 U.S. census listed only 100 laboratory technicians, all men.

Modern Medical/Clinical Laboratories

After World War I, laboratories grew in size and number and it soon became clear that there was a need for:

- Educating laboratory workers
- Defining educational requirements
- Identifying adequately trained persons

In 1926 the **American Society for Clinical Pathology (ASCP)**, a professional organization of physicians, appointed a Committee on Registration of Laboratory Technicians whose purpose was to identify qualified laboratory workers. With the formation of this committee the debate over terminology began, a debate that continues to this day. After much discussion the terms clinical laboratory technician and medical technician were discarded in favor of the terms *Medical Technologist* and *Laboratory Technician*.

By the 1930s, basic educational requirements had been established and schools of medical technology were training laboratory workers. Certifying examinations were given to measure the knowledge and ability of workers. In 1936, the Registry of Medical Technologists discontinued using the term "Registry of Medical Technicians," and designated a successful certificant as a **Medical Technologist (MT)**. In 1977, a newly formed credentialing agency, the **National Credentialing Agency for Laboratory Personnel (NCA)**, designated their successful certificants as **Clinical Laboratory Scientists (CLS)**. The term *scientist* was chosen over technologist in part because the term *technology* had come into wide use to refer to the broader medical field encompassing the rapid advances in improved medical devices and test and instrument designs.

Rapid changes in technology were incorporated into laboratory testing methods in the second half of the twentieth century. Laboratory tests became increasingly sophisticated. Specially trained laboratory workers made up a majority of the laboratory workforce, and laboratory tests came to play an even more essential role in medicine. Tests that were formerly tedious and time-consuming became obsolete as they were replaced by more efficient technologies. Laboratory workers no longer had to inoculate laboratory animals to diagnose certain infectious diseases. Tests that once required elaborate, multistep chemical assays became streamlined and miniaturized. The introduction of the computer into the laboratory increased efficiency and decreased errors. The array of analytes that could be tested increased dramatically.

The Clinical Laboratory in the Twenty-First Century

In all healthcare fields, today's technology provides a level of care only imagined a few years ago. New trends are emerging, such as emphases on wellness (preventive medicine), geriatric medicine, home health care, and hospice. These areas strive to keep patients healthy and at home, instead of requiring long hospital stays. Laboratory instruments incorporate state-of-the-art technologies such as microtechnology and nanotechnology components, flow cytometry, and laser imaging. These technologies allow rapid testing and portable testing.

In the twenty-first century, once again terminology regarding categories of laboratory professionals is in a state of change. The term *clinical laboratory science* largely replaced the term *medical technology* in the 1980s and 1990s. In 2009, another name change was proposed and accepted by the major laboratory professional certifying entities, the ASCP and NCA. Following unification in 2009 of the ASCP Board of Registry (BOR) and the NCA into one new certifying body called the **ASCP Board of Certification (ASCP BOC)**, the certification categories for laboratory professionals changed:

- Clinical laboratory scientist (CLS) became **medical laboratory scientist (MLS)**, and
- **Clinical laboratory technician (CLT)** once again became **medical laboratory technician (MLT)**.

Changes are continually occurring as the roles of laboratory professionals are redefined and as technology advances. The field of clinical and medical laboratory science continues to change and broaden in response to federal regulations, changes in healthcare needs, and new technologies. Laboratory professionals continue to adapt to these changes. What does not change is the primary goal of laboratory professionals, which is to provide relevant, timely, quality information that will be used to improve patient health and outcomes.

ROLE OF THE LABORATORY PROFESSIONAL

The laboratory professional is an integral partner in allied health care. Laboratory workers are found in many types of healthcare settings, from local health fairs to sophisticated laboratories such as those of the National Institutes of Health (NIH) and the Centers for Disease Control (CDC), where exotic, emerging diseases are studied. The most visible laboratory professional is the worker in the hospital laboratory. These workers interact daily with others on the healthcare team—physicians, nursing staff, therapists, infection prevention officers, and various other healthcare team members—to provide quality patient care.

The work of laboratory professionals is important whether they are employed in a large laboratory or a small one. Personnel staffing large laboratories include highly skilled professionals, such as clinical laboratory scientists (medical technologists and medical laboratory scientists) and clinical (medical) laboratory technicians (Figure 1-10). Smaller laboratories, especially those performing only waived tests, are often staffed by multiskilled personnel who are trained to perform some laboratory tests as well as nursing and office procedures. These personnel can be medical assistants, laboratory assistants, certified nursing assistants, and those who have varying levels of nursing training.

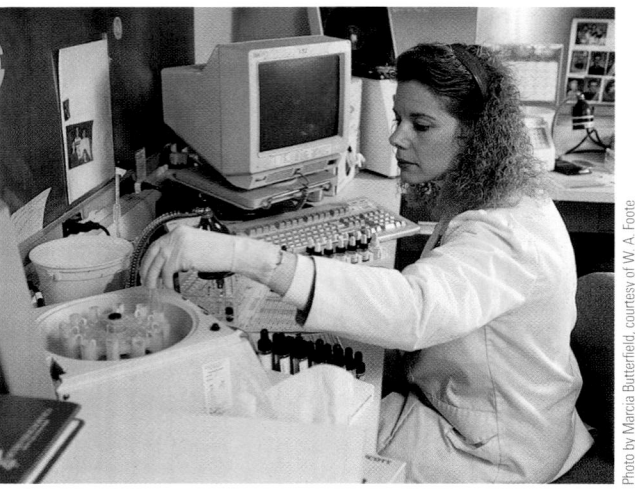

FIGURE 1-10 Blood bank technologist working in a clinical laboratory

Photo by Marcia Butterfield, courtesy of W. A. Foote Memorial Hospital, Jackson, MI

CERTIFICATION REQUIREMENTS FOR LABORATORY PERSONNEL

Completion of an approved course of study and successful completion of a national certifying examination are required to become a certified laboratory professional. Most large clinical and medical laboratories employ workers at several levels, each requiring different education, training, and skill levels. CLIA '88 defines the personnel qualifications required for laboratory personnel based on the job functions associated with the position. Some positions require only a high school education and documented on-the-job training. However, laboratories performing moderate- to high-complexity testing prefer to hire laboratory professionals who have completed a prescribed program of study in medical laboratory science and are qualified to work in any laboratory department.

Educational Programs and Accrediting Agencies

Several types of programs of study are available through hospitals, 2- and 4-year colleges, universities, technical schools, and private schools. The programs usually consist of an academic component and a clinical component.

Several organizations and agencies are involved in establishing and maintaining the principles and standards of the laboratory professions. Accredited educational programs must meet nationally established standards. The **National Accrediting Agency for Clinical Laboratory Sciences (NAACLS)** accredits educational programs that train MLS and MLT students. The **Commission on Accreditation of Allied Health Education Programs (CAAHEP)** provides accreditation for programs that train medical assistants and other allied health workers.

Educational Requirements

The majority of laboratory professionals have received one of two levels of education and training. The requirements for the two levels differ; the names of the programs or departments can also differ among institutions. Programs for educating medical laboratory personnal can be in departments of Medical Laboratory Science, Clinical Laboratory Science, or Medical Technology.

Medical Laboratory Scientist

The Medical Laboratory Scientist (MLS) generally has a baccalaureate degree from a college or university and has completed a specified period of on-site clinical training in an accredited medical laboratory science program. To become certified, the individual must pass a national examination. Individuals certified as an MLS are qualified to perform analyses in all departments of the laboratory; they can also be supervisors or work in other leadership positions in the laboratory. Certificants are entitled to cite their credentials following their name, such as Jane Doe, MLS(ASCP).

Medical Laboratory Technician

The Medical Laboratory Technician (MLT) generally has an associate's degree from a 2-year college or a certificate from an accredited MLT program and has completed a period of on-site clinical training. Upon passing a national certifying examination, the MLT is certified and can cite their credential as MLT(ASCP).

Areas of Specialization

Laboratory professionals can specialize in one area of laboratory work such as microbiology, hematology, or blood banking. To obtain specialist rank, such as specialist in hematology (SH) or specialist in blood bank (SBB), the professional must complete additional appropriate academic work, obtain the required number of years of clinical experience in the particular field, and pass an examination in the specialty area.

Credentialing and Certification

Credentialing (certifying) agencies are organizations that administer examinations for different categories of laboratory professionals. Two of these are the **ASCP Board of Certification (ASCP BOC)** and the **American Medical Technologists (AMT)** (Table 1-6). Professional titles used for equivalent training can differ depending on the organization offering certification. For instance, the qualifications are similar for MLS(ASCP) and MT(AMT) but certificants must cite their credentials according to the guidelines of their certifying organization. Table 1-7 gives the designations formerly used by the NCA and the equivalent new designations adopted in 2009 by the ASCP BOC. (Professional categories can sometimes be confusing because there are several certifying agencies, each with their own terminology. Information about specific eligibility requirements for certification categories can be obtained from the individual certifying agencies. Addresses of these organizations are given in Appendix D.)

TABLE 1-6. Selected credentialing/certifying agencies for clinical laboratory and other allied health personnel

AAB	American Association of Bioanalysts Board of Registry
AAMA	American Association of Medical Assistants
AMT	American Medical Technologists
ASCP BOC	American Society for Clinical Pathology Board of Certification
ASPT	American Society of Phlebotomy Technicians
NPA	National Phlebotomy Association

TABLE 1-7. Formerly used NCA certification categories and equivalent ASCP BOC certification categories with citation of credentials

NCA DESIGNATION	NEW ASCP BOC DESIGNATION
Clinical Laboratory Scientist, CLS(NCA)	Medical Laboratory Scientist, MLS(ASCP)
Clinical Laboratory Technician, CLT(NCA)	Medical Laboratory Technician, MLT(ASCP)
Clinical Laboratory Specialist, CLSp(NCA)	Specialist, S(ASCP)
Clinical Laboratory Supervisor, CLSup(NCA)	Diplomate in Laboratory Management, DLM(ASCP)
Clinical Laboratory Phlebotomist, CLPlb(NCA)	Phlebotomy Technician, PBT(ASCP)

Licensing of Laboratory Professionals

Although certification is usually sufficient to meet most employment requirements, some states regulate laboratory personnel by requiring workers to obtain a state license. Licensing laws vary from state to state and are nonexistent in some states. States can require a fee to obtain a license, or require that a test be taken before the license is issued; some states require both.

OTHER ALLIED HEALTH PERSONNEL IN THE CLINICAL LABORATORY

Along with the emergence of point-of-care testing (POCT) as an important part of the healthcare delivery system, a large number of CLIA waived tests have been developed. Waived tests are those tests determined to be simple enough that there is little risk for significant error. This has resulted in an expansion of the types

of personnel who can perform certain laboratory analyses. Where traditionally mostly baccalaureate-educated medical technologists performed these tests, waived testing is now being performed by allied health personnel such as paramedics, medical assistants, registered nurses, and licensed practical nurses. These individuals provide health care in a variety of settings from the patient's home to the physician's office and the hospital emergency room. Allied health personnel, other than nursing staff, who might perform certain laboratory tests include:

- Phlebotomist/Phlebotomy Technician (PBT)
- Certified Medical Assistant (CMA)
- Certified Nursing Assistant (CNA)
- Physician Office Laboratory Technician (POLT)
- Clinical Laboratory Assistant (CLA)
- Diagnostic Molecular Scientist
- Point-of-care Technician

The educational requirements, programs of study, and job responsibilities differ for each of these personnel. The programs for phlebotomists and medical assistants are briefly described in this lesson. Information on programs for other categories of personnel can be found by contacting the appropriate certifying agency (listed in Table 1-6 and Appendix D).

Phlebotomy Technicians

Phlebotomists are trained to collect blood specimens for laboratory testing (Figure 1-11). Training programs require a high school diploma or general equivalency diploma (GED) for

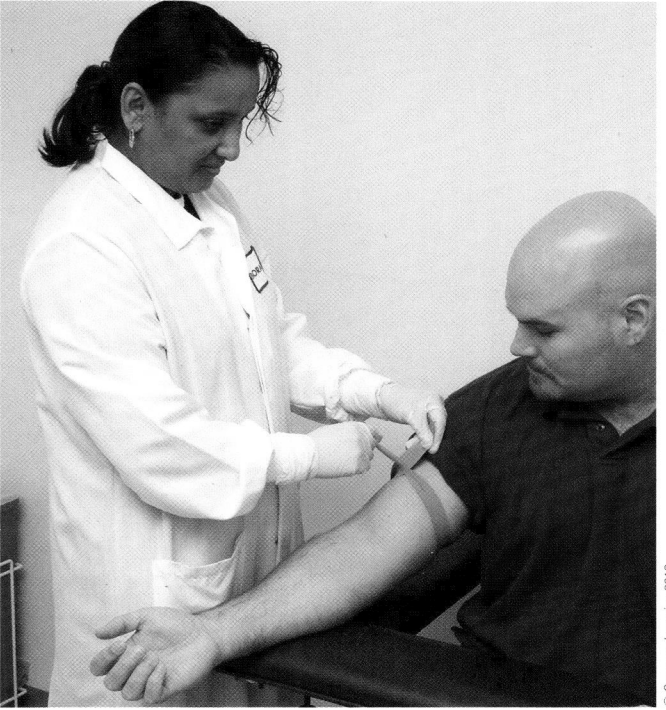

FIGURE 1-11 A phlebotomist preparing to perform a venipuncture in a POL

entrance. After the training program is complete, certification is available through several organizations following successful completion of a national examination. Examples of phlebotomist certifying organizations and the professional designations are:

- AMT (American Medical Technologists): Registered Phlebotomy Technician (RPT)
- ASCP BOC (ASCP Board of Certification): Phlebotomy Technician (PBT)
- ASPT (American Society of Phlebotomy Technicians): Phlebotomy Technician
- NPA (National Phlebotomy Association): Certified Phlebotomy Technician (CPT)

Certified Medical Assistant and Registered Medical Assistant

Medical assistants are allied health professionals frequently employed in ambulatory care settings such as physician office laboratories (POLs) and who have been trained in multiple areas, including administrative, clerical, nursing, and laboratory skills. The laboratory skills of medical assistants include collecting and processing blood specimens and performing waived tests such as hemoglobin, hematocrit, urine reagent strip tests, urine pregnancy tests, blood glucose, and fecal occult blood.

Training for medical assistants is available through community colleges and vocational-technical and private schools. A high school diploma or GED is required for entrance, and two levels of education are available for medical assistants. One level is a diploma program requiring 1 year of postsecondary education; the other is an associate of science degree, consisting of 2 years of postsecondary education. Upon completion of the course of study, certification is obtained by passing a national examination administered by a certifying organization. Two such organizations and their certification designations are:

- AAMA (American Association of Medical Assistants): Certified Medical Assistant (CMA)
- AMT (American Medical Technologists): Registered Medical Assistant (RMA)

ETHICS AND PROFESSIONALISM

Clinical laboratory personnel must subscribe to high ethical standards and exhibit professionalism in their work, behavior, and appearance.

Ethics and the Clinical Laboratory Professional

Clinical laboratory personnel are expected to observe **ethics**, a prescribed code of conduct and behavior. Organizations that credential healthcare professionals have codes of ethics to which their members are expected to subscribe. One example is the code of ethics for laboratory professionals adopted by the **American Society for Clinical Laboratory Science (ASCLS)**.

TABLE 1-8. Portion of Code of Ethics of the American Society for Clinical Laboratory Science (Reprinted with permission of American Society for Clinical Laboratory Science, Washington, DC)

As a clinical laboratory professional, I strive to:

- Maintain and promote standards of excellence in performing and advancing the art and science of my profession;
- Preserve the dignity and privacy of patients;
- Uphold and maintain the dignity and respect of our profession;
- Seek to establish cooperative and respectful working relationships with other healthcare professionals; and
- Contribute to the general well-being of the community

I will actively demonstrate my commitment to these responsibilities throughout my professional life.

A portion is shown in Table 1-8. Students might recite or sign a similar code of ethics when they begin their clinical rotation or at graduation.

The principles in this code stress that laboratory professionals have a duty to patients, colleagues, their profession, and society. Laboratory professionals have an obligation to the patient to:

- Provide a high quality of service and maintain high standards of practice
- Exercise sound judgment in establishing, performing, and evaluating laboratory testing
- Maintain strict confidentiality of patient information
- Safeguard the privacy and dignity of patients
- Strive to safeguard the patient from incompetent practice by others

Laboratory professionals have an obligation to their colleagues and to their profession to:

- Maintain a reputation of honesty, integrity, and reliability
- Maintain dignity and respect for the profession
- Contribute to the advancement of the profession
- Establish cooperative and respectful working relationships with other healthcare professionals

Laboratory professionals have a responsibility to society to:

- Use their professional competence to contribute to the general well-being of the community
- Comply with laws and regulations pertaining to the practice of clinical laboratory science
- Encourage all in the profession to meet high standards of care and practice

The principles and ideals expressed in the ASCLS code of ethics are applicable to ethical and professional behavior for all healthcare workers. By adhering to principles such as those given here, the foremost objective—maintaining the safety and well-being of the patient—can be achieved.

Qualities Desirable in Laboratory Professionals

Certain personal qualities are desirable in all healthcare professionals. These include honesty, integrity, dedication, dependability, cooperation, competence, discretion, and a caring attitude. Good communication skills and the ability to relate well to fellow workers are also desirable qualities. In addition, applicants to professional healthcare programs should expect that the application process will include a criminal background check and a drug test.

Additional personal qualities and physical capabilities are needed by laboratory personnel to succeed in the clinical laboratory profession. These include physical stamina, good eyesight, manual dexterity, a good intellect, and an aptitude for the biological sciences. Laboratory workers must be observant, motivated, capable of performing precise manipulations and calculations, and also must have good organizational skills.

Personal appearance and hygiene are important for all healthcare workers, including laboratory personnel. All personnel should present a clean, neat, and professional appearance. This inspires patients' confidence in the worker. Healthcare facilities and laboratories have rules of dress, and many of the rules relate directly to safety practices. For instance, closed-toed shoes are required—this prevents injury to the feet from accidental spills or breakage. Wearing loose, dangling jewelry is not permitted because it can cause patient injury, harbor microorganisms, or get caught in instruments. Other rules of dress are related to patient welfare; personnel are discouraged from wearing strongly scented personal products to prevent creating a problem for patients who are sensitive or allergic to strong scents. Lessons 1-4 and 1-5 contain specific information on appropriate laboratory apparel.

Patient Privacy/Confidentiality

Laboratory professionals carry out their duty to the patient by providing competent service and maintaining high standards. One important principle that *must* be adhered to is that of patient privacy. Patient information is confidential. It must only be discussed with healthcare employees directly related to the case who have a "need to know" in order to improve patient care. Elevators, cafeterias, or lounges are not appropriate places to discuss patient results or unusual findings.

The reliance on computers in health care has made access to patient information easier for healthcare workers. However, the use of computers also presents a risk of private information being improperly accessed. Although these advances make information transfer easier, appropriate security measures must be in place to protect patient data from inappropriate access and uses.

The privacy rule under the **Health Insurance Portability and Accountability Act (HIPAA)** describes the patient's right to privacy as well as the conditions under which patient information can be shared in order to provide the best possible care. Employees must be informed of their employer's privacy policies and procedures and must follow those procedures.

Interactions Between Laboratory Personnel and Patients

Often, the only contact patients have with the laboratory is through the laboratory technician, medical technologist, or phlebotomist who collects a blood sample from them. At best, it is not pleasant to have blood taken from a vein or finger. The laboratory professional should be aware at all times of the stress a patient is feeling when hospitalized or ill. The employee must be professional, courteous, patient, and considerate of patients.

Professional Organizations

Several professional societies for clinical laboratory professionals provide opportunities for professional growth and continuing education by offering workshops and seminars and by publishing journals (Table 1-9). Several journals and journal articles can be found online; other journals are available only in print. Some journals are *Laboratory Medicine, ADVANCE for Medical Laboratory Professionals* (free subscription), *Clinical Laboratory Science, Medical Laboratory Observer* (free subscription), and *ICT: Infection Control Today*.

Membership in a national society usually also includes membership in that society's state affiliate. A listing of several professional societies can be found in Appendix D. Membership and participation in professional society activities contribute to the continuing competence of the laboratory professional.

Laboratory professionals carry out their duty to colleagues and their profession through professional improvement activities, cooperation, and respect for their colleagues. Through competent practice of their profession, they contribute to the well-being of the community.

TABLE 1-9. Professional societies for clinical laboratory and other allied health personnel	
AAB	American Association of Bioanalysts
AABB	American Association of Blood Banks
AACC	American Association of Clinical Chemistry
AAMA	American Association of Medical Assistants
AMT	American Medical Technologists
APIC	Association for Professionals in Infection Control and Epidemiology
ASCLS	American Society for Clinical Laboratory Science
ASCP	American Society for Clinical Pathology
ASM	American Society for Microbiology
ASPT	American Society of Phlebotomy Technicians
CLMA	Clinical Laboratory Management Association
NPA	National Phlebotomy Association

CASE STUDY

Rob works in the laboratory at Bay Regional Hospital. Each work day before he begins his duties in the laboratory, he helps collect blood from hospital patients. On one occasion, the patient on his collection list was his friend Louis, who had been admitted to the hospital through the emergency department the night before. Rob collected blood from Louis for several laboratory tests and chatted with him briefly before returning to the laboratory.

After Rob got home that evening, he received a call from Susan asking for information about their mutual acquaintance Louis, who she heard was in the hospital. Susan said she had called the hospital but they would not release information about Louis and would not even confirm that he was a patient in the hospital. Susan asked Rob if he knew if Louis was hospitalized and if so, why.

1. How should Rob respond to Susan?
2. What are his obligations?
3. What are his options?

Role-play the conversation between Rob and Susan or Rob and Louis.

Employment Opportunities

Varied employment opportunities exist for clinical laboratory professionals. Many of the nation's clinical laboratory workers are employed in hospitals as technologists, supervisors, or laboratory directors or administrators. Other areas of employment include physician offices, clinics, public health agencies, reference laboratories, the military, research, education, veterinary medicine, and pharmaceutics. Laboratory professionals are also employed in sales, product development, and technical service departments of medical suppliers and instrument manufacturers.

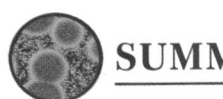

SUMMARY

Clinical laboratory professionals are key members of today's healthcare team. As in all other areas of health care, the field of medical laboratory science exists for the patient. Every day, nurses, physicians, and other healthcare workers rely on laboratory professionals to test blood and other body fluids, interpret test results, and help provide a complete picture of a patient's state of health. For a patient to receive the best possible care, a correct diagnosis must be made. Physicians rely on these laboratory analyses, along with information gained from the medical history, physical examination, and clinical symptoms to make a diagnosis. Therefore, it is imperative that laboratory analyses be performed carefully and accurately by well-trained, competent laboratory professionals.

Set rules and regulations govern health care in the United States. Healthcare agencies have very specific standards, rules, and regulations governing the educational requirements and job responsibilities of healthcare employees. In laboratories performing tests of moderate to high complexity, the personnel performing these tests are medical laboratory scientists or medical laboratory technicians. These laboratory professionals are required to complete a prescribed program of study and become certified through examination to qualify for this employment. Waived tests can be performed by other allied health personnel such as medical assistants and physician office assistants. All laboratory personnel are expected to strive to provide the best possible patient care, to protect patient privacy, and to exhibit professional and ethical behavior at all times.

Laboratory professionals work in a variety of settings, from hospitals, physician's offices, and community health fairs, to research laboratories. Whatever the setting, the laboratory professionals are working to improve patient care by providing precise and valuable information used in the diagnosis, treatment, and prevention of disease.

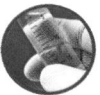

REVIEW QUESTIONS

1. What is clinical laboratory science? What other term is used for this field?
2. Describe the beginnings of medical technology.
3. Name five personal qualities desirable in clinical laboratory personnel.
4. What are the educational requirements for medical laboratory scientists? For medical laboratory technicians?
5. What is the purpose of accrediting agencies?
6. What are the functions of credentialing agencies?
7. List five places of employment for laboratory professionals other than in hospitals.

8. Explain the importance of ethical standards in the practice of medical laboratory science.

9. Explain the laboratory professional's obligation to the patient.

10. How do laboratory professionals become certified?

11. What is the value of professional societies to the laboratory professional?

12. Define American Association of Medical Assistants (AAMA), American Medical Technologists (AMT), American Society for Clinical Laboratory Science (ASCLS), American Society for Clinical Pathology (ASCP), American Society of Phlebotomy Technicians (ASPT), ASCP Board of Certification (ASCP BOC), clinical laboratory science, clinical laboratory scientist (CLS), clinical laboratory technician (CLT), Commission on Accreditation of Allied Health Education Programs (CAAHEP), ethics, Health Insurance Portability and Accountability Act (HIPAA), medical laboratory science,

medical laboratory scientist (MLS), medical laboratory technician (MLT), medical technologist (MT), medical technology, National Accrediting Agency for Clinical Laboratory Sciences (NAACLS), National Credentialing Agency for Laboratory Personnel (NCA), and National Phlebotomy Association (NPA).

 STUDENT ACTIVITIES

1. Complete the written examination for this lesson.

2. Use the interview fact sheet and interview a laboratory professional. Be sure to consider the following areas: job functions, relationship with coworkers and patients, advantages and disadvantages of job, satisfactions, dissatisfactions, salary, and opportunities for advancement. Describe the benefits of talking to the laboratory professional in person rather than reading the information in a book.

 WEB ACTIVITIES

1. Visit the web sites of three agencies or professional societies listed in Tables 1-6 and 1-9. List the programs they certify and the educational requirements of each program.

2. Search the Internet to find a school in your state (or nearby state) that offers training for laboratory scientists. Find out what required courses are listed in the curriculum.

3. Complete a career information fact sheet for medical laboratory technician and medical laboratory scientist. Use this text, other available texts, and the Internet to gather your information. For each career, include educational training, estimated cost of the program, nature of the job, advantages and disadvantages, employment opportunities, and salary range.

4. Use the Internet to find sources of current topics related to the clinical laboratory, such as online journals or newsletters. Request an email subscription to some of the free ones.

LESSON 1-2
The Clinical Laboratory Professional

(Answers from individual students will vary based on the interviews.)

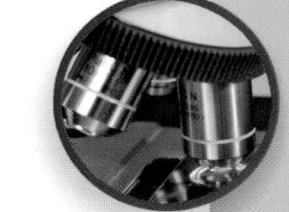

Name _____ Date _____

Interview a laboratory professional using this sheet as a guide to your questions.

Job title:

Education:

Approximate cost of education program:

Job functions:

Approximate salary:

Job satisfaction:

Job dissatisfaction:

Opportunities for advancement:

Options available to broaden employment opportunities:

© 2012 Delmar, Cengage Learning. Permission to reproduce for clinical use granted.

LESSON 1-2
The Clinical Laboratory Professional

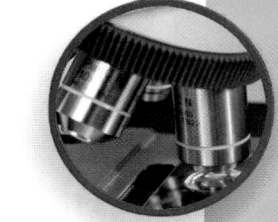

((Answers from individual students will vary based on resources used.)

Name _____ Date _____

Complete this fact sheet using information from this text, other texts, and the Internet.

Job title:

Legal requirement:

Name of program:

    Educational institution:

    Cost of program:

    Length of program:

    Admission requirements:

Nature of the job:

    Earnings:

    Advancement:

    Related occupation(s):

    Advantages:

    Disadvantages:

Potential sources of employment:

CAREER INFORMATION FACT SHEET

© 2012 Delmar, Cengage Learning. Permission to reproduce for clinical use granted.

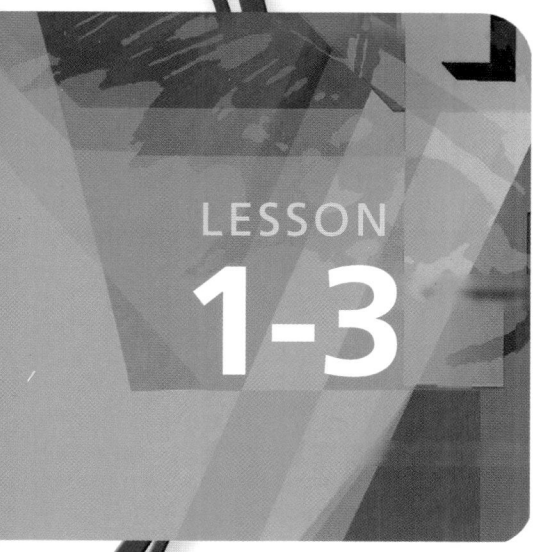

Medical Terminology

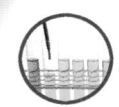

LESSON OBJECTIVES

After studying this lesson, the student will:

- ⊙ Discuss the importance of healthcare workers understanding and correctly using medical terms.
- ⊙ Define stem words from a selected list.
- ⊙ Define prefixes from a selected list.
- ⊙ Define suffixes from a selected list.
- ⊙ Identify common clinical laboratory abbreviations and acronyms from a selected list.
- ⊙ Pronounce commonly used medical terms from a selected list.
- ⊙ Recognize prefixes, stems, or suffixes in medical terms.
- ⊙ Analyze medical terms based on knowledge of prefixes, suffixes, and stems.
- ⊙ Define the glossary terms.

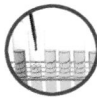

GLOSSARY

abbreviation / the shortening of a word, often by removing letters from the end of the word

acronym / combination of the first letters or syllables of a group of words to form a new group of letters that can be pronounced as a word

prefix / modifying word or syllable(s) placed at the beginning of a word

stem / main part of a word; root word; the part of a word remaining after removing the prefix or suffix

suffix / modifying word or syllable(s) placed at the end of a word

terminology / terms used in any specialized field

INTRODUCTION

Most specialized fields have a unique vocabulary or **terminology**. Medical terminology is the study of terms or words used in medicine. Healthcare workers must know, understand, and be able to correctly use medical terms to carry out instructions and communicate effectively.

Learning medical vocabulary is a long process. Knowledge and proper use of medical terms evolve and expand as the terms are used in the workplace. Confidence will be gained by frequently using medical terminology in daily activities.

This lesson is only an introduction to the structure of medical terms and to abbreviations and acronyms frequently used in the clinical laboratory—the lesson does not cover terminology used in nursing or other allied health fields.

STRUCTURE OF MEDICAL TERMS

Most medical terms are a combination of three word parts—prefixes, suffixes, and stems. The **stem** or root is the main part of the word. A **prefix** is a word or syllable(s) that modifies the stem and is placed at the beginning of the word. A **suffix** is a word or syllable(s) placed at the end of the word and usually describes what happens to the stem. The prefix and suffix are usually connected to the stem by a vowel (such as *a*, *i*, or *o*).

Most of the stems, prefixes, and suffixes used in medical terms are derived from Latin or Greek words and have specific meanings that provide clues to the meanings of the terms. By combining various prefixes, stems, and suffixes, many medical terms with precise meanings can be formed.

Not all terms have all three word parts. Some words have only a prefix and a stem or a stem and suffix. However, all terms will have a stem, or root, word.

If the meanings of commonly used word parts are known, then a new term can often be analyzed to determine the general idea of its meaning. For example, hyperproteinuria can be divided into three word parts: *hyper, protein, uria*. *Hyper* means an increased amount. *Uria* refers to in the urine. Therefore, the term refers to a condition in which an increased amount of protein is in the urine. By combining these parts to make a word, a medical shortcut has been created. One word describes a condition that would otherwise require a sentence or perhaps a paragraph.

Medical terms, although shorter than sentences, have precise meanings. Sometimes a slight modification, such as an alteration of one or two letters, can change the meaning of a word. For example, a *macrocyte* is a cell larger than normal, whereas a *microcyte* is a cell smaller than normal. With the change of just one letter, a term can be changed into another term with an opposite meaning. It is very important to spell, pronounce, and use medical terms correctly so the intended meaning is conveyed.

Prefixes

Prefixes placed before stem words give more information about the stem, such as location, time, size, or number. For example, *intra*vascular means inside the vessel and *pre*natal refers to something that happens before birth. Table 1-10 contains a list of commonly used prefixes and the definition of each. A sample term using the prefix is also given.

TABLE 1-10. Selected prefixes commonly used in medical terminology

PREFIX	DEFINITION	EXAMPLE OF USAGE	PREFIX	DEFINITION	EXAMPLE OF USAGE
a, an	absent, deficient	anemia	dys	bad, difficult, improper	dysphagia
ab	away from	absent	e, ecto, ex	out from	ectoparasite
ad	toward	adrenal	end(o)	inside, within	endoparasite
ambi	both	ambidextrous	enter(o)	intestine	enterotoxin
aniso	unequal	anisocytosis	epi	upon, after	epidermis
ante	before	antenatal	equi	equal	equilibrium
ant(i)	against	antibiotic	glyco	sweet	glycosuria
auto	self	autograft	hemi	half	hemisphere
baso	blue	basophil	hyper	above, excessive	hyperglycemia
bi	two	binuclear	hypo	under, deficient	hypoventilation
bio	life	biochemistry	infra	beneath	infracostal
brady	slow	bradycardia	inter	among, between	intercostal
circum	around	circumnuclear	intra	within	intracranial
co, com, con	with, together	concentrate	iso	equal	isotonic
contra	against	contraception	kilo	one thousand	kilogram
de	down, from	decay	macr	large	macrocyte
di	two	dimorphic	mal	bad, abnormal	malformation
dia	through	dialysis	medi	middle	medicephalic
dipl	double	diplococcus	mega	huge, great	megaloblast
dis	apart, away from	disease			

(Continues)

TABLE 1-10. Selected prefixes commonly used in medical terminology (*Continued*)

PREFIX	DEFINITION	EXAMPLE OF USAGE	PREFIX	DEFINITION	EXAMPLE OF USAGE
melan	black	melanoma	post	after	postoperative
meta	after, next	metamorphosis	pre, pro	before	prenatal
micro	small, one-millionth	microscope, microgram	pseudo	false	pseudoappendicitis
milli	one-thousandth	millimeter	psych(o)	mind	psychoanalyst
mon(o)	one, single	monocyte	py(o)	pus	pyuria
morph	shape	morphogenesis	quad(r)	four	quandrant
necro	dead	necrophobia	retro	backward	retroactive
neo	new	neoplasm	semi	half	semiconscious
neutro	neutral, neither	neutrophil	steno	narrow	stenothorax
olig	few	oliguria	sub	under	subcutaneous
orth	straight, normal	orthopedic	super, supra	above	superinfection
pan	all	pandemic	syn	together	synergistic
para	beside, accessory to	paramedic	tachy	swift	tachycardia
per	through	percutaneous	therm	heat	thermometer
peri	around	pericardium	trans	through	transport
phago	to eat	phagocyte	tri	three	trimester
poly	many	polyuria	uni	one	unicellular

Stems

The stem, or root, word gives the major subject of the term. For example, in the term *appendi*citis, the stem is "appendi." Therefore, appendicitis means an inflammation (*itis*) of the appendix.

In the term endo*card*itis, the root or stem is "card," referring to heart; the term literally means an inflammation (*itis*) within (*endo*) the heart. Commonly used stem words, their definitions, and examples of usage are listed in Table 1-11.

TABLE 1-11. Selected stems commonly used in medical terminology

STEM	DEFINITION	EXAMPLE OF USAGE	STEM	DEFINITION	EXAMPLE OF USAGE
adeno	gland	lymphadenitis	chol	bile, gall bladder	cholesterol
alg	pain	analgesic	chondr	cartilage	chondroplasia
arter	artery	arteriogram	chrom	color	chromogen
arthr	joint	arthritis	col(o)	colon	colonitis
audio	hearing	auditory	cran	skull	craniotomy
brachi	arm	brachial	cut	skin	subcutaneous
bronch(i)	air tube in lungs	bronchitis	cyan	blue	cyanosis
calc	stone	calcify	cyst	bladder, bag	cystocele
carcin	cancer	carcinogen	cyt(o)	cell	monocyte
card	heart	myocardium	dactyl	finger	arachnodactyly
caud	tail	caudate	dent, dont	tooth	orthodontist
ceph(al)	head	encephalitis	derm	skin	dermatitis

(*Continues*)

TABLE 1-11. Selected stems commonly used in medical terminology (*Continued*)

STEM	DEFINITION	EXAMPLE OF USAGE	STEM	DEFINITION	EXAMPLE OF USAGE
edema	swelling	edematous	os, osteo	bone	osteitis
erythro	red	erythrocyte	oto	ear	otitis
febr	fever	afebrile	path	disease	pathogen
gastr(o)	stomach	gastritis	phleb	vein	phlebitis
genito	reproductive	genital	phob	fear	phobia
gloss	tongue	glossitis	phot	light	photometer
hem(a), haem	blood	hematuria	pneum	air	pneumonitis
hepat(o)	liver	hepatitis	pod	foot	pseudopod
histo	tissue	histology	pulm	lung	pulmonary
hystero	uterus	hysterectomy	ren	kidney	adrenal
iatro	physician	podiatrist	rhin	nose	rhinoplasty
lip	fat	lipoma	scler	hard	sclerosis
lith	stone	cholelithiasis	sep	poison	septic
mening	membrane covering brain	meningitis	soma(t)	body	somatic
morph	shape, form	morphology	sperm	seed	spermatogenesis
myel	marrow	myelogram	stoma	mouth, opening	stomatitis
myo	muscle	myositis	thorac	chest	thoracotomy
nephro	kidney	nephrectomy	tome	knife	microtome
neur	nerve	neurectomy	tox(i)	poison	toxicology
onc	tumor	oncology	ur(o), uria	urine, urinary	urology
ophthal	eye	ophthalmologist	vas	vessel	intravascular
os	mouth	ostium	ven	vein	intravenous

Suffixes

Suffixes are modifiers attached to the end of a stem word. Suffixes usually tell what is happening to the subject of the stem. They often indicate a condition, operation, or symptom. In the term *appendectomy*, *ectomy* is a suffix that means to cut out or remove by excision. Therefore, an appendectomy is the surgical removal of the appendix. Commonly used suffixes, their definitions, and examples of usage are listed in Table 1-12.

PRONUNCIATION OF MEDICAL TERMS

It is not enough to just understand written medical terms. You must also be able to pronounce them correctly to communicate effectively with others. Correct pronunciation is relatively easy for some frequently used or short terms, but is often more difficult for longer terms.

Although most medical terms are derived from Greek or Latin, the Greek or Latin pronunciation is not always used.

Your medical dictionary can guide you, but different authors sometimes disagree on pronunciations. By listening to others who work with you, you can learn how words are commonly pronounced in your area. Practicing speaking terms out loud will improve your pronunciation and help you use medical terms with confidence.

ABBREVIATIONS AND ACRONYMS

An **abbreviation** is a shortening of a word, often achieved by removing letters from the end of the word, and sometimes followed by a period. For example, *diff* is the abbreviation for *differential count*. *Staph* is an abbreviation for *Staphylococcus*.

Some medical terms have more than one commonly used abbreviation. For example, *hematocrit* can be abbreviated by dropping the first two syllables and using the last syllable *crit*. This abbreviation is more common when speaking about the hematocrit result. Hematocrit can also be abbreviated *Hct*, and often appears this way on laboratory request forms. A common hematology request—the measurement of both hemoglobin and hematocrit—can be called *H & H*.

An **acronym** is a new pronounceable word created from the first letters or syllables of a group of words. *AIDS* is an acronym for *a*cquired *i*mmuno*d*eficiency *s*yndrome; *SIDS* is an acronym for *s*udden *i*nfant *d*eath *s*yndrome.

Abbreviations and acronyms are used commonly in medicine to avoid having to repeatedly write or say several syllables.

Some common abbreviations and acronyms used in the clinical laboratory are listed in Table 1-13. Many of these abbreviations will be used in other lessons in this text. Workers should be familiar with frequently used abbreviations and acronyms so physician's orders or instructions can be carried out correctly and patient records are interpreted correctly.

TABLE 1-12. Selected suffixes commonly used in medical terminology

SUFFIX	DEFINITION	EXAMPLE OF USAGE	SUFFIX	DEFINITION	EXAMPLE OF USAGE
algia	pain	neuralgia	opathy, pathia	disease	adenopathy
blast	primitive, germ	erythroblast	oscopy	observation, viewing	endoscopy
centesis	puncture, aspiration	amniocentesis	osis	state, condition, increase	leukocytosis
cide	death, killer	bactericide	ostomy	create an opening	ileostomy
ectomy	excision, cut out	gastrectomy	otomy	cut into	phlebotomy
emesis	vomiting	hematemesis	penia	lack of	leukopenia
emia	in, or of, the blood	bilirubinemia	phil	affinity for, liking	eosinophil
genic	origin, producing	pyogenic	phyte	plant	dermatophyte
ia	state, condition	anuria	plastic, plasia	to form or mold	hyperplasia
iasis	process, condition	amebiasis	poiesis	to make	hemopoiesis
iole	small	bronchiole	rrhage	excessive flow	hemorrhage
itis	inflammation	pharyngitis	rrhea	flow	diarrhea
lysis	free, breaking down	hemolysis	scope, scopy	view	arthroscope
oid	resembling, similar to	blastoid	stasis	same, standing still	hemostasis
(o)logy	study of	pathology	troph(y)	nourishment	hypertrophy
oma	tumor	hepatoma			

TABLE 1-13. Abbreviations and acronyms commonly used in clinical laboratories

A	absorbance		bacti	bacteriology
Ab	antibody		BBP	blood-borne pathogen
ACT	activated clotting time		BP	blood pressure
AFB	acid-fast bacillus		BSI	body substance isolation
Ag	antigen		BT	bleeding time
AHG	anti-human globulin		BUN	blood urea nitrogen
AIDS	acquired immunodeficiency syndrome		C	centigrade, Celsius
ALL	acute lymphocytic leukemia		CBC	complete blood count
ALP, AP	alkaline phosphatase		cc, ccm	cubic centimeter
ALT	alanine aminotransferase (formerly SGPT)		CC	critical care
AML	acute myelogenous leukemia		CCU	coronary care unit
ANA	antinuclear antibody		CFU	colony forming unit
APTT	activated partial thromboplastin time		CGL	chronic granulocytic leukemia
AST	aspartate aminotransferase (formerly SGOT)		chol	cholesterol
BA	blood agar			*(Continues)*

TABLE 1-13. Abbreviations and acronyms commonly used in clinical laboratories (*Continued*)

CK	creatine kinase	HCl	hydrochloric acid
Cl	chloride	HCO_3^-	bicarbonate
CLL	chronic lymphocytic leukemia	hs-CRP	high-sensitivity C-reactive protein
CLS	clinical laboratory scientist	Hct	hematocrit
CLT	clinical laboratory technician	HCV	hepatitis C virus
cm	centimeter	HDL chol	high-density lipoprotein cholesterol
CNS	central nervous system	HDN	hemolytic disease of newborn
CO	carbon monoxide	H & H	hemoglobin and hematocrit
CO_2	carbon dioxide	HIV	human immunodeficiency virus
CPD	citrate-phosphate-dextrose	HLA	human leukocyte antigen
CPK	creatine phosphokinase	H_2O	water
crit	hematocrit	HPF	high-power field
CRP	C-reactive protein	HSV	herpes simplex virus
C & S	culture and sensitivity	ICU	intensive care unit
CSF	cerebrospinal fluid	Ig	immunoglobulin
cu mm	cubic millimeter, mm^3	IgA	immunoglobulin A
DAT	direct antiglobulin test	IgE	immunoglobulin E
dL	deciliter	IgG	immunoglobulin G
DIC	disseminated intravascular coagulation	IgM	immunoglobulin M
diff	white blood cell differential count	IM	infectious mononucleosis
EBV	Epstein-Barr virus	IM, i.m.	intramuscular
EDTA	ethylenediaminetetraacetic acid	ITP	immune thrombocytopenic purpura
EIA	enzyme immunoassay	IU	international unit
EMB	eosin-methylene blue	IV, i.v.	intravenous
ESR	erythrocyte sedimentation rate	K	potassium
E.U.	Ehrlich units	kg	kilogram
F	Fahrenheit	L	liter
FBS	fasting blood sugar	LD, LDH	lactate dehydrogenase
FDP	fibrinogen degradation products	LDL chol	low-density lipoprotein cholesterol
fL	femtoliter	LPF	low-power field
FUO	fever of unknown origin	µg, mcg	microgram
g	gram	µL, µl	microliter
GC	gonococcus, gonorrhea	µmol	micromole
GFR	glomerular filtration rate	m	meter
GGT	gamma-glutamyltransferase	M	molar
GI	gastrointestinal	MCH	mean cell hemoglobin
GTT	glucose tolerance test	MCHC	mean cell hemoglobin concentration
GU	genitourinary	MCV	mean cell volume
HAV	hepatitis A virus	mEq	milliequivalent
Hb, Hgb	hemoglobin	mg	milligram
HbA1c	hemoglobin A1c	MI	myocardial infarction
HBV	hepatitis B virus	MIC	minimum inhibitory concentration
hCG	human chorionic gonadotropin	mIU	milli-international unit

(*Continues*)

TABLE 1-13. Abbreviations and acronyms commonly used in clinical laboratories (*Continued*)

mL, ml	milliliter		RDW	red (cell) distribution width
MLS	medical laboratory scientist		RF	rheumatoid factors
MLT	medical laboratory technician		RhIG	Rh immune globulin
mm	millimeter		RIA	radioimmunoassay
mmol	millimole		RNA	ribonucleic acid
mol	mole		rpm	revolutions per minute
MPV	mean platelet volume		RPR	rapid plasma reagin
MRI	magnetic resonance imaging		sed rate	erythrocyte sedimentation rate
MRSA	methicillin-resistant *Staphylococcus aureus*		SEM	scanning electron microscope
MSDS	material safety data sheet		SGOT	serum glutamic oxaloacetic transaminase
MT	medical technologist		SGPT	serum glutamic-pyruvic transaminase
N	normal, normality		SI	international units (Le Système International d'Unités)
Na	sodium			
NaCl	sodium chloride		SICU	surgical intensive care unit
nm	nanometer		SP	Standard Precautions
O.D.	optical density		sp. gr.	specific gravity
OGTT	oral glucose tolerance test		staph	*Staphylococcus*
O & P	ova and parasites		stat	immediately
OPIM	other potentially infectious material		STD	sexually transmitted disease
PCV	packed cell volume		STI	sexually transmitted infection
pg	picogram		strep	*Streptococcus*
pH	hydrogen ion concentration		STS	serological tests for syphilis
PLT	platelet		TEM	transmission electron microscope
PMN	polymorphonuclear neutrophil		TIA	transient ischemic attack
POC	point of care		TIBC	total iron-binding capacity
POCT	point-of-care test(ing)		TSH	thyroid stimulating hormone
POL	physician office laboratory		UA	urinalysis, uric acid
PP	postprandial		UP	Universal Precautions
PPE	personal protective equipment		URI	upper respiratory infection
PPM	parts per million		UTI	urinary tract infection
PRC	packed red cells		UV	ultraviolet
PSA	prostate specific antigen		VD	venereal disease
PT	prothrombin time, protime		VDRL	Venereal Disease Research Laboratory
QA	quality assessment		VLDL	very low density lipoproteins
QC	quality control		VRE	vancomycin-resistant *Enterococcus*
qns	quantity not sufficient		vWF	von Willebrand factor
qs	quantity sufficient		WBC	white blood cell
RA	rheumatoid arthritis		XDP	cross-linked fibrin degradation products
RBC	red blood cell			

Because of the wide range of topics in the field of health care, sometimes an abbreviation or acronym can have more than one meaning. Therefore, for correct interpretation, one must be careful to consider the context. For instance, to laboratory personnel *DAT* usually means *direct antiglobulin test*, whereas to nursing staff it can refer to *diet as tolerated*. *DAT* is also used to mean "drugs of abuse testing." Table 1-13 does not include abbreviations or acronyms used in prescriptions, nursing, or other areas of health care.

CASE STUDY 1

On a very busy day, Dr. Martin handed his medical assistant a handwritten preliminary diagnosis and an order for laboratory tests for his patient Mr. Jones. The medical assistant had difficulty reading Dr. Martin's handwriting and could not decide if the preliminary diagnosis was "temporary arthritis" or "temporal arteritis." Mr. Jones's major symptom was recurring headache and pain in the temple area of the head.

1. Which preliminary diagnosis is most likely the diagnosis written by Dr. Martin?
2. Discuss the importance of correctly spelling and understanding medical terms.

CASE STUDY 2

Mr. Benton went to the gastroenterologist because of abdominal pain and rectal bleeding. After examining Mr. Benton, the physician recommended an additional procedure be performed. After Mr. Benton arrived home, he became confused and could not remember if the test ordered was "colonoscopy" or "cholectomy."

Using only the stem and suffix tables, explain the differences between the two procedures.

CASE STUDY 3

Ms. Jackson consulted a urologist and described several symptoms. The urologist wrote a preliminary diagnosis of "paroxysmal nocturnal hemoglobinuria" and ordered several laboratory tests to help confirm the diagnosis.

1. Examine the name of the suspected condition. What symptom would the patient have reported to cause the physician to diagnose "hemoglobinuria?"
2. What other symptom(s) could have been reported based on the qualifiers "paroxysmal" and "nocturnal?"

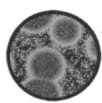

SUMMARY

Medical terminology encompasses a multitude of special terms with very precise meanings used in the field of medicine. Most medical terms are derived from Greek or Latin. Medical terms are formed by combining prefixes, stems, and suffixes that have specific meanings to produce a term with an exact definition. By learning the meanings of selected prefixes, stems, and suffixes, the worker can deduce the meanings of many medical terms, even if the terms are unfamiliar.

Clinical laboratory personnel need to understand and be able to use medical terms in both oral and written communications. In addition, personnel should be familiar with several abbreviations and acronyms that are in common use in the clinical laboratory and in laboratory reports. By becoming fluent in medical terminology, personnel will gain confidence in their communication skills.

REVIEW QUESTIONS

1. Why is it important for healthcare workers to understand medical terminology?
2. Most medical terms are derived from which languages?
3. How can one learn to correctly pronounce medical terms?
4. Name the stems for cell, heart, head, skin, chest, kidney, muscle, liver, and stomach.
5. Name 10 common suffixes and give a meaning for each.
6. Name 10 common prefixes and give a meaning for each.
7. List 10 abbreviations or acronyms frequently used in the clinical laboratory and give the meaning of each.
8. Define abbreviation, acronym, prefix, stem, suffix, and terminology.

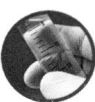

STUDENT ACTIVITIES

1. Complete the written examination for this lesson.

2. Practice pronouncing the word parts and medical terms in Tables 1-10 through 1-12. Look up pronunciations of 10 terms from each table and practice saying the terms out loud.

3. Study the definitions for prefixes, suffixes, and stems listed in the tables. Select 10 prefixes, suffixes, and stems from each of Tables 1-10, 1-11, and 1-12. Use each of the selected word parts in a word not on the list.

4. Prepare 20 flashcards using terms from tables in this lesson, a medical dictionary, or a textbook glossary. Write the term on the front and the definition on the back.

5. Obtain examples of laboratory requisition or report forms. Look for abbreviations or acronyms used on the forms.

WEB ACTIVITIES

1. Select five terms from each *usage* column in Tables 1-10, 1-11, and 1-12. Write your best definition of the term, using the definitions of stems, prefixes, and suffixes in the tables. Search an online medical dictionary for the terms, and compare your definitions with the dictionary definitions.

2. Search the Internet for free medical terminology tutorials or self-tests. Use these to enhance your knowledge of medical terms.

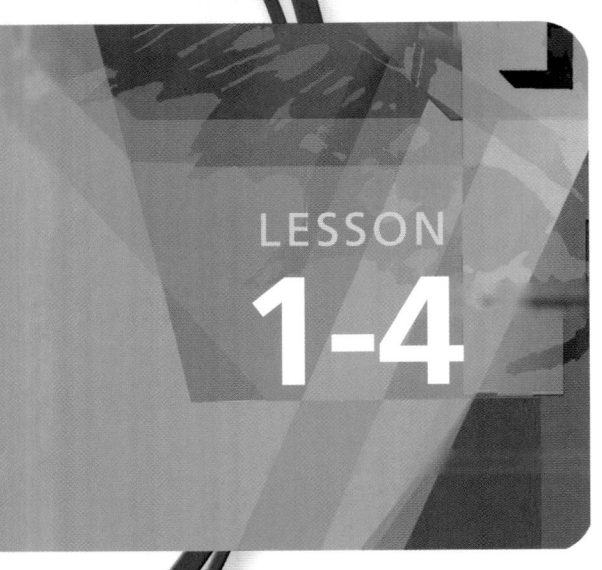

Biological Safety

LESSON OBJECTIVES

After studying this lesson, the student will:

- Explain the purpose of the Bloodborne Pathogens Standard.
- Explain the reason for issuing Standard Precautions in 1996.
- Explain what is meant by exposure control plan.
- List the components of an exposure control plan.
- Explain the evolution of safety laws and rules since the 1970s.
- Explain the roles of the Centers for Disease Control and Prevention (CDC) and the Occupational Safety and Health Administration (OSHA) in promoting safety in healthcare institutions.
- Explain the impact of the Needlestick Safety and Prevention Act of 2000.
- Discuss how work practice controls improve safety.
- Discuss how engineering controls improve safety.
- List types of personal protective equipment (PPE) commonly used in the clinical laboratory.
- Discuss infection prevention and healthcare-associated infections (HAIs).
- Demonstrate correct hand hygiene techniques.
- Demonstrate how to remove and discard contaminated gloves.
- Demonstrate the correct way to wear PPE such as face protection and fluid-resistant gowns or laboratory coats.
- Discuss how sterilization, disinfection, and antisepsis are used in the clinical laboratory.
- Explain the impact of human immunodeficiency virus (HIV) and hepatitis B and C viruses on safety practices in health care.
- List safety precautions that must be observed when handling biological materials.
- List additional safety precautions that must be observed when working in the microbiology laboratory.
- Define the glossary terms.

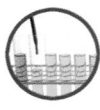

GLOSSARY

acquired immunodeficiency syndrome (AIDS) / a form of severe immunodeficiency caused by infection with the human immunodeficiency virus (HIV)

aerosol / liquid in the form of a very fine mist

alimentary tract / the digestive tube from the mouth to the anus

antiseptic / a chemical used on living tissues to control the growth of infectious agents

biohazard / risk or hazard to health or the environment from biological agents

biological safety cabinet / a special work cabinet that provides protection to the worker while working with infectious microorganisms

bloodborne pathogens (BBP) / pathogens that can be present in human blood (and blood-contaminated body fluids)

Bloodborne Pathogens (BBP) Standard / OSHA guidelines for preventing occupational exposure to pathogens present in human blood and body fluids, including, but not limited to, HIV and hepatitis B virus (HBV); final OSHA standard of December 6, 1991, effective March 6, 1992

community-acquired infection (CAI) / infection acquired through contact with friends, family, and the public or by contact with contaminated environmental surfaces

disinfectant / a chemical used on inanimate objects to kill or inactivate microbes

engineering control / use of available technology and equipment to protect the worker from hazards

exposure control plan / a plan identifying employees at risk for exposure to bloodborne pathogens and providing training in methods to prevent exposure

exposure incident / an accident, such as a needlestick, in which an individual is exposed to possible infection through contact with body substances from another individual

hand antisepsis / decontamination of hands using antiseptic soap or waterless antiseptic handrub

hand hygiene / a set of techniques that includes handwashing with soap and water, washing with antiseptic soap, or cleansing with a waterless antiseptic product

healthcare-associated infection (HAI) / infection acquired while being treated for another condition in a healthcare setting; synonym for healthcare-acquired infection; formerly called nosocomial infection

hepatitis B virus (HBV) / the virus that causes hepatitis B infection and is transmitted by contact with infected blood or other body fluids

hepatitis C virus (HCV) / the virus that causes hepatitis C infection and is transmitted by contact with infected blood or other body fluids

human immunodeficiency virus (HIV) / the retrovirus that has been identified as the cause of AIDS

isolation / the practice of limiting the movement and social contact of a patient who is potentially infectious or who must be protected from exposure to infectious agents; quarantine

other potentially infectious materials (OPIM) / any and all body fluids, tissues, organs, or other specimens from a human source

parenteral / any route other than by the alimentary canal; intravenous, subcutaneous, intramuscular, or mucosal

pathogenic / capable of causing damage or injury to the host

personal protective equipment (PPE) / specialized clothing or equipment used by workers to protect from direct exposure to blood or other potentially infectious or hazardous materials; includes, but is not limited to, gloves, laboratory apparel, eye protection, and breathing apparatus

Standard Precautions / a set of comprehensive safety guidelines designed to protect patients and healthcare workers by requiring that all patients and all body fluids, body substances, organs, and unfixed tissues be regarded as potentially infectious

sterilization / the act of eliminating all living microorganisms from an article or area

Transmission-Based Precautions / specific safety practices used in addition to Standard Precautions when treating patients known to be or suspected of being infected with pathogens that can be spread by air, droplet, or contact

Universal Precautions (UP) / a method of infection control in which all human blood and other body fluids containing visible blood are treated as if infectious

work practice controls / methods of performing tasks that reduce the worker's exposure to blood and other potentially hazardous materials

INTRODUCTION

Until the 1980s, clinical laboratory safety training concentrated primarily on using safety measures to protect from chemical and physical hazards and to protect from contagious diseases such as tuberculosis. However, the discovery of **acquired immunodeficiency syndrome (AIDS)**, caused by the **human immunodeficiency virus (HIV)**, and increases in **hepatitis B virus (HBV)** and **hepatitis C virus (HCV)** infections brought about an increased emphasis on biological safety and preventing exposure to and transmission of these agents.

As the modes of transmission of HIV, HBV, and HCV became known, it was realized that more stringent safety measures and work practices must be used to protect workers, patients, and the general public from exposure and infection. The Centers for Disease Control and Prevention (CDC) and the Occupational Safety and Health Administration (OSHA), as well as other government agencies, have taken the lead in developing safety guidelines to protect workers and the public from infectious agents. Over recent years, safety guidelines have been updated, improved, and expanded several times. Educational and training materials are available from several federal and state sources to help clinical sites implement good safety practices.

With this new emphasis on biological safety also came new terminology. The term **biohazard** came into use. A biohazard symbol was adopted and is now used widely to indicate the presence of a biological hazard or biohazardous condition (Figure 1-12). This symbol is used to warn that a risk or hazard to health or the environment from infectious agents exists. In this text, the symbol ⚙ alerts that a biological hazard can be present and the worker should use appropriate measures to prevent exposure.

This lesson describes the current status of biological safety regulations and recommendations intended to protect individuals from exposure to infectious agents both in the general healthcare setting and in the microbiology laboratory. By coordinating biological safety practices in this lesson with safety practices to protect against chemical and physical hazards (Lesson 1-5), the foundation of a comprehensive safety program can be formed. It should be emphasized that these lessons are merely an introduction to clinical laboratory safety practices. All details of safety procedures and practices are too extensive to be covered in full in this text.

EVOLUTION OF BIOLOGICAL SAFETY REGULATIONS AND GUIDELINES

As knowledge about transmission of infectious agents has grown, the guidelines for preventing exposure and infection have evolved. Table 1-14 gives a timeline of the major federal directives calling for improvements in safety practices. The directives included practices such as **isolation** techniques, Universal Precautions, Body Substance Isolation, Bloodborne Pathogens Standard, Standard Precautions, and Transmission-Based Precautions. Safety regulations continue to evolve.

In the first half of the twentieth century, the techniques used for dealing with infectious diseases changed significantly. At one time all infectious patients were quarantined together to try to stop disease from spreading to the public. It was common for infected patients to be sent to infectious disease or tuberculosis hospitals. However, patients infected or reinfected each other, leading to the use of isolation rooms or cubicles within these hospitals as a method of controlling disease spread. Also, aseptic procedures, such as washing hands, wearing gloves, and disinfecting patient-contaminated objects, came into wider use.

Isolation Techniques

By the 1960s, tuberculosis hospitals and infectious disease hospitals were closing as the methods of disease transmission became better understood. Infectious patients were placed in isolation rooms in regular hospitals in efforts to contain diseases and prevent their spread. To give guidance in infectious disease

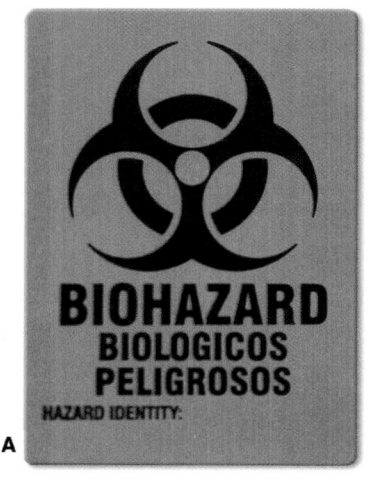
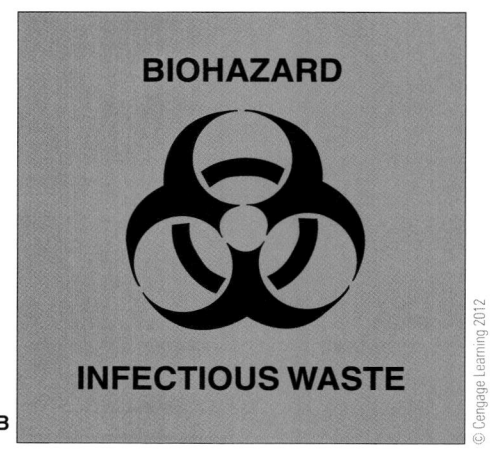

FIGURE 1-12 Examples of biohazard signs

© Cengage Learning 2012

TABLE 1-14. Timeline of federal guidelines and laws concerning biological safety

YEAR	ISSUING AGENCY/ ENTITY	GUIDELINE/LAW
1970	CDC	Published "Isolation Techniques for Use in Hospitals"
1975	CDC	Revised "Isolation Techniques" to include category-specific precautions and prohibition of recapping needles
1983	CDC	Issued nonbinding guidelines for isolation precautions in hospitals, designating seven isolation categories
1985	CDC	Introduced Universal Blood and Body Fluid Precautions (Universal Precautions or UP), primarily in response to HIV/AIDS epidemic
1987	CDC	Issued Body Substance Isolation guidelines
1988	U.S. Congress	Enacted Clinical Laboratory Improvement Amendments of 1988 (CLIA '88)
1991	OSHA	Issued Bloodborne Pathogens (BBP) Standard, mandating the use of UP
1996	CDC	Issued Standard Precautions, Transmission-Based Precautions, and synthesized UP and Body Substance Isolation
2000	U.S. Congress	Enacted Needlestick Safety and Prevention Act
2001	OSHA	Revised BBP Standard in response to Needlestick Safety and Prevention Act
2002	CDC	Guideline for Hand Hygiene in Healthcare Settings
2009	WHO	WHO Guidelines for Hand Hygiene in Healthcare

management, in 1970 the CDC outlined isolation techniques for hospitals and listed categories of isolation. In 1975, these guidelines were revised to include recommendations for specific safety precautions for each isolation category. Safe work practices, such as not recapping needles, were emphasized.

Universal Precautions

In 1983, the CDC issued guidelines for isolation precautions in hospitals that contained specific precautions for each communicable disease or condition. In 1985, in response to the growing HIV and AIDS epidemic, the CDC issued guidelines called *Universal Blood and Body Fluid Precautions*, commonly referred to as **Universal Precautions (UP)**. These precautions and practices were designed to protect the healthcare worker from exposure to blood and to body fluids containing visible blood. Universal Precautions were to be applied universally to *all* patients, regardless of whether they were suspected of being infectious. Universal Precautions were implemented by using **personal protective equipment (PPE)**, including gown, gloves, mask, and eye protection such as a full face shield or an acrylic splash shield.

Body Substance Isolation and Bloodborne Pathogens Standard

The limitations of the Universal Precautions were that they covered only blood and body fluids visibly contaminated with blood; they did not include all body fluids, secretions, or excretions or the possible need for isolation precautions. In 1987, the *Body Substance Isolation* (BSI) guidelines were issued, recommending the use of precautions for all body fluids and all moist and potentially infectious body substances (and for all patients). However, these guidelines still did not cover all isolation precautions needed to prevent all modes of disease transmission, such as airborne diseases.

In 1991, OSHA issued the **Bloodborne Pathogens (BBP) Standard**, mandating implementation of safety measures with the primary purpose of reducing or eliminating occupational exposure to HIV, HCV, and HBV. The Bloodborne Pathogens Standard outlined the requirements for protecting workers who could be exposed to **bloodborne pathogens** such as human blood or **other potentially infectious materials (OPIM)**. OPIM included all body fluids, open wounds, and microbiological cultures. The Bloodborne Pathogens Standard applied to employees in all healthcare facilities, as well as all other workers who could be at risk for exposure (Table 1-15).

TABLE 1-15. Workers who can be at risk for exposure to bloodborne pathogens*

Physicians	Dentists and other dental workers
Nurses	Blood donor facility personnel
Pathologists	Medical laboratory personnel
Phlebotomists	Laboratory research scientists
Dialysis personnel	Emergency medical technicians
Medical assistants	Morticians
Medical examiners	Paramedics
Some maintenance personnel	Some housekeeping personnel and laundry workers

*Exclusion of a job category here does not denote lack of risk.

Standard Precautions

Because of some confusion about how to implement Universal Precautions, Body Substance Isolation (BSI) guidelines, and the Bloodborne Pathogens Standard, in 1996, the CDC issued **Standard Precautions**, a comprehensive set of safety guidelines for healthcare workers, which included components of both Universal Precautions and BSI guidelines. Thus, "Standard Precautions" is the current terminology and the fundamental premise employed by healthcare personnel when rendering care to every patient. The intent of Standard Precautions is to protect patients and healthcare workers and to prevent **healthcare associated infections (HAIs)**, those infections acquired in a healthcare facility while being treated for another condition. All healthcare facilities are required to implement Standard Precautions and to insist that all workers comply with them.

The Standard Precautions guidelines also included a section on **Transmission-Based Precautions**, additional practices used with patients known or suspected to be infected with pathogens spread by air, droplets, or contact. Examples of these pathogens include the measles virus, tuberculosis bacterium, meningitis bacterium, and multidrug resistant organisms (MDROs). Lesson 7-9 contains a more complete discussion of Transmission-Based Precautions.

Needlestick Prevention

In 2001, OSHA revised the Bloodborne Pathogens Standard to emphasize safe practices to prevent accidental needlesticks in the workplace. This was in response to the Needlestick Safety and Prevention Act passed by Congress in 2000. Several designs of safety needles, lancets, syringes, sharps containers, and other devices are available to help workers reduce risk for needlestick injuries.

STANDARD PRECAUTIONS REGULATIONS

The use of Standard Precautions intensifies safety practices by requiring that every patient and every body fluid, body substance, organ, or unfixed tissue be regarded as potentially infectious. Standard Precautions must be applied:

- To *all* patients, regardless of their suspected infection status
- To *all* body fluids, excretions, and secretions
- To nonintact skin
- To mucous membranes
- To organs and unfixed tissue

Standard Precautions includes safe work practices such as the use of safety needles and other safety devices for blood collection and **hand hygiene** techniques, a set of techniques for decontamination of hands. Hand hygiene techniques include handwashing with soap and water and **hand antisepsis** using either **antiseptic** soaps or waterless antiseptics. The use of protective barriers such as gown, mask, gloves, and protection for eyes and mucous membranes (full face shield and/or acrylic splash shield) is also required. This added emphasis on exposure

prevention is important because, in addition to HIV, other bloodborne viruses such as HBV and HCV can cause severe disease. The safety practices that must be followed using the Standard Precautions guidelines are explained in Figure 1-13.

The Exposure Control Plan

Each facility is required to develop an **exposure control plan** (infection control plan) to identify all employees with potential for occupational exposure to human blood or OPIM. All employees must have access to an up-to-date safety manual containing specific biological safety guidelines for employees. The manual also includes safety education requirements and regulations for handling and disposal of contaminated materials.

A training program must be in place to inform employees of biological hazards, and the training must be documented. This training can be incorporated with general training on chemical, fire, and electrical safety, or it can be separate. The facility is required to update and document safety training annually. An example of a safety agreement form is shown in Figure 1-14.

The exposure control guidelines deal with safe handling of specimens, contaminated sharps, contaminated laundry, and regulated waste. OSHA guidelines must be consulted when the plan is being written. Each employee must have access to the plan. For example, a copy should be placed at each nursing station, in the laboratory, and in the housekeeping office. In the laboratory, the exposure control plan can be a separate document or included in the laboratory's standard operating procedure (SOP) manual.

Implementing an Exposure Control Plan

The employer has several responsibilities to the employee:

- The employer must provide employees with PPE appropriate for the tasks they perform.
- Warning labels and signs must be used to identify all biohazards.
- The exposure control plan must describe the control methods used to comply with the Bloodborne Pathogens Standard and Standard Precautions.
- The employer must provide free HBV immunization to workers at risk for exposure to bloodborne pathogens.

Identifying Employees at Risk

Employers must identify all employees who have occupational risk for exposure to blood or OPIM and provide training for them. Occupational exposure means reasonably anticipated contact with blood or other potentially infectious materials (Table 1-16). This contact can occur to the eyes, skin, or mucous membranes or through **parenteral** routes (routes other than the **alimentary tract**). An example of parenteral contact would be a needlestick. Laboratory personnel, nurses, and phlebotomists are not the only workers who require training. Dentists, dental technicians, dialysis personnel, some housekeeping and laundry workers, and others can be at risk (Table 1-15).

STANDARD PRECAUTIONS

Assume that every person is potentially infected or colonized with an organism that could be transmitted in the healthcare setting.

Hand Hygiene

Avoid unnecessary touching of surfaces in close proximity to the patient.

When hands are visibly dirty, contaminated with proteinaceous material, or visibly soiled with blood or body fluids, wash hands with soap and water.

If hands are not visibly soiled, or after removing visible material with soap and water, decontaminate hands with an alcohol-based hand rub. Alternatively, hands may be washed with an antimicrobial soap and water.

Perform hand hygiene:
    Before having direct contact with patients.
    After contact with blood, body fluids or excretions, mucous membranes, nonintact skin, or wound dressings.
    After contact with a patient's intact skin (e.g., when taking a pulse or blood pressure or lifting a patient).
    If hands will be moving from a contaminated-body site to a clean-body site during patient care.
    After contact with inanimate objects (including medical equipment) in the immediate vicinity of the patient.
    After removing gloves.

Personal protective equipment (PPE)

Wear PPE when the nature of the anticipated patient interaction indicates that contact with blood or body fluids may occur.

Before leaving the patient's room or cubicle, remove and discard PPE.

Gloves

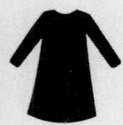

Wear gloves when contact with blood or other potentially infectious materials, mucous membranes, nonintact skin, or potentially contaminated intact skin (e.g., of a patient incontinent of stool or urine) could occur.

Remove gloves after contact with a patient and/or the surrounding environment using proper technique to prevent hand contamination. Do not wear the same pair of gloves for the care of more than one patient.

Change gloves during patient care if the hands will move from a contaminated body-site (e.g., perineal area) to a clean body-site (e.g., face).

Gowns

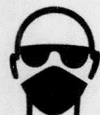

Wear a gown to protect skin and prevent soiling or contamination of clothing during procedures and patient-care activities when contact with blood, body fluids, secretions, or excretions is anticipated.

Wear a gown for direct patient contact if the patient has uncontained secretions or excretions.

Remove gown and perform hand hygiene before leaving the patient's environment.

Mouth, nose, eye protection

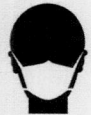

Use PPE to protect the mucous membranes of the eyes, nose and mouth during procedures and patient-care activities that are likely to generate splashes or sprays of blood, body fluids, secretions and excretions.

During aerosol-generating procedures wear one of the following: a face shield that fully covers the front and sides of the face, a mask with attached shield, or a mask and goggles.

Respiratory Hygiene/Cough Etiquette

Educate healthcare personnel to contain respiratory secretions to prevent droplet and fomite transmission of respiratory pathogens, especially during seasonal outbreaks of viral respiratory tract infections.

Offer masks to coughing patients and other symptomatic persons (e.g., persons who accompany ill patients) upon entry into the facility.

Patient-care equipment and instruments/devices

Wear PPE (e.g., gloves, gown), according to the level of anticipated contamination, when handling patient-care equipment and instruments/devices that are visibly soiled or may have been in contact with blood or body fluids.

Care of the environment

Include multi-use electronic equipment in policies and procedures for preventing contamination and for cleaning and disinfection, especially those items that are used by patients, those used during delivery of patient care, and mobile devices that are moved in and out of patient rooms frequently (e.g., daily).

Textiles and laundry

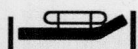

Handle used textiles and fabrics with minimum agitation to avoid contamination of air, surfaces and persons.

©2007 Brevis Corporation www.brevis.com

Courtesy Brevis Corp.

FIGURE 1-13 Guide to Standard Precautions for Infection Prevention, issued by the CDC in 1996

SAFETY AGREEMENT FORM

Safety training must be updated at least yearly. Verify safety training by initialing the items below:

_____ I have been informed about and received training concerning the chemical hygiene plan

_____ I have been informed of the location of the chemical hygiene plan and the MSDS folder

_____ I have been informed about and received training concerning the OSHA Bloodborne Pathogens Standard and Standard Precautions

_____ I understand that biological specimens and blood or blood products are potentially infectious

_____ I understand that even though diagnostic products and reagents are screened to prevent exposure to infectious agents such as HIV and HBV, no known test can offer 100% assurance that products derived from human blood cannot transmit disease

_____ I agree to follow all safety rules and regulations as required by the instructor, the supervisor and the institution.

_____

Name (Please Print)

_____   _____
Signature   Date

_____   _____
Supervisor/Safety Training   Date

© Cengage Learning 2012

FIGURE 1-14 Example of a safety agreement form

TABLE 1-16. Examples of substances recognized by the CDC as having the potential to transmit pathogens such as HBV, HCV, and HIV

Blood, including cord blood	Urine
	Breast milk
Blood products	Vaginal secretions
Semen	Pleural fluid
Peritoneal fluid	Pericardial fluid
Amniotic fluid	Unfixed tissue specimens
Cerebrospinal fluid	Organs
Saliva in dental settings where bleeding occurs	

Exposure Control Methods

Employee training must include training in exposure control methods, all the components determined as essential for a task to be completed safely for both the patient and the employee (Table 1-17).

TABLE 1-17. Control methods required as part of an exposure control plan

Standard Precautions	Treating all patients, body fluids, unfixed tissue, and organ specimens as if infectious
Personal protective equipment	Specialized clothing or equipment used by workers to protect from direct exposure to blood and other substances
Engineering controls	Devices that eliminate or minimize worker exposure
Work practice controls	The manner in which a task is performed to reduce the likelihood of exposure

These components include the use of:

- Standard Precautions
- PPE
- Engineering controls
- Work practice controls

Standard Precautions. Standard Precautions refers to a method of infection prevention in which *all* patients and *all* human blood and other body fluids or substances (including organs and unfixed tissues) are treated as if potentially infectious. Standard Precautions must be used each time a worker has contact with *every* patient and *every* specimen, even if the specimen is from a friend or a coworker.

Personal Protective Equipment. Personal protective equipment (PPE) is specialized apparel, devices, or equipment used by workers to protect from direct exposure to potentially infectious materials. This includes, but is not limited to, gloves, fluid-resistant gowns, full-face shields, masks, goggles, or safety glasses (Figures 1-15 and 1-16). Contact lenses should not be worn; if a splash of OPIM occurs, the material could lodge between the lens and the surface of the eye. The contact lenses would have to be removed before eye washing can begin, increasing the time that potentially infectious material is in contact with mucous membranes.

Engineering Controls. Engineering controls are devices and technology used to isolate the worker from hazards. An example is a benchtop acrylic splash shield to protect the worker from **aerosols,** fine mists of liquid. Aerosols can be created when a tube of blood is being uncapped or serum is being pipetted (Figure 1-17). Biohazard containers, appropriate surface **disinfectants** and hand antiseptics, puncture-resistant sharps containers, and safety needles are also engineering controls (Figures 1-17 and 1-18).

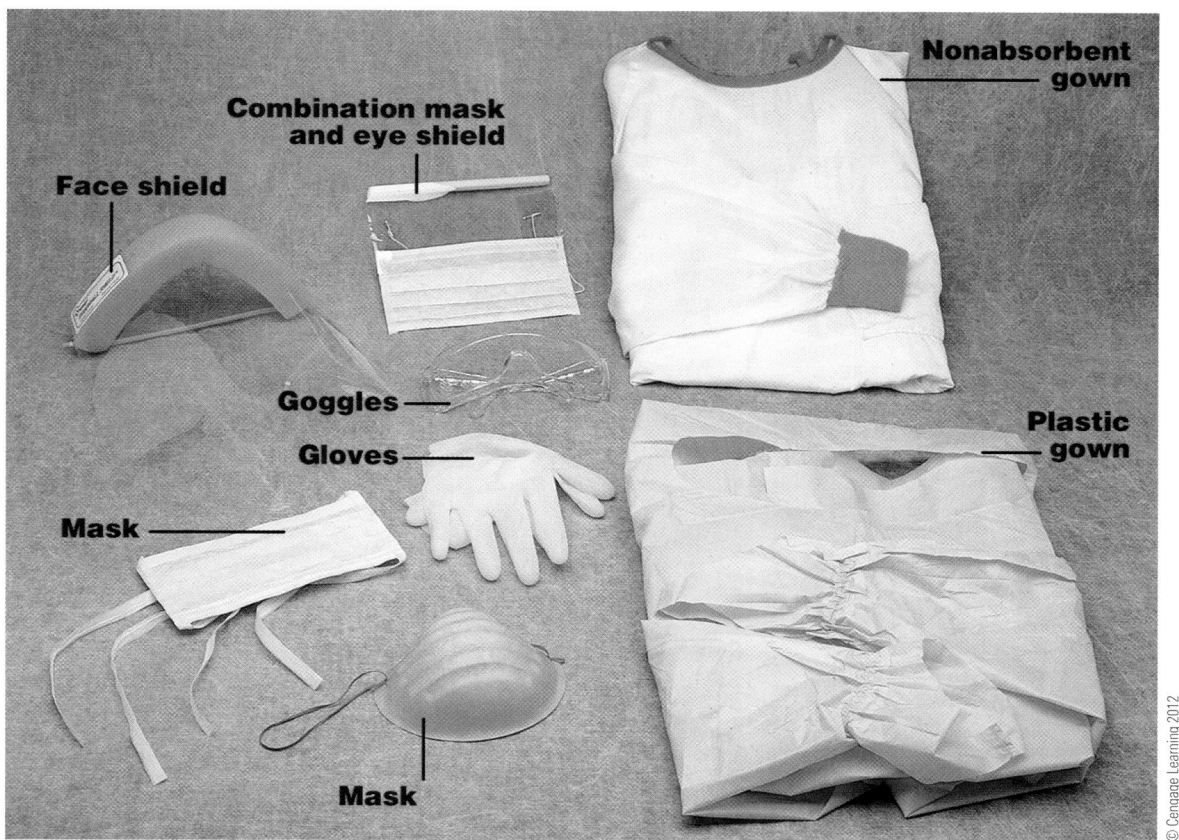

FIGURE 1-15 Personal protective equipment used to protect against biohazards

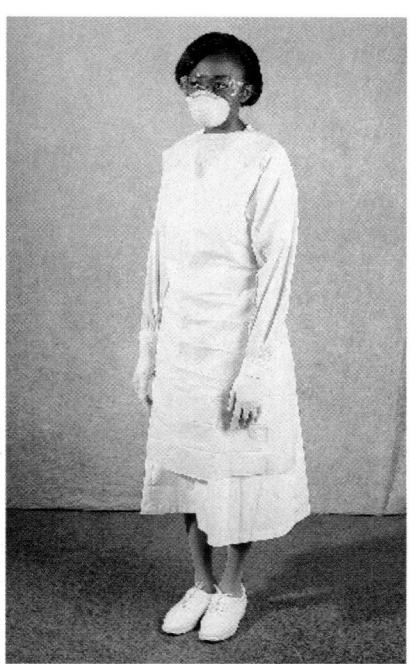
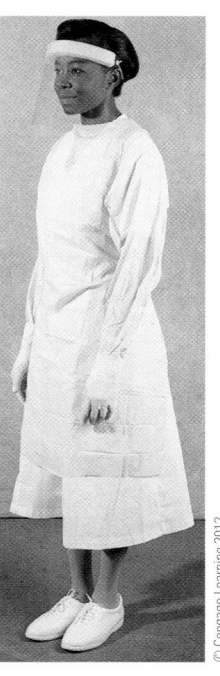

FIGURE 1-16 Worker wearing PPE including safety glasses and mask (left) and full face shield (right)

Work Practice Controls. Work practice controls refer to the manner in which the task is performed. The use of work practice controls is intended to reduce the likelihood of a worker being exposed to hazards (Figures 1-19 and 1-20). Many of these practices include commonsense work habits, such as (1) eating or drinking only in designated break areas; (2) storing food in refrigerators reserved for food products only; and (3) limiting personal grooming activities, such as applying cosmetics, to break rooms or restrooms. Computer keyboards and telephones within the laboratory work area are assumed to be contaminated, and gloves should be worn when using either of them. However, items such as keyboards and phones should be disinfected frequently as well as personal devices such as cell phones or pagers that might be carried during the work day.

Examples of mandated work practice controls include:

- Using hand hygiene practices such as washing hands with an appropriate antiseptic before donning gloves, after glove removal or any other time necessary (Figure 1-20)

- Wearing appropriate PPE when cleaning up biological spills

- Removing and disposing of PPE when leaving a work area or on completion of a task

- Using a surface disinfectant regularly, such as 10% chlorine bleach (hypochlorite), to clean the work area before and after each use, and anytime a spill occurs (Figure 1-19)

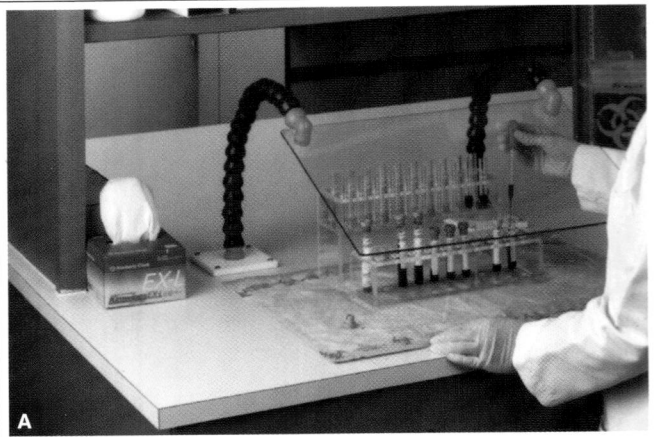

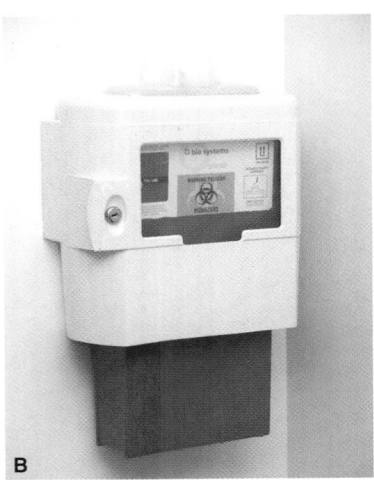

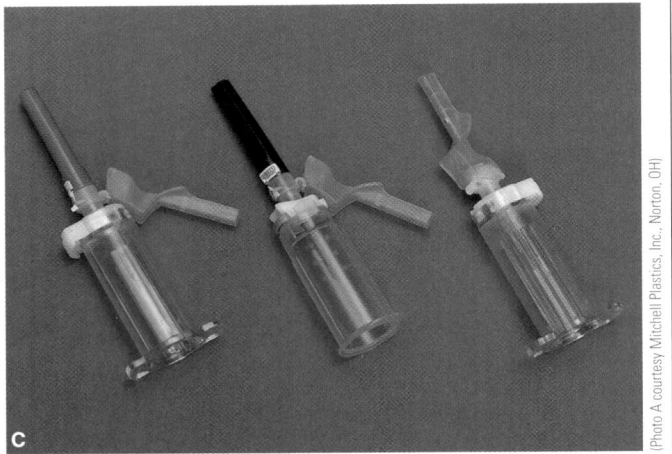

(Photo A courtesy Mitchell Plastics, Inc., Norton, OH)

FIGURE 1-17 Engineering controls: (A) acrylic safety shield to protect worker from splashes; (B) wall-hung sharps collector; (C) vacuum tube holders with safety needles

● Using approved needlestick prevention practices to prevent exposure to bloodborne pathogens through accidental needlesticks

Many of these work practice controls have been in place for some time. However, needlestick prevention practices have

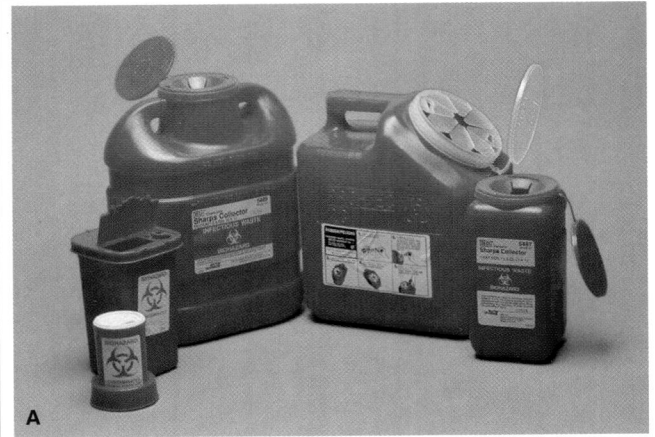

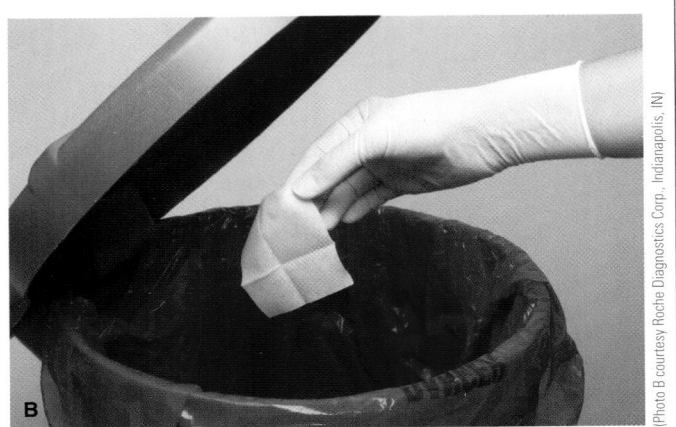

(Photo B courtesy Roche Diagnostics Corp., Indianapolis, IN)

FIGURE 1-18 Engineering controls: (A) rigid containers for disposal of contaminated sharps; (B) biohazard container for disposal of non-sharp objects

changed in recent years. The passage of the Needlestick Safety and Prevention Act in 2000 mandated that engineering controls such as safety needles and devices be used. It also required that immediately after needle use, the safety feature must be activated and the needle discarded into a readily accessible sharps container (Figure 1-19). This Act significantly changed phlebotomy practices.

COMPLYING WITH THE EXPOSURE CONTROL PLAN

The exposure control plan can differ slightly from one facility to another, but in general it will include specific information on the correct use of engineering controls, work practice controls such as hand hygiene, and appropriate use of PPE such as gloves, face protection, and fluid-resistant laboratory coats and gowns. Complying with an exposure control plan in the daily routine of the laboratory worker is not as difficult as it may seem. The example in Table 1-18 illustrates how a worker or student would use the plan while performing a venipuncture.

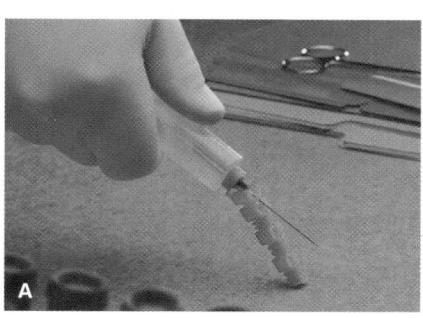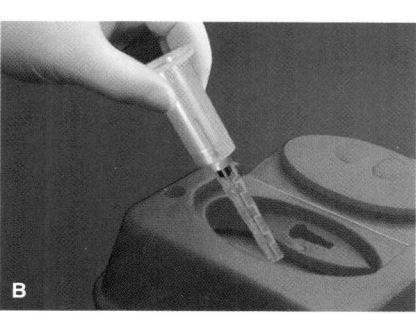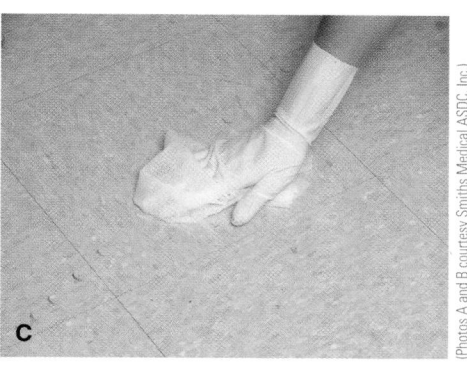

(Photos A and B courtesy Smiths Medical ASDC, Inc.)

FIGURE 1-19 Work practice controls: (A) engage safety shield on needle immediately after use; (B) discard used blood collecting devices into sharps container immediately after use; (C) clean up spills with disinfectant

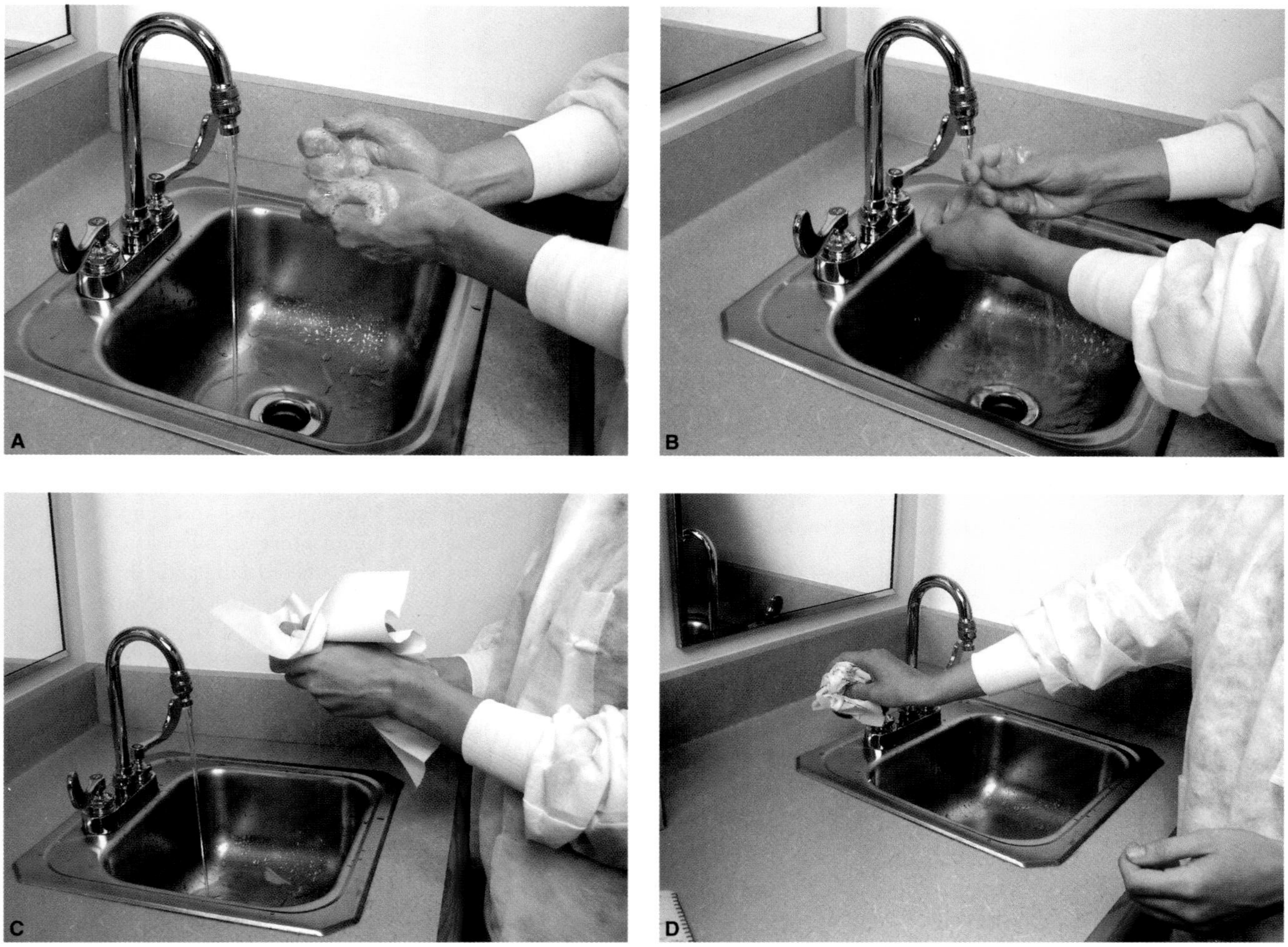

© Cengage Learning 2012

FIGURE 1-20 Handwashing technique: (A) with water running, soap hands thoroughly and rub together at least 15 seconds; (B) rinse hands and wrists thoroughly under running water; (C) dry hands with paper towel; and (D) use towel to turn off water

Infection Prevention

Healthcare-associated infections (HAIs) are infections acquired while being treated for another condition in a healthcare setting. HAIs can be a serious problem. A patient having a simple outpatient procedure can become infected through contact with contaminated environmental surfaces, a caregiver, or another patient. As a consequence the patient can require treatment or even subsequent hospitalization to treat the infection. However, if healthcare personnel follow the institution's protocol for infection prevention, these incidents can be eliminated.

TABLE 1-18. Example of using exposure control methods to protect against biohazards while performing a venipuncture

CONTROL METHOD	MECHANISM
Standard Precautions	Treat all patients and all specimens as if infectious
Personal protective equipment	Wear gloves to handle blood and all body fluids; wear fluid-resistant gown or laboratory coat; wear eye protection if splashes are possible
Engineering controls	Use appropriate surface disinfectants; sharps containers for contaminated sharps; separate biohazard containers for contaminated PPE and biohazardous waste
Work practice controls	Always wear gloves when working with blood; use safety needles and needle holders; never recap or remove needles from holders or syringes; immediately discard contaminated sharps; wash hands with antiseptic after removing gloves or any other time hands are contaminated

TABLE 1-19. Recommendations for hand hygiene

- Decontaminate hands before and after all procedures
- Use waterless antiseptic or antimicrobial soap and water for routine decontamination of hands in most clinical situations
- Wash visibly soiled hands with soap and water, followed by washing with antiseptic
- Wash hands with soap and water before and after eating and after using a restroom
- Wash hands with antiseptic soap and water after each 5 to 10 hand disinfections with a waterless antiseptic

Community-acquired infections (CAI) are infections acquired through contact with friends, family, the public, or contaminated environmental surfaces. These are the usual routes for infections spread in schools and other gathering places for the public. Infections can include a range of illnesses such as the common cold, influenza, communicable childhood diseases, bacterial infections, and parasitic infections.

Hand hygiene techniques are the single most important way of preventing both CAIs and HAIs. Studies show that the use of hand hygiene techniques significantly reduces HAIs. Failure to use appropriate hand hygiene is considered the leading cause of HAIs. Employees must follow their institution's hand hygiene policy. The intense campaign emphasizing proper and frequent handwashing was a huge factor in controlling the spread of H1N1 influenza in the 2009 to 2010 pandemic.

Several types and brands of antiseptic agents are available for use in hand hygiene practices. These agents include plain soaps, antimicrobial soaps, waterless antiseptic agents such as alcohol-based gels, and chemical antiseptics. The effectiveness of hand hygiene techniques depends on the amount of antiseptic agent used, the frequency and duration of the hand cleaning procedure, and the type of product used. General recommendations for routine hand hygiene are given in Table 1-19.

Using Waterless Hand Antiseptics

Waterless antiseptics are available in several forms, including rinses, alcohol-based gels, and foams. Products differ in efficacy so the manufacturer's recommendations for the correct volume and technique to use for effective hand antisepsis should be followed. Alcohol-based products are applied to the palm of one hand and the hands are vigorously rubbed together, covering all surfaces of hands and fingers. This procedure is continued for at least 30 seconds and until all alcohol has evaporated and the hands are completely dry. One advantage of the waterless antiseptics is that a sink is not required for hand decontamination.

Hand Antisepsis

Although the waterless antiseptics are convenient and quick, it is still necessary to frequently wash hands with water and antimicrobial or antiseptic soap. Hands should first be wet with warm or room temperature water and an amount of antiseptic recommended by the manufacturer applied to the hands. The hands and wrists should be lathered and hands should be rubbed together vigorously, covering all surfaces of the hands and fingers (Figure 1-20). Special attention should be given to cleaning fingernails and under rings. The arms or wrists and hands should be rinsed by holding the hands in a downward position and rinsing toward the tips of the fingers. The entire procedure should take 40–60 seconds. The hands should be dried thoroughly with a disposable towel. Hand-operated faucets should be turned on and off using a clean disposable towel to avoid contaminating hands with organisms or substances that can be present on faucet handles. The use of hot water during handwashing should be avoided because repeated exposure to hot water can increase the risk for dermatitis.

Using Personal Protective Equipment

Standard Precautions require that personnel wear PPE to protect against exposure to potentially infectious material. This PPE includes, but is not limited to, fluid-resistant laboratory coat, gloves, and protection for face and mucous membranes, such as safety glasses, goggles, face shields, and masks.

Gloves

Gloves must be changed frequently when working in the labora-tory, and hands must be washed with antiseptic between each glove change. Gloves that provide both chemical and biological protection should be worn. Gloves are put on by pulling the cuff or wrist area up so that all exposed skin is covered. Workers should not have long fingernails or wear sharp rings or jewelry that can puncture gloves. Situations requiring the use of sterile gloves are addressed in Lesson 7-9.

One way of removing contaminated gloves is shown in Figure 1-21. The outer surface of the cuff of one glove is grasped with the other gloved hand, and the glove is pulled off over itself. With the removed glove contained in the remaining gloved hand, the second glove is removed in the same manner, without touch-ing the outer glove surface with the bare hand. The gloves are then discarded into a biohazard container.

Face and Respiratory Protection

Full face protection should be worn when working in a situation in which aerosols or splashes can occur. This protection can be provided by wearing a disposable face shield that covers eyes, nose, and mouth or by wearing a combination of safety glasses and mask. It is not usually necessary to wear eye or respira-tory protection when working in a **biological safety cabinet**. Guidelines for wearing masks (including N95 respirator) to pro-tect against transmission of infectious diseases are discussed in Lesson 7-9.

Disposable Laboratory Coats or Gowns

Each institution will have a dress code describing the types of apparel permitted while working in the laboratory. Most require that workers wear some type of uniform or scrubs and a labora-tory coat or jacket to protect from contamination, spills, or stains. The use of disposable, fluid-resistant laboratory coats provides inexpensive protection and eliminates the need to launder con-taminated coats. Disposable gowns can also be worn to provide protection. In particular, disposable gowns are worn when a patient isolation room must be entered. Specific instructions for those cases are given in Lesson 7-9.

Exposure Incidents

The exposure control plan is designed to eliminate **exposure incidents**, accidental exposure to possible infectious agents through contact with body substances from another indi-vidual. Exposure incidents can include needlesticks, splashes onto mucous membranes, and exposure to aerosols of poten-tially infectious material. If any accident or exposure incident occurs, even if it seems insignificant, the employee should *immediately*:

- Flood the exposed area with water and clean any wound with antiseptic and water

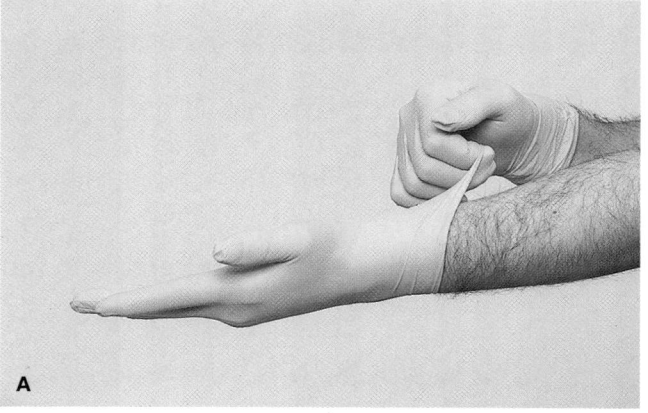
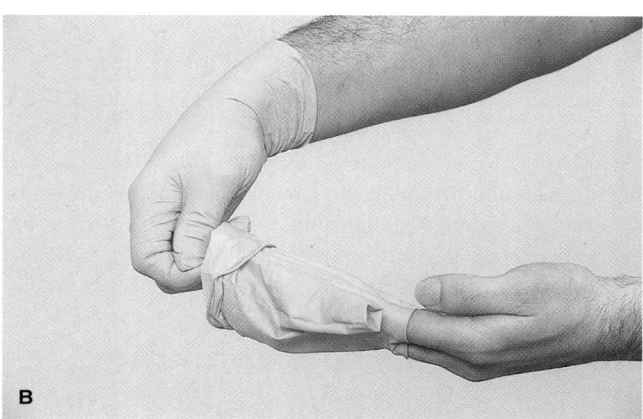
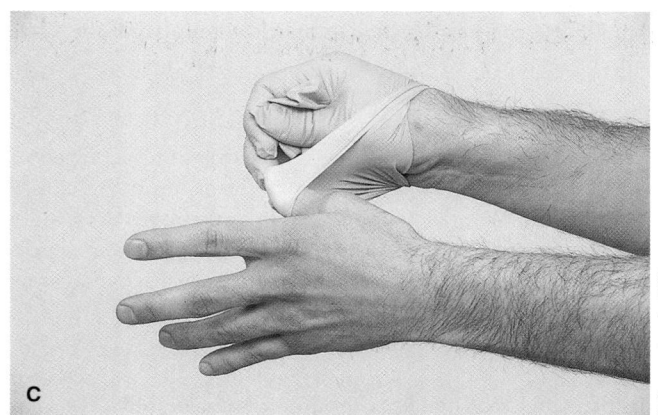

© Cengage Learning 2012

FIGURE 1-21 One method of removing contaminated gloves: (A) hold gloved hands over biohazard disposal container and grasp the outside of one glove cuff; (B) pull the glove down over the hand inside out and contain the removed glove in the palm of the remaining gloved hand; (C) insert bare fingers inside the remaining glove cuff, pull the glove inside out down over the hand taking care not to touch the outside of glove, and discard both gloves into biohazard container

- Report incident to supervisor or appropriate safety officer
- Seek immediate medical attention

The employer must provide a confidential, nonpunitive proce-dure for incident reporting, treatment, and follow-up.

ATTENTION!

ACTION TO TAKE IN CASE OF EXPOSURE INCIDENT

If you receive a needlestick or other injury from sharps, or if your eyes, nose, mouth, or broken skin are exposed to blood or OPIM:

1. Immediately flood the exposed area with water and clean skin with antiseptic and water.
2. Immediately report incident to supervisor or appropriate safety officer.
3. Seek immediate medical attention.

BIOLOGICAL HAZARDS OTHER THAN BLOODBORNE PATHOGENS

Clinical laboratory workers are exposed to biological hazards in addition to bloodborne pathogens. Clinical microbiology specimens can contain a variety of **pathogenic** microorganisms such as bacteria, viruses, fungi, or parasites. Students or workers in the laboratory must know how to protect themselves from these hazards.

Methods of Decontamination

Several methods are used in the clinical and microbiological laboratory to disinfect or decontaminate materials, surfaces, and skin. These can be classified as sterilization, disinfection, and antisepsis.

Sterilization

Sterilization refers to the killing or inactivation of all living organisms and viruses. In the laboratory, this is normally achieved by autoclaving contaminated materials. Autoclaves are used to decontaminate laboratory waste and to sterilize glassware, instruments, growth media for microbes, and reagents used in microbiology and other procedures requiring sterility.

Disinfection

Disinfectants are chemicals used on inanimate objects or surfaces, such as countertops, floors, instruments, or labware, to kill or inactivate microorganisms. Each type of disinfectant has advantages and disadvantages. The disinfectants selected should be effective against a wide range of microbes. The recommended shelf life, exposure time, and dilution for each disinfectant must be followed to achieve maximum disinfection. Some disinfectants can be skin, respiratory, or eye irritants, so precautions should be taken when using them. Disinfectants commonly used in the laboratory are:

- Dilute chlorine bleach (sodium hypochlorite), 1:10 dilution
- Alcohols, 70% to 90%
- Iodophors, 75 parts per million (ppm) or 4.5 mL/L of water
- Phenols
- Quaternary ammonium compounds

Iradecon (Decon Labs, Inc.) is a stabilized 10% sodium hypochlorite that retains efficacy over time, unlike in-house prepared 10% bleach solutions, which must be prepared fresh daily. Wipes such as Coverage Plus Germicidal Surface Wipes (Steris) can be used in appropriate situations. RelyOn antiseptic handwash products (DuPont) are available in both spray and wipes; they are effective against many viruses, including hepatitis A, B, and C viruses and HIV-I, and a variety of bacteria, including *Escherichia coli*, methicillin-resistant *Staphylococcus aureus* (MRSA) and the tuberculosis mycobacterium.

Antisepsis

Antiseptics are chemicals used on skin or tissue to inhibit growth of microbes. A variety of these are available, including alcohols, hydrogen peroxide, triclosan, chlorhexidine (Hibiclens), and iodine. They can be used for general skin cleaning, cleaning skin before injections or surgical procedures, or cleansing wounds. Many new hand antiseptics became available for healthcare workers, patients, and the public during the 2009-2010 H1N1 flu pandemic.

Microbiology Work Practices

Technologists in the microbiology laboratory must use Standard Precautions and follow the guidelines of the Bloodborne Pathogens Standard. Microbiology technologists must practice additional safety measures specific to the microbiology department, such as aseptic techniques. Microbiology work practices are described in more detail in Lesson 7-3.

Potential accidents in the microbiology laboratory that can expose the worker to risk include spills of culture material and formation of **aerosols**, fine mists that can form any time a cap is removed from a tube of liquid or a bacteriological loop is sterilized (Figure 1-22A). Gloves must be worn when working with specimens for microbiology testing to prevent exposure to any microorganisms that might be present in a patient's bacteriological specimen. Hands must be washed with antiseptic after the gloves are removed. When a task has been completed, work surfaces must be wiped with a disinfectant, such as 10% chlorine bleach. Examples of measures that can be taken to protect workers from hazards in the microbiology laboratory are listed in Table 1-20.

TABLE 1-20. Exposure control methods to protect against biological hazards in the microbiology laboratory

HAZARD	PROTECTIVE MEASURES
Blood or blood products	Wear gloves and a buttoned, fluid-resistant laboratory coat
Pathogenic microorganisms	Wear gloves and laboratory coat; work in biological safety cabinet
Hazardous aerosols	Place acrylic splash shield between worker and tubes when removing stoppers; wear mask, goggles, or face shield when disposing of urine
Contaminated work surfaces	Wipe with 10% chlorine bleach solution (or other surface disinfectant) before and after all procedures and at any other appropriate time
Needlesticks	Use safety needles or quick-release holders; never recap used needles

Some procedures in microbiology must be performed in a biological safety cabinet (Figure 1-22B). Positive air pressure in the cabinet keeps infectious materials inside the cabinet. Air inside the cabinet is drawn away from the worker, into a vent or special filter. A Class II biological safety cabinet is the type most commonly used in clinical laboratories.

CONTROL OF THE LABORATORY ENVIRONMENT

The laboratory must be a controlled environment. The air flow, humidity, room air exchange, and ambient temperature are all important considerations in the safety of the laboratory workers and optimum operation of the various instruments. Air quality parameters must be recorded daily or at specified intervals, and the records must be maintained for inspectors.

Air quality is an important aspect of laboratory safety. The components of air quality systems include heating, ventilating, and air conditioning. Several agencies regulate the air quality in buildings. Agencies that could evaluate healthcare settings include the CDC, National Institute of Occupational Safety and Health (NIOSH), Occupational Safety and Health Administration

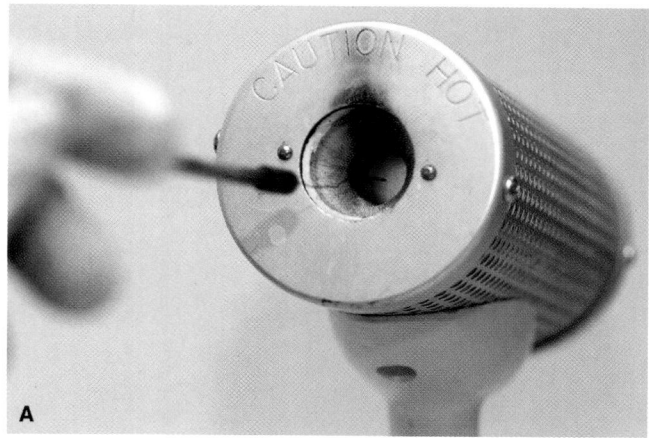
A

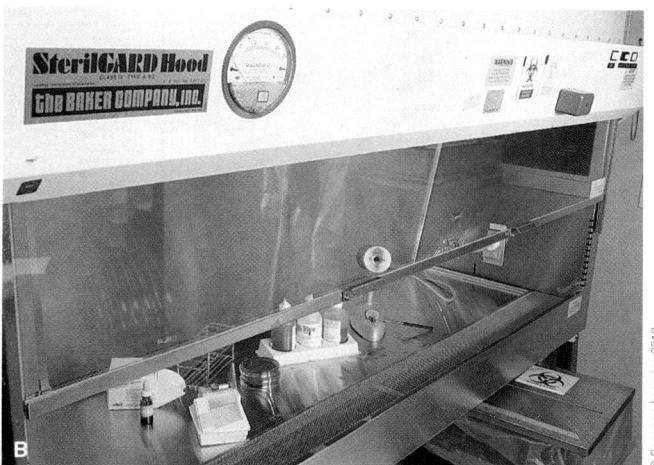
B

FIGURE 1-22 Work practice controls for microbiology: (A) use an electric incinerator to prevent aerosol formation when sterilizing a bacteriological loop; (B) use biological safety cabinet

© Cengage Learning 2012

(OSHA), and Joint Commission. These agencies can be called in to investigate and evaluate laboratory air flow and air quality. For instance, one of these agencies can perform an evaluation if there is suspicion that the ventilation system is carrying contaminated air from an area such as microbiology to other laboratory departments. It is important that the air pressure is always negative so that air in a contaminated area is not recirculated, which could pose a biological or chemical hazard to employees. Healthcare facilities must be certain that their air quality meets the specifications of the regulating and accrediting agencies.

CASE STUDY 1

Janie, a laboratory technician in a group practice clinic, frequently collects blood from clinic patients for laboratory tests. Janie's friend Bonnie came into the clinic for some blood tests. As Janie prepared to perform the venipuncture, Bonnie became offended when Janie put on gloves before collecting the blood.

1. How should Janie handle this situation?
2. Role-play this situation with a fellow student or coworker.

CASE STUDY 2

April is preparing serum chemistry control solutions for analysis in her department. She is wearing a laboratory coat and face shield. However, she does not like to wear gloves when handling the small control vials because she worries about dropping them.

1. Is it permissible for April to not wear gloves in this instance because patients are not involved?
2. What discussion should her supervisor have with her?

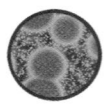

SUMMARY

Adherence to Standard Precautions and other biological safety rules is vitally important when working in the clinical laboratory. All patients and patient specimens present the potential risk for exposure to infectious agents. Laboratories are required to have in place a biological safety program that includes regular biosafety training, implementation, and monitoring.

    Standard Precautions and many other safety directives and guidelines issued by agencies such as the CDC and OSHA detail precise measures that workers can take to protect themselves and patients from exposure. An institution's exposure control plan outlines specific control measures and work practices that must be used to protect employees, patients, and visitors from exposure. Institutions must make safety supplies and devices available, such as hand hygiene stations, sharps disposal containers, and safety needles. Specific instructions, such as those for hand hygiene and the correct use of PPE, including gloves, masks, and gowns must be followed. Strict adherence to the biological safety plan provides a safe environment for patient and worker.

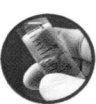

REVIEW QUESTIONS

1. How have biological safety rules changed in recent decades? Why have they become more stringent?

2. Explain the reason for the Bloodborne Pathogens Standard. Why was it revised in 2001?

3. What is meant by exposure control plan or infection control plan?

4. List the exposure control methods that are included in the exposure control plan.

5. What is meant by the terms Universal Precautions and Standard Precautions?

6. What additional safety rules and equipment are used in the microbiology laboratory?

7. What class of biological safety cabinet is most commonly used in medical laboratories?

8. Name three work practice controls that should be used in the laboratory workplace.

9. What are the OSHA rules regarding the handling and disposal of used needles?

10. What personal protective equipment is commonly worn when working in the biological laboratory?

11. Explain how to properly put on and take off gloves.

12. Discuss the advantages of wearing fluid-resistant disposable gowns or laboratory coats.

13. What action(s) should be taken in case of an exposure incident?

14. How does a disinfectant differ from an antiseptic?

15. Name four types of laboratory disinfectants and two antiseptics. Explain when and how antiseptics and disinfectants should be used.

16. Explain the proper technique for washing hands with antiseptic.

17. What is the purpose of a safety agreement?

18. Define acquired immunodeficiency syndrome, aerosol, alimentary tract, antiseptic, biohazard, biological safety cabinet, bloodborne pathogens, Bloodborne Pathogens Standard, community-acquired infection, disinfectant, engineering control, exposure control plan, exposure incident, hand antisepsis, hand hygiene, healthcare-acquired infection (HAI), hepatitis B virus, hepatitis C virus, human immunodeficiency virus (HIV), isolation, other potentially infectious materials (OPIM), parenteral, pathogenic, personal protective equipment (PPE), Standard Precautions, sterilization, Transmission-Based Precautions, Universal Precautions, and work practice controls.

STUDENT ACTIVITIES

1. Complete the written examination on this lesson.

2. Make a poster warning of a biological hazard.

3. Make a poster illustrating or describing proper hand hygiene techniques.

4. Practice the correct technique for removing contaminated gloves.

5. Practice correct hand hygiene techniques using waterless handrubs and antiseptic soaps.

6. Use the biological safety worksheet at the end of this lesson to evaluate the laboratory's biological safety policy.

WEB ACTIVITIES

1. Visit the CDC or OSHA web site to find information on the Needlestick Safety and Prevention Act. Look for publications or posters that emphasize safe practices.

2. Search the Internet for examples of engineering controls used to increase safety in the clinical laboratory. Obtain information on engineering controls such as safety needles, sharps containers, and acrylic splash shields.

3. Search the Internet for videos showing proper glove removal. Sketch the procedure in 4 or 5 simple drawings.

4. Report on the various types of gloves available for use in the clinical laboratory, using an online healthcare or laboratory supply catalog. Note which types provide chemical protection and which provide protection from infectious agents.

5. Access the CDC web site and find the October 25, 2002, *Morbidity and Mortality Weekly Report* (Vol. 51/No. RR-160). Read the "Guideline for Hand Hygiene in Health-Care Settings" and compare the CDC guidelines with your laboratory's written safety plan. Should your laboratory policy be strengthened? If so, how?

6. Search the Internet for safety videos demonstrating correct work practice controls and exposure control methods. Look for videos of hand hygiene, donning gloves, and cleaning work surfaces. Compare the techniques shown in the video with techniques you have learned from your instructor.

LESSON 1-4
Biological Safety

(Answers will vary based on available laboratory facilities.)

Name _____ Date _____

Use this worksheet to make a biological safety check of the laboratory.

SAFETY CHECK FOR BIOLOGICAL HAZARDS

I. Examine the laboratory for biological hazards

A. Are safety rules posted?   Yes ❑   No ❑

B. Are prominently labeled biohazard containers available?   Yes ❑   No ❑

C. Are safety needles used?   Yes ❑   No ❑

D. Are all sizes of gloves available for workers?   Yes ❑   No ❑

E. Are eye protection devices available?   Yes ❑   No ❑

Check which are available:

face shields ____ goggles ____ safety glasses ____ acrylic splash guards____

F. Are disposable, fluid-resistant gowns or coats available for tasks that might involve splashes or spills?   Yes ❑   No ❑

G. How are contaminated laboratory coats or gowns disposed of? _____

H. Is a policy in place to require countertops to be wiped with disinfectant at certain intervals and after every spill?   Yes ❑   No ❑

I. Where are used needles and other sharps discarded? _____

    1. Are containers puncture-resistant?   Yes ❑   No ❑

    2. Do containers have a biohazard labels?   Yes ❑   No ❑

Recommendation(s) for improvements: _____

_____

_____

II. Laboratory Safety Policy

Inquire about the laboratory's employee safety orientation and safety training policy.

A. Does the laboratory have a written exposure control plan?   Yes ❑   No ❑

B. Are Standard Precautions included in the exposure control plan?   Yes ❑   No ❑

C. Are hand hygiene stations conveniently located?   Yes ❑   No ❑

D. Have all employees considered at risk for exposure to bloodborne pathogens been offered the hepatitis B vaccination series at no charge?   Yes ❑   No ❑

E. Are written records kept of all employee safety training sessions?   Yes ❑   No ❑

F. Do employees sign forms acknowledging safety training?   Yes ❑   No ❑

G. Is safety training updated annually?   Yes ❑   No ❑

Recommendations or comments concerning the laboratory's safety program: _____

_____

_____

© 2012 Delmar, Cengage Learning. Permission to reproduce for clinical use granted.

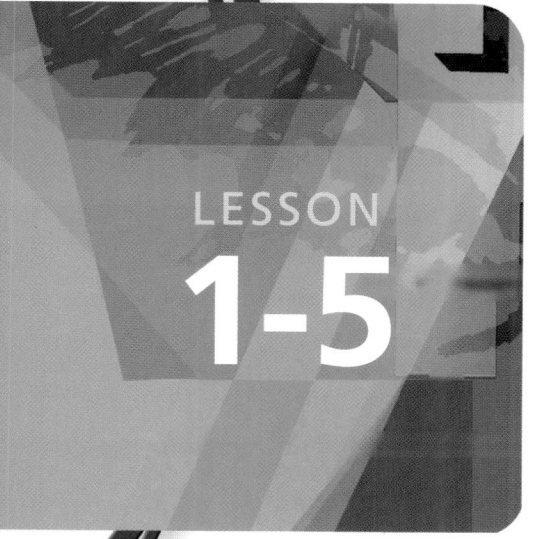

Chemical, Fire, and Electrical Safety

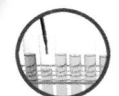

LESSON OBJECTIVES

After studying this lesson, the student will:

⊙ Describe the evolution of the Occupational Safety and Health Administration (OSHA) safety laws.

⊙ Explain the "right to know" provisions of OSHA.

⊙ Explain why safety rules must be observed.

⊙ List three general categories of laboratory hazards.

⊙ Give two examples of physical hazards and ways to prevent or correct each one.

⊙ Give two examples of chemical hazards and ways to prevent or correct each one.

⊙ List five components of a chemical hygiene plan.

⊙ Interpret and use the information on a material safety data sheet (MSDS).

⊙ Explain the importance of wearing appropriate clothing in the laboratory.

⊙ Discuss how personal protective equipment (PPE) is used in the laboratory.

⊙ List 16 laboratory safety work practices designed to protect against physical and chemical hazards.

⊙ Define the glossary terms.

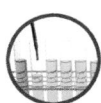

GLOSSARY

autoclave / an instrument that uses pressurized steam for sterilization

carcinogen / a substance with the potential to produce cancer in humans or animals

caustic / a chemical substance having the ability to burn or destroy tissue

centrifuge / instrument with a rotor that rotates at high speeds in a closed chamber

chemical hygiene plan / comprehensive written safety plan detailing the proper use and storage of hazardous chemicals in the workplace

fume hood / a device that draws contaminated air out of an area and either cleanses and recirculates it or discharges it to the outside

material safety data sheet (MSDS) / written safety information that must be supplied by manufacturers of chemicals and hazardous materials

mutagen / a substance or agent, such as radiation, certain chemicals, or some viruses, that causes a stable change in a gene that can then be passed on to offspring

National Institute for Occupational Safety and Health (NIOSH) / federal agency responsible for workplace safety research and that makes recommendations for preventing work-related illness and injury

(continues)

Occupational Safety and Health Act (OSH Act) / congressional act of 1970 created to help reduce on-the-job illnesses, injuries, and deaths and requiring employers to provide safe working conditions

Occupational Safety and Health Administration (OSHA) / the federal agency that creates workplace safety regulations and enforces the Occupational Safety and Health Act of 1970

personal protective equipment (PPE) / specialized clothing or equipment used by workers to protect from direct exposure to blood or other potentially infectious or hazardous materials

radioisotope / an unstable form of an element that emits radiation and can be incorporated into diagnostic tests, medical therapies, and biomedical research; radioactive isotope

teratogen / a substance or agent capable of causing birth defects by direct harm to a fetus or embryo, or by interfering with normal fetal development

INTRODUCTION

Safety in health care should be a priority of all healthcare providers. Employers and employees must provide quality patient care in an environment that is safe for both workers and patients. Creating a safe workplace is not optional, it is required by law.

Clinical laboratory workers encounter unique safety hazards that can be classified in three categories:

- Physical hazards
- Chemical hazards
- Biological hazards

This lesson identifies some physical and chemical hazards that can be present in the laboratory and outlines safety practices mandatory for safe and legal operation of a clinical laboratory. Throughout this textbook, the symbol ① is used to alert that a physical hazard can be present when performing an activity or using the instrument or equipment. The symbol ⚠ alerts that a chemical hazard can be present in a procedure or situation. Safety procedures concerned primarily with biological hazards ⬡ were addressed in Lesson 1-4.

WORKPLACE SAFETY

Rules to protect workers against physical and chemical hazards have existed for decades. Laboratories operate under both federal and state safety regulations and guidelines.

Federal Regulations

In 1970, Congress enacted the **Occupational Safety and Health Act (OSH Act)** to try to reduce workplace illnesses, injuries, and deaths. The act required employers to provide safe working conditions and to inform and train workers about hazardous conditions present in their workplace. The **Occupational Safety and Health Administration (OSHA)**, a part of the Department of Labor, is the agency that establishes the rules and enforces adherence to the OSH Act.

OSHA's Hazard Communication Rule

In 1983, OSHA issued a rule intended to provide further protection to workers from hazardous chemical exposure. This rule was called the *Hazard Communication* and applied only to the manufacturing industry. However, in 1987, the rule was expanded to include the nonmanufacturing sector. The rule places the burden on the employer to keep workers informed and protected by providing safety training, approved safety apparel, and a safe work environment.

Enforcement of the OSH Act

OSHA has responsibility for general workplace safety. OSHA inspectors can arrive unannounced and inspect the safety conditions in a workplace. If safety violations are found, they are noted and violators are subject to being fined.

Agencies such as the Centers for Disease Control and Prevention (CDC), Centers for Medicare and Medicaid Services (CMS), and the **National Institute for Occupational Safety and Health (NIOSH)** are also involved in ensuring that best safety practices are used. These agencies provide free safety educational materials and training, make recommendations for best safety practices, and conduct workplace safety research.

State Safety Codes

In addition to the OSH Act of 1970, and expanded rules of 1983 and 1987, most states have enacted additional safety codes to ensure that employers provide safe work environments. Under these state laws, the employer, supervisor, or educator has the responsibility to provide safety orientation and training to employees and students.

Safety Training

Each laboratory is required to have an up-to-date procedure manual that contains specific safety guidelines covering biological, chemical, and physical hazards. The location of the manual must be posted so that anyone can find it. The manual must include standard operating procedures (SOPs); regulations for the safe handling, storage, and disposal of chemicals; and strategies to follow in case of fire or chemical accident. It must also include general laboratory safety rules and guidelines for employee safety training.

Students and employees must be trained in safe laboratory practices, correct use of safety equipment, and the Hazard Communication. The safety training must be completed and documented in writing before the employee or student is allowed to perform procedures in the laboratory. Both trainer and trainee must sign, verifying that training was given or received and that the trainee understood the training. An example of a safety agreement form is included in Lesson 1-4, Figure 1-14.

Refresher safety training sessions must be provided for employees at least once per year to reinforce the importance of using safe practices. It is the responsibility of the employer, supervisor, and educator to monitor employee or student adherence to safety regulations. It is the employee's responsibility to follow safety rules and comply with the institution's safety guidelines and regulations so that the employee or fellow workers are not endangered.

Personal Protective Equipment

Employers must provide employees or students with **personal protective equipment (PPE)** to protect against identified hazards in the laboratory. Safety equipment appropriate to protect against physical and chemical hazards can include:

- Eye, face, mucous membrane, and skin protection such as masks, goggles, face shield, or acrylic splash shield
- Fume hood to protect against inhalation of fumes
- Gloves to protect skin of hands and arms

In addition, workers should wear clothing that can be easily decontaminated, such as uniforms or scrubs and a fluid-resistant laboratory coat or apron.

PHYSICAL HAZARDS

Several physical hazards are present in ordinary laboratory equipment and surroundings. Electrical equipment, laboratory instruments, and glassware can be hazardous if used improperly. Warning signs should be posted in appropriate places throughout the laboratory as a constant reminder to employees to use safe work practices (Figure 1-23).

Electrical Safety

Electricity can be a major physical hazard. Employees must follow the guidelines in the safety manual for safe operation of all electrical equipment. Examples of good safety practices

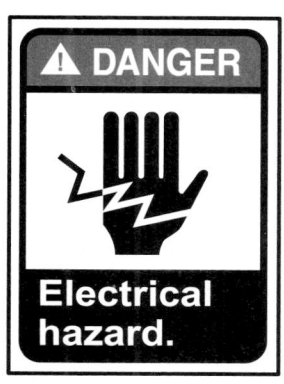

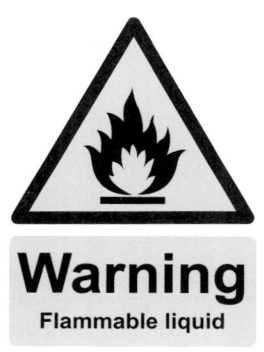

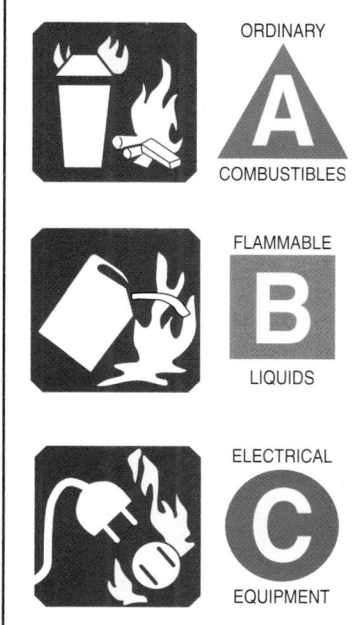

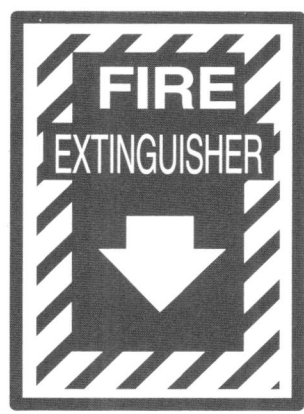

© Cengage Learning 2012

FIGURE 1-23 Examples of fire safety signs showing location and correct use of fire extinguishers and warning signs for electrical hazards and flammable liquids

include: (1) grounding of all electrical equipment, following the manufacturer's instructions and according to electrical codes; (2) disconnecting instruments from the power supply before attempting instrument repair, even minor repair such as replacing microscope light bulbs; (3) keeping electrical cords and plugs in good repair, with no frayed cords or exposed wires; (4) avoiding overloading electrical circuits that can create a fire hazard and can also cause equipment damage; and (5) avoiding the use of extension cords

Fire Safety

Fire is another potential danger in the workplace. Fortunately, laboratory fires are rare. When possible, open flames (such as from alcohol lamps or Bunsen burners) should not be used in the clinical laboratory. Most laboratory procedures can be modified to use laboratory hotplates, microwave ovens, electric incinerators, and slide warmers instead of open flames. If a flame is required for a procedure, care must be taken to keep loose clothing and long hair away from the flame.

Flammable chemicals should be stored in a flame-proof cabinet, away from heat sources and in a well-ventilated area. In the case of fire, a flameproof chemical cabinet protects flammable chemicals from flames until firefighters arrive and also allows workers more time to escape.

Fire extinguishers must be located in several accessible sites in the laboratory; a fire blanket should also be accessible in case clothing ignites (Figure 1-24). All workers must know the locations of fire extinguishers and how to use them. In some laboratories the acronym PAS (pull, aim, and squeeze) is taught during fire safety training and is also on a sign near the extinguisher.

Fire extinguishers must be inspected periodically by the fire department or a certified fire safety company and the date of inspection recorded. Fire drills must be held frequently to be sure that workers know the escape route and the procedure to follow if that exit is blocked (Figure 1-25).

Laboratory Equipment Safety

Laboratory equipment must be used only as the manufacturers' instructions dictate. Any instrument that has moving parts, or operates at high speed, such as a **centrifuge**, must be operated with special attention to safety. Centrifuges should be equipped with safety latches that prevent the centrifuge from being opened during operation or being turned on unless the lid is latched. No attempt should be made to open a centrifuge lid until the rotor has come to a complete stop.

Autoclaves, which use pressurized steam to sterilize surgical instruments, glassware, and other materials, present special hazards. Manufacturers' instructions should be followed carefully to prevent explosions and burns. Insulated gloves should be worn when removing hot items from the autoclave. Lesson 1-6 contains additional information on the safe operation of common laboratory equipment and instruments.

Glassware Safety

In most laboratory procedures, glassware has been replaced with disposable polycarbonate, polyethylene, or polystyrene labware. However, glass is required for some procedures. Glassware that

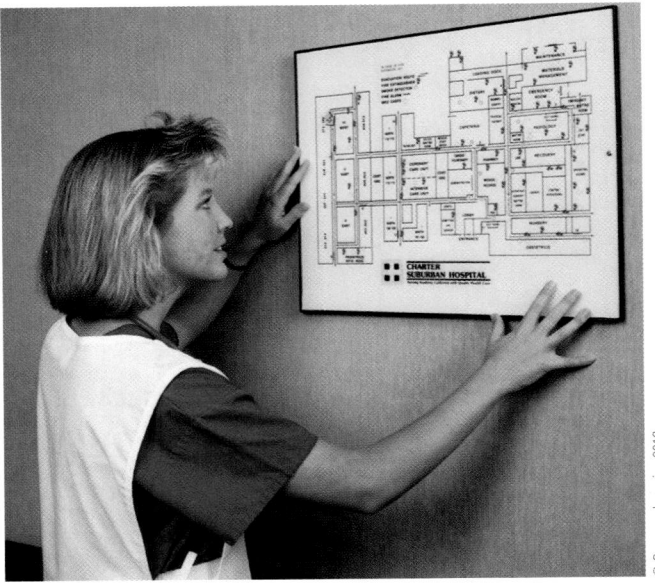

FIGURE 1-25 Employees must be familiar with their facility's fire escape route and emergency plan

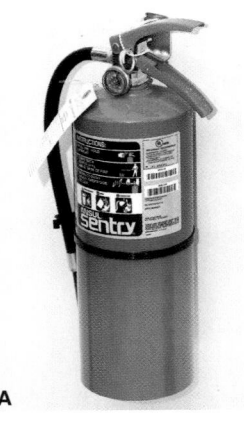
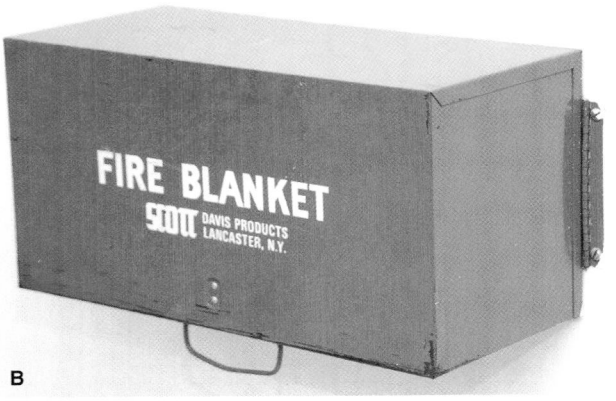

FIGURE 1-24 Fire safety: (A) fire extinguisher; (B) fire blanket

is to be subjected to heat should be heat-resistant glass, such as Kimax or Pyrex. Only glassware that is free of chips and cracks should be used. Damaged glassware is weakened and can break, causing injury. Broken glass should be cleaned up with a brush and dustpan, not with bare hands. Glass should not be discarded into regular trashcans, but into rigid thick-walled cardboard or plastic containers. Additional information on the safe use of glassware can be found in Lesson 1-6.

CHEMICAL HAZARDS

Chemicals present a variety of hazards. Chemicals can be flammable, toxic, caustic, corrosive, carcinogenic, or mutagenic. A hazardous chemical is any liquid, solid, or gas that could present a physical or health hazard to an employee.

Most routine clinical laboratory procedures use either nonhazardous chemicals or chemicals that present few serious hazards. When possible, safer chemicals are substituted for more hazardous chemicals in laboratory procedures. Several test methods minimize the need for chemical handling by enclosing chemicals in test cassettes or cartridges, providing extra worker protection from chemical contact. However, it is still sometimes necessary to pipet or work with a hazardous reagent. Technicians should always avoid direct skin contact with chemicals and inhalation of chemical fumes or dust.

Chemical Hygiene Plan

OSHA mandates that a comprehensive, written safety plan for the use of hazardous chemicals be implemented at each workplace. This is often called the **chemical hygiene plan** and must be readily available to all employees. The plan sets forth specific work practices, procedures, and PPE that must be used to ensure that employees are protected from the health hazards associated with chemicals used in that particular laboratory. The chemical hygiene plan should include the following components:

- Standard operating procedures for the safe use of hazardous chemicals
- Measures to reduce exposure to hazardous chemicals, including the use of PPE and hand hygiene practices

- Specifications for safe function of protective equipment and fume hoods
- Specific hazard information for all hazardous chemicals
- Provisions for employee education and training

After handling and using chemicals, gloves should be removed carefully, avoiding touching bare skin with the outer glove surfaces (Figure 1-26). Any chemicals that do contact the skin should be washed off immediately with water for at least 5 minutes unless the container label says otherwise. A safety shower must be available in case large quantities of chemicals are spilled on a worker (Figure 1-27A). An eyewash station must be accessible to workers who accidently have chemicals splashed into the eyes (Figure 1-27B).

Material Safety Data Sheets

Manufacturers are required by law to provide a **material safety data sheet (MSDS)** for every chemical. This information describes the hazard(s) of the chemical, the PPE required, and the body organs that could be adversely affected following exposure to the chemical. Additional information is included describing first aid techniques and any further medical treatment required if exposure to the chemical occurs.

The MSDS must be kept on file in the laboratory where every employee has access to them. Each employee who uses a chemical must read the MSDS for that chemical and understand hazards associated with the chemical, measures to prevent injuries from exposure, and first aid procedures. The MSDS format is somewhat standardized among all manufacturers so that chemical reactivity, physical characteristics, transportation requirements, and other safety information are easily located on each MSDS. Categories of information included in MSDS are listed in Table 1-21.

Chemical Labels

Chemicals must be labeled with detailed hazard information, including exposure symptoms, appropriate first aid procedures on exposure, and spill response procedures (Figure 1-28). The

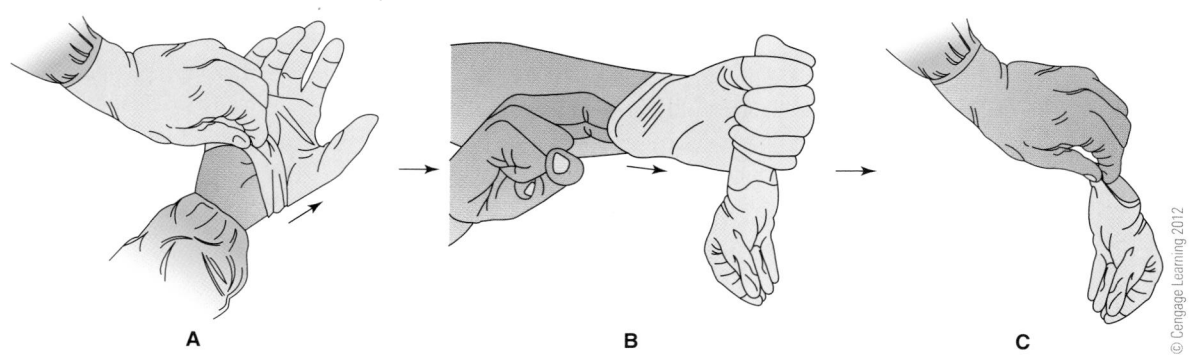

A   B   C

© Cengage Learning 2012

FIGURE 1-26 Illustration of removing contaminated gloves: (A) touching only the outside of the glove, grasp the glove cuff and pull the glove down over the hand turning the glove inside out; (B) hold the removed glove in the palm of the gloved hand and pull the remaining glove off (inside-out) by touching only the inside of the glove with the bare hand; (C) discard gloves into appropriate container

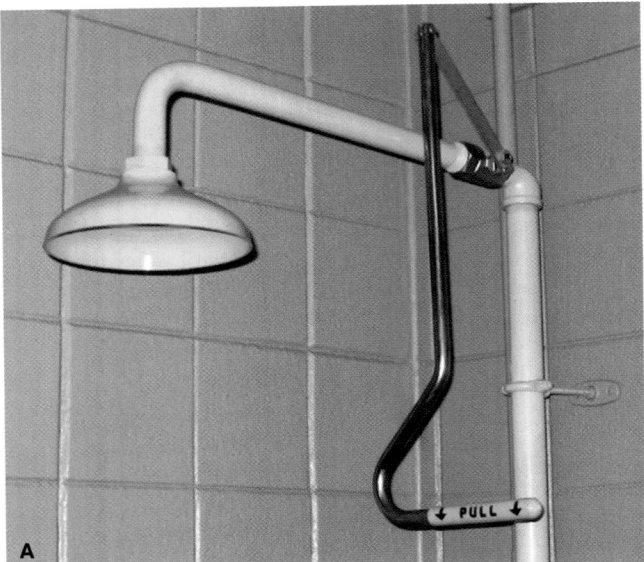

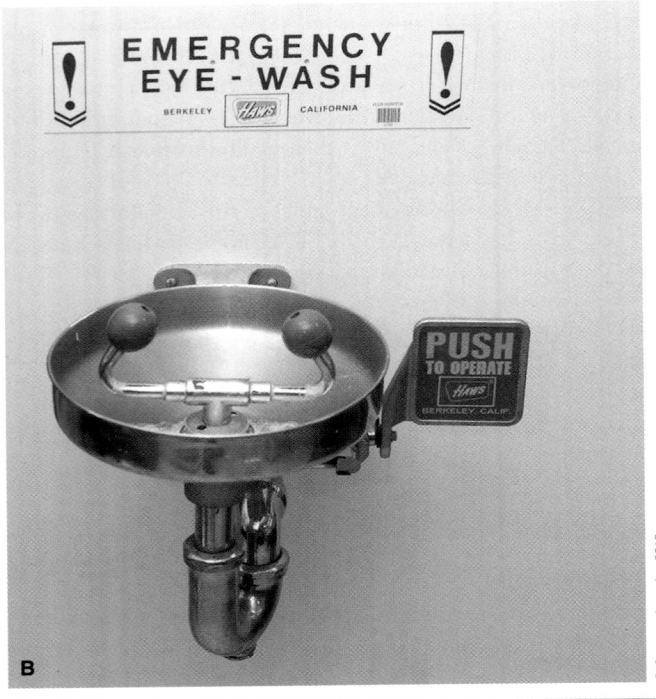

FIGURE 1-27 (A) Safety shower; (B) eyewash station

National Fire Protection Association (NFPA) uses four colors on chemical labels to indicate the type of hazard a chemical presents (Figure 1-29). The label is diamond-shaped and divided into four smaller diamonds: blue, red, yellow, and white. Each color is associated with a specific class of hazards. The NFPA color codes are:

- **Blue**—indicates health hazards or toxicity
- **Red**—indicates fire hazard or flammability
- **Yellow**—indicates reactive or unstable chemicals such as oxidizers
- **White**—indicates reactivity with water or a contact hazard

    For each blue, red, and yellow color, a number system (0 to 4) rates the relative risk for hazard associated with that category. A *0* means no unusual hazard is present in that category; a *4*

TABLE 1-21. Examples of information provided in an MSDS

Product identification
Hazardous ingredients
Physical characteristics
Fire and explosion hazards
Reactivity
Health hazard
Spill or leak procedures
Transportation data (for DOT classification)
Precautions for safe handling and use
Special precautions

indicates the highest hazard level for that category (see Safety Worksheet II at the end of this lesson). The white hazard category uses a lettering system to denote water reactivity, contact hazard (such as acid, corrosive), or a code for the type of PPE required when using the chemical. These ratings are also present on the MSDS. Additionally, certain symbols are widely used to warn of specific chemical hazards (Figure 1-30).

Caustic Chemicals

Some chemicals used in the laboratory are **caustic**, meaning they are strong acids or bases capable of causing severe skin burns (Figure 1-30). Fumes or vapors from caustic chemicals can burn mucous membranes; caustic chemicals must be used in a **fume hood**, a special cabinet that draws the fumes away from the worker (Figure 1-31A). Potassium hydroxide (KOH), sodium hydroxide (NaOH), sulfuric acid (H_2SO_4), nitric acid (HNO_3), and concentrated sodium hypochlorite (chlorine bleach) are examples of caustic chemicals. Goggles or a face shield, chemical-resistant gloves, and a protective apron should be worn to protect against injury from splashes and spills when working with strong chemicals (Figure 1-31B). Appropriate PPE must be worn when cleaning up chemical spills.

Toxic Chemicals

Some laboratory chemicals, such as those containing heavy metals, are toxic or poisonous either through skin contact or by respiratory exposure. When using these chemicals, the worker must follow special safety precautions. Chemical-resistant gloves and protective rubber or vinyl sleeves can be used to protect skin from contact. If a chemical produces harmful fumes, it should be used only in a fume hood (Figure 1-31).

Carcinogens, Mutagens, Teratogens, and Radioisotopes

Some procedures require the use of hazardous chemicals such as **carcinogens** (cancer-causing substances), **mutagens** (substances that cause stable gene changes), **teratogens** (substances that can harm a fetus or embryo), or **radioisotopes** (elements that can emit radiation). These categories of chemicals require special handling and disposal.

© Cengage Learning 2012

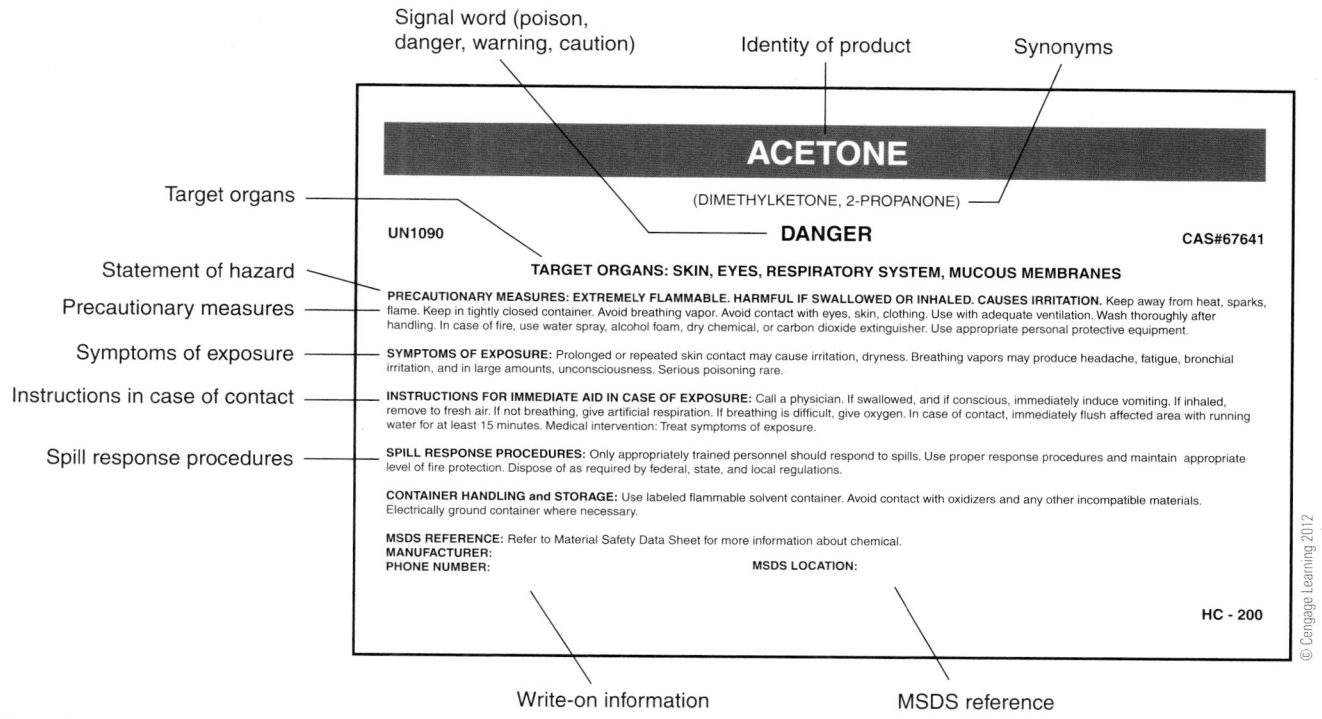

Signal word (poison, danger, warning, caution)

Identity of product

Synonyms

Target organs

Statement of hazard

Precautionary measures

Symptoms of exposure

Instructions in case of contact

Spill response procedures

ACETONE

(DIMETHYLKETONE, 2-PROPANONE)

UN1090   **DANGER**   CAS#67641

TARGET ORGANS: SKIN, EYES, RESPIRATORY SYSTEM, MUCOUS MEMBRANES

PRECAUTIONARY MEASURES: EXTREMELY FLAMMABLE. HARMFUL IF SWALLOWED OR INHALED. CAUSES IRRITATION. Keep away from heat, sparks, flame. Keep in tightly closed container. Avoid breathing vapor. Avoid contact with eyes, skin, clothing. Use with adequate ventilation. Wash thoroughly after handling. In case of fire, use water spray, alcohol foam, dry chemical, or carbon dioxide extinguisher. Use appropriate personal protective equipment.

SYMPTOMS OF EXPOSURE: Prolonged or repeated skin contact may cause irritation, dryness. Breathing vapors may produce headache, fatigue, bronchial irritation, and in large amounts, unconsciousness. Serious poisoning rare.

INSTRUCTIONS FOR IMMEDIATE AID IN CASE OF EXPOSURE: Call a physician. If swallowed, and if conscious, immediately induce vomiting. If inhaled, remove to fresh air. If not breathing, give artificial respiration. If breathing is difficult, give oxygen. In case of contact, immediately flush affected area with running water for at least 15 minutes. Medical intervention: Treat symptoms of exposure.

SPILL RESPONSE PROCEDURES: Only appropriately trained personnel should respond to spills. Use proper response procedures and maintain appropriate level of fire protection. Dispose of as required by federal, state, and local regulations.

CONTAINER HANDLING and STORAGE: Use labeled flammable solvent container. Avoid contact with oxidizers and any other incompatible materials. Electrically ground container where necessary.

MSDS REFERENCE: Refer to Material Safety Data Sheet for more information about chemical.
MANUFACTURER:
PHONE NUMBER: **MSDS LOCATION:**

HC - 200

© Cengage Learning 2012

Write-on information   MSDS reference

FIGURE 1-28 Chemical label containing hazard information

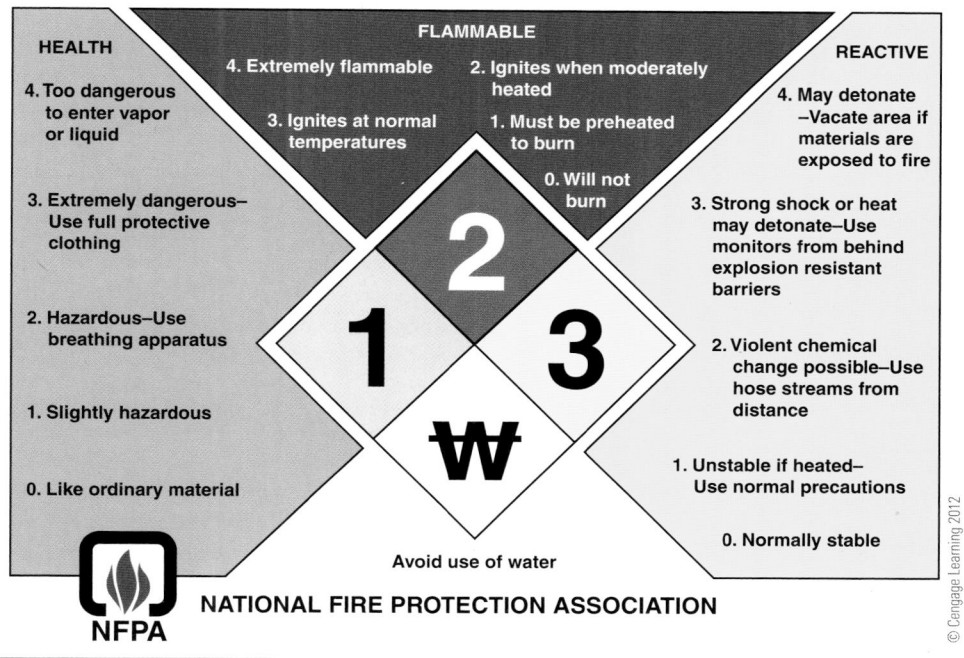

HEALTH

4. Too dangerous to enter vapor or liquid

3. Extremely dangerous– Use full protective clothing

2. Hazardous–Use breathing apparatus

1. Slightly hazardous

0. Like ordinary material

FLAMMABLE

4. Extremely flammable

3. Ignites at normal temperatures

2. Ignites when moderately heated

1. Must be preheated to burn

0. Will not burn

REACTIVE

4. May detonate –Vacate area if materials are exposed to fire

3. Strong shock or heat may detonate–Use monitors from behind explosion resistant barriers

2. Violent chemical change possible–Use hose streams from distance

1. Unstable if heated– Use normal precautions

0. Normally stable

2

1   3

W

Avoid use of water

NATIONAL FIRE PROTECTION ASSOCIATION

NFPA

© Cengage Learning 2012

FIGURE 1-29 National Fire Protection Association's color-coded labeling system for identifying and warning of chemical hazards

Carcinogens must be handled with care, following all recommended safety precautions and wearing appropriate PPE. Procedures that use mutagens or teratogens must be clearly identified so that females of childbearing age can avoid exposure (Figure 1-30). Occasionally, diagnostic or laboratory procedures use radioisotopes, which present the potential of exposure to radioactivity. Workers must complete special radiation safety training before working with radioisotopes; gloves and appropriate radiation shields must be used when handling radioisotopes. Special radioisotope disposal is required and is regulated by state and federal guidelines.

Chemical Storage

Flammable liquids, concentrated acids, concentrated bases, and other hazardous chemicals should be stored in the original containers in special chemical cabinets. In the past, chemicals

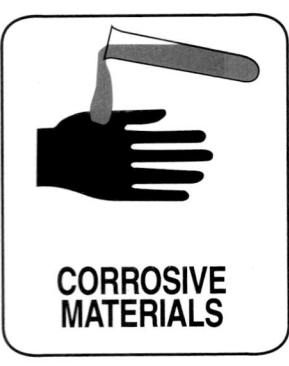 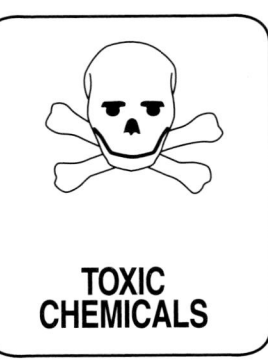 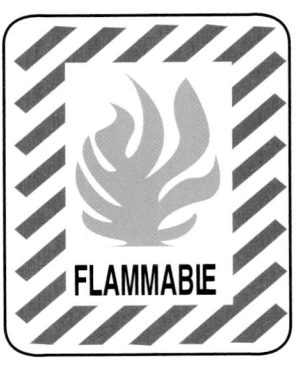 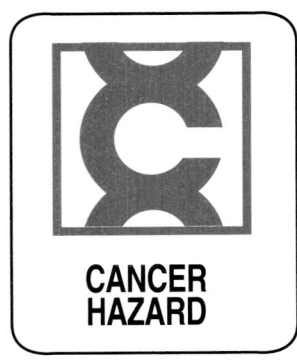

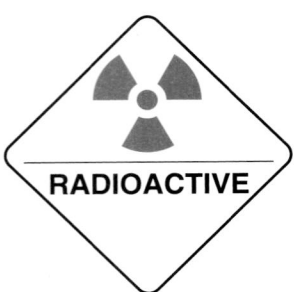 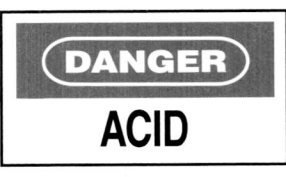 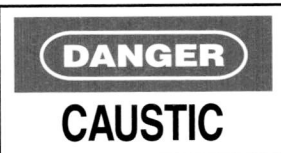 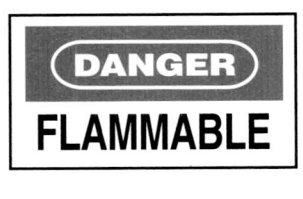

FIGURE 1-30 Examples of symbols and signs warning of chemical hazards

were stored in alphabetical order to make them easier to locate. However, this storage method sometimes placed incompatible chemicals near each other.

Chemical manufacturers offer reliable safety guides that can be used to plan safe chemical storage. Information on color-coded labels on chemical containers also indicates proper chemical storage conditions. Examples of some chemicals that should not be stored near each other are shown in Table 1-22.

Chemical Disposal

All chemicals and reagents must be disposed of according to specific regulations. Many laboratory reagents can be safely poured down the drain, followed by large amounts of water to dilute them. However, some reagents, for example, those containing

heavy metals such as mercury, lead, or chromium, require special disposal by toxic waste personnel and must never enter the sewer system. Therefore, it is very important that laboratory supervisors or instructors provide explicit instructions and receptacles for appropriate chemical and reagent disposal.

The types of chemicals used in a method should be considered when adopting laboratory procedures. Efforts should be made to adopt test methods that minimize or eliminate the use of hazardous chemicals when possible or practical, as long as the quality of test results is not adversely affected. The use of safe chemicals eliminates problems associated with disposal of hazardous chemicals, such as increased costs from special disposal requirements.

LABORATORY CLOTHING

Each employer will have a written policy describing rules and standards of appropriate laboratory clothing, types of PPE, and guidelines for selecting the appropriate PPE for the task (Table 1-23). Because laboratory work has its own particular set of hazards, rules of dress for laboratory personnel are usually slightly different than those for other healthcare workers.

Some dress rules are intended to reduce risk for injury. Loose jewelry, such as long chains, bracelets, and dangling earrings should not be worn because they can become caught in moving equipment and cause serious injury. In addition, metal jewelry can contact electrical parts in equipment and cause injury or death by electrical shock. Shoes should be comfortable and stable and must have closed toes to protect skin from spills or injury from sharp objects. Long hair should be pulled back to prevent contact with moving equipment parts or chemicals.

Laboratory workers can be required to wear a uniform or scrubs covered by a buttoned, knee-length, and fluid-resistant laboratory coat to protect skin and clothing from spills and splashes

TABLE 1-22. Examples of some incompatible chemicals*

CHEMICAL	DO NOT STORE NEXT TO ANY OF THESE
Acetic acid	Hydroxides (NaOH, KOH), nitric acid
Acetone	Concentrated sulfuric or nitric acids
Flammable liquids	Chromic acid, hydrogen peroxide, nitric acid
Sodium azide	Copper (in plumbing drains)

* This is only a partial listing; for details, consult a safety handbook and the labels on the chemical containers

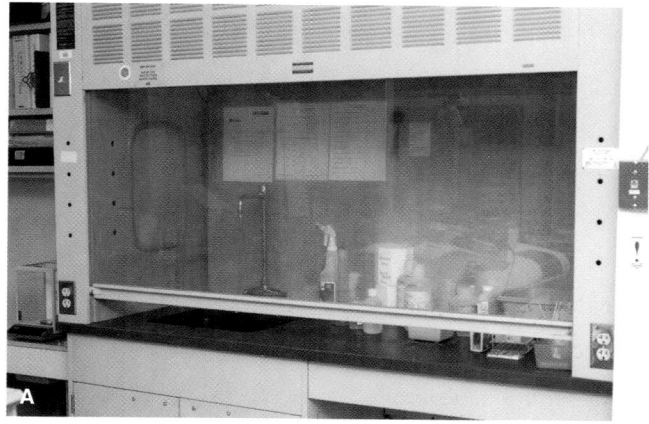

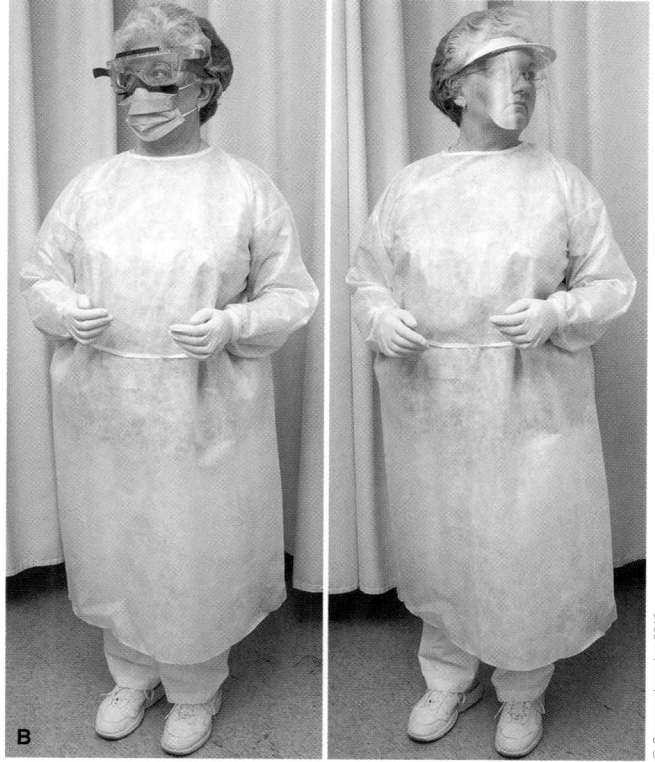

FIGURE 1-31 Chemical safety: (A) fume hood; (B) worker wearing appropriate PPE including face protection, fluid-resistant gown, and gloves

of chemicals, stains, or hazardous material. A rubberized or other special type of apron can be worn when working with strong chemicals such as concentrated acids (Table 1-23). Protective eyewear such as laboratory safety goggles or face shield must be worn or an acrylic splash shield used if splashes are possible. Contact lenses should not be worn in the laboratory (Table 1-23). Chemicals in the form of fumes or splashes can get under the lenses and cause damage to the eyes before the lenses can be removed.

Chemical-resistant gloves must be worn when hazardous chemicals are handled. MSDS information includes the types of gloves appropriate for the chemical, and many scientific supply catalogs contain charts to aid in glove selection. Nitrile or vinyl gloves are good choices for routine laboratory use because they are nonreactive, nonallergenic, and resistant to most chemicals. Latex gloves should not be worn when working with strong chemicals, because chemicals can penetrate latex, allowing the chemicals to contact the skin. In addition, latex sensitivity can develop in some individuals, causing dermatitis or more severe allergic reactions.

SAFETY RESOURCES

Official OSHA guidelines must always be consulted to ensure the laboratory is in compliance. A copy of OSHA guidelines can be found in the *Federal Register* in the local library or on various web sites such as those of the CDC, OSHA, and NIOSH. (See Appendix D.) In addition, universities or state public health laboratories often have safety consultants who will provide advice by phone or send printed information.

TABLE 1-23. Exposure control methods to protect against physical and chemical hazards in the laboratory

HAZARD	EXPOSURE CONTROL METHOD
Spills and splashes on the skin	Wear laboratory coat, apron, gloves
Strong acids	Wear rubberized apron, acid-resistant gloves
Splashes into eyes	Use face shield and/or ANSI*-approved goggles; do not wear contact lenses in the laboratory
Toxic fumes or chemical dust	Use chemical fume hood
Electrical shock	Disconnect equipment from power supply before repair

* American National Standard Institute

GENERAL LABORATORY SAFETY RULES

 Despite certain safety hazards, the clinical laboratory can be a safe work environment. Each worker must be responsible, use safe work practices, and observe all safety rules.

No set of safety rules can cover every situation that might arise. Also, nothing can replace the use of common sense when working with laboratory equipment and chemicals. General safe work practices to protect against physical and chemical hazards include the following:

1. Report any accident immediately to the supervisor.
2. Be familiar with MSDS information before working with a chemical or reagent.
3. Do not eat, drink, chew gum, or apply cosmetics in the work area.
4. Wear a laboratory apron or buttoned fluid-resistant laboratory coat and closed-toe shoes.
5. Pin long hair back to prevent contact with chemicals or moving equipment.
6. Do not wear chains, bracelets, large rings, or other loose jewelry.
7. Use chemical-resistant gloves when working with hazardous chemicals.
8. Clean the work area before and after laboratory procedures and any other time it is needed.
9. Wash hands before donning gloves, after removing gloves, and any other time necessary.
10. Wear safety glasses, goggles, and face shield or use a countertop acrylic splash shield to protect from splashes into eyes or mucous membranes; do not wear contact lenses in the laboratory.
11. Wipe up spills promptly, using the appropriate procedure for the type of spill.
12. Use a fume hood or appropriate mask or respirator when working with chemicals or other materials that create dust or emit fumes.
13. Follow manufacturers' instructions for operating all equipment; handle all equipment with care and store properly.
14. Report any broken or frayed electrical cords, exposed electrical wires, or any damage to equipment.
15. Use a broom or brush and dustpan to pick up broken glass; discard into special rigid, thick-walled containers.
16. Allow visitors in the laboratory work area only if institution policy permits.

 CASE STUDY 1

Michelle, a phlebotomist in the laboratory of a small clinic, arrived at work a few minutes early dressed neatly in scrubs and new sandals. After putting on her laboratory coat and buttoning it, she began work. Within the hour her supervisor told her she was inappropriately dressed.

What do you think is the problem?

 CASE STUDY 2

Doug began preparing laboratory surface disinfectant from chlorine bleach. He put on a chemical resistant apron and gloves and then removed the bleach container from the special chemical cabinet. He carefully placed the container on the laboratory benchtop and began to add the chlorine bleach to distilled water. Nearby workers began complaining of burning eyes. Doug was reprimanded by the supervisor.

Explain why.

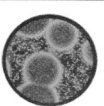

SUMMARY

The modern era of workplace safety began with the 1970 OSH Act. This federal legislation and subsequent rules mandated increased attention to safety in workplaces. OSHA is the agency that enforces the OSH Act and oversees workplace safety.

The clinical laboratory workplace has special hazards—physical, chemical, and biological. Physical hazards include fire, electrical hazards, and hazards associated with laboratory equipment. Chemical hazards are associated with the use of chemicals in laboratory procedures. Each laboratory is required to have a comprehensive written safety plan, readily available to all employees, that explains workplace hazards and provides specific information about safe work practices. A chemical hygiene plan gives information about the use of MSDS and the safe handling, storage, and disposal of chemicals.

All laboratory employees must receive documented safety training at regular intervals, at least once a year. New employees must complete safety training before being allowed to perform laboratory procedures. Employees are required to use PPE such as gloves, full face protection, and fluid-resistant laboratory coats or aprons to protect from chemical exposure. The safety program should include training on fire prevention and the use of different types of fire extinguishers. All personnel should know the escape route from the department.

Although laboratory procedures do have associated hazards, the laboratory can be made a safe workplace. It is the employer's responsibility to provide a safe work environment and all necessary safety equipment and supplies. It is each employee's responsibility to follow the safety rules.

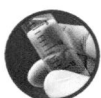

REVIEW QUESTIONS

1. What are the three categories of laboratory hazards?

2. Give two examples of physical hazards and tell how each might be avoided or corrected.

3. Give two examples of chemical hazards and tell how each might be avoided or corrected.

4. Why is it important to conduct frequent fire drills?

5. Why must safety rules be strictly observed?

6. Name the governmental agency responsible for enforcing safety regulations in the workplace.

7. Describe the type of clothing that should be worn by laboratory workers.

8. State 16 general laboratory safety rules and explain the rationale for each.

9. Discuss the importance of reading and understanding the MSDS information for each chemical used.

10. Define autoclave, carcinogen, caustic, centrifuge, chemical hygiene plan, fume hood, material safety data sheet (MSDS), mutagen, National Institute for Occupational Safety and Health (NIOSH), Occupational Safety and Health (OSH) Act, Occupational Safety and Health Administration (OSHA), personal protective equipment, radioisotope, and teratogen.

STUDENT ACTIVITIES

1. Complete the written examination for this lesson.

2. Make a poster warning of a physical or chemical hazard.

3. Use the Chemical, Fire, and Electrical Safety Worksheet I at the end of this lesson to inspect the laboratory for physical or chemical hazards. Check for frayed cords, exposed wires, fire extinguisher, safety posters, and posting of fire exit routes.

4. Practice the procedure to follow in case of fire and the use of the fire extinguisher; learn the fire escape route.

5. Inspect the chemicals in the laboratory and make a report using Chemical, Fire, and Electrical Safety Worksheet I. Are chemicals labeled with appropriate information? Do chemical labels contain instructions for accidental exposure? Note the procedure to follow in case of skin contact or chemical spill.

6. Make an inventory of six chemicals in your laboratory, using the inventory form on Chemical, Fire, and Electrical Safety Worksheet II at the end of this lesson. Consult the MSDS to determine the hazard class and type of PPE required when using each chemical.

WEB ACTIVITIES

1. Use the Internet to find MSDS information for NaOH, HCl, and Clorox (hypochlorite). Report on the reactivity, flammability, and health hazard of each; list the PPE that should be worn when working with each of these chemicals.

2. Visit the OSHA or NIOSH web site and find out what safety information is available. Look for free safety posters or brochures and order or download and print free copies for your laboratory or class.

3. Search the Internet for videos or tutorials demonstrating chemical, fire, and electrical safety practices.

4. Search the Internet for tutorials or self-tests covering laboratory safety.

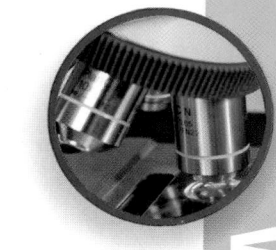

LESSON 1-5
Chemical, Fire, and Electrical Safety

(Answers will vary depending on available laboratory facilities.)

Name _____ Date _____

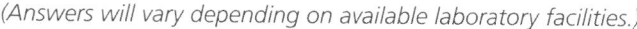

Make a safety check of the laboratory. For each item listed below, determine if the current laboratory conditions are satisfactory (safe), **S**; or unsatisfactory (unsafe), **U**. If unsatisfactory (U), recommend correction(s) in the spaces indicated.

I. Safety Check for Physical Hazards

A. Examine all electrical instruments (microscopes, spectrophotometers, etc.) for frayed wires and proper storage conditions (storage away from water and harsh chemicals, use of dust covers, etc.). Evaluate conditions and record recommendations for each instrument examined.

Instrument	S	U	Observation/Recommendation
_____	____	____	_____
_____	____	____	_____
_____	____	____	_____
_____	____	____	_____

B. Make a fire safety check of the laboratory.

1. Are fire extinguishers present? _____

   When was the last inspection date? _____

   Do extinguishers have instructions for their use posted with them? _____

   Fire extinguishers: S_____ U_____

2. Is the fire exit route posted? _____

   Is it up to date? _____

   Walk the fire exit route. Was it easy to follow? _____

   Could all exit doors be opened? _____

   Fire exit route: S_____ U_____

   Recommendation(s) for improving fire safety: _____

   _____

   _____

   _____

II. Safety Check for Chemical Hazards

A. Examine the chemicals in the laboratory.

1. Are all clearly labeled? _____

2. Do the labels contain information on storage, disposal, and procedure in case of spills or accidental exposure? _____

3. Are chemicals labeled "flammable" stored in a flameproof cabinet? _____

© 2012 Delmar, Cengage Learning. Permission to reproduce for clinical use granted.

WORKSHEET I

4. Where are concentrated acids and bases stored? _____

   Chemical storage: S ____ U ____

B. Is a fume hood present? _____

   When was last air flow inspection? _____

   Is air flow unimpeded by items stored in fume hood? _____

   Fume hood: S ____ U ____

C. Is an eyewash station present? _____

   Are instructions for its use posted? _____

   Are eyewash solutions changed at appropriate intervals _____

   Eyewash station: S ____ U ____

   Recommendation(s) for improving chemical safety: _____

   _____

   _____

   _____

III. Laboratory Safety Policy

Inquire about the laboratory's policy regarding employee safety orientation and training.

A. Is a written safety manual available in the laboratory? _____

   Is the location of the safety manual posted? _____

B. Does the laboratory administration follow appropriate "employee right-to-know" policies in the safety orientation and training programs? _____

C. Are written records kept of employee safety training sessions? _____

D. Are all employees required to sign safety agreement forms after safety training? _____

E. Is a(n) MSDS on file for each chemical? _____

   Laboratory safety policy: S _____ U _____

   Recommendation(s) for improving safety policy: _____

   _____

   _____

   _____

© 2012 Delmar, Cengage Learning. Permission to reproduce for clinical use granted

LESSON 1-5
Chemical, Fire, and Electrical Safety

(Answers will vary depending on laboratory facilities available.)

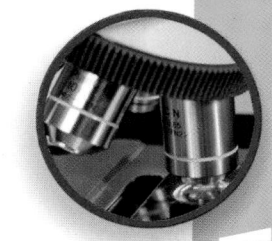

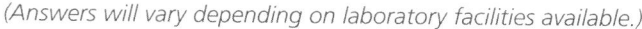

Name _____ Date _____

Make an inventory of six chemicals in your laboratory using the inventory form below. Consult the chemical labels and MSDS to determine the hazard class and type of PPE required when using each chemical.

CHEMICAL INVENTORY FORM

Name _____ Date _____

Location _____ Date _____

Chemical Name	Catalog #	Quantity	Physical State	Hazard Class				Manufacturer	Comments
				H	F	R	P		

(H) Health Hazard
0 - Minimal/None
1 - Slightly hazardous
2 - Hazardous
3 - Extreme
4 - Deadly

(F) Fire Hazard/Flashpoint
0 - Will not burn
1 - Slight, above 200°F
2 - Moderate, below 200°F
3 - Serious, below 100°F
4 - Extreme, below 73°F

(R) Reactivity Hazard
0 - Stable, not reactive with water
1 - Slight, unstable if heated
2 - Water reactive
3 - Shock or heat may detonate
4 - May detonate

(P) Protection Required
A - Goggles
B - Goggles/Gloves
C - Goggles/Gloves/Apron
D - Face shield/Gloves/Apron
E - Goggles/Gloves/Mask
F - Goggles/Gloves/Apron/Mask
X - Gloves

© 2012 Delmar, Cengage Learning. Permission to reproduce for clinical use granted.

WORKSHEET II

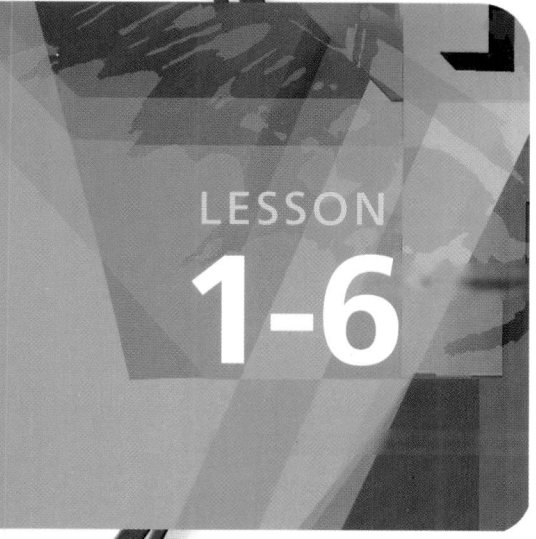

LESSON
1-6

General Laboratory Equipment

LESSON OBJECTIVES

After studying this lesson, the student will:

⊙ Identify five basic types of containers used in the laboratory and explain the use of each.

⊙ Explain the differences between critical and noncritical measurements.

⊙ Identify glassware that can be used for critical measurements.

⊙ Identify heat-resistant glassware.

⊙ Discuss the advantages and disadvantages of using plastic containers in the laboratory.

⊙ Describe the proper care of and cleaning procedures for laboratory glassware and plasticware.

⊙ Explain how the condition of labware can affect the outcome of test procedures.

⊙ Explain the proper use of a centrifuge.

⊙ Explain the function of a pH meter.

⊙ Discuss the operation of an autoclave.

⊙ List four rules for using a laboratory balance.

⊙ Explain how temperature-controlled chambers are used in the laboratory.

⊙ Discuss safety precautions that must be followed when using labware and laboratory equipment such as centrifuges, autoclaves, pH meters, and balances.

⊙ Explain the importance of performing regular equipment maintenance and keeping maintenance and repair records.

⊙ Define the glossary terms.

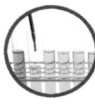

GLOSSARY

autoclave / a device that uses pressurized steam for sterilization

beaker / a wide-mouthed, straight-sided container with a pouring spout formed from the rim and used to make estimated measurements

borosilicate glass / nonreactive glass with high thermal resistance commonly used to make high-quality labware

centrifuge / an instrument with a rotor that rotates at high speeds in a closed chamber

critical measurements / measurements made when the accuracy of the concentration of a solution is important; measurements made using glassware manufactured to strict standards

flask / a container with an enlarged body and a narrow neck

(continues)

flint glass / inexpensive glass with low resistance to heat and chemicals

graduated cylinder / an upright, straight-sided container with a flared base and a volume scale

labware / article(s) or container(s) intended for laboratory use

meniscus / the curved upper surface of a liquid in a container

microfuge / a centrifuge that spins microcentrifuge tubes at high rates of speed; microcentrifuge

National Institute for Standards and Technology (NIST) / a federal agency that promotes international standardization of measurements; formerly the National Bureau of Standards

noncritical measurements / estimated measurements; measurements made in containers that estimate volume (such as beakers)

pH / a measurement of the hydrogen ion concentration expressing the degree of acidity or alkalinity of a solution

pipet / a slender calibrated tube used for measuring and transferring liquids

polyethylene / plastic polymer of ethylene used for containers

polypropylene / lightweight plastic polymer of propylene that resists moisture and solvents and withstands heat sterilization

polystyrene / clear, colorless polymer of styrene used for labware

quartz glass / expensive glass with excellent light transmission; glass used for cuvettes; silica glass

reagent / substance or solution used in laboratory analyses; substance involved in a chemical reaction

rotor / the part of a centrifuge that holds the tubes and rotates during the operation of the centrifuge

serological centrifuge / a centrifuge that spins small tubes such as those used in blood banking; serofuge

solute / the substance dissolved in a given solution

solvent / a dissolving agent, usually a liquid

tare / in chemical analysis, a determination of the net weight of a chemical by subtracting the weight of the container from the overall weight of the container and the chemical being weighed

INTRODUCTION

Several types of glassware, plasticware, and general laboratory equipment are used in clinical laboratories to prepare and store reagents and specimens. The types of equipment found in a clinical laboratory are determined by the size of the laboratory and the number and nature of tests performed. A small laboratory might have only a microscope, a few pieces of equipment, and **pipets**, calibrated tubes used to measure and transfer liquids. Large laboratories have an assortment of general equipment including glassware, pipetters, pH meters, autoclaves, balances, incubators, water baths, and analyzers.

The quality of laboratory test results is based on several factors, including the equipment used in the testing process. This lesson introduces some general guidelines for the use, care, and maintenance of common laboratory equipment and labware. In this text, the symbol ⬢ is used to alert that temperature is important to the procedure or to the operation of an instrument. The symbol ⬢ is used to remind that timing is an essential consideration when performing a procedure or using an instrument.

Laboratory safety rules as explained in Lessons 1-4 and 1-5 must be followed when using all laboratory equipment. However, special safety concerns can be associated with particular types of equipment. Manuals provided by equipment manufacturers must be consulted to determine the correct use and limits of each piece of equipment.

Types of pipets and pipetting techniques are explained in Lesson 1-8, along with a discussion of the types of reagent water and instructions for preparing different types of solutions. Lesson 1-10 contains detailed information about the use and care of the microscope.

GENERAL LABWARE

Laboratory glassware has many functions and comes in many shapes and sizes. Glassware can be used in a specific test procedure or in preparing or storing **reagents**, solutions used in laboratory analysis. In recent years, it has become common to use plastic laboratory containers as well as glass. Because of this, the term **labware** is used to include glassware and plasticware. Much of today's labware is designed to be used only once and then discarded. This eliminates the possibility of using a container that is contaminated with residue from previous use. Types of general labware include bottles, beakers, flasks, test tubes, graduated cylinders, and pipets.

Glassware

Laboratory glassware can be made of flint glass, borosilicate glass, or quartz/silica glass.

- **Flint glass** is inexpensive but has low resistance to heat and chemicals. Disposable test tubes are often made of flint glass.

- **Borosilicate glass** is nonreactive with most chemicals, is resistant to both heat and cold shock, and can be heat sterilized. Pyrex and Kimax are brands of borosilicate glass commonly used for beakers, flasks, and other reusable laboratory glassware.

- **Quartz glass**, or silica glass, is an expensive glass that is used when glass must have excellent light transmission without distortion, such as in cuvettes for spectrophotometers.

Plasticware

Plastic containers are useful because they are lightweight and impact- and corrosion-resistant. Plastics are unaffected by most aqueous solutions. Plastics do not release ions into solution as some types of glass do, but some plastics can bind and release (leach) solutes.

Three common plastics used to make labware are **polyethylene, polypropylene,** and **polystyrene.** Containers made of polyethylene and polystyrene are clear, inexpensive, and disposable but are not heat resistant. Polypropylene containers usually have a milky or opaque appearance, are heat resistant, and can be heat sterilized.

TYPES AND FUNCTIONS OF LABWARE

The functions of labware are determined by the design and manufacturing standards of the items. Some labware, such as bottles, beakers, test tubes, and certain flasks, are used to make **noncritical measurements,** measurements that are estimated or approximate. Noncritical glassware can be divided into two groups: *approximate* glassware which includes beakers and certain flasks; and *measuring* glassware, which includes graduated cylinders and serological pipets.

Other labware is designed to strict standards to allow **critical measurements** requiring precision and accuracy to be made. This glassware, called Class A glassware, or *precise* glassware, is manufactured and calibrated to standards prescribed by the **National Institute for Standards and Technology (NIST)** and comes with a certificate of calibration. Class A glassware includes volumetric flasks and volumetric pipets and is marked with capacity tolerance limits (error limits). Class A glassware is used for reconstituting controls and standards and preparing solutions.

Bottles

Reagent bottles are available in a variety of sizes and types. Plastic bottles should be used for all reagents that do not interact with plastic. Reagents should not be stored for long periods in low-quality glass containers that can slowly release ions into the solutions. The reagent bottle should be only slightly larger than the volume of reagent. Brown plastic or glass bottles are used for storing light-sensitive reagents.

Test Tubes

Test tubes are used in many laboratory procedures and are available in various types of plastic and glass and a variety of sizes and shapes (Figure 1-32). Test tubes function as containers for liquids such as blood, urine, plasma and serum. Even though some test tubes have graduated markings they are not calibrated to accurately measure liquids.

In some procedures, the analysis is performed in a test tube. Sometimes a test method requires that the contents be heated in the test tube. This must be done with caution, using a test tube made of heat-resistant glass, such as Kimax or Pyrex. Only test

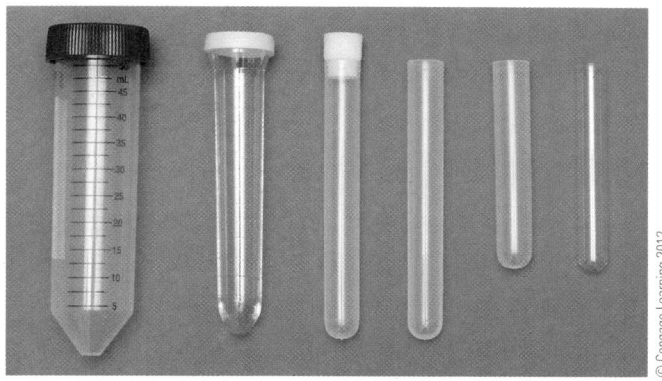

FIGURE 1-32 Test tubes

tubes rated to withstand the force of centrifugation should be used to centrifuge samples.

Beakers

Beakers are wide-mouthed, straight-sided containers with a pouring spout formed from the rim (Figure 1-33). They are used for *estimating* volumes of liquids, mixing solutions, or simply holding liquids. Each beaker is labeled to indicate the approximate capacity in milliliters and the estimated accuracy of the capacity markings. For instance a 250-mL beaker marked ±5% indicates that, when the beaker is filled to the 250 mL mark, the actual volume in the beaker could be between 237 mL (–5%) and 263 mL (+5%). A beaker with capacity nearest the volume to be measured should be selected. For instance, a 1000-mL beaker should not be used to measure 100 mL.

Graduated Cylinders

A **graduated cylinder** is an upright, straight-sided container with a flared base and a volume scale. Graduated cylinders are somewhat more accurate than beakers and flasks but are not used for precise measurements. Graduated cylinders are commonly used to measure the volume of 24-hour urine specimens

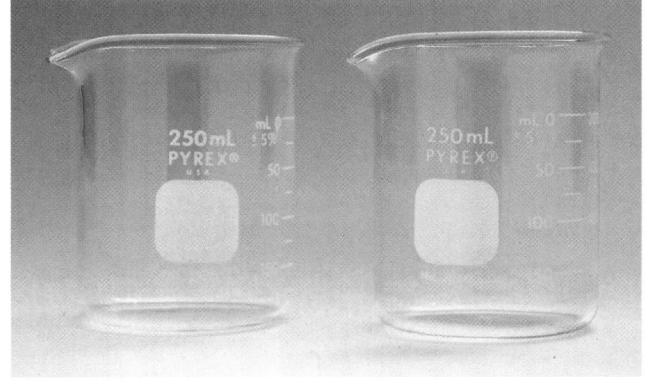

FIGURE 1-33 Beakers with markings

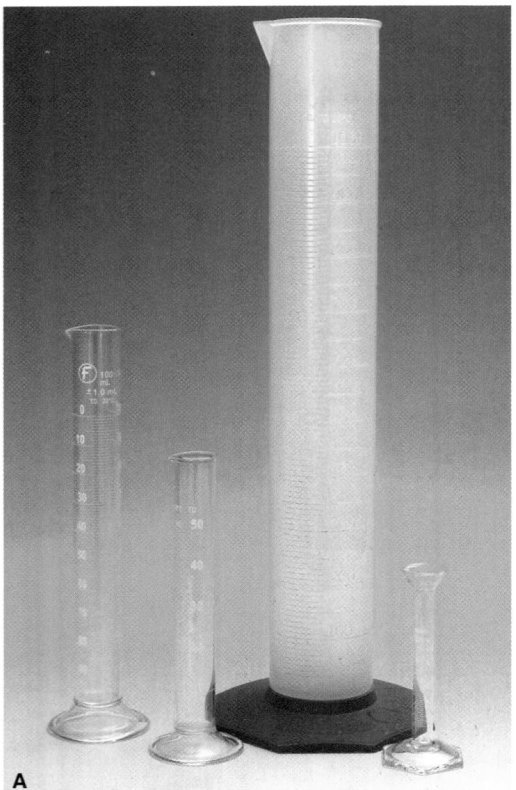

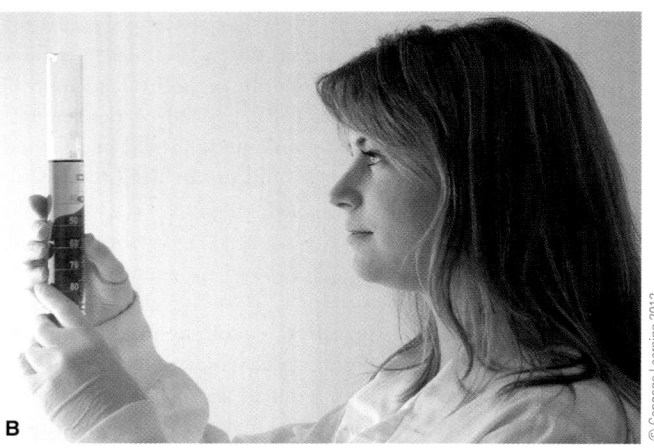

FIGURE 1-34 Graduated cylinders: (A) graduated cylinders with markings; (B) observing the meniscus in a graduated cylinder

(Figure 1-34A). Graduated cylinders are available in capacities ranging from 5 to 2000 mL. Liquids are measured in a graduated cylinder by pouring the liquid into the cylinder and reading the volume at the lowest point of the **meniscus**, the curved liquid surface (Figure 1-34B).

Flasks

A **flask** is a container with an enlarged body and a narrow neck. Two common flasks are Erlenmeyer flasks and volumetric flasks (Figure 1-35). The *Erlenmeyer flask* has a flat bottom

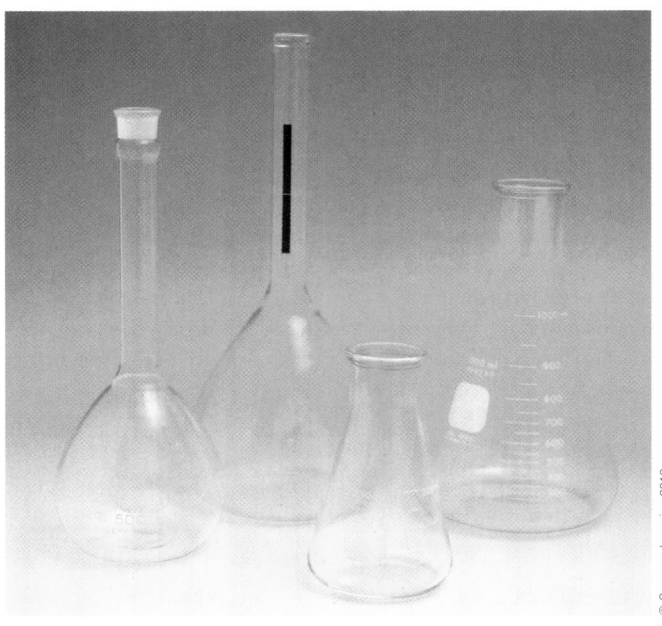

FIGURE 1-35 Flasks: left, volumetric flasks; right, Erlenmeyer flasks

and sloping sides that gradually narrow in diameter so the top opening is bottle-like. The opening can be plain, so it can be stoppered with a cork, or can have threads for a screw-on cap. Erlenmeyer flasks range from 10 mL to 4000 mL capacity. They are used to hold liquids, mix solutions, or measure noncritical volumes. Markings on the side indicate the approximate capacity in milliliters. Flasks that have increment marks are called "graduated flasks" and are convenient for estimating volumes (noncritical measurements).

The *volumetric flask* is a pear-shaped flask used for making critical measurements. Volumetric flasks are available in a variety of sizes, ranging from 5 mL to 1000 mL. They are manufactured to strict standards and are guaranteed to contain a certain volume at a particular temperature. A line is etched in the neck of the flask to indicate the correct fill level. The capacity (in milliliters) is marked on the flask along with the tolerance limit.

To prepare a reagent using a volumetric flask, the flask is filled one-half to two-thirds full with **solvent.** An exact amount of **solute** is measured into the flask, and the solute is allowed to dissolve. Solvent is then added until it approaches the fill line. The last portion of solvent is added slowly (dropwise) until the lowest point of the meniscus is level with the fill line when viewed at eye level (Figure 1-36).

CARE AND CLEANING OF LABWARE

Good-quality glassware is expensive and must be handled with care. Clean labware should be stored protected from dust and accidental breakage.

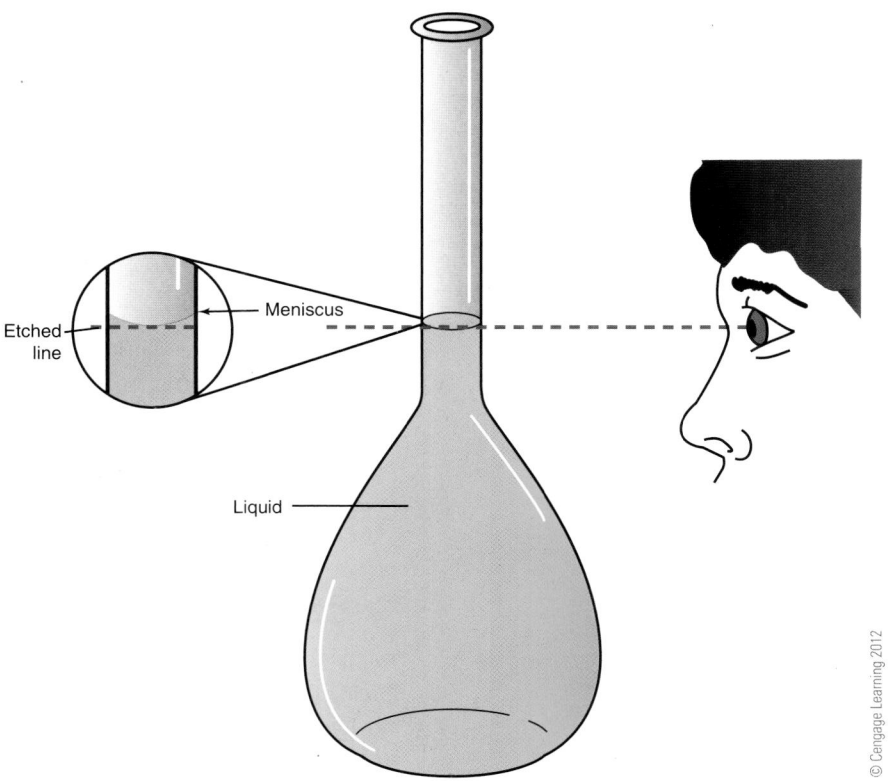

FIGURE 1-36 Observing the meniscus at the fill line of a volumetric flask

Routine Cleaning

  Disposable labware is intended to be used once and then discarded. The use of disposable plastic labware when a procedure permits reduces the hazards associated with washing of labware.

Reusable labware must be cleaned thoroughly after each use. Most cleaning problems, such as dried reagents, can be avoided if labware is rinsed with water immediately after use and soaked in a laboratory detergent solution such as Sparkleen or Cytoclean until it can be washed. Stubborn deposits can usually be removed by soaking the container overnight.

Labware can be washed in an automatic dishwasher; however, some plastics are weakened by frequent washing and drying in automatic dishwashers because of the high heat. Labware can also be washed by hand in laboratory detergent, followed by several rinses. Heavy-duty gloves must be worn when hand-washing glassware. The grade of water called Autoclave and Wash Water (formerly called type III) can be used for washing and rinsing glassware. Clinical Laboratory Reagent Water (CLRW) or Instrument Feed Water (formerly type I and type II) should be used as the final rinse for glassware. (The various types of laboratory water and their preparation are explained in Lesson 1-8.) An indication that glassware is clean is that the water will "sheet" or uniformly wet the glassware. After washing, heat-resistant labware can be dried in a drying oven.

Cleaning Contaminated Labware

   Labware that has come in contact with any serum control, blood, body fluid, patient specimen, or other potentially infectious material (OPIM) must be decontaminated before it is washed. This is usually accomplished by soaking the labware in a disinfectant solution, such as dilute chlorine bleach, quaternary ammonium detergent, or a phenol-based solution such as Amphyl for at least 1 hour or overnight. Following decontamination, the items should be rinsed free of disinfectant and then washed as described earlier for the routine cleaning of glassware. In some cases, labware must be sterilized by autoclaving before it can be washed.

SAFETY PRECAUTIONS

Labware Safety

  The use of labware presents several hazards, such as the potential for spills, splashes, aerosol formation, or injury from broken or chipped glass. Injuries can be prevented by using careful technique and wearing appropriate PPE. Whenever possible, plastic labware should be used to reduce the possibility of injury from broken glass. Each item of glassware should be inspected for chips or cracks before use and should not be used if these are present. If damaged glassware cannot be repaired, it should be discarded into rigid, puncture-proof containers.

Standard Precautions must be observed and appropriate PPE must be worn when handling labware containing blood or other body fluids or substances. Disposable contaminated labware must be discarded into appropriate biohazard or sharps containers. Reusable labware that has been contaminated with blood or other potentially infectious materials (OPIM) must be decontaminated by soaking in a disinfectant before washing.

Heavy-duty gloves and other appropriate PPE must be worn when cleaning glassware. Glassware marked with the Kimax or Pyrex trade name is heat-resistant, can be used for boiling solutions, and can be sterilized by autoclaving. Glassware not manufactured of heat-resistant glass must not be heated over direct heat or autoclaved.

Equipment Safety

The use of laboratory equipment can present certain hazards, such as the presence of high-voltage electrical current and exposure to moving equipment parts, steam, or hot liquids. Certain instruments can also present the risk for exposure to blood or OPIM. The hazards differ according to the type of equipment and how it is used.

All equipment must be operated in a safe manner, following the manufacturers' directions. Preventive maintenance should be performed carefully, adhering to Standard Precautions and other recommended safety practices. Only trained persons should repair equipment. Additional equipment-specific safety information is included in the section describing the function and operation of each type of equipment.

QUALITY ASSESSMENT

Labware

Labware must be used appropriately because the type and quality of labware can affect test outcome. Critical measurements must be made using certified volumetric glassware. Containers such as beakers and Erlenmeyer flasks should only be used for noncritical measurements. When making estimated volume measurements, containers that have a capacity close to the volume being measured should be used.

Whenever possible, disposable labware should be used. For reusable labware, only clean, dry items free from chemical residues or detergents should be used in test procedures or for reagent storage. Accurate measurements cannot be made using glassware that is not clean and the solutions that are being measured or stored can become contaminated.

Laboratory Equipment

As part of the overall quality assessment program, regular maintenance, calibration, and performance checks must be performed for all laboratory equipment, including refrigerators, water baths, centrifuges, autoclaves, pH meters, and balances. The results of these procedures must be documented. Any problems detected must be corrected before the equipment is used for laboratory work. The laboratory SOP manual will specify the frequency and types of checks that must be performed for each piece of laboratory equipment.

COMMON LABORATORY EQUIPMENT

Types of equipment and instruments commonly found in the laboratory include centrifuges, autoclaves, laboratory balances, pH meters, and various temperature-controlled chambers, such as refrigerators, freezers, and waterbaths or heat blocks. Procedures for the correct use and quality control checks required for each of these will be specified in the SOP manual. These procedures must be followed for safe and accurate use of the instrument(s).

Centrifuges

Centrifuges are instruments that spin samples at high speeds, forcing the heavier particles to the bottom of the container (usually a tube). The part of the centrifuge that holds the tubes and rotates during operation is the **rotor**. Centrifuges are frequently used to separate the cellular components of blood from serum or plasma and to centrifuge urine to obtain urine sediment. Centrifuges vary in size, capacity, and speed capability. *Clinical centrifuge* is the name given to models that can be used for urinalysis or serum separation (Figures 1-37 and 1-38). Clinical centrifuges can be large floor models or small enough to fit on a benchtop. These usually have a speed capacity of 0 to 3000 rpm (revolutions per minute), and hold tubes ranging in size from 5 to 50 mL, depending on the rotor or tube carriers. A **serological centrifuge** is a centrifuge used in blood banking to spin small tubes (approximately 2 to 3 mL capacity).

Microcentrifuges, or **microfuges**, are widely used in the clinical laboratory to spin special microtubes (0.5 to 1.5 mL capacity) at high speeds, up to 14,000 rpm (Figure 1-39). The microhematocrit centrifuge is a variation of the microfuge; it spins capillary tubes at high speeds for measuring microhematocrits.

Other types of centrifuges include high-speed refrigerated centrifuges that have speed capabilities up to 20,000 rpm, and ultracentrifuges that are capable of speeds over 50,000 rpm. These centrifuges are specially equipped to keep samples cool during centrifugation. Ultracentrifuges are often used in research laboratories but not usually required for clinical laboratory samples.

Centrifuge Safety

Centrifuges present several safety hazards. Because they are used to process biological specimens, Standard Precautions must be observed and appropriate PPE must be worn when operating a centrifuge. All centrifuge surfaces (interior and exterior) must be cleaned using surface disinfectant any time spills or splashes occur.

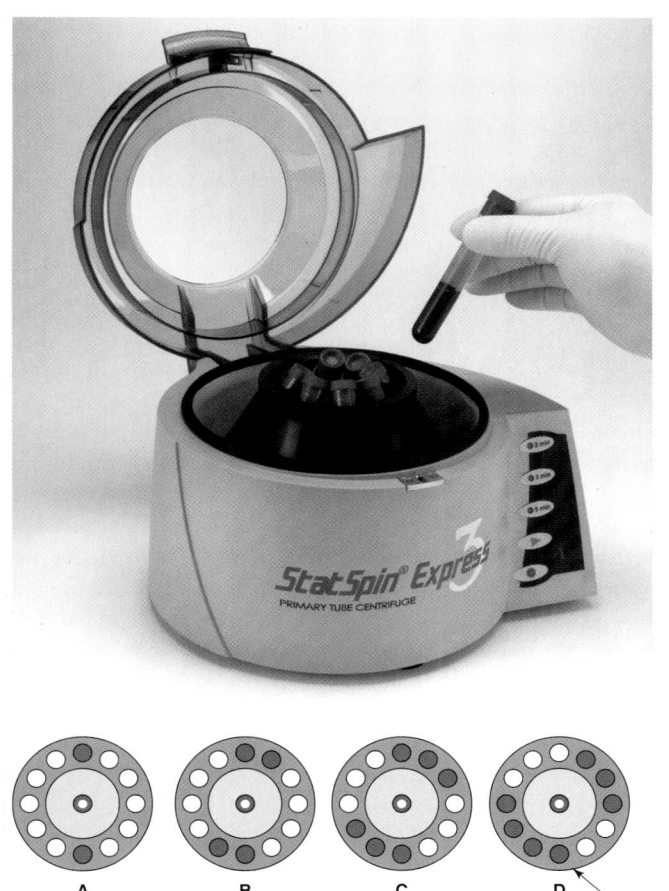

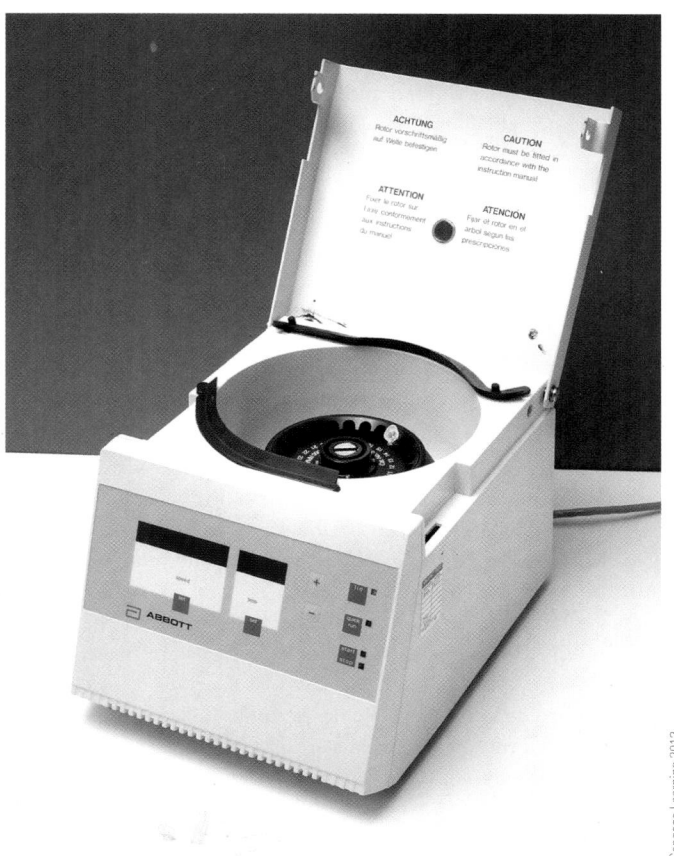

FIGURE 1-39 Microcentrifuge and microtubes (in foreground)

FIGURE 1-37 Correct way to balance tubes in a centrifuge rotor: Top, placing tubes in the rotor of a tabletop clinical centrifuge; Bottom, A-C, diagrams showing correct placement of tubes (small, dark blue circles) in rotor and, D, incorrect placement of tubes (Photo A courtesy of Iris Sample Processing, Westwood, MA)

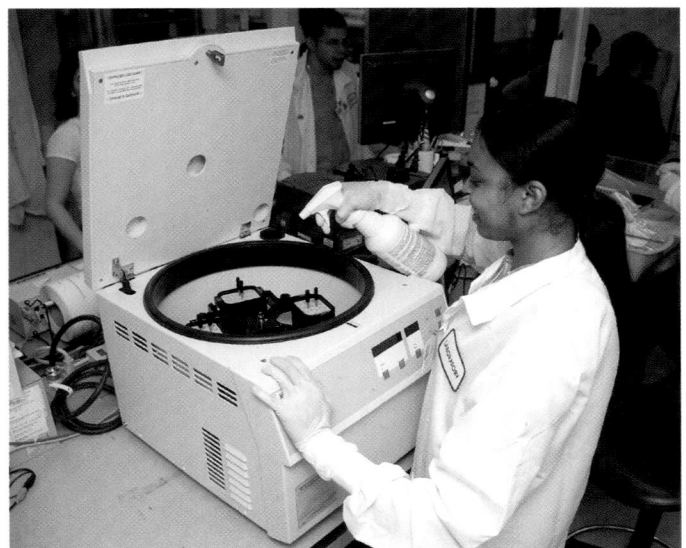

FIGURE 1-38 Disinfecting a clinical centrifuge

Centrifuge safety requires that a centrifuge be operated only when the rotor contains a balanced load. Imbalanced loads can cause damage to centrifuge rotors or the centrifuge. To balance a load, specimen tubes of equal size, volume contained, and density of liquid in the tubes are placed directly opposite each other in the rotor (Figure 1-37B). If an uneven number of tubes are to be spun, a balance tube is loaded opposite the last sample tube. The balance tube must be identical to the sample tubes, containing the same volume and liquid density as the tube being balanced.

Manufacturer's instructions must always be followed when using a centrifuge. Some general rules to follow include:

1. Load must be balanced before centrifuge operation.

2. Tubes should remain capped during centrifugation to prevent aerosol formation.

3. Only tubes rated as appropriate for the particular centrifuge and speed should be used.

4. The centrifuge must not be opened while the rotor is spinning. Centrifuges should be equipped with safety latches called cover interlocks that keep the centrifuge lid locked during centrifuge operation and prevent the operation of the centrifuge unless the lid is locked.

5. Spills must be cleaned immediately with surface disinfectant (Figure 1-38).

Quality Assessment

The rotation speeds and accuracy of centrifuge timers must be verified and documented at specific intervals, usually monthly or quarterly.

Autoclaves

Autoclaves use steam under pressure to sterilize items such as dental and surgical instruments, solutions, and materials to be used in microbiology (Figure 1-40). Autoclaves are also used to decontaminate materials such as blood specimens, bacterial cultures, or filled biohazard containers before disposal.

Autoclaves can range in size from large (refrigerator size) to tabletop size. Large autoclaves obtain steam from either an internal steam generator or a connection to the facility's steam plant. Smaller ones create their own steam by heating water.

Items to be sterilized or decontaminated are placed in bags, wrapped in paper, or placed in heat-proof autoclave pans. An indicator such as autoclave tape is used on packages and glassware in each run; this tape changes color when the proper temperature is reached in the autoclave. Items are placed inside the autoclave, and the autoclave door is closed and locked. The temperature, length of cycle, and pounds of steam pressure are set. Typical autoclave conditions are 121° C for 15 to 20 minutes at 15 pounds per square inch (psi). Steam is admitted into the chamber and timing begins when the temperature and pressure reach preset levels. Autoclaves have temperature and pressure gauges, and most have a chart or digital recorder that records the temperature of each autoclave cycle. At the end of the cycle, the pressure and temperature will drop; the autoclave is safe to open when the chamber pressure gauge reads zero (0) psi.

Autoclave Safety

Because of the pressurized steam generated by an autoclave, great care must be used during autoclave operation. The autoclave door must never be opened unless the chamber pressure is zero (0) psi. Regularly scheduled safety inspections by a qualified autoclave service technician are required. To prevent burns, tongs and/or heat-proof gloves must be used to remove items from the autoclave. When liquids are sterilized, they must be in loosely capped, heat-resistant containers that are no more than half full. These containers must be placed in an autoclavable tray or pan to catch overflow. Chamber pressure must be reduced slowly at the end of a "liquid run" to prevent the liquids from boiling over because of rapid decreases in pressure.

Quality Assessment

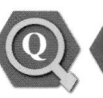 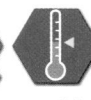

It is important that autoclaves work properly, since nonsterile items could endanger both worker and patient or could cause problems in a test procedure requiring sterile solutions or components. Indicator strips containing spores from the bacterium *Bacillus stearothermophilus* can be used to check the effectiveness of the steam sterilization process. The strips are autoclaved with a normal load, removed, and incubated in a tube of bacterial growth medium. Lack of bacterial growth confirms the efficiency of sterilization; growth of bacteria indicates the sterilization method was inadequate and the items in that run are not sterile. Temperature, pressure, and time controls must then be checked to determine the cause of failure.

Daily records must be kept of sterilization times, temperatures, chamber pressures, and indicator strip results. The temperature chart recorder must be changed at specified intervals and the charts maintained in the equipment logbook.

Laboratory Balances

Several types of balances or scales are used in the laboratory. They differ in the maximum amount they can accurately weigh, their sensitivities, and basic design (Figure 1-41). Measurements that require sensitivity to 0.10 g can be made using inexpensive double- or triple-beam balances. Measurements of as little as 0.0001 g (10^{-4} g) or even 0.00001 g (10^{-5} g) can be made using an analytical balance with sufficient sensitivity. Most critical weighing is done using electronic top-loading balances (Figure 1-41A) or analytical balances (Figure 1-41B).

Laboratory Balance Safety

Because balances are used to weigh chemicals, appropriate chemical safety precautions must be used to prevent exposure to the chemical or chemical dust. Technicians should observe basic safety rules, know the hazards of the chemicals they are working with, and wear appropriate PPE. Care should be taken that chemical dusts are not created during transfer of chemicals. Work practice controls should include:

- Wear eye protection to avoid getting chemicals in the eyes.
- Wear a mask to avoid breathing in chemical dusts that can be respiratory irritants.
- Wear gloves and a laboratory coat to avoid chemical contact with skin and clothing.
- Clean up spills around the balance to keep the work area safe.

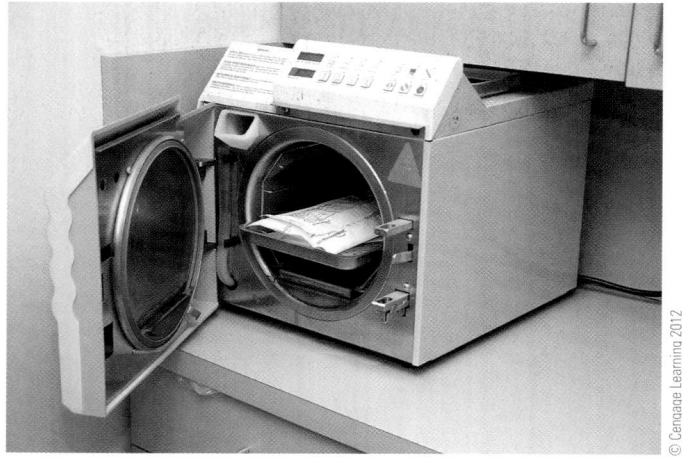

FIGURE 1-40 A tabletop autoclave

© Cengage Learning 2012

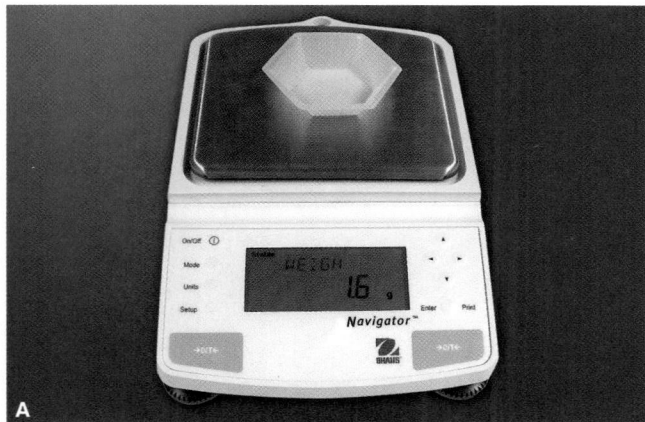

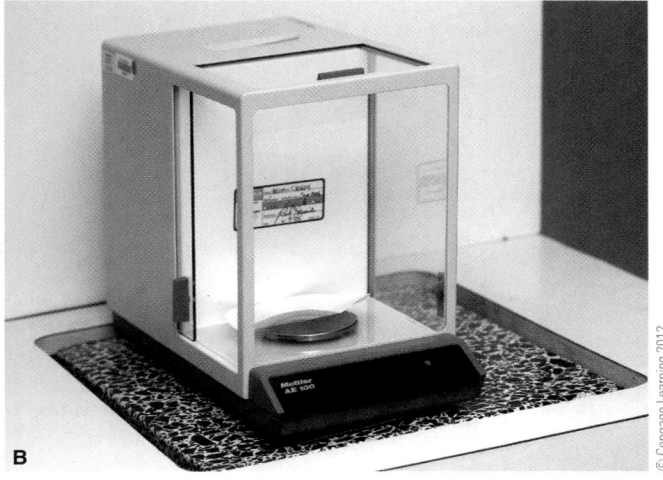

FIGURE 1-41 Laboratory balances: (A) top-loading balance; (B) analytical balance

Quality Assessment

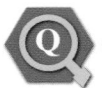   Chemicals must be weighed accurately to prepare reagents correctly. The manufacturer's instruction manual must be followed for the particular balance being used. Purchased sets of calibration weights can be used to calibrate balances. These weights must be kept protected from dust and only handled with forceps, never touched with the bare hands. Some general rules to follow to protect the balance and ensure quality results are:

- Keep balances clean and wipe up any spills immediately.
- Protect the balance from jarring, sudden shocks, and temperature extremes.
- Keep the balance in the same location; do not move it from place to place.
- Level the balance by adjusting balance legs.
- Position the balance in a location free of drafts and vibrations. Special stabilizing tables are available if vibrations are a problem.
- Check zero adjustment; scale should read zero (0) when the weigh pan is empty.

- Always use a container for weighing chemicals; do not place chemicals directly on balance pan.
- Tare the balance (place the empty weighing container on the balance and set the balance weight to zero).
- Observe the sensitivity limits of the balance; do not try to weigh 0.001 g on a balance that is accurate only to 0.01 g.
- Calibrate balances on a regular schedule; perform yearly maintenance or contract to have the services done.

pH Meters

The pH of reagents is critical to many laboratory procedures. The **pH** is a measure of the hydrogen ion (H^+) concentration of a solution. It indicates the acidity or alkalinity of a solution. The pH scale is 0 to 14.0. A pH of 7.0 is neutral; at pH 7, the hydrogen ion (H^+) concentration equals the hydroxyl ion (OH^-) concentration. pH values below 7.0 indicate acid solutions; values above 7.0 indicate alkaline solutions. Lemon juice, vinegar, and hydrochloric acid (HCl) are examples of acids; solutions of baking soda, sodium hydroxide (NaOH), and potassium hydroxide (KOH) are examples of alkaline solutions.

A pH electrode connected to the pH meter detects the hydrogen ion concentration of a solution by comparing it to a reference electrode. The meter measures the potential across a membrane inside the electrode. Most meters use a single combination electrode that contains both the detecting electrode and reference electrode in one probe. When an unknown solution is tested, the potential of the unknown solution is compared to the potential created in the reference electrode. The measurement is converted to pH and displayed on the dial or digital screen of the pH meter (Figure 1-42A). If the pH of a reagent is too low, it can be made more alkaline by adding a few drops of a concentrated alkaline solution, usually NaOH. If the pH is too high, a concentrated acid such as hydrochloric acid or acetic acid can be used to lower the pH.

pH can be estimated using special papers treated with indicator solutions. These papers are dipped into the solution to be

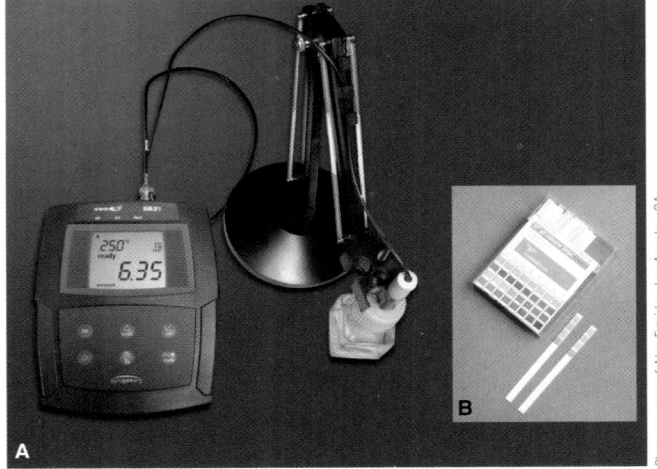

FIGURE 1-42 Measuring pH: (A) pH meter; (B, inset) pH indicator strips for estimating pH

tested, and the color that develops is compared to a color chart to determine the pH (Figure 1-42B). This method is suitable for measuring urine pH, but is not sensitive enough for preparing most laboratory reagents.

pH Meter Safety

  Care should be used when performing pH measurements. Caustic or acid solutions must be handled carefully. Chemical spills must be wiped up immediately. The pH meter should be disconnected from the electrical source before attempting any repair.

Quality Assessment

  Special care must be taken in handling, maintaining, and storing the pH electrode so it will not dry out or be broken. The electrodes must always be rinsed with distilled or reagent water between samples, but never stored in water. Manuals that come with the meters give detailed instructions for use and storage of electrodes.

Electrodes must be calibrated using solutions of known pH values, usually 4.0, 7.0, and 10.0, which should be stored at room temperature. The electrodes are immersed in the known solutions, and the meter is calibrated. Reagents should be at room temperature before attempting to measure pH.

Temperature-Controlled Units

Most test procedures, specimens, and reagents require testing or storage at specific temperatures. Many reagents must be stored refrigerated or frozen; patient specimens are refrigerated or frozen; and microbiological cultures and some chemistry tests require special incubation conditions. To accomplish these tasks, several types of temperature-controlled chambers are used in the clinical laboratory. These include:

- Ovens for drying labware
- Microbiology incubators
- Water baths and heating blocks
- Refrigerators
- Freezers
- Microwaves

Microbiology incubators are commonly set near body temperature (37° C) for optimum growth of most bacterial pathogens. Water baths provide controlled heat above ambient (room) temperature. These can be used as test incubation chambers or to thaw frozen reagents. Microwaves can be used for thawing or heating some solutions. Refrigerated units are used occasionally for tests that must be performed in the cold, but are more commonly used to store reagents and patient specimens such as anticoagulated blood or serum and plasma (Figure 1-43). Freezers are used to store certain reagents and sera. Table 1-24 lists standard permissible temperature ranges for various temperature-controlled chambers.

Temperature-Controlled Chamber Safety

   Temperature-controlled units such as refrigerators, freezers, and water baths, must be used only for

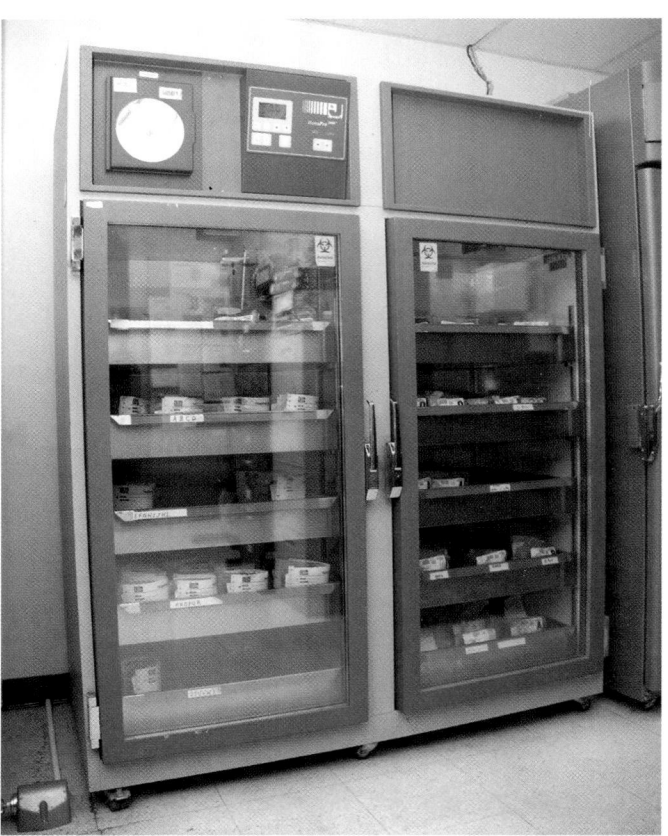

FIGURE 1-43 Blood bank refrigerator, a temperature-controlled chamber in the hospital laboratory

TABLE 1-24. Permissible temperature ranges for common laboratory equipment

EQUIPMENT	TEMPERATURE (° C)	PERMISSIBLE RANGE (° C)
Refrigerator	6 ± 2	4 to 8
Freezer	−20 ± 5	−15 to −25
Ultracold freezer	−70 ± 5	−65 to −75
Microbiology incubator	36 ± 1	35 to 37
Water bath	36 ± 1	35 to 37

laboratory purposes, not for storing or heating food. Because biological specimens are stored or used in these chambers, Standard Precautions must be followed when using and cleaning the units. Stable racks and trays should be used to secure specimens and prevent tipping, spilling, or breakage. Cooling units should be cleaned regularly inside and out with a surface disinfectant. Units such as water baths must be emptied and cleaned frequently using surface disinfectant, followed by wiping with 70% alcohol or dilute (3% to 6%) hydrogen peroxide to prevent growth of microorganisms. Bacteriostatic chemicals or copper wire can be placed in the water of water baths to inhibit bacterial and fungal growth.

Quality Assessment

 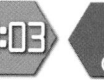 Laboratory air flow, room air exchange, and laboratory temperature maintenance influence the operation of temperature-controlled units. Increased air flow over waterbaths will contribute to more rapid water evaporation. Fluctuating room temperatures and increased air flow can also make it more difficult for temperature-controlled units to maintain their set temperatures. All temperature-controlled units must be monitored regularly to be sure they are operating at the correct temperature. Temperatures must be recorded daily and checked before each use of a unit.

Thermometers.
Certified thermometers calibrated with NIST-certified thermometers must be used for measuring temperatures. A thermometer should be kept in each unit so that the temperature can be checked frequently.

Temperature Stability.
Water baths must be filled to the appropriate level to ensure that specimens will heat properly. The laboratory environment must be kept stable, without abrupt temperature changes or drafts. Either of these conditions can cause temperature-controlled units to be unable to maintain their set temperatures.

Freezers and refrigerated units are fitted with alarms to alert when the temperature fluctuates outside the permissible range. Critical temperature units such as freezers or blood bank refrigerators are also usually connected to accessory (generator) power in case of power outage.

Equipment Maintenance Records

The laboratory's SOP procedure manual will outline the required maintenance and performance checks for each piece of equipment. Log sheets are used for recording maintenance, service, repairs, and performance checks. An example of an equipment maintenance and performance checklist is given at the end of this lesson. A common schedule of performance checks in a small laboratory would include:

- Monitor and record room temperature and temperatures of water baths, refrigerators, and incubators once each shift, or at least daily.
- Check temperature and chamber pressure record of autoclave after each use.
- Measure centrifuge timer and centrifuge rpm every 3 months.
- Calibrate pH meter daily and check with standard solutions before each use.

SAFETY REMINDERS

- Review Safety Precautions sections before using equipment or labware.
- Disinfect contaminated glassware before washing.
- Inspect glassware for chips and cracks before using.
- Unplug electrical equipment before attempting repairs.
- Use care when operating equipment with moving parts.
- Wipe up all spills promptly and appropriately.

PROCEDURAL REMINDERS

- Review Quality Assessment sections before using equipment or labware.
- Use the correct glassware for the task.
- Use equipment according to manufacturer's instructions and facility SOP.
- Record all equipment maintenance and repairs.

 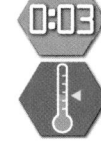

CRITICAL THINKING

June was working in clinical chemistry when a blood specimen came in with orders for STAT (immediate) testing. The main clinical centrifuge was in use, so June located the backup centrifuge. However, a sign was on the backup centrifuge stating that the interlock was broken. June considered using the centrifuge anyway, but decided to wait the 5 minutes until the main centrifuge was available.

Because the test was ordered STAT, and the result was needed as soon as possible, did June do the right thing? Explain your answer.

CASE STUDY

Jamie was in training in the Specimen Collection and Processing section of a small hospital laboratory. One of the laboratory employees asked him to measure the volume of a 24-hour urine specimen received in the laboratory that morning. At the work area were a 1000-mL beaker, a 1000-mL Erlenmeyer flask, and a 1000-mL graduated cylinder.

1. Which item(s) would give the most accurate measurement of volume? Explain your answer.
2. Which of the three items available can be used for critical measurements?

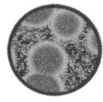

SUMMARY

Many types of glassware and plasticware having a variety of functions are used in the laboratory. These include bottles, beakers, flasks, test tubes, graduated cylinders, and pipets. Test tubes can be used as reaction vessels in laboratory tests. Some items, such as bottles and beakers, are used only to hold or contain reagents. Other items such as graduated cylinders, volumetric flasks, and pipets, are used to estimate and measure volumes.

Laboratory glassware is manufactured to different standards of precision and accuracy, indicated by tolerance markings on the items. Selecting the proper container for the task and using the container correctly can be critical to accurate laboratory results.

Reusable labware must be properly disinfected and cleaned after use, using special attention to Standard Precautions as well as following safety practices for chemical and physical hazards. Disposable labware should be used when possible.

Several types of general equipment are used in clinical laboratories, including refrigerators, freezers, water baths, centrifuges, autoclaves, pH meters, and laboratory balances. Although these types of equipment are not high-tech, they require regular maintenance and performance checks to be sure they are operating optimally. For instance, a refrigerator temperature that is just a few degrees out of the acceptable temperature range can cause reagent failure or specimen degradation either by accidental freezing or by allowing products or specimens to become too warm and deteriorate.

Each piece of equipment carries its own set of operating procedures, maintenance instructions, calibration methods, and operating hazards. The manufacturer's safety and operating instructions should always be followed for each piece of equipment. These instructions will be incorporated into the laboratory SOP manual. Laboratory equipment such as refrigerators, freezers, and centrifuges are usually not directly involved in laboratory analyses, but they indirectly affect test results because they are used for reagent preparation, specimen processing, and specimen and reagent storage.

REVIEW QUESTIONS

1. Name five types of containers used to hold liquids.
2. Name two types of laboratory flasks.
3. Which types of glassware are used to make critical measurements?
4. Why is it important that damaged glassware not be used?
5. Why should reusable glassware be immediately rinsed after use?
6. Why is it important that glassware be rinsed until it is free of detergent?
7. How do flint glass and borosilicate glass differ?
8. Name three types of plastics commonly used in the laboratory and give characteristics of each.
9. What is the procedure for cleaning labware that is contaminated with blood or OPIM?
10. What rules should be followed when using a laboratory balance?
11. A solution with a pH of 8.5 is _____ (acidic, neutral, alkaline).
12. Give five general rules to follow when operating a centrifuge.
13. Name three types of centrifuges that can be found in a clinical laboratory.
14. Explain how autoclaves operate.
15. Why is it important to be careful when using an autoclave?
16. What quality assessment procedures are used for temperature control chambers?
17. Explain why equipment maintenance records are important.
18. Why is it important to maintain a stable laboratory environment?
19. Name a hazard associated with autoclave, centrifuge, pH meter, and laboratory balance.

20. Define autoclave, beaker, borosilicate glass, centrifuge, critical measurements, flask, flint glass, graduated cylinder, labware, meniscus, microfuge, National Institute for Standards and Technology, noncritical measurements, pH, pipet, polyethylene, polypropylene, polystyrene, quartz glass, reagent, rotor, serological centrifuge, solute, solvent, and tare.

STUDENT ACTIVITIES

1. Complete the written examination on this lesson.

2. Measure 100 mL of water in a beaker and transfer it to another beaker or flask. Does it measure 100 mL in the second container?

3. Measure 100 mL of water in an Erlenmeyer flask and transfer it to a 100-mL volumetric flask. Is the volume exactly 100 mL?

4. Practice measuring volumes using a graduated cylinder: Hold cylinder with desired volume marking at eye level and carefully pour water into the cylinder until it reaches the volume marking. Observe the meniscus: the lowest point should be level with the volume marking (Figures 1-34 and 1-36). If necessary, adjust volume by adding or removing solution dropwise until the meniscus is at the proper level. Repeat procedure using a different size cylinder.

5. Practice measuring volumes using a volumetric flask: identify the fill line in the neck of the flask; pour water into the flask slowly until the fluid level nears the fill line; hold the flask so the fill line is at eye level and use a transfer pipet to deliver water dropwise until the low point of the meniscus is level with the fill line.

6. Depending on the instruments available, complete activities 6a to 6c. Read the instruction manual carefully before attempting to use an instrument. Then be sure to follow the instructions carefully when using that instrument.

   a. If a pH meter is available, practice measuring the pH of solutions such as 0.9% saline and 0.9% buffered saline. Note how the pH changes when a drop or two of 0.1% HCl or 0.1% NaOH is added to each solution. Dilute the solution by adding 1 part water to 1 part solution. Now measure the pH. Did it change? How can the result be explained? How does the pH of the nonbuffered saline differ from that of the buffered saline?

   b. If a balance is available, practice weighing a nontoxic chemical or a substance such as NaCl (salt) or glucose (sugar). Be sure to zero the balance before beginning and tare the balance with the empty weighing container on the pan. Note the capacity of the balance; what is the largest weight that can be measured? What is the smallest increment that can be read (1 g, 0.1 g, 0.01 g, etc.)?

   c. If a centrifuge is available, practice centrifuging a sample, using appropriately sized tubes and balance tubes. Note the speed scale; what is the maximum rpm the centrifuge can achieve? What size tubes can the centrifuge handle safely? Does the centrifuge have a cover interlock?

7. Use the general laboratory equipment worksheet at the end of this lesson to record the performance and maintenance of any available equipment.

WEB ACTIVITIES

1. Search the product listing of an online laboratory supply catalog for information about types of centrifuges that are available. Compare three sizes including maximum speed, types of tubes, and type of rotor.

2. Visit the NIST web site. Find information on certified glassware.

3. Look in online scientific catalogs for calibrators or standards for general laboratory equipment:

   a. Find examples of thermometers for use in clinical refrigerators, freezers, and incubators. List the various designs available. Are the thermometers NIST certified?

   b. Determine what devices are available for calibrating centrifuge speed and how they are used.

   c. Find examples of calibration weight sets for use with laboratory balances. How are the weight sets used to calibrate a laboratory balance?

   d. Find information on pH standard solutions for calibrating pH meters.

4. Search the Internet for instrument calibration services for clinical equipment such as centrifuges and laboratory balances. What calibration service intervals are recommended for different types of equipment?

5. Search the Internet for online videos or tutorials demonstrating the correct use of laboratory glassware such as graduated cylinders or beakers.

6. Search the Internet for online videos or tutorials demonstrating the safe and correct use of laboratory equipment such as centrifuges or laboratory balances. Try to find demonstration videos for the type of instruments available in your laboratory.

LESSON 1-6
General Laboratory Equipment

(Answers may vary based on laboratory facilities available.)

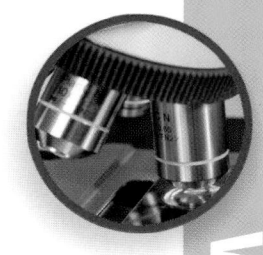

Name _____ Date _____

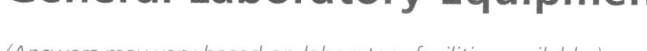 Use this form to record general laboratory equipment maintenance and performance. Identify each piece of equipment on the sheet. Locate instruction manuals for the equipment and determine the recommended maintenance and/or calibration procedures and schedules.

I. Temperature-Controlled Units

A. Record the temperatures of refrigerators, freezers, water baths, or incubators in the laboratory. In a working laboratory, this must be done at least daily. If a thermometer is not built-in or permanently installed in the equipment, place one inside for 20 to 30 minutes, then record the temperature while the thermometer is still in place. Refrigerator thermometers can be stored with the bulb immersed in water or propylene glycol in a stoppered bottle to approximate the temperature of liquids in the refrigerator. If the temperature is not within acceptable range, make the necessary adjustment and remeasure or inform the supervisor or instructor.

Equipment I.D.	Range (° C)	Temperature Observed	Date	Comment/Signature
Freezer	−20 ± 5	_____	_____	_____
Refrigerator	6 ± 2	_____	_____	_____
Water bath	36 ± 1	_____	_____	_____
Incubator	36 ± 1	_____	_____	_____

B. Record the daily ambient temperature of the laboratory over a 1-week period. Does the temperature remain constant within a small range (±3 degrees)? Yes_____ No_____

Day 1 _____   Day 5 _____
Day 2 _____   Day 6 _____
Day 3 _____   Day 7 _____
Day 4 _____

II. Autoclave

During or after each run of the autoclave, check to see that the preset temperature and chamber pressure were reached. Each run should be given a number.

Autoclave: Run # _____ Temp ° C _____ Chamber pressure _____
Autoclave: Run # _____ Temp ° C _____ Chamber pressure _____

III. pH meter

Calibrate the pH meter before each use with two calibration solutions, one near the pH of the solution to be measured. (Commercial pH calibration solutions usually are pH 4.0, pH 7.0, and pH 10.0.) Check to see that the pH electrode is always stored in the appropriate solution when not in use.

Date	Calibration Solution	Comment/Signature
_____	_____	_____
_____	_____	_____
_____	_____	_____

© 2012 Delmar, Cengage Learning. Permission to reproduce for clinical use granted.

WORKSHEET

IV. Centrifuges

Use a stopwatch to check the timer on the centrifuge. If available, use a tachometer to check rpm. *Do not attempt to check the speed unless the centrifuge lid is closed and the lid has an opening in the center or a see-through cover.*

I.D.	Date	Timer Check	RPM Check	Comment/Signature
Serofuge	_____	_____	_____	_____
Microfuge	_____	_____	_____	_____
Clinical	_____	_____	_____	_____
Centrifuge	_____	_____	_____	_____

V. Balances

Check balances to see that they are clean and located on a stable counter in a draft-free site. If available, use standard weights (available from scientific equipment companies) to check the calibration of the balances, following the balance manufacturer's instructions.

Balance I.D.	Sensitivity Limit	Date Balance Checked	Comment/Signature
_____	_____	_____	_____
_____	_____	_____	_____

© 2012 Delmar, Cengage Learning. Permission to reproduce for clinical use granted.

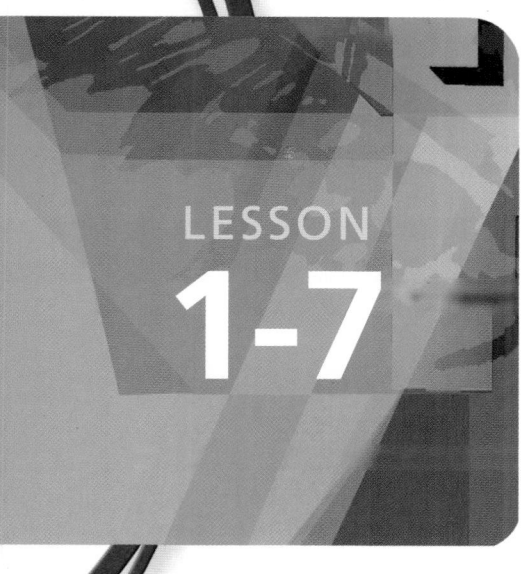

The Metric System

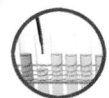

LESSON OBJECTIVES

After studying this lesson, the student will:

- ⊙ Discuss the importance of understanding metric units and using the metric system in the laboratory.
- ⊙ Name common prefixes used to denote small and large metric units.
- ⊙ Convert English units to metric units.
- ⊙ Convert metric units to English units.
- ⊙ Convert units within the metric system.
- ⊙ Perform measurements of distance, volume, and weight (mass) using the metric system.
- ⊙ Make temperature conversions between the Fahrenheit and Celsius scales.
- ⊙ Define the glossary terms.

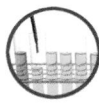

GLOSSARY

Celsius (C) scale / temperature scale having the freezing point of water at 0° C and the boiling point at 100° C

centi / prefix used to indicate one-hundredth (10^{-2}) of a unit

Clinical and Laboratory Standards Institute (CLSI) / an international institute composed of representatives from government, industry, and patient-testing professions that develops and publishes standards and guidelines for regulatory agencies and accrediting bodies; formerly National Committee for Clinical and Laboratory Standards (NCCLS)

deci / prefix used to indicate one-tenth (10^{-1}) of a unit

English system of measurement / system of measurement in common use in the United States for nonscientific measurements; sometimes called U.S. customary system

Fahrenheit (F) scale / temperature scale having a freezing point of water at 32° F and boiling point at 212° F

femto / prefix used to indicate 10^{-15}

gram (g) / basic metric unit of weight or mass

kilo / prefix used to indicate 1000 (10^{3}) units

liter (L) / basic metric unit of volume

meter (m) / basic metric unit of length or distance

metric system / the decimal system of measurement used internationally for scientific work

micro / prefix used to indicate one-millionth (10^{-6}) of a unit

milli / prefix used to indicate one-thousandth (10^{-3}) of a unit

nano / prefix used to indicate one-billionth (10^{-9}) of a unit

(continues)

National Institute of Standards and Technology (NIST) / a federal agency that promotes international standardization of measurements; formerly the National Bureau of Standards

pico / prefix used to indicate 10^{-12} of a unit

SI units / standardized units of measure; international units

INTRODUCTION

Units of measurements are used frequently in medicine. They are used to measure vital statistics such as height, weight, and body temperature; the amount of fluid intake and output; and dosages of medication. The clinical laboratory uses measurements in almost all aspects of its operations.

Measurements commonly made in the laboratory include:

- Concentration or numbers of substances or cells
- Weight of a substance or object
- Volume of a solution or object
- Size or length of an object
- Temperature
- Time

In the laboratory, time and temperature are most often used to monitor test conditions or procedures. Test results report measurements of concentration, number, weight, volume, and size when indicating numbers and types of cells or indicating quantities of substances in a patient's blood, serum, or other body fluids. These measurements are then compared to reference (normal) values to aid in assessing a patient's condition.

Measurements made in the clinical laboratory have a direct impact on the quality of patient care. Laboratory results can be a basis for establishing a diagnosis and are also used to follow the course of disease and prescribe appropriate treatment. The measurements must be reliable, accurate, precise, and easily standardized. For this reason, the metric system is used to make laboratory measurements. In this text the ⚛ icon will be used to emphasize that calculations or correct use of units is an important part of the procedure.

SYSTEMS OF MEASUREMENTS

In the United States, two systems of measurements are in common use, the *metric system* and the *English system of measurement,* sometimes called *U.S. customary system.*

English System of Measurement

In everyday life in the United States, the **English system of measurement** is still used for most measurements and observations. Weight is reported in pounds and height in feet and inches. Cooks use measures such as teaspoon, cup, and pint. Speed is measured in miles per hour. However, the English system of measurement is cumbersome and is not accurate enough for most scientific measurements.

The Metric System

The **metric system** of measurement has been used internationally for scientific work for decades. In most countries the metric system is also used in everyday life. Gasoline is purchased by the liter, body weight is measured in kilograms, and distance is expressed in meters or kilometers. Figure 1-44 compares a metric ruler showing centimeters and millimeters with an English style ruler, which shows measurements in inches and fractions of inches.

The metric system is based on a fundamental unit of distance, the **meter (m)**. In this system, the **gram (g)** is the basic unit used to measure mass or weight, and the **liter (L)** is the basic unit used to measure volume. Because the metric system is based on a decimal system, very small quantities can be measured accurately and easily. In the decimal system, units are divided into increments of 10. This means that units larger or smaller than the basic units (meter, liter, and gram) can be obtained by multiplying or dividing by increments of 10.

Although the metric system has been used internationally for laboratory measurements, the units used to report results can differ from country to country or even within countries and among institutions. For example, the concentration of protein can be expressed as grams per liter (g/L) in one laboratory and as grams per deciliter (g/dL) in another. This can be confusing when comparing data among laboratories.

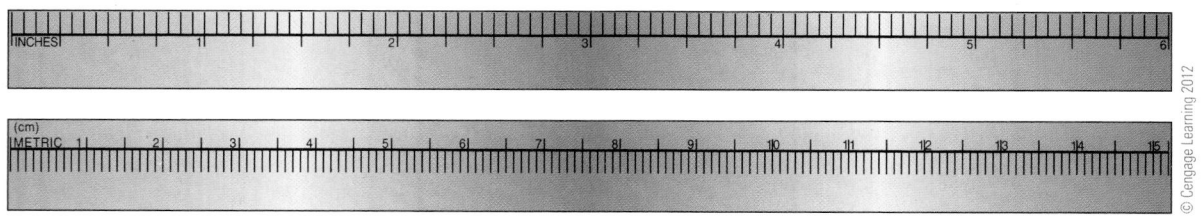

© Cengage Learning 2012

FIGURE 1-44 Comparison of nonmetric or English-style ruler (top) with metric ruler (bottom)

International System of Units (SI Units)

In an effort to standardize scientific measurements worldwide, most countries have adopted the use of **SI units**, from the *International System of Units*, the modern metric system of measurement. The United States adopted this system in 1991, mandating its use in all federal agencies and departments. The **National Institute of Standards and Technology (NIST)**, formerly known as the National Bureau of Standards, is the government agency responsible for assisting in this transition to the uniform use of SI units.

The International System of Units comes from the 200-year old French *Le Système International d'Unités* (hence the abbreviation SI). SI units are derived from the metric system and are based on seven fundamental units, from which commonly used units are derived (Table 1-25). These seven units have internationally agreed-upon values and were selected because they make possible more precise, reproducible measurements.

METRIC SYSTEM TERMINOLOGY

The SI units most commonly used in medicine are the liter (L), gram (g), meter (m), and mole (mol). By adding prefixes to these terms, one can indicate larger or smaller units (Table 1-26).

For example, **kilo** means 1000. Therefore, a *kilometer* (km) is 1000 meters or 10^3 meters, a *kilogram* (kg) is 1000 grams, and a *kiloliter* (kL) is 1000 liters. Although "kilo" is the prefix most commonly used for large units, "deca" can be used to indicate the unit times 10, as in decaliter. "Hecto" indicates the unit times 100. The prefixes and their definitions are the same for the three basic units.

In laboratory analyses, it is more common to measure units smaller than the basic units. Table 1-26 lists the prefixes and the multiples of the basic unit that each represents. Three common prefixes are **milli**, which means one-thousandth (0.001 or 10^{-3}); **centi**, which means one-hundredth (0.01 or 10^{-2}); and **deci**, which means one-tenth (0.1 or 10^{-1}). A *milliliter* is 0.001 liter, or 10^{-3} liter. In chemistry, solutions can be made by adding *milligrams* (mg) of substances to milliliters (mL) of solvent. Analytes can be measured in grams per deciliter (g/dL) or milligrams per deciliter (mg/dL). Cell counts can be reported as number of cells per microliter (μL) or per liter (L).

Other prefixes commonly used to denote size are **micro**, which denotes one-millionth or 10^{-6}; **nano**, which is 10^{-9}; **pico**, which is 10^{-12}; and **femto**, which is 10^{-15}. Small samples are measured in microliters (μL), which is 10^{-6} liter. Wavelengths of light are measured in nanometers (nm), or 10^{-9} meter.

TABLE 1-25. The seven basic SI units

PROPERTY	UNIT NAME	ABBREVIATION (SYMBOL)
Length	meter	m
Mass	kilogram	kg
Time	second	s
Electric current	ampere	A
Temperature	Kelvin	K
Luminous intensity	candela	cd
Quantity of substance	mole	mol

TABLE 1-26. Commonly used prefixes in the metric system

PREFIX	SYMBOL/ ABBREVIATION	MEANING	FACTOR (MULTIPLE OF BASIC UNIT)	WEIGHT, GRAM (G)	LENGTH, METER (M)	VOLUME, LITER (L)
giga	G		10^9			
mega	M		10^6			
kilo	k	1000	10^3	kg	km	kL
hecto	h	100	10^2	hg*	hm*	hL*
deca	da	10	10^1	dag*	dam*	daL*
deci	d	0.1	10^{-1}	dg*	dm*	dL
centi	c	0.01	10^{-2}	cg*	cm	cL*
milli	m	0.001	10^{-3}	mg	mm	mL
micro	μ	0.000001	10^{-6}	μg	μm	μL
nano	n		10^{-9}	ng	nm	nL*
pico	p		10^{-12}	pg	pm*	pL*
femto	f		10^{-15}			fL

* Units not commonly used in the laboratory

CONVERSION FACTORS

 It is sometimes necessary to convert units within the metric system or to convert English units to metric or metric units to English.

English to Metric Conversions

To make English to metric conversions, it is helpful to have a general idea of the metric equivalents of commonly used English measures. Some of these equivalents are listed in Tables 1-27 and 1-28. To convert units from one system to another, simply multiply by the factor listed. For example, because 1 inch is equal to 2.54 centimeters (cm), 12 inches would equal 12 × 2.54, or 30.48 cm (Table 1-27). To convert metric units to English units, use Table 1-28 in the same manner. Because 1 kg equals 2.2 pounds, the weight in pounds of a patient weighing 70 kg is determined by multiplying 70 × 2.2 to equal 154 pounds.

Converting Units Within the Metric System

In laboratory work, it is more common to need to convert units within the metric system. To make these conversions, the worker needs to know equivalents, such as how many milliliters or microliters are in a liter or how many milligrams are in a gram. These conversions can be made by using the information in Table 1-29.

Converting to Larger Units

To convert metric units to larger units, such as grams to kilograms or milliliters to liters, the decimal in the original unit is moved to the left for the appropriate number of spaces. For example, to

TABLE 1-27. Conversion of English units to metric units

	ENGLISH UNIT	ENGLISH ABBREVIATION	MULTIPLY BY	TO GET METRIC UNIT	METRIC ABBREVIATION
Distance	1 mile	mi	= 1.6	kilometers	km
	1 yard	yd	= 0.9	meters	m
	1 inch	in	= 2.54	centimeters	cm
Mass	1 pound	lb	= 0.454	kilograms	kg
	1 pound	lb	= 454	grams	g
	1 ounce	oz	= 28	grams	g
Volume	1 quart	qt	= 0.95	liters	L
	1 fluid ounce	fl oz	= 30	milliliters	mL
	1 teaspoon	tsp	= 5	milliliters	mL

TABLE 1-28. Conversion of metric units to English units

	METRIC UNIT	METRIC ABBREVIATION	MULTIPLY BY	TO FIND ENGLISH UNIT	ENGLISH ABBREVIATION
Distance	1 kilometer	km	= 0.6	miles	mi
	1 meter	m	= 3.3	feet	ft
	1 meter	m	= 39.37	inches	in
	1 centimeter	cm	= 0.4	inches	in
	1 millimeter	mm	= 0.04	inches	in
Mass	1 gram	g	= 0.0022	pounds	lb
	1 kilogram	kg	= 2.2	pounds	lb
Volume	1 liter	L	= 1.06	quarts	qt
	1 milliliter	mL	= 0.03	fluid ounces	fl oz

TABLE 1-29. Common metric equivalents

Mass	10^{-3} kg	= 1 g	= 10^3 mg	= 10^6 μg (mcg)
	10^{-3} g	= 1 mg	= 10^3 μg	= 10^6 ng
	10^{-9} g	= 1 ng	= 10^3 pg	
Volume	10^{-3} kL	= 1 L	= 10^3 mL	= 10^6 μL
	10^{-3} L	= 1 mL	= 10^3 μL	= 10^6 nL
	10^{-1} L	= 1 dL	= 10^2 mL	
Length	10^{-3} km	= 1 m	= 10^3 mm	= 10^6 μm
	10^{-3} m	= 1 mm	= 10^3 μm	= 10^6 nm
	10^{-2} m	= 1 cm	= 10 mm	= 10^4 μm
	10^{-3} mm	= 1 nm	= 10 Å	

TABLE 1-30. SI equivalents recommended for use in the clinical laboratory

OLD USAGE	SI EQUIVALENT
micron (μ)	micrometer (μm; 10^{-6} meter)
cubic micron (μ³)	femtoliter (fL; 10^{-15} liter)
micromicrogram (μμg)	picogram (pg; 10^{-12} gram)
microgram (mcg)	microgram (μg; 10^{-6} gram)
angstrom (Å)	nm × 10^{-1}
millimicron (mμ)	nanometer (nm; 10^{-9} meter)
lambda (λ)	microliter (μL; 10^{-6} liter)

TABLE 1-31. Examples of reporting laboratory test results using SI units

TEST	OLD UNIT	SI UNIT
Cell counts	cells/mm³ or cells/cu mm	cells/μL or cells/L
Hematocrit	%	percentage expressed as decimal
Hemoglobin	g/dL	g/L
MCV	μ³	fL
MCH	μμg	pg
MCHC	%	g/dL (or g/L)

convert 50 g to kg, multiply by 0.001, or move the decimal to the left three places: 50 g = 0.050 kg. To convert centimeters to meters, multiply by 0.01, or move the decimal two places to the left: 160 cm = 1.6 m.

Converting to Smaller Units

To convert metric units to smaller units, such as grams to milligrams or liters to microliters, the decimal in the number is moved to the right the appropriate number of spaces. For example, to convert 5.0 g to milligrams (mg), multiply by 1000, or move the decimal to the right three places: 5.0 g = 5000 mg. Scientific notation is often used to make numbers less bulky and easier to compute. For example, 5.0 g equals 5,000,000 μg which is 5.0×10^6 μg.

STANDARDIZED REPORTING OF LABORATORY RESULTS

The **Clinical and Laboratory Standards Institute (CLSI)** has published guidelines for uniform reporting of clinical laboratory results using SI units. (The address for CLSI is given in Appendix D.) By phasing out some previously used metric units and using SI units when reporting laboratory values, data are standardized regionally, nationally, and internationally. These older traditional units still appear in texts, manuals, and laboratory reports; therefore, it is important to understand the SI equivalents of these units. Tables 1-30 and 1-31 show SI equivalents for formerly used laboratory units.

The correct units of measurement must be included when reporting all laboratory results. This is especially important during the transition from using traditional units to using SI units. A number by itself is meaningless; it must be accompanied by the unit of measure. For example, the normal blood glucose range has traditionally been listed as 70 to 100 mg/dL. However, in SI units, glucose is reported as millimoles per liter (mmol/L), and glucose of 5.6 mmol/L is in the normal range. A glucose reported simply as 5.6 (omitting the mmol/L unit) would alarm someone accustomed to blood glucose measurements reported in milligrams per deciliter.

In other examples, blood cell counts have traditionally been expressed as the number of cells per cubic millimeter (cu mm) of blood. In the SI system, however, cell counts are expressed as number of cells per liter or microliter of blood. Chemical substances such as bilirubin or protein, which are expressed as milligrams per deciliter (dL) or per 100 mL, are recommended to be reported as milligrams or grams per liter or as micromoles (μmol) or millimoles (mmol) per liter.

TIME AND TEMPERATURE

  Units of time and temperature are not reported in metric or SI units. In everyday life the time is usually reported using a 12-hour clock (AM/PM). In laboratory reports, time is often recorded in military time (24-hour clock). Twelve-hour clock and equivalent 24-hour clock times are shown in Table 1-32.

Temperature is measured using either the **Fahrenheit (F) scale** or the **Celsius (C) scale** (Figure 1-45). The Fahrenheit temperature scale has a boiling point of 212° F and a freezing point of 32° F. In the United States, the Fahrenheit scale is used

TABLE 1-32. Twelve-hour clock times and equivalent 24-hour clock (military) times

TIME	24-HOUR TIME	TIME	24-HOUR TIME
12:30 AM	0030	12:30 PM	1230
1:30 AM	0130	1:30 PM	1330
2:30 AM	0230	2:30 PM	1430
3:30 AM	0330	3:30 PM	1530
4:30 AM	0430	4:30 PM	1630
5:30 AM	0530	5:30 PM	1730
6:30 AM	0630	6:30 PM	1830
7:30 AM	0730	7:30 PM	1930
8:30 AM	0830	8:30 PM	2030
9:30 AM	0930	9:30 PM	2130
10:30 AM	1030	10:30 PM	2230
11:30 AM	1130	11:30 PM	2330
Noon	1200	Midnight	2400

TABLE 1-33. Temperature conversion chart

°F =	°C	°F =	°C	°F =	°C
23	−5	101	38.3	115	46.1
32	0	102	38.9	116	46.7
70	21.1	103	39.4	117	47.2
75	23.9	104	40	118	47.8
80	26.7	105	40.6	119	48.3
85	29.4	106	41.1	120	48.9
90	32.2	107	41.7	125	51.7
95	35	108	42.2	130	54.4
96	35.6	109	42.8	135	57.2
97	36.1	110	43.3	140	60
98	36.7	111	43.9	150	65.6
98.6	37	112	44.4	212	100
99	37.2	113	45	230	110
100	37.8	114	45.6		

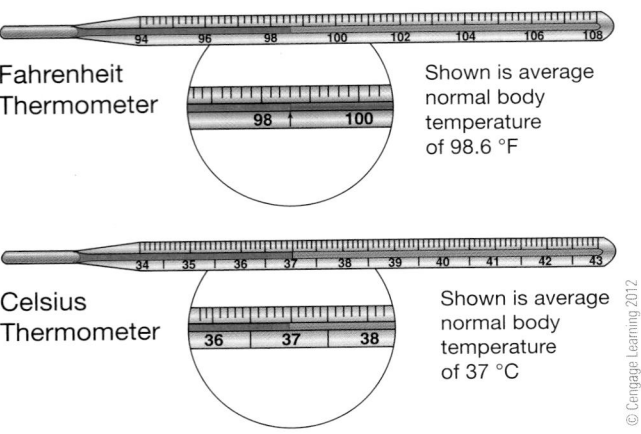

Fahrenheit Thermometer

Shown is average normal body temperature of 98.6 °F

Celsius Thermometer

Shown is average normal body temperature of 37 °C

© Cengage Learning 2012

FIGURE 1-45 Comparison of Fahrenheit (top) and Celsius (bottom) thermometers showing normal body temperature on each

for cooking, measuring body temperature, and reporting weather conditions. The Celsius scale has a boiling point of 100° C and a freezing point of 0° C. It is used for making most scientific temperature measurements such as temperatures of reactions, incubation, and boiling points. Most countries other than the United States use the Celsius scale in everyday life as well as for making scientific measurements.

It is sometimes necessary to convert temperatures from Fahrenheit to Celsius, or vice versa. Although many texts contain a temperature conversion chart such as the one in Table 1-33, this information is not always readily available. Formulas for temperature conversion and an example of using each are shown in Figure 1-46. Two common conversions are for body temperature (98.6° F to 37° C) and the freezing point of water (32° F to 0° C).

Problem A: Convert 98.6°F (normal body temperature) to Celsius (C) degrees.	**Problem B:** Convert 37°C to Fahrenheit (F) degrees.
Formula: $C = \dfrac{5}{9}\,(F - 32)$	Formula: $F = \dfrac{9}{5}\,(C) + 32$
Solution: $C = \dfrac{5}{9}\,(98.6 - 32)$	Solution: $F = \dfrac{9}{5}\,(37) + 32$
$C = \dfrac{5}{9}\,(66.6)$	$F = 66.6 + 32$
$C = 36.99$ or 37	$F = 98.6$
Answer: 98.6°F is equal to 37°C	Answer: 37°C is equal to 98.6°F

© Cengage Learning 2012

FIGURE 1-46 Examples of using formulas to convert Fahrenheit temperature to Celsius temperature (Problem A), and convert Celsius temperature to Fahrenheit temperature (Problem B)

PROBLEM 1

  Jeremy was the only person working the night shift in his town's hospital laboratory. As he prepared to perform a chemistry test, he noticed that the waterbath thermometer was missing. The reagent he needed was frozen, and the instructions were to thaw at 30° C to 32° C. He located a thermometer, but it was in Fahrenheit scale.

What Fahrenheit temperature range would be acceptable for thawing his reagent?

PROBLEM 2

  Shirley was on duty when laboratory test results were called in for Dr. Simpson's patient. The results, reported in SI units, were as follows: total protein, 70.0 g/L; hemoglobin, 150.0 g/L; and WBC count, 9.5×10^9/L. Shirley related the test results to Dr. Simpson, but he asked her to give him the results using the "old" units (total protein and hemoglobin in g/dL, and WBC count in cells/μL).

Convert the SI units.

Total protein 70.0 g/L = _____ g/dL
Hemoglobin 150.0 g/L = _____ g/dL
WBC count 9.5×10^9/L = _____ cells/μL

 ## SUMMARY

Although English units such as pound, gallon, and mile are used in everyday life in the United States, it is not possible to make small measurements with accuracy using these units. The metric system is used around the world in clinical laboratories because it enables precise, accurate measurements to be made, a requirement for quality laboratory results.

The metric system has been used for years in clinical laboratories, but the reporting methods were not standardized until recent years. Laboratories are transitioning from reporting results using traditional metric units, such as cubic millimeters (cu mm) or milligrams per deciliter (mg/dL), to using standardized SI units.

Laboratory results are used to help assess a patient's health status, establish a diagnosis, prescribe therapy, and monitor effects of therapy. Therefore, it is important that all measurements are made correctly and accurately. Laboratory personnel must know, understand, and be able to correctly use the metric system and SI units in making laboratory observations, measurements, and calculations.

 ## REVIEW QUESTIONS

1. What is the basic metric unit of distance or length?

2. What is the basic metric unit of volume?

3. What is the basic metric unit of weight?

4. What are the meanings of deca and hecto?

5. Why is the metric system preferred over the English system for scientific measurements?

6. Use the tables in this lesson to convert the following English measurements to metric units:

   3 inches = _____ cm or _____ mm

   5 qt = _____ L or _____ mL

   64 oz = _____ g or _____ kg or _____ mg

7. Convert the following units:

   12 mg = _____ μg or _____ g

   50 mL = _____ μL or _____ cc or _____ dL

8. Convert the following temperatures using the formulas in Figure 1-46:

    101° F = _____ °C

    25° C = _____ °F

9. Define Celsius (C) scale, centi, Clinical and Laboratory Standards Institute (CLSI), deci, English system of measurement, Fahrenheit (F) scale, femto, gram, kilo, liter, meter, metric system, micro, milli, nano, National Institute of Standards and Technology (NIST), pico, and SI units.

STUDENT ACTIVITIES

1. Complete the written examination for this lesson.

2. Practice measuring metric volumes, lengths, and weights and converting metric units using Worksheets I, II, and III.

3. Obtain a laboratory report form from a clinical laboratory in your area. Are reference ranges listed? Are SI units used?

WEB ACTIVITIES

1. Search the Internet for information on the International System of Units. Find information about using SI units in reporting laboratory results. Determine what units are used to report results of laboratory tests such as platelet counts, blood urea nitrogen, potassium, sodium, and bilirubin.

2. Use the Internet to locate lists of reference ranges for laboratory tests. Examine each list to determine what system of measurement is used to report results. Are SI units used?

3. Search the Internet for metric system tutorials, practice exercises, or self-tests and use these to enhance and test your knowledge.

LESSON 1-7
The Metric System

(Answers to question 7 can vary from student to student.)

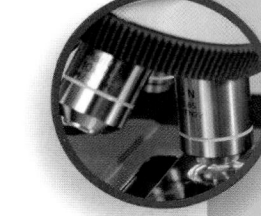

Name _____   **Date** _____

$\frac{n}{x}$ Obtain a meter stick or metric ruler and an English ruler from the instructor. Use the information in Tables 1-26 through 1-29 to answer the questions below.

1. Look at the meter stick. Locate the cm and mm divisions. How many centimeters are in a meter? _____ How many mm in a cm? _____ How many mm in a meter? _____

2. Draw the indicated length of line beside each number, beginning at the dot.
    35 mm   •
    6 cm   •

3. Measure the lines above (question 2) using a ruler marked in English units (inches):
    35 mm = _____ inches
    6 cm   = _____ inches
    Which of the measurements (English or metric) do you feel is the most accurate? _____

4. How many mm in 1 inch? _____   1 mm = _____ inch
    How many cm in 1 inch? _____   1 cm = _____ inch

    Convert the following units:
    4 inches   = _____ cm
    0.5 inches = _____ cm
    38 cm   = _____ inches
    7 cm   = _____ inches

5. How many inches are in a meter? _____

6. What English unit of measurement is closest in size to the meter? _____

7. Measure your height or the height of another student using the meter stick. What is the height in cm? _____ in meters? _____

    Convert the height in cm to inches: _____ Now measure the height in inches and compare the results.

© 2012 Delmar, Cengage Learning. Permission to reproduce for clinical use granted.

LESSON 1-7
The Metric System

(Answers to question 9 can vary from student to student.)

Name _____   Date _____

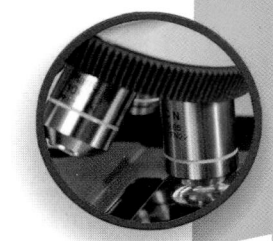

$\dfrac{n}{x}$ Use Tables 1-26 through 1-29 to answer the questions below.

1. What is the basic metric unit of weight? _____

2. How many mg in a g? _____ How many μg in a g? _____
    How many g in a kg? _____

3. Convert the following units:
    80 g   = _____ kg
    300 mg = _____ g   = _____ kg
    50 mg   = _____ g   = _____ kg
    4000 mg = _____ g   = _____ kg
    200 μg = _____ mg = _____ g
    750 μg = _____ mg
    What decimal rule did you follow to make the conversions? _____
    _____

4. Convert the following units:
    0.4 kg = _____ mg = _____ μg
    0.6 g   = _____ μg
    15 mg   = _____ μg = _____ pg
    280 mg = _____ μg = _____ ng
    What decimal rule did you follow to make the conversions? _____
    _____

5. A man who weighs 165 pounds would weigh _____ kg.

6. A child who weighs 32 pounds would weigh _____ kg or _____ g.

7. Is a man who is 178 cm tall and weighs 135 kg overweight, underweight, or of normal weight?
    _____

8. If a balance is available, weigh a container, add 10 mL of water, and weigh again. How much does
    the water weigh? _____
    Does 1 mL of water weigh approximately 1 g? Yes _____ No_____

9. Weigh yourself or another student. What is the weight in g? _____ in kg? _____

© 2012 Delmar, Cengage Learning. Permission to reproduce for clinical use granted

LESSON 1-7
The Metric System

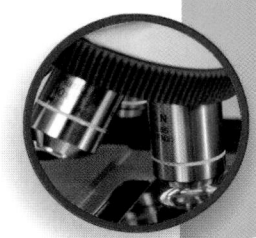

Name _____ Date _____

$\dfrac{n}{x}$ Obtain a medicine cup, a 50-mL graduated cylinder, and a 50-mL beaker from the instructor. Use Tables 1-26 through 1-29 to answer the questions below.

1. What is the basic unit of volume in the metric system? _____

2. How many milliliters in a liter? _____ How many deciliters in a liter? _____
   How many microliters in a liter? _____

3. Convert the following units:
   550 mL = _____ L
   4 dL   = _____ L
   60 mL   = _____ L = _____ dL
   0.1 dL   = _____ L
   6700 mL = _____ L
   What decimal rule did you follow to make the conversions? _____
   _____

4. Convert the following units:
   0.3 L = _____ dL = _____ mL
   5 L   = _____ mL
   3 dL   = _____ mL = _____ µL
   0.1 dL = _____ mL
   What decimal rule did you follow to make the conversions? _____
   _____

5. What English unit is closest in volume to the liter? _____

6. Convert the following English units:
   3.5 pints = _____ mL = _____ L
   3 quarts = _____ mL = _____ L
   5 fl. oz. = _____ mL = _____ L

7. If gasoline is $2.20 per gallon at station A and 60 cents per liter at station B, which has the cheapest gasoline? _____

8. Fill the medicine cup to the 1 fl oz mark with water. Then transfer the water to a 50-mL graduated cylinder. How many milliliters of water are in 1 fl oz? _____

   Fill the medicine cup again with 1 fl oz of water and transfer to a 50-mL beaker. Which gives the most accurate measurement, the beaker or the graduated cylinder? _____

© 2012 Delmar, Cengage Learning. Permission to reproduce for clinical use granted.

WORKSHEET III — VOLUME

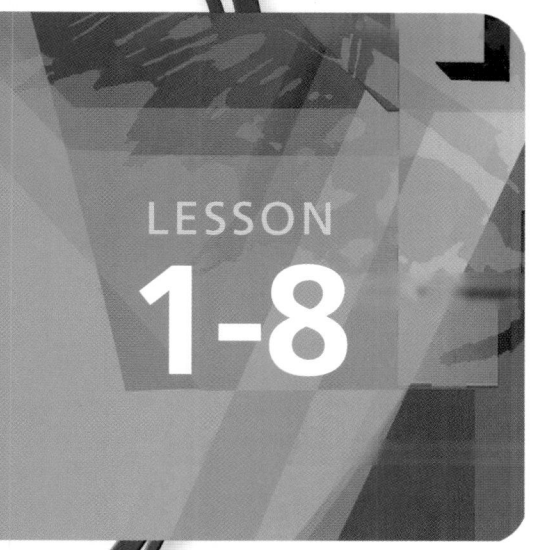

LESSON 1-8

Laboratory Math and Reagent Preparation

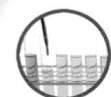

LESSON OBJECTIVES

After studying this lesson, the student will:

⊙ Identify volumetric and graduated pipets and explain the correct use of each.

⊙ Measure and transfer liquids using pipets and micropipetters.

⊙ Discuss the use of pipets in the preparation of reagents.

⊙ Describe the differences between pipets and micropipets.

⊙ Explain how distilled water and deionized water are made.

⊙ List the types of water used in the laboratory and discuss their correct uses.

⊙ Prepare percent solutions.

⊙ Prepare a reagent using ratio or proportions.

⊙ Prepare dilutions of a reagent.

⊙ State the formula for preparing a dilute solution from a concentrated solution.

⊙ Prepare molar (mol/L) solutions.

⊙ Explain the difference between molar and normal solutions.

⊙ Perform serial and compound dilutions.

⊙ Discuss safety precautions that must be observed when pipetting and when preparing laboratory reagents.

⊙ Explain the quality assessment procedures that should be used to ensure high-quality laboratory reagents.

⊙ Define the glossary terms.

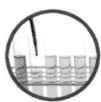

GLOSSARY

Beral pipet / a disposable plastic pipet with a built-in bulb on one end that usually can deliver up to 2 mL and can have a graduated stem; also called a transfer pipet

deionized water / water that has had most of the mineral ions removed

diluent / a liquid added to a solution to make it less concentrated

dilution / a solution made less concentrated by adding a diluent; the act of making a dilute solution; the degree to which a solution is made less concentrated

dilution factor / reciprocal of the dilution

distilled water / the condensate collected from steam after water has been boiled

(continues)

formula weight (F.W.) / the sum of the atomic weights of the atoms in a compound; molecular weight

gram equivalent weight / the number obtained by dividing the formula weight by the valence

lyophilize(d) / remove water from a frozen solution under vacuum; freeze-dry

micropipet / a pipet that measures or holds 1 milliliter or less

micropipetter / a mechanical pipetter that can measure or deliver very small volumes, usually 1 mL or less

molar solution (M) / solution containing 1 mole of solute per liter of solution

mole / formula weight of a substance expressed in grams

molecular weight (M.W.) / the sum of the atomic weights of the atoms in a molecule or compound; formula weight

normality (N) / the number of gram equivalents of a compound per liter of solution

percent solution / a solution made by adding units of solute per 100 units of total solution

physiological saline / 0.85% (0.15 M) sodium chloride solution

pipet / a slender calibrated tube used for measuring and transferring liquids

proportion / relationship in number or amount of one portion compared to another portion or to the whole; ratio

ratio / relationship in number or degree between two things

reagent / substance or solution used in laboratory analyses; substance involved in a chemical reaction

reverse osmosis / purification of water by forcing water under high pressure through a semi-permeable membrane

solute / the substance dissolved in a given solution

solution / a homogeneous mixture of two or more substances

solvent / a dissolving agent, usually a liquid

TC / on pipets, a mark indicating *to contain*

TD / on pipets, a mark indicating *to deliver*

titer / in serology, the reciprocal of the highest dilution that gives the desired reaction; the concentration
      of a substance determined by titration

valence / the positive or negative charge of a molecule; a number representing the combining power of an atom

INTRODUCTION

Reagents are chemical solutions or substances used in laboratory analyses. Most clinical laboratory reagents are purchased in the required concentrations; however, there can be times when reagents or solutions must be prepared in the laboratory. To do this correctly, it is necessary to have knowledge of some basic chemistry terms and simple math. Moreover, knowing how to perform these mathematical operations allows the laboratory scientist to recognize when a certain instrument, such as a micropipetter, is not working correctly.

Most laboratory reagents are **solutions**, homogeneous mixtures of two or more substances. Solutions are made by combining a **solute**, the substance being dissolved, with a **solvent**, a dissolving agent. Water is the most familiar and widely used solvent. Laboratory procedures can require dilution of a reagent or a serum. A **dilution** is a solution that is made less concentrated by adding a solvent.

Math is involved in the preparation of laboratory solutions. Each laboratory's standard operating procedure (SOP) manual should contain instructions for preparing commonly-used reagents. However, there are also situations in which the technologist must determine how to prepare a specific solution and directions are not given. In these situations, simple formulas and calculations are used. The calculations for making most reagents are not difficult but can require step-by-step

clarification at first. It is important that reagents be made accurately because they can directly influence test results and personnel safety.

This lesson introduces methods of preparing solutions using ratio and proportions, dilution, percent, moles/liter, and normality. Information on types of pipets, pipetting techniques, and types of reagent water is also presented. The icon $\frac{n}{x}$ is used in this text to indicate that an activity or procedure requires math skills.

COMMON LABORATORY REAGENTS

Several common laboratory solutions, such as surface disinfectants and dilute acids, are easily prepared by making simple dilutions. *Stock* (concentrated) solutions can be diluted to a *working* concentration. Some tests require that serial dilutions of serum be tested. Percent solutions or molar solutions of saline can be made.

Lyophilized controls and standards are reagents with the liquid removed. These are rehydrated by adding the diluting fluid recommended by the manufacturer. Examples of lyophilized reagents include chemistry standards and controls, positive and negative serum and plasma immunology controls, and urine chemistry controls.

CHEMICAL PURITY

Several levels or grades of chemical purity are available for use in the laboratory. The American Chemical Society (ACS) has set specifications for *reagent* or *analytical reagent* grade chemicals. Chemicals in these two grades are suitable for both quantitative and qualitative work. An ultrapure grade is required for analytical methods that require even greater purity; this grade can be described by terms such as "spectrograde," "nanograde," and "HPLC pure." Lower grades of chemicals labeled "purified," "practical," "technical," or "commercial" should never be used in clinical laboratory reagents but can be used for non-clinical purposes.

TYPES OF LABORATORY REAGENT WATER

Several grades of water are used in the laboratory. The Clinical and Laboratory Standards Institute (CLSI) has established specifications for Clinical Laboratory Reagent Water (CLRW). Formerly, the College of American Pathologists (CAP) and CLSI had established three levels of water purity: type I, type II, and type III, with type I being the most pure. All three of these types were made from deionized, distilled, or reverse osmosis water. However, in 2010 and 2011 CLSI issued new guidelines for clinical laboratory water purity; these guidelines also specify the types of tests required to guarantee the purity of each water grade (Table 1-34).

In the former classification scheme, only type I water could be designated Clinical Laboratory Reagent Water (CLRW). In the new regulations CLRW can be used in any task that previously called for types I and II waters. The grades of purified water for use in the clinical laboratory in the 2011 guidelines are:

- Clinical Laboratory Reagent Water
- Special Reagent Water
- Instrument Feed Water
- Water supplied by a method manufacturer
- Autoclave and wash water
- Commercially bottled purified water

Each grade of reagent water has a role in the laboratory. The grade of water used depends on the task and will be specified in the SOP manual. The goal of all laboratories is to produce accurate results, and water purity plays a large part in attaining this goal.

Distilled, Deionized, and Reverse Osmosis Water

All grades of water begin as distilled, deionized, or reverse osmosis water. **Distilled water** is the condensate collected from steam created when water is boiled. This process removes most of the common minerals such as iron, calcium, and magnesium but does not remove volatiles such as carbon dioxide, chlorine, and ammonia.

Deionized water is prepared by passing tap or distilled water through a resin column containing charged particles. The unwanted impurities in the water bind to these charged particles and are removed from the water. However, not all organic substances, particulate matter, or microorganisms are removed.

Reverse osmosis (RO), a process that forces water through a semi-permeable membrane, can also be used as an initial water purification step. RO removes nearly all bacteria, colloidal silica, particulates, organics, and a large percentage of ionic contaminants from water. However, water that passes through the RO membrane still contains small amounts of contaminants and will not meet CLSI/CAP specifications for CLRW, special reagent water, or instrument feed water unless treated further.

Clinical Laboratory Reagent Water (CLRW)

To make CLRW from RO water, the RO water is passed through a high-quality resin to remove remaining ions and through a small-pore filter (0.22 µm) to exclude any remaining bacteria from the water. CLRW can also be obtained by processing deionized water using membrane filters to remove microorganisms and insoluble matter and charcoal absorption to remove organic matter. Distilled water must be passed over resin and then be membrane-filtered to become CLRW.

CLRW is the purest grade and is used to prepare standards, control solutions, and buffers for analytical procedures. Many of the standards and controls used in the laboratory are lyophilized (freeze-dried) material. CLRW is used to

---

TABLE 1-34. Specifications for purity of laboratory water

PARAMETER	TEST/CHARACTERISTIC	SPECIFICATION
Resistivity	Lack of conductivity of electricity	$\geq$10 MΩ/cm at 25° C
Microbiological content	Colony-forming units (CFU) per mL	$\leq$10 CFU/mL
Particulate matter	Contaminants	Pass through 0.2-µm filter
Organics (TOC)	Organic molecules	Pass over activated charcoal resin
Silicate* mg SIO$_2$/L	Contaminants from glass	$\leq$0.05 mg/L

* Has been removed from some regulations

reconstitute (bring into solution) these materials because it does not contain substances that can interfere with the analysis being performed. CLRW and Special Reagent Water are used for special analyses such as trace metals, electrolytes, and enzymes. CLRW should not be stored, but should be prepared just before use to prevent the absorption of gases such as carbon dioxide.

Instrument Feed Water

Instrument feed water was formerly called type II. It can be used for procedures in which the presence of small numbers of bacteria ($\leq$100 per liter) will not affect results. It can be used to make reagents for most procedures in hematology, immunology, and qualitative chemistry. It can be used in microbiology if it is *sterilized*.

Autoclave and Wash Water

This grade of water was formerly called type III; it can be used for some laboratory analyses such as routine urinalysis. The major use is for washing and rinsing glassware and for water used to make steam in the autoclave. Tap water can be used for initial washing of labware, but is never used for final rinsing of labware or preparing laboratory reagents. Only CLRW or Instrument Feed Water (old type I or type II) should be used as the final rinse for glassware.

Purity grades of Instrument Feed Water (formerly type II) and Autoclave and Wash water (formerly type III) can be stored in tightly capped borosilicate glass or polyethylene containers. Analyses performed by high performance liquid chromatography (HPLC) require ultrapure water that can be prepared by passing CLRW or Special Reagent Water through a final 0.1-μm membrane.

Water Testing Requirements

Laboratory waters must be tested a minimum of once per week. The characteristics tested include resistivity, total organic carbon (TOC), plate counts and particulate contamination (Table 1-34). Resistivity refers to the resistance caused by lack of ions in the water. TOC indicates the amount of organic contamination. Viable plate counts (bacterial colony counts) indicate level of bacterial contamination. Two additional tests, epi-fluorescence and endotoxin testing, are recommended to replace bacterial plate counts. The epi-fluorescence and endotoxin tests give more rapid results than the bacterial culture tests, which can take several days.

PIPETS

Pipets are open-ended glass or plastic tubes used to measure and transfer precise volumes of a liquid. It is important to know the different types of pipets, select the appropriate pipet for the task, and use each type correctly. Pipets are manufactured to strict specifications and calibrated to transfer or deliver specified volumes, which are marked on the pipets (Figure 1-47). Many types and sizes of pipets are used in laboratory work. Pipets can range in capacity from 1.0 mL to 50 mL; volumes of 1.0 ml or less are usually delivered by **micropipet** and **micropipetters**. One important advantage of micropipetters is the plastic, disposable tips that eliminate the possibility of cross-contamination (Figure 1-48).

Plastic pipets can be open-ended like glass pipets or can have a built-in bulb. The bulb type, shown at far left of Figure 1-48, is called a transfer pipet or **Beral pipet**. Transfer pipets are cheap, disposable, and very useful in the laboratory for delivering a few drops of a reagent or transferring small amounts of liquid when the volume does not need to be measured.

Pipets are filled by suction with the aid of mechanical pipet-aids, bulb-type pipet-aids (Figure 1-49A), or handheld electric or battery-powered pipet filler-dispensers (Figure 1-49B). The "mouth" or wide end of the pipet is fitted into the pipet-aid or pipet filler held in the operator's hand. Trigger-type buttons activate a pump that controls aspirating and dispensing by the pipet filler-dispenser. These devices are easy to use and can be used with pipets of various sizes and volumes. No matter which type of pipet is used, it is *never* permissible to mouth-pipet.

Pipets can be categorized according to their design and accuracy as:

- *Volumetric* pipets or
- *Serological* or *graduated* pipets

To Deliver (TD) Pipets

Pipets are also marked to indicate how they are to be used to deliver liquids. A *to deliver* pipet is marked with the letters **TD** near the top of the pipet (Figure 1-47A). This means that the pipet is calibrated to deliver the volume marked on the pipet in a specified time and at a specified temperature when the pipet is emptied by gravity drainage (Figure 1-47). When used correctly,

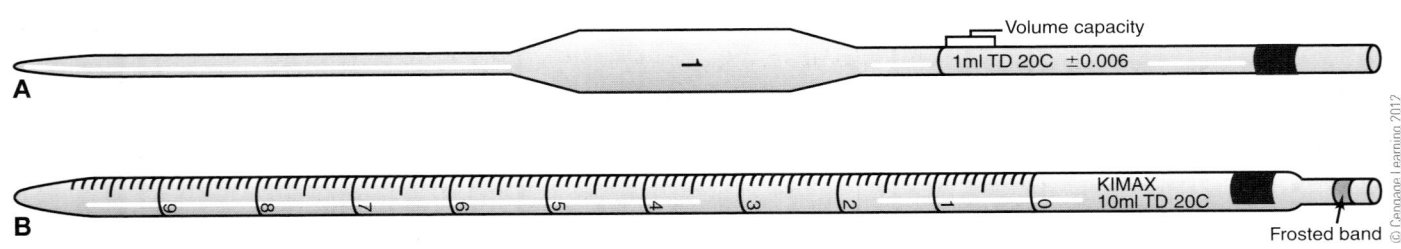

FIGURE 1-47 Pipets: (A) volumetric pipet; (B) serological pipet. Both pipets are TD and bottom pipet is blowout type (frosted band)

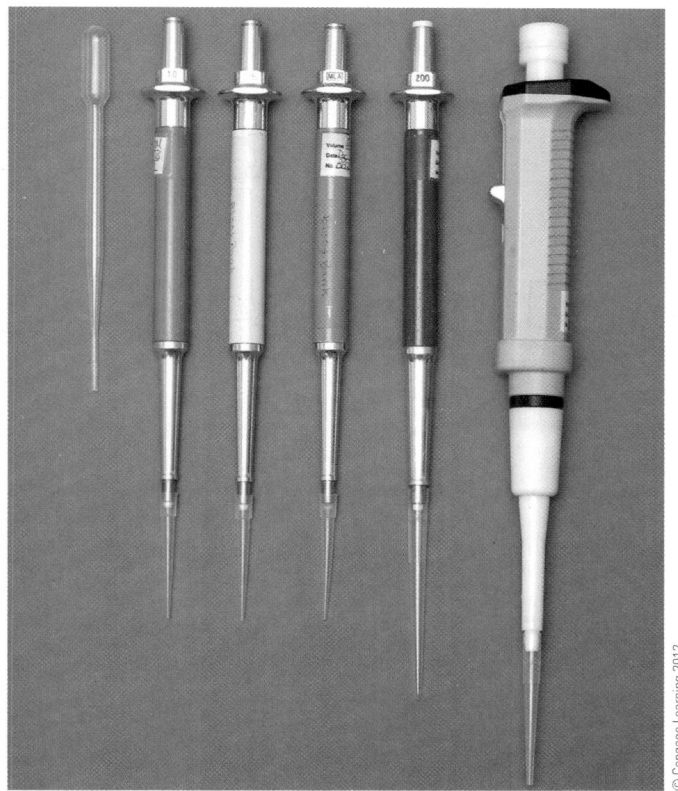

FIGURE 1-48 Micropipetters with disposable tips and disposable transfer (Beral) pipet on far left

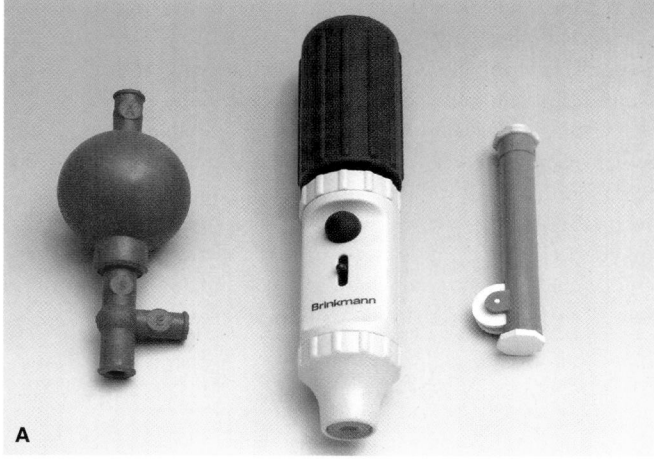

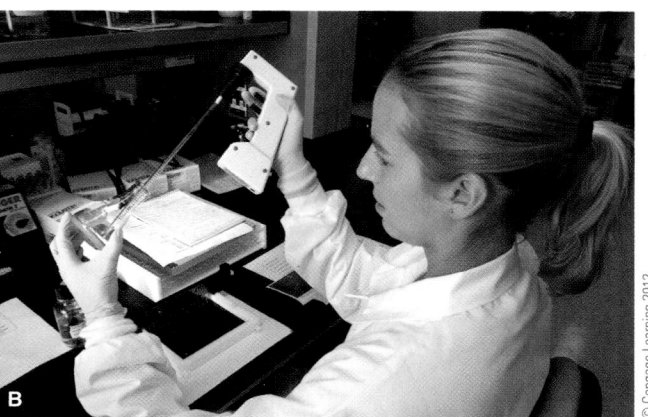

FIGURE 1-49 Pipet aids: (A) three types of manual pipetting aids; (B) using a battery-operated pipet filler-dispenser to transfer a liquid

the TD pipet delivers the specified volume of fluid, leaving a small drop of fluid in the pipet tip.

A TD pipet with a frosted band etched around the top of the pipet is called a *blowout* pipet (Figure 1-47B). To correctly deliver the stated volume using a blowout pipet, the last drop remaining in the tip must be expelled or "blown out" using a pipet-aid or pipet filler-dispenser.

To Contain (TC) Pipets

A *to contain* pipet has the letters **TC** near the top of the pipet, indicating that the pipet is calibrated to contain the volume marked on the pipet. Because liquid will cling to the inner walls of the pipet, the pipet must be rinsed to be sure the stated volume is delivered. Most micropipetters are used in the same manner as TC pipets.

Volumetric Pipets

Volumetric pipets have a wide opening on the suctioning end, an oval bulb in the center, and a tapered tip on the dispensing end (Figure 1-47A). Volumetric pipets are usually labeled TD and are used when critical measurements are required, such as when preparing standards. Each volumetric pipet is marked and calibrated to deliver only one volume.

Volumetric pipets are used by attaching a suctioning aid or pipet filler to the top of the pipet (Figure 1-49). The liquid is suctioned into the pipet to slightly above the etched line. The liquid level is carefully lowered until the meniscus is even with the etched line. The outside of the pipet tip is wiped with tissue, using care that the tissue does not contact fluid inside the tip. The pipet is held nearly vertical, and the tip is placed against the inner wall of the container into which the liquid is to be transferred. Suction is released and the liquid is allowed to flow into the container. The tip is left in contact with the container wall a few seconds to completely drain the pipet. A small drop will remain in the pipet tip.

Serological or Graduated Pipets

Serological or graduated or pipets have a total capacity marking near the suction end and are usually labeled TD. Serological pipets are graduated to the tip, with markings indicating uniform increments. These pipets can be used to transfer total capacity or partial volume. The pipets are usually marked TD and have a frosted band (Figure 1-47B). Graduated pipets with a frosted band around the top of the pipet are used by forcing out the last drop of liquid after the contents are drained.

To use a TD serological pipet with a frosted band, a suctioning device is attached. The liquid is suctioned up to just above the desired mark and then the level is lowered to the desired volume mark as with the volumetric pipet. The pipet tip is wiped dry with tissue. To deliver the total volume from the pipet, the liquid is allowed to drain out while the pipet is held almost vertically. The last remaining drops are forced out using the pipetting aid. Fluid is dispensed more accurately when it is dispensed between two marks on the pipet, rather than dispensing the entire contents in the tip. To illustrate, if 3 mL is to be delivered from a 5-mL pipet, fluid delivery will be more accurate if fluid is drawn up to the zero (0) mark and dispensed down to the 3-mL mark than if drawn up to the 2-mL mark and then all of the liquid dispensed.

Micropipets and Micropipetters

Measuring and transferring very small volumes (microliter range) requires the use of precisely manufactured pipets or pipetting systems and careful technique. Capillary micropipets are calibrated glass capillary tubes that deliver volumes as small as 5 µL. Examples of these are the small glass capillaries used to make blood dilutions for manual blood cell counts. Most capillary micropipets are TC types, meaning that the contents of the capillary are rinsed in the diluting fluid.

Micropipetters are mechanical pipets manufactured by several companies in various designs (Figure 1-48). Micropipetters are used to perform most manual pipetting tasks in the clinical laboratory. A single-use disposable plastic tip is used for each sampling. The volume is aspirated or delivered when the operator depresses and releases a plunger on the micropipetter. Most micropipets are used in the manner of TC pipets. Once the volume is delivered with the micropipet, the pipet tip is rinsed a standard number of times in the receiving liquid by gently depressing and releasing the plunger.

The instructions accompanying each type of micropipette must be followed for pipetting accuracy and precision; correct use can differ slightly depending on pipet design. Micropipetters must be calibrated at regular intervals to ensure accurate volume delivery. Some micropipetters are preset to deliver just one volume while others are adjustable within a narrow range, such as 1 to 20 µL or 20 to 100 µL. The use of micropipetters provides better accuracy than manual pipetting and eliminates the need for pipet-aids or safety bulbs. Many laboratory analyzers aspirate and dispense samples automatically, which eliminates errors resulting from variation in pipetting techniques among workers.

SAFETY PRECAUTIONS

 The preparation of laboratory reagents can be associated with potential chemical, physical, and biological hazards. The chemical container label and material safety data sheet (MSDS) must be consulted before using a chemical and the recommended personal protective equipment (PPE) and work practice controls must be used. Chemicals that produce fumes must be used only in a fume hood. (Chemical safety is discussed in detail in Lesson 1-5.) The use of plastic labware eliminates the possibility of injury from broken or chipped glass.

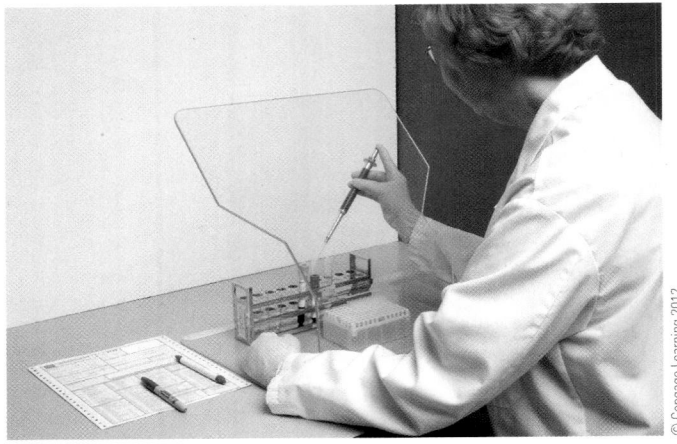

FIGURE 1-50 Using a micropipetter behind an acrylic safety shield

Standard Precautions must always be observed when pipetting patient specimens and other biological materials. Pipet-aids or pipet filler-dispensers must be used when measuring and dispensing liquids using pipets, and work can be performed using an acrylic splash shield (Figure 1-50). Mouth pipetting must *never* be done.

QUALITY ASSESSMENT

 Reagents should be prepared using chemically clean, dry, nonreactive containers. The measuring container must be appropriate for the task. The correct formulas and calculations for preparing various types of reagents must be used. Markings on beakers and Erlenmeyer flasks are only approximate; therefore, only certified glassware such as volumetric flasks must be used for critical measurements. The correct grade of reagent water must be selected for the reagent being prepared.

Correct pipetting techniques must be used to measure and transfer liquids. Pipetting errors made in the preparation of a reagent can affect all analyses in which the reagent is used.

The pipet used should be appropriate for the task; volumetric pipets should be used when making critical measurements, such as preparing standards and controls. Micropipetters must be calibrated at set intervals that will be specified in the SOP manual.

Standards and controls are usually stored refrigerated; other reagents might be stored at room temperature. Before using any laboratory reagent, the reagent should be inspected for signs of deterioration, such as color change, precipitation, or turbidity. Laboratory reagents have a limited shelf life and should not be used beyond the expiration date. Fresh reagents should be made before the existing reagent runs out or reaches the expiration date. Many procedures require that the new reagent be tested along with the one already in use to be sure equivalent results are obtained.

PREPARING LABORATORY SOLUTIONS

 There are several methods of preparing laboratory solutions, including dilutions, ratios, percent solutions, and molar solutions. When preparing any solution, the technician must follow all safety rules and quality assessment guidelines.

Using Proportion to Make Dilutions

Dilutions are often required in laboratory procedures. A dilution is usually expressed as a ratio, **proportion**, or fraction. For example, if a serum has been diluted 1:5, it means that 1 part of the serum has been combined with 4 parts of a **diluent** to create 5 total parts. A simple formula for calculating dilutions is:

$$\frac{(A)}{(A) + (B)} = C$$

where   A = parts or volume of substance being diluted
          B = parts or volume of diluent added, and
          C = the dilution, expressed as a fraction
          (A and B must be in the same units of volume)

An example of using proportion to prepare a reagent is shown in Figure 1-51A.

Preparing a Dilute Solution from a Concentrated Solution

Sometimes it is necessary to prepare a dilute solution from a concentrated solution. For instance, 0.1 M HCl can be made from a concentrated solution of HCl, such as a 1 M solution (Figure 1-51B). The general formula is:

$$C_1 \times V_1 = C_2 \times V_2$$

or

$$V_1 = \frac{C_2 \times V_2}{C_1}$$

where C_1 = concentration of the solution of greater
                concentration
          V_1 = volume required of the solution of greater
                concentration
          C_2 = concentration of final (dilute) solution
          V_2 = volume of final (dilute) solution

Solve for V_1, volume of concentrated solution needed to prepare the dilute solution.

Using Ratios to Prepare Dilutions

A **ratio** is the relationship in number or degree between two things. Dilutions, which are ratios, express the relationship between a part of a solution and the total solution. Dilutions are used frequently in the laboratory, especially in hematology and immunology.

Problem A:	A buffer is made by adding 2 parts of "solution A" to 5 parts of "solution B." How much of solution A and solution B would be required to make 70 mL of the buffer?
Formula:	$\dfrac{\text{Total volume required (C)}}{\text{parts of "A" + parts of "B"}}$ = volume of one part (V)
Solution:	$\dfrac{70 \text{ mL required}}{2 \text{ parts "A" + 5 parts "B"}}$ = volume of one part $\dfrac{70}{7}$ = 10 mL = volume of one part (V) 2 parts of solution "A" = 2 × 10 = 20 mL 5 parts of solution "B" = 5 × 10 = 50 mL
Answer:	The buffer would be made by mixing 20 mL of solution A with 50 mL of solution B to give a total volume of 70 mL.

Problem B:	Prepare 100 mL of 0.1 M HCl using 1 M HCl.
Formula:	$C_1 \times V_1 = C_2 \times V_2$
Solution:	(1 M) (V_1) = (100 mL) (0.1 M) $V_1 = \dfrac{100 \text{ mL} \times 0.1}{1}$ $V_1 = 10$ mL
Answer:	10 mL of 1M HCl is added to 90 mL of H_2O to make 100 mL of 0.1 M HCl solution.

© Cengage Learning 2012

FIGURE 1-51 Prepare dilute solutions from concentrated solutions: (Problem A) preparing a solution using proportion; (Problem B) using the formula $C_1 \times V_1 = C_2 \times V_2$ to prepare a solution

One procedure for performing the white blood cell (WBC) count requires that a 1-to-100 (1:100) dilution of the blood sample be made. This is accomplished by adding 0.02 mL (20 µL) blood to 1.98 mL diluent. The total volume is equal to 2.0 mL and represents a 1:100 dilution. Likewise, if a 2 M solution is diluted 1:5, the dilution factor is 5, and the concentration of the dilution is 0.4 M.

$$\frac{2\ M}{5} = 0.4\ M$$

The general rule for calculating the concentration of a diluted solution is to *divide* the concentration of the original solution by the **dilution factor**, which is the reciprocal of the dilution. A reciprocal is one of a pair of numbers that has a product equaling 1. For instance, 100 is the reciprocal of 1/100, and conversely 1/100 is the reciprocal of 100.

This rule can also be used to find the original concentration of a diluted solution. For example: the albumin concentration of a 1:10 serum dilution was measured as 4 g/L. By *multiplying* the concentration by the dilution factor, the albumin concentration of the original sample is found to be 40 g/L:

$$4g/L \times 10 = 40\ g/L$$

Preparing Percent Solutions

One type of expression of concentration is the **percent solution**. A percent solution refers to the weight of solute per 100 weight units or volume units of solution. Percent refers to parts per 100 parts. A penny is 1% of a dollar—one part (cent) per 100 parts (cents). A nickel is 5% of a dollar—5 cents per 100 cents.

In the laboratory, percent solutions usually refer to grams of solute per 100 mL of solution. This is because the solvent used most frequently in the laboratory is water and 1 mL of water weighs approximately 1 gram. So a 1% solution would contain 1 g of solute per 100 mL (or 100 g) of solution. Three ways to prepare percent solutions are weight to volume (w/v), volume to volume (v/v), and weight to weight (w/w).

Weight/Volume (w/v) Solutions

Percent solutions can be made by dissolving a specific weight of a solute (chemical) in 100 mL of solution (water or other liquid). This is called a *weight-to-volume (w/v) solution*.

One example is the 0.85% **physiological saline** solution used in many serological and bacteriological procedures. Using the definition of a percent solution, 100 mL of 0.85% saline contains 0.85 g of sodium chloride (NaCl) in 100 mL of solution. This would be prepared by placing approximately 50 mL of CLRW into a 100-mL volumetric flask, adding 0.85 g NaCl, mixing thoroughly until the NaCl dissolves, and then adding CLRW to the flask's fill line. In a similar fashion, 500 mL of 0.85% saline could be prepared as shown in Figure 1-52A.

Volume/Volume (v/v) Solutions

Another type of percent solution is called a *volume-to-volume (v/v) solution*, in which a certain volume of one liquid is added to a specific volume of another. One hundred milliliters (mL) of a 10% solution of bleach can be prepared by adding 10 mL of chlorine bleach (sodium hypochlorite) to 90 mL of water, for a total volume of 100 mL. Figure 1-52B shows how 500 mL of a v/v solution would be prepared.

Weight/Weight (w/w) Solutions

A percent solution can also be prepared by weighing both the solute and the solvent. For these types of solutions, the laboratory balance must be zeroed (tared) with the empty container on the

Problem A:	Prepare 500 mL of 0.85% (w/v) saline.

Solution:	1. A 0.85% (w/v) solution contains 0.85 g of the solute in every 100 mL of solution.
	2. To prepare 500 mL, 5 × 0.85 g, or 4.25 g, of sodium chloride (NaCl) must be used.
	3. To prepare the solution:
	   a. Weigh out 4.25 g of NaCl.
	   b. Fill a 500 mL volumetric flask approximately half full with water.
	   c. Add 4.25 g of NaCl and swirl gently to dissolve.
	   d. Add water to the flask's fill line.

Problem B:	Prepare 500 mL of 10% (v/v) bleach solution.

Solution:	1. A 10% (v/v) solution of bleach contains 10 mL bleach (hypochlorite) per 100 mL of solution.
	2. 500 mL of solution would contain 50 mL of bleach (5 × 10 mL).
	3. To prepare the solution:
	   a. Measure 450 mL of water and place into a flask or bottle.
	   b. Add 50 mL of bleach and mix.

© Cengage Learning 2012

FIGURE 1-52 Preparing percent solutions: (Problem A) weight-to-volume (w/v) percent solution; (Problem B) volume-to-volume (v/v) percent solution

balance pan. The solution volume is determined by its weight. For example, a 5% solution would require that approximately 90 g of water be added to the empty container (with the scale set to zero). Five grams of a chemical would then be added to the container. With the container still on the balance, water is added until the total solution weight is 100 g. This type of percent solution is rarely used in the clinical laboratory.

Preparing Molar Solutions

Concentrations of chemical solutions are expressed as moles per liter (mol/L), which is replacing the older term molarity. A solution containing 1 mole of a substance per liter is a **1 molar solution**. A **mole** of a pure compound is the **formula weight (F.W.)** or **molecular weight (M.W.)** of that compound expressed in grams. For instance, NaCl is composed of sodium atoms and chloride atoms. Sodium has a weight of 23 and chloride has a weight of 35.4, making the formula weight of NaCl 58.4. A moles per liter (mol/L) solution is made by adding the required weight of chemical to enough solvent to make a total volume of one liter. *Note that 1 liter is not added to the solute; instead the volume is brought up to 1 liter after the solute is dissolved.*

A formula for calculating mol/L of a solution is:

$$\frac{Grams(g)}{1\ liter} \times \frac{1\ mole}{F.W.(g)} = \frac{moles}{L} = M$$

Simplified, to calculate the number of moles, divide the weight of chemical in a solution (the solute) by the formula weight of the chemical. For example: 1 liter of a solution contains 60 g of NaOH (formula weight 40). Determine the moles per liter of the solution:

$$\frac{Grams\ of\ solute}{F.W.(g)} = \frac{moles}{L} = mol/L$$

$$\frac{60\ g\ NaOH}{40\ (F.W.)} = 1.5\ mol/L\ (or\ 1.5\ M)$$

An example of preparing a mol/L solution is in Figure 1-53.

Preparing Normal Solutions

Another term for expressing the concentration of a solution is **normality (N)**. Although still occasionally used, it has largely been replaced by the use of moles per liter (formerly called molarity [M]) solutions.

Normality gives an indication of the reactivity of chemicals; it has been used primarily to describe reactivity of acids and salts because these chemicals dissociate into reactive entities in solution. For example, NaCl in solution dissociates into Na^+ and Cl^-. NaCl is said to have a **valence** or *charge* of 1. A salt such as $MgCl_2$ in solution will dissociate into two Cl^- ions and has a valence of 2. Normality is not used for molecules such as glucose, which do not dissociate in solution.

To determine normality, the valence or charge of a chemical must be known. The gram molecular weight of a chemical divided by the valence equals the **gram equivalent weight** of the compound. Normality (N) is the number of gram equivalents of a compound per liter of solution.

$$Gram\ equivalents = \frac{gram\ molecular\ weight}{valence}$$

$$N\ (normality) = \frac{gram\ equivalents}{liter\ solution}$$

For chemicals with a valence of 1, such as NaCl, a normal solution and a moles per liter solution contain the same amount of NaCl per liter. For a solution with a valence of 2, a 1 N solution contains only half the amount of chemical per liter as a 1 mol/L solution. For an acid such as sulfuric acid (H_2SO_4, MW = 98) the valence is 2^+. Therefore, 98 g of sulfuric acid in a liter of solution is 1 M, but the normality is 2 N because the equivalent weight is equal to 98/2. Containers of concentrated acids include the normality on the chemical label.

Preparing Serial Dilutions

The concept of dilutions was introduced in the section on proportions. In those examples, only single dilutions were made. However, in some cases laboratory workers have to make *serial dilutions* of a sample to find the **titer** of a particular component in the sample. The titer of a component is the measure of reactivity or strength of the component and is reported as the reciprocal of the highest dilution giving a reaction. (An example of reciprocals is: 16 is the reciprocal of 1/16, and 1/16 is the reciprocal of 16. In other words, if a tube containing a 1/16 dilution is the last one showing a reaction, the titer is 16.)

Titers are useful when a component cannot be easily analyzed using available chemical methods. Titers are often used in immunology to indicate the level of a particular antibody in a serum sample. Dilutions of serum are used in certain tests such as the rheumatoid factor (RF) test for rheumatoid arthritis or tests measuring levels of antibodies to infectious agents.

Problem:	Prepare one liter of a 2 M (mol/L) solution of NaOH.
Formula:	M Solution = $\dfrac{\text{gram formula weight (GFW)}}{\text{Liter}}$
Solution:	1. A 2 M Solution contains 2 GFW per liter 2. The GFW of NaOH is 40 3. A 2 M solution of NaOH = 2 x 40 g/L 4. 80 g NaOH are required to make a 2 M solution

© Cengage Learning 2012

FIGURE 1-53 Preparing a 2 M (mol/L) NaOH solution

1. Set up 9 tubes, each containing one mL of diluent.
2. Transfer one mL of patient serum to tube 1.
3. Mix the serum and diluent, and transfer one mL of the mixture to tube 2.
4. Repeat the procedure, transferring one mL each time after mixing with diluent.
5. Discard one mL from the last tube.
6. When dilution series is complete, each of the nine tubes should contain one mL.

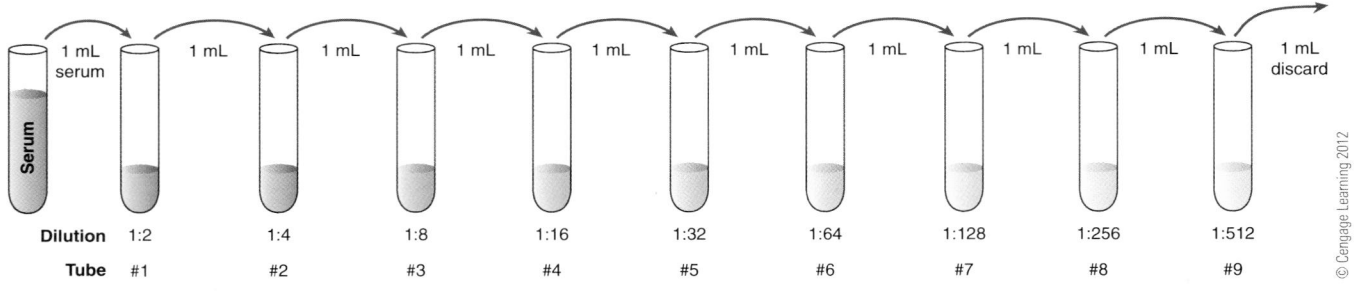

FIGURE 1-54 Preparing a two-fold dilution series

Making a Two-Fold Serial Dilution

In a serial dilution, a sample is diluted a number of times by the same dilution factor. In a two-fold dilution (also called doubling dilution) series, each dilution is two times as dilute as the previous dilution. Figure 1-54 shows one example of how a nine-tube two-fold serial dilution would be performed. Nine tubes are set up, each containing 1 mL of diluent. A serum sample is diluted in half (1:2) by adding 1 mL of serum to the 1 mL of diluent in tube 1 and mixing. Then 1 mL from tube 1 (1:2 dilution) is transferred to tube 2 and mixed with the 1 mL of diluent in tube 2. This creates a two-fold dilution in tube 2 (two times more dilute than tube 1). Tube 2 now contains a 1:4 dilution of the original serum.

The dilution series is continued by sequentially transferring 1 mL to the next tube in the series until the last tube is reached. After the 1 mL transferred from tube 8 has been mixed with the diluent in tube 9, 1 mL of the mixture in tube 9 is discarded. This leaves all tubes in the series containing 1 mL each, and provides serum dilutions ranging from 1:2 in tube 1 to 1:512 in tube 9. This means that in tube 9, only 1 part in 512 parts is serum from the original sample.

Each tube of the dilution series would then be used as a separate sample in the test procedure. The last tube in the series that shows a reaction is the end-point of the test and determines the titer. For instance, in a test in which tubes 1 through 6 were reactive, but tubes 7 through 9 were not, the highest dilution showing a reaction would be 1:64. The titer, the reciprocal of the highest dilution giving the desired reaction, would be reported as 64.

Making a Compound Dilution

Sometimes it is necessary to dilute a concentrated reagent or a patient sample. If the dilution needs to be large, it can be made more accurately by performing a series of small dilutions, rather than just a one-step dilution. For instance, a worker might need to make 10 mL of a 0.001 M solution from a 1 M stock (concentrate) solution. The first step is to find the dilution required to make the 0.001 M solution; the desired concentration of the final

solution (0.001 M) is divided by the concentration of the starting solution (1 M) and the fraction is converted to whole numbers:

$$\frac{0.001}{1} = \frac{1}{1000} = \text{desired dilution}$$

Therefore, the 1 M solution needs to be diluted 1:1000 to make the 0.001 M solution. This can be done by adding 1 part of the concentrate to 999 parts of diluent (or adding 0.01 mL to 9.99 mL). However, transferring a small volume such as 0.01 mL to 9.99 mL in one step does not usually create an accurate dilution. A more accurate way to make the 1:1000 dilution is by using a compound dilution series as shown in Figure 1-55. In this example, a three-tube, 10-fold dilution series was set up. The first dilution made is a 1:10 dilution (in our example, 1.0 mL would be added to 9 mL; it is easier to accurately pipet 1.0 mL than 0.01 mL). Then two more 1:10 dilutions are made to achieve the final 1:1000 dilution. The dilution in tube 4 (the final dilution) is calculated by multiplying the dilutions of each tube.

Prepare a 0.001 M solution from a 1 M solution using a 10-fold compound dilution:

1. Set up 3 tubes, each containing nine mL of diluent.
2. Transfer 1 mL of 1.0 M solution to tube 1 (creating a 1:10 or 0.1 M solution)
3. Mix tube 1 contents well and transfer 1 mL of the mixture to tube 2 (creating a 1:10 dilution of original solution or a 0.01 M solution)
4. Mix tube 2 contents well and transfer 1 mL to tube 2, creating 10 mL of a 0.001 M solution (1:1000 dilution of original solution)

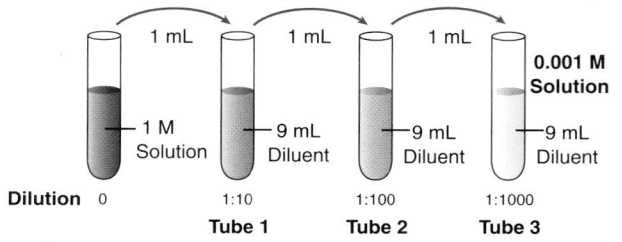

FIGURE 1-55 Making a 10-fold compound dilution series

SAFETY REMINDERS

- Review Safety Precautions section before beginning procedure.
- Wear appropriate PPE.
- Consult MSDS information for safe handling of chemicals.
- Use care to prevent injuries when using glassware.

PROCEDURAL REMINDERS

- Review Quality Assessment section before beginning procedure.
- Check calculations before proceeding with a task.
- Weigh and measure chemicals accurately.
- Use correct pipetting technique.
- Do not use pipets with broken or chipped tips.
- Use the correct type of water for the task.

$\frac{n}{x}$

CASE STUDY 1

Carl is reconstituting clinical chemistry standards. He needs them in a hurry and there is no CLRW water in the chemistry department. He sees a full container of Autoclave and Wash Water and decides to use it.

1. Is Carl's action acceptable?
2. What are the possible consequences?

CASE STUDY 2

Jody, a medical assistant in a small clinic, ran out of surface disinfectant while cleaning the counters in the clinic laboratory. The label of the disinfectant bottle she was using contained instructions for preparing the surface disinfectant from the concentrated stock solution. The instructions read "Dilute the concentrate 1:50 with water." Jody was using a disinfectant bottle with a 500 mL capacity.

1. Jody should prepare the replacement surface disinfectant by:
   a. Adding 1 mL of concentrate to 50 mL of water
   b. Adding 10 mL of concentrate to 500 mL of water
   c. Adding 10 mL of concentrate to 100 mL of water
   d. Adding 10 mL of concentrate to 490 mL of water
2. Justify your answer.

CASE STUDY 3

A laboratory scientist made a serial dilution of a patient's serum sample to determine the titer of an antibody. She found that the end-point, the last dilution in which a reaction occurred, was in the tube with the 1/128 serum dilution.

What is the titer of the test?

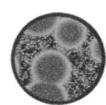

SUMMARY

Pipets and micropipetters are used in the laboratory to measure and deliver liquid volumes. The use of mechanical micropipetters with disposable tips increases pipetting accuracy. These micropipetters require calibration at regular intervals. The choice of the correct types of pipets and other glassware is critical to successful reagent preparation. Safety rules appropriate for the procedure must be followed.

Although most laboratory analyzers use prepackaged reagents or reagents contained in a reaction cartridge or strip, sometimes reagent or solution preparation is still necessary. The technician should be familiar with the principles involved in preparing reagents and making dilutions. Examples include:

- Preparing reagents such as or buffers or saline
- Diluting patient specimens for testing
- Preparing dilute solutions such as disinfectants or alcohols from concentrated solutions

Correct preparation of laboratory reagents is not difficult if the type of preparation (ratio, proportion, percentage, molar, or dilution) is considered carefully and the correct technique is used. Calculations must be made and checked for accuracy because errors in preparing reagents used in analyses can adversely affect test results.

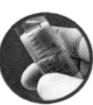

REVIEW QUESTIONS

1. Name two types of glass pipets and explain the differences between them.
2. The last drop is forced out of which kind of pipet?
3. Explain how a volumetric pipet is used.
4. List the three basic types of water used to prepare reagent water.
5. What grade of water is used to make or reconstitute laboratory standards and controls?
6. What are the advantages of micropipetters? How are they used?
7. Give an example of a percent solution used in the laboratory.

8. What dilution is created when one part of concentrate is added to nine parts solvent?
9. What formula is used to prepare a dilute solution from a concentrated solution?
10. How is a 1% (v/v) solution prepared?
11. How is a 5% (w/v) solution prepared?
12. Explain how to prepare 1 liter of 0.1 M potassium hydroxide (KOH). (Molecular weight 56; valence is 1). What is the normality (N) of the solution?
13. List three safety precautions that must be followed when preparing reagents.
14. In what circumstances must Standard Precautions be used when preparing laboratory reagents?
15. Define Beral pipet, deionized water, diluent, dilution, dilution factor, distilled water, formula weight, gram equivalent weight, lyophilize(d), micropipet, micropipetter, molar solution, mole, molecular weight, normality, percent solution, physiological saline, pipet, proportion, ratio, reagent, reverse osmosis, solute, solution, solvent, TC, TD, titer, and valence.

STUDENT ACTIVITIES

1. Complete the written examination for this lesson.
2. Practice the calculations for percent solutions, proportions, ratios, normality, and molarity using the laboratory math and reagent preparation worksheet.
3. Find examples of solutions prepared using percent, dilutions, or ratios in a chemistry or similar textbook. Examine labels of reagents and solutions in the laboratory and find different types of solutions (percent, dilution, molar, etc.).
4. If materials are available, practice preparing some of the solutions and serial dilutions from the worksheet as directed by the instructor.
5. Practice pipetting techniques following the procedure in the Student Performance Guide.

WEB ACTIVITIES

1. Find MSDS information about the following chemicals using the Internet: sodium hydroxide, potassium hydroxide, sodium carbonate, ammonium hydroxide, dextrose, and glutamic acid. For each chemical, list the molecular weight and state the precautions that should be used when working with the chemical or solutions containing the chemical.
2. Use the Internet to find tutorials or videos demonstrating pipetting techniques or preparation of solutions.

LESSON 1-8
Laboratory Math and Reagent Preparation

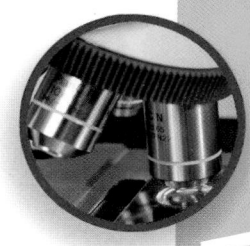

Name _____ Date _____

1. A 1% solution of hydrochloric acid is required for a procedure. A 5% solution is available. How much of the 5% solution will be required to make 500 mL of a 1% solution?

2. A procedure calls for acetic acid and water, with the proportions being one part acetic acid to three parts water. One hundred milliliters are needed. How much acetic acid and water are required? _____ What dilution is made?_____

3. One liter (L) of 70% alcohol is needed. How much 90% alcohol is required to make the 70% solution?

4. How would 1 liter (L) of a 10% solution of chlorine bleach be prepared?

5. How could 250 mL of a 4.0 N solution of hydrochloric acid (HCl) be prepared from a 10.0 M solution of HCl?

6. Give the instructions for preparing a two-fold serial dilution of serum from 0.5 mL serum and using 0.5 mL saline in each of five numbered tubes.

7. A 1-to-25 dilution of blood is required for a procedure. How can it be prepared?

8. How could a 1:10 dilution of serum be prepared?

9. What is the dilution when 0.5 mL is diluted to a total of 100 mL?

10. Give instructions for preparing 500 mL of a 0.15 M solution of NaCl (FW 58).

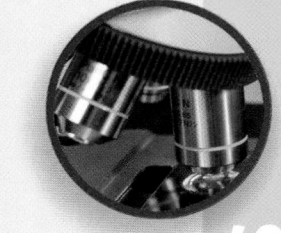

LESSON 1-8
Laboratory Math and Reagent Preparation

(Activities can vary depending on available laboratory resources and equipment.)

Name _____ Date _____

INSTRUCTIONS

1. Practice using pipets and micropipetters following the step-by-step procedure.

2. Demonstrate the procedures satisfactorily for the instructor, using the Student Performance Guide. Your instructor will explain the procedures for evaluating and grading your performance. Your performance may be given a number grade, letter grade, or satisfactory (S)/unsatisfactory (U) depending on course or institutional policy.

MATERIALS AND EQUIPMENT

- gloves
- hand antiseptic
- full-face shield (or equivalent PPE)
- pipets, volumetric and serological
- pipet-aids
- pipet filler-dispenser (optional)
- micropipetters with disposable tips and manufacturer's instructions for use
- small beakers
- small test tubes or microtubes
- distilled water or saline solution
- dilute solution of food coloring (optional)
- disposable plastic transfer pipets
- laboratory tissue or paper towels
- surface disinfectant (such as 10% chlorine bleach)
- biohazard container
- sharps container

PROCEDURE

Record in the comment section any problems encountered while practicing the procedure (or have a fellow student or the instructor evaluate your performance).

S = Satisfactory
U = Unsatisfactory

You must:	S	U	Evaluation/Comments
1. Wash hands with antiseptic			
2. Put on gloves and face protection			
3. Assemble materials and equipment: obtain pipetting systems including pipets, pipet-aid and/or pipet filler-dispenser, micropipetter and tips; beakers, test tubes or microtubes, disposable plastic transfer pipets, and nontoxic solution such as water or saline			

(Continues)

© 2012 Delmar, Cengage Learning. Permission to reproduce for clinical use granted.

You must:	S	U	Evaluation/Comments
4. Obtain a beaker of solution, an empty beaker, a TD pipet, and pipet-aid or pipet filler-dispenser			
5. Examine the pipet to determine if it is TD or TD blowout (frosted band). Observe the volume markings			

6. **For TD pipet (nonblowout):** Practice using a TD (to deliver) graduated pipet to measure and transfer volumes following steps 6-a through 6-f
NOTE: Adjust procedure to fit equipment available. Pipet-aids come in several designs. Consult directions on correct use of pipet-aid
a. Fit the pipet-aid securely to the top of the pipet
b. Keep the pipet vertical and insert the pipet tip well below the surface of the fluid in the beaker
c. Draw up fluid slowly into the pipet using the pipet-aid, filling the pipet to slightly above the desired volume marking
d. Remove the pipet from the solution, keep it in the vertical position, and wipe the outside of the pipet tip quickly with tissue to remove excess fluid, being careful not to allow the tissue to touch the opening in the pipet tip
e. Touch the pipet tip to the inner wall of the beaker and slowly lower the fluid level using the pipet-aid, until the lowest point of the meniscus touches the desired volume marking
f. Move the pipet and hold it vertically over the empty beaker
  1) Place the pipet tip against the inner wall of the empty beaker
  2) Release the suction on the pipet-aid and allow the liquid to drain from the pipet by gravity drainage
  3) Leave the pipet tip in contact with the inner wall of the container 1 to 3 seconds to allow the correct volume to be delivered
  4) Examine the pipet tip—a small drop of fluid should remain in the tip			

7. **For TD pipet (blowout):** Practice using a TD blowout pipet, following steps 6-a through 6f-3 **then** use the pipet-aid to force out the last drop of solution from the pipet tip into the beaker			
8. Continue practicing transferring liquids using both TD and TD blowout pipets			

© 2012 Delmar, Cengage Learning. Permission to reproduce for clinical use granted.

You must:	S	U	Evaluation/Comments
9. **Volumetric TD pipets:** Practice using volumetric TD pipets to measure and transfer volumes.			
a. Obtain a beaker of solution, empty beaker, volumetric pipet, and pipet-aid or pipet filler-dispenser			
b. Examine the pipet to check that it is a TD pipet and locate the single fill line on the pipet			
c. Fit the pipet-aid securely to the top of the pipet			
d. Keep the pipet vertical and insert the pipet tip well below the surface of the fluid in the beaker			
e. Draw up fluid into the pipet using the pipet-aid, filling the pipet to slightly above the fill line			
f. Remove the pipet from the solution, keep it in the vertical position, and wipe the outside of the pipet tip quickly with tissue to remove excess fluid, being careful not to allow the tissue to touch the opening in the pipet tip			
g. Touch the pipet tip to the inner wall of the beaker and slowly lower the fluid level in the pipet using the pipet-aid, until the lowest point of the meniscus touches the etched line on the pipet			
h. Hold the pipet vertically over the empty beaker			
i. Place the pipet tip against the inner wall of the beaker			
j. Release the suction on the pipet-aid and allow the liquid to drain from the pipet by gravity drainage			
k. Leave the pipet tip in contact with the side of the container 1 to 3 seconds to allow the correct volume to be delivered			
l. Examine the pipet tip—a small drop of fluid should remain in the tip			
m. Continue practicing transferring liquids using volumetric pipets			
10. **Micropetters:** Practice using a micropipetter to deliver liquids following steps 10-a through 10-j and the instructions that accompany the micropipetter			
a. Seat pipet tip firmly on the micropipetter before pipetting			
b. Adjust volume before pipetting if using an adjustable volume micropipetter			
c. Hold micropipetter vertically and depress plunger			

(Continues)

STUDENT PERFORMANCE GUIDE

© 2012 Delmar, Cengage Learning. Permission to reproduce for clinical use granted.

125

You must:	S	U	Evaluation/Comments
d. Place the lower portion of the pipet tip beneath the surface of the fluid to be pipetted. e. Release the plunger slowly and smoothly to fill pipet tip **NOTE:** Do not allow bubbles to enter the pipet tip as liquid is aspirated and do not immerse shaft of micropipetter into liquid f. Observe pipet tip while it fills to be sure liquid is not aspirated into the micropipetter shaft g. Dispense liquid into test tube or microtube by slowly depressing plunger with pipet tip placed against inside wall of the tube h. Use the two dispensing "stops" (if applicable) i. Eject the used pipet tip into a sharps container j. Continue practicing transferring liquids using the micropipetter			
11. Place used glassware in appropriate cleaning solution and return unused equipment to storage			
12. Clean micropipetter as recommended by manufacturer			
13. Clean work surface with disinfectant			
14. Remove gloves and discard into biohazard container			
15. Wash hands with antiseptic			

Instructor/Evaluator Comments:

Instructor/Evaluator _____ Date _____

© 2012 Delmar, Cengage Learning. Permission to reproduce for clinical use granted.

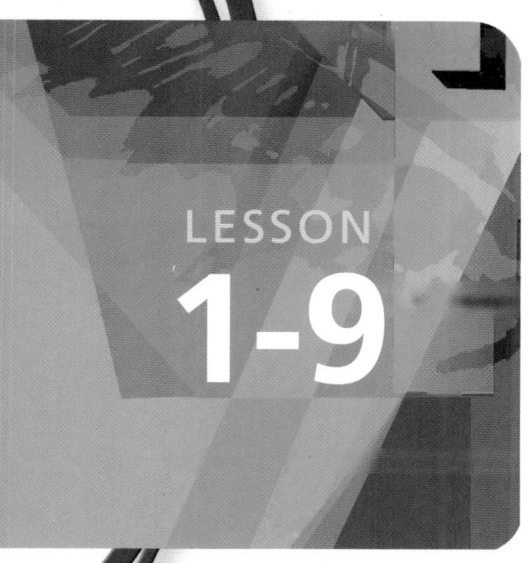

LESSON 1-9

Quality Assessment

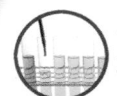

LESSON OBJECTIVES

After studying this lesson, the student will:

- ⊙ Explain the importance of quality assessment programs in the laboratory.
- ⊙ Explain the importance of quality assessment programs in point-of-care testing.
- ⊙ Discuss the use of standards and controls.
- ⊙ Explain the differences between external controls and equivalent controls.
- ⊙ Discuss the role of CLIA '88 in mandating laboratory quality assessment programs.
- ⊙ Explain the difference between accuracy and precision.
- ⊙ Discuss preanalytical, analytical, and postanalytical factors.
- ⊙ Explain how preanalytical, analytical and postanalytical factors can affect the reliability of test results.
- ⊙ Determine the mean value for a set of test results.
- ⊙ Calculate the standard deviation for an analytical method.
- ⊙ Describe how a Levey-Jennings chart is used.
- ⊙ Detect a result that is out-of-control.
- ⊙ Explain how to detect the development of a trend in a method.
- ⊙ Explain how to calculate a coefficient of variation and discuss its usefulness.
- ⊙ Describe safety procedures that must be followed when performing quality assessment procedures.
- ⊙ Define the glossary terms.

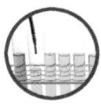

GLOSSARY

accuracy / the closeness of agreement of a measured value with the true value

average / the sum of a set of values divided by the number of values in the set; the mean

blind sample / an assayed sample that is provided as an unknown to laboratories participating in proficiency testing programs

calibration / the process of checking, standardizing, or adjusting a method or instrument so that it yields accurate results

coefficient of variation (CV) / a calculated value that compares the relative variability between different sets of data

controls / commercially available assayed solutions that are chemically and physically similar to the unknown and are tested in the same manner as the unknown to monitor the precision of a test method

(continues)

Gaussian curve / a graph plotting the distribution of values around the mean; normal frequency curve

Levey-Jennings chart / a quality control chart used to record daily quality control values

mean / the sum of a set of values divided by the number of values in the set; the average

population / the entire group of items or individuals from which the samples under consideration are presumed to have come

precision / reproducibility of results; the closeness of obtained values to each other

quality assessment (QA) / in the laboratory, a program that monitors the total testing process with the aim of providing the highest quality patient care; formerly called quality assurance

quality control (QC) / a system that verifies the reliability of analytical test results through the use of standards, controls, and statistical analysis

quality systems (QS) / in an institution, a comprehensive program in which all areas of operation are monitored to ensure quality with the aim of providing the highest quality patient care

random error / error that is inconsistent and whose source cannot be definitely identified

sample / in statistics, a subgroup of a population

shift / an abrupt change from the established mean indicated by the occurrence of all control values on one side of the mean

standard / a chemical solution of a known concentration that can be used as a reference or calibration substance

standard deviation (s) / a measure of the spread of a population of values around the mean

statistics / the branch of mathematics that deals with the collection, classification, analysis, and interpretation of numerical data; a collection of quantitative data

systematic error / error that is introduced into a test system and is not a random occurrence

trend / an indication of error in the analysis, detected by a progressive drift of control values in one direction for at least 5 consecutive runs

variance (s^2) / the square of the standard deviation; mean square deviation

Westgard's rules / a set of rules used to determine when a method is out of control

INTRODUCTION

Clinical laboratories are required to have programs in place that continually assess the quality of the laboratory's performance. Over the years, programs concerned with quality have been given a variety of names. A few decades ago the common term was **quality control (QC)**. QC programs were mostly concerned with ensuring that the test procedures provided as accurate results as possible. Then the term *quality assurance* came into use. Quality assurance programs included QC programs but also evaluated and monitored a broader range of factors affecting quality, such as specimen collection and results reporting. Other terms, such as Total Quality Management (TQM) and Continuous Quality Improvement (CQI), have also been used to refer to comprehensive quality programs; these programs can be institution-wide and not just limited to a laboratory.

In the final CLIA '88 regulations (Final Rule) published by the CDC and CMS and which became effective in 2003, new terminology was introduced. The term **quality assessment (QA)** replaced quality assurance; the term **quality systems (QS)** was designated to be used to refer to all policies, procedures, and processes needed to achieve quality testing. The ultimate purposes of quality programs are to provide quality health care that is safe, effective, timely, equitable, and patient-centered. Quality programs help achieve these goals by ensuring performance excellence and reliable laboratory test results.

Under the final regulations of CLIA '88, all laboratories are required to have programs in place to evaluate quality and ensure that laboratories provide the highest quality of patient care. This directive required few operational changes for hospital and larger laboratories, because in order to be accredited they already had rigorous QA programs in place. However, some smaller laboratories and those located in physician offices might have had insufficient QA programs. These laboratories are now required to put a QA program in place and to document the results. The goal of CLIA '88 is to provide patients with the best possible care by ensuring that results from all laboratories, large and small, are as reliable as possible.

This lesson describes the basic components of laboratory quality programs and introduces the reader to elementary statistical concepts. Throughout this text, the (Q) symbol is used to call attention to quality assessment components in a procedure or activity.

COMPONENTS OF A QUALITY SYSTEMS PROGRAM

A comprehensive quality systems program is designed to follow a specimen all the way through the testing process, from the time a test is ordered, through specimen collection and testing to reporting, charting, and delivery and use of results. The scope of QS programs differs among laboratories, but in general QS programs are broad, ongoing, and encompass evaluation of:

- Personnel qualifications, training, and competency
- Quality Assessment components including
  - Preanalytical (before test) factors
  - Analytical factors and QC methods
  - Postanalytical (after test) factors
- Proficiency testing

Personnel Qualifications and Training

Quality systems programs specify the education and training required for individuals performing the different levels of testing. Training of testing personnel must be up-to-date. Attendance at training sessions, continuing education seminars, and verification of competency in a test method must be documented and kept on file.

Quality Assessment

 Quality assessment (QA) is a component of a QS program and is an essential part of every laboratory's daily operations. QA programs are designed to ensure that reliable laboratory results are obtained and reported in the shortest possible time. Errors can occur at many points during a laboratory test procedure, but a QA program is designed to eliminate or minimize this possibility. A comprehensive quality assessment program includes evaluation of preanalytical, analytical, and postanalytical factors that can affect test outcomes. Preanalytical and postanalytical factors are factors outside of the test procedure that can influence the results. Analytical factors are associated with the actual test procedures.

Preanalytical Factors

Preanalytical factors are factors affecting specimen quality before the specimen is analyzed. Preanalytical factors that can affect test outcome include:

- Patient identification procedure
- Selection of the appropriate specimen and specimen collection method for the test ordered
- Specimen collection technique
- Specimen labeling and transport
- Handling and processing of specimen at testing site

In this era of near-patient testing, specimen collection is often performed by nonlaboratory personnel. It is important that laboratory personnel, especially the QA officer, establish good communication channels with off-site personnel who collect specimens. It must be emphasized that the manner in which a specimen is collected and handled has a direct effect on test results.

Methods to prevent preanalytical errors include (1) using two patient identifiers; (2) maintaining an up-to-date specimen collection manual; (3) using correct specimen selection, collection, and handling techniques; (4) establishing and following specimen rejection criteria; and (5) maintaining ancillary equipment, such as specimen storage refrigerators and freezers, in good working order.

Use of bar-coded patient ID numbers and matching bar-coded specimen labels reduces misidentification of patients and patient specimens. Selecting appropriate test methods, having qualified and trained testing personnel, and regular updating of procedure manuals are also steps that can reduce preanalytical problems.

Postanalytical Factors

Postanalytical errors occur primarily in the reporting and charting of test results. Many postanalytical errors have been eliminated because of the increased use of computers and improved labeling technology such as barcodes on patient identification armbands, laboratory request forms, preprinted labels, and specimen containers. These same practices also help prevent preanalytical errors. An example of a postanalytical error would be a test that is performed correctly and yields an accurate result, but the result is accidentally entered into the wrong patient chart. A postanalytical error could also occur by entering an incorrect patient identification number in the computer. The interfacing of laboratory analyzers and computers with patient records helps eliminate transcription and clerical errors.

Analytical Factors Affecting Laboratory Test Results

Quality assessment programs also evaluate analytical factors that can affect the actual test procedure. Many of these factors fall under the umbrella of QC. Analytical factors include:

- Instrument maintenance and calibration
- Use of standards and procedural controls
- Techniques and test components associated with performing the test procedure (reagents, laboratory water, pipetting, timing, etc.)
- Interfering substances or conditions
- Statistical analysis of control results

An example of an analytical error is inaccurate sampling caused by problems with an instrument's automatic sampler, perhaps because of dirt or protein buildup in the sampling probe. The error might be detected when control values show an abrupt or steady change. Such an error can usually be prevented by performing recommended maintenance tasks.

Proficiency Testing

Proficiency testing (PT) is another component of laboratory quality programs. Laboratories that perform nonwaived procedures are required to subscribe to an external PT program. At regular intervals during the year, the PT agency sends **blind samples** to the laboratory. These are samples that have been assayed multiple times by the PT agency. The subscribing laboratory analyzes these blind samples and sends the results to the PT agency. The subscribing laboratory's results are then compared to the PT agency's assayed values and to the results of peer laboratories participating in the PT program. Participating laboratories receive a report evaluating their performance.

QUALITY CONTROL: A COMPONENT OF QUALITY ASSESSMENT

Quality control procedures are an important part of the QA program and are sometimes the most visible part of the program. The principles and statistics that are part of QC programs can be complicated; this lesson includes just a brief introduction to some statistical concepts that are basic to QC programs. Laboratories are required to have a documented QC program in place.

Although not every technologist is responsible for actually performing statistical calculations, QC terminology and basic QC concepts must be understood and used by all testing personnel.

Safety Precautions

   Laboratory personnel can be exposed to bloodborne pathogens while using instrument calibrators and control solutions. Most controls are of human origin. Although control materials are screened for certain pathogens during the manufacturing process, they should still be considered potentially infectious. Standard Precautions must be followed while performing all control procedures in the same manner as when working with patient samples. Instrument maintenance procedures must only be performed by qualified personnel, with special attention to potential electrical and chemical hazards, as well as biological hazards.

External Controls

A major part of a QC program includes the daily use of controls. **Controls** are commercially available assayed solutions that contain the same constituents as those being analyzed in the patient sample. They are chemically and physically similar to the unknown and are tested in the same manner as the unknown to monitor the accuracy of a test method. Most controls are commercially produced from pools of human or plasma; some can be from sheep or pig. The manufacturer analyzes each control lot for a variety of components, such as glucose, sodium, cholesterol, and potassium. A list of the assayed values and acceptable ranges for all components in a control is included with each lot of controls. The laboratory must confirm these ranges using their own analytical systems.

Controls must be analyzed at the same time as patient samples, using identical methods, test conditions, and reagents. For nonwaived tests, at least two levels of controls must be used, and these must be run a minimum of once each day. These are called external controls. One control must contain constituents that fall within the normal range—this is called the *normal control*. The other control must contain constituents that are outside the normal range (either lower or higher than normal), commonly called the *abnormal control*.

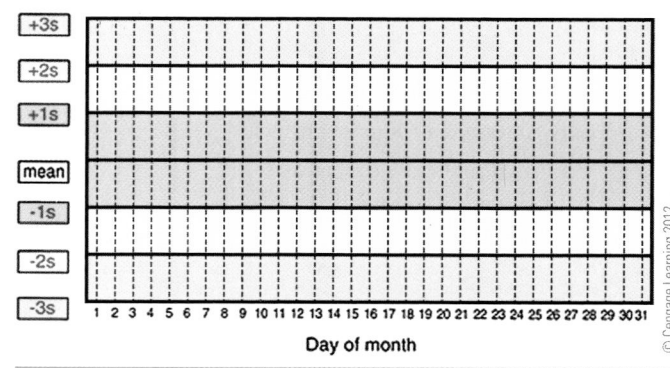

FIGURE 1-56 A form used to construct a Levey-Jennings chart

A single control might contain all the constituents tested on a certain chemistry profile and therefore be suitable to be included in all the chemistry assays the laboratory performs. If a single control does not meet these criteria, the laboratory will have to use a combination of controls to be sure that procedures such as chemistry profiles incorporate control(s) that contain each substance analyzed in the profile. In large laboratories, certain controls must be analyzed with each batch of patient samples, at least once per shift, any time patient results seem questionable, after instrument repair or calibration, and when reagents are changed. The frequency and types of controls required for each analytical procedure will be specified in the standard operating procedure (SOP) manual.

Each day's control results are used to construct a QC record called a **Levey-Jennings chart** (Figure 1-56). These daily control results are used in laboratory statistics. The records of the control assays must be retained and be available during laboratory inspections.

Equivalent or Internal Controls

Advances in instrument technologies have led to the manufacture of test systems that include internal monitoring systems and do not require operator calibration or standardization at every use. These are called internal, electronic, or procedural controls. The type of monitoring performed by the instrument differs according to the instrument—the color detection system might be monitored, or the electronics can go through a self-check.

For certain test systems, regulations allow laboratories to reduce the number or frequency of using external controls if an instrument can be shown to have internal monitoring systems that are reliable. Use of these internal check systems is called *equivalent QC*. To be permitted to use equivalent QC, the laboratory must demonstrate to the Centers for Medicare and Medicaid Services (CMS) that the test system is reliable. The use of equivalent QC is most common in small point-of-care (POC) instruments.

Standards and Calibration

Standards are also an essential part of a QC program. A **standard** is a substance that has an exact known composition and that, when accurately weighed or measured, can produce a solution

© Cengage Learning 2012

of an exact concentration. Standards are also called *reference materials*. Standards are often more expensive than controls and are usually not used on a daily basis. Standards are used to calibrate newly purchased instruments and recalibrate instruments after repair, at manufacturer's recommended intervals, or if a problem is suspected with a test method.

Calibration refers to the process of checking, standardizing, or adjusting a method or instrument so that it yields accurate results. Some instruments are calibrated using a standard; for others calibration can be accomplished electronically or by using a calibration strip or cartridge provided by the instrument manufacturer. All analytical instruments must be calibrated at set intervals, controls must be run regularly to verify calibration, and these actions must be documented.

Accuracy and Precision

In any discussion of QC, the terms *accuracy* and *precision* must be considered. The terms have two very different meanings. The worker's goal should be to achieve both precision and accuracy in the laboratory analyses performed (Figure 1-57).

Accuracy refers to the closeness of a measured value to the actual, or true, value. Results nearer the true value are more accurate than ones further away. For example, suppose that the true value for an individual's serum protein is 75 g/L. Then suppose that the individual's serum was analyzed three times by one method yielding results of 71, 79, and 75 g/L, and three times by another method yielding results of 66, 69, and 68 g/L. Imagine that the true value (75 g/L) is the center of a bull's eye target. Accurate values placed on the target would be clustered closely around the true value (target center) as shown in Figure 1-57A. The set of analyses of 71, 79, and 75 g/L would be more accurate than the other set because they are closer to the true value.

The term **precision** refers to the reproducibility of results or the closeness of obtained values to each other. Precision can be understood by again examining the two sets of protein values discussed under accuracy. The values 66, 69, and 68 g/L vary little from each other, so they are considered to show precision. However, they are not near the true value. These values, if placed on the same bull's eye target (where the true value, or target center, is 75 g/L), would be grouped very closely together but would be away from the true value (Figure 1-57B).

Test procedures can yield precise results without accuracy. In other words, a test can yield results close in value to each other, but because of error the values can be inaccurate, that is, not near the true value. QC procedures are designed to detect errors such as these.

Random and Systematic Errors

One critically important goal of a QA/QC program is to detect errors before test results leave the laboratory. Analytical errors occurring during the test procedure can be random or systematic. **Random errors** are errors for which the source cannot be definitely identified. The possibility of this type of error is always present in any system. Random errors can occur as a result of temporary variations in voltage, temperature changes, pipetters, dispensers, air bubbles in a reagent line, or differences in technique among workers. Random errors can also be caused by interfering substances in patient specimens occurring because of diet, medication, disease or other factors.

Systematic error is a variation that can make results consistently higher or lower than the actual value. Factors that can cause this type of error are deteriorated, contaminated, or out-of-date reagents; mechanical trouble in an instrument; or a peculiarity in a worker's technique, such as pipetting.

QUALITY PROGRAMS IN POINT-OF-CARE TESTING

Point-of-care testing (POCT) is also regulated by CLIA '88. Several types of laboratory tests performed in the United States are CLIA-waived tests that can be performed at POC. Waived tests are not subject to the rigorous use of controls required for nonwaived (moderate and high complexity) tests. However, manufacturer's instructions for an instrument or test kit must be kept on file, and their procedural recommendations, including use of controls, must be followed consistently.

Some POCT procedures are moderately complex and are subject to more stringent regulations. Personnel performing these tests must be adequately trained, and their training must be documented. Having the test kit and instrument manufacturer's instructions on file is not sufficient—the procedure for each test must be written in a procedure manual and records must be kept of control results. In addition, the laboratory must participate in a proficiency testing program covering the moderately complex tests performed.

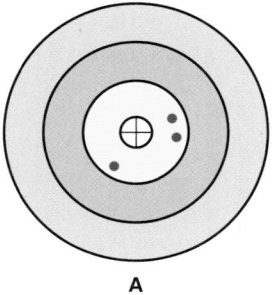 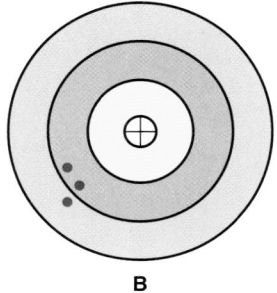 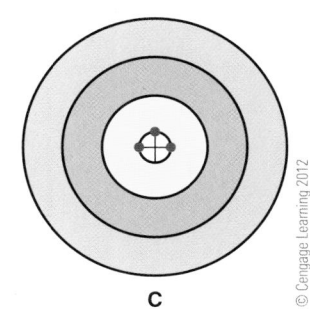

A   B   C

© Cengage Learning 2012

FIGURE 1-57 Illustration of accuracy (A) vs. precision (B); (C) shows both accuracy and precision

BASIC STATISTICS

Quality control programs use **statistics**, the branch of mathematics that deals with collecting, classifying, analyzing, and interpreting numerical data. An entire group or collection of observations is called a **population**. In laboratory statistics, a subgroup of the population (a group of specimens) is called a **sample**. The statistics involved in a good QC program can be very complicated; therefore, only the fundamentals will be covered in this lesson.

Calculating the Mean, Variance, and Standard Deviation

$\dfrac{n}{x}$ The calculations for mean, variance, and standard deviation for test procedures are the foundations of a laboratory QC program. The **mean** is the **average** of a set of values. The **standard deviation**, a measure of the scatter of the sample values around the mean, is derived from the calculation of the **variance**, the mean square deviation. Therefore, once the mean of a set of values has been determined, it is possible to determine the acceptable variation in the results of that analytical method.

Calculating the Mean

The mean is calculated by finding the sum of all the values in the set and dividing this by the number of values in the set; in other words, by calculating the average of a set of numbers (Figure 1-58). For example, 10 values obtained in repeated analyses of a glucose control were: 82, 85, 89, 85, 91, 90, 81, 85, 93, and 89 (mg/dL). The formula for determining the mean is

$$\overline{X} = \frac{\Sigma X}{n}$$

where
$\overline{X}$ = the mean
X = each individual value in the set
ΣX = the sum of all the individual values in the set
n = the number of values in the set

Column One	Column Two	Column Three
Test Value (mg/dL) X	Deviation from Mean $\overline{X} - X$	Deviation Squared $(\overline{X} - X)^2$
82	5	25
85	2	4
89	2	4
85	2	4
91	4	16
90	3	9
81	6	36
85	2	4
93	6	36
89	2	4
sum = 870		sum = 142

mean = $\dfrac{870}{10}$ = 87

© Cengage Learning 2012

FIGURE 1-58 Using a set of 10 values to calculate the deviation from the mean and the deviation squared

Substituting the 10 glucose values into the formula, the mean is found to be 87:

$$\overline{X} = \frac{82 + 85 + 89 + 85 + 91 + 90 + 81 + 85 + 93 + 89}{10}$$

$$\overline{X} \text{ (mean)} = \frac{870}{10} = 87$$

Calculating the Variance

The variance (s^2) is calculated by subtracting each value in the set from the mean, squaring this number, and calculating the sum of the squares. That sum is then divided by $n - 1$, which is the number of individual values in the set *minus one*. The formula for variance is:

$$\text{Variance} \, (s^2) = \frac{\Sigma(\overline{X} - X)^2}{n - 1}$$

An example of how to find the deviation from the mean and the deviation squared is shown in Figure 1-58. The values in column two are obtained by subtracting each value in column one from the mean. Therefore, the first entry in column two is negative ($-$) 5. This is obtained by subtracting 82, the first value in column one, from the mean, 87. It does not matter if some of the differences are negative numbers, because squaring them makes them positive numbers. From the example in Figure 1-58, the following substitutions can be made in the variance formula:

$$s^2 \text{(variance)} = \frac{142}{9} = 16$$

Calculating the Standard Deviation

The standard deviation is denoted by s (in italics), σ (the Greek symbol for sigma), or sometimes just **SD**. The standard deviation (s) is obtained by taking the square root of the variance:

$$s = \sqrt{16} = 4$$

Therefore, the standard deviation (s or $1s$) for this glucose mean is 4. Glucose values between 83 and 91 would lie within $\pm$ $1s$ of the mean (87). For this particular glucose control then $2s = 8$, and $3s = 12$.

These calculations seem complicated, but software in most analyzers includes a program that automatically calculates statistics from control values.

Using the Standard Deviation in the Laboratory

When a set of values with a normal distribution is plotted on a graph, the distribution of the values around the mean forms a **Gaussian curve** (Figure 1-59). This curve is also known as a normal frequency or normal distribution curve. In a set of numbers that have normal distribution, half of the values are greater than the mean and half are less than the mean. There are also more values close to the mean than values away from the mean.

To better understand normal distribution, suppose that the heights of 100 second-grade students in a school were measured, and the average (mean) height was determined. If this information

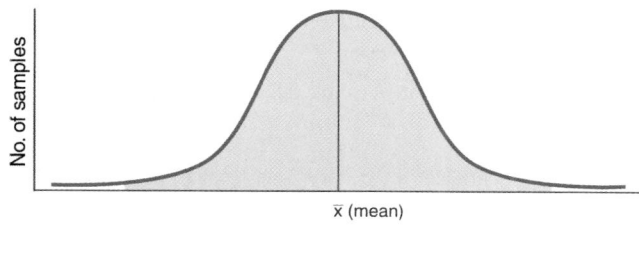

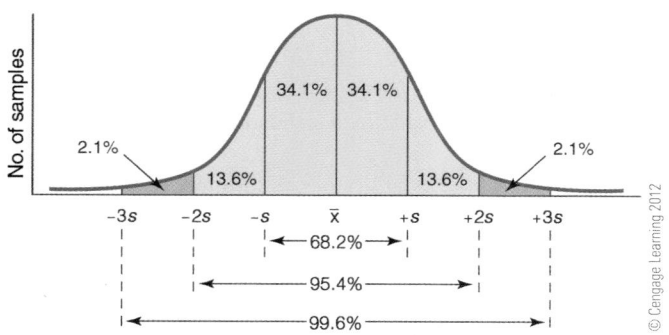

© Cengage Learning 2012

FIGURE 1-59 Normal distribution curves: (A) Gaussian curve showing normal frequency distribution around the mean; (B) Gaussian curve showing the proportion of the population falling between the mean and ± 1*s*, ± 2*s*, and ± 3*s*

was plotted in a graph like that shown in Figure 1-59A, it should produce a normal distribution curve. The height of most of the second graders would be near the mean height. Only a few of the students would be expected to be very tall or very short—values that would lie away from the mean.

Once the standard deviation has been determined, the curve can be divided into percentage divisions as shown in Figure 1-59B. This figure shows that, in a normally distributed population, 68.2% of all results obtained for this method of glucose analysis will fall between 1*s* below the mean to 1*s* above the mean. In other words, 68.2% of the values will fall between 83 (87 − 4) and 91 (87 + 4) in this particular example, which has a mean of 87. In addition, 95.4% of the values will fall between 2*s* below the mean to 2*s* above the mean, or between 79 (87 − 8) and 95 (87 + 8). If 3*s* is used, 99.6% of the values will be between 75 (87 − 12) and 99 (87 + 12).

Clinical laboratories must establish the allowable control limits for each analytical method, based on the component being analyzed and the method of analysis. A two-standard-deviation limit is a common choice. This is sometimes called the *confidence limit*. In this example, using a control with a mean of 87 mg/dL, the laboratory expects analysis of that control to be within ±2*s* (between 79 and 95 mg/dL) 95% of the time when it is analyzed along with patient samples. The confidence limit should not be confused with the *reference range* or the *reportable range* for a test method.

1. The confidence limit defines the upper and lower limits of values that are acceptable when a control is analyzed. This limit is usually the mean of the normal control ± 2 standard deviations. A control value falling outside the confidence limit is called an *outlier*.

2. The reference range, sometimes called the normal range, defines the upper and lower limits within which test results from a normal population would be expected to fall. The reference range will appear on laboratory report forms that contain patient test results. The reference range of an analyte must be reevaluated when a method changes or the patient population changes.

3. The *reportable range* or *linear range* is a range of values defining the limits of reliability and accuracy of a particular test method. The linear range defines the upper and lower limits that can be directly measured in a method without diluting the sample. For instance, a glucose meter might have the capability to accurately measure glucose only up to 400 mg/dL. A test result that is above that level (such as 450 mg/dL) cannot be reported; the specimen would have to be diluted and retested so that the result falls within the instruments' ability to give an accurate measurement. The value obtained on the diluted sample would then be adjusted to compensate for the degree of dilution.

QUALITY CONTROL CHARTS

QC charts called Levey-Jennings charts can be constructed for each analytical method and each control based on the calculated mean and standard deviation. Levey-Jennings charts display the confidence limits of a test method as determined by establishing the mean and standard deviation of a control. The charts are used to evaluate a method's accuracy and precision and as a way to detect problems in a test system.

The QC chart shown in Figure 1-60A was constructed using the mean and standard deviation calculated from the glucose data in Figure 1-58. The mean obtained was 87; therefore, the mean line is labeled 87. The lines on either side of the mean represent 1*s*, 2*s*, and 3*s*. In this method, the confidence limit was determined to be ± 2*s* (or 87 ± 8). As control data are obtained each day, they should be entered on the chart. The chart form has divisions for 31 days, so it can be used for any month. In a hospital laboratory, a control would be plotted at least daily. In an office laboratory, controls might only be run 5 days per week. Figure 1-60B is an example of a quality control chart with control values plotted for 15 days.

Trend

A **trend** occurs when a series of control values consistently increases or decreases in the same direction for at least five consecutive days (Figure 1-60B). A trend is a signal that something has gone wrong in the procedure—in the instrument, the technique, the reagents, or the control sera. The problem might be something as simple as deterioration of a control or a reagent, which can be discovered by testing a new reagent or control lot. Or the problem can be more complicated, requiring instrument recalibration or service. The technologist must investigate, find the source of error, and correct the problem before patient results can be reported.

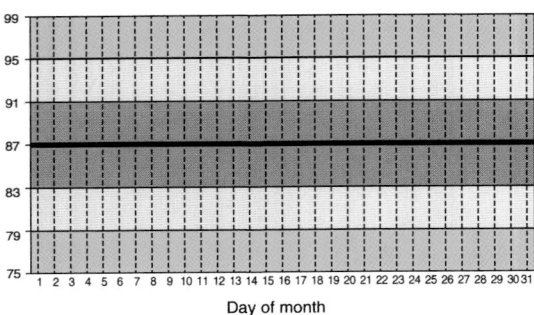

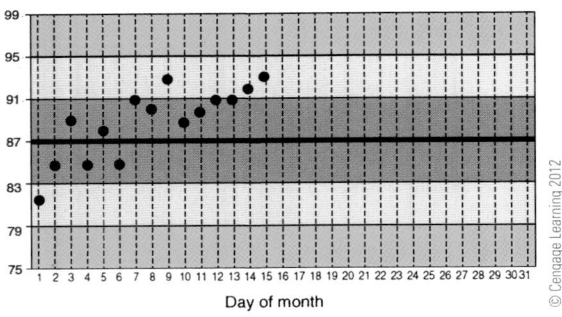

© Cengage Learning 2012

FIGURE 1-60 Levey-Jennings quality control charts: (A) chart constructed using the mean and standard deviation obtained from glucose control values; (B) plot of 15 daily control values, showing a normal distribution in values on days 1-6 and a "trend" on days 10-15

Shift

Normally, control results randomly fluctuate above and below the mean. When the control results for at least five consecutive days are distributed on one side of the mean, but remain at a constant level, a **shift** has occurred. This also signals error; the reagents and the instrument must be investigated for the cause.

Westgard's Rules

Each QC program has an established set of guidelines that are used to determine if a method is *in control* or *out of control*. Patient results can only be reported when test methods are in control. When a method is out of control, problems in the test method exist and must be investigated and corrected before patient tests can be run or results reported. One such set of QC guidelines is called **Westgard's rules**. These rules list specific limits about how much variation is acceptable in control values before patient test results are rejected. To use these rules, the laboratory must analyze two different levels of control sera (normal and abnormal) along with each set of patient samples. A *run* (set of samples) is considered out of control, and the patient results must be rejected if any of the following is true:

1. Both controls are outside the ±2s limit

2. The same control level is outside the ±2s limit in two successive runs

3. Controls in four consecutive runs have values greater than ±1s all in the same direction

4. Ten consecutive control values fall on one side of the mean

COEFFICIENT OF VARIATION

When a laboratory changes from one method of analysis to another, the precision of the new method must be compared to that of the old one. This can be done by calculating the **coefficient of variation (CV)** for each method. The CV is a calculated value that compares the relative variability between two different sets of values by expressing each standard deviation as a percentage of the mean.

For example, if a laboratory is purchasing a new blood glucose analyzer, the means and the standard deviations of the controls run on both the old and new analyzers would be used to calculate the CV for each instrument. Suppose that the mean glucose for the normal control using the first (old) analyzer is 98.5 mg/dL with a standard deviation (*s*) of 2.5 mg/dL and the mean glucose control value using the second (new) analyzer is 96 mg/dL with a standard deviation of 2.3 mg/dL. The CV's for the two methods would be calculated as shown below:

1st method

$$CV = \frac{s}{\overline{x}} \times 100$$

$$CV = \frac{2.5 \text{ mg/dL}}{98.5 \text{ mg/dL}} \times 100$$

$$CV = 2.5\%$$

2nd method

$$CV = \frac{s}{\overline{x}} \times 100$$

$$CV = \frac{2.3 \text{ mg/dL}}{96 \text{ mg/dL}} \times 100$$

$$CV = 2.4\%$$

In this comparison, the CVs are about the same, so the precision of the methods is similar. However, if a third analyzer gave a control mean of 95 mg/dL and *s* of 5.0 mg/dL, the CV would be calculated as follows:

3rd method

$$CV = \frac{s}{\overline{X}} \times 100$$

$$CV = \frac{5.0 \text{ mg/dL}}{95 \text{ mg/dL}} \times 100$$

$$CV = 5.3\%$$

The CV of the third method is 5.3%, indicating that the third analyzer yields less precise results than the first two analyzers.

SAFETY REMINDERS

- Review Safety Precautions section.
- Observe Standard Precautions.
- Wear appropriate PPE when handling samples, calibrators, or control sera.
- Observe safety rules when operating instruments or performing maintenance.

PROCEDURAL REMINDERS

- Follow instructions for calibration procedures.
- Keep QC charts and records up-to-date.
- Examine QC charts daily to detect out-of-control results.
- Follow instructions for reconstituting control sera.

CASE STUDY

Karen was working the day shift in the hematology laboratory. The laboratory's protocol called for three levels of blood cell controls to be run at the following times: (1) at the beginning of the shift, (2) within each run of patient samples during the day, and (3) any time reagents were changed. The mean for the low (abnormal) control for the red blood cell count was given as 2.00×10^{12}/L, the standard deviation was 0.15, and the confidence limit (acceptable control range) was 2.00×10^{12}/L $\pm 2\,s$ (or ± 0.3).

The first morning low control result was 2.10 ($\times 10^{12}$/L). In five subsequent runs, the low control results were 2.16, 2.19, 2.20, 2.22, and 2.25.

1. These values represent:
   a. a shift
   b. a trend
   c. neither shift nor trend
2. Should Karen be concerned about these values? Explain.
3. Does Karen need to take any action?

CRITICAL THINKING 1

Is it possible for an analytical procedure to be "out of control" if all of the control values fall within the 95% confidence range? Explain your answer.

CRITICAL THINKING 2

What are the 95% confidence limits for a control mean of 140 mg/dL and a standard deviation (*s*) of 2.5 mg/dL?

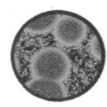

SUMMARY

Programs for improving the quality of laboratory testing have been in place for years. These programs have gone through many name changes, but the overall goal has not changed—to provide high-quality patient care by performing procedures in a manner that ensures that test results are reliable. CLIA '88 mandates the way in which laboratories accomplish this goal and requires that the laboratory's Quality Assessment (QA) procedures and results must be documented.

In current laboratory practice, quality control statistics programs are usually incorporated into the computer software that operates automated analyzers. Charts of control results can be printed directly from the analyzer for the technologist's review. Analyzers can be programmed to alert the operator when control results are suspect and even display messages giving trouble-shooting steps.

Programs that assess quality in the laboratory are an essential part of every laboratory's daily operations. QC charts are used daily in assessing the reliability of results from automated analyzers. Most technologists are not required to personally calculate QC statistics. However, they must understand the QC principles and concepts. This allows them to interpret the QC information produced by the analyzers, recognize problems, and troubleshoot any problems that become evident in QC reports.

Although laboratory personnel are intensely focused on performing their duties within the laboratory setting, the overall aim of health care personnel should always be to provide quality health care to the patient. Laboratory workers have the ethical and legal responsibility to perform to their highest level of ability and to ensure that work performed in the laboratory is of the highest quality.

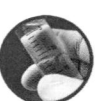

REVIEW QUESTIONS

1. What is the importance of quality assessment and quality control in the laboratory?

2. Explain the use of standards and controls in the laboratory's daily operation.

3. How and when are equivalent controls used?

4. Explain how results can be precise but not accurate.

5. How is the mean of a set of values determined?

6. Describe how to calculate the standard deviation.

7. How are Levey-Jennings charts used in the laboratory?

8. Explain the differences in confidence limits, reportable range, and reference range.

9. Explain how an out-of-control result can be detected.

10. Explain how to detect a trend in a procedure.

11. How can the coefficient of variation be used to compare methods of analysis?

12. What is the CV when the mean = 290 g/dL and one (1) $sD = 12$

13. What is the purpose of Westgard's rules?

14. What are preanalytical and postanalytical factors? Give an example of each.

15. What are the differences in systematic error and random error?

16. Define accuracy, average, blind sample, calibration, coefficient of variation, controls, Gaussian curve, Levey-Jennings chart, mean, population, precision, quality assessment, quality control, quality systems, random error, sample, shift, standard, standard deviation, statistics, systematic error, trend, variance, and Westgard's rules.

STUDENT ACTIVITIES

1. Complete the written examination for this lesson.

2. Calculate the standard deviation using this group of 10 numbers: 10, 9, 15, 10, 12, 11, 10, 12, 14, and 12.

3. Using the results of the calculations from activity 2, construct a Levey-Jennings quality control chart showing the mean, $+1s$, $+2s$, $+3s$, $-1s$, $-2s$, and $-3s$.

4. Complete the quality assessment worksheet at the end of this lesson.

WEB ACTIVITIES

1. Use the Internet to find information about quality control. One source site is www.westgard.com.

2. Search terms such as Levey-Jennings chart, trend, and shift using the Internet. From the information in your text and on the web, write a brief set of rules for determining when a control value for an instrument available in your laboratory is "out of control." Give a list of remedies or checks to perform to identify the problem.

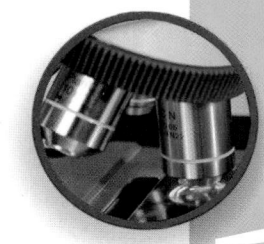

LESSON 1-9
Quality Assessment

WORKSHEET

Name _____   Date _____

A. Calculate the Mean and the Standard Deviation

1. Use this worksheet to calculate the mean and the standard deviation of a set of red blood cell (RBC) counts performed using a RBC control: 3.2, 3.3, 3.5, 3.2, 3.0, 3.4, 3.8, 3.5, 3.4, and 3.3.

2. Write the formula for finding the mean _____

3. Substitute the values (from A-1) into the formula. The mean of the red cell counts is _____

4. Following the example in Figure 1-58, calculate the deviation squared for each of the RBC values (from A-1).

5. Calculate the sum of the deviation squared of the 10 values: _____

6. Write the formula for variance _____

7. Determine the variance using the answer in step 5. _____

8. Write the formula for determining the standard deviation _____

9. Substitute the value from step 7 into the formula: _____

10. What is the standard deviation (s)? _____ What is ± 2 s? _____ What is ± 3 s? _____

B. Construct a Levey-Jennings Chart

1. Use the chart below and the mean and standard deviation (s) from part A to construct a Levey-Jennings chart. Indicate the mean value, ±1s, ±2s, and ±3s (from part A) on the appropriate lines.

2. Plot the following control values obtained for days 1 to 10 on the chart: Day 1 = 3.2, Day 2 = 3.3, Day 3 = 3.5, Day 4 = 3.2, Day 5 = 3.0, Day 6 = 3.4, Day 7 = 3.8, Day 8 = 3.5, Day 9 = 3.4, and Day 10 = 3.3.

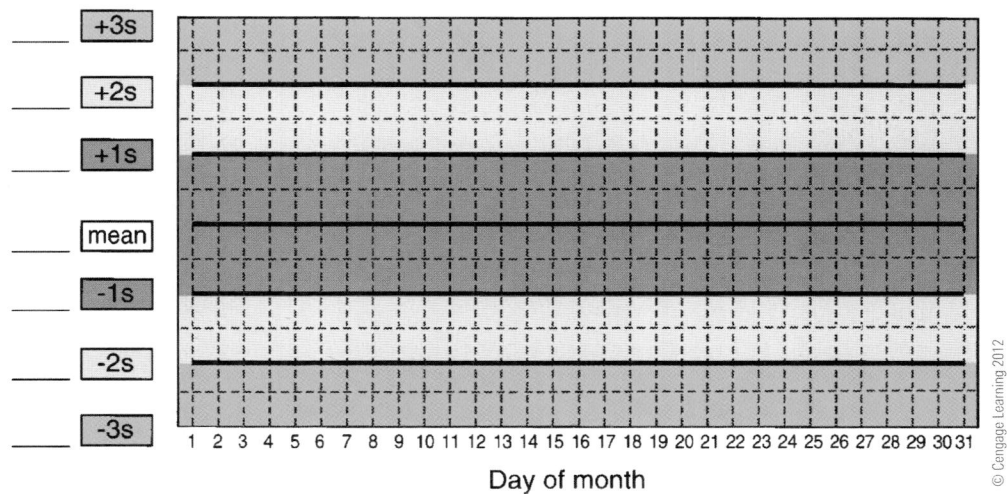

Day of month

© Cengage Learning 2012

© 2012 Delmar, Cengage Learning. Permission to reproduce for clinical use granted.

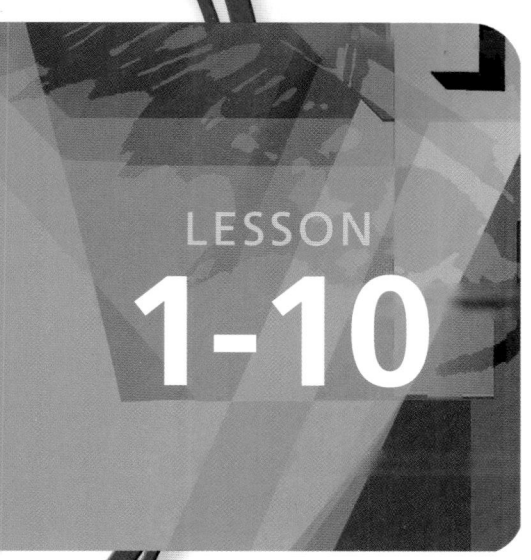

LESSON 1-10   The Microscope

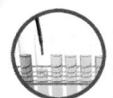

LESSON OBJECTIVES

After studying this lesson, the student will:

- ⊙ Locate and name the parts of a bright-field microscope.
- ⊙ Explain the function of each part of the bright-field microscope.
- ⊙ Explain the correct use of the coarse and fine adjustments.
- ⊙ Adjust the condenser and iris diaphragm.
- ⊙ Use Köhler illumination to align the microscope light path.
- ⊙ Explain how to perform dioptic and interpupillary distance adjustments.
- ⊙ Use the low-power objective to view a specimen.
- ⊙ Use the high-power objective to view a specimen.
- ⊙ Use the oil-immersion objective to view a specimen.
- ⊙ Explain when Standard Precautions and personal protective equipment (PPE) should be used while using the microscope.
- ⊙ Explain how light microscopes differ from electron microscopes.
- ⊙ Discuss the differences in the images produced by the two types of electron microscopes.
- ⊙ Explain why electron microscopes are not used in the typical clinical laboratory.
- ⊙ Discuss situations requiring use of the epi-fluorescence microscope.
- ⊙ Compare the differences in designs and uses of microscopes equipped with dark field, phase contrast, polarizing, and differential interference contrast (DIC) optics.
- ⊙ Explain how the use, care, and storage of the microscope can affect the quality of results.
- ⊙ Define the glossary terms.

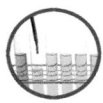

GLOSSARY

binocular / having two oculars or eyepieces

birefringence / the characteristic of double refraction; the characteristic of being able to split a beam of polarized light into two light beams

coarse adjustment / control that adjusts position of microscope objectives and is used to initially bring objects into focus

condenser / apparatus located below the microscope stage that directs light into the objective

(continues)

confocal laser scanning microscope / a microscope using a laser as the light source and producing images of very high resolution

differential interference contrast (DIC) microscope / a microscope equipped with special Nomarski optics that enhance contrast in unstained, transparent specimens, producing a three-dimensional image

electron microscope / a microscope using an electron beam to create images from a specimen and that is capable of much greater magnification and resolving power than a light microscope

eyepiece / ocular

field diaphragm / adjustable aperture attached to microscope base

fine adjustment / control that adjusts position of microscope objectives and is used to sharpen focus

fluor / a substance that absorbs short wavelength (exciting) light and emits longer wavelength (emitting) light

iris diaphragm / device that regulates the amount of light striking the specimen being viewed through the microscope

Köhler illumination / alignment of illuminating light for microscopy; double diaphragm illumination

lens / a curved transparent material that spreads or focuses light

lens paper / a special nonabrasive material used to clean optical lenses

magnification / in microscopy, the size of the image produced compared to the actual size of the object being viewed

micrometer / a ruled device for measuring small objects

microscope arm / the portion of the microscope that connects the lenses to the base

microscope base / the portion of the microscope that rests on the table and supports the microscope

monocular / having one ocular or eyepiece

nosepiece / revolving unit to which microscope objectives are attached

numerical aperture (N.A.) / a mathematical expression of the resolving power of a lens

objective / magnifying lens closest to the object being viewed with a microscope

ocular / eyepiece of the microscope that contains a magnifying lens

ocular micrometer / a clear glass disk that fits in the microscope eyepiece, is etched with a precise scale, and is used to measure objects viewed with the microscope; also called ocular reticle

parfocal / having objectives that can be interchanged without varying the instrument's focus

resolving power / the ability of a microscope to produce separate images of two closely spaced objects

reticle / a glass circle etched with a pattern of calibrated grids, lines, or circles and inserted into a microscope eyepiece to allow the etched pattern to be imposed on the field of view

stage / platform that holds the object to be viewed microscopically

stage micrometer / a transparent glass slide marked with a precise scale in micrometers and used to calibrate ocular micrometers by aligning the ocular scale with the stage scale

working distance / distance between the microscope objective and the microscope slide when the object is in sharp focus

INTRODUCTION

Microscopes are used in many clinical laboratory departments to evaluate stained blood smears and tissue sections, perform cell counts, examine urine sediment, observe cellular reactions, and interpret smears containing microorganisms. The microscopist must be skilled in microscope use if maximum information is to be gained from procedures using the microscope.

This lesson is an introduction to microscopy and includes descriptions of several types of microscopes used in medicine and research. The correct use of the bright-field clinical microscope is described in detail. Because the microscope is a delicate, expensive instrument, special care must be taken in its use, cleaning, and storage.

TYPES OF MICROSCOPES

Microscopes come in various sizes, prices, designs, and capabilities. Microscopes can be divided into two broad categories based on the type of illumination used. Clinical microscopes fall into the classification of *light microscopes*. Light microscopes use visible light, ultraviolet light, or lasers as the light sources to illuminate specimens. Tungsten, halogen, and light-emitting diode (LED) light sources emit a full spectrum of visible light (white light); mercury lamps emit light in the ultraviolet range. High-resolution microscopes called confocal microscopes use focused laser beams of very narrow wavelength to illuminate specimens.

The other major category of microscopes is the *electron microscopes*. These are named because specimens are visualized by focusing an electron beam on the specimen rather than light waves. Electron microscopes are discussed in the Current Topics section of this lesson.

Light Microscopes: The Bright-field Microscope

Modern light microscopes are also called *compound* light microscopes because they have two lens systems, one system in the oculars and one system in the objectives. The most common type of light microscope in the clinical laboratory is the bright-field microscope (Figure 1-61).

The bright-field microscope is the workhorse of the clinical laboratory. The microscope is named bright-field because the object being viewed is seen against a *bright field* of view. Routine clinical laboratory tests requiring a microscope are usually performed using the bright-field microscope. Bright-field microscopes are especially well suited for viewing stained specimens, such as stained blood smears or stained bacterial smears. Figure 1-62A shows stained blood cells as seen with a bright-field microscope.

Modifications of the Light Microscope

Although the bright-field microscope is the most common microscope in the clinical laboratory, several modifications of the light microscope have special uses in the laboratory. Other types of light microscopes include the phase-contrast microscope, polarizing microscope, dark-field (DF) microscope, differential interference contrast (DIC) microscope, epi-fluorescence microscope, and confocal laser scanning microscope (CLSM).

Phase-Contrast Microscope

The phase-contrast microscope provides an improved way of viewing unstained cells, which are nearly transparent when viewed by bright-field microscopy. By installing special phase objectives and a phase condenser, bright-field microscopes can be equipped for phase-contrast microscopy. Some bright-field microscopes will have one or two phase objectives, so the microscope can be used as either bright-field or phase, depending on the need.

Phase contrast is useful for viewing unstained specimens such as urine sediments and for performing white blood cell and platelet counts using the hemacytometer. With phase-contrast microscopy, the background (field) appears gray and the specimen is bright. Figure 1-62B shows unstained cells in urine sediment viewed with phase-contrast microscopy.

Dark-Field Microscope

In the DF microscope, the light in the center of the condenser is blocked to cause light to hit the specimen at a high angle, scattering the light rays. The image obtained is a bright specimen against a dark field. The resolution is typically not as good as in bright-field microscopy, but images are of high contrast and

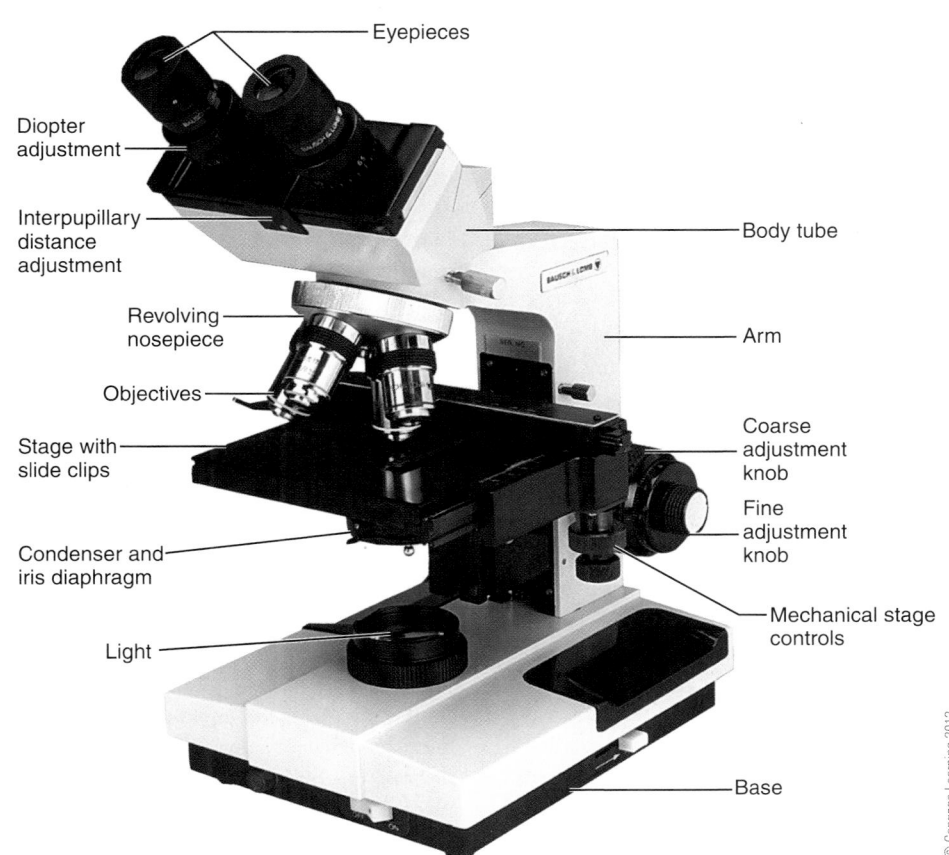

FIGURE 1-61 Binocular bright-field microscope with parts labeled

Eyepieces
Diopter adjustment
Interpupillary distance adjustment
Revolving nosepiece
Objectives
Stage with slide clips
Condenser and iris diaphragm
Light
Body tube
Arm
Coarse adjustment knob
Fine adjustment knob
Mechanical stage controls
Base

© Cengage Learning 2012

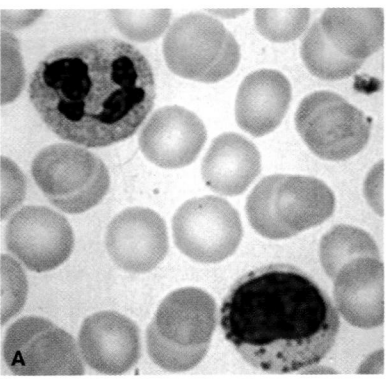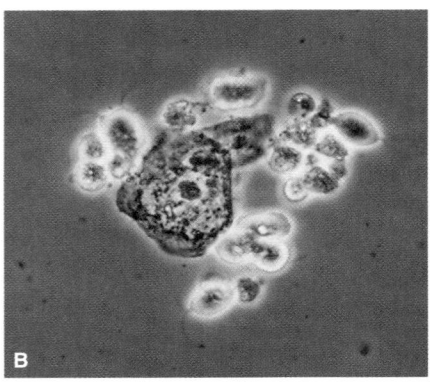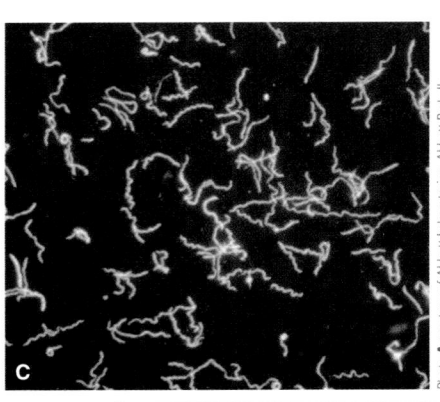

Photo **A** courtesy of Abbott Laboratories, Abbott Park, IL; photo **B** courtesy of CDC, Atlanta, GA

FIGURE 1-62 Light microscopy images: (A) stained blood cells viewed with a bright-field microscope; (B) phase-contrast image of urine sediment; (C) *Borrelia burgdorferi* stained with fluorescent antibody and viewed with epi-fluorescence microscopy

unstained cells, particularly living or moving cells such as sperm or parasites, are easily seen.

Polarizing and Differential Interference Contrast (DIC) Microscopes

Polarizing microscopes produce a bright image on a dark background. These microscopes are useful in identifying substances that have the characteristic of **birefringence**, which means that a beam of polarized light is split into two light beams by the substance. This is also called double refraction.

Polarizing microscope optics work much like polarizing sunglasses—polarizing lenses in the condenser and in the objective are crossed (positioned at a 90-degree rotation to each other). The crossed polarizers allow no light to pass, but birefringent specimens "rotate" light striking them and allow the objects to be seen. Polarizing microscopy can reveal information about the structure and composition of substances and can be especially useful in identifying urine crystals.

Light microscopes equipped with **differential interference contrast (DIC)** optics (sometimes called *Normarski* optics), produce three-dimensional images of unstained specimens. DIC optics provide excellent resolution and contrast and make it possible to view cell membranes and compartments within unstained cells, such as cell nuclei.

Epi-fluorescence Microscope

Epi-fluorescence microscopes use ultraviolet light to illuminate the specimen. The epi-fluorescence microscope enables the microscopist to view objects that have been stained with fluorescent dyes. A **fluor** or fluorescent dye is a substance that absorbs short-wavelength (exciting) light and emits longer wavelength (emitting) light. Filters between the light source and the specimen exclude all but the exciting wavelength from reaching the specimen. This excitation light is deflected by a prism onto the specimen, causing excitation of the fluor used to stain the specimen. The light emitted from the specimen is then collected by a prism and passes through another filter that excludes all but the excitation wavelength from reaching the eyepiece. This produces a high-resolution image that appears as a brightly stained specimen against a black field. No condenser is needed for this microscope

because light is applied from above the specimen—hence the name *epi*-fluorescence.

When fluors are attached to specific labels, such as antibodies, it is possible to identify particular areas of reaction within a cell or on a cell surface. The epi-fluorescence microscope can be used to identify microorganisms such as mycobacteria, and to detect the presence of antibodies in certain diseases such as syphilis and lupus erythematosus. Figure 1-62C shows *Borrelia burgdorferi*, the bacterium that causes Lyme disease. The bacteria are stained with a fluorescent-labeled antibody and viewed with epi-fluorescence microscopy.

Confocal Laser Scanning Microscopes

Confocal laser scanning microscopes (CLSM), sometimes called confocal microscopes, are one of the most powerful light microscopes (Figure 1-63). As the name implies, lasers are used as the illumination source, and images of excellent resolution are produced. Confocal microscopes can be used to examine fluorescently stained specimens but also have other applications. Specimens can be viewed and scanned in different planes of focus to create a series of images that are captured digitally. These images can then be merged to create 3-D or stereo images that can be digitally rotated or otherwise manipulated (Figure 1-63B).

PARTS OF THE MICROSCOPE

Microscope design can differ slightly from one model to another. However, some parts are common to all microscopes. Figure 1-61 shows a bright-field microscope with the parts labeled.

Oculars

A microscope can be **monocular** or **binocular**. Monocular microscopes have only one **ocular**, or **eyepiece**. Because of this, most people find it difficult to use them without eyestrain. Binocular microscopes have two eyepieces to allow viewing with both eyes, resulting in less eyestrain (Figure 1-61).

The oculars, or eyepieces, located at the top of the microscope, are attached to a barrel or tube connected to the

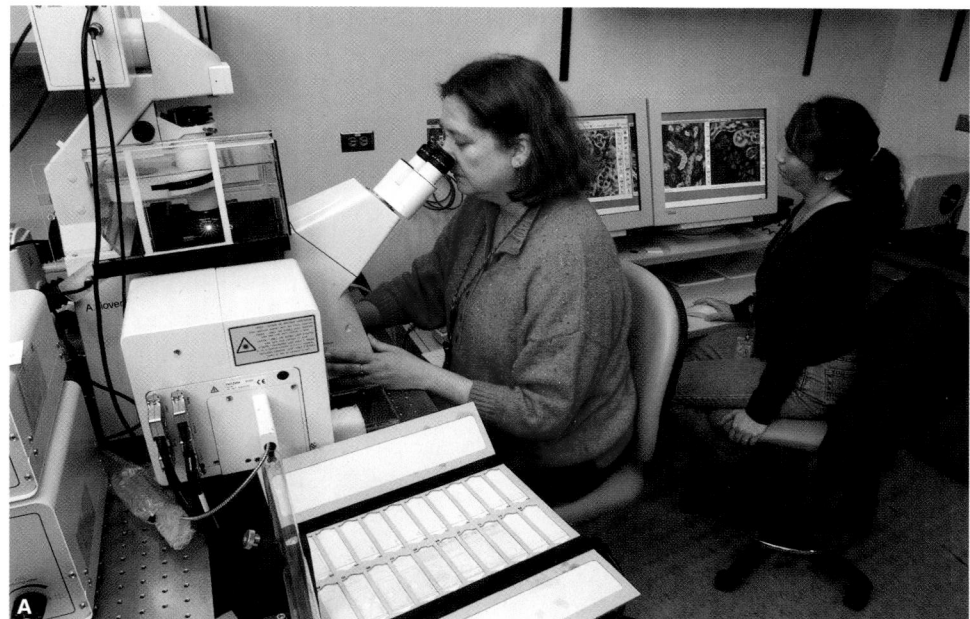

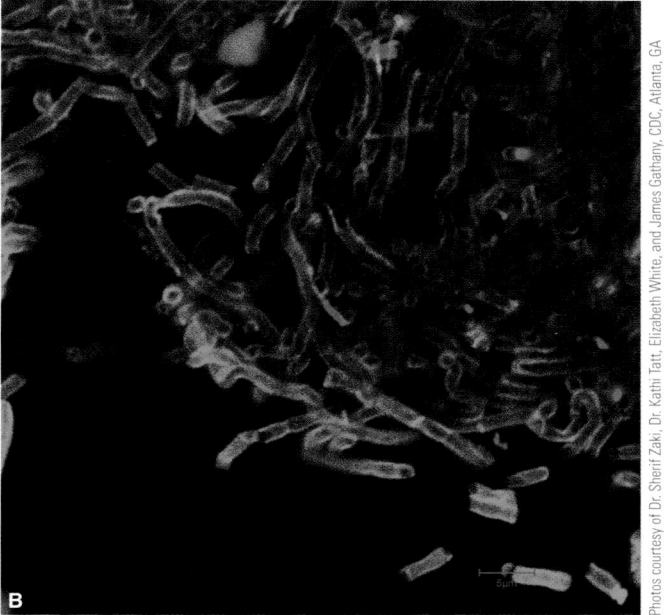

Photos courtesy of Dr. Sherif Zaki, Dr. Kathi Tatt, Elizabeth White, and James Gathany, CDC, Atlanta, GA

FIGURE 1-63 Confocal microscope: (A) confocal microscopes use lasers to illuminate specimens and images are displayed on computer monitors; (B) 3-dimensional colorized confocal image *of Bacillus anthracis*—cell walls appear green and spores appear red

microscope arm. Each ocular, through which the object is viewed, contains a magnifying **lens**. The usual magnification is 10 times (10×), but oculars are also available in 15× and 20×.

One ocular of a microscope is often fitted with **reticle** such as an **ocular micrometer**, used for accurately measuring the size of cells, parasitic ova, or any other structures of interest viewed with the microscope. An ocular micrometer is a clear glass disk etched with a precise scale (Figure 1-67). The ocular micrometer scale must be calibrated for each objective by focusing on a **stage micrometer**, a glass slide placed on the microscope stage that has a scale divided in divisions as small as 10 μm.

Objective Lenses

The underside of the microscope arm contains a revolving **nosepiece** to which the **objectives** are attached. Most microscopes are equipped with at least three objectives or magnifying lenses and these are available in a variety of magnifications. The low-power objective usually magnifies 10× or 20×; the high-power objective magnifies 40×, 43×, or 45×; and the oil-immersion objective magnifies 95×, 97×, or 100×. Each objective is marked with color-coded bands and the exact power of magnification.

Magnification refers to the size of the image produced compared to the actual size of the object. To determine the degree of magnification, the magnification listed on the ocular (usually 10×) is multiplied by the magnification listed on the objective being used (Table 1-35). For example, an object viewed with a 10× ocular and high-power (43×) objective would be

CURRENT TOPICS

ELECTRON MICROSCOPES

Electron microscopes provide much greater magnification and resolving power than light microscopes. The image from an electron microscope is created by exposing specimens to an electron beam, rather than illuminating them with a light source. Electron microscopes have been used in medical research for several years, but have been limited for the most part to pathology and virology. However, with new knowledge and techniques, their use in clinical medicine is increasing.

With the electron microscope, objects as small as 0.001 mm (too small to be seen with light microscopes) can be viewed. The two types of electron microscopes are the *transmission electron microscope* (TEM) and the *scanning electron microscope* (SEM), shown in Figures 1-64 and 1-65.

Objects are visualized in the TEM by passing an electron beam through the specimen. The image is displayed on a phosphorescent screen and viewed through protective glass or projected onto a monitor (Figure 1-64). Minute details inside a cell, such as nuclear structure, can be seen (Figure 1-66A). In the SEM, the electron beam is scanned over the surface of the specimen, which has been coated with a metal, causing the electrons to bounce off the specimen (rather than pass through the specimen as in the TEM). These deflected electrons are measured with a detector and converted into a three-dimensional image similar to an image on a television screen. Figure 1-66B is a color-enhanced scanning electron microscope image of blood cells.

Electron microscopes are very expensive and require special expertise to operate. Specimen preparation requires the use of special instruments and hazardous chemicals, and can take hours to several days to complete. The electron microscope technician needs much skill and experience to prepare a high-quality specimen as well as to operate the microscopes. Reference laboratories, medical schools, and large teaching hospitals are the most likely clinical locations for electron microscopes.

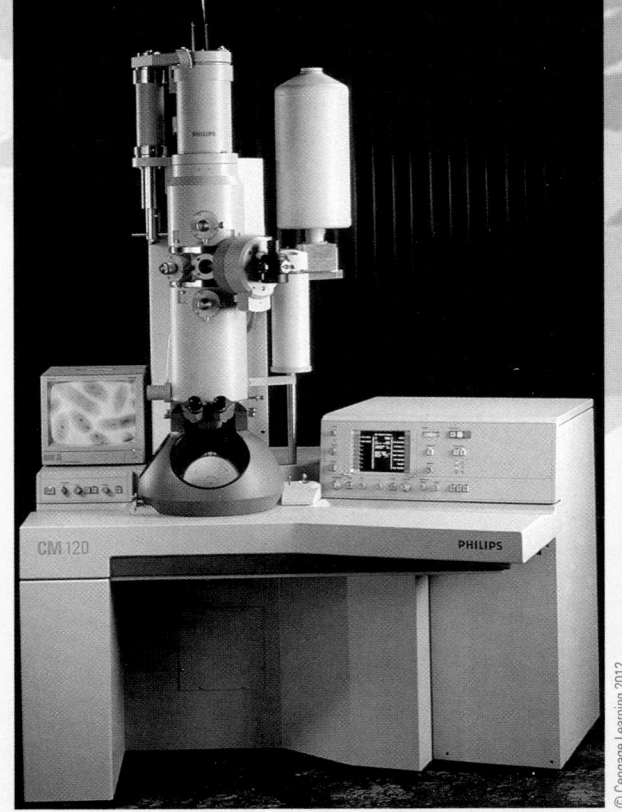

© Cengage Learning 2012

FIGURE 1-64 Transmission electron microscope

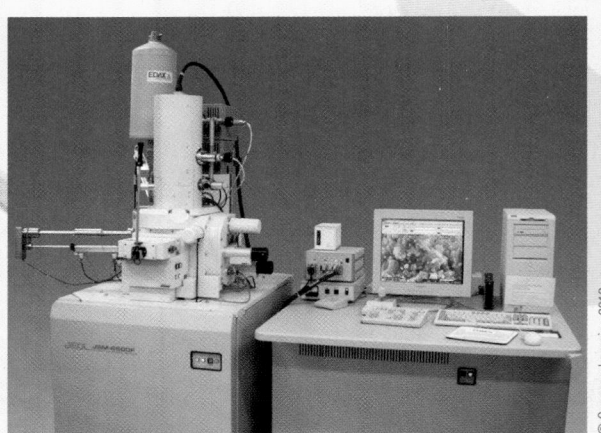

© Cengage Learning 2012

FIGURE 1-65 Scanning electron microscope

CURRENT TOPICS (Continued)

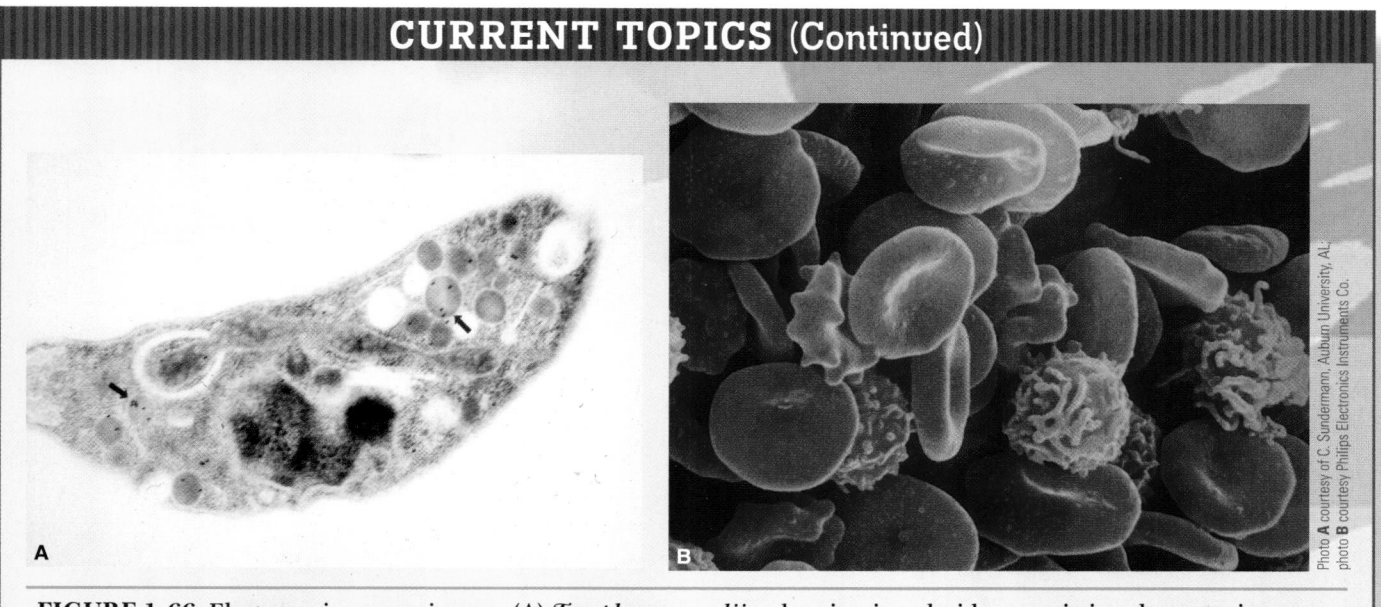

FIGURE 1-66 Electron microscopy images: (A) *Toxoplasma gondii* tachyzoite viewed with transmission electron microscope and showing numerous cell organelles; (B) color enhanced scanning electron microscope image of blood cells

magnified 430 times (430×). An object viewed with a 10× ocular and the oil-immersion objective (97×) would be magnified 970 times.

Numerical Aperture

Besides magnification power, several other characteristics of objective lenses affect the quality of the images produced. There is a limit to the degree of magnification that can be obtained with a light microscope and still yield a clear image.

The ability of a microscope to produce separate images of closely spaced details in the object being viewed is called its **resolving power**, and is determined by the quality of the objective lenses. The **numerical aperture (N.A.)** is a mathematical expression that indicates the resolving power of a lens based on the light-gathering capacity of the lens. Microscope objectives, particularly oil-immersion objectives, and sometimes condenser lenses, are marked with the factory-determined N.A. The larger the N.A. number, the better the resolving power

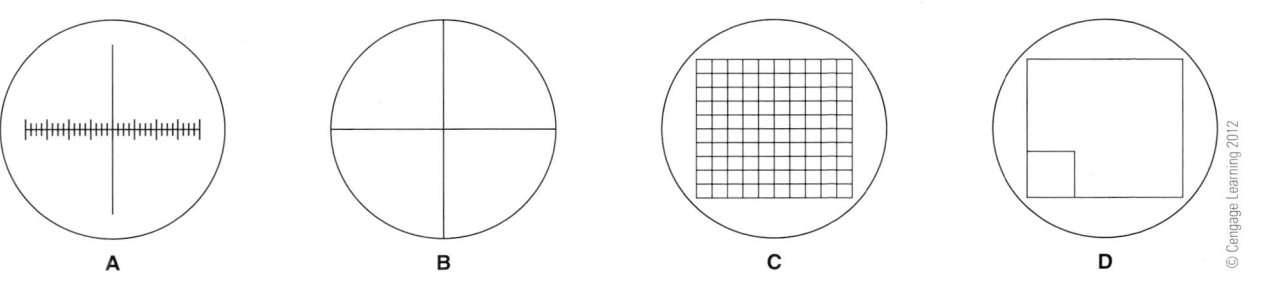

FIGURE 1-67 Types of eyepiece reticles: (A) ocular micrometer; (B) crossline reticle; (C) grid reticle; (D) Miller reticle

TABLE 1-35. Calculation of total magnification in a compound microscope

OBJECTIVE LENS	MAGNIFICATION STRENGTH	×	OCULAR STRENGTH	=	TOTAL MAGNIFICATION
Low power	10×	×	10×	=	100×
High power	40×	×	10×	=	400×
Oil immersion	100×	×	10×	=	1000×

of the lens, the more crisp and sharp the image, and the more expensive the objective lens.

Plan and Achromatic Lenses

Two other characteristics of objective lenses are often marked on the side of the objective, especially the oil-immersion objective. Lenses that are *achromatic* are designed to correct for the tendency of light to separate into colors when passing through glass. Therefore, achromatic lenses produce a more accurate color image of the object being viewed.

Because lenses are curved, there is also a tendency for images to be in sharp focus in the center of the field of view but slightly out of focus nearer the edges of the field of view. *Plan* lenses correct for focusing errors caused by this field curvature, which is most noticeable at high magnification. Achromatic objectives only have sharp focus quality for 60% to 70% of the field of view. Semi-plan lenses provide a larger area of sharp focus and plan lenses should have 100% of the field of view in focus at one time. The best quality objective lenses are marked "plan achromatic."

Light Source, Condenser, and Diaphragm

The microscope arm connects the objectives and eyepiece(s) to the **microscope base**, which supports the microscope. The base also contains the light, which illuminates the object viewed. Some microscopes have fixed light intensity, whereas others have a rheostat that allows light intensity to be adjusted. Microscopes that use tungsten lamps often have a blue filter placed over the light to correct for the yellow color of the light from the lamp.

Located above the light is the moveable condenser and iris diaphragm (Figures 1-61 and 1-68). The **condenser** focuses or directs the available light into the objective as it is raised or lowered, enhancing specimen contrast. The **iris diaphragm**, located in the condenser unit, regulates the amount of light that strikes the object being viewed (much like the shutter of a camera). The iris diaphragm can be adjusted by a movable lever. Microscopes can also have an adjustable **field diaphragm**, located just over the light source. The field diaphragm is used to help align or focus the light in a procedure called **Köhler illumination** (Figure 1-69).

Coarse and Fine Focus Adjustments

The two focusing knobs are usually located on the sides of the microscope base. The **coarse adjustment** is used to focus with the low-power objective only. The **fine adjustment** is used to give a sharper image after the object is brought into view with the coarse adjustment (Figure 1-61). The coarse and fine adjustment knobs are often in a *coaxial* configuration in which one knob is centered on top of another so that the center of each knob is on the same axis (Figure 1-61).

The **working distance** is the distance between the objective and the specimen slide when the object is in sharp focus.

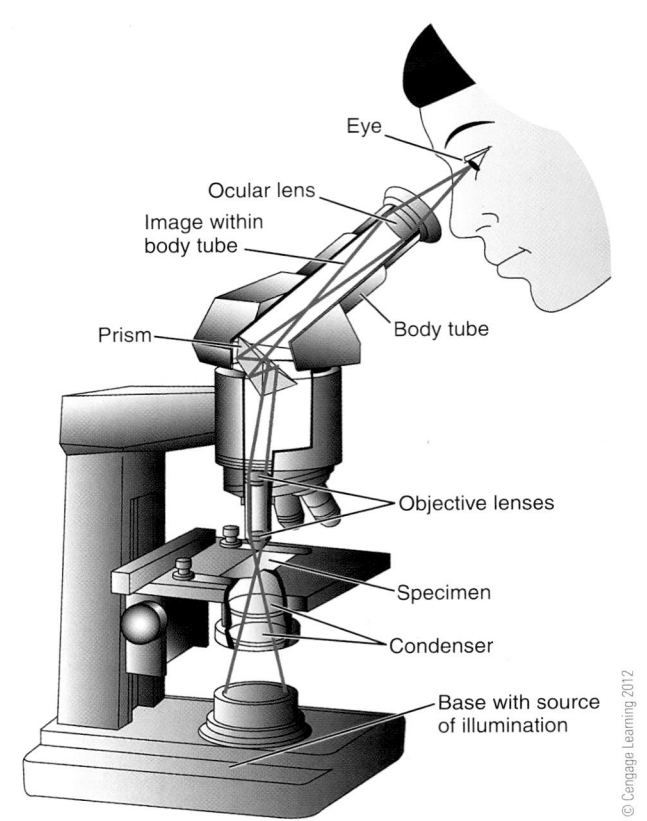

FIGURE 1-68 Diagram of light path in a compound microscope

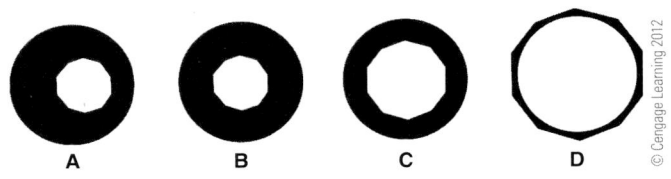

FIGURE 1-69 Köhler illumination: (A) closed, off-center field diaphragm; (B) closed, centered field diaphragm; (C) partially open and centered field diaphragm; (D) open, centered field diaphragm

The higher the magnification of the objective, the shorter the working distance will be. The coarse adjustment should *not* be used when using the higher magnification lenses to prevent the objective from accidentally striking the slide and becoming damaged.

Stage

The **stage** of the microscope is supported by the microscope arm and is located between the nosepiece and the light source. The stage serves as the support for the object being viewed and has a stage clip to keep slides stationary. The stage, called a mechanical stage, can be moved by using coaxial controls located just below the stage. These move the stage in a horizontal plane left and right or backward and forward (Figure 1-61).

HOW THE IMAGE IS PRODUCED

To see an image through the microscope oculars, the image must be magnified, focused, and directed into the oculars (Figure 1-68). The light in the microscope base is directed upward through the condenser, which focuses the light beam on the specimen. Some light striking the specimen is absorbed, some is deflected, and some is transmitted (passes through the specimen). The transmitted light enters the lens of the objective, which magnifies the image. The light then strikes a prism or mirror located between the objective and ocular. This prism deflects or bends the light (image) to direct it into the oculars. The oculars contain magnifying lenses that enlarge the image again and allow the eye to focus on the image. The combination of these two magnifying lens systems is the basis for the compound microscope.

USING THE BRIGHT-FIELD MICROSCOPE

The bright-field microscope is the one most frequently used in the clinical laboratory. Much practice is required to become competent and adept in its use in clinical microscopy. Microscopists must be proficient in making all of the adjustments required to achieve an optimal image of various types of biological specimens. They must also use appropriate safety measures and cleaning and maintenance techniques to keep the microscope operating at maximum capacity. The microscope should be on a sturdy, nonvibrating table at a comfortable height for the technician.

Microscope Safety

 Safety rules for electrical equipment must be followed when using the microscope. Electrical cords must be in good condition and should be plugged into grounded receptacles. Liquids must be kept away from cords. The microscope must be unplugged before attempting any maintenance, repairs, or bulb replacement.

Glass slides should be handled carefully to avoid the chance of chipping or breaking. If unfixed (living) or fluid biological specimens (such as urine sediment) are to be examined, Standard Precautions must be observed and appropriate PPE such as gloves must be worn. The microscope stage must be disinfected after examining such specimens.

Quality Assessment

 The microscopist should follow good microscopy practice in the care and use of the microscope to prevent damage to the instrument. Patient results should only be reported by experienced microscopists who have demonstrated the required level of competency.

Care and Cleaning of Lenses

The amount and quality of information that can be gained from microscopic examination of a specimen is dependent on the condition of the lenses. Lenses that become damaged or cloudy should be replaced. Cloudy, scratched, or otherwise damaged lenses can interfere with image clarity, possibly preventing the microscopist from observing important details in specimens being examined. Oculars and objective lenses should be cleaned before and after each use with **lens paper** and following the microscope manufacturer's instructions.

Immersion Oil

The use of immersion oil improves resolution by filling the space between the objective and the specimen with oil rather than air. Several types of immersion oil are available; the qualities of the objectives and the microscopy application must be considered when choosing the appropriate oil. The two most common oils for bright-field microscopy are type A (low viscosity) and type B (high viscosity). Type A or B oils that also have low fluorescence should be used for fluorescent techniques.

Only immersion oil manufactured for microscopy should be used with the oil-immersion objective. Immersion oil should never be allowed to touch the low- or high-power objectives. After the oil-immersion objective is used, the objective lenses and condenser should be cleaned to remove any residual oil. It is especially important that lenses never be left with oil on them, because oil can soften the cement that holds the lens in place in the objective. Lens cleaner, similar to a glass-cleaning solution, can be used with lens paper to remove oil from objectives.

Focusing with the Low-Power Objective

The low-power objective is used to initially locate objects and view large objects. The coarse adjustment focus knob is used to bring the objective and the slide as close together as possible. Then, while looking through the ocular, the coarse adjustment is used to move the objective and slide apart until the object on the slide comes into focus. (Note: The coarse and fine adjustments work by either raising and lowering the stage or raising and lowering the revolving nosepiece. Many microscopes are fitted with an adjustable *rack stop*, a safety feature that prevents the lens from striking the stage or condenser by limiting the degree of movement as a result of using the coarse adjustment knob.)

The fine focus adjustment knob can then be used to bring the image into sharp focus. When viewing objects using the low-power objective, the light intensity and iris diaphragm should be adjusted for optimum viewing.

Adjusting the Oculars

Once the object is in view, the oculars should be adjusted to accommodate each microscopist's eyes. Two adjustments are made, the *interpupillary distance adjustment* and the *dioptic adjustment*.

The interpupillary distance is adjusted by sliding the oculars either closer together or further apart until only one image is seen when looking through both oculars. This adjustment is like the one made when adjusting binoculars to your eyes.

Once the interpupillary distance is correct, then the dioptic adjustment should be made. This adjustment compensates for the microscopist's vision. The microscopist should look through the right ocular with the right eye (left eye closed) and use the coarse adjustment to bring the object into sharp focus. Then the microscopist should look through the left ocular with the left eye (right eye closed) and use the knurled collar (Figure 1-61) on the ocular (*not* the coarse focus adjustment) to bring the specimen into focus.

Alignment of Illumination

The path of light through the microscope must be properly aligned to have good resolution. Incorrect alignment causes poor resolution, artifacts, and unevenly lit field of view. The illumination alignment of many student and clinical microscopes is preset during manufacture, and realignment is done periodically by a professional microscope repair and service company. In these cases the microscopists do not perform the alignment procedure; it has been done for them.

Clinical microscopes that have an adjustable field diaphragm built into the light source allow the microscopist to manually align the illumination. The technique of centering and aligning or focusing the light path using the field diaphragm is called Köhler illumination and must be performed each time the microscope is used before viewing specimens with the microscope.

A specimen slide is placed on the microscope stage (specimen-side up) and positioned so that the specimen is directly beneath the low-power objective lens. The microscope light is turned on, and the specimen is brought into focus. The field diaphragm is closed as much as possible, and the edges of the diaphragm are brought into focus by raising or lowering the condenser. Both the specimen and diaphragm edge should be in focus, and the diaphragm outline should be centered in the field of view (Figure 1-69B). If the diaphragm outline is off-center, the image of the diaphragm outline is centered using the condenser centering knobs. The field diaphragm is then opened so that the edges of the image lie at the edge of the field of view (Figure 1-69D). The condenser iris diaphragm is adjusted to produce the desired contrast. Once these adjustments are made, the light intensity is adjusted using the voltage control (rheostat) without further adjusting the condenser or iris diaphragm. The microscope is now correctly adjusted and ready for viewing specimens.

Using the High-Power Objective

The high-power (40×) objective is used when greater magnification is needed, such as for cell counts and viewing urine sediments. After initial focusing using the low-power objective

and aligning illumination (if applicable) has been completed, the high-power objective is carefully rotated into position. The fine adjustment is used to bring the object into sharp focus. Most microscope objectives are **parfocal** and therefore require only slight changes in the fine adjustment when rotating between objectives. Most microscope objectives are also *parcentric*, meaning that specimens in the center of the field of view with one objective will also be centered when viewed with another objective.

Because the working distance between the slide and the high-power objective is so small, only the fine adjustment should be used when the high-power objective is in place. This avoids the possibility of the objective striking the slide and possibly damaging the objective or the slide.

To view unstained specimens using the high-power objective, the light intensity and iris diaphragm should be adjusted to provide proper lighting and contrast. When viewing most stained preparations with the high-power objective, the condenser should be raised, the diaphragm opened, and light intensity increased.

Using the Oil-Immersion Objective

The oil-immersion objective is used to view stained blood cells, tissue sections, and stained slides containing microorganisms. This objective gives the highest magnification of the bright-field objectives. After initial focusing with the low-power objective, the objective is slightly rotated to the side. A drop of immersion oil is placed on the slide directly over the condenser. The oil-immersion objective is then carefully rotated into the drop of oil, taking care that no other objectives contact the oil and that the oil-immersion objective does not strike the slide (Figure 1-70A). The object is then brought into sharp focus using only the fine adjustment. *The coarse adjustment should never be used when the oil-immersion objective is in position.* When viewing specimens with the oil-immersion objective, the condenser should be raised to its highest position (almost touching the bottom of the slide). The iris diaphragm should be open and maximum light should be used.

After completing examination of the slide, the low-power objective is rotated into position and the slide is removed from the stage. All oil must be cleaned from the oil-immersion objective with lens paper. The stage and condenser should be cleaned if necessary.

Transporting and Storing the Microscope

Microscopes should be left in a permanent position on a sturdy table where they cannot be jarred. However, if a microscope must be moved, it should be held securely, with one hand supporting the base and the other holding the arm (Figure 1-70B). The microscope should be placed gently to avoid jarring.

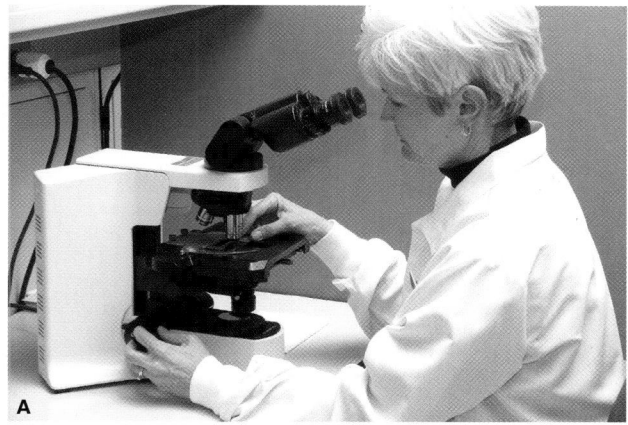

When the microscope is not being used, it should be left with the low-power objective in position and the nosepiece in the lowest position. The stage should be centered so that it does not project from either side of the microscope. The microscope should be stored under a dust-proof cover.

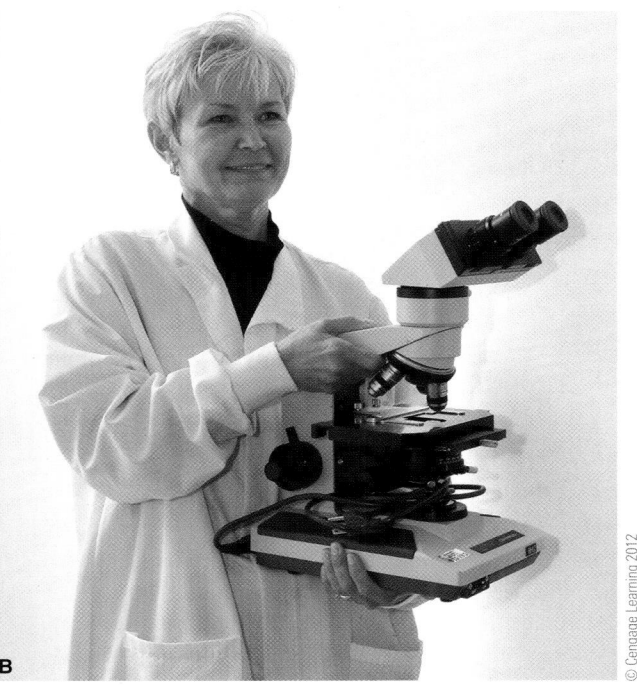

A

B

© Cengage Learning 2012

FIGURE 1-70 Use and care of the microscope: (A) observe the slide and objectives when changing from high-power to oil-immersion objective; (B) correct way to transport a microscope

SAFETY REMINDERS

- Review Microscope Safety before using microscope.
- Use Standard Precautions when examining unfixed biological materials.
- Disinfect microscope stage after examining unfixed biological samples.
- Disconnect the microscope from power source before performing repair.

PROCEDURAL REMINDERS

- Review Quality Assessment before using the microscope.
- Clean oculars and objectives before and after each use.
- Use coarse adjustment with the low-power objective only.
- Use immersion oil with the oil-immersion objective only.
- Make interpupillary distance and dioptic adjustments.
- Avoid jarring or bumping the microscope.
- Transport the microscope properly.

CRITICAL THINKING 1

Cheryl was performing urine microscopic examinations when the light went out on her microscope. She removed the microscope slide, turned the microscope over, and opened up the light compartment. She removed the light bulb with difficulty, saw that the filament was broken, and replaced the bulb. As soon as the bulb was fitted into the holder, the microscope light came on.

Comment on Cheryl's microscope repair technique.

CRITICAL THINKING 2

Roberta needed to use a microscope to examine a blood smear. She cleaned the oculars and the 10×, 40×, and 100× oil-immersion objectives with lens paper, using a clean section of lens paper for each objective. The lens paper used to clean the oil-immersion objective revealed oil on the objective. Roberta mentioned this to Jack, a technician who worked regularly with that microscope, and he replied that it was only necessary to remove oil from the objective once a shift because the objective might be used as many as 10 to 12 times during the day.

Is Jack correct? Explain your answer.

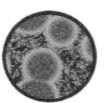

SUMMARY

The microscope is a valuable instrument used in many departments in the clinical laboratory. A large clinical laboratory will usually have several bright-field microscopes and also can have microscopes equipped with special optics such as phase-contrast or DIC optics. Epi-fluorescence microscopes are used in many clinical laboratories but electron microscopes are still used primarily in research.

Urine sediments, blood and bacterial smears, and various other specimens are examined and evaluated using the microscope. Specialized tests such as fluorescent antibody techniques also can require microscope use. Microscopists must become skilled in the proper operation of the microscope. Because microscopes are expensive, precision instruments, the technician must use the microscope with care, maintain the microscope in good working order, and be sure that it is cleaned and stored properly after each use. Much practice is required to become a competent microscopist.

REVIEW QUESTIONS

1. Explain the functions of the iris diaphragm and condenser.
2. Name the three objectives commonly used on a clinical microscope.
3. Explain the uses of the coarse and fine adjustments.
4. Describe the proper method of cleaning a microscope after use.
5. How should a microscope be stored when not in use?
6. When is the oil-immersion objective used?
7. When is immersion oil used on a slide? What is the function of the immersion oil?
8. Explain how to adjust the interpupillary distance on a binocular microscope.
9. What is the purpose of making a dioptic adjustment? Explain how the adjustment is made.

10. How is total magnification calculated in the compound microscope?
11. How do electron microscopes differ from light microscopes?
12. When must Standard Precautions be used with the microscope?
13. What is Köhler illumination? How is it performed?
14. Why is a condenser not used in epi-fluorescence microscopes?
15. Why are electron microscopes not in routine use in clinical laboratories?
16. Explain how the image formed in the TEM differs from that formed in the SEM.
17. Explain the difference between objective lenses that are parfocal and those that are parcentric.
18. Define binocular, birefringence, coarse adjustment, condenser, confocal laser scanning microscope, differential interference contrast microscope, electron microscope, eyepiece, field diaphragm, fine adjustment, fluor, iris diaphragm, Köhler illumination, lens, lens paper, magnification, micrometer, microscope arm, microscope base, monocular, nosepiece, numerical aperture, objective, ocular, ocular micrometer, parfocal, resolving power, reticle, stage, stage micrometer, and working distance.

STUDENT ACTIVITIES

1. Complete the written examination for this lesson.
2. Obtain a microscope and locate and identify the following parts: oculars, condenser, condenser adjustment knob, condenser centering knobs, field diaphragm, iris diaphragm, light, light intensity control, nosepiece, arm, base, stage, stage controls, coarse and fine adjustment knobs, and diopter adjustment ring. Note which (if any) parts are not found on your microscope.
3. Obtain a stained slide from your instructor. View the specimen with the low-power, high-power, and oil-immersion objectives. Draw the structure(s) you see when using each

objective. Observe the specimen when the condenser is raised and when it is lowered, and with the iris diaphragm wide open and closed. Discuss the differences in the image you see in each of these conditions. Which conditions or microscope adjustments reveal the most information about your specimen?

4. If you live near a university or a large research laboratory, find out if they have an electron microscope or a confocal laser scanning microscope. If so, try to arrange a visit to the facility to tour the microscope laboratory.

5. Practice using a microscope following the procedure outlined in the Student Performance Guide.

WEB ACTIVITIES

1. Find images taken with transmission and scanning electron microscopes using the Internet.

2. Use the Internet to find information about various types of light microscopes. Try to find examples of images obtained with phase-contrast, polarizing, DIC, epi-fluorescence, and confocal microscopes. Compare these images to the way stained images appear with the bright-field microscope in your laboratory.

3. Search the Internet for tutorials or videos describing the correct use and care of the bright-field microscope.

LESSON 1-10
The Microscope

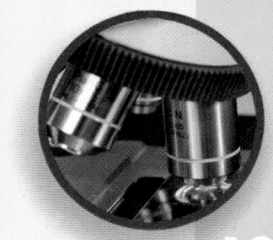

STUDENT PERFORMANCE GUIDE

Name _____ Date _____

INSTRUCTIONS

1. Practice using the microscope following the step-by-step procedure.

2. Demonstrate the correct use of the microscope satisfactorily for the instructor using the Student Performance Guide. Your instructor will explain the procedures for evaluating and grading your performance. Your performance may be given a number grade, letter grade, or satisfactory (S) / unsatisfactory (U) depending on course or institutional policy.

NOTE: Procedure will vary slightly according to microscope design. Consult operating procedure in microscope manual for specific instructions.

MATERIALS AND EQUIPMENT

- hand antiseptic
- microscope and microscope dust cover
- lens paper
- lens cleaner
- prepared slides (commercially available)
- immersion oil
- paper towels or laboratory tissue
- surface disinfectant (such as 10% chlorine bleach)

PROCEDURE

Record in the comment section any problems encountered while practicing the procedure (or have a fellow student or the instructor evaluate your performance).

S = Satisfactory
U = Unsatisfactory

You must:	S	U	Evaluation/Comments
1. Wash hands with antiseptic			
2. Clean work surface and obtain microscope and other needed materials			
3. Clean the microscope oculars and objectives with lens paper			
4. Use the coarse adjustment to raise the nosepiece unit			
5. Raise the condenser as far as possible by adjusting the condenser knob			
6. Rotate the low-power (10×) objective into position, so it is directly over the condenser			
7. Turn on the microscope light			
8. Open the iris diaphragm until maximum light comes up through the condenser			

(Continues)

© 2012 Delmar, Cengage Learning. Permission to reproduce for clinical use granted.

You must:	S	U	Evaluation/Comments
9. Place slide on stage (specimen side up) and secure. Position the condenser so it is almost touching the bottom of the slide			
10. Locate the coarse adjustment			
11. Look directly at the stage and low-power (10×) objective and turn the coarse adjustment until the objective is as close to the slide as it will go. Stop turning when the objective no longer moves NOTE: Do not move any objective toward a slide while looking through the oculars			
12. Look into the ocular(s) and slowly turn the coarse adjustment in the opposite direction (from step 11) to raise the objective (or lower the stage) until the object on the slide comes into focus			
13. Locate the fine adjustment and use it to sharpen the focus of the image			
14. Adjust the oculars for your eyes (steps 14a and 14b) a. Adjust interpupillary distance by adjusting distance between oculars so one image is seen (as when using binoculars) b. Make dioptic adjustment: 1) Use coarse and fine adjustments to bring object into focus while looking through the right ocular with right eye (and with left eye closed) 2) Close the right eye, look into the left ocular with left eye, and use the knurled collar on the left ocular to bring the object into sharp focus. (Do not turn coarse or fine adjustment at this time.) 3) Look into oculars with both eyes to observe that object is in clear focus. If not, repeat step 14			
15. If field diaphragm is present, perform Köhler illumination, following steps 15a–15g. If field diaphragm is not present, go to step 16 a. Stop down (close) the field diaphragm located on the microscope base b. Bring the edge of the diaphragm into focus using the condenser adjustment knob (which raises and lowers the condenser) c. Confirm that both the specimen and the diaphragm edge are in focus d. Center the image of the field diaphragm using the condenser-centering knobs e. Open the centered and focused field diaphragm so the edges lie just beyond the field of view f. Adjust the condenser iris diaphragm to increase or decrease image contrast; the proper position depends on the specimen g. Adjust light intensity by adjusting the voltage to the light source with the rheostat			

© 2012 Delmar, Cengage Learning. Permission to reproduce for clinical use granted.

You must:	S	U	Evaluation/Comments
16. Scan the slide using the stage controls to move the slide in a left and right or back and forth pattern while looking through the oculars			
17. Rotate the high-power (40×) objective into position while observing the objective and the slide to see that the objective does not strike the slide			
18. Look through the oculars to view the object on the slide			
19. Locate the fine adjustment			
20. Look through the oculars and turn the fine adjustment until the object is in sharp focus. Do not use the coarse adjustment			
21. Check alignment of Köhler illumination. Repeat steps 15a–15g if necessary			
22. Scan the slide as in step 16, using the fine adjustment if necessary to keep the object in focus			
23. Rotate the oil-immersion objective slightly to the side			
24. Place one drop of immersion oil on the portion of the slide directly over the condenser			
25. Rotate the oil-immersion objective into position, being careful not to rotate the high-power (40×) objective through the oil. Look to see that the oil-immersion objective is touching the drop of oil			
26. Look through the oculars and slowly turn the fine adjustment until the image is in sharp focus. Use only the fine adjustment to focus the oil-immersion objective. Scan the slide as in step 16			
27. Rotate the low-power (10×) objective into position; do not allow high-power (40×) objective to touch oil			
28. Remove the slide from the microscope stage, gently blot oil from slide, and return slide to slidebox			
29. Clean the oculars, low-power (10×) objective, and high-power (40×) objective with clean lens paper and lens cleaner			
30. Clean the oil-immersion objective with lens paper and lens cleaner to remove all oil			
31. Clean all oil from the microscope stage and condenser			
32. Turn off the microscope light and disconnect the microscope from power source			
33. Position the nosepiece in the lowest position using the coarse adjustment			

(Continues)

STUDENT PERFORMANCE GUIDE

© 2012 Delmar, Cengage Learning. Permission to reproduce for clinical use granted.

You must:	S	U	Evaluation/Comments
34. Center the stage so it does not project from either side of the microscope			
35. Place dust cover on microscope and return microscope to storage			
36. Clean work area with disinfectant			
37. Wash hands with antiseptic			

Instructor/Evaluator Comments:

Instructor/Evaluator _____ Date _____

© 2012 Delmar, Cengage Learning. Permission to reproduce for clinical use granted.

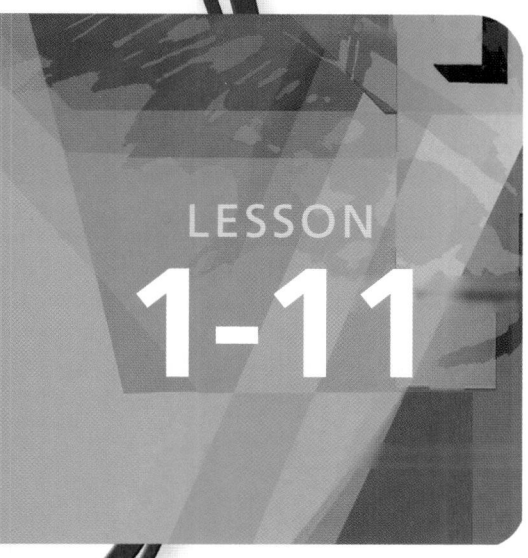

Capillary Puncture

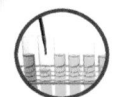

LESSON OBJECTIVES

After studying this lesson, the student will:

- ⊙ Explain why a capillary puncture is performed.
- ⊙ Identify suitable sites for capillary punctures.
- ⊙ Discuss capillary puncture in infants, children, and adults.
- ⊙ Choose and prepare a site for capillary puncture.
- ⊙ Perform a capillary puncture.
- ⊙ Collect a blood specimen from a capillary puncture.
- ⊙ Discuss how collection procedure affects capillary specimen quality.
- ⊙ List the safety precautions to be observed when performing a capillary puncture.
- ⊙ Define the glossary terms.

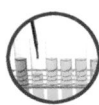

GLOSSARY

capillary / a minute blood vessel that connects the smallest arteries to the smallest veins and serves as an oxygen exchange vessel

capillary action / the action by which a fluid enters a tube because of the attraction between the fluid and the tube

capillary tube / a slender glass or plastic tube used for laboratory procedures

heparin / an anticoagulant used therapeutically to prevent thrombosis; also used as an anticoagulant in certain laboratory procedures

lancet / a sterile, sharp-pointed blade used to perform a capillary puncture

lateral / toward the side

INTRODUCTION

Capillary puncture, also called dermal puncture, is a safe, rapid, and efficient means of collecting a blood specimen. To perform capillary puncture, a small sterile **lancet** or blade is used to puncture the skin and **capillaries** to create a blood flow. Capillary punctures are performed when only a small amount of blood is required, when obtaining blood from infants, or when the patient has a condition that makes venipuncture difficult.

In the clinical laboratory, capillary blood has been used only in special situations, because of the small sample volume and potential for rapid clotting of the sample. However, the increased use of small, portable, easy-to-use instruments that require only a drop or two of blood, has made capillary blood the specimen of choice for these analyzers. The rapid increase in the use of these instruments in bedside testing, physician office laboratories (POLs), and other point-of-care (POC) testing sites has increased the need to train a variety of medical personnel in correct capillary puncture techniques.

THE CAPILLARY PUNCTURE

Factors that must be considered in performing a capillary puncture are the age of the patient, type of lancet required, and type of container used to collect the blood.

Capillary Puncture Sites

The usual site for capillary puncture in adults and children is the fingertip (Figure 1-71). In adults, the ring finger is often selected because it usually is less calloused. For newborns and infants, capillary blood can be obtained from the **lateral** or side portion of the heel pad (Figure 1-72). Once an infant begins to walk (about the age of 1 year) blood should be collected from a fingerstick.

Capillary Puncture Equipment

Equipment required for capillary puncture includes lancets and a variety of collection containers.

Lancets

Several designs of disposable, sterile safety lancets are available for capillary puncture. These lancets make punctures of uniform depth at the touch of a button and are available in several blade lengths for use in different situations (Figure 1-73). Special pediatric lancets that produce a shallow puncture should be used with infants.

Capillary Collection Containers

Capillary blood can be collected in capillary tubes or collection vials. Capillary blood can also be applied directly to a test strip, cuvette, or cartridge for use in POC instruments.

Capillary Tubes. Capillary tubes are slender tubes used primarily for microhematocrit measurements. Several types of capillary tubes are available: plain, heparinized, precalibrated, flexible, and self-sealing. Tubes coated with the anticoagulant **heparin** have a red ring on one end. These are used to prevent clotting of the blood during the collection of capillary blood samples. Precalibrated tubes are usually heparinized and are intended to be used only in the special microhematocrit centrifuges designed for them. Non-heparinized (blue ring) capillary tubes are used with venous blood that has been previously collected in an anticoagulant.

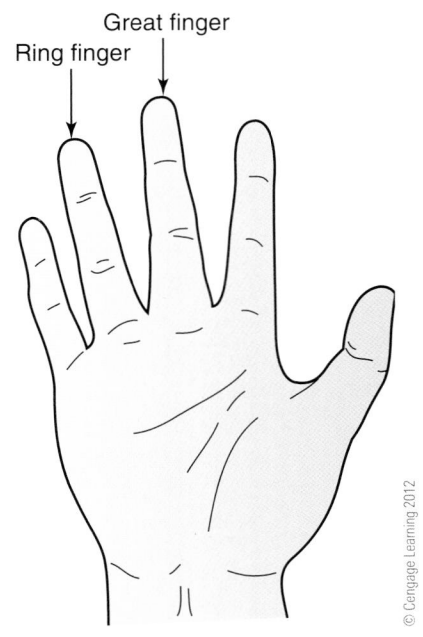

FIGURE 1-71 Capillary blood collection sites for adults and children

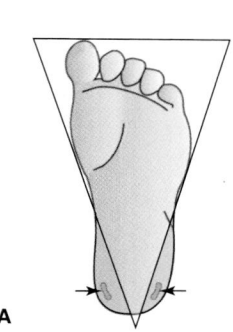

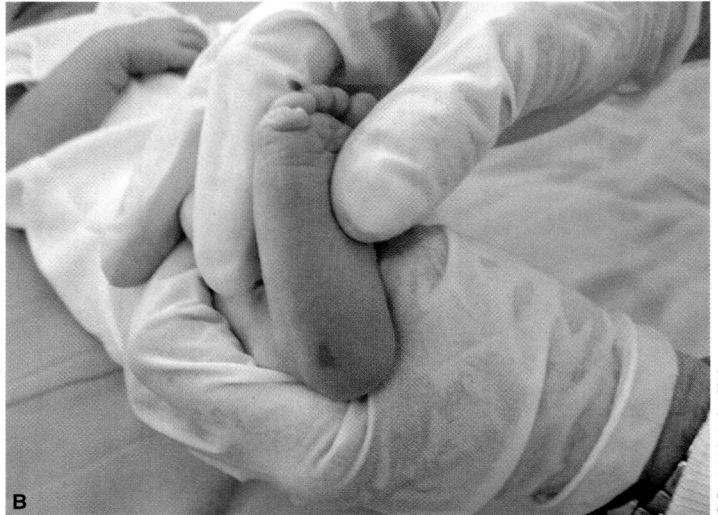

FIGURE 1-72 Pediatric capillary blood collection sites: (A) the lateral surface of the heel is used for newborns and small infants (correct puncture sites are green areas lying outside the triangle as shown); (B) collecting blood from the heel pad of a newborn

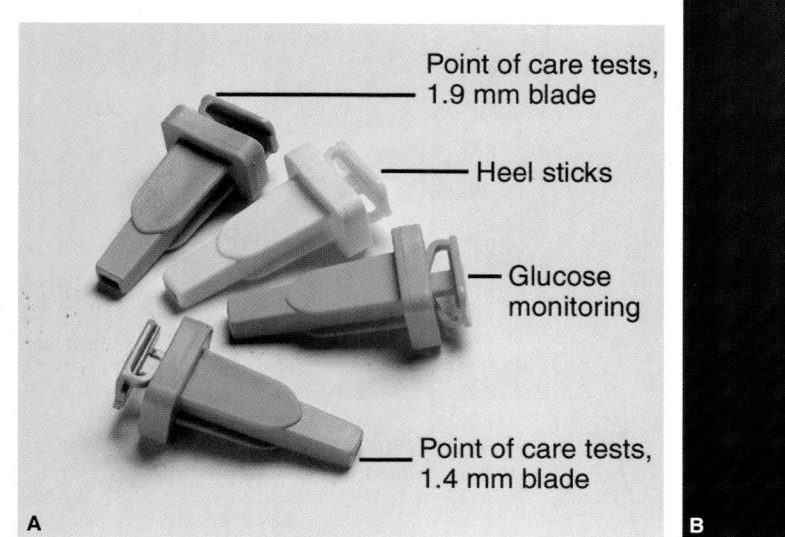

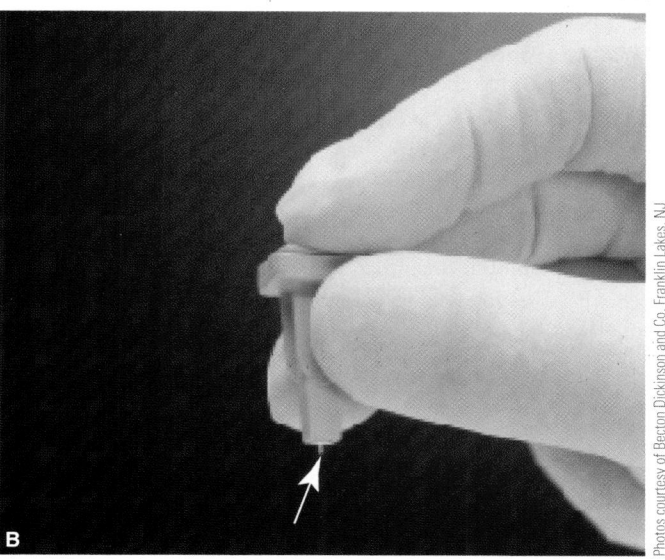

FIGURE 1-73 Single-use lancets: (A) lancets of different lengths; (B) lancet with blade (arrow) exposed

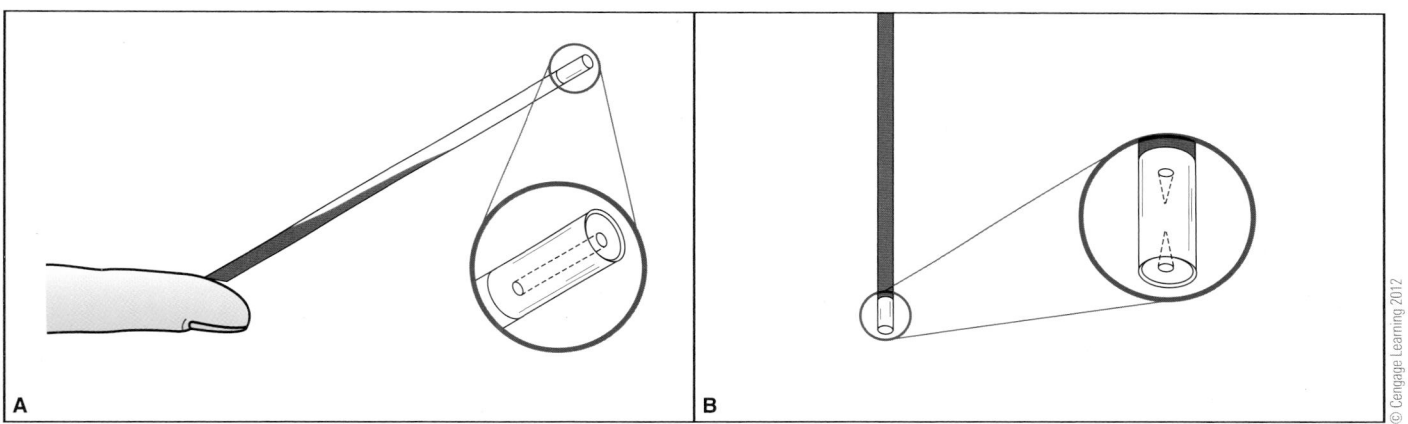

FIGURE 1-74 Self-sealing Mylar-wrapped capillary tubes: (A) sealing plug has channel that allows air to escape while the tube is being filled; (B) channel seals automatically when blood contacts plug

In an effort to prevent injury and possible exposure to infectious agents from capillary tube breakage, the Occupational Safety and Health Administration (OSHA) and National Institute for Occupational Safety and Health (NIOSH) recommended that glass tubes not be used unless sheathed in a plastic protective film. To minimize exposure risk, glass tube alternatives such as flexible plastic tubes or Mylar-wrapped tubes with self-sealing plugs should be used when possible. Self-sealing tubes have a plug at one end with a channel that allows air to escape while the tube is filled; the plug expands and seals when blood touches the plug (Figure 1-74).

Capillary Collection Vials. Capillary blood required for tests other than microhematocrit, such as chemistry tests, can be collected in special vials with a capillary or other extension for directing the blood into the vial (Figure 1-75). These vials are available plain or with anticoagulant. Using these vials, a small quantity of whole blood, plasma, or serum can be obtained

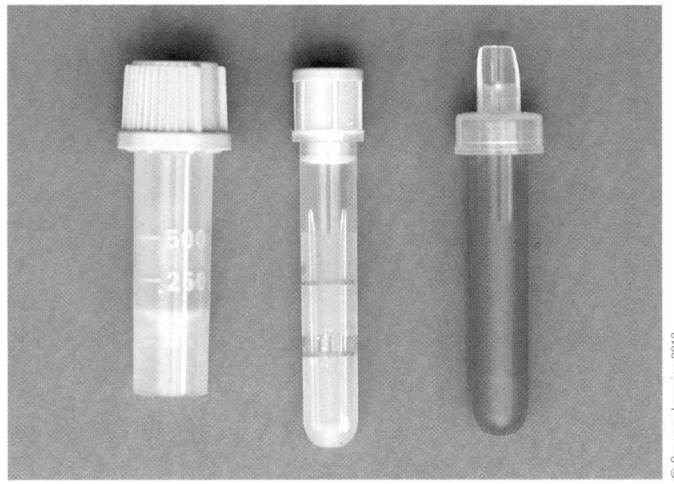

FIGURE 1-75 Capillary collection vials

without performing venipuncture, which is particularly useful with pediatric patients.

Procedures That Use Capillary Blood

Several hematology procedures such as blood cell counts, hemoglobin, microhematocrit, and the blood smear can be performed using capillary blood. Small handheld analyzers in POLs and a variety of POC testing sites also use capillary blood for coagulation, immunology, glucose, and other chemistry tests.

PERFORMING CAPILLARY BLOOD COLLECTION

Although the capillary blood collection procedure appears to be simple, the technician must consider several factors. Careful technique must be used to collect a quality specimen.

Safety Precautions

  Standard Precautions must always be observed when collecting capillary blood. Gloves and other appropriate personal protective equipment (PPE), such as a full-face shield or eye protection, must be worn by the technician. Plastic or Mylar-sheathed tubes should be used to minimize risk for injury from broken capillary tubes and prevent potential exposure to bloodborne pathogens. Used lancets and tubes must be discarded into biohazard sharps containers. Other blood-contaminated materials such as cotton or gauze must be disposed of in biohazard containers.

Quality Assessment

   Personnel who perform capillary puncture must be adequately trained in correct collection techniques. This includes the correct use of collection equipment, collection procedures, and specimen handling. The capillary puncture procedure must be completed quickly so that blood will not clot during the collection process. The puncture site must not be squeezed excessively; instead, the site selected for puncture should be gently warmed or massaged before the puncture is made. Proper sampling technique is the first step toward obtaining reliable patient test results with capillary blood.

Selecting the Puncture Site

All materials should be assembled within easy reach of the phlebotomist (Figure 1-76). The capillary puncture procedure should be explained to the patient. The patient's fingertips should be examined for a suitable site that is not calloused and has good blood circulation. Patients whose work involves physical labor can have very calloused fingertips and the technician must take extra care to find a suitable site. Warm skin indicates adequate circulation; cool

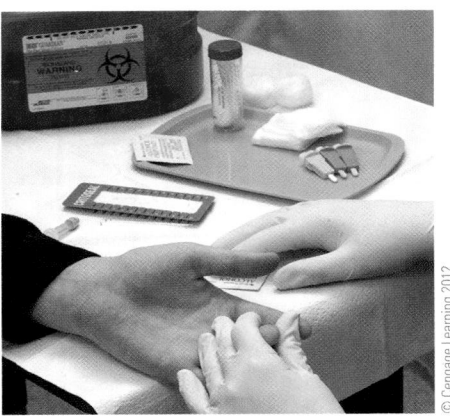

FIGURE 1-76 Assemble equipment and examine patient's fingers to locate the best puncture site

skin indicates decreased circulation. A patient's hands can be gently massaged briefly to enhance circulation. Recent puncture sites should be avoided, especially in pediatric patients.

Preparing the Puncture Site

An alcohol swab should be used to cleanse the puncture site. The site must then be allowed to air-dry or can be wiped dry with sterile gauze. A puncture should not be made on moist skin because the blood will not form a good drop.

Performing the Puncture

The patient's hand and finger should be held so the puncture site is readily accessible. Using a safety lancet, the puncture is made at the tip of the fleshy pad and slightly to the side (Figure 1-77A). A lancet with a longer blade can be used for fingertips that are calloused or have thickened skin. The lancet should be discarded into a nearby sharps container (Figure 1-78).

Collecting the Blood Sample

The first drop of blood should be wiped away with dry, sterile gauze. This first drop contains tissue fluid, which dilutes the blood drop and can also activate clotting. The second and following drops of blood are used for the test sample. A well-rounded drop of blood should be allowed to form before collection begins (Figure 1-77B). The hand can be gently massaged to increase blood flow, but excessive pressure near the puncture site should be avoided. (Squeezing the fingertip can force tissue fluid into the blood sample.)

Capillary blood should be collected as quickly as possible to prevent clotting. The capillary tube should be held in an almost horizontal position, or tilted slightly downward; the blood collecting vial should be held vertically so blood will flow down into the tube (Figure 1-77C, D). When the tip of the capillary tube is touched to the blood drop, blood will enter the tube by **capillary action** because of the attraction between the liquid and the tube. Capillary tubes should be filled three-quarters full.

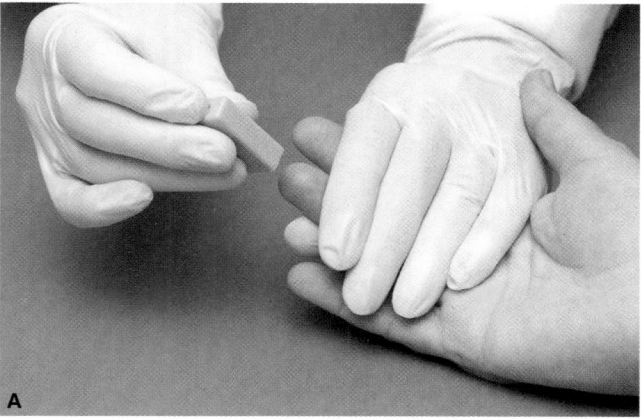
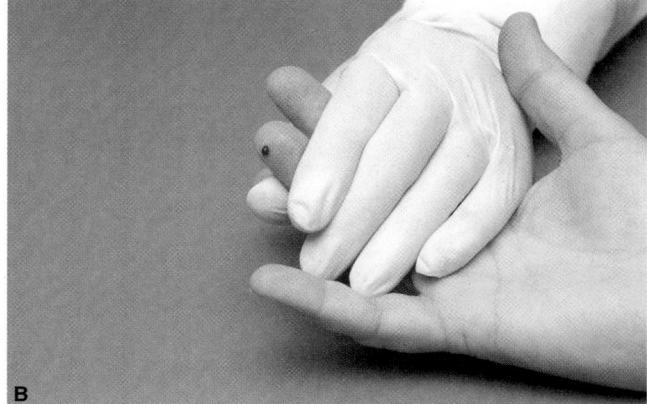
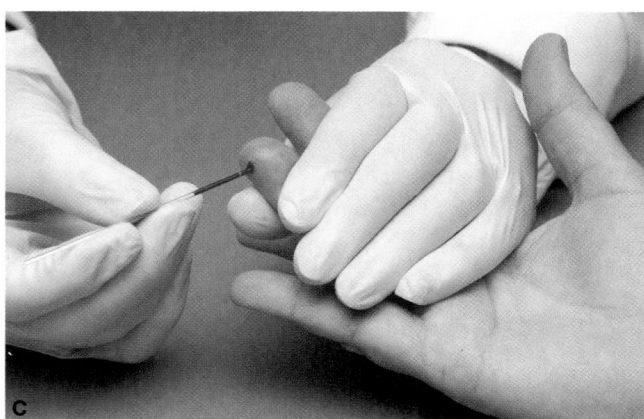
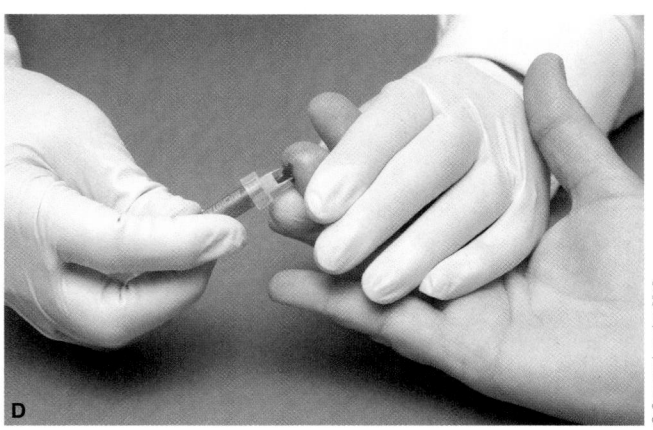

FIGURE 1-77 Performing the capillary puncture: (A) perform puncture on cleansed fingertip; wipe away first blood drop and (B) allow rounded drop of blood to form; (C) collect blood into capillary tube or (D) collection vial

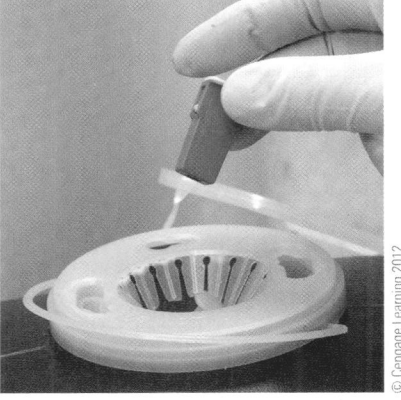

FIGURE 1-78 Discard used lancet into sharps container

Test strips or cartridges are filled following the manufacturer's directions.

Caring for the Puncture Site

After the blood has been collected, sterile gauze or a cotton ball should be placed on the puncture site and pressure applied until bleeding stops. A small adhesive bandage can be applied if necessary.

SAFETY REMINDERS

- Review Safety Precautions section before performing puncture.
- Observe Standard Precautions.
- Wear appropriate PPE.
- Use plastic or Mylar-sheathed capillary tubes.

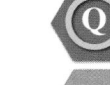
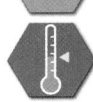

PROCEDURAL REMINDERS

- Review Quality Assessment section before beginning procedure.
- Select a puncture site with good circulation.
- Allow puncture site to dry before performing puncture.
- Wipe away the first drop of blood.
- Do not squeeze the finger excessively.

CASE STUDY 1

Mr. Stewart, a construction worker, came into the clinic for a blood cholesterol test. When Robert, the laboratory technician, performed a capillary puncture on him, he was unable to obtain the amount of blood needed for the procedure ordered.

Explain the steps Robert can take to obtain adequate capillary blood flow before he repeats the capillary puncture.

CASE STUDY 2

In the multiphysician office a young couple is told to take their 4-month-old infant to the laboratory to have blood taken. The requested test requires just two drops of blood. Jackie, the laboratory technician, is not sure if she should collect the blood from the baby's heel or finger.

1. Which site should she use?
2. Explain your answer.

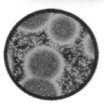

SUMMARY

Capillary puncture is used to obtain blood when only a small quantity is needed or when blood must be collected from children and infants. Capillary puncture is performed using a disposable lancet. Blood is usually collected into capillary tubes, special capillary collection containers, or can be applied directly onto the test strip or cartridge of a POC instrument. Although capillary puncture is a relatively easy procedure to perform, care must be taken to use proper techniques so that a quality sample is obtained. Because capillary blood clots very rapidly, the technician must have the competency to complete the task quickly. The quality of the capillary specimen will have a direct impact on the quality and reliability of the test results.

Capillary puncture has become more common because of the increased use of compact analyzers that require only small quantities of blood for testing. These analyzers are used for POC testing, such as at the bedside, in the emergency room, or in the physician's office, to perform several tests formerly only done in the hematology and chemistry laboratories. Because the tests are usually complete within just a few minutes, the healthcare provider can receive the test results quickly, improving patient care.

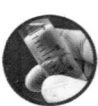

REVIEW QUESTIONS

1. What is a capillary puncture?
2. Why are capillary punctures performed?

3. What are the usual puncture sites for adults and for infants?
4. How is a capillary puncture site prepared?
5. What is the procedure if circulation seems poor at the selected site?
6. Why is the first drop of blood wiped away?
7. List the safety precautions that must be observed when performing a capillary puncture.
8. When is a capillary tube with a blue band used?
9. When is a capillary tube with a red band used?
10. Why must the blood from capillary puncture be used quickly?
11. What is the advantage of using plastic capillary tubes?
12. List three important aspects of quality assessment in capillary puncture.
13. Define capillary, capillary action, capillary tube, heparin, lancet, and lateral.

STUDENT ACTIVITIES

1. Complete the written examination for this lesson.
2. Practice performing a capillary puncture as outlined on the Student Performance Guide.
3. Find out how capillary punctures are performed on newborns in a local hospital nursery.

WEB ACTIVITIES

1. Search online laboratory supply catalogs to find examples of plastic or Mylar-coated capillary tubes.
2. Search the Internet for reliable sources offering tutorials or videos that demonstrate capillary or dermal puncture techniques.

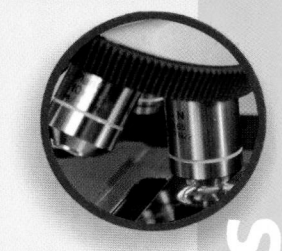

LESSON 1-11
Capillary Puncture

Name _____ Date _____

INSTRUCTIONS

1. Practice the procedure for performing a capillary puncture following the step-by-step procedure.

2. Demonstrate the procedure for capillary puncture satisfactorily for the instructor, using the Student Performance Guide. Your instructor will explain the procedures for grading and evaluating your performance. Your performance may be given a number grade, a letter grade, or satisfactory (S) or unsatisfactory (U) depending on course or institutional policy.

NOTE: Follow manufacturer's instructions for the type of capillary tubes or collection vials used.

MATERIALS AND EQUIPMENT

- gloves
- hand antiseptic
- full-face shield (or equivalent PPE)
- sterile, disposable lancets
- sterile cotton balls or gauze squares
- alcohol swabs
- small adhesive bandage (finger-size)
- Mylar-coated, self-sealing capillary tubes (heparinized and plain)
- precalibrated capillary tubes (optional)
- capillary collection vials
- sealant pad (optional)
- paper towels
- surface disinfectant (such as 10% chlorine bleach)
- biohazard container
- sharps container

PROCEDURE

Record in the comment section any problems encountered while practicing the procedure (or have a fellow student or the instructor evaluate your performance).

S = Satisfactory
U = Unsatisfactory

You must:	S	U	Evaluation/Comments
1. Wash hands with antiseptic and put on gloves and face protection			
2. Assemble materials and equipment			
3. Explain the procedure to the patient			
4. Select and warm the puncture site			
5. Cleanse the puncture site with alcohol			
6. Allow the site to air-dry or wipe dry with sterile gauze or cotton			

(Continues)

© 2012 Delmar, Cengage Learning. Permission to reproduce for clinical use granted.

You must:	S	U	Evaluation/Comments
7. Position the puncture site, holding the skin taut with one hand and holding the lancet in the other hand			
8. Perform the capillary puncture; press the lancet firmly against the selected site and activate trigger mechanism			
9. Wipe away the first drop of blood with sterile gauze or cotton			
10. Massage the hand gently to produce a well-formed second drop of blood			

11. Collect the blood specimen into capillary tubes following steps 11a and 11b or steps 12a–12d for collection vial:
   a. Fill a capillary tube three-quarters full (fill to the line if using precalibrated tubes; follow manufacturer's directions for the type of tube used)
   b. Fill a second tube in the same manner and seal the tubes			

12. Collect capillary blood into a collection vial:
   a. Select the correct capillary collection vial
   b. Follow manufacturer's directions for the type of collection vial used
   c. Touch the vial opening to a well-formed drop of blood and allow the container to fill, working quickly to prevent clotting
   d. Seal the vial			

13. Apply pressure to the puncture site by pressing with dry sterile gauze or cotton ball. Instruct patient to continue applying pressure; apply small adhesive bandage if necessary			
14. Discard sharps into sharps container			
15. Discard all other contaminated materials into biohazard container			
16. Return supplies to proper storage			
17. Wipe the work surface with disinfectant			
18. Remove gloves and discard into biohazard container			
19. Wash hands with antiseptic			

Instructor/Evaluator Comments

Instructor/Evaluator _____   Date _____

© 2012 Delmar, Cengage Learning. Permission to reproduce for clinical use granted.

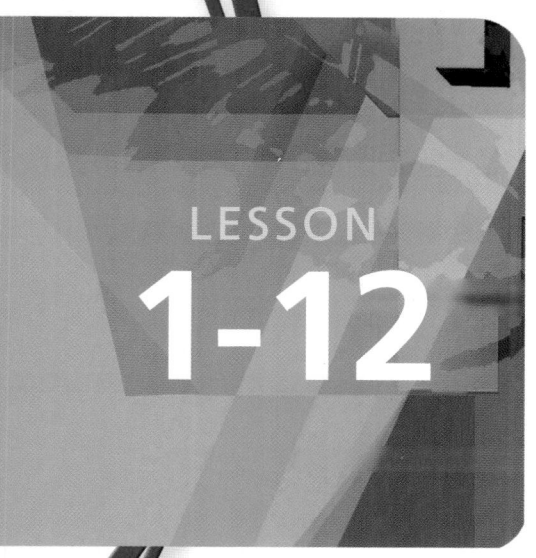

Routine Venipuncture

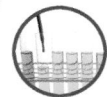

LESSON OBJECTIVES

After studying this lesson, the student will:

- ⦿ Explain why venipuncture is performed.
- ⦿ Describe the venipuncture procedure.
- ⦿ Discuss three methods for performing venipuncture.
- ⦿ Select the equipment necessary to perform a venipuncture.
- ⦿ Apply a tourniquet.
- ⦿ Select a proper venipuncture site.
- ⦿ Perform a venipuncture.
- ⦿ List the safety precautions to be observed when performing a venipuncture and give the rationales.
- ⦿ Discuss factors that can affect the quality of a blood specimen obtained by venipuncture.
- ⦿ Name three common anticoagulants in blood collecting tubes and state why they are used.
- ⦿ Explain the reasons why the order of draw is important.
- ⦿ Define the glossary terms.

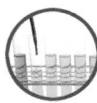

GLOSSARY

basilic vein / large vein on inner side ("pinky" side) of arm

cephalic vein / a superficial vein of the arm (thumb side) commonly used for venipuncture

gauge / a measure of the internal diameter (or bore) of a needle

ethylenediaminetetraacetic acid (EDTA) / an anticoagulant commonly used in hematology

hematoma / the swelling of tissue around a vessel resulting from leakage of blood into the tissue

hemoconcentration / increase in the concentration of cellular elements in the blood

hemolysis / rupture or destruction of red blood cells resulting in the release of hemoglobin

hypodermic needle / a hollow needle used for obtaining fluid specimens or for injections

lumen / the open space within a tubular organ or tissue

median cubital vein / a superficial vein located in the bend of the elbow (cubital fossa) that connects the cephalic vein to the basilic vein

order of draw / a prescribed order for filling vacuum tubes during blood collection to prevent contaminating one tube with the additive of another

palpate / to examine by touch

(continues)

phlebotomy / venipuncture; entry of a vein with a needle

syringe / a hollow, tube-like container with a plunger, used for withdrawing fluids or for injections

tourniquet / a band used to constrict blood flow

vein / a blood vessel that carries deoxygenated blood from the tissues to the heart

venipuncture / entry of a vein with a needle; a phlebotomy

winged collection set / a short, small-gauge needle with attached plastic tabs (wings), six or more inches of tubing and a Luer-Lok or vacuum tube holder connector; sometimes called "butterfly" set

INTRODUCTION

Venipuncture is a common method of obtaining blood for laboratory examination. The venipuncture is a quick way to obtain a large sample of blood on which many different analyses can be performed. In a venipuncture, also called a **phlebotomy**, a superficial **vein** is punctured with a **hypodermic needle** and blood is collected into a vacuum tube or **syringe.**

Performing a venipuncture involves several important steps that must be thoroughly understood before the procedure is attempted:

- Observing Standard Precautions and other safety measures throughout procedure
- Selecting the proper equipment
- Identifying the patient using two identifiers
- Preparing the patient for venipuncture
- Selecting and preparing the puncture site
- Applying and removing the tourniquet
- Obtaining the blood
- Caring for the puncture site
- Observing the patient for adverse reaction
- Labeling blood specimens immediately following blood collection

The venipuncture is a safe procedure when performed correctly by trained personnel. These personnel can include phlebotomists, medical assistants, nursing staff, physicians, medical laboratory technicians, and medical laboratory scientists. The venipuncture must be performed carefully to preserve the condition of the vein. Much observation and practice under the supervision of an experienced phlebotomist is required to become skilled and self-confident in the art of venipuncture.

VENIPUNCTURE MATERIALS AND SUPPLIES

Venipuncture can be performed using a safety needle/collection tube holder assembly (Figure 1-79), a safety needle and syringe (Figure 1-80), or a **winged collection set** with tubing and tube holder (Figure 1-81). Other materials required for venipuncture include evacuated blood collecting tubes, alcohol swabs, sterile gauze, disposable tourniquet, and small adhesive bandage (Figure 1-79).

Needles

The length and **gauge** (internal diameter) of the needle used for venipuncture vary. Venipuncture needles can be from 3/4 inch

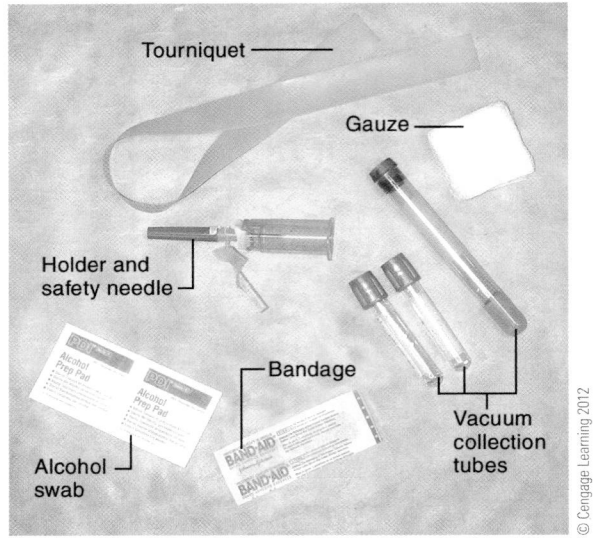

FIGURE 1-79 Venipuncture supplies

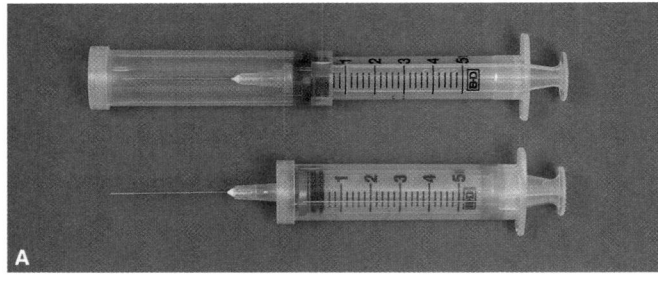

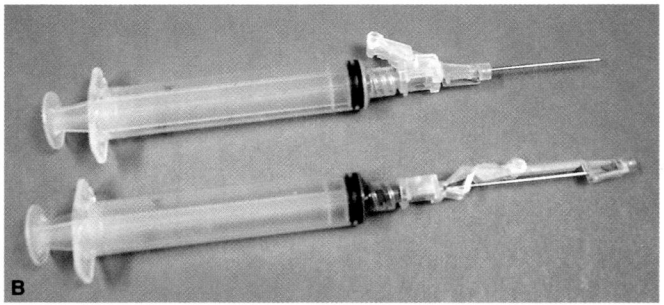

FIGURE 1-80 Safety syringes: (A) with sliding plastic sheath covering needle; (B) with sliding needle cap

to 1½ inches in length. For routine venipuncture, 21-gauge × 1- or 1½-inch needles are used. (The higher the gauge number, the smaller the needle internal bore.) Larger bore needles are required for collection of blood donor units.

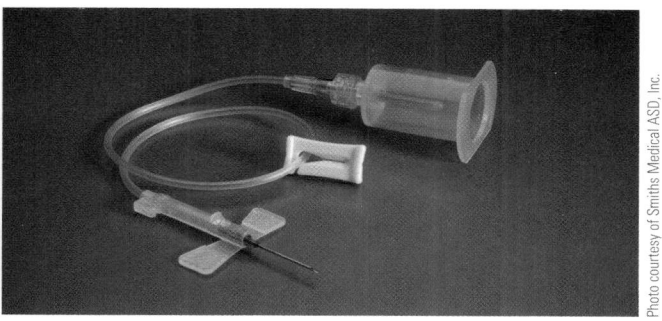

FIGURE 1-81 Saf-T Wing® Blood collection set with pre-attached Saf-T Holder® device

Photo courtesy of Smiths Medical ASD, Inc.

Venipuncture needles used with vacuum tube holders are double-ended. The short, rubber-sheathed end of the needle inside the tube holder is used to pierce the top of the vacuum tube during blood collection (Figure 1-82B). The long end of the needle, covered by a removable plastic cap, is used to puncture the vein.

Safety devices must be used when performing venipuncture. In response to the mandates to use safer methods to minimize or prevent accidental needlesticks, manufacturers of phlebotomy supplies have modified designs of needles, vacuum tube systems, syringes, and winged collection systems to include a variety of safety features (Figures 1-80 and 1-82). One system uses safety needles with in-vein activation, meaning that the needle is retracted as it is removed from the vein. Other systems use a standard needle and a disposable needle/tube holder with needle guard. After venipuncture, the guard snaps over the exposed needle, and the entire unit is discarded (Figure 1-82D). Improved designs are continually being developed.

Vacuum Tubes

Vacuum tubes, blood collecting tubes from which most of the air has been evacuated, are available in a variety of types and sizes. The majority of vacuum tubes are plastic. Each tube is

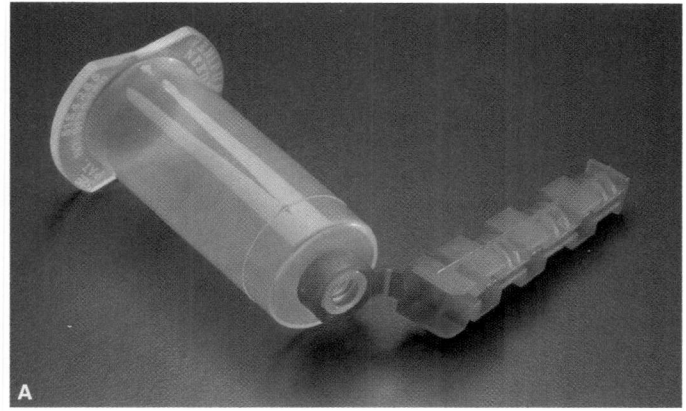

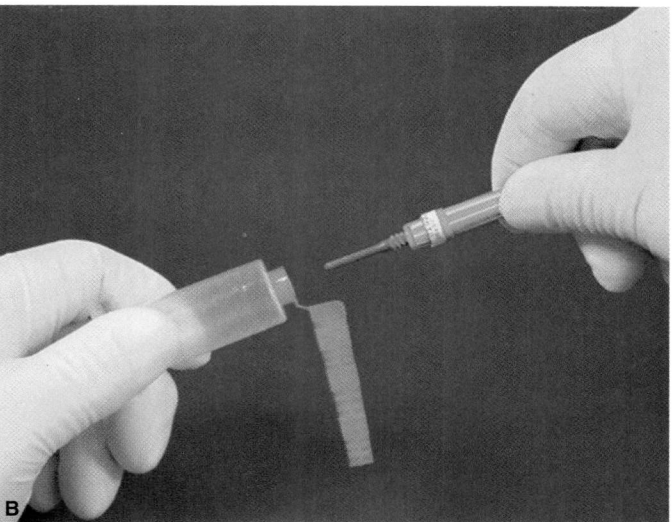

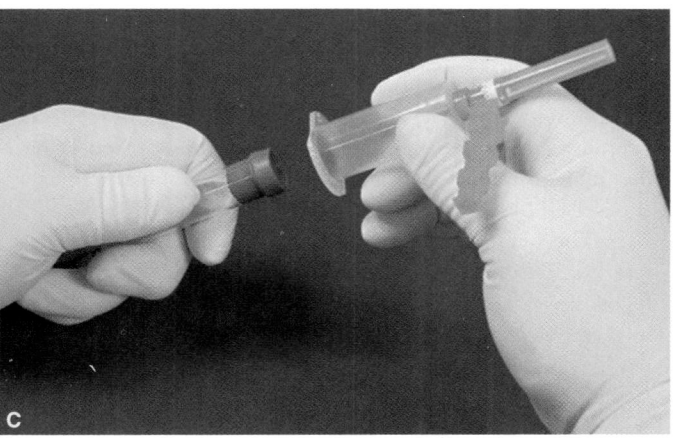

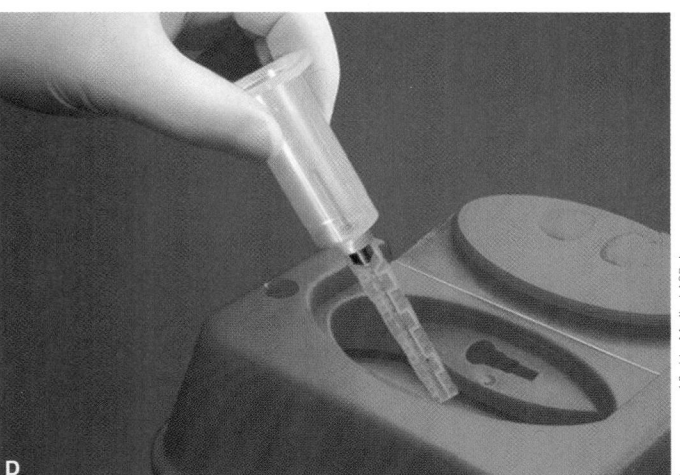

Photo courtesy of Smiths Medical ASD, Inc.

FIGURE 1-82 Vacuum tube blood collecting system incorporating a safety device: (A) disposable needle holder with needle safety guard; (B) inserting sheathed short end of needle into needle holder; (C) assembled holder and needle accepting blood collecting tube; (D) discarding entire used needle/holder assembly into sharps container

manufactured to draw a specific volume of blood; common vacuum tube total capacities are 2, 3, 4, 5, 6, and 8.5 mL.

Tubes are sealed with color-coded stoppers. The stoppers can be recessed within a color-coded plastic guard cap that protects the worker from contact with blood when the tube is opened.

Anticoagulants and Additives

The standard operating procedure (SOP) manual will include a list of tests performed and the type and size of vacuum tube that should be used when collecting blood for each test. The cap colors of the blood collection tubes designate which, if any, anticoagulant or additive is present (Figures 1-83 and 1-84). In some cases, the color coding for tubes with plastic stopper shields is slightly different from the stopper colors of tubes without the shield. A color guide should be on hand for the phlebotomist to reference when necessary.

When multiple tubes must be filled during a venipuncture, a particular **order of draw**, such as shown in Figure 1-84, must be used. Filling tubes in the correct order prevents cross contamination of anticoagulants between tubes, which could adversely affect test results. (A more comprehensive order of draw list is in Lesson 6-2.)

When the tube stopper or cap is pierced by the blunt end of the venipuncture needle, the vacuum draws the blood into the tube. It is important that tubes be filled to their stated capacities because an incorrect blood:anticoagulant ratio can alter cell morphology and cause erroneous test results, especially in coagulation tests. Some tubes have a fill line marked on the tube to easily determine if blood volume is sufficient. For certain tests, tubes with anticoagulant can still be used for tests if they are not completely filled but are at least 70% full. The laboratory's SOP

manual will specify the tests for which the level of tube fill is critical. For example, one requirement for coagulation specimen acceptability is that citrate tubes must be filled to at least 90% capacity.

Red-top tubes contain no anticoagulant and are used for tests that are performed on serum, primarily blood chemistries. Tubes with red-gray stoppers, called serum separator tubes, contain clotting activators to initiate clotting along with a gel serum separator. During centrifugation, the red cells displace the gel as a result of the centrifugal force, moving the gel from the tube bottom to a position separating cells from serum.

For procedures that use plasma, blood is collected with a specific anticoagulant. Tubes with lavender tops contain **ethylenediaminetetraacetic acid (EDTA)**, the anticoagulant used for most hematology studies such as cell and differential counts. Tubes with light blue tops contain sodium citrate, the anticoagulant used for most coagulation studies. Gray-top tubes containing potassium oxalate anticoagulant and sodium fluoride (to inhibit glycolysis) are used for glucose tests and blood alcohol level tests. Green-top tubes containing heparin anticoagulant are used for several types of chemistry analyses and special hematology tests. Heparinized tubes with plasma separator gels are also available; these are centrifuged to separate red cells from plasma in the same manner as serum separator tubes.

PERFORMING A VENIPUNCTURE

Venipuncture is performed using a vacuum-tube system, a syringe, or a winged collection set. The safety guidelines and quality assessment considerations are the same for all venipuncture methods.

Safety Precautions

  The phlebotomist must observe Standard Precautions and wear gloves when performing venipuncture. The phlebotomist should wear personal protective equipment (PPE), such as a buttoned, fluid-resistant laboratory coat and face protection. Phlebotomy trays used to transport or hold blood-collecting supplies should never be placed on the patient's bed or over-bed table. Students learning to perform venipuncture must be supervised by a qualified instructor.

The venipuncture site must be carefully chosen. The laboratory's SOP manual will have instructions for the procedure to follow if venipuncture attempts are unsuccessful. The phlebotomist can be tempted to use the **basilic vein** in these cases. (The basilic vein is on the "pinkie" side of the arm when the palm is facing upward and is often readily visible). However, the basilic vein should *not be used* for venipuncture because of the potential for causing damage to the nerves and tendons in this area. The patient can suffer permanent nerve damage and continuing pain from improperly performed basilic vein venipuncture, and the phlebotomist can be held liable.

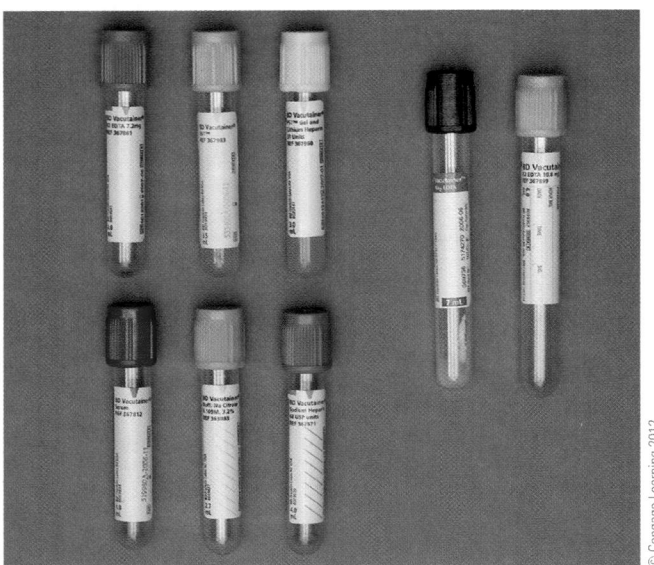

© Cengage Learning 2012

FIGURE 1-83 Plastic vacuum tubes with color-coded Hemogard® caps

ORDER OF DRAW		Cap Color	Use	Additive	Special Directions
First		Special	Blood culture	Culture media	Must draw first; Use sterile technique
		Clear (Discard tube)	Fill before filling blue-top tube when using butterfly set	None	Discard tube
		Light blue	Coagulation studies	Sodium citrate	Invert 3-4 times
		Red	Chemistry	No anticoagulant (glass), Silicon coating (palstic)	Do not invert (glass) Invert 5 times (plastic)
		Red/gray	Chemistry	Clot activatior, gel separator	Invert 5 times
		Gold (SST)	Chemistry	Gel separator, clot activator	Invert 5 times
		Green	Chemistry	Heparin	Invert 8 times
		Lavender	Hematology, hemoglobin A1c	EDTA	Invert 8 times
Last		Gray	Blood alcohol	Potassium oxalate, Sodium fluoride	Do not cleanse site with alcohol, Invert 8-10 times
		Gray	Glucose	Potassium oxalate, Sodium fluoride	Invert 8-10 times

© Cengage Learning 2012

FIGURE 1-84 Order of draw and color guide to blood collection tubes

Venipuncture products with enhanced safety designs should be used. Several types of safety needles, needle holders, syringes, and winged collection sets are available (Figures 1-79, 1-80 and 1-81). Used needles must never be recapped. After use, the needle safety feature must be immediately engaged and the used needle discarded into a rigid, puncture-proof biohazard sharps container (Figure 1-82D). The correct use of engineering controls such as safety needles should decrease the incidence of accidental needlesticks and possible transmission of bloodborne pathogens associated with needlesticks. However, workers must continue to be aware of the potential for injury since no system is 100% safe 100% of the time.

Quality Assessment

 Specimen collection is the first step in ensuring quality test results on blood samples. Specimen collection parameters required for each laboratory test are described in the laboratory procedure manual and must be followed.

The phlebotomist must identify the patient using two patient identifiers, select the correct tubes for blood collection, collect the specimen under the proper conditions, label the tubes appropriately, and deliver the specimen to the testing site within the specified time limits. Tubes should not be prelabeled, to prevent the possibility of using a prelabeled tube for the wrong patient. Specimen quality can be compromised because of improper venipuncture technique as well as the improper handling, transport, or storage of the specimen. Some test procedures require special collection and handling, such as immediate placement of the blood specimen in an ice bath or protecting the specimen from light.

Two conditions that can occur as a result of improper blood collection technique are hemolysis of the specimen and hemoconcentration in the venous circulation. Either of these two conditions will adversely affect test results. **Hemolysis**, the rupture of red blood cells, can cause erroneous hematology and blood chemistry results. Specimen hemolysis can occur if the gauge of the collection needle is too small. Hemolysis can also be caused by slowing of blood flow into the collection tube because of incorrect positioning of the needle in the vein. **Hemoconcentration** can occur when the tourniquet is left on too long before the venipuncture is performed. This can cause localized stasis in the vein and artificially alter the concentration of blood constituents in the blood specimen.

Performing a Venipuncture Using a Vacuum-Tube System

The vacuum tube blood collection system consists of a double-ended safety needle, needle holder, and evacuated blood tube. The safety needle and holder should be selected and assembled and the correct vacuum tube(s) selected. Phlebotomy supplies should be within easy reach of the phlebotomist. Supplies can be organized on a table adjacent to the phlebotomy chair or in a portable phlebotomy tray (Figure 1-85), so that supplies are readily accessible at patient bedside. A portable phlebotomy tray should hold a sharps disposal container, gloves, and face protection, in

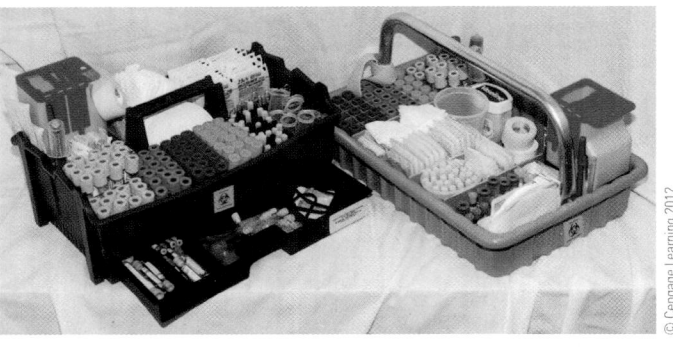

FIGURE 1-85 Phlebotomy trays stocked with specimen collection supplies and sharps container

addition to the required venipuncture supplies. Because portable phlebotomy trays can become contaminated, they should not be placed on surfaces that patients use, such as beds or overbed tables.

Preparing the Patient

The patient should be identified using two patient identifiers. For outpatient testing, the phlebotomist can ask the patient's name and verify the name on the laboratory request form. If the patient is hospitalized, the phlebotomist should ask the patient's name, and check the patient's identification band against the request form and any preprinted labels. For some critical procedures, such as collecting blood for pretransfusion testing, the phlebotomist can place an additional identification wristband on the patient that is coded to the labels placed on the blood-collection tubes.

The venipuncture procedure should be fully explained to the patient to minimize apprehension. The patient should be lying down or seated in a chair that has arm supports. The patient's arm must be fully extended and firmly supported so that it will remain still during the venipuncture. The phlebotomist should be trained in first aid procedures to be prepared for the occasional patient who might faint.

Applying the Tourniquet

A **tourniquet** is applied to the arm to make the veins more prominent. Disposable nonlatex tourniquets are preferred, because they eliminate both the need to disinfect tourniquets that contact blood as well as exposure of sensitive patients to latex.

The tourniquet is placed under the arm 2 to 4 inches above the elbow and the two ends of the tourniquet are stretched and crossed over the top of the arm. The tourniquet end that is to the front is stretched, and a portion is tucked behind the back end of the tourniquet to secure the tourniquet (Figure 1-86). The loop should extend downward, and the ends of the tourniquet should be directed away from the venipuncture site. When the

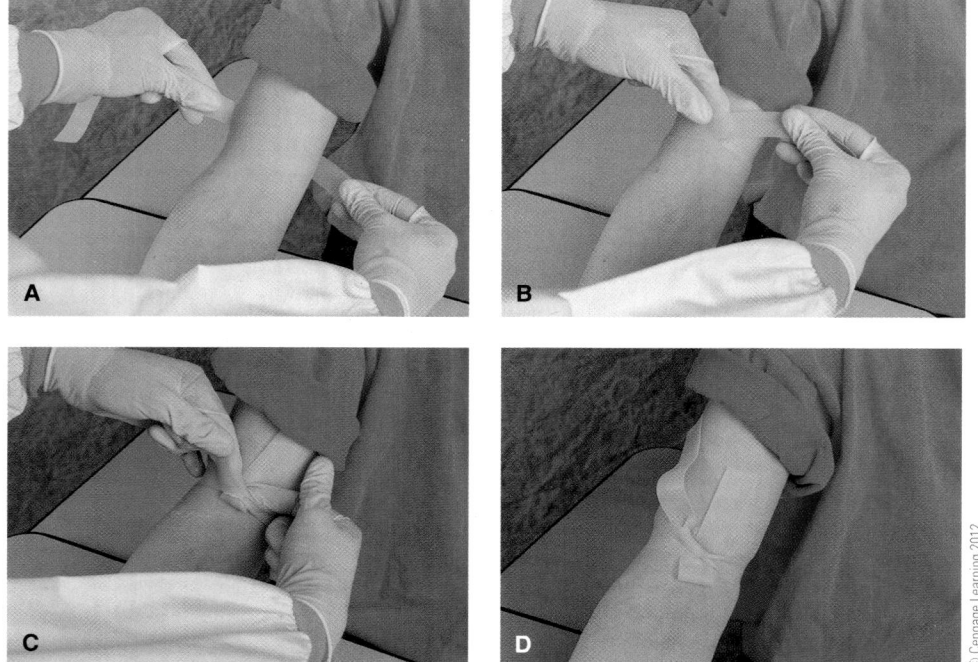

FIGURE 1-86 Applying a tourniquet: (A) place tourniquet under arm 2-4 inches above venipuncture site; (B) bring two ends of tourniquet around front of arm, stretching the two ends tight and crossing over the arm; (C) maintain tension on the tourniquet ends and tuck a portion of the front tourniquet under the back forming a loop; (D) the ends of the tourniquet are directed away from the venipuncture site

tourniquet is secured in this manner, it will release easily with a gentle pull on one end. *The tourniquet should never be tied tight enough to compromise circulation.* The tourniquet should be left in place for no more than 1 minute during venipuncture procedure.

Selecting the Venipuncture Site

The puncture site should be selected after inspecting both arms to locate the best vein. The tourniquet can be applied to aid in selection of the puncture site, but it should be released while the site is cleansed, and retied before the puncture is performed. The veins most frequently used are the **median cubital vein** and the **cephalic vein** of the forearm (Figure 1-87); the basilic vein should not be used (see Safety Precautions section).

The phlebotomist should **palpate** the vein by gently pressing the fingertip along the vein to determine its direction and estimate its size and depth (Figure 1-88). The vein will have a *bouncy* feel to it. Veins that have scarring or bruising or that have

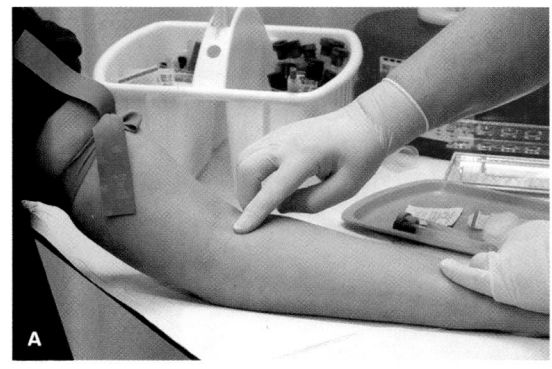

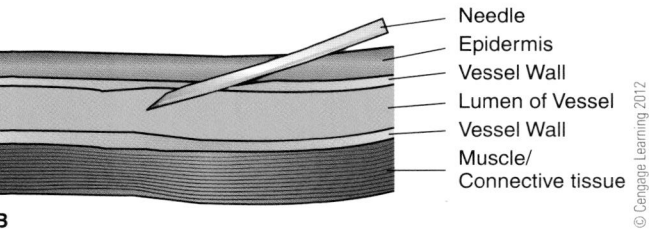

FIGURE 1-88 (A) Palpating a vein with fingertip; (B) illustration of proper angle of needle insertion into lumen of vein

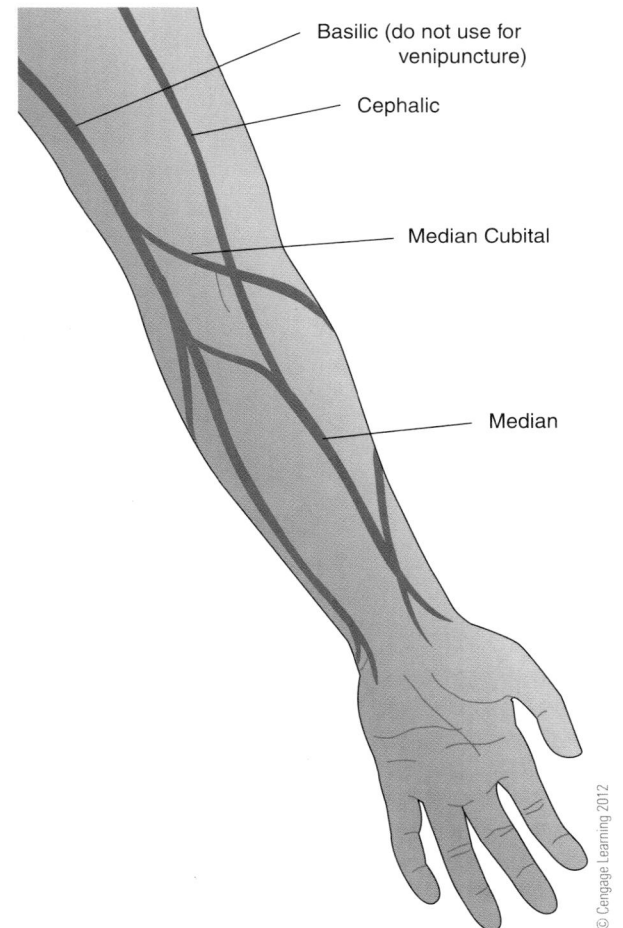

FIGURE 1-87 Cephalic or median cephalic veins are commonly used for venipuncture (left arm shown); use of the basilic vein for venipuncture is not recommended

had recent venipuncture should not be used. Blood should not be collected from an arm with an intravenous line or from the arm of a patient who has had a mastectomy (breast removal) on that side.

Preparing the Venipuncture Site

The venipuncture procedure using a vacuum tube system is illustrated in Figure 1-89. The area around the puncture site should be cleansed thoroughly in a circular motion from the center outward with a 70% alcohol swab (Figure 1-89A). The site should then be allowed to air-dry or be wiped dry with sterile gauze. Once the site is cleansed, it should not be touched again except to enter the vein with the sterile needle. If the vein must be palpated again, the skin must be recleansed.

Obtaining the Blood

When the puncture site has been cleansed, the tourniquet should be reapplied to the arm, taking care that it does not touch the cleansed area. The needle/holder assembly should be held in one hand with the needle bevel facing up and the needle shaft lined up with the vein (Figure 1-89B).

The phlebotomist should hold the patient's forearm and place the thumb on the arm 1 to 1½ inches below the selected puncture site to anchor the vein (Figure 1-89B). The skin should then be pressed and pulled taut toward the phlebotomist. Holding the needle/holder at a 15- to 20-degree angle, the skin and vein should be entered in one smooth motion until the needle is in the **lumen** of the vein (Figure 1-89C). Penetration of the vein should be at a low angle (Figure 1-87B) to prevent piercing the

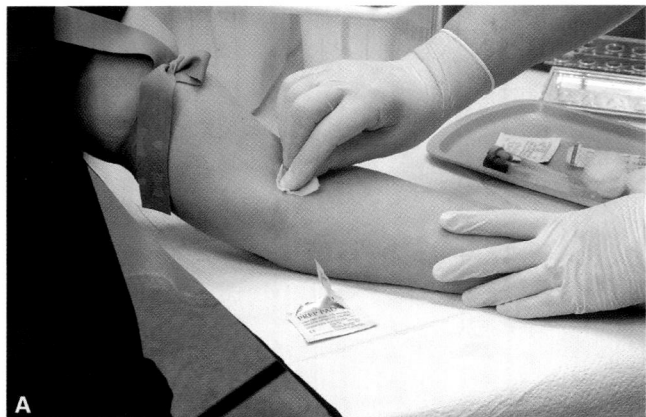

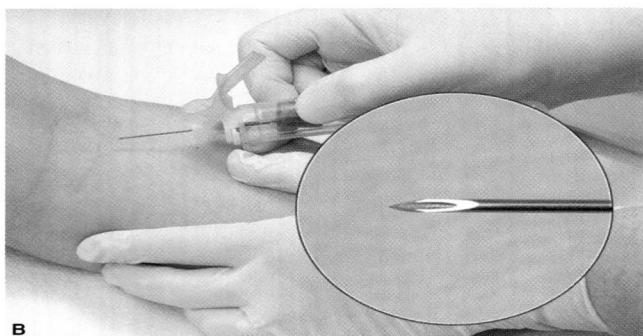

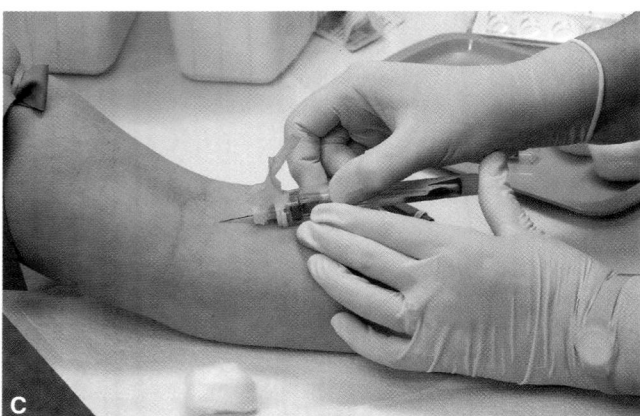

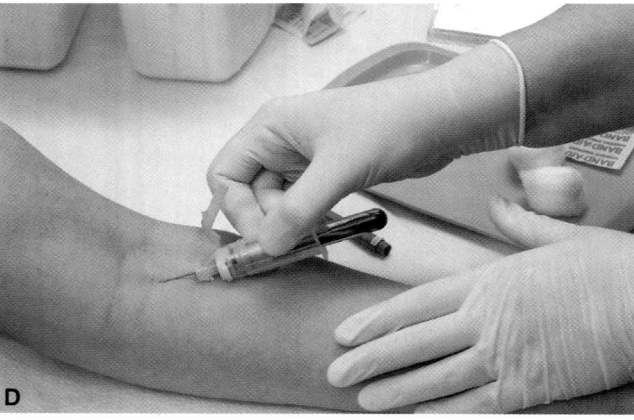

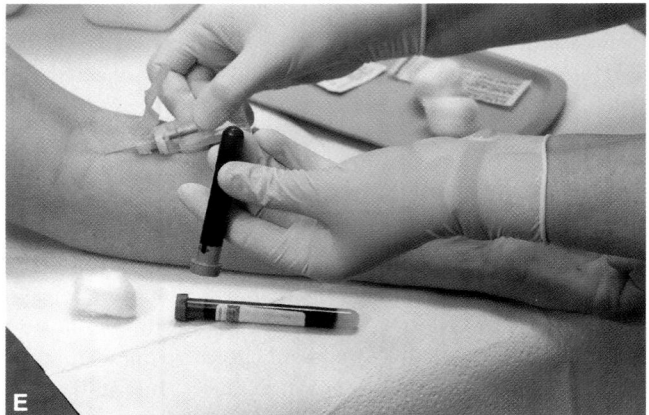

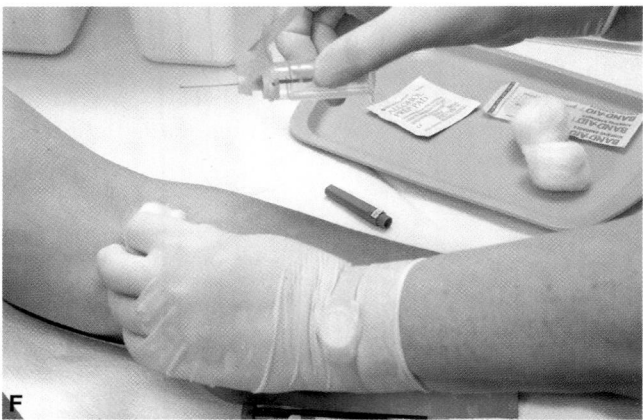

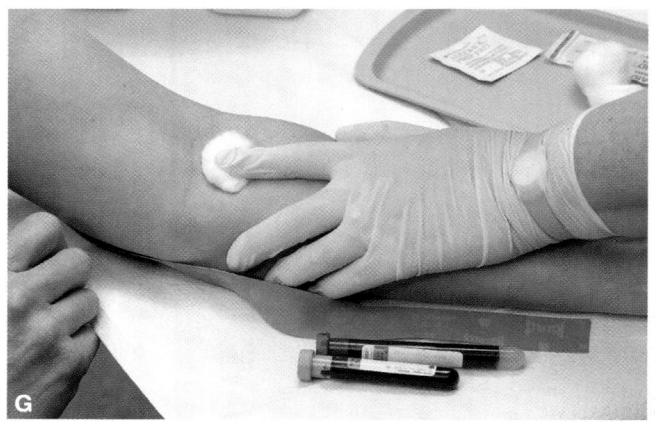

FIGURE 1-89 Performing a venipuncture using a safety needle, vacuum tubes, and tube holder: (A) Cleanse the puncture site with alcohol using a circular motion; (B) line up needle with vein, needle bevel up; (C) pierce skin and vein in one smooth motion and insert tube into holder to puncture cap of vacuum tube; (D) allow tube to fill; (E) fill additional tubes, inverting tubes to mix blood and anticoagulant; (E-F) release tourniquet and withdraw vacuum tube from holder before withdrawing needle from vein; (G) apply pressure to puncture site, keeping patient's arm extended

© Cengage Learning 2012

bottom wall of the vein, and possibly causing a **hematoma**, or swelling. *If a hematoma begins to form during the procedure, the tourniquet should be immediately released, the needle withdrawn, and gauze and pressure applied to the puncture site.*

Once the needle is in the vein, the needle holder should be steadied with one hand while the vacuum tube is gently pushed onto the sheathed needle inside the holder, allowing blood to be drawn into the tube by vacuum (Figure 1-89D). When the tube is full, it is removed from the holder. If more than one tube is needed, the second tube is then gently pushed onto the needle in the holder. The rubber sheath on the needle (inside the tube holder) prevents blood leakage between tube changes. If a citrate tube (light blue top) is to be collected, it must be filled first. Otherwise, the serum tube (red top) must be filled before tubes containing anticoagulants other than citrate. This prevents contamination of the serum tubes with anticoagulants. Tubes containing anticoagulant should be inverted gently (not shaken) a few times immediately after filling to mix the blood with the anticoagulant (see Figure 1-89E). The last tube should be removed from the needle holder before the needle is withdrawn from the vein (Figure 1-89F).

Completing the Venipuncture and Caring for the Patient

When the necessary blood has been collected, the tourniquet should be released. (Or, once the vein is entered and good blood flow is obtained, the tourniquet can be released while the remainder of blood is collected.) The tourniquet is *always* released before the needle is withdrawn from the vein to prevent hematoma formation at the venipuncture site.

As the needle is withdrawn from the vein, sterile gauze should be immediately placed over the puncture site and pressure applied (Figure 1-89G). The patient should be instructed to press the gauze on the puncture site with the arm extended to ensure that bleeding stops and a hematoma does not form.

The needle safety feature must immediately be activated as soon as the needle is withdrawn from the vein so that an accidental needlestick is not possible. Needles must not be recapped or removed from the needle holder by hand. The needle/holder unit is then discarded into a biohazard sharps container. The phlebotomist should then apply patient labels to the tubes in the presence of the patient. The labels must contain patient information, date and time of collection, and phlebotomist's name or initials.

The venipuncture site should be checked and pressure continued if the site is still bleeding. The phlebotomist should not leave the patient until bleeding has ceased. A small bandage should be applied when bleeding stops. Most sites will stop bleeding within 1 to 2 minutes.

Performing a Venipuncture Using A Syringe

Syringes can be used to obtain blood from elderly patients or patients with small veins that make routine venipuncture with vacuum tubes difficult. Table 1-36 gives some guidelines for

TABLE 1-36. Guidelines for choosing a venipuncture method		
INDICATIONS FOR USE	**METHOD**	**ADVANTAGE(S)**
Good vein	Vacuum tube system or winged collection set	Fast; fills multiple tubes for different types of tests
Elderly patients Difficult draws	Syringe or winged collection set	Less likely to collapse veins
Hand vein or other small vein in adults and small children	Winged collection set	Lower angle of needle, safer transfer of blood to vacuum tubes (compared to syringe)

choosing the appropriate venipuncture method. The phlebotomist should use syringes and/or needles designed with safety features to prevent needlesticks. Disposable syringe/needle units are available that have a retractable needle or a sliding shield to cover the needle after use. Alternatively, a safety needle with a protective sheath can be attached to a disposable syringe. The syringe plunger should be pushed up and down to be sure that it moves freely. It should then be left pushed completely into the barrel so that no air remains in the syringe. The syringe should be held so that the bevel of the needle faces up.

The syringe venipuncture procedure is the same as with the vacuum tube system except that instead of the vacuum tube drawing the blood automatically, the phlebotomist must steady the syringe with one hand while the other hand gently pulls back on the plunger to draw blood into the syringe (Figure 1-90). The needle should be observed while the syringe is filling to be sure it is not accidentally pulled out of the vein. After the syringe is filled and the tourniquet released, the needle is withdrawn from the vein, the needle safety feature is activated, and blood is transferred to a vacuum tube using a special transfer device, such as the BD Vacutainer Blood Transfer Device (Figure 1-91). After the blood is transferred, the filled collection tube is removed from the holder, and the syringe and transfer device are discarded into a biohazard sharps container.

Performing a Venipuncture Using A Winged Collection Set

Winged collection sets can be used for routine venipuncture of the median cubital or cephalic veins, providing these veins are not located deep under the skin. Winged collection sets, also called butterfly sets, are especially useful for obtaining

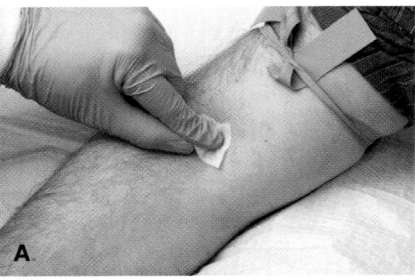

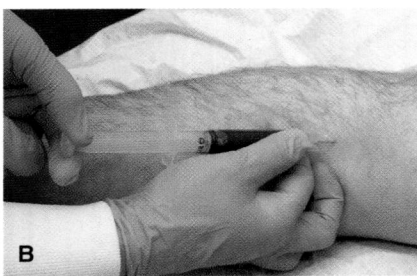

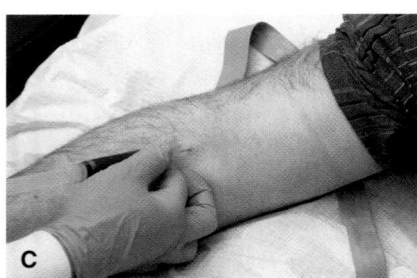

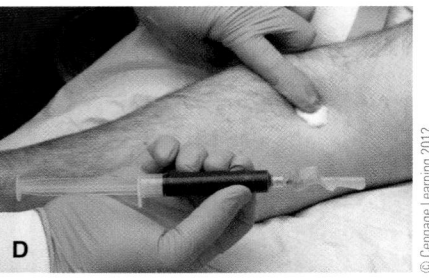

FIGURE 1-90 Performing venipuncture using syringe: (A) cleanse puncture site, anchor vein and insert needle; (B) hold syringe with one hand while pulling back on plunger with the other hand; (C) release tourniquet and (D) apply pressure to site immediately after removing needle

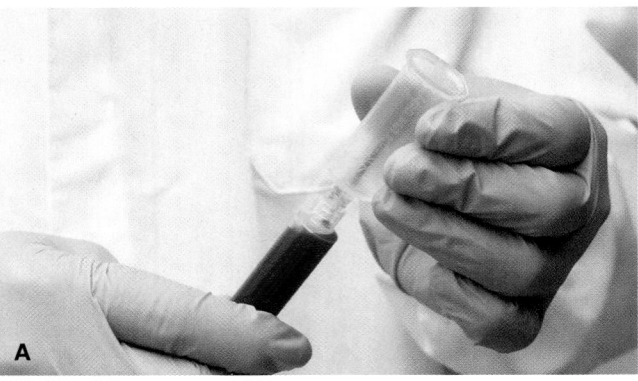

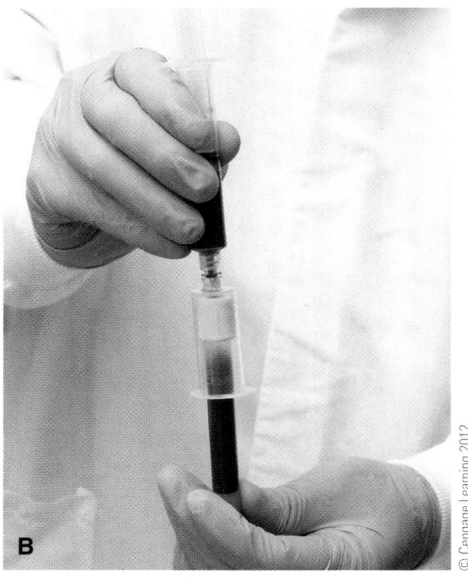

FIGURE 1-91 Using a needleless transfer device to transfer blood from syringe to blood collection tube: (A) attach transfer device to Luer lock of syringe; (B) push collecting tube into holder

blood from small children, elderly patients or other patients with small veins or veins that tend to roll, and from veins of the hand or wrist (Table 1-36).

The winged collection set has a small gauge needle attached to a length of tubing which has a connector for syringe or vacuum tube holder on the opposite end of the tubing (Figures 1-81 and 1-92). The winged set incorporates a needle safety feature to prevent accidental needlestick.

Venipuncture using a winged collection system is similar to the procedure using a vacuum tube system. The tube holder is attached to the collection set tubing and the collection tube is selected. The puncture site is selected and cleansed, and the needle shield is removed. The needle is inserted into the vein at a very low angle, holding the needle unit by grasping the plastic "wings" together (Figure 1-92B) or by holding the body of the needle unit behind the wings. When the vein is successfully entered, a flash of blood will be seen (Figure 1-92C). The collection tube is inserted into the tube holder and allowed to fill. When blood collection is complete, the needle is retracted into the device by depressing the button as the needle is withdrawn from the vein (Figure 1-92D). Pressure is applied to the puncture site and the entire collection set is discarded into a biohazard sharps disposal container (Figure 1-92G).

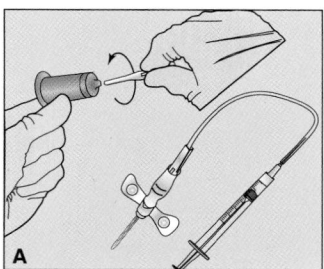
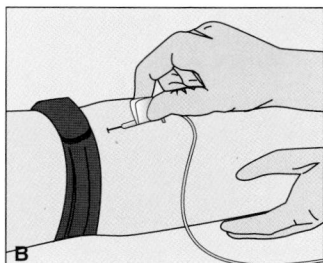
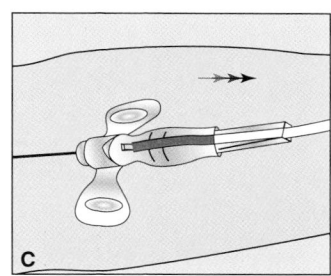
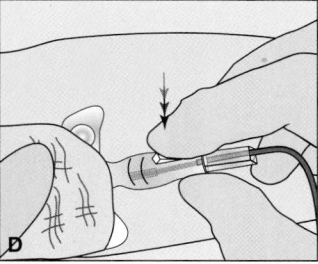
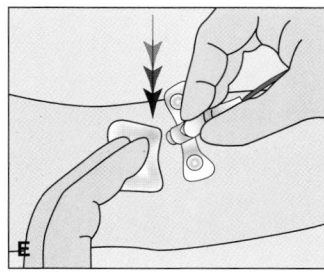
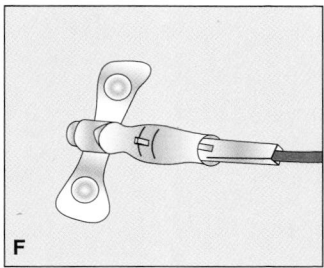
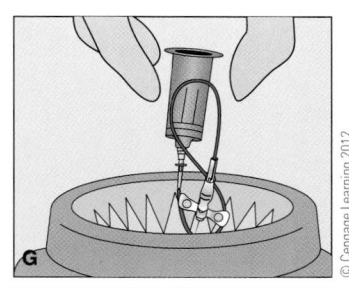

© Cengage Learning 2012

FIGURE 1-92 Performing venipuncture using a winged collection system: (A) attach tube holder or syringe to collection set; (B) remove shield and insert needle into vein by grasping wings together or holding body of device; (C) observe "flash" of blood behind "wings"; (D) when blood collection is complete, activate safety feature while needle is still in vein by depressing button with index finger; (E) apply pressure to venipuncture site; (F) confirm that needle is retracted; and (G) discard entire set into sharps disposal container

ATTENTION!

ACTION TO TAKE IN CASE OF EXPOSURE INCIDENT

 In case of needlestick, other injury from sharps, or if eyes, nose, mouth, or broken skin are exposed to blood or other potentially infectious material (OPIM):

1. Immediately flood the exposed area with water and clean skin with antiseptic soap and water.
2. Report accident immediately to supervisor or appropriate safety officer.
3. Seek immediate medical attention.

SAFETY REMINDERS

- Review Safety Precautions section before performing venipuncture.
- Observe Standard Precautions.
- Use safety needles and other safety devices.
- Do not attempt to recap needles.
- Discard sharps into sharps container.
- Check patient and venipuncture site before leaving patient.

PROCEDURAL REMINDERS

- Review Quality Assessment before beginning the procedure.
- Review venipuncture procedure before attempting venipuncture.
- Identify patient using two identifiers.
- Fill collection tubes to capacity.
- Label filled tubes as soon as venipuncture is completed.

CASE STUDY 1

Jerry was completing his fourth week of MLS internship at Pleasant Valley Hospital. All interns were required to collect blood from 8 to 10 patients each morning before beginning the day's clinical rotation. Jerry had completed his phlebotomy rotation the previous week, so he was collecting blood on his own (without supervision). One of the patients on his collection list was 72 years old. Jerry saw only one adequate vein in the patient's left arm but was unable to obtain blood when he attempted venipuncture.

1. What should Jerry do?
    a. Stick the same vein again
    b. Try a different vein using a syringe or winged collection set
2. Discuss factors that cause venipuncture to be difficult and explain how these venipunctures can be handled.

CASE STUDY 2

Katie, a medical assistant in a POL, is asked to collect blood for transport to a reference laboratory. After consulting the specimen collection manual, she determined that she will need to collect a gray-capped tube, an EDTA tube, and a serum tube.

1. Which is the correct order of draw for filling these tubes?
    a. gray first, then lavender, then red
    b. red first, then lavender, then gray
    c. red first, then green, then gray
    d. lavender first, then gray, then red
2. If the orders had included collection of a citrate tube for coagulation studies, what would the order of draw be for the four tubes?

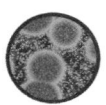

SUMMARY

Venipuncture is a common method of obtaining blood for routine laboratory analysis. The procedure is safe when performed by personnel trained in phlebotomy techniques. Venipuncture can be performed using a vacuum tube collecting system, a syringe, or a winged collection system. The phlebotomist must use the proper technique to obtain the blood, the correct tubes must be selected for the tests ordered, and special handling conditions must be followed. This information is provided in the laboratory's SOP manual.

The phlebotomist must follow Standard Precautions and wear appropriate PPE when performing venipuncture. The development of safety needles and safety collection devices and the use of sharps disposal containers have increased the safety level for the phlebotomist by decreasing the risk for accidental needlesticks. However, these measures do not lessen the responsibility of the phlebotomist to use the utmost care to prevent accidental needlestick. These safety devices as well as safe work practices must be used when performing venipuncture.

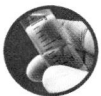

REVIEW QUESTIONS

1. Why is a venipuncture performed?
2. What is the purpose of a tourniquet?
3. How long can a tourniquet be left on?
4. Name five precautions that must be observed when performing a venipuncture.
5. How can hemoconcentration affect the quality of the blood specimen?
6. List the steps in performing a venipuncture.
7. What is the most common venipuncture site?
8. Why must the tourniquet be released before removing the needle from the vein?

9. How should the puncture site be cared for after the needle is removed?

10. Explain briefly the vacuum system of obtaining venous blood.

11. What precautions should the phlebotomist take to avoid exposure to blood when performing a venipuncture?

12. Name three anticoagulants used in collecting blood. Which one is most commonly used in hematology?

13. Why is it important to verify patient identification before performing a venipuncture?

14. Name a situation that might require the use of a syringe or winged collection set for venipuncture.

15. Explain the advantages of using a winged collection set for venipuncture.

16. List the three actions that must be taken in case of an exposure incident.

17. Define basilic vein, cephalic vein, ethylenediaminetetraacetic acid, gauge, hematoma, hemoconcentration, hemolysis, hypodermic needle, lumen, median cubital vein, order of draw, palpate, phlebotomy, syringe, tourniquet, vein, venipuncture, and winged collection set.

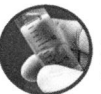 **STUDENT ACTIVITIES**

1. Complete the written examination for this lesson.

2. Practice applying a tourniquet and locating suitable veins for venipuncture.

3. Practice performing a venipuncture as outlined in the Student Performance Guides. NOTE: You must be supervised during venipuncture practice until the Instructor has approved your technique.

WEB ACTIVITIES

1. Use the Internet to find information on three safety devices used for venipuncture. Explain how each type protects the worker from accidental needlesticks.

2. Visit web sites of agencies such as the Centers for Disease Control and Prevention, Occupational Safety and Health Administration, and National Institute for Occupational Safety and Health. Look for information on preventing needlestick or sharps injury. Try to find free brochures, PowerPoint presentations, or other safety information that can be downloaded.

3. Search the Internet for videos or tutorials showing how to apply a tourniquet or how to perform a venipuncture. Use reliable sources such as phlebotomy equipment manufacturers, healthcare education programs, government sites, or online phlebotomy resources.

4. Search the Internet for videos showing how to activate various types of safety needles used for venipuncture.

LESSON 1-12
Venipuncture—Vacuum Tube Method

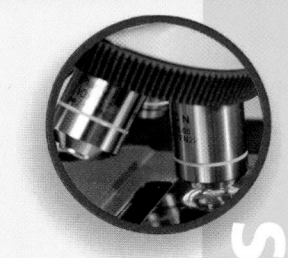

Name _____ Date _____

INSTRUCTIONS

1. Practice performing a venipuncture using a vacuum tube system and following the step-by-step procedure. *Practice this procedure only under the supervision of your instructor or a designated experienced phlebotomist.*

2. Demonstrate the venipuncture procedure using a vacuum tube system satisfactorily for the instructor, following the Student Performance Guide. Your instructor will explain the procedures for evaluating and grading your performance. Your performance may be given a number grade, letter grade, or satisfactory (S) or unsatisfactory (U) depending on course or institutional policy.

NOTE: If necessary, adjust procedure according to available venipuncture supplies

MATERIALS AND EQUIPMENT

- gloves
- hand antiseptic
- full-face shield (or equivalent PPE)
- tourniquet
- sterile gauze or cotton
- 70% alcohol or alcohol swabs
- adhesive bandage
- vacuum-tube holder with safety needle (and manufacturer's instructions for use)
- vacuum blood-collection tubes
- test tube rack
- paper towels
- sharps container
- surface disinfectant (such as 10% chlorine bleach)
- biohazard container

STUDENT PERFORMANCE GUIDE

PROCEDURE

NOTE: Perform this procedure only under your instructor's supervision.
Your instructor will evaluate your performance and record in the comment section any problems encountered while performing the procedure.

S = Satisfactory
U = Unsatisfactory

You must:	S	U	Evaluation/Comments
1. Wash hands with antiseptic and put on gloves and face protection			
2. Assemble equipment and materials			
3. Place venipuncture equipment and supplies within easy reach			

(Continues)

© 2012 Delmar, Cengage Learning. Permission to reproduce for clinical use granted.

You must:	S	U	Evaluation/Comments
4. Use two identifiers to identify the patient			
5. Explain venipuncture procedure to the patient and position the patient			
6. Obtain needle holder with sterile, capped needle (assemble if necessary)			
7. Insert vacuum-collection tube into needle holder, but do not pierce stopper with inner sheathed needle			
8. Ask the patient to extend the arm and tie the tourniquet around the patient's arm 2 to 4 inches above the elbow. It should be just tight enough to make the veins more prominent, but not so tight that it is extremely uncomfortable			
9. Inspect the arm to locate a suitable vein			
10. Palpate the vein to determine its direction, and estimate its size and depth. NOTE: The vein most frequently used is the median cubital vein of the forearm			
11. Release the tourniquet			
12. Cleanse the puncture site in a circular motion from the center out using an alcohol swab and allow alcohol to dry			
13. Retie the tourniquet, being careful not to touch the cleansed puncture site CAUTION: Do not allow the tourniquet to remain on for more than 1 minute to avoid causing hemoconcentration			
14. Uncap the needle and visually inspect it to see that the point is smooth and sharp			
15. Hold the needle/tube holder assembly so the bevel of the needle is facing upward (toward ceiling). With the thumb of your other hand placed 1 to 2 inches below the puncture site, press and hold the skin taut to anchor the vein			
16. Hold the needle at a 15- to 20-degree angle to the arm and insert it into the vein			
17. Push the vacuum tube gently onto the holder's inner sheathed needle while steadying the needle holder with the other hand			
18. Watch for blood flow into the tube			
19. Release the tourniquet when the desired amount of blood is obtained			
20. Remove the vacuum tube from the needle holder			

© 2012 Delmar, Cengage Learning. Permission to reproduce for clinical use granted.

You must:	S	U	Evaluation/Comments
21. Place a dry, sterile gauze over the puncture site and withdraw the needle from the vein, activating needle safety feature and taking care not to press down on the needle (safety needles operate differently according to brand; be sure to follow package insert directions); DO NOT ATTEMPT TO RECAP THE NEEDLE			
22. Instruct the patient to apply pressure to the puncture site keeping the arm extended			
23. Discard safety needle and tube holder into the sharps container.			
24. Label the collection tube			
25. Check puncture site for bleeding. If bleeding has not ceased, continue pressure until bleeding stops and apply bandage			
26. Discard other used supplies appropriately			
27. Discard all sharps into sharps container			
28. Discard all contaminated materials into biohazard container			
29. Return unused supplies to storage			
30. Clean the work area with disinfectant			
31. Remove gloves and discard into biohazard container			
32. Wash hands with antiseptic			

Instructor/Evaluator Comments

Instructor/Evaluator _____ Date _____

© 2012 Delmar, Cengage Learning. Permission to reproduce for clinical use granted.

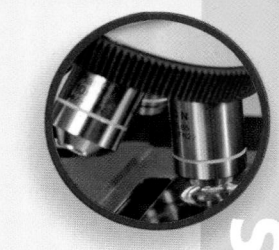

LESSON 1-12

Venipuncture—Syringe Method

Name _____ Date _____

INSTRUCTIONS

NOTE: Do not perform this procedure unless a safety adapter for transferring blood from a syringe to a vacuum tube is available!

1. Practice performing a venipuncture using a syringe following the step-by-step procedure. *Practice this procedure only under the supervision of your instructor or a designated experienced phlebotomist.*

2. Demonstrate the venipuncture procedure using a syringe satisfactorily for the instructor, following the Student Performance Guide. Your instructor will explain the procedures for evaluating and grading your performance. Your performance may be given a number grade, a letter grade, or satisfactory (S) or unsatisfactory (U) depending on the course or institutional policy.

MATERIALS AND EQUIPMENT

- gloves
- hand antiseptic
- full-face shield (or equivalent PPE)
- tourniquet
- sterile gauze or cotton
- 70% alcohol or alcohol swabs
- adhesive bandage
- disposable 10- to 12-mL syringe/safety needle assembly
- sterile, disposable 21-gauge safety needle (if syringe is not equipped with needle)
- vacuum collection tubes
- test tube rack
- safety adapter for transferring blood from syringe to vacuum tube
- paper towels
- surface disinfectant (such as 10% chlorine bleach)
- biohazard container
- sharps container

PROCEDURE

NOTE: Perform this procedure only under your instructor's supervision. Your instructor will evaluate your performance and record in the comment section any problems encountered while performing the procedure.

S = Satisfactory
U = Unsatisfactory

You must:	S	U	Evaluation/Comments
1. Wash hands with antiseptic and put on gloves and face protection			
2. Assemble equipment and materials			
3. Place venipuncture equipment and supplies within easy reach			

(Continues)

© 2012 Delmar, Cengage Learning. Permission to reproduce for clinical use granted.

You must:	S	U	Evaluation/Comments
4. Identify patient using two identifiers			
5. Explain venipuncture procedure to patient and position patient			
6. Attach the capped safety needle to the syringe, maintaining sterility (if required)			
7. Slide the plunger up and down in the barrel of the syringe to be sure it moves freely			
8. Push the plunger to the bottom of the barrel so no air remains in the syringe			
9. Ask the patient to extend the arm and tie the tourniquet around the patient's arm 2 to 4 inches above the elbow. It should be just tight enough to make the veins more prominent, but not so tight that it is extremely uncomfortable			
10. Inspect the arm to locate a suitable vein			
11. Palpate the vein with the fingertip to determine its direction and estimate its size and depth (a glove can be removed to more easily feel the vein)			
12. Release the tourniquet (put glove back on, if removed)			
13. Cleanse the puncture site in a circular motion from the center out using an alcohol swab and allow alcohol to dry			
14. Retie the tourniquet, being careful not to touch the cleansed puncture site CAUTION: Do not allow the tourniquet to remain on for more than 1 minute			
15. Instruct the patient to keep the arm extended			
16. Uncap the needle and inspect it to see that the point is smooth and sharp			
17. Hold the syringe so the volume markings on the syringe and the bevel of the needle are in full view (facing toward the ceiling). With thumb of the other hand, hold skin taut 1 to 2 inches below puncture site, anchoring the vein			
18. Hold the needle at a 15- to 20-degree angle to the arm and insert it into the vein			
19. Watch for blood flow into the syringe and use one hand to pull the plunger back slowly, filling the syringe while steadying the syringe and needle with the other hand			
20. Release the tourniquet when the desired amount of blood is obtained			

© 2012 Delmar, Cengage Learning. Permission to reproduce for clinical use granted.

You must:	S	U	Evaluation/Comments
21. Place a dry, sterile gauze over the puncture site and withdraw the needle from the vein, activating needle safety feature and taking care not to press down on the needle (safety needles operate differently according to brand; be sure to follow package insert directions)			
22. Instruct the patient to apply pressure to the puncture site while keeping the arm extended			
23. Use blood transfer device to transfer blood from syringe to vacuum tube			
24. Label the blood collection tube			
25. Discard sharps into sharps container			
26. Check puncture site to be sure bleeding has stopped; continue pressure if necessary or apply bandage if bleeding has ceased. Do not leave patient until bleeding has ceased			
27. Discard all contaminated materials into biohazard container			
28. Return unused supplies to storage			
29. Wipe the work surface with disinfectant			
30. Remove gloves and discard into biohazard container			
31. Wash hands with antiseptic			

Instructor/Evaluator Comments

Instructor/Evaluator _____ Date _____

© 2012 Delmar, Cengage Learning. Permission to reproduce for clinical use granted.

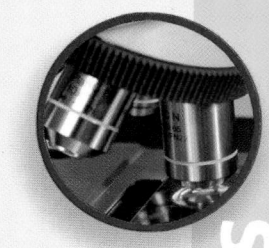

LESSON 1-12
Venipuncture—Winged Collection Method

Name _____ Date _____

INSTRUCTIONS

1. Practice performing a venipuncture using a winged collection set following the step-by-step procedure. *Practice this procedure only under the supervision of your instructor or a designated experienced phlebotomist.*

2. Demonstrate the venipuncture procedure using a winged collection set satisfactorily for the instructor, following the Student Performance Guide. Your instructor will explain the procedures for evaluating and grading your performance. Your performance may be given a number grade, a letter grade, or satisfactory (S) or unsatisfactory (U) depending on the course or institutional policy.

MATERIALS AND EQUIPMENT

- gloves
- hand antiseptic
- full-face shield (or equivalent PPE)
- tourniquet
- sterile gauze or cotton
- 70% alcohol or alcohol swabs
- adhesive bandage
- winged collection set with safety needle and vacuum tube adapter
- vacuum collection tubes
- test tube rack
- paper towels
- surface disinfectant (such as 10% chlorine bleach)
- biohazard container
- sharps container

PROCEDURE

NOTE: Perform this procedure only under your instructor's supervision. Your instructor will evaluate your performance and record in the comment section any problems encountered while performing the procedure.

S = Satisfactory
U = Unsatisfactory

You must:	S	U	Evaluation/Comments
1. Wash hands with antiseptic and put on gloves and face protection			
2. Assemble equipment and materials			
3. Place venipuncture equipment and supplies within easy reach			
4. Identify patient using two identifiers			
5. Explain venipuncture procedure to patient and position the patient			

(Continues)

© 2012 Delmar, Cengage Learning. Permission to reproduce for clinical use granted.

You must:	S	U	Evaluation/Comments
6. Remove winged collection set from package; attach vacuum tube holder (if necessary)			
7. Ask patient to extend arm and tie the tourniquet around the patient's arm 2 to 4 inches above the elbow. It should be just tight enough to make the veins more prominent, but not so tight that it is extremely uncomfortable			
8. Inspect the arm to locate a suitable vein			
9. Palpate the vein to determine its direction and estimate its size and depth (a glove can be removed to more easily feel the vein)			
10. Release the tourniquet (put glove back on, if removed)			
11. Cleanse the puncture site in a circular motion from the center out using an alcohol swab and allow alcohol to dry			
12. Retie the tourniquet, being careful not to touch the cleansed puncture site CAUTION: Do not allow the tourniquet to remain on for more than 1 minute			
13. Instruct the patient to keep arm extended			
14. Position the appropriate collection tube for easy access			
15. Grasp the plastic "wings" of the collection set between your thumb and forefinger and remove the needle cover			
16. Hold the needle at a low angle (5 to 10 degrees) with bevel facing up and slide the needle into the vein. Watch for flash of blood			
17. Push the vacuum tube into the tube holder so the blunt needle pierces the cap and blood is drawn into the tube			
18. Release the tourniquet when the desired amount of blood is obtained			
19. Place a dry, sterile gauze pad over the puncture site and activate the retractable needle as the needle is withdrawn from the vein, taking care not to press down on the needle.			
20. Instruct the patient to apply pressure to the puncture site with the arm extended			
21. Discard used winged collection set into sharps container, needle end first			
22. Label the blood collection tube(s)			
23. Check puncture site to be sure bleeding has stopped; continue pressure if necessary or apply bandage if bleeding has ceased. Do not leave patient until bleeding has ceased			

© 2012 Delmar, Cengage Learning. Permission to reproduce for clinical use granted.

You must:	S	U	Evaluation/Comments
24. Discard all contaminated materials into biohazard container			
25. Return unused supplies to storage			
26. Wipe the work surface with disinfectant			
27. Remove gloves and discard into biohazard container			
28. Wash hands with antiseptic			

Instructor/Evaluator Comments

Instructor/Evaluator _____ Date _____

© 2012 Delmar, Cengage Learning. Permission to reproduce for clinical use granted.

UNIT 2

Basic Hematology

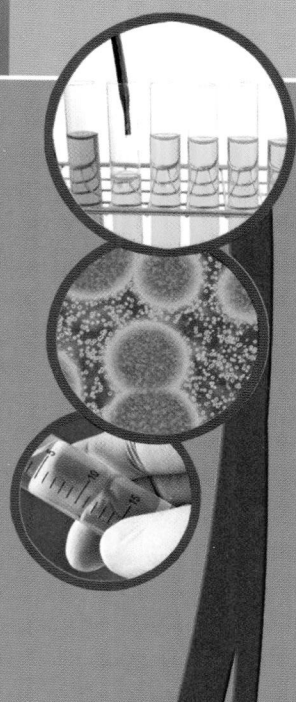

UNIT OBJECTIVES

After studying this unit, the student will:

- Explain the functions of the hematology laboratory.
- Explain how blood is formed.
- Describe the composition of blood and the function of the blood components.
- Perform a hemoglobin determination.
- Perform a microhematocrit.
- Use a hemacytometer.
- Perform a manual red blood cell count.
- Perform a manual white blood cell count.
- Perform a manual platelet count.
- Prepare and stain a peripheral blood smear.
- Identify normal blood cells from a stained blood smear and visual aids.
- Perform a white blood cell differential count.
- Explain the principles of automated cell counters.
- Interpret the information available from automated differential counts.
- Identify selected abnormal blood cells from stained smears and visual aids.
- Calculate the red blood cell indices and explain their significance.
- Perform a reticulocyte count.
- Perform an erythrocyte sedimentation rate test.
- Discuss the importance of adhering to laboratory safety policies when performing hematology procedures.
- Discuss quality assessment procedures in the hematology laboratory.

Hematology is the area of medicine involving the study of the cellular elements of blood and the blood-forming tissues. Unit 2 is an introduction to several basic procedures commonly performed in the hematology laboratory. The unit begins with a discussion of the discipline of hematology in Lesson 2-1. This includes basic information about the circulatory system, the origin of blood cells, blood composition, blood diseases, and analytical methods used in the hematology laboratory.

Information and step-by-step instructions for manually performing the tests comprising the CBC (complete blood count), one of the most frequently requested hematology tests, are spread over several lessons. The CBC has traditionally included the hemoglobin, hematocrit, red blood cell (RBC) count, white blood cell (WBC) count, WBC differential count, and RBC indices. Several additional parameters are measured and reported from a blood sample when a CBC is performed using automated cell counters or hematology analyzers.

A discussion of the theory of hemoglobin measurement and the procedure for using a hemoglobin analyzer is included in Lesson 2-2, Hemoglobin. Lesson 2-3, Microhematocrit, explains the procedure for determining the centrifuged hematocrit, also called the microhematocrit.

In Lesson 2-4, The Hemacytometer, the student learns the principles and techniques of using the hemacytometer before going on to Lesson 2-5, Manual Red Blood Cell and White Blood Cell Counts. Manual platelet counts are covered in Lesson 2-6. Although the platelet count is included on the menu of most hematology analyzers, extremely low counts are sometimes verified by a manual count.

Lesson 2-7, Preparing a Blood Smear, lays the foundation for later lessons by explaining the procedures for producing and staining a blood smear and emphasizing the importance of these techniques. Lesson 2-8 describes normal blood cell morphology and details morphological features to consider when identifying blood cells. After basic blood cell identification is mastered, the student can proceed to Lesson 2-9, White Blood Cell Differential Count.

Lesson 2-10, Principles of Automated Hematology, explains the two major principles used in hematology cell counters and analyzers. The lesson also includes information about interpreting results obtained from hematology analyzers. Red blood cell indices are routinely calculated by most cell counters and reported as part of the CBC. The formulas for calculating the RBC indices using the RBC count, hemoglobin, and hematocrit values are included in Lesson 2-10. The red cell indices estimate the size and hemoglobin content of a RBC population. Indices values are useful in studies of red cell morphology and conditions affecting RBC production and development.

Lesson 2-11, Abnormalities in Blood Cell Morphology, is intended as an introduction to a complex topic. Lesson 2-11 also explains how RBC indices can be used in the evaluation of RBC morphology. The Reticulocyte Count, explained in Lesson 2-12, is useful in evaluating the patient's response to treatment for anemia. The principles and procedures of the erythrocyte sedimentation rate (ESR) are presented in Lesson 2-13. Erythrocyte sedimentation rate results are used to help the clinician detect inflammation and evaluate treatment of some inflammatory disease processes.

Results of hematology laboratory tests provide important information used in diagnosing and treating blood diseases such as anemias and leukemias. Information from hematology tests also aids in the diagnosis and management of diseases that originate in other body systems. Practice and skill are required to perform basic hematology procedures in a reliable manner. The tests must be performed with accuracy, precision, and the utmost attention to procedure, safety, and quality assessment.

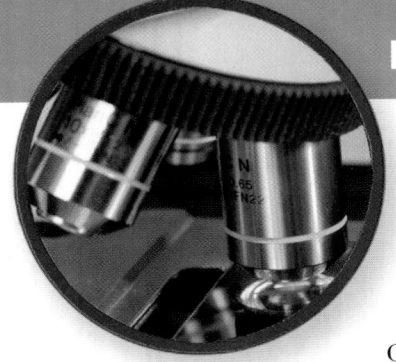

General

Baker, F. J., et al. (2001). *Baker & Silverton's introduction to medical laboratory technology.* (7th ed.). Oxford, UK: Oxford University Press.

Greer, J. P., et al. (Eds.). (2008). *Wintrobe's clinical hematology.* (12th ed.). Philadelphia, PA: Lippincott Williams & Wilkins.

Harmening, D. M. (2008). *Clinical hematology and fundamentals of hemostasis.* (5th ed.). Philadelphia: F. A. Davis Co.

HemoCue. Manufacturer's instructions. Lake Forest, CA.

Hillman, R .S., et al. (2005). *Hematology in clinical practice.* (4th ed). New York: McGraw-Hill Medical Publishing Division.

Kaushansky, K., et al. (Eds.) (2010). *Williams hematology.* (8th ed.). Columbus, OH: McGraw-Hill.

Lindh, W. Q., et al. (2010). *Delmar's clinical medical assisting.* (4th ed.). Clifton Park, NY: Delmar Cengage Learning.

McKenzie, S. B. (2009). *Clinical laboratory hematology.* (2nd ed.). Upper Saddle River, NJ: Prentice Hall.

McPherson, R. A. & Pincus, M. R. (Eds.) (2007). *Henry's clinical diagnosis & management by laboratory methods.* (21st ed.). Philadelphia: Saunders.

Rizzo, D. C. (2009). *Fundamentals of anatomy and physiology.* (3rd ed.). Clifton Park, NY: Delmar Cengage Learning.

Rodak, B. F., et al. (2011). *Hematology: clinical principles and applications.* (4th ed.). Philadelphia: Saunders.

Scott, A. S. & Fong, E. (2009). *Body structures and functions.* (11th ed.). Clifton Park, NY: Delmar Cengage Learning.

Simmers, L. (2008). *Introduction to health science technology.* (2nd ed.). Clifton Park, NY: Delmar Cengage Learning.

Turgeon, M. L. (2004). *Clinical hematology theory and procedures.* (4th ed.). Philadelphia, PA: Lippincott Williams & Wilkins.

Turgeon, M. L. (2011). *Linne & Ringsrud's clinical laboratory science: The basics and routine techniques.* (6th ed.). St. Louis, MO: Mosby.

Blood Cell Morphology, Atlases

Bain, B. J. (2006). *Blood cells: a practical guide.* Oxford, UK: Blackwell Publishing.

Bain, B. J. (2004). *A beginner's guide to blood cells.* (2nd ed.). Oxford, UK: Blackwell Publishing.

Bell, A. & Sallah, S. (2005). *The morphology of human blood cells.* (7th ed.). Abbott Park, IL: Abbott Laboratories.

Carr, J. H. & Rodak, B. F. (2004). *Clinical hematology atlas.* (2nd ed.). Philadelphia: W. B. Saunders Co.

Löffler, H., et al. (2004). *Atlas of clinical hematology.* (6th ed.). Berlin: Springer-Verlag.

Phlebotomy

Garza, D. & Becan-McBride, K. (2009). *Phlebotomy handbook: Blood specimen collection from basic to advanced.* (8th ed.). Upper Saddle River, NJ: Prentice Hall.

Hoeltke, L. B. (2006). *The complete textbook of phlebotomy.* (3rd ed.). Clifton Park, NY: Delmar Cengage Learning.

Kalanick, K. A. (2004). *Phlebotomy technician specialist.* Clifton Park, NY: Delmar Cengage Learning.

Web Sites of Interest

Centers for Disease Control and Prevention, www.cdc.gov

Clinical Laboratory Improvement Amendments, www.cma.gov/clia/

Digital blood cell morphology software such as CellAtlas iphone application, available free through itunes store at www.apple.com

Federal Drug Administration, www.fda.gov

National Institutes of Health, www.nih.gov

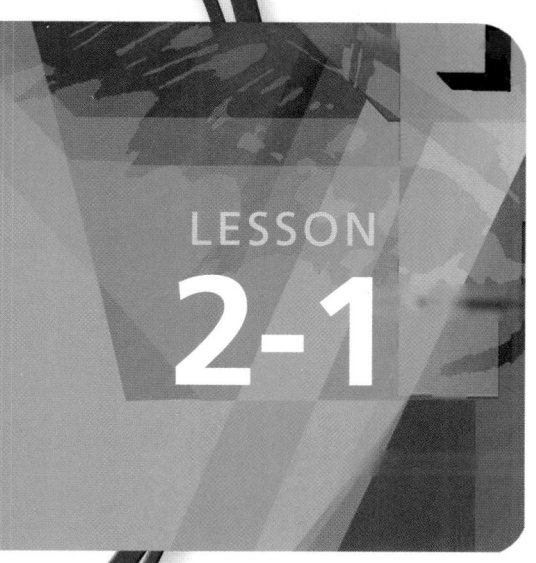

LESSON 2-1 Introduction to Hematology

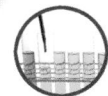

LESSON OBJECTIVES

After studying this lesson, the student will:

⊙ Explain the differences in the cardiopulmonary circulation and systemic circulation.

⊙ Discuss the origin of blood cells.

⊙ List five components of plasma.

⊙ Name the three types of formed elements in blood.

⊙ Describe the appearance of the three types of formed elements of blood and state the function of each.

⊙ List the five types of white blood cells.

⊙ Name the preferred specimens for most hematology tests.

⊙ Name eight tests that are included in the complete blood count (CBC).

⊙ Explain safety precautions that must be observed in the hematology laboratory.

⊙ Discuss the importance of quality assessment (QA) programs in hematology.

⊙ Name two inherited hematological diseases.

⊙ Define secondary or acquired hematological disease.

⊙ Discuss why stem cells can be useful in treating disease.

⊙ Define the glossary terms.

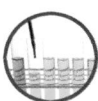

GLOSSARY

anemia / a condition in which the red blood cell count or hemoglobin level is below normal; a condition resulting in decreased oxygen-carrying capacity of the blood

anticoagulant / a chemical or substance that prevents blood coagulation

arteriole / a small branch of an artery leading to a capillary

artery / a blood vessel that carries oxygenated blood from the heart to the tissues

capillary / a minute blood vessel that connects the smallest arteries to the smallest veins and serves as an oxygen exchange vessel

cardiopulmonary circulation / the system of blood vessels that circulates blood from the heart to the lungs and back to the heart

complete blood count (CBC) / a commonly performed grouping of hematological tests

deoxyhemoglobin / the hemoglobin formed when oxyhemoglobin releases oxygen to tissues

(continues)

EDTA / ethylenediaminetetraacetic acid; an anticoagulant commonly used in hematology

erythrocyte / red blood cell; RBC

Ethylenediaminetetraacetic acid (EDTA) / an anticoagulant commonly used in hematology

granulocyte / a white blood cell containing granules in the cytoplasm; any of the neutrophilic, eosinophilic, or basophilic leukocytes

hematology / the study of blood and the blood-forming tissues

hematopoietic stem cell / see hemopoietic stem cell

hemoglobin (Hb, Hgb) / the major functional component of red blood cells that is the oxygen-carrying molecule

hemopoiesis / the process of blood cell formation and development; hematopoiesis

hemopoietic stem cell / an undifferentiated bone marrow cell that gives rise to blood cells; also called hematopoietic stem cell

hemostasis / the process of stopping bleeding, which includes clot formation and clot dissolution

leukemia / a chronic or acute disease involving unrestrained increase in leukocytes

leukocyte / white blood cell; WBC

megakaryocyte / a large bone marrow cell from which platelets are derived

oxyhemoglobin / the form of hemoglobin that binds and transports oxygen

plasma / the liquid portion of blood in which the blood cells are suspended; the straw-colored liquid remaining after blood cells are removed from anticoagulated blood

platelet / a formed element in circulating blood that plays an important role in blood coagulation; a small disk-shaped fragment of cytoplasm derived from a megakaryocyte; a thrombocyte

red blood cell (RBC) / blood cell that transports oxygen (O_2) to tissues and carbon dioxide (CO_2) to the lungs; erythrocyte

stem cell / an undifferentiated cell

systemic circulation / the system of blood vessels that carries blood from the heart to the tissues and back to the heart

thrombocyte / a blood platelet

vein / a blood vessel that carries deoxygenated blood from the tissues to the heart

venule / a small vein connecting a capillary to a vein

white blood cell (WBC) / blood cell that functions in immunity; leukocyte

INTRODUCTION

Hematology is the branch of medicine concerned with studying the formed elements of blood (blood cells) and the blood-forming tissues. The formed elements of blood—red blood cells, white blood cells, and platelets—are examined in the hematology laboratory. The tests can be qualitative, such as observing and recording blood cell morphology, or quantitative, such as performing white blood cell (WBC) or red blood cell (RBC) counts or determining the hematocrit. The study of **hemostasis**, the process of stopping bleeding, which includes both clot formation (coagulation) and clot dissolution (fibrinolysis), is included in the study of hematology.

Hematological tests can give important information about a patient's general well-being. The hematology laboratory also performs tests to detect diseases such as anemias, leukemias, and inherited blood disorders such as hemophilia and sickle cell anemia. Hematological test results can be used to evaluate the success of treatments for conditions such as anemias, leukemias, and cancer. Common tests performed in the hematology laboratory are presented in this Unit. Hemostasis principles and coagulation tests are covered in Unit 3, Basic Hemostasis.

THE CIRCULATORY SYSTEM

The circulatory system performs several vital functions, including

- delivery of oxygen (O_2), nutrients, water, and hormones to tissues and cells
- removal of carbon dioxide (CO_2) and other waste products from tissues and cells
- regulation of body temperature
- protection against infection

These functions are carried out by the *blood*, the fluid that circulates through the vessels of the circulatory system and bathes the tissues.

In the **cardiopulmonary circulation**, blood circulates from the heart to the lungs and back to the heart. Oxygen exchange occurs in the lungs when O_2 is picked up by the blood and CO_2 is released (Figure 2-1). In the **systemic circulation**, blood is carried from the heart to the tissues and back to the heart, providing O_2 to tissues and cells in exchange for CO_2, a waste product (Figure 2-2).

Blood is circulated by three major types of vessels: arteries, capillaries, and veins. The average adult human body contains

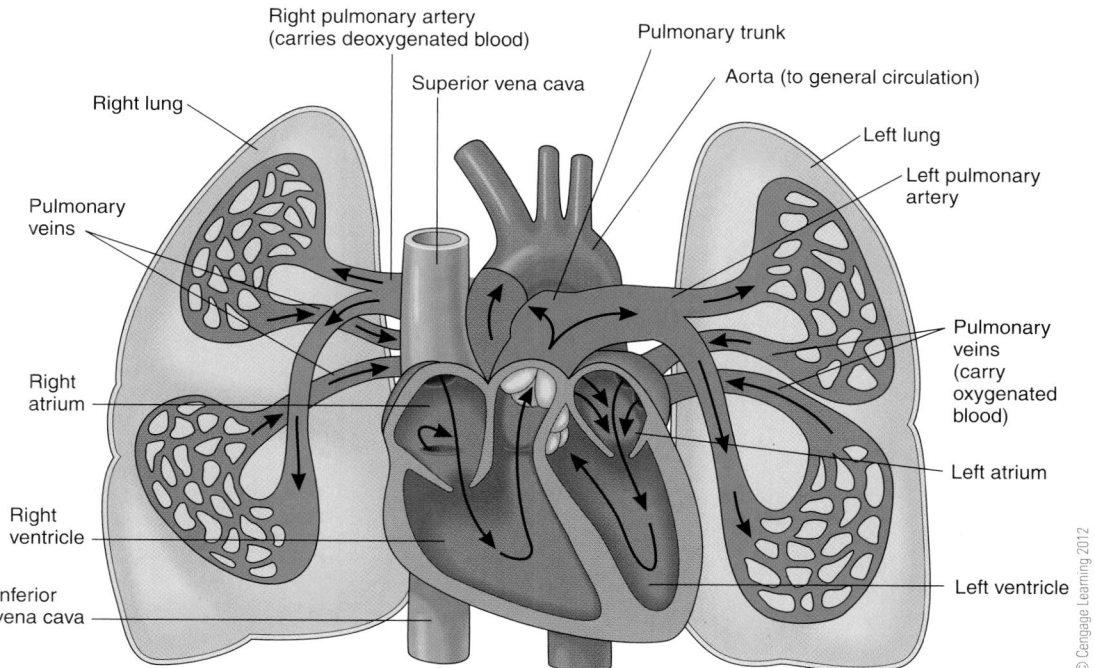

FIGURE 2-1 Diagram of cardiopulmonary circulation

about 60,000 miles of blood vessels. In general, arteries carry oxygenated blood and veins carry deoxygenated blood.

Arteries are thick-walled, elastic, and muscular and are the strongest type of blood vessel (Figure 2-2). The aorta is the largest artery in the body. Blood flows from the heart through the aorta into a series of successively smaller arteries and **arterioles** (small branches of arteries) that eventually diverge to form a network of capillaries (Figure 2-3).

Capillaries are the smallest of the blood vessels and connect the smallest arterioles with the smallest veins, called **venules** (Figure 2-3). Capillaries have thin walls allowing fluid, nutrients, and waste products to easily pass through these walls to or from the tissue cells. Oxygenated and deoxygenated blood are both present in capillary beds, the site of O_2–CO_2 exchange.

Veins carry deoxygenated blood from the capillaries to the heart. Capillaries expand into venules and then into veins that eventually converge to larger and larger vessels and form the largest vein, the vena cava. The walls of veins are not as thick, muscular, or elastic as those of arteries (Figure 2-2). Veins have valves that allow blood flow in only one direction—toward the heart.

COMPOSITION OF BLOOD

Blood makes up 6% to 8% of total body weight. A normal adult's blood volume is approximately 5 L, or 10 times the volume of a blood donor unit. Blood is composed of cellular elements suspended in a complex fluid, **plasma** (Figure 2-4). Approximately 50% to 60% of blood volume is plasma; the rest is primarily red blood cells.

Plasma

Plasma is more than 90% water; the remainder is dissolved solids, including proteins such as albumin and antibodies, lipids, carbohydrates, amino acids, hormones, and electrolytes. Most of these substances are measured in the clinical chemistry department. Plasma also contains blood coagulation proteins necessary for normal blood clotting and for dissolving blood clots.

Cellular Elements of Blood

The cellular elements of blood are commonly called blood cells. These include **red blood cells (erythrocytes)**, **white blood cells (leukocytes)**, and **platelets** (also called **thrombocytes**). Most hematology tests are designed to evaluate or measure a characteristic or function of one or more of the three blood cell types (Figure 2-5).

Red Blood Cells

Red blood cells (RBCs) are the most numerous blood cell (Figure 2-5). Each microliter (μL) of blood contains approximately 5 million red blood cells; that means *1 drop* of blood contains about 250 million red cells! Red blood cells live an average of 120 days in the circulation and remain in the vessels of the circulatory system for their entire life span. Senescent (old) red blood cells are removed from circulation by the phagocytic cells in the spleen and components such as iron are recycled to make hemoglobin for new red blood cells.

The primary function of red blood cells is to transport O_2 to the tissues and CO_2 to the lungs. This function is performed by the **hemoglobin** molecules, the major component of RBCs.

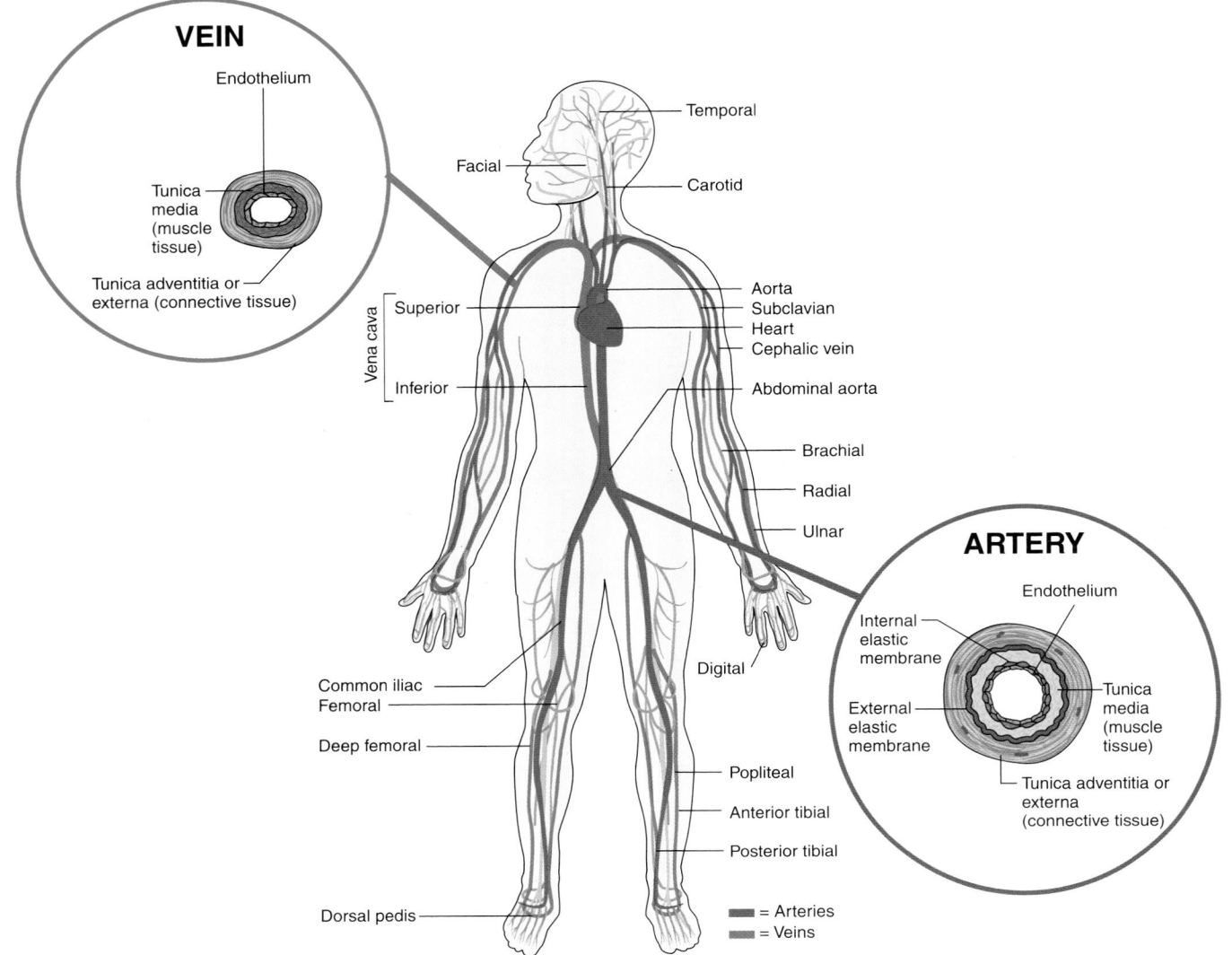

FIGURE 2-2 Systemic circulation showing the differences in the structure of veins and arteries

Hemoglobin gives blood its red color. Arterial blood is bright red because of the **oxyhemoglobin**, hemoglobin that has bound O_2. Venous blood is dark red because of the presence of **deoxyhemoglobin**, hemoglobin that has released O_2.

White Blood Cells

White blood cells (WBCs) are the least numerous cell in peripheral blood (Figure 2-5). Each microliter of blood contains approximately 5,000 to 10,000 WBCs, which equals 5.0×10^9 to 10.0×10^9 per liter of blood.

Five types of WBCs are present in normal blood: *neutrophils, basophils, eosinophils, lymphocytes,* and *monocytes.* The neutrophils, basophils, and eosinophils are called **granulocytes** because of granules present in the cell cytoplasm.

White blood cells have varied life spans, from a few days to several years. Each type of white cell has unique functions, but all are associated with immunity or defense against infection, foreign substances, or tumor cells. White blood cells perform most of their functions in the tissues and use blood as a means of transport from one part of the body to another.

Platelets

Platelets are not complete cells but instead are fragments of cytoplasm that have been released into circulating blood from large cells in the bone marrow called **megakaryocytes** (Figure 2-5). Platelets average about 300,000 per microliter of blood and have a life span of approximately 10 days in the blood. Platelets are important in several stages of hemostasis. They help stop bleeding by forming a plug in injured or damaged vessel walls. They also release chemicals and enzymes that are important in another stage of hemostasis, the coagulation cascade.

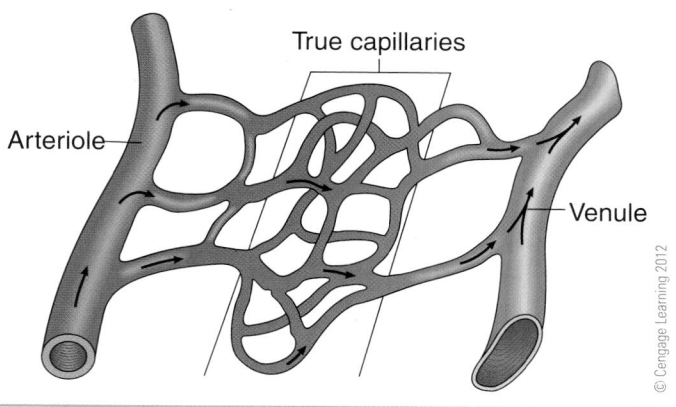

FIGURE 2-3 Capillary bed connecting an arteriole with a venule

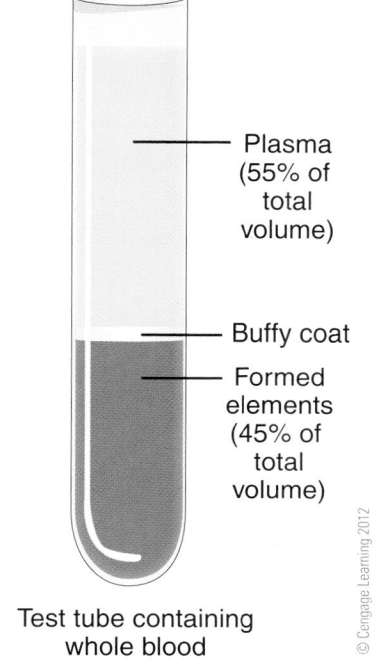

FIGURE 2-4 Diagram of a tube of blood showing separation of formed elements from plasma

ORIGIN OF BLOOD CELLS

Hemopoiesis (also called hematopoiesis) is the formation and development of blood cells. In the young fetus, blood cells are made in the fetal liver. As the fetus develops, the bone marrow begins to take over this function. In adults, the cellular elements of blood are produced in the bone marrow. Lymphocytes are produced in bone marrow and also in secondary lymphoid tissue such as the spleen and lymph nodes. After a period of development and maturation in the bone marrow, mature blood cells are released into the circulating blood, where they function in respiration (RBCs), immunity (WBCs), and hemostasis (platelets). (See Figure 2-5.)

Blood cells require the same basic growth factors and nutrients for their synthesis as other cell types. In addition, because red blood cells are very specialized, they require iron, vitamin B_{12}, and folic acid for proper formation and maturation.

Blood cells are continuously produced throughout an individual's life. All blood cells are derived from an undifferentiated bone marrow cell called the **hemopoietic**, or **hematopoietic**, **stem cell**. These cells continuously replicate and differentiate into all of the blood cell types, thus replenishing the body's blood cells (Figure 2-6).

The presence of stem cells in bone marrow is the basis for using bone marrow transplants to treat hematological disorders such as leukemia and aplastic anemia, and to combat the damaging effects of cancer chemotherapy on blood cell production. The fact that the umbilical cord blood of newborns is rich in stem cells provides an additional donor source of stem cells. Because cord blood is routinely collected when the umbilical cord is cut at birth, it is now possible to harvest these cells and use them for transplantation.

HEMATOLOGICAL DISEASES

Many diseases involve primarily the blood cells. Some of these diseases are caused by faulty or insufficient production of a cell type. In **anemia**, red cell numbers are below normal. Anemia can be due to decreased red cell production, such as might be seen when a person has an iron deficiency. Anemia can also result when blood loss is more rapid than bone marrow blood cell production, such as when a person has a bleeding ulcer. For example, in **leukemia**, too many white blood cells are produced. *Thrombocytopenia*, a low platelet count, can lead to bleeding problems. Thrombocytopenia can have several causes including viral infections, drug interactions, and *hypersplenism*, a complex condition in which the spleen is overactive in removing cells from circulation.

Hematological diseases can also be due to defective cell function. Often, a disease is due to a combination of improper cell production and defective function, as with most anemias and leukemias. For example, in iron-deficiency anemia the patient does not produce enough red blood cells and the cells that are produced do not function properly because they do not contain enough hemoglobin. This results in fatigue, pallor, and shortness of breath, typical symptoms of anemia caused by decreased oxygen available to the tissues. In leukemia, although the patient has many leukocytes, the cells have not matured properly and cannot provide immunity. The leukemia patient can be highly susceptible to infections, even though the white blood cell count is high.

Inherited Hematological Diseases

Some hematological diseases, such as *hemophilia*, are inherited. People who have hemophilia have bleeding problems either because they lack one of the coagulation factors required for blood to clot or because one of the coagulation factors is defective. In other inherited hematological diseases, patients can have abnormal hemoglobin function, such as that

	White Blood Cell (Leukocyte)	Red Blood Cells (Erythrocytes)	Platelets (Thrombocytes)
Function	Immunity (extravascular)	Transport of oxygen and carbon dioxide (intravascular)	Stoppage of bleeding
Formation	Bone marrow, lymphatic tissue	Bone marrow	Bone marrow
Size	9–18 micrometers	6–8 micrometers	1–4 micrometers
Shape	Nuclear shape varies	Bioconcave disc	Varied
Life span	Varies, 24 hours–years	100–120 days	8–12 days
Numbers	4,500–11,000/ microliter	4–6 million/ microliter	150,000–400,000/ microliter

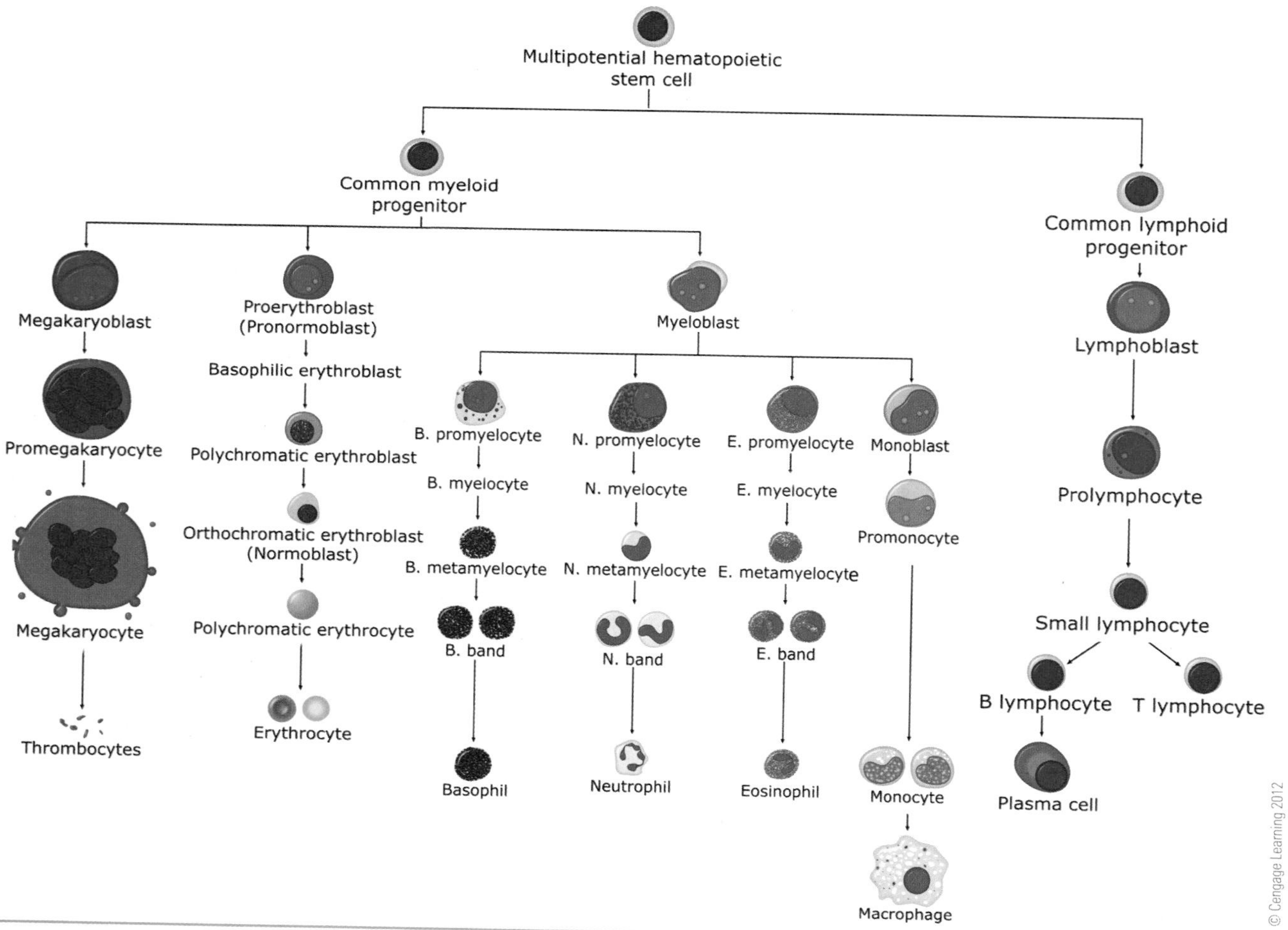

© Cengage Learning 2012

FIGURE 2-5 Characteristics of white blood cells, red blood cells, and platelets

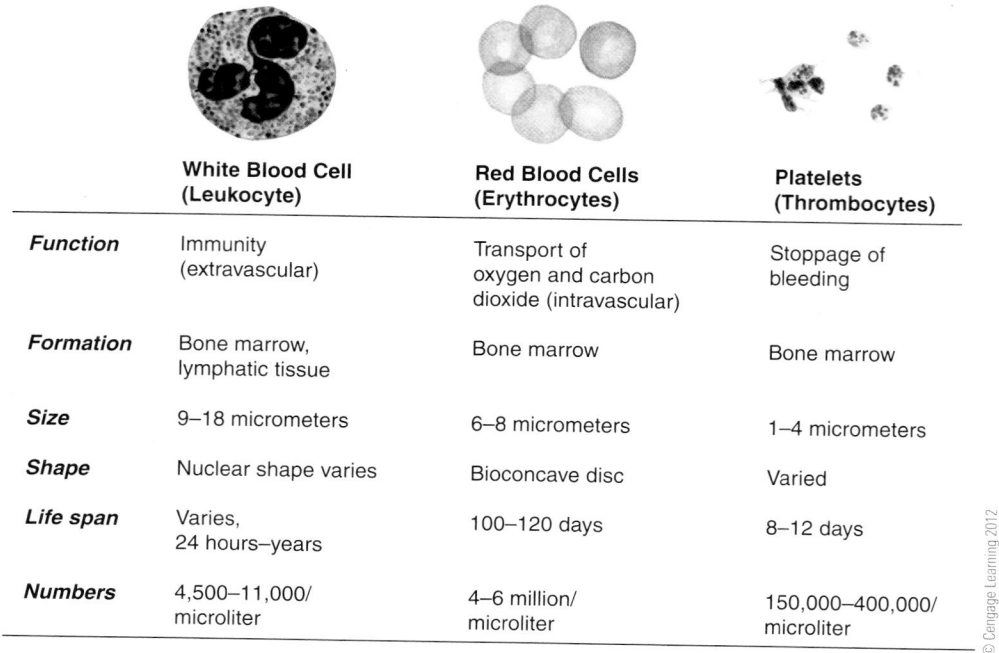

FIGURE 2-6 Origin and maturation of blood cells

© Cengage Learning 2012

caused by the abnormal structure of hemoglobin in *sickle cell anemia.*

Secondary or Acquired Hematological Diseases

Abnormalities in blood cells can also occur because of a condition or disease originating in another organ system. These are called secondary or acquired conditions. For example, abnormal-appearing red blood cells can be present in patients with severe hypertension or renal failure because the cells become damaged as they circulate through small blood vessels. In infectious mononucleosis, a viral disease, lymphocytes develop an "atypical" appearance that can be observed when a stained blood smear is examined microscopically.

Blood cells can be affected by treatments or medications directed at nonhematological conditions. For example, aspirin inhibits platelet function for the life of the platelet. Normal platelet function only returns several days after aspirin is discontinued, when the body has had time to produce new platelets. Chemotherapy and radiation treatments designed to stop the growth of cancer cells can also affect blood cell precursors in the bone marrow and therefore inhibit blood cell production. Patients being treated for cancer must have regular blood cell

counts to be sure their blood cell concentrations do not fall to dangerously low levels.

THE HEMATOLOGY LABORATORY

Methods of Analysis in the Hematology Laboratory

Routine hematology tests are usually performed using one of the many types of hematology analyzers available, but tests can also be performed manually. Some analyzers are designed for small facilities such as physician office laboratories (POLs) and perform only a few different tests. Other analyzers suitable for large laboratories can perform several analyses on hundreds of samples daily. Lesson 2-10 contains information about the principles of hematology analyzers and gives examples of types of results available.

Laboratories that use hematology analyzers must also have backup systems for performing analyses in the event of instrument malfunction. Larger laboratories usually have a small backup instrument to perform analyses while the main instrument is being repaired. However, it is always advisable that personnel be trained in manual techniques for the most basic and frequently requested tests.

CURRENT TOPICS

WHAT ARE STEM CELLS?

Stem cells are often in the news, in relation either to controversy over funding for research or scientific or medical news about stem cells as a potential cure for a disease or a genetic defect. But what are stem cells, what is their origin, where are they found, and why are they important?

What are stem cells? Stem cells are undifferentiated cells that have the ability to renew themselves by cell division and also have potential to develop into many different types of specialized cells that make up the tissues and organs of the body. The ability of stem cells to replicate themselves means that they can sometimes be grown in the laboratory and studied. Stem cells cannot give rise to a complete organism.

What is the origin of stem cells? Where are they found? Researchers work with two types of stem cells: adult stem cells and embryonic stem cells. These have different sources and different characteristics.

Adult stem cells—Although termed *adult,* adult stem cells are found in low numbers in various tissues and organs of animals and humans of all ages. Typically they can give rise to specialized cells of the organ in which they reside. They are also called *multipotent* cells, meaning they have the potential (potent) to develop into several (multi) cell types. Within our bodies, adult stem cells are our repair systems, constantly working to replenish our damaged cells.

The *hematopoietic stem cells* found in the bone marrow are examples of adult stem cells. They can develop into several types of blood cells (such as red cells, white cells, or megakaryocytes) but normally cannot become cells of other tissues, such as kidney or muscle. Bone marrow transplants are successful because the adult stem cells within the transplanted marrow colonize and reproduce to form new blood cells in the transplant recipient. Hematopoietic stem cells can also be harvested from *umbilical cord blood* and used for transplant. An advantage of cord blood transplant over bone marrow transplant is that

(Continues)

CURRENT TOPICS (Continued)

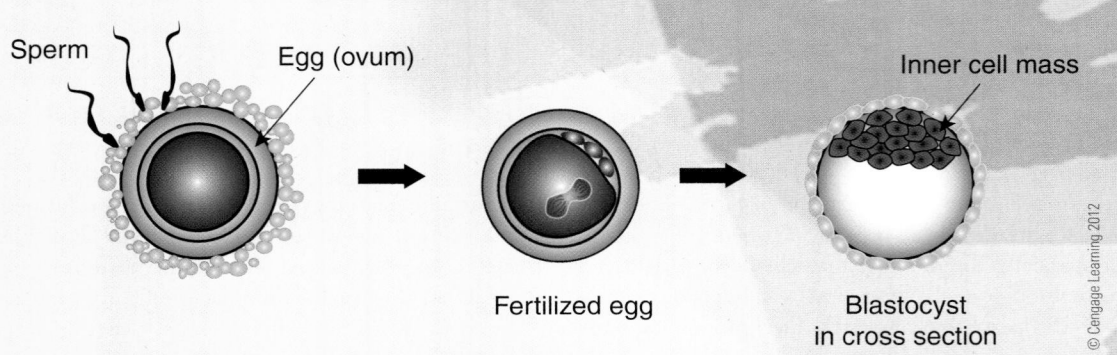

Blastocyst formation

cord blood cells are less likely to be rejected by the recipient because cord blood stem cells have not yet developed markers that could stimulate rejection by the recipient.

Embryonic stem cells—When a sperm fertilizes an egg, a single cell is formed, the fertilized egg (see diagram). This single cell has the potential to form an entire organism; that is, the cell is *totipotent*. A few hours after fertilization, this cell divides into several identical cells, any of which still has the potential to develop into an organism. After about 4 days and several cell divisions, the cells become more specialized (pluripotent). A *blastocyst* is formed, with an outer layer of cells (the trophoblast) and an *inner cell mass* of about 30 to 150 cells (see diagram). The cells in the inner mass have the potential to produce a complete fetus if implantation and development proceed normally. Once removed from the blastocyst, they no longer have the potential to form an individual even though they remain *pluripotent*, meaning they have the potential to give rise to all the tissues of the organism. Embryonic stem cells are derived from this inner cell mass of the blastocyst.

In vitro fertilization clinics store fertilized eggs at the blastocyst stage, and blastocysts that are not to be used can be donated to research. Embryonic stem cells obtained from the inner cell mass can be cultured (grown) in the research laboratory under conditions in which the cells continue to divide but do not differentiate or specialize. Cells that survive several months of laboratory growth and replication, and that remain pluripotent and genetically normal, can be used as *embryonic stem cell lines*.

Why are stem cells important? Stem cell researchers foresee almost unlimited possibilities for using stem cells to treat disease, injuries, and genetic disorders—these are called *cell-based therapies*. With further research to learn how to direct the specialization of stem cells, patients who need organ transplants may be able to be treated instead with stem cells. Stem cells could generate new heart tissue when transplanted into a heart; diabetics could grow new insulin-producing cells by receiving stem cell transplants; and Parkinson's disease could be treated by transplants of stem cells that could be induced to become dopamine neurons. Stem cells could also be used as a renewable source of cells to treat diseases and injuries such as spinal cord injury, stroke, Alzheimer's disease, burns, and arthritis, as well as a way to test new drugs. Stem cells are fascinating and somewhat miraculous in their innate ability to respond to stimulation and develop into a predictable precursor of certain tissues or cells.

Safety Precautions

   Standard Precautions must be observed at all times in the hematology laboratory. These practices are detailed in the laboratory or facility safety manual.

Personnel must use appropriate work practice controls to prevent spills, splatters, aerosol formation, or other exposure to blood and body fluids. Benchtop acrylic safety shields or face shields can be used in the blood-collecting area as well as the testing area to protect against splashes. Lesson 1-4 contains detailed laboratory biosafety information.

In many facilities, the hematology department is responsible for blood collection as well as hematology testing. Personnel must wear gloves and other appropriate protective clothing such as fluid-resistant laboratory coats and face protection when collecting blood specimens. Safety needles must be used for venipuncture. These needles have safety guards or shields that, when activated after use, cover the needles, reducing the potential for needlesticks (Lesson 1-4). All used needles and other sharps must be discarded into rigid, puncture-proof sharps containers.

Hematology personnel can have greater potential for exposure to bloodborne pathogens than personnel in some other laboratory departments. A blood sample tube used to perform a CBC, blood smears, and sedimentation rate—three separate tests—might have to be opened as many as three times, creating three potential exposure events. This type of exposure potential can be minimized by using instruments that automatically sample through the cap of the collection tube.

Quality Assessment

Each laboratory will have a standard operating procedure (SOP) manual containing detailed information about test methods, quality assessment procedures, and the types of control materials, standards and calibrators required. In clinical chemistry departments, certified standards for substances such as glucose or sodium are easily obtained. In hematology, however, stable standards are not as widely available. Standard solutions have an exact assayed concentration and are stable over several weeks to months. This is not possible with blood cells, because they are living tissues. For example, because red blood cells live in circulation approximately 120 days and each day 1/120 of the cells are replaced, a sample of red blood cells would contain cells of all "ages" and some cells would die each day. The red cell count on such a sample would not be consistent from day to day, and the sample could not be used as a standard.

The hemoglobin standard is the only true hematology standard that is available for use in calibrating hematology analyzers. Cell counts and differential counts are calibrated using *control solutions*. Controls for cell counts and automated differentials are made with stabilized cells and have a limited shelf-life of a few months in the unopened vial but sometimes as short as 5 days once the vial is opened. Controls made with suspensions of latex particles can have a shelf-life up to 24 months in the unopened vial but only 30 days once the vial is opened. Hematology controls are available for cell counts, automated differential counts, and more specialized analyses such as flow cytometry (explained in Lesson 2-10). Because true blood cell standards are not available, many hematology procedures and analyzers require more complex calibration and standardization procedures than analyzers in other laboratory departments.

Specimens for Hematology Testing

Both capillary and venous blood can be used for most routine hematological procedures. Blood obtained by capillary puncture (Lesson 1-11) is good for procedures such as blood smears because no chemicals are added to the sample to alter cell appearance. However, because only a small sample volume is obtained by capillary puncture, tests cannot be repeated unless another sample is obtained.

When a larger sample is required, blood is obtained by venipuncture (Lesson 1-12). Venous blood samples for hematology tests are collected in a tube containing an **anticoagulant** to prevent clotting. The anticoagulant most frequently used in the hematology laboratory is **ethylenediaminetetraacetic acid (EDTA)**. Sodium citrate is the anticoagulant commonly used for coagulation tests.

The Complete Blood Count

One of the most frequently requested procedures in the hematology laboratory is the **complete blood count (CBC)**. (An example of a hematology requisition is shown in Figure 2-7.) The CBC is performed on hematology cell counters or hematology analyzers from one blood specimen. The number and types of tests included in the CBC are determined by the instrument used, but can include from a few tests to dozens of tests. The CBC includes at a minimum:

- Red blood cell count
- White blood cell count
- Hemoglobin
- Hematocrit
- Red blood cell indices
- White blood cell differential count
- Platelet count or platelet estimate
- Evaluation of blood cell morphology

Methods for performing the basic hematology tests included in the CBC are explained in the remaining lessons of this unit. After completing this unit, the student should be able to perform these tests and discuss their uses.

Coagulation Tests and Special Hematology Tests

Many tests other than those included in the CBC are performed in the hematology laboratory. Some of these, such as the erythrocyte sedimentation rate and reticulocyte count, are included in this unit. Basic coagulation tests such as the prothrombin time are explained in Unit 3, Basic Hemostasis. Other hematology tests beyond the scope of this book include special stains for blood and bone marrow cells to classify leukemias; identification of hemoglobin variants, such as the hemoglobin that causes sickle cell anemia; assessment of iron status; and tests of leukocyte function to help diagnose immune deficiencies.

HEMATOLOGY

CBC			HEMA LOG #		INSTR. OPER	
HGB & HCT					X2	
WBC						
PLATELET CT.						

TEST NO.

SA		OP CODES	NORMAL VALUES	
	•	WBC x10³	M	7.8±3
			F	
	•	RBC x10³	M	5.4±0.7
			F	4.8±0.6
	•	Hgb g/dl	M	16.0±2
			F	14.0±2
	•	Hct %	M	47±5
			F	42±5
	•	MCV μm³	M	87±7
			F	90±9
	•	MCH pg	M	29±2
			F	
	•	MCHC g/dl	M	35±2
			F	
	•	RDW %	M	13±1.5
			F	
	•	PLT x10³	M	130-400
			F	
	•	MPV μm³	M	8.9±1.5
			F	
	•	LYMPH %	M	28±13
			F	
	•	LYMPH x10³	M	2.0±1
			F	

42474

SEGS		NORMAL RBC			
BANDS		MORPH	1	2	3 4
LYMPHS		POLYCHROM			
MONOS		HYPOCHROM			
EOS		POIK			
		TARGET			
BASOS		SPHERO			
ATYP LYMPHS		ANISO			
META		MICRO			
MYELO		MACRO			
PRO		SICKLE CELLS			
		BASO STIP			
BLAST					
		TOXIC GRAN			
NRBC/100 WBC		1. SLIGHT			
WBC CT CORRECTED FOR NRBC's		2. MODERATE 3. MOD TO MARKED 4. MARKED			
PLATELETS CK'd					

Ordering Physician

Nurse/Ward Clerk

Date Ordered

To Be Done:
☐ STAT
☐ Routine   AM
☐ Time _____ PM

COMMENTS:

REMARKS (For Lab Use Only)

COLLECTED BY	REPORTED	CALLED
TECH/NURSE	TECH	BY
		TO
DATE	DATE	DATE
TIME	TIME	TIME
☐AM ☐PM	☐AM ☐PM	☐AM ☐PM

HEMATOLOGY I

© Cengage Learning 2012

FIGURE 2-7 Hematology requisition form

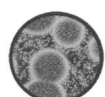

SUMMARY

Hematology is the study of the formed elements of the blood and the blood-forming tissues. Knowledge of the circulatory system, the blood vessels, and the composition of blood is necessary when studying or working in hematology.

Blood is composed of the cellular elements suspended in plasma, the fluid portion of blood. The cellular elements are commonly called blood cells and include the red blood cells, the white blood cells, and the platelets. The red cells function in respiration, the white cells in immunity, and the platelets in hemostasis. Hemopoiesis, the formation and development of blood cells, begins in the liver in the early fetus. By the time of birth, the bone marrow has taken over blood cell production. Blood cells are derived from hemopoietic stem cells and continue to be produced throughout an individual's life.

Tests performed in the hematology laboratory can be qualitative, such as observation and evaluation of blood cell morphology, or quantitative, such as the red blood cell and white blood cell counts or determination of the hematocrit. The majority of testing is performed using instrumentation. However, manual methods are sometimes required when the main instrument malfunctions or is being repaired and a backup instrument is not available.

Safety and quality assessment programs are important in hematology. Standard Precautions must always be observed. Hematology personnel can have increased chance of exposure to potentially infectious specimens compared to personnel in some other areas of the laboratory. A comprehensive quality assessment program is essential to ensure that test results are accurate and reliable.

Hematology tests can give much information about the general well-being of a patient. In addition, hematology test results can be used to monitor the effects of therapies such as chemotherapy or radiation treatments and to provide information critical to the diagnosis of conditions such as anemias, leukemias, and coagulation disorders.

REVIEW QUESTIONS

1. Where are red blood cells produced?
2. Where are white blood cells produced?
3. What is the most primitive blood cell called?
4. What are the three groups of formed elements in the blood? What are the functions of each group?
5. Name the five types of white blood cells found in the blood and state which are granulocytes.
6. Name five components of plasma.
7. What two types of blood specimens are used for most hematological tests?
8. What anticoagulant is used for most hematological tests?

9. What anticoagulant is used for most coagulation tests?

10. Name the three major types of blood vessels and explain the differences among them.

11. Name three ways workers can lessen the chance of exposure to blood and body fluids in the hematology laboratory.

12. Which specific blood component is responsible for oxygen exchange?

13. Name an inherited hematological disease.

14. What is meant by a secondary or acquired hematological condition?

15. Explain the differences in adult stem cells and embryonic stem cells.

16. Discuss the uses of stem cells.

17. What tests are usually included in a complete blood count (CBC)?

18. How does hematology QA differ from QA methods in clinical chemistry?

19. Define anemia, anticoagulant, arteriole, artery, capillary, cardiopulmonary circulation, complete blood count, deoxyhemoglobin, EDTA, erythrocyte, ethylenediamenetetraacetic acid, granulocyte, hematology, hematopoietic stem cell, hemoglobin, hemopoiesis, hemopoietic stem cell, hemostasis, leukemia, leukocyte, megakaryocyte, oxyhemoglobin, plasma, platelet, red blood cell, stem cell, systemic circulation, thrombocyte, vein, venule, and white blood cell.

 # STUDENT ACTIVITIES

1. Complete the written examination for this lesson.

2. Visit a hematology laboratory in the community. Find out what tests are performed there; ask for a copy of a hematology report form.

WEB ACTIVITY

Research a hematological disease using the Internet. Report on the cause of the disease, the laboratory tests that can be used for diagnosis, and the appropriate treatment. Possible sources are the web sites of the National Institutes of Health, medical schools, or universities.

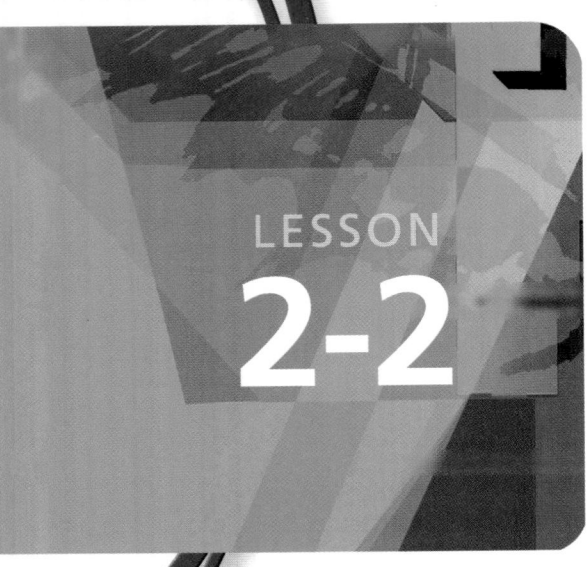

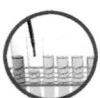

LESSON OBJECTIVES

After studying this lesson, the student will:

- List the two main components of hemoglobin.
- Describe the structure of hemoglobin.
- State the function of hemoglobin.
- List the hemoglobin reference values for children and adults.
- Perform a hemoglobin determination using a hemoglobin analyzer.
- Explain the principle of hemoglobin measurements using hemoglobin analyzers.
- Discuss physiological factors that can affect the hemoglobin value.
- List the safety precautions to observe when performing a hemoglobin determination.
- Discuss factors that can affect the quality of a hemoglobin result.
- Define the glossary terms.

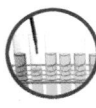

GLOSSARY

azidemethemoglobin / a stable compound formed when azide combines with methemoglobin

cyanmethemoglobin / a stable colored compound formed when hemoglobin is reacted with Drabkin's reagent; hemiglobincyanide (HiCN)

Drabkin's reagent / a hemoglobin diluting reagent that contains iron, potassium, cyanide, and sodium bicarbonate

globin / the protein portion of the hemoglobin molecule

heme / the iron-containing portion of the hemoglobin molecule

hemiglobincyanide (HiCN) / cyanmethemoglobin

hemoglobin (Hb, Hgb) / the major functional component of red blood cells that is the oxygen-carrying molecule

INTRODUCTION

The measurement of blood hemoglobin is one of the most common clinical laboratory tests. **Hemoglobin (Hb or Hgb)** is the primary component of red blood cells (RBCs) and is the oxygen

carrying molecule. Hemoglobin binds oxygen (O_2) and transports it from the lungs to the tissues. In the tissues oxygen is released and hemoglobin binds carbon dioxide (CO_2) and carries it back to the lungs to be discharged from the body (Figure 2-8). Therefore, the measurement of blood hemoglobin indirectly

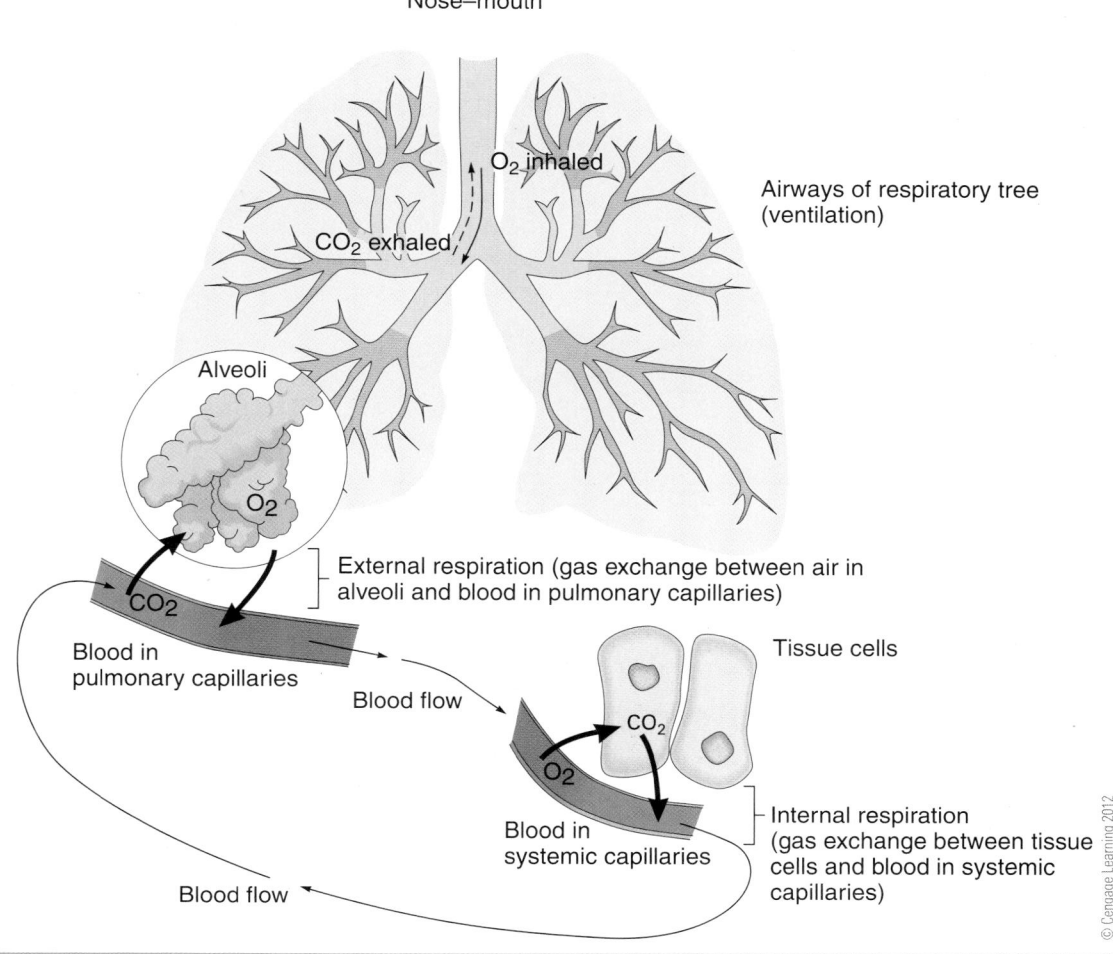

Nose–mouth

O_2 inhaled

CO_2 exhaled

Airways of respiratory tree (ventilation)

Alveoli

O_2

CO_2

External respiration (gas exchange between air in alveoli and blood in pulmonary capillaries)

Blood in pulmonary capillaries

Blood flow

Tissue cells

CO_2

O_2

Blood in systemic capillaries

Internal respiration (gas exchange between tissue cells and blood in systemic capillaries)

Blood flow

© Cengage Learning 2012

FIGURE 2-8 Diagram of lungs showing sites of oxygen exchange in the alveoli and capillaries

evaluates the oxygen-carrying capacity of the blood. This makes the hemoglobin test an important aid in the detection of blood loss and anemia and in monitoring the treatment of certain red cell disorders.

The hemoglobin determination can be performed using either capillary or venous blood and is requested as an individual test or as part of a complete blood count (CBC). The hemoglobin test is precise, simple to perform, and easily standardized. It can be performed using a dedicated hemoglobin instrument or a hematology analyzer.

CHARACTERISTICS OF HEMOGLOBIN

Hemoglobin makes up over 98% of red blood cell protein content. The hemoglobin molecule gives the characteristic red color to the red cells and to blood.

Hemoglobin Structure

The hemoglobin molecule is composed of two parts, **heme** and **globin**. The globin portion of hemoglobin contains four protein chains (Figure 2-9). The structure of these chains is genetically determined.

Hemoglobins are named according to the structure of the protein chains present. Hemoglobin A (Hb A) is the normal adult hemoglobin for most ethnic groups, but there are hundreds of variant hemoglobins, caused by slight variations in the structure of one or more of the globin chains (see Current Topic). Some of these changes are benign, but others are debilitating or fatal. For example, hemoglobin S (Hb S), present in sickle cell anemia, has a different protein structure than normal adult hemoglobin (Hb A).

Each hemoglobin molecule contains four heme groups, one heme group associated with each protein chain (Figure 2-9). Each heme group in a hemoglobin molecule contains iron; therefore, iron is required for hemoglobin synthesis. More than two-thirds of the body's iron is contained in hemoglobin and in a similar molecule in muscle, myoglobin. Iron is highly conserved by the body; as old red blood cells die, the iron in heme is recycled to make new heme molecules. If sufficient iron is not available in the body, hemoglobin production will decrease, causing the red blood cells to be deficient in hemoglobin. When this happens, the oxygen-carrying capacity of the blood is decreased and the individual will develop symptoms of anemia, such as fatigue and pallor. For example, in situations such as a bleeding ulcer, excessive blood loss can cause iron loss to exceed

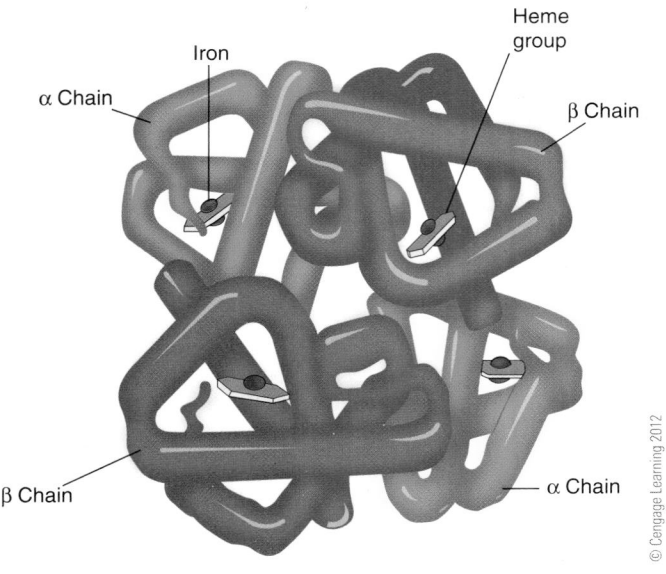

FIGURE 2-9 Structure of the hemoglobin molecule

the intake of dietary iron, eventually causing decreased hemoglobin production and leading to anemia.

Hemoglobin Reference Values

The hemoglobin reference values vary with age and gender. The hemoglobin value at birth normally ranges from 16 to 23 g/dL. In early childhood, the value declines, and 10 to 14 g/dL is normal. When children begin the rapid growth associated with adolescence, hemoglobin values increase until adult levels are reached. Adult males usually have hemoglobin values in the range of 13 to 17 g/dL, and females have values ranging from 12 to 16 g/dL. The elderly usually have hemoglobin values in the lower adult reference ranges.

Hemoglobin reference ranges are listed in Table 2-1. A rule-of-thumb is that the hemoglobin value should be approximately one-third the hematocrit value (see Lesson 2-3). Therefore, an individual with a hematocrit of 45% would be expected to have a hemoglobin value of approximately 15 g/dL.

Hemoglobin can be reported in g/dL or in SI units (g/L or mmol/L). To convert g/dL to grams per liter, the Hb (g/dL) is multiplied by a factor of 10 (Table 2-1). To convert to mmol/L, the Hb (g/dL) is multiplied by a factor of 0.6206.

Physiological Factors Affecting Hemoglobin Levels

Hemoglobin concentration is affected by physiological factors such diet and lifestyle. The diet must contain adequate amounts of iron for red cells to make hemoglobin. Some foods are higher in iron than others; for example, red meat has more iron than cow's milk. If the diet is deficient in iron, the body will use its storage iron until it is depleted and then *iron deficiency anemia* can develop.

People who have an active lifestyle that includes frequent exercise are more likely to have hemoglobin values in the upper range of normal than those who are inactive. The altitude at which people live can also affect hemoglobin values. In areas located at high altitude, such as the Rocky Mountains in the United States, the thin air (reduced oxygen pressure) stimulates increased production of red blood cells, resulting in residents at these altitudes often having hemoglobin levels (and red cell counts) above the reference values.

PRINCIPLES OF HEMOGLOBIN DETERMINATION

Various methods of determining hemoglobin have been used over the years. Current methods include the specific gravity technique and chemical methods such as the cyanmethemoglobin and azidemethemoglobin methods.

Specific Gravity Technique

The specific gravity method of measuring hemoglobin is only an estimate of hemoglobin concentration. A drop of blood is dropped into a copper sulfate ($CuSO_4$) solution with a specific gravity of 1.052 to 1.054. This specific gravity is the same specific gravity as that of blood with a hemoglobin concentration at the low end of the reference range. If the drop falls through the solution rapidly, the specific gravity of the blood is greater than the specific gravity of the copper sulfate solution. Blood with the normal amount of hemoglobin falls rapidly; blood with a low hemoglobin concentration falls slowly or floats (does not drop).

The specific gravity technique of estimating hemoglobin has primarily been performed in the United States in past years as a hemoglobin-screening method for potential blood donors. Most blood donation centers now measure hemoglobin by hemoglobinometer or estimate hemoglobin indirectly by performing a microhematocrit.

Chemical Methods

Measurement of **cyanmethemoglobin** is a widely used chemical method of determining blood hemoglobin. In this method, blood is reacted with **Drabkin's reagent**, which contains iron, potassium, cyanide, and sodium bicarbonate. The Drabkin's and the hemoglobin combine to form a stable colored end-product, cyanmethemoglobin, also called **hemiglobincyanide (HiCN)**. This product is measured photometrically using a hematology analyzer or hemoglobinometer.

AGE/ GENDER	HEMOGLOBIN REFERENCE RANGE		
	g/dL	CONVERSION FACTOR	g/L (SI UNITS)
Newborn	16–23	×10	160–230
Children	10–14	×10	100–140
Adult males	13–17	×10	130–170
Adult females	12–16	×10	120–160

TABLE 2-1. Hemoglobin reference ranges

CURRENT TOPICS

VARIATIONS IN HEMOGLOBIN STRUCTURE

Several forms of hemoglobin exist, determined by variations in structure of the globin portion of the hemoglobin molecule. Red blood cells from a normal adult contain three types of hemoglobin:

- Hemoglobin A_1—Hb A_1 contains two alpha (α) globin chains and two beta (β) globin chains and makes up 95% to 98% of hemoglobin in adults. It is called adult hemoglobin (Figure 2-9).

- Hemoglobin A_2—Hb A_2 has two α and two delta (δ) chains and makes up 2% to 3% of hemoglobin in adults.

- Hemoglobin F—Hb F has two α and two gamma (γ) chains and makes up 2% of hemoglobin in adults. It is the primary hemoglobin produced by the fetus during gestation. Its production usually falls to a low level shortly after birth and to adult levels by 1 to 2 years of age.

Abnormal or variant forms of hemoglobin can occur when a mutation occurs in a gene that codes for a globin chain, causing a change in the amino acid structure of the chain. Besides affecting hemoglobin structure, these changes can affect the function, rate of production, or stability of the hemoglobin. The mutation is usually in the gene for the β globin chain. Hundreds of hemoglobin variants have been discovered, but only a few are widely distributed or clinically significant.

Individuals inherit one copy of each globin gene from each parent. If one abnormal gene and one normal gene are inherited, the person is said to be heterozygous for the abnormal gene and is considered a carrier. That is, they can pass the gene on to offspring but do not generally have health problems from the abnormal gene themselves. If two abnormal genes of the same type are inherited, the person is homozygous for the abnormal hemoglobin and will always pass an abnormal gene on to offspring.

Three of the more common abnormal hemoglobins are:

- Hemoglobin S: This is the primary hemoglobin in people with sickle cell (Hb S) disease. Hb S molecules have two β^S chains and two normal α chains. Individuals who inherit two genes for the β^S chain are homozygous for the sickle Hb gene and have sickle cell disease. Individuals who are heterozygous for the Hb S gene have sickle cell trait. Approximately 0.15% of African Americans are homozygous for β^S and have sickle cell disease;

8% are heterozygous and have sickle cell trait. Statistics show that the homozygous form is present in approximately 4.0% of populations of sub-Saharan Africa. Hb S causes the red blood cells to deform and assume a sickle shape when oxygen is decreased, such as during exercise. Sickle shaped red blood cells can block small blood vessels causing impaired circulation, pain, and organ damage. Sickling decreases the oxygen-carrying capacity of the red blood cell and decreases the red cell's life span, causing sickle cell anemia.

- Hemoglobin E: Hb E is one of the most common hemoglobin variants in the world. It is present in certain parts of Southeast Asia and some individuals of Southeast Asian descent. Those who are homozygous for Hb E have two copies of the gene coding for the β^E globin chain and can have mild hemolytic anemia, microcytosis (small red blood cells), and slight enlargement of the spleen.

- Hemoglobin C: Approximately 2% to 3% of people of West African descent are heterozygous for Hb C—that is they have Hb C trait. Hb C disease (homozygous for the gene) is rare and relatively mild. It usually causes mild hemolytic anemia and mild to moderate enlargement of the spleen.

There are several other less common hemoglobin variants. Some cause no symptoms, whereas others affect the function of the hemoglobin molecules. Hemoglobin H (Hb H) is a hemoglobin composed of four β globin chains and is produced in response to a severe shortage of α chains. Although each of the β globin chains is normal, hemoglobin with four β chains does not function normally. Hb H has an increased affinity for oxygen, holding onto it instead of releasing it to the tissues and cells. Examples of other variants include Hb D, Hb G, Hb J, and Hb M.

The role of Hb F in the fetus is to provide efficient transport of oxygen in the low-oxygen environment of the uterus. Hb F can remain elevated after birth in several congenital disorders. Hereditary persistence of fetal hemoglobin (HPFH) is a rare condition in which Hb F levels remain increased after infancy with no observed hematological or clinical features.

Thalassemias are a group of inherited disorders in which an imbalance of α to β chains occurs, causing decreased production of normal hemoglobin. The majority of thalassemias are found in people of Mediterranean descent. Thalassemia patients often have increased amounts of minor hemoglobins such as Hb F or Hb A_2. Symptoms of thalassemia can be mild to severe, depending on the globin chain affected.

Some hemoglobin analyzers use a hemoglobin method in which **azidemethemoglobin** is measured. The azidemethemoglobin reagent contains a lysing chemical such as sodium deoxycholate, an oxidizing chemical such as sodium nitrite, and azide. In this method, oxyhemoglobin (which contains ferrous iron) is oxidized to ferric iron to form methemoglobin. The methemoglobin then combines with azide to form azidemethemoglobin, a stable compound that can be measured photometrically.

PERFORMING THE HEMOGLOBIN DETERMINATION

Several point-of-care analyzers include hemoglobin measurements in their test menus. Other analyzers, sometimes called dedicated hemoglobinometers, measure only hemoglobin and are inexpensive, easy to use, and accurate. Most hemoglobinometers have been granted CLIA waived status. One advantage of hemoglobinometers is that the procedures usually require only a drop or two of blood obtained by capillary puncture.

Safety Precautions

Standard Precautions must be observed when performing hemoglobin measurements. Work practice controls include wearing appropriate PPE, working in a well-ventilated area, disposing of used reagents correctly, and wiping up all spills with surface disinfectant. In addition, because hemoglobin reagents contain hazardous chemicals such as cyanide or azide, care must be taken when performing the tests and handling the reagents.

Quality Assessment

The use of Drabkin's reagent to form the stable compound cyanmethemoglobin was an important advancement in hematology because it made reliable hemoglobin standards available for the first time. A hemoglobin solution made with Drabkin's is stable for at least 6 months and provides laboratories a reliable standard to use for standardizing hemoglobin assays.

Hemoglobinometers and hematology analyzers must be calibrated at regular intervals as specified by the manufacturers. Appropriate controls must be run following the laboratory's standard operating procedure (SOP) manual, control results must be recorded, and the records must be maintained. Reagents must not be used beyond their expiration date. Each instrument will have its own particular checks that must be performed and documented.

HemoCue Hemoglobin Analyzer

The HemoCue Hb 201+ is a small handheld analyzer for use in point-of-care testing. The analyzer is simple to use and provides quality results in less than one minute from a small blood sample. Hemoglobin determination is CLIA-waived when using the HemoCue Hb 201+ analyzer. Capillary or venous blood can

be used with the HemoCue Hb 201+. For capillary puncture, the first drop of blood must be wiped away before collecting the sample. Venous anticoagulated blood must be well-mixed before sampling. The blood sample is collected into a special cuvette that automatically draws up the correct amount of blood (Figure 2-10). Reagents coating the inside of the cuvette mix with the blood to form azidemethemoglobin. The cuvette is inserted into the analyzer and a dual-wavelength photometer in the analyzer measures the absorbance of the solution (Figure 2-11). The absorbance is converted into the hemoglobin value and the result is displayed in grams per deciliter or grams per liter. The dual-wavelength photometer allows results to be corrected for blood samples that

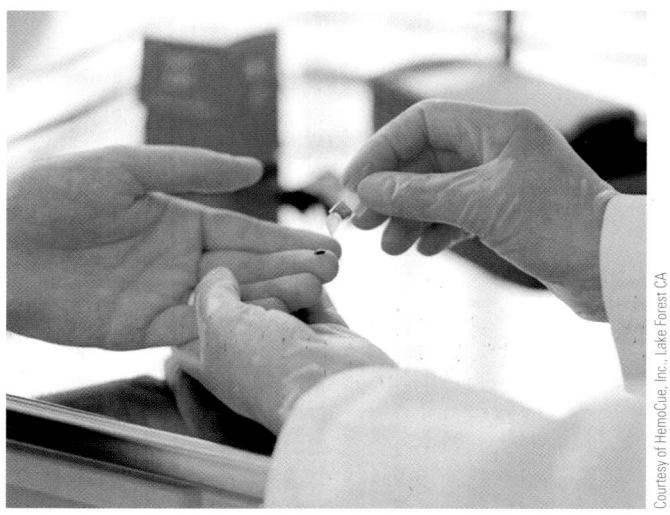

Courtesy of HemoCue, Inc., Lake Forest CA

FIGURE 2-10 Filling the cuvette for the HemoCue Hb 201+ analyzer

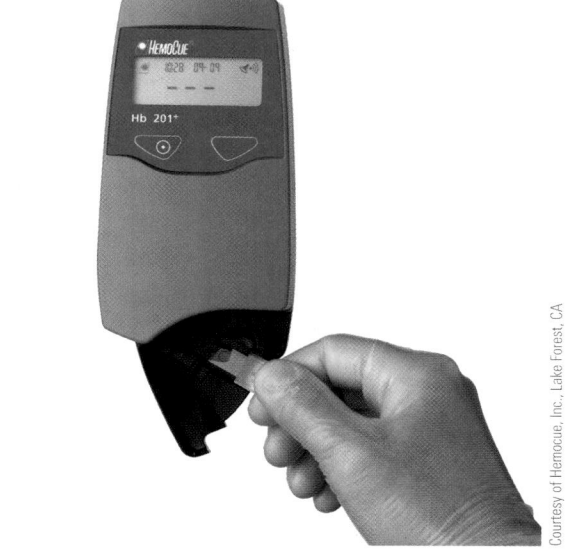

Courtesy of Hemocue, Inc., Lake Forest, CA

FIGURE 2-11 Inserting cuvette into the HemoCue Hb 201+ analyzer

have lipemia, leukocytosis, or other causes of turbidity that could interfere with the readings. The HemoCue Hb 201+ has an internal electronic self-test to automatically verify performance.

STAT-Site M Hgb Meter

The STAT-Site M Hgb Photometer (Stanbio Laboratory) is a CLIA-waived system designed to measure hemoglobin in settings such as physician office laboratories (POLs), blood donation centers, health centers, and emergency departments. The system includes a palm-size, battery-operated hemoglobin meter; test cards; and a CODE key (calibration cartridge). The meter can measure hemoglobin from a single drop of blood in just a few seconds. The test method is also based on the azidemethemoglobin method, and capillary blood or venous anticoagulated blood can be used. A lot-specific CODE key is provided in each package of test cards (Figure 2-12A). When a test card is inserted into the meter, it is checked and coded to the CODE key. A drop of blood is added to the card and the sample is detected by the meter and analyzed. Within a few seconds the hemoglobin result is displayed in conventional units (g/dL), as shown in Figure 2-12B, or in SI units (mmol/L). This meter can measure hemoglobin in the range of 6 to 21 g/dL and can be used for hemoglobin measurements in infants, children, and adults.

Hgb Pro

The Hgb Pro (International Technidyne Corporation) is another small handheld hemoglobin meter (Figure 2-13). The instrument requires a very small blood sample. A test strip is inserted into the meter and a drop of blood is applied to the strip. The hemoglobin value is read on the display. The Hgb Pro comes with quality

control solutions that are analyzed in the same manner as patient samples.

Automated Hemoglobin Analyzers

Automated cell counters and hematology analyzers perform hemoglobin determinations (Lesson 2-10). These instruments require a venous anticoagulated blood specimen. In many instruments, the sample can be aspirated from the blood collection tube by a probe that penetrates the collection tube cap, improving efficiency and worker safety. Several clinical chemistry analyzers are also capable of performing hemoglobin assays.

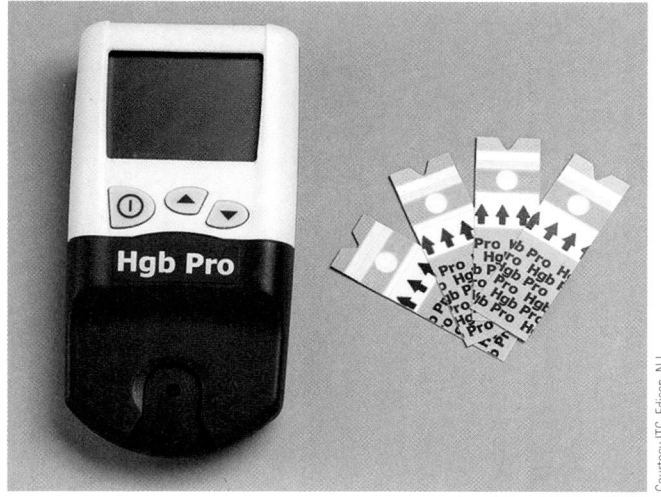

Courtesy ITC, Edison, NJ

FIGURE 2-13 Hgb Pro

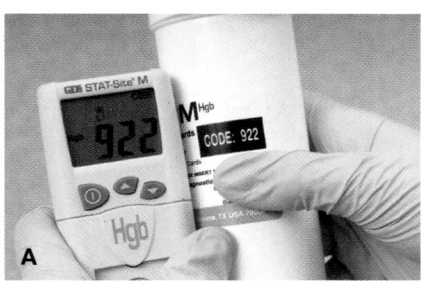

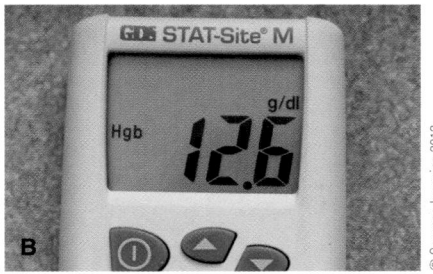

© Cengage Learning 2012

FIGURE 2-12 STAT-Site M Hemoglobin meter: (A) meter must be calibrated for each new package of test cards; (B) hemoglobin result is displayed a few seconds after applying blood to test card

SAFETY REMINDERS

- Review Safety Precautions section before beginning procedure.
- Observe Standard Precautions.
- Wear appropriate PPE.
- Dispose of reagents according to facility guidelines.

PROCEDURAL REMINDERS

- Review Quality Assessment before beginning procedure.
- Follow method in SOP manual.
- Use appropriate controls and standards.
- Store supplies as recommended by the manufacturer.
- Do not use reagents beyond the expiration date.

CRITICAL THINKING

Jennifer was transferred from her company's Virginia Beach office to Colorado Springs. Before moving, she flew to Colorado Springs for a week of new employee orientation. After being there only a few days, she had to seek medical attention for extreme fatigue and shortness of breath. The physician ordered a hemoglobin test along with other tests.

1. Which of the following is most likely?
   a. Jennifer is depressed because she will be moving away from family.
   b. Jennifer has not had sufficient rest because of stress from the new job.
   c. Jennifer is having problems acclimating to the altitude.
   d. Jennifer does not like her new job.
2. Explain your answer.

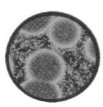

SUMMARY

Hemoglobin is the primary constituent of red blood cells. Each hemoglobin molecule is composed of four globin chains, each chain associated with a heme molecule. The structure of the globin portion of hemoglobin is determined by inherited genes. Hemoglobin is responsible for oxygen delivery to the tissues; the hemoglobin result is used along with the hematocrit result to estimate the oxygen-carrying capacity of the blood. Production of hemoglobin is affected by diet, age, gender, and certain physiological factors.

The hemoglobin determination is part of the CBC. The hemoglobin test can be performed using a handheld hemoglobin analyzer, such as the ones described in this lesson, or using an automated hematology analyzer. All quality assessment steps must be followed to ensure valid results. Standard precautions for safe handling of blood samples must always be observed for the protection of personnel and patients.

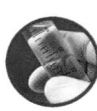

REVIEW QUESTIONS

1. What are the two main components of hemoglobin?
2. Describe the structure of the hemoglobin molecule.
3. Explain the function of hemoglobin.

4. What was the significance of the development of the cyanmethemoglobin method?
5. Explain the principle of the specific gravity technique of estimating hemoglobin concentration.
6. Explain the principle of the HemoCue hemoglobin method.
7. Give hemoglobin reference ranges for children and adults.
8. Discuss how diet, age, gender, and living at high altitude can affect the hemoglobin value.
9. List safety precautions to be observed when measuring hemoglobin.
10. List three factors that can affect the quality of hemoglobin test results.
11. Define azidemethemoglobin, cyanmethemoglobin, Drabkin's reagent, globin, heme, hemiglobincyanide, and hemoglobin.

STUDENT ACTIVITIES

1. Complete the written examination for this lesson.
2. Inquire at physician offices, blood donation centers, or community anemia screening clinics about the methods of hemoglobin determination used.
3. Practice the procedure for determining blood hemoglobin concentration as listed in the Student Performance Guide.

WEB ACTIVITIES

1. Use the Internet to find information about abnormal forms of hemoglobin (such as Hb S, E, C, or H). Choose one to research: describe the condition, disorder, or disease associated with the abnormal hemoglobin and the laboratory test(s) used to detect and confirm it.
2. Use the Internet to find two brands of hematology analyzers. Find information about how the instruments measure hemoglobin. Request or download free product information describing the test methods.

LESSON 2-2
Hemoglobin

(Results can vary from student to student depending on available blood specimens.)

Name _____ Date _____

INSTRUCTIONS

1. Practice the procedure for determining blood hemoglobin concentration using a hemoglobin analyzer and following the step-by-step procedure.

2. Demonstrate the hemoglobin determination procedure satisfactorily for the instructor, using the Student Performance Guide. Your instructor will explain the procedures for evaluating and grading your performance. Your performance may be given a number grade, letter grade, or satisfactory (S) or unsatisfactory (U) depending on course or institutional policy.

NOTE: Consult manufacturer's instructions for specific procedure.

MATERIALS AND EQUIPMENT

- gloves
- hand antiseptic
- full-face shield (or equivalent PPE)
- acrylic safety shield (optional)
- capillary puncture supplies
- HemoCue Hemoglobin Analyzer, or other hemoglobin analyzer with supplies appropriate for the analyzer
- hemoglobin controls
- paper towels
- laboratory tissue
- surface disinfectant (such as 10% chlorine bleach)
- biohazard container
- sharps container

PROCEDURE

Record in the comment section any problems encountered while practicing the procedure (or have a fellow student or the instructor evaluate your performance).

S = Satisfactory
U = Unsatisfactory

You must:	S	U	Evaluation/Comments
1. Wash hands with antiseptic and put on gloves			
2. Put on face protection (or position acrylic safety shield)			
3. Assemble materials and equipment			
4. Follow steps 5a–5j if using the HemoCue 201+. If using a different brand of hemoglobin analyzer, go to step 6			
5. For the HemoCue 201+: a. Turn on instrument to warm up; wait until electronic calibration is completed			

(Continues)

You must:	S	U	Evaluation/Comments
b. Remove a cuvette from vial and immediately replace the vial cap			
c. Perform a capillary puncture observing Standard Precautions			
d. Wipe away the first drop of blood			
e. Touch the pointed tip of the cuvette to a well-rounded drop of blood and allow the cuvette to fill in one continuous motion			
f. Wipe excess blood from outside of cuvette, being careful not to touch the open end of the cuvette			
g. Insert the filled cuvette into the holder within 10 minutes of filling the cuvette			
h. Push the holder into the analyzer to the measuring position			
i. Read hemoglobin value from display and record			
j. Repeat steps 5e–5i using the hemoglobin control			
6. If using another hemoglobin analyzer, follow the manufacturer's instructions for calibration and for performing a hemoglobin determination			
7. Discard contaminated sharps into sharps container			
8. Discard other contaminated materials into biohazard container			
9. Turn off instrument(s), wipe up any spills, and return all equipment to storage			
10. Wipe the work area with disinfectant			
11. Remove gloves and discard into biohazard container			
12. Wash hands with antiseptic			

Instructor/Evaluator Comments:

Instructor/Evaluator _____ Date _____

© 2012 Delmar, Cengage Learning. Permission to reproduce for clinical use granted.

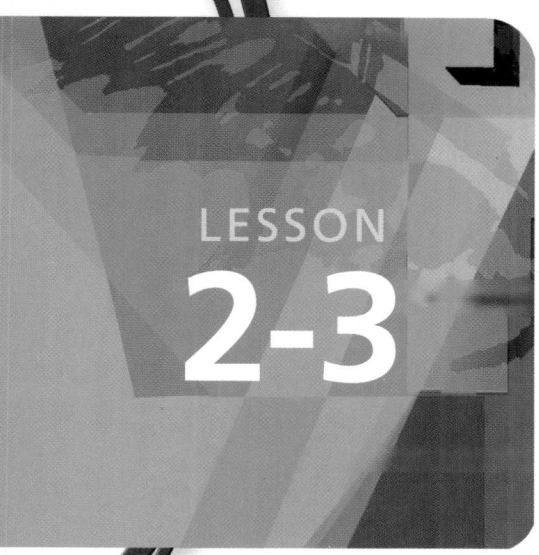

LESSON
2-3

Microhematocrit

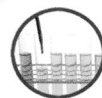

LESSON OBJECTIVES

After studying this lesson, the student will:

⊙ Explain the principle of the microhematocrit test.

⊙ List the reference values for the hematocrit.

⊙ List five diseases or conditions that can affect the hematocrit value.

⊙ Perform a microhematocrit and interpret the result.

⊙ Correlate hematocrit results with hemoglobin results.

⊙ Correlate hematocrit results to patient clinical symptoms.

⊙ Discuss factors that affect the quality of microhematocrit results.

⊙ List safety precautions that should be observed in performing the microhematocrit.

⊙ Define the glossary terms.

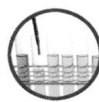

GLOSSARY

buffy coat / a light-colored layer of white blood cells and platelets that forms on top of the red blood cell layer when a sample of blood is centrifuged or allowed to stand undisturbed

capillary tube / a slender glass or plastic tube used in laboratory procedures

hematocrit / the volume of red blood cells packed by centrifugation in a given volume of blood and expressed as a percentage; packed cell volume (PCV)

microhematocrit / a hematocrit performed in capillary tubes using a small quantity of blood; packed cell volume (PCV)

microhematocrit centrifuge / an instrument that spins capillary tubes at a high speed to rapidly separate cellular components of the blood from the liquid portion of blood

packed cell column / the layers of blood cells that form when a tube of whole blood is centrifuged

INTRODUCTION

The **hematocrit** is a commonly performed test that provides the clinician with an estimate of the patient's red cell volume and, thus, the blood's oxygen-carrying capacity. The hematocrit measurement is useful in screening for anemia, screening potential blood donors, evaluating anemia therapies, and estimating blood loss following hemorrhage or trauma.

There are two methods of determining the hematocrit. The manual method is called a **microhematocrit** and requires only a small volume of blood. It is a simple procedure in which whole blood is centrifuged in slender **capillary tubes**.

The microhematocrit (also called spun hematocrit) is a CLIA-waived test.

The hematocrit can also be determined using a hematology analyzer. It is performed as part of a complete blood count (CBC). Hematocrits performed on automated counters or analyzers are electronically calculated from the red blood cell (RBC) count and RBC volume. Measurements made using hematology analyzers are called hematocrits; those made using the centrifuge are called microhematocrits. In practice, the terms are interchangeable and the results are comparable. Both methods provide rapid, reliable results.

PRINCIPLE OF THE MICROHEMATOCRIT TEST

The microhematocrit test is based on the principle of separating the cellular elements of blood from plasma by centrifugation. After the blood is centrifuged in a capillary tube, the red cells are at the bottom of the tube, the white cells and platelets form a thin layer on top of the red cells, and the plasma is at the top (Figure 2-14). This layered arrangement following centrifugation is called the **packed cell column**. The layer containing white cells and platelets has a whitish-tan appearance and is commonly referred to as the **buffy coat** (Figure 2-14).

The microhematocrit is determined by comparing the volume of red cells to the total volume of the whole blood sample. This volume of red cells is the packed cell volume (PCV) and is reported as the microhematocrit in percentage. Laboratory personnel often refer to a microhematocrit as a *crit* or abbreviate it with the letters *Hct*.

Microhematocrit Centrifuges

Several types of **microhematocrit centrifuges** are available for performing spun hematocrits (Figure 2-15). Some centrifuges are multifunctional and can spin urinalysis, coagulation, and

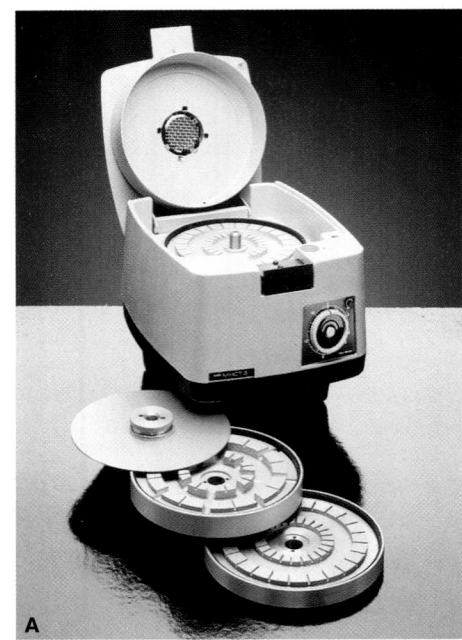

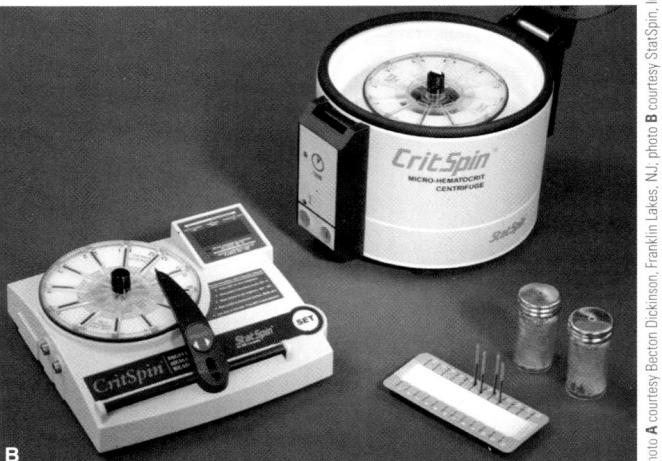

FIGURE 2-15 Microhematocrit centrifuges: (A) Adams MHCT 2; (B) CritSpin with reader

blood chemistry tubes as well as microhematocrit tubes. Other centrifuges, such as the StatSpin CritSpin from Iris Sample Processing are used only for microhematocrits and will spin only capillary tubes (Figure 2-15B).

Microhematocrit centrifuges can have built-in microhematocrit readers that require the use of precalibrated capillary tubes. For other centrifuges, a separate microhematocrit reader is used that can read both noncalibrated and precalibrated tubes.

The STAT-CRIT is a small, portable instrument that assays blood hemoglobin and hematocrit in 30 seconds. The test is performed by collecting blood from a capillary puncture into a disposable blood-sample carrier. The carrier is inserted into the instrument, analyzed, and the result is displayed digitally.

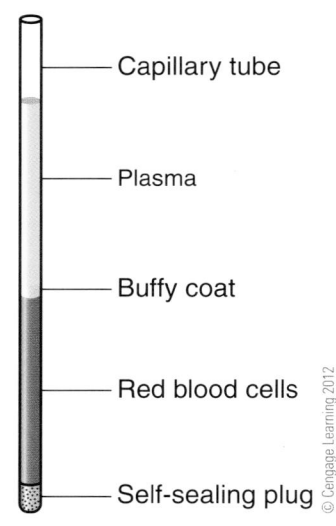

FIGURE 2-14 Diagram of packed cell column in a microhematocrit tube showing separation of cells and plasma after centrifugation

- Capillary tube
- Plasma
- Buffy coat
- Red blood cells
- Self-sealing plug

Microhematocrit Tubes

Several types of capillary tubes are available for microhematocrit determinations. The tubes are from 0.5 to 1 mm in internal diameter and come in two lengths, 40 mm and 75 mm. The length of tube must be appropriate for the type of microhematocrit centrifuge to be used. Heparinized tubes with a red ring are used for capillary blood; plain (unheparinized) tubes (blue ring) are used for venous blood that already has an anticoagulant added (Figure 2-16). Mylar-wrapped glass tubes or flexible plastic capillary tubes should be used, because they are less likely to break than unwrapped glass tubes. Self-sealing tubes are available that eliminate the need for sealant pads. (Lesson 1-11 contains additional information about capillary tubes.)

HEMATOCRIT REFERENCE VALUES

The hematocrit value varies with the gender and age of the patient (Table 2-2). The values range from a low of 32% for a 1-year-old to a high of 61% for a newborn. Hematocrits for females are usually lower than for males. The SI value for the

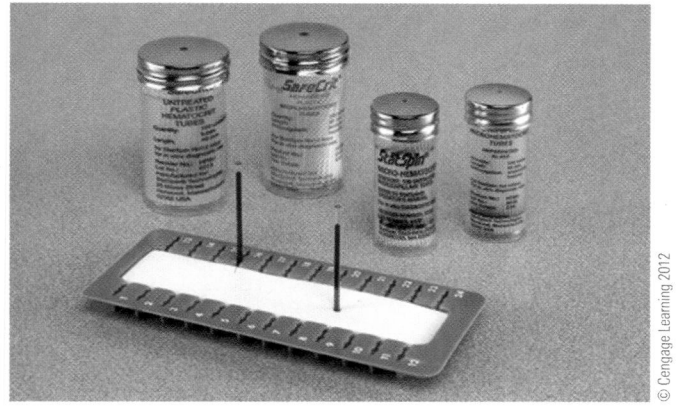

FIGURE 2-16 Microhematocrit tubes and sealant pad

© Cengage Learning 2012

hematocrit is obtained by multiplying the hematocrit percentage by a factor of 0.01. The result is expressed in SI units as liter of packed cells per liter of whole blood (L/L). A hematocrit of 32% would be expressed as 0.32 L/L.

CORRELATING HEMATOCRIT RESULTS TO PATIENT HEALTH

The hematocrit value is influenced by both physiological and pathological factors (Table 2-3). A hematocrit value below the normal range can indicate a condition such as anemia or the presence of bleeding in a patient. A hematocrit value above the normal range can be due to a physical cause such as dehydration or by an uncommon condition such as polycythemia.

The hematocrit reference ranges are different for males and females and also vary with age, so the reference range appropriate for the patient must be considered when determining the significance of hematocrit results. Because of these factors, it is important that identification labels on specimens be complete and include patient age and gender. For instance, suppose a technician performs a hematocrit on a specimen and the results are read as 37%. If the patient were an adult female or a child, this value would be within the reference range and would not require any special attention. However, if the patient were a healthy middle-aged male the value is well below the reference range, and the result should be flagged as low (L) on the laboratory report. A general rule is that, in healthy individuals, the hematocrit result should equal the hemoglobin result multiplied by three (3). Thus a blood sample having a hemoglobin of 12 g/dL (120 g/L) should have a hematocrit of approximately 36% or 0.36 L/L.

The appearance of the blood sample in a spun hematocrit can also give clues to a patient's health. Normal blood samples centrifuged in a microhematocrit tube will have a characteristic appearance—the plasma portion will be pale yellow and transparent and the buffy coat will be a narrow whitish tan layer above the red cell layer. Plasma that is very yellow could indicate the patient

TABLE 2-2. Hematocrit reference ranges					
	AVERAGE			**RANGE**	
	PERCENT (%)	**SI UNITS* (L/L)**		**PERCENT (%)**	**SI UNITS* (L/L)**
Adults					
Males	47	0.47		42–52	0.42–0.52
Females	42	0.42		36–48	0.36–0.48
Children					
Newborn	56	0.56		51–61	0.51–0.61
1 year	35	0.35		32–38	0.32–0.38
6 years	38	0.38		34–42	0.34–0.42
*SI Units = International System of Units					

TABLE 2-3. Conditions and factors affecting hematocrit values

CONDITION/ FACTOR	EFFECT ON HEMATOCRIT VALUE
Age	
Newborns	Increased
Children	Less than adult value
Older adults	Decreased from adult value
Gender	Adult female value less than adult male value
Residence at high altitudes	Increased
Severe dehydration	Increased
Anemias	Decreased
Polycythemia	Increased
Leukemias	Decreased
Bleeding, such as bleeding ulcer	Decreased

has an elevated bilirubin level; plasma that is opaque could indicate a high fat (triglyceride) level. A prominent buffy coat layer could indicate that the patient has an elevated white blood count. It is the responsibility of the technician to be observant and report unusual findings such as these.

PERFORMING THE MICROHEMATOCRIT TEST

Safety Precautions

Standard Precautions must be observed when performing microhematocrit measurements. Plastic or Mylar-coated self-sealing tubes should be used to reduce chance of injury. Only capillary tubes approved for the available centrifuge should be used. Alternatives to sealant pads should be used when possible.

Special care must be taken when operating the centrifuge. The centrifuge interior should be cleaned frequently with disinfectant. The microhematocrit centrifuge operates at high speeds; the internal and external lids must be locked in place before operating the instrument. The rotor must come to a complete stop before the centrifuge is opened.

Quality Assessment

Reliable microhematocrit results require correct specimen collection and test setup, calibrated centrifuges, and careful reading and reporting of microhematocrit values. Although the test is

relatively simple, variations in technique and several other factors can affect the results. Measures that should be followed to ensure reliable results include:

- Follow the procedure in the standard operating procedure (SOP) manual.
- Run hematology controls daily and chart the results.
- Mix venous blood specimens before filling capillary tubes.
- Follow correct capillary blood collection techniques.
- Collect capillary blood in heparinized capillary tubes.
- Fill microhematocrit tubes three-fourths full.
- Run each patient sample in duplicate; the two results should agree within $\pm 2\%$.
- Repeat the test if results do not agree within $\pm 2\%$.

The centrifuge speed and accuracy of the timer must be checked at regular intervals and the results documented. Periodic preventive maintenance must be performed and documented. The centrifuge speed and time directly affect the microhematocrit values—failure to spin tubes at the correct speed and for the correct time can cause erroneous results. Samples spun at speeds slower than specified or for a shorter time will have falsely increased microhematocrit values. Spinning the samples at speeds higher than specified or for a longer time than specified can falsely decrease microhematocrit values as a result of excessive RBC packing or RBC hemolysis.

Obtaining and Preparing the Specimen

The blood sample for a microhematocrit can be obtained from a capillary puncture (Figure 2-17A) or from a tube of venous blood to which the anticoagulant ethylenediaminetetraacetic acid (EDTA) has been added (Figure 2-17B). Capillary blood should be collected into heparinized capillary tubes. Before sampling from tubes of venous anticoagulated blood, the blood must be gently mixed by either inverting the tube approximately 60 times, or placing it on a mechanical mixer for a minimum of 2 minutes (Figure 2-18).

Blood is drawn by capillary action into capillary tubes, which are then sealed. Self-sealing tubes are preferred. These have a dry plug in one end that expands to form a seal when it contacts blood. If a sealant pad is used it should be treated as a biohazard (Figure 2-16).

Centrifuging the Samples

Sealed capillary tubes are placed into the rotor of the microhematocrit centrifuge, with the sealed ends against the rubber gasket (toward the outer rim of the rotor). Tubes must be balanced in the rotor. Centrifuge lids must be carefully secured, following all manufacturer and facility safety precautions. The length of centrifugation is determined by the type of centrifuge, its calibration, and the procedure manual for each facility.

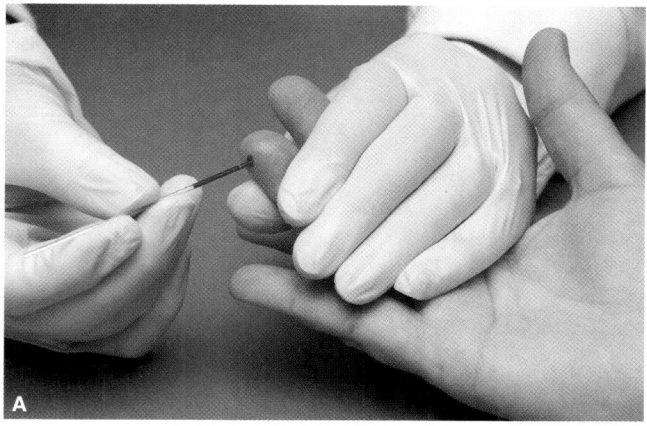

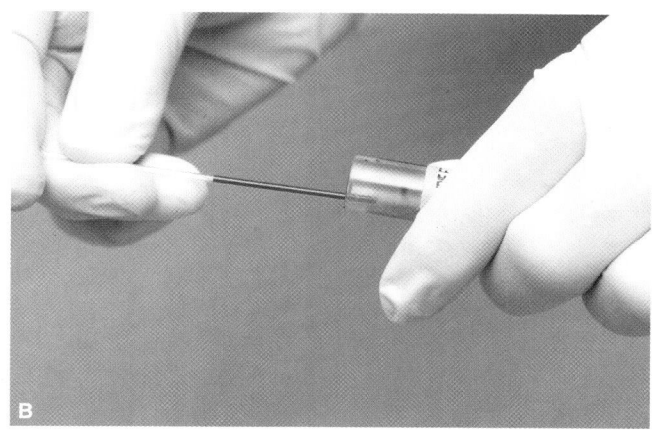

FIGURE 2-17 Fill a capillary tube: (A) from a capillary puncture; (B) from a tube of EDTA blood

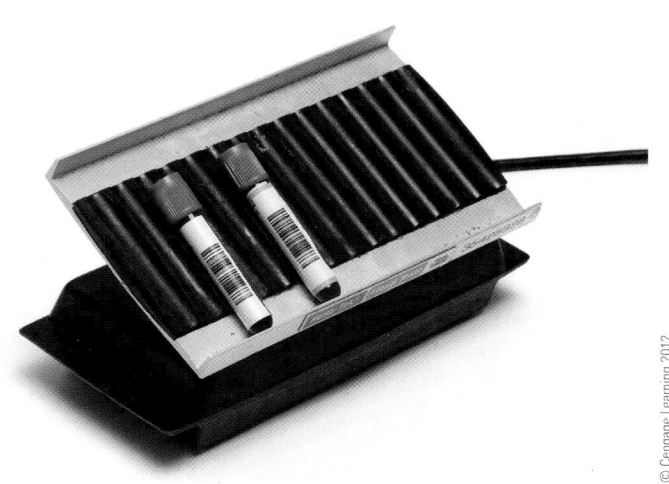

FIGURE 2-18 Mixer for hematology specimens

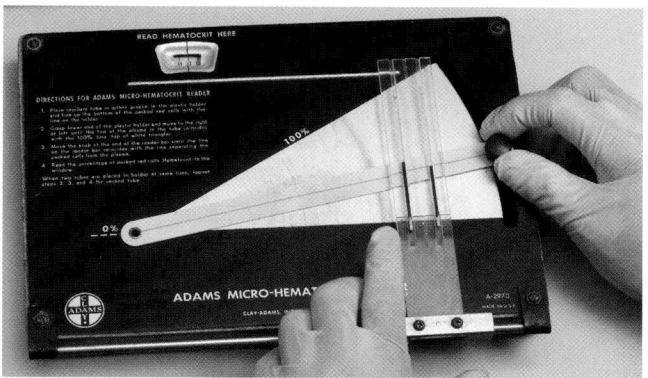

FIGURE 2-19 Using a microhematocrit reader

Generally, microhematocrit tubes are spun for 2 to 4 minutes at 10,000 rpm.

Reading and Reporting the Microhematocrit Value

The percent of red blood cells in the blood sample is determined using a microhematocrit reader. After centrifugation, the tubes should be inspected to see that no leakage occurred during centrifugation and then placed on the microhematocrit reader (Figure 2-19). The instructions for the type of reader being used must be followed carefully to ensure correct reading of the microhematocrit. Only the red blood cell portion of the packed cell column is measured (Figure 2-14); neither the buffy coat nor the sealant plug should be included in the measurement. The microhematocrit reading should be determined for each of the duplicate tubes. The values from the two tubes should not vary by more than ±2%. The average of the two readings is reported.

SAFETY REMINDERS

- Review Safety Precautions section before beginning procedure.
- Observe Standard Precautions.
- Use plastic or Mylar-coated self-sealing tubes.
- Balance tubes correctly on the rotor.
- Lock centrifuge lid(s) securely.
- Never open a centrifuge until the rotor has stopped.

PROCEDURAL REMINDERS

- Review Quality Assessment section before beginning the procedure.
- Follow the SOP manual.
- Mix anticoagulated blood before filling capillary tubes.
- Read the microhematocrit value at the top of the red cell layer.

CASE STUDY 1

A hematocrit test was ordered on a 52-year-old man who went to the physician because of feeling tired. Following his facility's SOP, Stephen, the laboratory technician, prepared duplicate microhematocrit tubes from a tube of the patient's venous blood. During centrifugation one capillary tube leaked; the microhematocrit on the remaining tube was 38% (0.38 L/L). Stephen hurriedly found the patient's sample and filled two additional tubes. After centrifugation the hematocrit value for each tube was 32% (0.32 L/L).

1. Which of the following is probably true?
   a. There was no need to repeat the test; the value of 38% should have been reported.
   b. The 32% value can be reported because the duplicate tubes agree with each other.
   c. Stephen should review his actions; perhaps he failed to thoroughly mix the venous blood before he performed the second microhematocrit.
2. What should the laboratory technician do next?
   a. Report the 32% value
   b. Report the 38% value
   c. Mix the venous blood sample thoroughly and fill two capillary tubes to repeat the centrifugation
3. Can Stephen make any conclusions about the patient's condition from the available information? Explain your answer.

CASE STUDY 2

$\frac{n}{x}$ A female patient's hematocrit is 42% (0.42 L/L), and her red blood cell count is $4.5 \times 10^6/\mu L$.

What should her hemoglobin be?

CASE STUDY 3

A hemoglobin and hematocrit performed in a pediatric clinic on a 2-year-old gave results of 120 g/L hemoglobin and 0.35 L/L hematocrit.

1. Do these results agree?
2. Are these results in the normal range for his age?

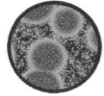

SUMMARY

The hematocrit is performed as part of the CBC but is also frequently ordered as a single test. The results are relied upon to quickly assess a patient's oxygen-carrying capacity, such as to evaluate magnitude of blood loss or to follow recovery from blood loss. The hematocrit can be performed by centrifugation or using a hematology analyzer or cell counter. The centrifuged hematocrit is called a microhematocrit. Automated hematology instruments do not measure the hematocrit by centrifugation but calculate the hematocrit from the hemoglobin value and red blood cell count results. Microhematocrit

results are influenced by specimen collection techniques, length and speed of centrifugation, and reading of the results. Standard Precautions must be observed, and all policies of quality assessment must be followed when performing the microhematocrit procedure.

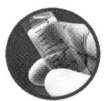

REVIEW QUESTIONS

1. What does the hematocrit measure?
2. Give the hematocrit reference values for males, females, and newborns.

3. What are advantages of the microhematocrit test?

4. Name a condition that could cause a decreased hematocrit value.

5. Explain the microhematocrit procedure.

6. Blood enters the capillary tube by what action?

7. Why must the capillary tube be sealed securely?

8. What is the usual length of time for centrifugation of microhematocrit tubes?

9. What is the correlation between a healthy person's hematocrit value and their hemoglobin value?

10. What safety precautions should be observed when performing a microhematocrit?

11. What technical factors can affect the quality of microhematocrit results?

12. Define buffy coat, capillary tube, hematocrit, microhematocrit, microhematocrit centrifuge, and packed cell column.

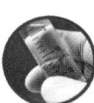

STUDENT ACTIVITIES

1. Complete the written examination for this lesson.

2. Practice performing the microhematocrit test on several blood samples as outlined in the Student Performance Guide.

3. Perform a microhematocrit on a blood sample. Repeat the microhematocrit procedure on the blood sample, lengthening or shortening the centrifugation time by 1 to 3 minutes. Record the results and discuss differences between these results and the initial microhematocrit result.

4. Demonstrate the importance of using well-mixed blood: perform a microhematocrit on a well-mixed sample; allow the sample tube to stand upright 15 minutes and perform another microhematocrit without remixing the blood. Compare the results and discuss.

WEB ACTIVITIES

1. Search the Internet for information about hematology analyzer technology. Find out how the hematocrit is performed on a hematology analyzer.

2. Search the Internet for videos demonstrating the microhematocrit procedure. Compare the procedure shown in the video with the procedure explained by your instructor.

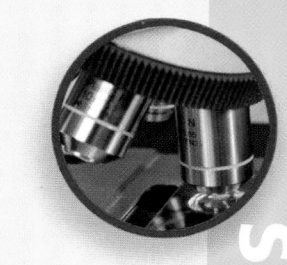

LESSON 2-3
Microhematocrit

(Answers will vary from student to student depending on the types of specimens provided by the instructor.)

Name _____ Date _____

INSTRUCTIONS

1. Practice the microhematocrit procedure following the step-by-step instructions.

2. Demonstrate the microhematocrit procedure satisfactorily for the instructor, using the Student Performance Guide. Your instructor will explain the procedure for grading and evaluating your performance. Your performance may be given a number grade, a letter grade, or satisfactory (S) or unsatisfactory (U) depending on course or institutional policy.

NOTE: Consult manufacturer's instructions for the centrifuge being used and the laboratory procedure manual for the specific procedure being performed. Microhematocrit tubes are available in different sizes; use tubes specified as appropriate for the centrifuge in use.

MATERIALS AND EQUIPMENT

- gloves
- hand antiseptic
- full-face shield (or equivalent PPE)
- acrylic safety shield (optional)
- microhematocrit centrifuge and reader
- plastic or Mylar-coated capillary tubes, heparinized and plain, self-sealing preferred
- precalibrated capillary tubes (if required for type of microhematocrit centrifuge available)
- sealant pad (if self-sealing tubes are unavailable)
- tube of anticoagulated venous blood
  - test tube rack
  - mechanical mixer
- capillary puncture supplies
  - alcohol swabs
  - sterile gauze or cotton balls
  - sterile, disposable lancets
- laboratory tissue
- paper towels
- surface disinfectant (such as 10% chlorine bleach)
- biohazard container
- sharps container

PROCEDURE

Record in the comment section any problems encountered while practicing the procedure (or have a fellow student or the instructor evaluate your performance).

S = Satisfactory
U = Unsatisfactory

You must:	S	U	Evaluation/Comments
1. Wash hands with antiseptic and put on gloves and face protection			
2. Assemble equipment and materials for capillary puncture and microhematocrit			

(Continues)

© 2012 Delmar, Cengage Learning. Permission to reproduce for clinical use granted.

You must:	S	U	Evaluation/Comments
3. Fill two capillary tubes from a capillary puncture (steps 3a–3g): a. Perform a capillary puncture b. Wipe away the first drop of blood c. Touch one end of a heparinized capillary tube to the second drop of blood d. Allow the tube to fill at least three-fourths full by capillary action, holding the tube at a slight downward angle. If using precalibrated tubes, fill to the line e. Fill a second tube in the same manner f. Wipe the outside of the filled capillary tube with soft tissue, if necessary, to remove excess blood g. Seal the tubes (if not self-sealing)			
4. Fill two capillary tubes using a tube of EDTA anticoagulated blood following steps 4a–4g (If not available, proceed to step 5): a. Mix the blood thoroughly by gently inverting the tube 50 to 60 times or mixing for 2 minutes using a mechanical mixer b. Remove cap from tube carefully to avoid creating aerosol (wearing face protection or with tube positioned behind acrylic safety shield) c. Tilt the tube so the blood is very near the mouth of the tube d. Insert the tip of a plain capillary tube into the blood and fill three-quarters full by capillary action. If using precalibrated tubes, fill to the line. e. Wipe the outside of the filled capillary tube with tissue, if necessary, to remove excess blood f. Seal the capillary tube g. Fill a second tube in the same manner and seal			
5. Place tubes into the microhematocrit centrifuge with sealed ends placed securely against the gasket; balance the load by placing the tubes directly opposite each other			
6. Fasten both lids securely			
7. Set the timer (and adjust the speed if necessary)			
8. Centrifuge for the prescribed and at the correct speed			
9. Allow centrifuge to come to a complete stop and unlock lids			

(Continues)

© 2012 Delmar, Cengage Learning. Permission to reproduce for clinical use granted.

You must:	S	U	Evaluation/Comments

10. Determine the microhematocrit values using one of the following methods:
  a. For a centrifuge that requires precalibrated tubes and has a built-in scale:
    (1) Position the tubes as directed by the manufacturer's instructions
    (2) Read the microhematocrit value from the scale
  b. For a centrifuge without a built-in reader:
    (1) Remove capillary tubes from centrifuge rotor carefully
    (2) Place tubes on the microhematocrit reader
    (3) Follow instructions on the reader to obtain the microhematocrit value. The values must agree within ±2%			

11. Average the readings from the two tubes and record the microhematocrit			
12. Discard all sharps into sharps containers			
13. Discard all contaminated materials into a biohazard container			
14. Disinfect equipment and return unused supplies to storage			
15. Wipe the work area with disinfectant			
16. Remove gloves and discard into biohazard container			
17. Wash hands with antiseptic			

Instructor/Evaluator Comments:

Instructor/Evaluator _____ Date _____

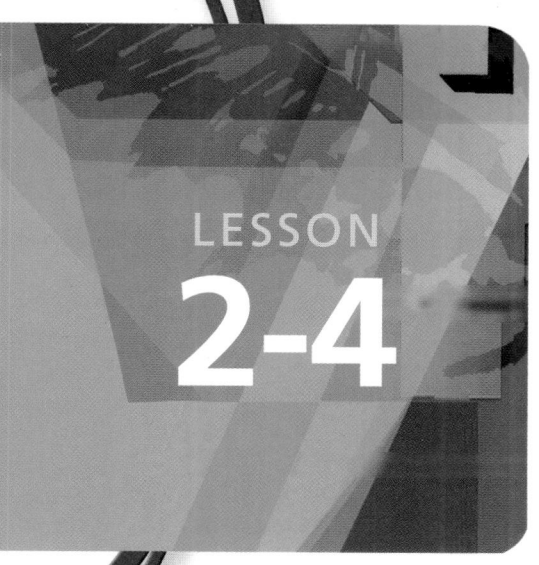

LESSON 2-4

The Hemacytometer

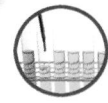

LESSON OBJECTIVES

After studying this lesson, the student will:

⊙ Identify the parts of a hemacytometer.

⊙ Use the microscope to identify the ruled areas of the hemacytometer used to count red blood cells (RBCs), white blood cells (WBCs), and platelets.

⊙ Load the hemacytometer using a micropipet or capillary tube.

⊙ Explain the boundary rules and counting pattern used with the hemacytometer.

⊙ Write and use the general formula for calculating cell counts using a hemacytometer.

⊙ List the safety precautions to observe when using the hemacytometer.

⊙ Discuss quality assessment issues associated with manual cell counts using the hemacytometer.

⊙ Define the glossary terms.

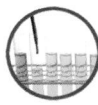

GLOSSARY

cell diluting fluid / a solution used to dilute blood for cell counts

hemacytometer / a heavy glass slide made to precise specifications and used to count cells microscopically; a counting chamber

hemacytometer coverglass / a special coverglass of uniform thickness used with a hemacytometer

micropipet / a pipet that measures or holds 1 mL or less

INTRODUCTION

Blood cell counts are routinely performed using automated cell counters or hematology analyzers. However, when cell counters are not available or when blood cell counts are extremely low, manual blood cell counts can be performed microscopically using the **hemacytometer**, a special counting chamber. The hemacytometer is also used to count cells in cerebrospinal fluid and other body fluids and to count sperm in fertility testing.

Hemacytometers are manufactured to meet the specifications of the National Institute of Standards and Technology (NIST). The use of the hemacytometer, explanations of the ruled areas, and the method of calculating cell counts are explained in this lesson. Procedures for performing WBC and RBC counts and a brief discussion of automated cell counters are outlined in Lesson 2-5.

THE HEMACYTOMETER

The hemacytometer is a precision-made slide for performing manual cell counts using the microscope. The hemacytometer is sometimes called a counting chamber. The hemacytometer counting chamber contains two microscopic ruled areas marked off by precise lines. The arrangement of lines in the ruled area can vary according to the type hemacytometer being used. Most hematology laboratories use hemacytometers with improved *Neubauer*-type design for blood cell counts.

Glass Hemacytometers

The traditional hemacytometer is a heavy glass slide with two counting areas. When viewed from the top, two polished raised platforms are surrounded by moats (troughs) on three sides (Figure 2-20A) form the shape of an *H*. Each raised platform contains a ruled counting area.

The hemacytometer must be used with a **hemacytometer coverglass** of uniform thickness (0.4 mm) that has been manufactured to meet NIST specifications. The hemacytometer coverglass is positioned so that it covers both ruled areas of the hemacytometer (Figure 2-20). The coverglass creates a chamber, confines the fluid when the chamber is loaded, and regulates the depth of the fluid. The chamber depth in the Neubauer-type hemacytometer is 0.1 mm with the coverglass in place. Hemacytometer and coverglass are both reusable, but must be disinfected between uses.

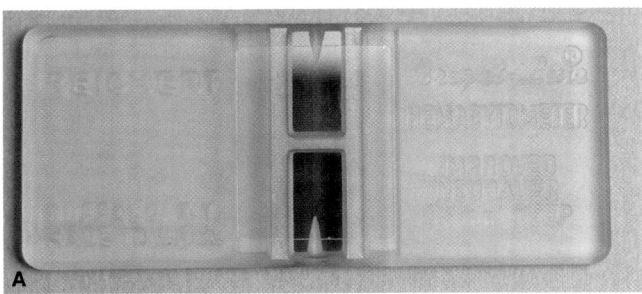

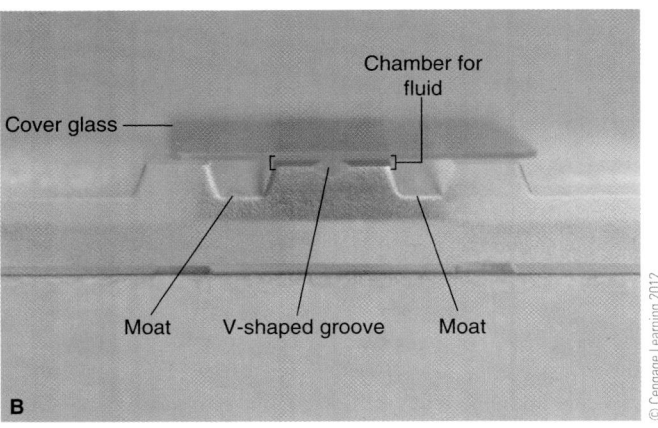

FIGURE 2-20 The hemacytometer: (A) top view of hemacytometer with coverglass in place; (B) side view of hemacytometer with coverglass in place

Disposable Hemacytometers

Efforts to improve efforts to improve laboratory biosafety have resulted in several single-use disposable products being developed for laboratory use. Disposable plastic hemacytometers designed to be used like the standard glass hemacytometer are available. An integral part of the design is a plastic "coverglass" to confine the fluid and standardize the volume (Figure 2-21). Disposable hemacytometers can be purchased with Neubauer rulings as well as other types for rulings used for a variety of purposes, such as bacterial counting. The use of disposable products increases cost but also increases safety.

Ruled Counting Areas

The hemacytometer contains two identical ruled areas composed of etched lines that define squares of specific dimensions. In the Neubauer-type hemacytometer, the total ruled area on each side consists of a large square, 3×3 mm, divided into nine equal squares (Figure 2-22), each 1-mm square (mm²). The total area of the large square is 9 mm². When the coverglass is in place and fluid is introduced into the chamber, the fluid volume in the ruled area can be calculated. For example, if the depth is 0.1 mm, the total volume is equal to 0.1 mm $\times$ 9 mm² or 0.9 mm³.

White Blood Cell Counting Area

The area counted for a WBC count is determined by the degree of blood dilution used for the count. The facility's standard operating procedure (SOP) manual will provide detailed instructions. For blood diluted 1:100, all nine large squares of the ruled area are counted. The cells in the four large corner squares (Figure 2-23) are counted when using a 1:20 dilution.

Red Blood Cell and Platelet Counting Areas

The large center square is used for platelet counts and RBC counts (Figure 2-23). This center square is divided into 25 smaller squares, which are each subdivided into 16 squares.

The entire large center square (circled) is used to count platelets (Figure 2-23). For RBC counts, only five of the 25 squares in the center square are counted. These can be the four corner

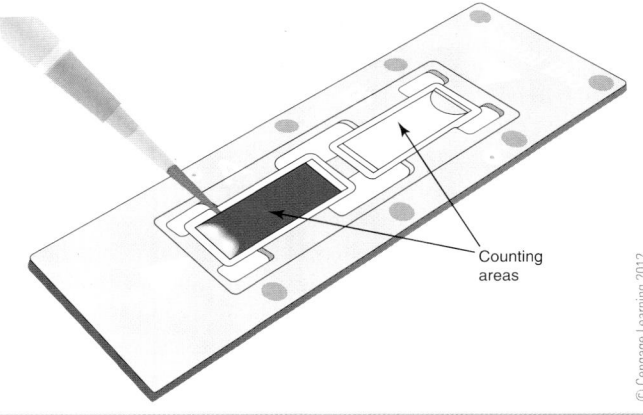

FIGURE 2-21 Diagram of disposable hemacytometer showing counting areas and sample loading points

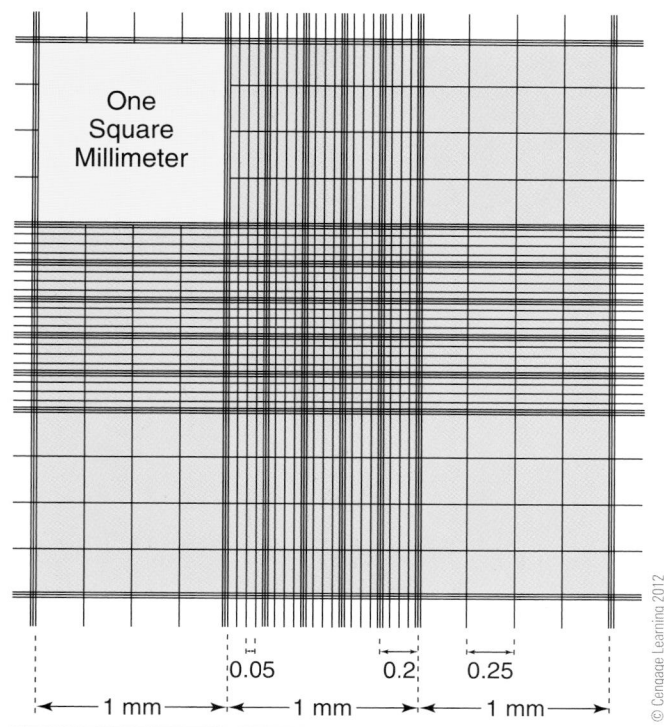

FIGURE 2-22 Ruled area of a hemacytometer chamber showing the dimensions

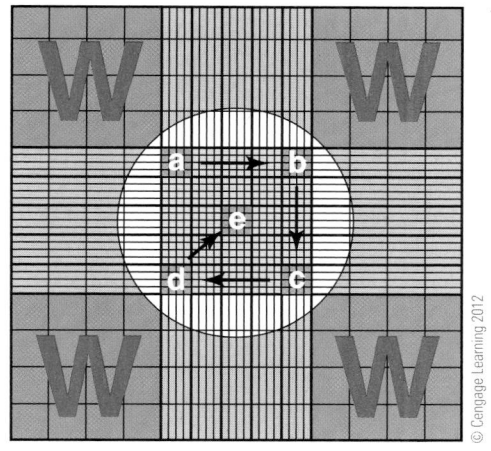

FIGURE 2-23 Cell counting areas: Cells in the four large corner squares (shown in blue) are counted for the white blood cell count; all cells in the entire center square (yellow, circled) are counted for the platelet count; the four red corner squares and center red square within the large center square (labeled a-e) are used for the red blood cell count

squares and the center square (a through e) or five squares in a diagonal line within the large center square (Figure 2-23).

USING THE HEMACYTOMETER

Laboratory personnel should be skilled in microscope use before using the hemacytometer. Instructions for using the microscope are in Lesson 1-10.

Safety Precautions

Standard Precautions must be observed and appropriate PPE worn when performing counts on blood or any body fluid. The hemacytometer and coverglass should be handled carefully to prevent personal injury or damage to the hemacytometer such as chips or breakage. The slide and coverglass must be disinfected after each use by soaking in a disinfectant such as a 10% chlorine bleach solution. Both can then be carefully washed in a solution of laboratory detergent, thoroughly rinsed, dried, and stored. Use of disposable hemacytometers eliminates the hazards associated with disinfecting and cleaning glass hemacytometers, as well as the potential for damage to the glass hemacytometer from frequent handling and use.

Quality Assessment

Cell counting procedures described in the laboratory's SOP manual must be followed. Counting procedures can differ slightly depending on the cell diluting systems available. Because few blood cell standards are available for manual cell counts in hematology, quality assessment for hemacytometer counts is primarily concerned with technique. Specimen collection and preparation, cell count procedures, and calculations are all areas in which good technique and attention to detail are very important.

The hemacytometer and coverglass are delicate pieces of equipment that must be carefully handled. The hemacytometer and coverglass should be stored covered in a dust-free location to prevent an accumulation of dust and grit that could scratch the surfaces. Before the chamber is loaded, the polished surfaces and the coverglass should be cleaned with lens paper and 90% or 95% ethanol to remove fingerprints or debris. This prevents erroneous results caused by counting debris as cells. Care must be taken to avoid overloading the sides of the chamber, which would allow the fluid to overflow into the moats and alter the cell distribution. If the fluid overflows, the hemacytometer must be cleaned and reloaded.

Once the hemacytometer has been loaded, the cells must be allowed to settle before counting. Cell counts must be performed using the correct ruled areas, and calculations must be performed accurately. Counting must be completed within 10 minutes of loading the hemacytometer, before evaporation can occur and alter cell distribution. If the total number of cells counted on each side of the chamber differs by more than 10%, it is an indication that the loading could have been uneven. If this occurs a clean hemacytometer must be loaded and the counts repeated.

Dilutions and Cell Diluting Fluids

The first step in manual blood cell counts is to dilute the blood using the appropriate **cell diluting fluid**. The degree of dilution and the type of cell diluting fluid used depends on the cell type to be counted.

Red cells are the most numerous blood cells (in the millions per microliter [μL] of blood); white cells are the least numerous (in the thousands per microliter); and platelets fall in between (in the hundreds of thousands per microliters). For red cell counts, blood is diluted 1:200. The red cell diluting fluid must be isotonic to protect the delicate red blood cells from hemolysis.

A common white cell diluting fluid is dilute ammonium oxalate, which lyses red cells while leaving white cells intact. White cell diluting fluids often contain a dye to make the white cell nuclei more prominent and the cells easier to count. Blood for white cell counts is diluted 1:100 using the LeukoChek system (Biomedical Polymers, Inc.). The Leuko-TIC system (bioanalytic GmbH) uses a blood dilution of 1:20 for white cell counts.

Blood for platelet counts must also be diluted in a fluid that lyses red blood cells. The dilute ammonium oxalate solution used for WBC counts is commonly used for platelet counts; the platelet dilution is 1:100. Table 2-4 summarizes some of the major differences in counting procedures for RBCs, WBCs, and platelets.

Loading the Hemacytometer

Once the blood dilution is made, the hemacytometer is loaded. A clean hemacytometer coverglass should be positioned so that it covers both ruled areas of a clean hemacytometer. The hemacytometer is loaded by touching a filled capillary tube or **micropipet** to the point where the coverglass and the raised platform meet (Figure 2-24). Approximately 10 µL of fluid from the pipet is allowed to flow into one side of the chamber. The other side is loaded in the same manner. Some hemacytometers have a V-shaped groove on each platform to guide the placement of the pipet tip when loading the chamber (Figure 2-20A).

The fluid should flow into the chamber in a smooth unbroken stream. *The fluid should not be allowed to overflow into the moats (troughs), and no air bubbles should be present.* After the both sides of the chamber have been correctly loaded, the hemacytometer should stand undisturbed for at least 2 minutes to allow the cells to settle.

Viewing the Ruled Areas

The hemacytometer is placed on the microscope stage with the low power (10×) objective in place, and a ruled area of one side of the chamber is positioned over the light source. The coarse adjustment knob is then used to locate the ruled area, and the fine adjustment is used to bring the etched lines into sharp focus. This

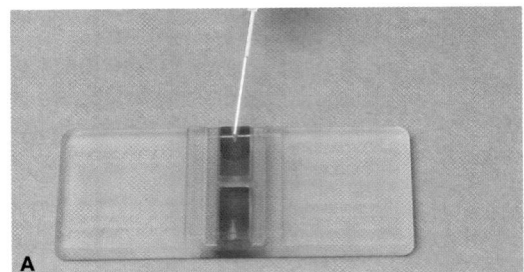
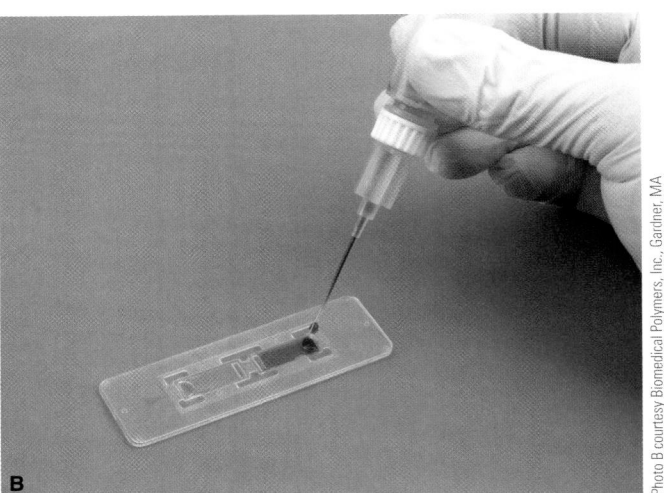

FIGURE 2-24 Loading the hemacytometer: (A) reusable glass hemacytometer loaded using capillary pipet; (B) single-use, disposable hemacytometer loaded using BMP LeukoChek

Photo B courtesy Biomedical Polymers, Inc., Gardner, MA

must be done carefully so that the objective does not touch the coverglass. The etched lines are more easily viewed when the microscope condenser and light intensity are adjusted for best contrast.

When the ruled area is in sharp focus, the counting areas should be located and identified by moving the stage. Depending on the blood dilution system used, the four large corner squares or the entire nine large squares are used for WBC counts. After the WBC area has been observed, the central square used for RBC counts should be located. The high power (40×) objective

TABLE 2-4. Comparison of manual red blood cell, white blood cell, and platelet counting procedures

CELL TYPE	CHARACTERISTIC OF DILUTING FLUID	BLOOD DILUTION MADE	DILUTION FACTOR	RULED SQUARES COUNTED	AREA COUNTED (mm²)
Red blood cells	Isotonic for RBCs	1:200	200	5 squares within large center square	0.2
White blood cells (Leuko-TIC method)	RBC lysing	1:20	20	4 large corner squares	4.0
White blood cells (LeukoChek method)	RBC lysing	1:100	100	Entire ruled area (9 large 1 × 1 mm squares)	9.0
Platelets	RBC lysing	1:100	100	Entire large center square	1.0

should be carefully rotated into place. *If the microscope is parfocal, the ruled area will be brought into focus with only a slight rotation of the fine adjustment. The oil-immersion objective is never used with a hemacytometer.* The large center square used for platelet counts and the five small squares used for an RBC count should be located (Figure 2-23).

Once all parts of the ruled area of one side of the chamber have been located, the low-power objective should be rotated into place and the stage control should be used to move the hemacytometer to bring the ruled area in the second side of the chamber into view.

The Cell Counting Pattern and Boundary Rule

A definite counting pattern should be followed to ensure that cells are counted only once. The count should begin in the upper left corner of a square and proceed in a serpentine manner (Figure 2-25). Single, double, or triple boundary lines divide the squares. When triple lines are present, the center line is the boundary. When double lines are present, the outer line is the boundary.

All cells that lie completely within a square, and those that touch the left boundary of the square, or touch the top boundary of the square, are considered to be in that square and are counted. Cells that touch the right boundary or lower boundary of a square should not be counted in that square even if they lie mostly within the square (Figure 2-25).

The cells in the appropriate squares should be counted on both sides of the chamber. The results for the two sides are totaled and an average calculated. The average is used in the formula to calculate the cell counts.

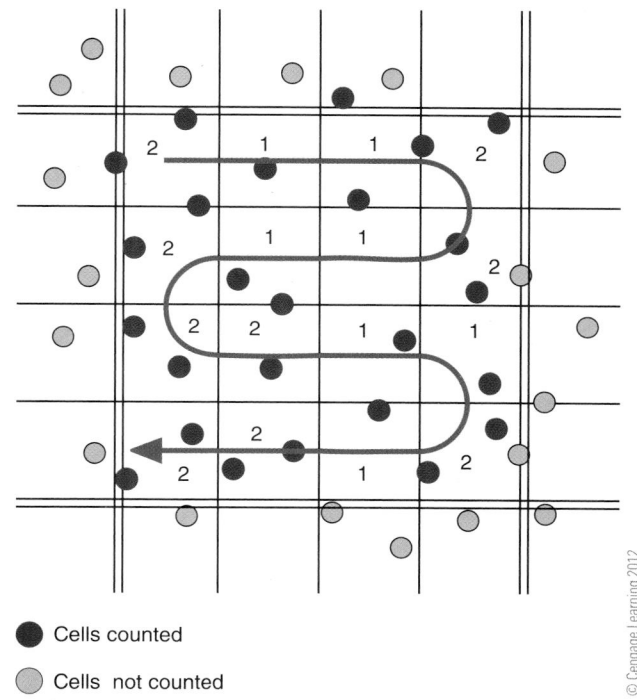

● Cells counted

○ Cells not counted

© Cengage Learning 2012

FIGURE 2-25 Counting pattern: A sample hemacytometer square containing 16 small squares and showing cells to include in a count (red circles) and cells excluded from the count (green circles). The square has double boundary lines; any cells touching the upper or left lines are counted. The count should begin in the square at the upper left corner and follow the serpentine counting pattern indicated by the arrow. In the diagram shown, the cell count is 25

---

1. Count the cells:

	Side 1			Side 2	
Square	**Cells counted**		**Square**	**Cells counted**	
a	110		a	105	
b	100		b	115	
c	90		c	100	
d	95		d	106	
e	105		e	94	
Total	500		Total	520	

2. Compute the average:
   A. 500 + 520 = 1020 cells
   B. 1020 ÷ 2 = 510 average

3. Calculate the count:

$$\text{RBC} = \frac{\text{Average \# cells counted} \times \text{Dilution factor}}{\text{Area counted (mm}^2) \times \text{D(0.1 mm)}}$$

$$\text{RBC} = \frac{510 \times 200}{0.2 \ \text{mm}^2 \times 0.1 \ \text{mm}}$$

$$\text{RBC} = 510 \times 10{,}000/\text{mm}^3 \ (\text{or } \mu\text{L})$$

$$\text{RBC} = 5{,}100{,}000/\mu\text{L} \ (\text{reported as } 5.1 \times 10^6/\mu\text{L or } 5.1 \times 10^{12}/\text{L})$$

© Cengage Learning 2012

FIGURE 2-26 Sample calculation of a red blood cell count using a 1:200 dilution

CALCULATING THE CELL COUNTS

A general formula for calculating hemacytometer cell counts is:

$$\text{Cells/}\mu\text{L} = \text{Cells/mm}^3 = \frac{\text{avg} \times \text{DF}}{\text{A (mm}^2) \times \text{D (0.1 mm)}}$$

Where

$$\text{Cells/}\mu\text{L} = \text{Final cell count/}\mu\text{L}$$
$$\text{avg} = \text{sum of cells counted on both sides of hemacytometer divided by 2}$$
$$\text{DF} = \text{dilution factor (reciprocal of dilution)}$$
$$\text{A (mm}^2) = \text{area counted}$$
$$\text{D (0.1 mm)} = \text{depth of chamber, a constant (always 0.1 mm)}$$

The *area* (A) counted is calculated using the dimensions of the particular ruled area. The area counted will vary depending on which cell type is being counted. The dilution factor is determined by the blood dilution used for the cell count being performed. The *dilution factor* (DF) is the reciprocal of the dilution. For instance, if a 1:200 dilution is made (by combining 1 part blood + 199 parts diluting fluid), the *dilution factor* is 200 and is the number used in the formula. The *depth* (D) is always 0.1 mm because the chamber is 0.1 mm deep when the coverglass is in place. A sample calculation for a red blood cell count is shown in Figure 2-26.

SAFETY REMINDERS

- Review Safety Precautions section before beginning procedure.
- Observe Standard Precautions.
- Disinfect hemacytometer and coverglass after each use.

PROCEDURAL REMINDERS

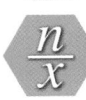

- Review Quality Assessment section before beginning procedure.
- Follow facility SOP manual for the counting system used.
- Complete counts within 10 minutes of loading chamber.
- Use serpentine counting pattern and observe boundary rules.
- Use correct values in the formula and make accurate calculations.

CALCULATION PROBLEMS

1. Write the formula to use for a manual RBC count using the hemacytometer.
2. A manual RBC count was performed using a 1:200 dilution. If 310 cells were counted on side 1 and 332 on side 2 of the hemacytometer, what cell number should be used in the formula to calculate the RBC count?
3. Use the formula and the answer for question #2 to calculate the RBC count. Report it in conventional units (cells/μL) and SI units (cells/L).

CRITICAL THINKING

Melissa had just completed a manual blood cell count. After she reported the result she found that there was also a manual platelet count to be done. The laboratory had only one hemacytometer. What is the appropriate action?

Melissa should:
a. Wipe the hemacytometer and coverglass with lens paper before using them again
b. Disinfect hemacytometer and coverglass and wash in detergent before use
c. Wash hemacytometer and coverglass in a laboratory detergent before disinfecting them
d. Wipe the hemacytometer and coverglass with sterile gauze before using them

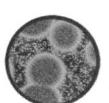

SUMMARY

Most blood cell counts are performed using cell counters or hematology analyzers. However, there are instances when it can be necessary to count blood cells manually. Cells from other body fluids can also be counted manually.

Manual cell counts are performed using a hemacytometer, a glass counting chamber divided into precise areas for counting cells and used with a special coverglass that defines the volume of fluid contained in the chamber. Exact procedures for diluting the sample, loading the hemacytometer, and counting the cells are described in the facility SOP manual and must be followed. The correct values from the count must be entered into the formula, calculations must be performed accurately, and correct units must be used for reporting the count result. The hemacytometer and coverglass must be disinfected and cleaned correctly to keep them free from dust, dirt, or oil which could interfere with cell counts. The use of disposable hemacytometers lessens the hazards associated with performing manual counts using glass equipment. It is important for the laboratory to have a technician who is competent in using the hemacytometer for cases when manual cell counts must be performed.

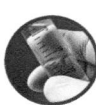

REVIEW QUESTIONS

1. How are blood cells routinely counted in the hematology laboratory?
2. Explain the importance of knowing how to perform a manual blood cell count.
3. Name the special slide used to perform manual cell counts.
4. Diagram the hemacytometer and its parts.

5. Draw a hemacytometer ruled area; indicate the areas used for the WBC, RBC, and platelet counts.
6. List the three functions of the coverglass when it is in place on the hemacytometer.
7. Explain how to position the coverglass on the hemacytometer.
8. What dilution is used for RBC count? Why is the WBC dilution different?
9. Why is the type of cell diluting fluid important?
10. Explain how to load a hemacytometer using a micropipet or capillary tube.
11. What are the advantages of using a disposable hemacytometer?
12. Why is it important to ensure that fluid does not overflow into the moats?
13. What procedure should be used to clean the hemacytometer and coverglass after use?
14. Write the general formula used to calculate cell counts when using the hemacytometer. Explain A, Avg, D, DF, and C/µL.
15. Define cell diluting fluid, hemacytometer, hemacytometer coverglass, and micropipet.

STUDENT ACTIVITIES

1. Complete the written examination for this lesson.
2. Practice loading the hemacytometer and microscopically viewing the counting areas using the Student Performance Guide.
3. Use the general formula to calculate the cells/µL for the following RBC averages: 412, 450.

WEB ACTIVITIES

1. Search the Internet for laboratory regulatory web sites to find out if cell counts performed using the hemacytometer are CLIA-waived tests.
2. Use the Internet to find information about other designs of counting chambers, such as the Petroff-Hausser counting chamber. Compare the features of the Neubauer hemacytometer to those of one or more other counting chamber designs. Discuss the importance of knowing the type of counting chamber being used when performing and calculating cell counts.

LESSON 2-4

The Hemacytometer

Name _____ Date _____

INSTRUCTIONS

1. Practice using the hemacytometer following the step-by-step procedure.

2. Demonstrate the use of the hemacytometer satisfactorily for the instructor, using the Student Performance Guide. Your instructor will explain the procedures for evaluating and grading your performance. Your performance may be given a number grade, letter grade, or satisfactory (S) or unsatisfactory (U) depending on course or institutional policy.

MATERIALS AND EQUIPMENT

- gloves
- hand antiseptic
- hemacytometer (Neubauer type)
- hemacytometer coverglass
- lens paper
- lens cleaner
- 90% or 95% ethanol
- micropipetter (10 to 20 µL capacity) with disposable tips, or capillary tubes
- distilled water (optional: dilute food coloring or a cell diluting fluid)
- microscope
- laboratory tissue
- laboratory detergent
- paper towels
- surface disinfectant (such as 10% chlorine bleach)
- sharps container

PROCEDURE

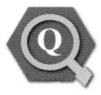

Record in the comment section any problems encountered while practicing the procedure (or have a fellow student or the instructor evaluate your performance).

S = Satisfactory
U = Unsatisfactory

You must:	S	U	Evaluation/Comments
1. Wash hands with antiseptic and put on gloves			
2. Assemble equipment and materials			
3. Use lens paper and 90% or 95% ethanol to carefully polish the hemacytometer and coverglass			
4. Place the coverglass over the ruled areas of the hemacytometer			
5. Use a capillary tube to load the hemacytometer following steps 5a through 5e. If a micropipet is used skip to step 6			

(Continues)

© 2012 Delmar, Cengage Learning. Permission to reproduce for clinical use granted.

You must:	S	U	Evaluation/Comments
a. Fill a capillary tube ½ full with distilled water (or with dilute food coloring or cell diluting fluid) b. Hold the capillary tube at a 30- to 45-degree angle and touch the tip to the point where the coverglass and the hemacytometer meet, taking care not to move the coverglass c. Control fluid delivery and allow fluid to slowly flow into one side of the chamber d. Load the chamber in one smooth motion without allowing air bubbles to enter chamber or fluid to overflow into the moats e. Load the other side of the chamber in the same manner			
6. Use a micropipetter to load the hemacytometer following steps 6a through 6e: a. Draw distilled water into the micropipetter (approximately 10 μL will be needed for each side of the chamber). *Optional*: Use very diluted food coloring or a cell diluting fluid instead of distilled water. b. Hold the micropipetter or capillary tube at a 30- to 45-degree angle and touch the tip to the point where the coverglass and the hemacytometer meet, taking care not to move the coverglass c. Control fluid delivery and allow fluid to slowly flow into one side of the chamber. d. Load the chamber in one smooth motion without allowing air bubbles to enter chamber or fluid to overflow into the moats e. Load the other side of the chamber in the same manner			
7. Position the low-power (10×) objective in place			
8. Place the hemacytometer on the microscope stage securely with one ruled area over the light source			
9. Look directly at the hemacytometer (not through the microscope eyepiece) and turn the coarse-adjustment knob to bring the microscope objective and the hemacytometer close together, continuing until the objective is almost touching the coverglass NOTE: Use focusing knobs with care to prevent striking the hemacytometer coverglass with the objective			
10. Look into the eyepiece and slowly turn the coarse-adjustment knob in the opposite direction until the etched lines come into view			
11. Rotate the fine-adjustment knob until the lines are in clear focus			
12. Locate the nine large squares of the ruled area by moving the stage			

(Continues)

© 2012 Delmar, Cengage Learning. Permission to reproduce for clinical use granted.

You must:	S	U	Evaluation/Comments
13. Locate the four large corner squares of the ruled area by moving the stage			
14. Scan squares using left-to-right, right-to-left serpentine pattern and note boundary lines			
15. Locate the large center square used for the platelet count			
16. Rotate the high-power (40×) objective carefully into position, and use the fine-adjustment knob to adjust the focus until the etched lines appear distinct			
17. Locate the four smaller corner squares and the center square (within the large center square) used for the RBC count (each small square will contain 16 smaller squares divided with single etched lines)			
18. Scan the counting area using left-to-right, right-to-left pattern and note the boundary lines			
19. Rotate the low power (10×) objective into position and view the second ruled area, repeating steps 11–18			
20. Rotate the low-power objective into position			
21. Remove the hemacytometer carefully from the microscope stage and clean the microscope lenses with lens paper			
22. Clean the hemacytometer and the coverglass carefully using 90% or 95% ethanol and lens paper			
23. Dry the hemacytometer and coverglass with lens paper			
24. Clean and return all equipment to proper storage			
25. Discard sharps into sharps container			
26. Discard used materials appropriately			
27. Wipe work area with disinfectant			
28. Remove and discard gloves; wash hands with antiseptic			

Instructor/Evaluator Comments:

Instructor/Evaluator _____ Date _____

© 2012 Delmar, Cengage Learning. Permission to reproduce for clinical use granted

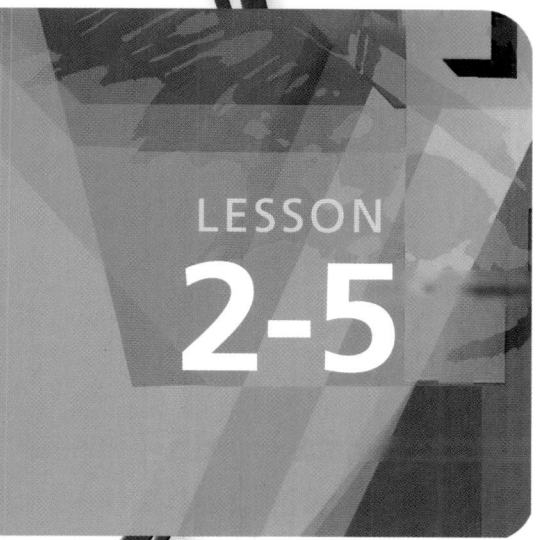

LESSON 2-5

Manual Red Blood Cell and White Blood Cell Counts

LESSON OBJECTIVES

After studying this lesson, the student will:

⊙ Write the general formula for calculating cell counts using the hemacytometer.

⊙ Compare the properties of cell diluting fluids used for red and white blood cell counts.

⊙ List the red blood cell reference values for adult men, adult women, and newborns.

⊙ Name a condition or disease associated with an increased red blood cell count and one associated with a decreased red blood cell count.

⊙ Perform a manual red blood cell count and calculate the results.

⊙ List the white blood cell reference values for adults, children, and newborns.

⊙ Name a condition that causes leukocytosis and one that causes leukopenia.

⊙ Perform a manual white blood cell count and calculate the results.

⊙ Discuss the safety issues involved in performing manual blood cell counts.

⊙ Discuss the importance of quality assessment in performing manual blood cell counts.

⊙ Define the glossary terms.

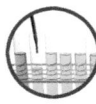

GLOSSARY

anemia / a condition in which the red blood cell count or blood hemoglobin level is below normal; a condition resulting in decreased oxygen-carrying capacity of the blood

aperture / an opening

erythrocytosis / an excess of red blood cells in the peripheral blood; sometimes called polycythemia

hemolysis / the rupture or destruction of red blood cells, resulting in the release of hemoglobin

immunity / resistance to disease or infection

isotonic solution / a solution with the same concentration of dissolved particles as the solution or cell with which it is compared

leukemia / a cancer of white blood cells characterized by an abnormal increase of white blood cells and their precursors in bone marrow, tissue, and peripheral blood

leukocytosis / increase above normal in the number of leukocytes (white blood cells) in the blood

leukopenia / decrease below normal in the number of leukocytes (white blood cells) in the blood; leukocytopenia

INTRODUCTION

The red blood cell (RBC) count and the white blood cell (WBC) count are parts of the routine complete blood count (CBC). RBCs are the most numerous of the blood cells. The RBC count approximates the number of circulating RBCs and thus gives an indirect estimate of the blood's oxygen-carrying capacity (hemoglobin). The RBC count is helpful in the diagnosis and treatment of many diseases, especially **anemia**, a condition in which there is a decrease below normal in the RBC count or hemoglobin level.

WBCs are less numerous in the peripheral blood than RBCs. All WBCs play important roles in **immunity**, the body's ability to resist disease. The WBC count gives general information concerning a patient's ability to fight infection.

BLOOD DILUTING SYSTEMS FOR MANUAL CELL COUNTS

Although blood cell counts are routinely performed using instrumentation, situations can arise in which manual cell counts must be performed. For years the Unopette systems (Becton Dickinson) provided a standardized way of performing manual cell counts. These systems are being discontinued in the United States, but materials for manual cell counts are available from other manufacturers.

This lesson provides instructions for performing hemacytometer counts using disposable blood collecting and diluting systems from two manufacturers.

- Biomedical Polymers, Inc. markets the LeukoChek for WBC and platelet counts

- Bioanalytic GmbH offers three systems, the
  - Ery-TIC system for RBC counts
  - Leuko-TIC system for WBC counts
  - Thrombo-TIC system kit for platelets (covered in Lesson 2-6, Platelet Count.)

The Ery-TIC and Leuko-TIC systems consist of calibrated capillary tubes that hold a precise blood volume and vials of pre-measured diluting fluid specific for the type of cells to be counted (Figure 2-27). Once the appropriate blood dilution is made, manual counts are performed by loading the blood dilution into a hemacytometer (Lesson 2-4) and viewing and counting the cells using the microscope.

The LeukoChek (Biomedical Polymers, Inc.) system is designed to replace the Unopette WBC/Platelet system (Becton Dickinson) for counting WBCs and platelets. This system is used in the same way that the Unopette system was used (Figure 2-28).

Dilutions for Red Blood Cell Counts

The Ery-TIC system for RBC counts includes a vial containing 995 μL (0.995 mL) of Hayem's RBC diluting fluid consisting of a buffered NaCl solution plus a preservative. The RBC diluting fluid is an **isotonic solution** to prevent **hemolysis**, or destruction, of the delicate red cells. The capillary pipet for measuring the blood sample is manufactured to contain 5 μL (0.005 mL). When 5 μL is added to the 995 μL of diluting fluid, the blood is diluted 1 part blood plus 199 parts diluting fluid. This equals a 1:200 dilution (1 part blood in a total of 200 parts).

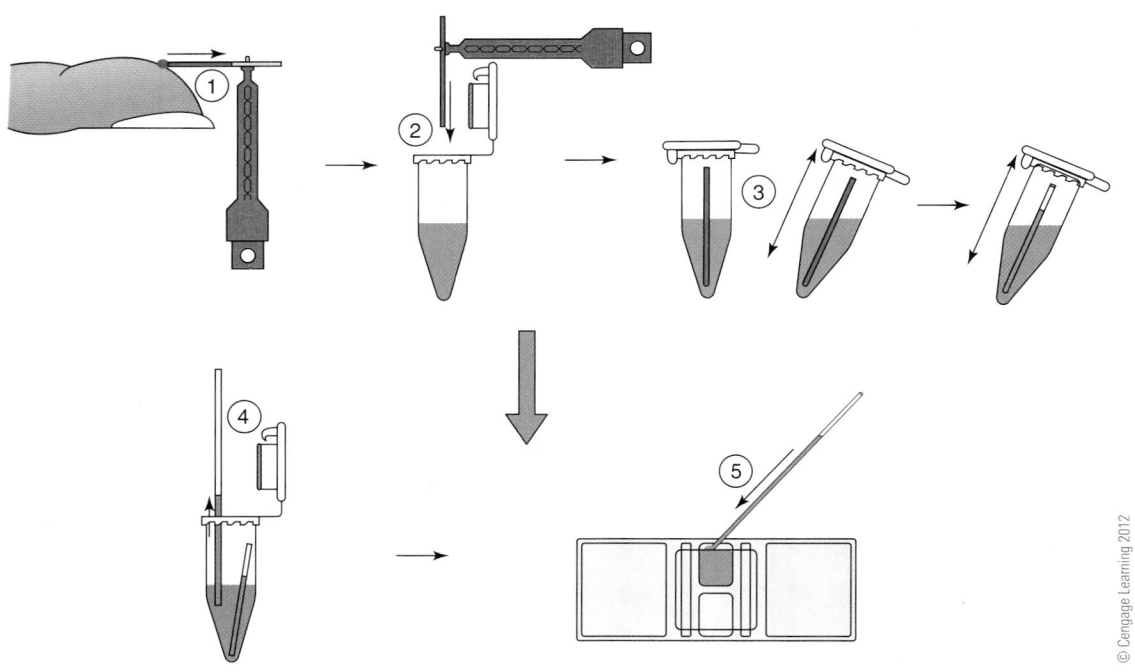

© Cengage Learning 2012

FIGURE 2-27 Illustration of bioanalytic GmbH Ery-TIC® and Leuko-TIC® blood dilution procedures: (1) collect blood in capillary using capillary holder; (2) drop capillary into diluting fluid; (3) cap vial and mix by inversion; (4) withdraw sample and (5) load hemacytometer

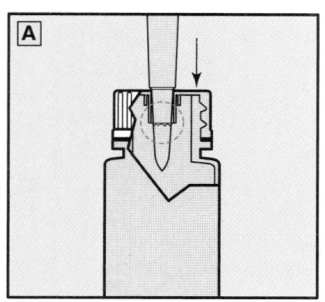 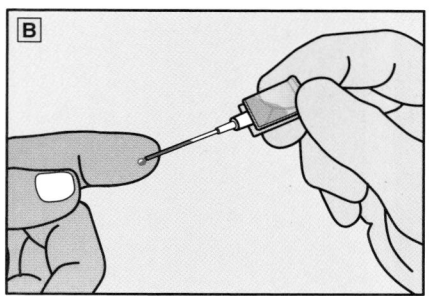 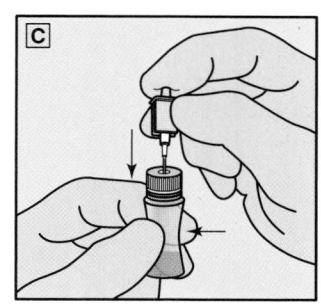

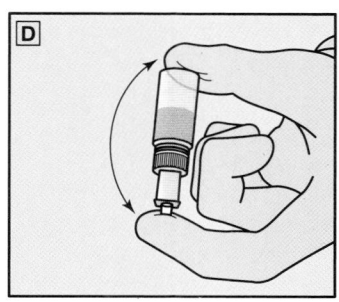 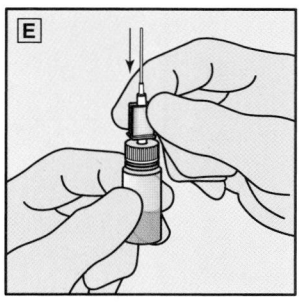

FIGURE 2-28 Illustration of BMP LeukoChek™ blood dilution procedure

Dilutions for White Blood Cell Counts

Leuko-TIC

The Leuko-TIC system for WBC counts consists of a vial containing 380 μL (0.38 mL) of WBC diluting fluid and a 20 μL (0.02 mL) capacity capillary. The WBC diluting fluid is an acetate buffer to lyse the RBCs without harming the white blood cells. The buffer also contains gentian violet to stain WBC nuclei so they are easily seen with the microscope. When the 20 μL of blood is added to the 380 μL of diluting fluid, the dilution is 1:20 (1 part blood plus 19 parts diluting fluid).

LeukoChek

The LeukoChek system for WBC counts consists of a sealed reservoir containing 1.98 mL of WBC diluting fluid and a 0.02 mL (20 μL) capillary pipet with pipet shield. The diluting fluid is a buffered ammonium oxalate solution that lyses the RBCs. This system can also be used for counting platelets (see Lesson 2-6). When 0.02 mL of blood is added to the 1.98 mL of diluting fluid, the blood is diluted 1:100 (1 part blood plus 99 parts diluting fluid).

PERFORMING MANUAL RBC AND WBC COUNTS

The procedures for preparing the blood dilutions for the RBC and WBC counts are the same except for the sample size and type and volume of diluting fluid used. Safety issues and quality assessment issues apply to all manual cell counts. The procedures given in this section are general. Step-by-step instructions for performing both counts are in the Student Performance Guides at the end of this lesson.

Safety Precautions

   Standard Precautions must be observed when performing manual cell counts on blood or any other body fluid. The technician must wear appropriate personal protective equipment (PPE). Special care must be taken to avoid creating aerosols when opening blood tubes. All contaminated materials must be discarded into appropriate biohazard or sharps containers. The hemacytometer and coverglass must be disinfected after each use by soaking in disinfectant such as 10% chlorine bleach, then carefully washed in detergent, rinsed, and dried.

Quality Assessment

   Cell counting procedures in the laboratory's standard operating procedure (SOP) manual must be followed for the system used. Manual cell counts are less accurate and precise than counts performed using automated cell counters. Good technique with attention to detail is crucial in all aspects of the procedure, including specimen collection, preparation of cell dilutions, counting methods, and calculation of results.

Hemacytometers and coverglasses must be carefully cleaned with lens paper saturated with 90% or 95% ethanol before each use to be sure no fingerprints or debris are present on the polished surfaces containing the ruled areas. Any debris present can cause uneven loading or be mistaken for cells when a count is performed. Care must be taken to avoid overloading the hemacytometer, which would allow the fluid to flow into the moats and alter the cell distribution in the counting area.

The difference in the total number of cells counted on each side of the hemacytometer should not be more than 10%. A larger difference indicates that cell distribution was not uniform between the two sides, and the count should be repeated after loading a clean hemacytometer. The difference among counts in squares on the same side of the hemacytometer also should not differ by more than 10%.

Performing a Manual Red Blood Cell Count

The Ery-TIC method for performing a cell count is illustrated in Figure 2-27. The 5-µL capillary is filled with blood from a capillary puncture or from a tube of well-mixed EDTA-anticoagulated blood. A capillary holder is used to secure and stabilize the capillary during filling. Laboratory tissue is used to carefully remove any blood from the outside of the capillary. The filled capillary is then released from the holder and dropped into a vial containing 995 µL of red cell diluting fluid. The vial is capped securely, and the contents are mixed well by gently inverting the sealed vial several times to ensure that all blood is rinsed from the capillary. The resulting blood dilution is 1:200. The count can be performed immediately; however, the blood dilution is stable for up to 8 hours.

Loading the Hemacytometer

A clean coverglass is positioned on a clean hemacytometer to cover both counting areas. The blood dilution is mixed thoroughly but gently, and a micropipetter is used to remove 10 to 15 µL. The pipet tip is touched to the edge of the coverglass, and one side of the hemacytometer is loaded by capillary action (Figure 2-29). The cell dilution is again mixed, 10 to 15 µL is drawn into the micropipetter, and the opposite side of the hemacytometer is loaded in the same manner. If fluid overflows into the moat around the platforms or if air bubbles occur, the hemacytometer must be cleaned, dried, and reloaded.

Counting the Red Blood Cells

The loaded hemacytometer should remain undisturbed for 2 to 3 minutes to allow cells to settle. The hemacytometer is then placed on the microscope stage and the RBC ruled area is located using the low-power (10X) objective. The high-power (40×) objective is then carefully rotated into place to perform the count. Figure 2-30 illustrates the appearance of RBCs on the hemacytometer using the 40× objective.

The RBC count is performed using the center square of the ruled area as shown in Figure 2-31. Within the center square are 25 smaller squares. Of these 25 squares, only 5 are used for the count—the 4 corner squares and the center square, marked "a–e" in Figure 2-31. (Alternatively, 5 squares in a diagonal line from the top left corner to the bottom right corner of the center square can be used.)

Each of the 5 squares contains 16 smaller squares in four rows of four. All cells within each of the small five squares are counted using the left-to-right, right-to-left serpentine counting pattern. The cells touching either the top or left boundaries of the squares are included in the count. (Where triple boundary lines are present, the middle line is used as the boundary.) Cells touching the right boundary and the cells touching the lower boundary of each square are not counted. Cells lying beyond these boundaries are *not* counted (Figure 2-32).

A hand tally counter is used to tabulate the red cells as they are counted. The cell numbers for each of the five squares are recorded separately and then totaled. A count is then performed in five squares on the second side of the hemacytometer in the same manner. If good technique was used, the number of cells in a square should not vary from any other square on the same side of the hemacytometer by more than 10%.

Calculating the Red Blood Cell Count

The general formula to use for the hemacytometer is

$$\text{Cells}/\mu L = \frac{\text{Avg} \times \text{DF}}{A\,(\text{mm}^2) \times D\,(0.1\,\text{mm})}$$

To calculate the RBC count using the Ery-TIC method, the formula is used in the following manner:

1. The average number of cells is obtained by totaling the counts for the five squares on each side of the hemacytometer and dividing the total by two. This gives the average.

2. The dilution made is 1:200. Therefore the dilution factor (DF) is 200.

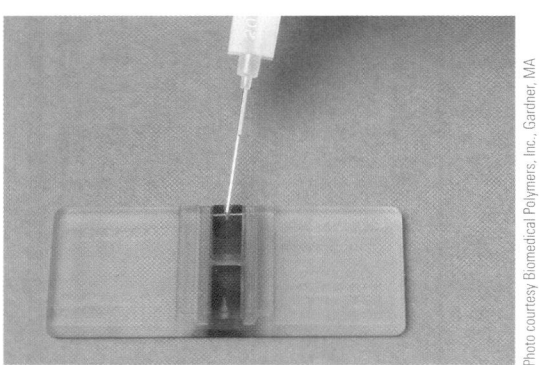

FIGURE 2-29 Loading the hemacytometer

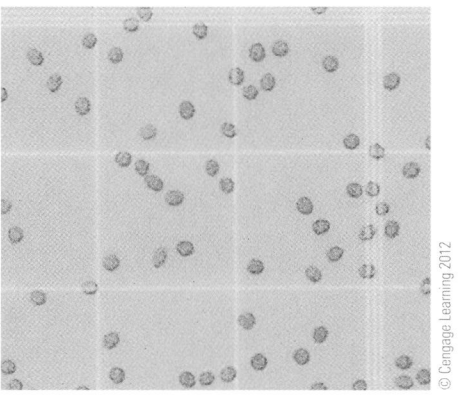

FIGURE 2-30 Photomicrograph of red blood cells as they appear on a hemacytometer

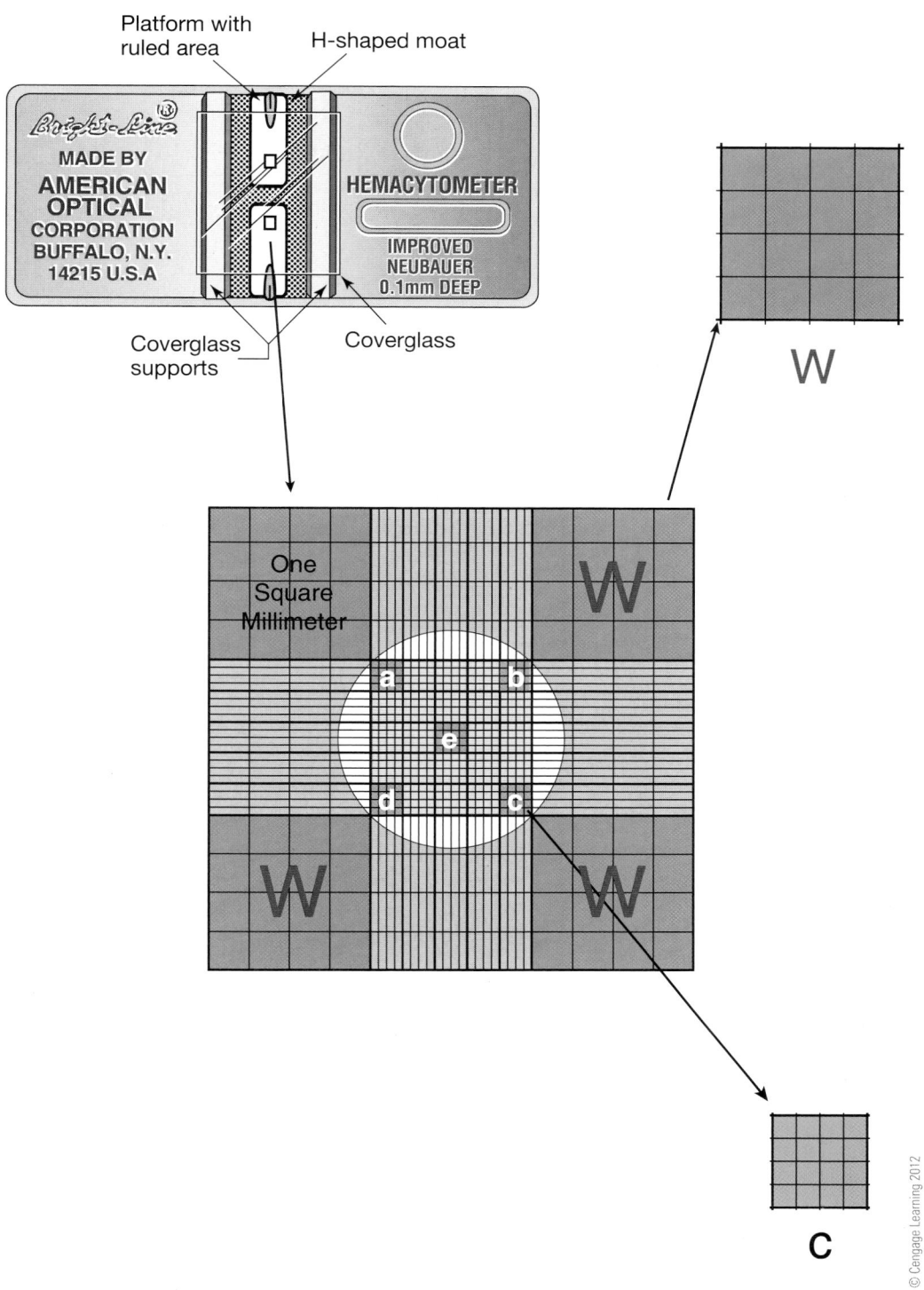

FIGURE 2-31 RBC and WBC counting areas: Cells in the four large corner squares (shown in blue) are counted for the white blood cell count; the four red corner squares and center red square within the large center yellow square are used for the red blood cell count

3. The depth (D) of the chamber is 0.1 mm, a constant.

4. The area (A) counted is 0.20 mm². (Each of the five squares within the large central square has a length of 0.2 mm and a width of 0.2 mm, making the area of each small square 0.04 mm². Because five squares are counted, the area is 5 × 0.04 mm², or 0.20 mm².) Substitute these numbers into the formula as shown:

$$\text{RBC/}\mu\text{L} = \frac{\text{Average} \times 200}{0.20 \text{ mm}^2 \times 0.1 \text{ mm}}$$

$$\text{RBC/}\mu\text{L} = \text{Average \# cells} \times 10,000$$

When an RBC count is performed this way, the number of cells per microliter can be calculated by simply adding four zeroes to the average number of cells counted (the same as

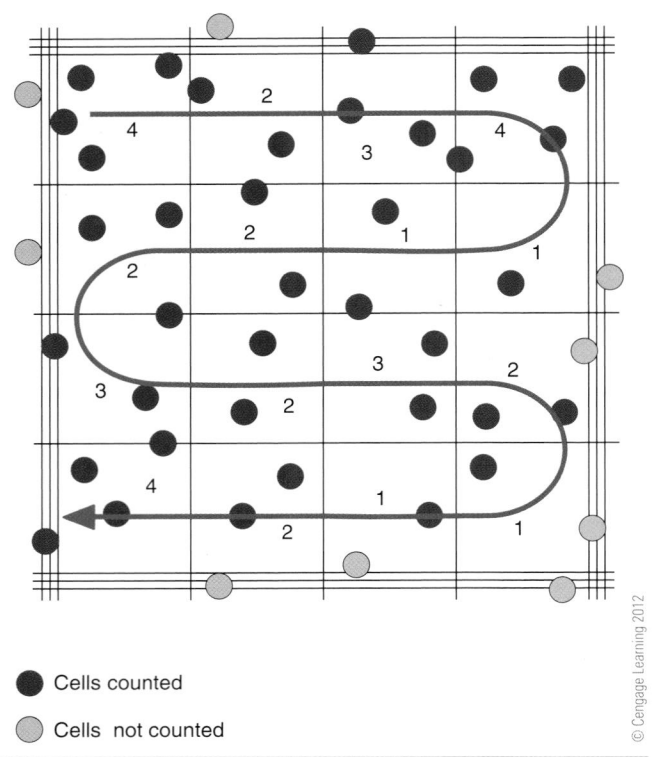

● Cells counted

○ Cells not counted

FIGURE 2-32 Counting method: A sample hemacytometer square with triple boundary lines showing cells to count; cells colored red should be counted and green cells should not be counted

multiplying by 10,000). A sample calculation is shown in Figure 2-33.

Reference Ranges for Red Blood Cell Counts

The reference values for RBC counts range from approximately 4 million per microliter of blood ($4.0 \times 10^6/\mu L$) to 6 million per microliter ($6.0 \times 10^6/\mu L$), depending on age and gender.

TABLE 2-5. Reference ranges for red blood cell counts

AGE/GENDER	REFERENCE RANGES CONVENTIONAL UNITS CELLS/µL	SI UNITS CELLS/L
Adult male	$4.5–6.0 \times 10^6/\mu L$	$4.5–6.0 \times 10^{12}/L$
Adult female	$4.0–5.5 \times 10^6/\mu L$	$4.0–5.5 \times 10^{12}/L$
Newborn	$5.0–6.3 \times 10^6/\mu L$	$5.0–6.3 \times 10^{12}/L$

Males have slightly higher RBC counts than females (Table 2-5). Newborns have elevated RBC counts that decline during early childhood and then increase to adult levels at puberty.

RBC counts can be reported as either the number of cells per microliter (µL) or per liter (L) of blood. For example, a count of 5.6×10^6 RBC/µL reported in SI units is 5.6×10^{12} RBC/L.

Performing a Manual White Blood Cell Count

The specific instructions contained in the package inserts included with the system being used and the instructions in the facility SOP manual should be followed.

Diluting the Blood

Leuko-TIC Method. The Leuko-TIC 20-µL capillary is filled with blood from a capillary puncture or from a tube of well-mixed EDTA blood. A capillary holder is used to secure and stabilize the capillary tube while filling (Figure 2-27). Blood from the outside of the capillary is carefully removed using laboratory tissue. The filled capillary is then released from the holder and dropped into a vial containing 380 µL of white cell diluting fluid. The vial is capped securely, and the contents are mixed well by

1. Count the cells:

	Side 1			Side 2	
Square	Cells counted		Square	Cells counted
a	100		a	97
b	95		b	95
c	90		c	90
d	90		d	96
e	105		e	88
Total	480		Total	466

2. Compute the average:
   A. 480 + 466 = 946 cells
   B. 946 ÷ 2 = 473 average

3. Calculate the count:

$$RBC = \frac{\text{Average \# cells counted} \times \text{Dilution factor}}{\text{Area counted (mm}^2) \times D\ (0.1\ mm)}$$

$$RBC = \frac{473 \times 200}{0.2\ mm^2 \times 0.1\ mm}$$

$$RBC = 4,730,000/\mu L \text{ (reported as } 4.73 \times 10^6/\mu L \text{ or } 4.73 \times 10^{12}/L)$$

FIGURE 2-33 Sample calculation for red blood cell count

© Cengage Learning 2012

CURRENT TOPICS

CLINICAL SIGNIFICANCE OF RED BLOOD CELL COUNTS

The primary function of RBCs is to facilitate oxygen exchange in the tissues. If the RBC count is low, less oxygen is available to body tissues. Significant decreases in the number of red cells can cause several physical symptoms, such as fatigue, weakness, headache, pallor, and increased heart rate. This condition is called anemia, and there can be many causes. In order to successfully treat anemia, the cause of the anemia must be discovered.

Two general causes of anemia are:

• Decreased RBC production
• Increased RBC loss or destruction

Anemia caused by decreased RBC production can be due to a deficiency in one or more of the substances or factors required to synthesize hemoglobin or to produce RBCs. For instance, because iron is required for heme synthesis, iron deficiency can cause anemia. The lack of iron can be due to poor diet or poor iron absorption. Vitamins such as B_{12} and folic acid (Table 2-6) are other factors required for RBC synthesis, so deficiencies in either of these can result in low RBC counts and symptoms of anemia.

Anemia caused by increased RBC loss or destruction can be caused by acute or chronic blood loss, such as from a bleeding ulcer. It can also be due to inherited conditions, such as sickle cell anemia, in which the life span of RBCs is shortened because of the presence of hemoglobin S in the cells.

TABLE 2-6. Examples of conditions affecting red blood cell counts

CONDITION	EFFECT ON RBC COUNT
Anemias	Decreased
Iron deficiency	
Sickle cell	
B_{12} deficiency	
Folic acid deficiency	
Acute or chronic blood loss	Decreased
Erythrocytosis	Increased
Polycythemia vera	Increased
Living at high altitude	Increased

At the other end of the scale is **erythrocytosis**—an RBC count above normal. Erythrocytosis can have physiological or pathological causes. People who live at very high altitudes have increased RBC levels because the lower oxygen content of the air stimulates RBC production. For instance, the RBC reference ranges for a population living in a region such as the Andes would be higher than the ranges for a population living near sea level. Heavy smokers also sometimes have increased RBC counts. *Polycythemia vera* is a disease in which the RBC count is greatly increased. Patients with polycythemia vera can require phlebotomy at regular intervals to remove excess RBCs.

---

inverting the sealed vial several times to ensure that all blood is rinsed from the capillary. The resulting blood dilution is 1:20. This blood dilution can be used after waiting a few minutes to allow time for RBCs to lyse and WBC nuclei to become stained. The diluted cell mixture is stable for up to 8 hours.

LeukoChek Method. The LeukoChek reservoir cap is pierced using the pipet shield. The 0.02 mL (20-µL) capillary is removed from the shield and the capillary is filled with blood from capillary puncture or from a tube of well-mixed ethylenediaminetetraacetic acid (EDTA) blood (Figure 2-28). While pressing lightly on the sides of the reservoir to expel some of the air, the filled capillary pipet is inserted into the reservoir. Pressure on the sides of the reservoir is released, drawing the blood into 1.98 mL of diluting fluid and creating a 1:100 blood dilution. Blood is rinsed from the pipet by gently squeezing the reservoir a few times (Figure 2-28). The capillary pipet is removed, inverted, and

seated into the top of the cap so that the capillary extends upward. This changes the pipette assembly from a collection device to a dropper. The mixture must stand for a few minutes before loading the hemacytometer, to allow time for the RBCs to be lysed.

Loading the Hemacytometer

A clean coverglass is positioned on a clean hemacytometer to cover both counting areas. The blood dilution is mixed thoroughly. For the Leuko-TIC method, a micropipetter is used to remove 10 to 15 µL. The pipet tip is touched to the edge of the coverglass, and one side of the hemacytometer is loaded by capillary action (Figure 2-29). The cell dilution is again mixed, 10 to 15 µL is drawn into the micropipetter, and the opposite side of the hemacytometer is loaded in the same manner.

For the LeukoChek method, the reservoir is swirled to mix the contents and a few drops are expelled from the capillary pipet tip and discarded. The capillary pipet is then used to load both sides of the hemacytometer (Figure 2-29).

For both methods, if fluid overflows into the depression around the platforms or if air bubbles occur, the hemacytometer must be cleaned and reloaded. Cells are allowed to settle for 2 minutes in the loaded hemacytometer.

Counting the White Blood Cells

Once cells have settled, the hemacytometer is placed securely onto the microscope stage for counting. The low-power objective (10×) is used to locate the ruled area. The WBCs will appear more distinct if the microscope's light level is reduced by adjusting the condenser, iris diaphragm, and light intensity.

- Leuko-TIC Counting Method (1:20 dilution)—cells in the four large corner squares of the ruled area are counted (as shown in Figure 2-31) using the 10× objective (100× magnification).

- LeukoChek Counting Method (1:100 dilution)—cells in the entire ruled area (all nine of the large squares) are counted using the 10× objective (100× magnification).

A. Perform white blood cell count using 1:20 dilution:

1. Count the cells:

	Side 1			Side 2	
Square	Cells counted		Square	Cells counted	
1	30		1	36	
2	29		2	32	
3	33		3	33	
4	32		4	35	
Total	124		Total	136	

2. Compute the average:

$$\frac{124 + 136}{2} = 130$$

3. Calculate the count:

$$WBC = \frac{\text{Average cells counted} \times \text{Dilution factor}}{\text{Area counted (mm}^2\text{)} \times \text{Depth (0.1mm)}}$$

$$WBC = \frac{130 \times 20}{4 \text{ mm}^2 \times 0.1\text{mm}}$$

$WBC = 130 \times 50 / \text{mm}^3$ (or μL)

$WBC = 6{,}500/$ μL (reported as $6.5 \times 10^3/$ μL or $6.5 \times 10^9/$ L)

B. Perform white blood cell count using 1:100 dilution:

1. Count the cells:

	Side 1		Side 2
Square	Cells counted		Cells counted
1	8		9
2	7		9
3	8		7
4	9		10
5	6		8
6	8		7
7	9		7
8	8		9
9	7		10
Total	70		Total 76

2. Compute the average:

$$\frac{70 + 76}{2} = 73$$

3. Calculate the count:

$$WBC = \frac{\text{Average cells counted} \times \text{Dilution factor}}{\text{Area counted (mm}^2\text{)} \times \text{Depth (0.1mm)}}$$

$WBC = [\text{Average counted} + (0.1 \times \text{average counted})] \times 100 / \text{mm}^3$ (or μL)

$WBC = [73 + (.10) \, 73] \times 100/$μL

$WBC = (73 + 7.3) \times 100/$μL

$WBC = (73 + 7) \times 100/$μL

$WBC = 80 \times 100/$μL

$WBC = 8000/$μL (or $8 \times 10^3/$μL)

$WBC = 8.0 \times 10^9/$L

© Cengage Learning 2012

FIGURE 2-34 Sample calculations for white blood cell counts: (A) using a 1:20 dilution and (B) using 1:100 dilution

The WBCs will appear as refractile round objects with a definite outline and a blue nucleus. The WBCs lying are counted using the left-to-right, right-to-left pattern (Figure 2-32). All cells touching either the upper or left boundary of the square are counted. Cells touching the lower or right boundary of the square are not counted. The counts from side 1 are recorded, and the procedure is repeated for side 2. The totals of sides 1 and 2 are added together and divided by two to obtain the average.

Calculating the White Blood Cell Count

The total number of WBCs per microliter of blood can be calculated using the average number of cells counted, the depth of the counting chamber, the area counted, and the dilution.

Leuko-TIC Method. The dilution made with the Leuko-TIC is 1:20, so the dilution factor is 20. The total area (A) counted is 4.0 mm²; the volume counted is 0.4 μL (depth × area = volume; 0.1 mm × 4 mm² = 0.4 mm³ = 0.4 μL). The WBC count is reported as cells per microliter or cells per liter using the following formula:

$$\text{WBC/μL} = \frac{\text{average \# cells} \times 20}{0.4\ \text{μL}}$$

$$\text{WBC/μL} = \text{average \# cells} \times 50$$

$$\text{WBC/L} = \text{average \# cells} \times 50{,}000$$

A sample WBC calculation using 1:20 dilution is shown in Figure 2-34A.

LeukoChek Method. The dilution made with the Leu-koChek system is 1:100, so the dilution factor is 100. The total area counted is 9.0 mm²; the volume counted is 0.9 μL (depth × area = volume; 0.1 mm × 9 mm² = 0.9 mm³ = 0.9 μL). However, the WBC count is reported as cells per microliter (or cells per liter). To correct for this, the following formula is used:

$$\text{WBC/μL} = \text{average \# cells} + (0.1 \times \text{average \# cells}) \times 100$$

A sample WBC calculation using a 1:100 dilution is shown in Figure 2-34B.

Reference Ranges for the White Blood Cell Count

The WBC reference range varies according to age (Table 2-7). WBC counts for newborns range from 9,000 to 30,000/μL. Within a few weeks after birth, the count drops rapidly and approaches the one-year old reference range of 6,000 to 14,000/μL. By adulthood, the normal count is in the range of 4,500 to 11,000/μL.

AUTOMATED CELL COUNTERS

Most blood cell counts are performed by automation, using instruments that range from relatively simple cell counters to complex hematology analyzers. Small analyzers can be used in a physician office laboratory (POL) or a small clinic (Figure 2-35). More elaborate equipment can be found in large hospitals and

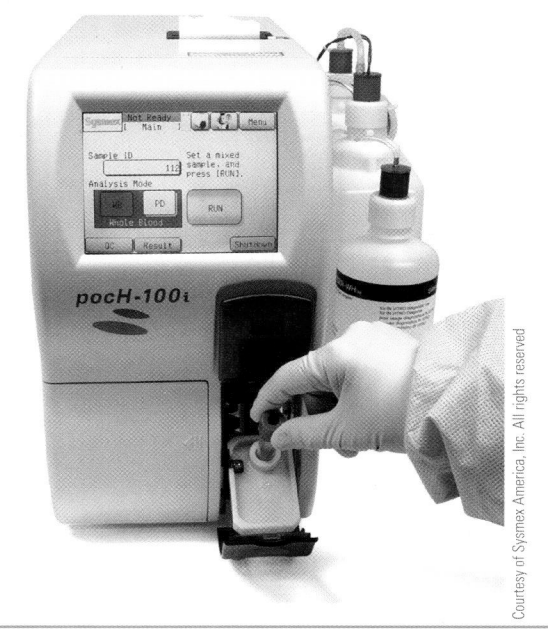

Courtesy of Sysmex America, Inc. All rights reserved

FIGURE 2-35 The pocH-100i cell counter is suitable for small laboratories and has the safety feature of through-the-cap sampling

	AVERAGE		RANGE	
AGE	**CONVENTIONAL UNITS (CELLS/μL)**	**SI UNITS (CELLS/L)**	**CONVENTIONAL UNITS (CELLS/μL)**	**SI UNITS (CELLS/L)**
Newborn	18,000	1.8×10^{10}	9,000–30,000	9.0–30.0×10^9
One year	11,000	1.1×10^{10}	6,000–14,000	6.0–14.0×10^9
Six years	8,000	8.0×10^9	4,500–12,000	4.5–12.0×10^9
Adult	7,400	7.4×10^9	4,500–11,000	4.5–11.0×10^9

TABLE 2-7. Reference ranges for white blood cell counts

CURRENT TOPICS

CLINICAL SIGNIFICANCE OF WHITE BLOOD CELL COUNTS

WBCs play important roles in the body's ability to fight infection. Each type of WBC has specific roles. For example, one role of lymphocytes is to respond to viral infections. Eosinophils and basophils increase in response to allergic conditions. Neutrophils and monocytes participate in defense against microorganisms such as bacteria. In response to stimuli such as bacterial by-products, neutrophils cluster or *marginate* on the walls of venules and capillaries. These marginating neutrophils then migrate through narrow spaces between the endothelial cells in the capillary walls and enter the site of infection in the tissues.

Leukocytosis, an increase in the WBC count, can be caused by many factors. Physiological factors such as stress, exercise, anesthesia, and even a cold shower can cause the WBC count to increase temporarily (Table 2-8). Changes in the WBC count as a result of disease are called pathological changes and continue until the illness or condition is under control. Bacterial infections usually cause an increase in the WBC count. The increase can be slight, such as in appendicitis, in which the WBC count usually does not go above 15 × 10⁹/L. In some other bacterial infections, the WBC count can reach 30 × 10⁹/L.

Two other conditions accompanied by leukocytosis are **leukemia** and *leukemoid reaction*. In leukemia— a cancer of WBCs and their precursors—an increase in the total WBC count is seen but it is usually caused by an increase in only one cell line, such as the one of the granulocytes or the lymphocytes.

Patients with leukemia can have WBC counts of 200 × 10⁹/L, and the WBC count can even reach 1,000 × 10⁹/L. In a leukemoid reaction the total WBC count can be 50 × 10⁹/L or higher, but is due to an infection or other noncancerous condition.

A decrease below normal in the total number of WBCs is called **leukopenia** (leukocytopenia). Leukopenia can be caused by certain viral infections or exposure to ionizing radiation, certain chemicals, and chemotherapy drugs. Infection by the human immunodeficiency virus (HIV) is an example of a viral disease that causes a decrease in the WBC count (Table 2-8).

TABLE 2-8. Some causes of leukocytosis and leukocytopenia

CAUSES OF LEUKOCYTOSIS	CAUSES OF LEUKOCYTOPENIA
Pathological	Some viral infections
Infection	including HIV
Leukemias	Ionizing radiation
	Certain chemicals
Polycythemia	Chemotherapy drugs
Physiological	
Exercise	
Exposure to sunlight	
Obstetric labor	
Stress	
Anesthesia	

TABLE 2-9. Comparison of manual red blood cell, white blood cell, and platelet counting procedures

CELL TYPE	CHARACTERISTIC OF DILUTING FLUID	BLOOD DILUTION MADE	DILUTION FACTOR	RULED SQUARES COUNTED	AREA COUNTED (MM²)
Red blood cells	Isotonic for RBCs	1:200	200	5 squares within large center square	0.2
White blood cells (Leuko-TIC)	RBC lysing	1:20	20	4 large corner squares	4.0
White blood cells (LeukoChek)	RBC lysing	1:100	100	All 9 large squares	9.0

reference laboratories. Most instruments at a minimum perform RBC and WBC counts, hemoglobin, hematocrit, platelet counts, RBC indices, and automated WBC differentials.

Automated cell counters operate on one of two principles. In some instruments, the cells to be counted are diluted in a fluid that conducts an electrical current. The cells are aspirated through a special narrow opening called an **aperture**. As the cells flow through the aperture, they interrupt the flow of electrical current across the opening. Each interruption is recorded and counted as a cell.

In another type of hematology instrument, the diluted blood sample is aspirated into a special channel that permits only one cell to pass through at a time. As each cell passes through the channel, it interrupts a laser beam. Each interruption of the beam is counted as a cell. Lesson 2-10 explains in more detail the principles of hematology instrumentation.

SAFETY REMINDERS

- Review Safety Precautions section before beginning procedure.
- Observe Standard Precautions.
- Observe electrical safety when using the microscope.

PROCEDURAL REMINDERS

- Review Quality Assessment section before beginning procedure.
- Follow manufacturer's instructions and facility SOP manual.
- Do not allow microscope objectives to touch the hemacytometer coverglass.
- Complete cell counts within 10 minutes of loading hemacytometer.
- Use correct values in formula and perform calculations accurately.

CASE STUDY

Hank was performing manual blood cell counts in hematology. He performed a WBC count on Mrs. Rodriguez using the BMP LeukoChek kit. He examined nine large squares of the ruled area on each side of the hemacytometer and counted 78 WBCs on one side of the hemacytometer and 82 cells on the other side.

1. Calculate the WBC count per liter.
2. Is the count within the reference range for an adult woman?

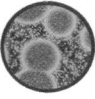

SUMMARY

The results of RBC and WBC counts provide valuable information about the state of a patient's health and wellness. These two cell counts are routinely performed as part of a CBC. The WBC count is also often ordered as a separate test because the results can be used to diagnose and follow the progress of an infection or to evaluate the effect of certain drug or radiation therapies.

Manual cell counts are performed using a hemacytometer and a special coverglass. Procedures for diluting the sample, loading the hemacytometer, and counting the cells must be carefully followed and are slightly different depending on the type of blood cell being counted and the type of kit or materials available to perform the counts. Differences in the WBC and RBC cell counting procedures are summarized in Table 2-9.

Use of automated cell counters has improved cell count accuracy and laboratory efficiency. Although automated cell counters are essential in even small laboratories, there can be times when manual counts are performed. The laboratory should have supplies for manual counts available and technicians who are proficient in performing manual counting procedures.

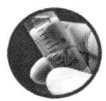

REVIEW QUESTIONS

1. Diagram and label the ruled area of the hemacytometer. Indicate which areas are counted for a WBC count and for an RBC count.
2. Explain how to prepare a 1:200 dilution of blood.
3. What is the proper procedure for cleaning the hemacytometer and coverglass after use?
4. What is the general formula used to calculate cell counts when using the hemacytometer?
5. What are the reference RBC counts for an adult man, an adult woman, and a newborn?

6. What are the reference WBC values for newborns, children, and adults?

7. Name three diseases or conditions in which the RBC count is usually abnormal. For each condition listed, state whether an increased or decreased RBC count would be expected.

8. What is one requirement of an RBC diluting fluid?

9. Name three causes of leukocytosis.

10. Name three factors that can cause leukopenia.

11. What are the functions of the WBC diluting fluid?

12. Define anemia, aperture, erythrocytosis, hemolysis, immunity, isotonic solution, leukemia, leukocytosis, and leukopenia.

STUDENT ACTIVITIES

1. Complete the written examination for this lesson.

2. Practice performing and calculating RBC counts as outlined in the Student Performance Guide, using the RBC worksheet.

3. Practice performing and calculating WBC counts as outlined in the Student Performance Guides.

LESSON 2-5

Manual Red Blood Cell Count

(Answers will vary based on blood specimens available and variations in student techniques.)

Name _____ Date _____

INSTRUCTIONS

1. Practice performing red blood cell (RBC) counts following the step-by-step procedure.

2. Demonstrate the RBC count procedure satisfactorily for the instructor, using the Student Performance Guide. Your instructor will explain the procedures for evaluating and grading your performance. Your performance may be given a number grade, letter grade, or satisfactory (S) or unsatisfactory (U) depending on course or institutional policy.

NOTE: The following is a general procedure for performing a manual RBC count using Ery-TIC (bioanalytic GmbH). Consult the laboratory procedure manual and package insert for specific instructions for the counting method used.

MATERIALS AND EQUIPMENT

- gloves
- hand antiseptic
- full-face protection (or equivalent PPE)
- acrylic safety shield (optional)
- materials for capillary puncture, or tube of venous blood anticoagulated with EDTA
- laboratory tissue
- hemacytometer with coverglass (or disposable plastic hemacytometer)
- test tube rack

- Ery-TIC supplies for RBC count including
  - 5-µL capillary
  - vial containing 995 µL RBC diluting fluid
  - capillary holder
  - chamber-loading capillary (optional)
  - manufacturer's instructions or package insert
- if Ery-TIC is not available, supplies required include
  - disposable capped vial containing 995 µL isotonic RBC diluting fluid
  - 5-µL capillary (such as Drummond capillary)
  - 10- to 20-µL micropipetter with disposable tips
- 10- to 100-µL micropipetter with disposable tips
- microscope
- lens paper and lens cleaner
- ethanol (90% or 95%)
- timer
- hand tally counter
- paper towels
- surface disinfectant (such as 10% chlorine bleach)
- biohazard container
- sharps container
- RBC worksheet
- calculator (optional)

© 2012 Delmar, Cengage Learning. Permission to reproduce for clinical use granted.

PROCEDURE

Record in the comment section any problems encountered while practicing the procedure (or have a fellow student or the instructor evaluate your performance).

S = Satisfactory
U = Unsatisfactory

You must:	S	U	Evaluation/Comments
1. Wash hands with antiseptic and put on gloves			
2. Put on face protection or work behind acrylic safety shield			
3. Assemble equipment and materials			
4. Place a clean hemacytometer coverglass over a clean hemacytometer			
5. Attach a capillary holder to a 5-µL end-to-end capillary (open holder and attach to capillary about 2/3 of distance from end of capillary used to collect blood drop)			
6. Obtain blood from capillary puncture or from a tube of well-mixed venous EDTA anticoagulated blood. For capillary puncture, wipe away the first drop of blood; for anticoagulated blood, mix tube contents well before removing sample			
7. Fill the end-to-end capillary with capillary blood or venous EDTA-anticoagulated blood. The pipet will fill by capillary action and will stop filling automatically. Be sure no air bubbles are present in micropipet NOTE: Hold capillary at a slight (5 degree) upward angle to avoid overfilling			
8. Wipe excess blood from the outside of the capillary with soft laboratory tissue being careful not to remove any blood volume from inside the capillary NOTE: Do not allow tissue to touch capillary tip			
9. Drop the capillary into the vial of diluting fluid, close vial securely, and mix vial contents by inversion until all blood is rinsed from capillary			
10. Mix contents of vial again and immediately remove 10 to 15 µL using a chamber-loading capillary or a micropipetter with disposable tip			
11. Load one side of the hemacytometer, using care not to overload			
12. Mix vial contents again, remove 10 to 15 µL immediately after mixing, and load the second side of the hemacytometer			

© 2012 Delmar, Cengage Learning. Permission to reproduce for clinical use granted.

You must:	S	U	Evaluation/Comments
13. Allow hemacytometer to remain undisturbed for 2 minutes for cells to settle			
14. Place the hemacytometer on the microscope stage carefully and secure			
15. Use the low-power (10×) objective to bring the ruled area into focus			
16. Locate the large central square			
17. Rotate the high-power (40×) objective into position carefully and focus with the fine adjustment knob until the ruled lines are in focus			
18. Adjust the light or condenser so RBCs are visible			
19. Count the red cells in the four corner squares and one center square within the larger center square of the counting area, using the left-to-right, right-to-left counting pattern			
20. Record the results for each of the five squares (four corners and one center)			
21. Repeat the count on the other side of the hemacytometer, completing the entire count within 10 minutes of loading the chamber			
22. Use the worksheet to calculate the RBC count			
23. Disinfect the hemacytometer and coverglass and then wash them			
24. Discard or store the venous specimen as directed by instructor			
25. Discard used sharps into sharps container and other contaminated materials into appropriate biohazard container			
26. Disinfect microscope stage; clean microscope lenses and return equipment to storage			

(Continues)

© 2012 Delmar, Cengage Learning. Permission to reproduce for clinical use granted.

You must:	S	U	Evaluation/Comments
27. Clean work area with disinfectant			
28. Remove gloves and discard into biohazard container			
29. Wash hands with antiseptic			

Instructor/Evaluator Comments:

Instructor/Evaluator _____ Date _____

© 2012 Delmar, Cengage Learning. Permission to reproduce for clinical use granted.

LESSON 2-5
Manual Red Blood Cell Count

(Answers will vary based on the blood specimens tested and variations in student techniques.)

WORKSHEET

Name _____   Date _____

Specimen I.D. _____

$\dfrac{n}{x}$

SIDE 1	NUMBER OF CELLS COUNTED
Square 1	_____
Square 2	_____
Square 3	_____
Square 4	_____
Square 5	_____
Total cells counted side 1 =	_____

SIDE 2	NUMBER OF CELLS COUNTED
Square 1	_____
Square 2	_____
Square 3	_____
Square 4	_____
Square 5	_____
Total cells counted side 2 =	_____
Total of sides 1 and 2 =	_____
Average of two sides (total divided by two) =	_____
Multiply average number of cells by 10,000	_____ = RBC/µL
Convert to SI units by multiplying RBC/µL by 10^6	_____ = RBC/L

© 2012 Delmar, Cengage Learning. Permission to reproduce for clinical use granted.

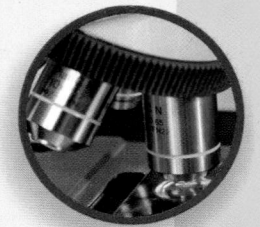

LESSON 2-5

Manual White Blood Cell Count: LeukoChek Method

(Answers will vary based on the blood specimens available and variations in student techniques.)

Name _____ Date _____

INSTRUCTIONS

1. Practice performing and calculating a WBC count using the LeukoChek (Biomedical Polymers, Inc.) system.

2. Demonstrate the WBC count procedure satisfactorily for the instructor, using the Student Performance Guide. Your instructor will explain the procedures for evaluating and grading your performance. Your performance may be given a number grade, letter grade, or satisfactory (S) or unsatisfactory (U) depending on course or institutional policy.

NOTE: The following is a general procedure for using the LeukoChek WBC/platelet system (Biomedical Polymers, Inc.). Consult the package insert for specific instructions. (This general procedure can also be followed for the BD Unopette WBC/Platelet system.)

MATERIALS AND EQUIPMENT

- gloves
- hand antiseptic
- full-face protection (or equivalent PPE)
- acrylic safety shield (optional)
- laboratory tissue
- tube of EDTA blood or supplies for a capillary puncture
- LeukoChek kit, including capillary, prefilled reservoir and instructions
- hemacytometer with coverglass (or disposable, plastic hemacytometer)
- hand tally counter
- 90% or 95% ethanol
- microscope
- lens paper and lens cleaner
- timer
- calculator
- paper towels
- surface disinfectant (such as 10% chlorine bleach)
- sharps container
- biohazard container

PROCEDURE

Record in the comment section any problems encountered while practicing the procedure (or have a fellow student or the instructor evaluate your performance).

S = Satisfactory
U = Unsatisfactory

You must:	S	U	Evaluation/Comments
1. Assemble equipment and materials; obtain a LeukoChek system for WBC counts			
2. Put on face protection or set up acrylic safety shield			
3. Wash hands with antiseptic and put on gloves			
			(Continues)

© 2012 Delmar, Cengage Learning. Permission to reproduce for clinical use granted.

You must:	S	U	Evaluation/Comments
4. Place a clean hemacytometer coverglass on a clean hemacytometer			
5. Pierce the seal of the LeukoChek reservoir with the pipet shield			
6. Remove the shield from the pipet assembly			
7. Fill the capillary pipet from a capillary puncture or from a tube of well-mixed EDTA blood			
8. Allow the blood to flow into the capillary until it automatically stops; be sure no air bubbles are in pipet			
9. Wipe any excess blood from the outside of the pipet using laboratory tissue, being careful not to touch the capillary tip with the tissue			
10. Squeeze the reservoir lightly, being careful not to expel any of the liquid			
11. Maintain pressure on the reservoir and insert the capillary pipet into the reservoir, seating the pipet firmly in the neck of the reservoir. Do not expel any of the liquid			
12. Release the pressure on the reservoir, drawing the blood out of the capillary into the diluent			
13. Squeeze the reservoir gently 3 or 4 times to rinse the remaining blood from the capillary pipet. NOTE: Do not allow the blood-diluent mixture to flow out the top			
14. Mix contents of the reservoir by gently swirling the reservoir or tilting it from side to side			
15. Let the reservoir sit for 10 minutes (but no longer than an hour) to allow the RBCs to be lysed			
16. Remove the pipet from the reservoir and seat it into the neck of the reservoir so the pipet tip extends upward from the reservoir			
17. Mix the contents of the reservoir thoroughly, invert the reservoir, and gently squeeze to discard 4 or 5 drops onto laboratory tissue			
18. Touch the tip of the pipet to the edge of the coverglass and hemacytometer; load both sides of the hemacytometer and wait 2 minutes for cells to settle			
19. Place the hemacytometer on the microscope stage carefully and secure it			
20. Use the low-power (10×) objective to bring the ruled area into focus.			

© 2012 Delmar, Cengage Learning. Permission to reproduce for clinical use granted.

You must:	S	U	Evaluation/Comments
21. Identify the nine WBC squares			
22. Count the WBCs lying within all nine squares, using the boundary rule and the serpentine counting pattern			
23. Record the results			
24. Count the cells on the other side of the hemacytometer, and record the results			
25. Obtain the average count by adding the results from the two sides together and dividing by two			
26. Calculate 10% of the average and add that to the average. Then multiply that total by 100 to determine the number of WBCs per microliter			
27. Disinfect hemacytometer and coverglass, wash, rinse, and dry carefully with lens paper			
28. Discard sharps into a sharps container and discard other contaminated materials into appropriate biohazard container			
29. Return tube of blood to storage or discard as directed by instructor			
30. Clean microscope lenses, disinfect microscope stage, and return equipment to proper storage			
31. Clean work area with disinfectant			
32. Remove gloves and discard into biohazard container			
33. Wash hands with antiseptic			

Instructor/Evaluator Comments:

Instructor/ Evaluator _____ Date _____

© 2012 Delmar, Cengage Learning. Permission to reproduce for clinical use granted.

LESSON 2-5

Manual White Blood Cell Count: Leuko-TIC Method

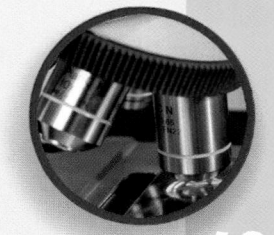

(Answers will vary based on the blood specimens available and variations in student techniques.)

Name _____   Date _____

INSTRUCTIONS

1. Practice performing and calculating a WBC count following the step-by-step procedure.

2. Demonstrate the WBC count procedure satisfactorily for the instructor, using the Student Performance Guide. Your instructor will explain the procedures for evaluating and grading your performance. Your performance may be given a number grade, letter grade, or satisfactory (S) or unsatisfactory (U) depending on course or institutional policy.

NOTE: The following is a general procedure for performing a WBC count using the Leuko-TIC system (bioanalytic GmbH). Consult the laboratory procedure manual and package insert for specific instructions.

MATERIALS AND EQUIPMENT

- gloves
- hand antiseptic
- full-face protection (or equivalent PPE)
- acrylic safety shield (optional)
- laboratory tissue
- tube of EDTA venous blood or supplies for a capillary puncture
- test tube rack

- Leuko-TIC supplies for WBC count including
  - 20-µL capillary
  - vial containing 380 µL WBC diluting fluid
  - capillary holder
  - chamber-loading capillary (optional)
  - manufacturer's instructions or package insert
- if Leuko-TIC is not available, supplies required include
  - disposable capped vial containing 380 µL WBC diluting fluid (such as Turk's solution)
  - 20-µL capillary (such as Drummond capillary) or 20-µL micropipetter with disposable tips
- 10- to 100-µL micropipetter with disposable tips
- microscope
- hemacytometer with coverglass (or disposable plastic hemacytometer)
- hand tally counter
- 90% or 95% ethanol
- microscope
- lens paper and lens cleaner
- timer
- calculator (optional)
- paper towels
- surface disinfectant (such as 10% chlorine bleach)
- biohazard container
- sharps container

PROCEDURE

Record in the comment section any problems encountered while practicing the procedure (or have a fellow student or the instructor evaluate your performance).

S = Satisfactory
U = Unsatisfactory

You must:	S	U	Evaluation/Comments
1. Wash hands with antiseptic and put on gloves			
2. Put on face protection or work behind acrylic safety shield			
3. Assemble equipment and materials for WBC count			
4. Place a clean hemacytometer coverglass on a clean hemacytometer			
5. Attach a capillary holder to a 20-μL end-to-end capillary (open holder and attach to capillary about 2/3 of distance from end of capillary used to collect blood drop)			
6. Obtain blood from capillary puncture or from a tube of well-mixed venous EDTA anticoagulated blood. For capillary puncture, wipe away the first drop of blood; for anticoagulated blood, mix tube contents well before removing sample			
7. Fill the end-to-end capillary with blood; the capillary will fill by capillary action; be sure no air bubbles enter capillary NOTE: Hold capillary at a slight (5 degree) upward angle to avoid overfilling			
8. Wipe excess blood from the outside of the capillary with soft laboratory tissue being careful not to remove any blood from inside the capillary. NOTE: Do not allow tissue to touch the capillary tip			
9. Drop the capillary into the vial of diluting fluid, close vial securely, and mix vial contents by inversion until all blood is rinsed from capillary			
10. Allow vial to stand 2 to 5 minutes for RBCs to lyse			
11. Mix vial contents thoroughly, and immediately remove 10 to 15 μL using a chamber-loading capillary or a micropipetter with disposable tip			
12. Load one side of the hemacytometer, using care not to overload			
13. Mix vial contents again, immediately remove 10 to 15 μL and load the second side of the hemacytometer			
14. Leave hemacytometer undisturbed for 2 minutes to allow cells to settle			

© 2012 Delmar, Cengage Learning. Permission to reproduce for clinical use granted.

You must:	S	U	Evaluation/Comments
15. Place the hemacytometer on the microscope stage carefully and secure it			
16. Use the low-power (10×) objective to bring the ruled area into focus. Locate the four large corner squares used to count white cells			
17. Adjust the condenser and light to provide best contrast to see WBCs (WBC nuclei should stain blue)			
18. Count the WBCs lying within all four large corner squares, using the boundary rule. Use fine adjustment focus and high power (40×) objective to identify any questionable cells			
19. Record the results			
20. Repeat the count on the other side of the hemacytometer and record the results			
21. Obtain the average by adding the counts from the two sides together and dividing by two			
22. Multiply the average by 50 to find the number of WBCs per microliter			
23. Disinfect hemacytometer and coverglass, wash, rinse, and dry carefully with lens paper			
24. Discard used sharps into sharps container and other contaminated materials into appropriate biohazard container			
25. Return tube of blood to storage area or discard as directed by instructor			
26. Clean microscope lenses, clean and disinfect microscope stage, and return equipment to proper storage			
27. Clean work area with disinfectant			
28. Remove gloves and discard into biohazard container			
29. Wash hands with antiseptic			

Instructor/Evaluator Comments:

Instructor/Evaluator _____ Date _____

© 2012 Delmar, Cengage Learning. Permission to reproduce for clinical use granted.

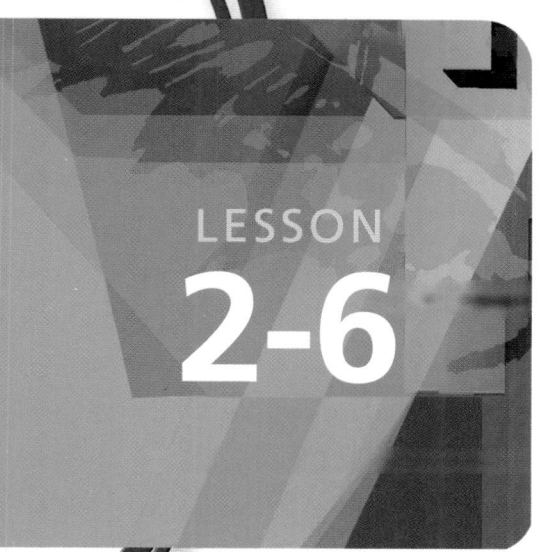

LESSON
2-6

Platelet Count

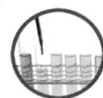

LESSON OBJECTIVES

After studying this lesson, the student will:

⊙ Discuss the origin and functions of platelets.

⊙ Name two pathological conditions in which the platelet counts can be outside the reference range.

⊙ Discuss medical complications that can accompany extremely high or low platelet counts.

⊙ Perform a manual platelet count.

⊙ Calculate the results of a platelet count.

⊙ State the platelet count reference range.

⊙ List three safety precautions that must be observed when performing a platelet count.

⊙ Discuss the importance of quality assessment in platelet counts.

⊙ Discuss the usefulness of platelet counts in diagnosis and treatment.

⊙ Define the glossary terms.

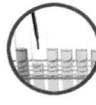

GLOSSARY

immune thrombocytopenic purpura (ITP) / a blood disorder characterized by purpura in skin and mucous membranes and low platelet count caused by the destruction of platelets by antiplatelet autoantibodies; also called idiopathic thrombocytopenic purpura.

petri dish / a shallow, round covered dish made of plastic or glass primarily used to culture microorganisms

thrombocytopenia / abnormally low number of platelets in the blood

thrombocytosis / abnormally high number of platelets in the blood; thrombocythemia

thromboembolism / blockage of a blood vessel by a clot (thrombus) that formed in another vessel

INTRODUCTION

Platelets are the smallest of the formed elements in the blood. They are not complete cells but are fragments of the cytoplasm of megakaryocytes, large cells in the bone marrow (Figure 2-36). Platelets play an important role in hemostasis by helping to initiate blood clotting following injuries to blood vessels. Therefore the platelet count can be used to investigate and assess some bleeding and clotting disorders. Platelets are counted on hematology cell counters, and the platelet count is included in the complete blood count (CBC) report.

Some drug and radiation therapies affect the bone marrow, causing the production of platelets (as well as other blood cells) to be decreased. The platelet count can be used to monitor the toxic effects of these therapies. Lessons 3-1 and 3-2 contain additional information about the functions of platelets and platelet disorders.

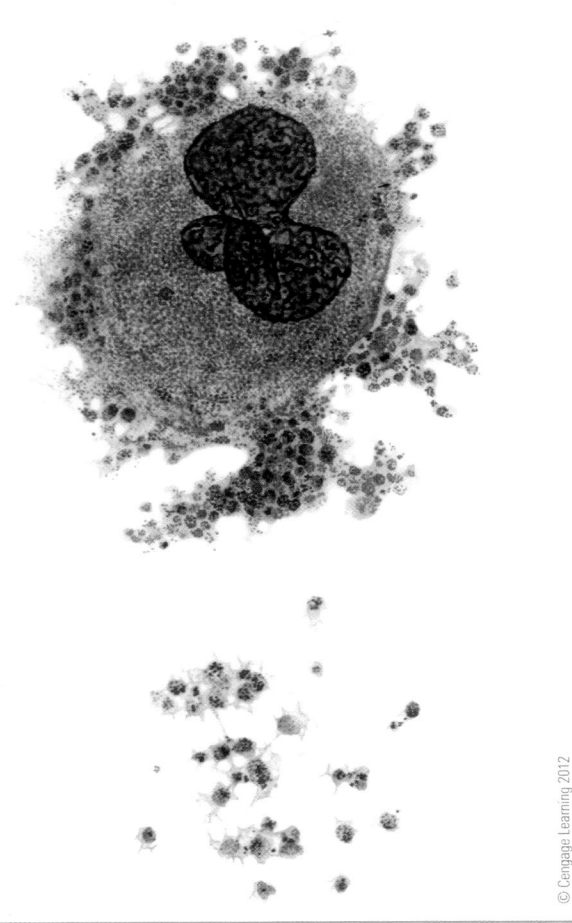

FIGURE 2-36 Megakaryocyte and platelets

REFERENCE RANGE FOR PLATELET COUNT

The reference range for platelet counts in adults is 150,000 to 400,000 platelets per microliter of blood. (This is $1.50 \times 10^5/\mu L$ to $4.0 \times 10^5/\mu L$.) In SI units the range would be expressed as $1.5 \times 10^{11}/L$ to $4.0 \times 10^{11}/L$. The reference range is the same for males and females. The platelet reference range must be established by each laboratory, using the technology available in the laboratory.

PERFORMING A MANUAL PLATELET COUNT

Manual platelet counts are performed by diluting blood in a solution that lyses red blood cells (RBCs) while leaving platelets and WBCs unharmed. The dilution can be made by manually pipetting platelet diluting fluid and blood or by using kits such as the LeukoChek (Biomedical Polymers, Inc.) system (Figure 2-37) or the Thrombo-TIC (bioanalytic GmbH) system (Figure 2-38). Both of these kits include vials of premeasured diluting fluid and calibrated capillaries for measuring the blood sample.

Safety Precautions

Standard Precautions must be observed when performing platelet counts. Laboratory personnel must wear appropriate PPE; in addition, technicians should wear face protection or work behind an acrylic safety shield when opening tubes of blood and pipetting blood. All spills must be wiped up with surface disinfectant. Contaminated equipment, such as

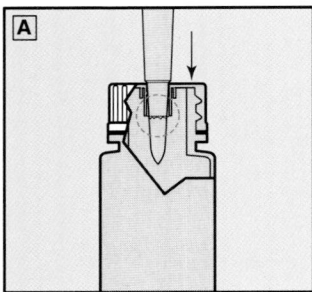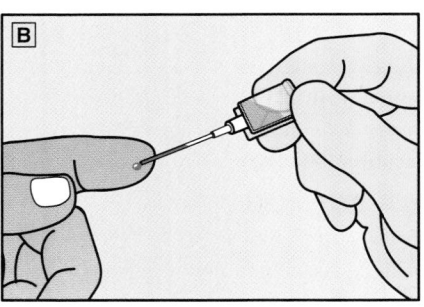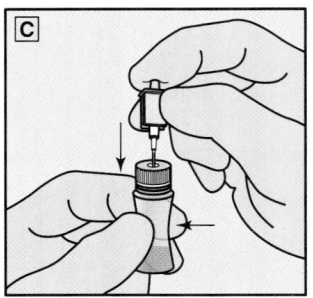
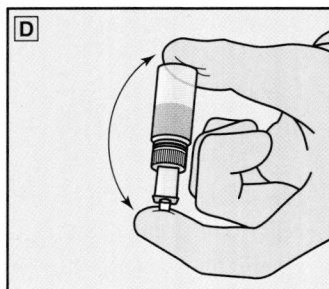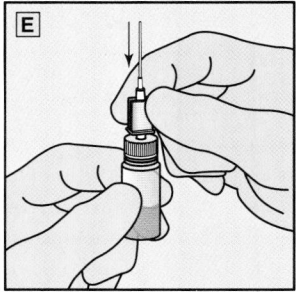

FIGURE 2-37 Illustration of BMP LeukoChek™ dilution procedure for platelet count

CURRENT TOPICS

CLINICAL SIGNIFICANCE OF PLATELET COUNTS

Platelets help control bleeding by forming a sticky plug to seal damaged vessel walls. Platelets also help initiate a series of enzymatic reactions that result in formation of the fibrin clot. Platelet counts higher or lower than the reference range can affect the normal clotting mechanisms, causing excessive clotting (high platelet count) or bleeding (low platelet count).

Thrombocytosis, an increase above normal in platelet numbers, can occur in normal physiological conditions such as after strenuous exercise or when living at high altitudes. Diseases or conditions such as polycythemia, myeloproliferative disorders, hemolytic anemias, or surgical removal of the spleen (splenectomy) can also be associated with thrombocytosis. If platelet numbers are extremely high, spontaneous clot formation can occur, which is a serious situation and can lead to thromboembolism.

Several conditions and diseases cause thrombocytopenia, a decrease below normal in platelet numbers. Any condition that is toxic to the bone marrow can cause decreased platelets; this is often seen following chemotherapy and radiation therapy. Thrombocytopenia can also occur in some anemias and leukemias, as well as in several other conditions. Immune thrombocytopenic purpura (ITP), also called idiopathic thrombocytopenic purpura,

---

TABLE 2-10. Conditions that can cause thrombocytopenia or thrombocytosis

Thrombocytopenia
  Bone marrow damage
  Sequestration of platelets by enlarged spleen
  Disseminated intravascular coagulation (DIC)
  Chronic alcoholism
  Immune thrombocytopenic purpura (ITP)
Thrombocytosis
  Polycythemia vera
  Bleeding disorders
  Hemolytic anemias
  Inflammatory reactions
  Chronic granulocytic leukemia

---

is a blood disorder with low platelet count caused by the destruction of platelets by antiplatelet autoantibodies. If platelet numbers fall to critical levels, 10,000 to 20,000/μL (10×10^9/L to 20×10^9/L), uncontrolled bleeding can occur and can quickly create a life-threatening situation. When this happens, several platelet transfusions can be required to return the platelet numbers to a safe level. Table 2-10 lists examples of conditions that can cause thrombocytosis or thrombocytopenia.

---

the hemacytometer and coverglass, must be soaked in disinfectant and then washed with laboratory detergent. Use of disposable hemacytometers eliminates the hazards associated with reusing the hemacytometer and coverglass.

Quality Assessment

   The platelet counting procedure in the laboratory's standard operating procedure (SOP) manual must be followed. Careful attention must be paid to maintaining good technique when performing hemacytometer counts. The hemacytometer and coverglass must be clean to avoid mistaking dirt particles for platelets, which are very small. Care must be taken to avoid overloading the hemacytometer this would allow the fluid to flow into the moat and alter the platelet distribution in the counting chamber.

Because of the tendency of platelets to clump, attention must be paid to the distribution of the platelets in the counting

chamber. If clumping is seen, the hemacytometer should be cleaned and reloaded. If clumping is still seen, a new blood dilution should be prepared, or the blood sample should be recollected if it was from a capillary puncture.

After the hemacytometer is loaded, the platelets must be allowed to settle for 10 minutes in a moist chamber before performing the count. If counts vary by more than 10% between the two sides of the hemacytometer, the procedure should be repeated.

Collecting the Blood Specimen

Venous blood collected in ethylenediaminetetraacetic acid (EDTA) is the preferred specimen for platelet counts. Capillary blood can be used for platelet counts, but venous anticoagulated blood gives better results because platelets tend to clump rapidly in a capillary sample. If capillary blood is used, the first blood drop appearing after the puncture must be wiped away; blood collection should begin with the second drop.

Diluting the Blood Specimen

Blood for manual platelet counts is diluted 1:100. The most common platelet diluting fluid is dilute (1%) buffered ammonium oxalate. Platelet counts should be performed within 3 hours after the blood is diluted (or following kit manufacturer's recommendation).

LeukoChek Method

The blood dilution made with the LeukoChek system is 1:100. It is made by filling the 0.02 mL (20-μL) capillary with blood and diluting it in the reservoir containing 1.98 mL of diluting fluid (Figure 2-37).

The cap diaphragm of the reservoir is pierced with the protective pipet shield, making an opening large enough for the capillary pipet. The 0.02 mL capillary is filled from a tube of well-mixed EDTA blood (preferable) or a capillary puncture and excess blood is carefully wiped from the outside of the pipet. Pressure is applied to the sides of the reservoir to expel some of the air. While the pressure is maintained, the filled capillary pipet is inserted into the reservoir, and pressure is released from the reservoir, allowing the blood to be drawn into the reservoir and mixed with the diluting fluid (Figure 2-37). The reservoir is gently squeezed and released a few times to rinse the remaining blood out of the pipet and into the diluting fluid. The pipet assembly is removed and reinserted in the reservoir with the pipet extending upward. The reservoir contents are mixed by swirling and then the mixture is allowed to stand for at least 10 minutes, but no longer than 3 hours, to allow the RBCs to be lysed.

Thrombo-TIC Method

For the Thrombo-TIC method, a 10-μL end-to-end capillary is inserted into the capillary holder; the capillary is then filled from either a tube of well-mixed EDTA blood (preferable) or from a capillary puncture (Figure 2-38). A tissue is used to carefully wipe blood from the outside of the capillary, being careful not to remove any blood from inside the capillary. The filled capillary is released into the vial of premeasured diluting fluid (990 μL), the cap is closed securely, and the vial contents are mixed several times by inversion until all blood is rinsed from inside the capillary (Figure 2-38). The resulting dilution is 1:100 (10 μL added to 990 μL). The vial is allowed to stand for at least 5 minutes (but no more than 3 hours) to allow the RBCs to be lysed.

Loading the Hemacytometer

A clean hemacytometer coverglass is placed on a clean hemacytometer so that both sides of the counting chamber are covered by the coverglass. The contents of the dilution vial are again mixed well. For the LeukoChek method, the reservoir is swirled to mix the contents, a few drops are expelled and discarded from the capillary tip, and the hemacytometer is loaded by touching the tip of the capillary to the edge of the coverglass. For the Thrombo-TIC method, 10 to 20 μL of well-mixed blood dilution is withdrawn from the vial with a micropipetter and the hemacytometer is loaded.

Because platelets are so small, it takes them longer to settle in the hemacytometer than larger RBCs and WBCs. The loaded hemacytometer should be placed into a moist chamber to prevent evaporation while allowing time (5 to 10 minutes) for the platelets to settle so they can be more accurately counted (Figure 2-39). A moist chamber can be created by placing moistened filter paper in the bottom of a **petri dish**, placing two wooden applicator sticks on top of the filter paper, and then resting the hemacytometer on the applicator sticks. The cover should then be placed on the petri dish and it should remain undisturbed for 5 to 10 minutes.

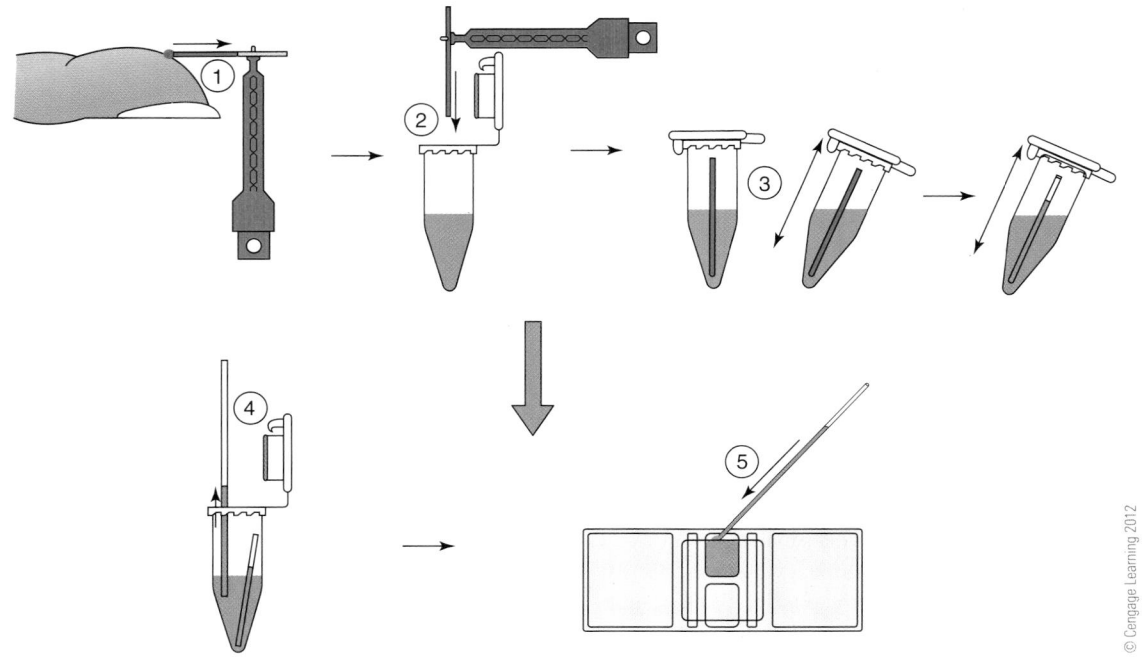

© Cengage Learning 2012

FIGURE 2-38 Illustration of bioanalytic GmbH Thrombo-TIC® dilution procedure for platelet count

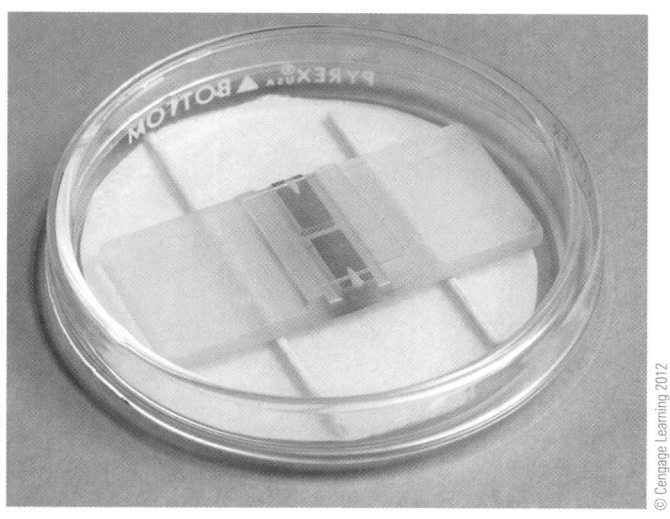

FIGURE 2-39 Hemacytometer in moist chamber

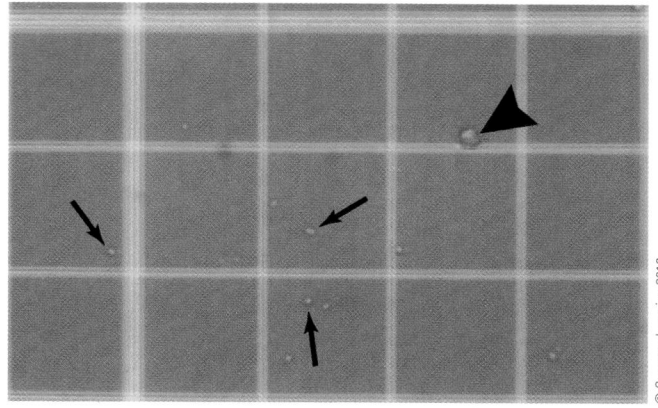

FIGURE 2-41 Photomicrograph of platelets (arrows) as they appear on a hemacytometer (large arrowhead points to a WBC)

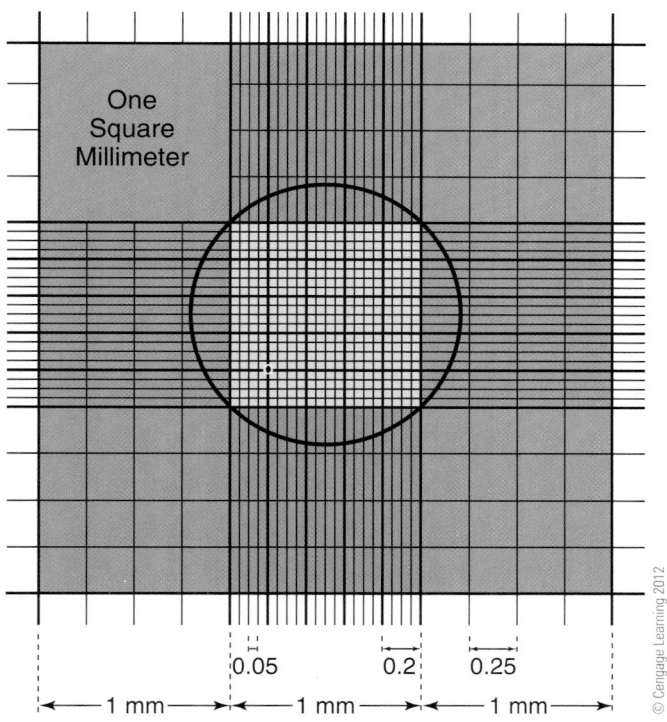

FIGURE 2-40 Platelet counting area: count platelets in all 25 squares inside the large center square (circled)

Counting the Platelets

To perform the platelet count, the hemacytometer is removed from the moist chamber and placed on the microscope stage. The low-power (10×) objective is used to locate the counting area. Platelets *in all 25 small squares of the large center square* (1 mm²) are counted (Figure 2-40) using the high-power (40×) objective. The count is performed on both sides of the hemacytometer, and the average of the two sides is calculated.

The number of platelets counted on each side of the chamber should not differ by more than 10%.

Manual platelet counts are best performed using a phase-contrast microscope. If a bright-field microscope is used, the platelets can be seen more easily by adjusting the condenser and the light level to create the best contrast. The platelets will appear as shiny refractile objects that darken when the fine-adjustment knob is rotated (Figure 2-41).

Calculating the Platelet Count

The number of platelets per microliter of blood is calculated using the general formula:

$$\text{platelets/}\mu L = \frac{\text{Avg} \times \text{DF}}{\text{A (mm}^2) \times \text{D (0.1 mm)}}$$

To simplify, use the following numbers:

1. The platelet average (Avg) is computed using counts from both sides of the hemacytometer.

2. The dilution factor (DF) is 100.

3. The area (A) counted is 1 mm².

4. The depth is 0.1 mm.

These numbers are substituted into the formula as follows:

$$\text{platelets/}\mu L = \frac{\text{Average \# of platelets} \times 100}{1 \times 0.1}$$

$$\text{platelets/}\mu L = \text{Average \# of platelets} \times 1000$$

Using this counting method for a 1:100 blood dilution, the platelet count can be calculated by simply multiplying the average number of platelets by 1000 (or by adding three zeroes). A sample calculation of a platelet count is shown in Figure 2-42.

Perform platelet count using 1:100 dilution:

1. Count the platelets in the entire large center square (1 mm²):

    Side 1 = 166   Side 2 = 170

2. Compute the average:
    A. 166 + 170 = 336 platelets
    B. 336 ÷ 2 = 168 average

3. Calculate the count:

$$\text{Platelets} = \frac{\text{Average \# platelets} \times \text{Dilution factor}}{\text{Area counted (mm}^2) \times D \text{ (0.1 mm)}}$$

$$\text{Platelets} = \frac{168 \times 100}{1 \times 0.1} / \text{mm}^3 \text{ (or } \mu L)$$

$$\text{Platelets} = 168 \times 1000 / \mu L$$

$$\text{Platelets} = 168,000 \text{ (or } 1.68 \times 10^5) / \mu L$$

$$\text{Platelets} = 1.68 \times 10^{11} / L$$

© Cengage Learning 2012

FIGURE 2-42 Sample calculation of a platelet count

AUTOMATED PLATELET COUNTS

Platelets are routinely counted by automated cell counters. Hematology analyzers perform platelet counts, other tests included in the CBC, and several other blood cell parameters. Lesson 2-10 contains more information on hematology automation.

SAFETY REMINDERS

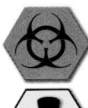  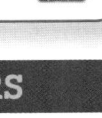

- Review Safety Precautions section before beginning procedure.
- Observe Standard Precautions.
- Disinfect hemacytometer and coverglass after each use.

PROCEDURAL REMINDERS

  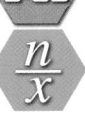

- Review Quality Assessment section before beginning procedure.
- Follow procedure in SOP manual.
- Allow platelets to settle in moist chamber before performing the count.
- Count platelets using the high-power (40×) objective.
- Adjust light for best contrast.

CASE STUDY

$\frac{n}{x}$ Dr. Jones ordered a manual platelet count on Mrs. Rogers, who reported frequent bruising. Marco, the technician, counted the platelets in five small squares within the large center square of the hemacytometer and got the following numbers on one side: 13, 14, 12, 15, and 14. On the second side he counted: 13, 12, 16, 14, and 15. Using the standard formula for counting platelets, Marco determined the patient's platelet count was $6.9 \times 10^{10}/L$.

Because of the results of the count, Marco reviewed the platelet count procedure in his facility's standard operating procedure manual, and then he immediately repeated the platelet count. His total from side 1 was 350, and the total from side 2 was 346.

1. Is the first count normal, high, or low?
2. Calculate the repeat platelet count.
3. Explain why the two counts are different. Which is the correct count? Is the correct count low, normal, or high?

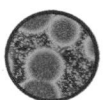

SUMMARY

The platelet count is important because of the role of platelets in stopping bleeding. Platelets can be counted on hematology cell counters and can also be counted manually. Quality assessment policies must be followed to ensure accurate results. Standard Precautions for handling blood must be observed.

Several factors can affect platelet numbers and cause increases or decreases in the platelet count. Low platelet counts can be seen in several disease states; low counts can also be present in patients undergoing chemotherapy or radiation therapy. An extremely low platelet count can cause a bleeding tendency and create a potentially life-threatening situation, making the accuracy of such counts critical. Increased platelet counts can be associated with increased tendency to form blood clots.

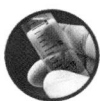

REVIEW QUESTIONS

1. Where do platelets originate?

2. What is the function of platelets?

3. Name a condition in which thrombocytosis can occur.

4. Name a cause of thrombocytopenia.

5. Why is it important to thoroughly clean the coverglass and hemacytometer before performing the platelet count?

6. What is the purpose of placing the loaded hemacytometer in the moist chamber?

7. What area of the hemacytometer is used to count platelets?

8. State the formula for calculating a platelet count.

9. What blood dilution is used for a platelet count using the Thrombo-TIC system? What dilution is used for the Leuko-Chek system?

10. What PPE must be worn while performing manual platelet counts?

11. Define immune thrombocytopenic purpura, petri dish, thrombocytopenia, thrombocytosis, and thromboembolism.

STUDENT ACTIVITIES

1. Complete the written examination for this lesson.

2. Practice performing a platelet count as outlined in the Student Performance Guide.

3. Read more about the function of platelets in Lessons 3-1 and 3-2.

WEB ACTIVITY

Research thrombocytopenia using the Internet: Report on a condition selected from Table 2-10; include cause, symptoms, laboratory findings, treatment, and prognosis. Or find a condition causing thrombocytopenia that is not listed in Table 2-10 and report on it.

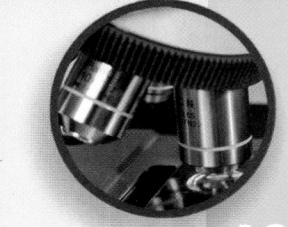

LESSON 2-6
Platelet Count

(Answers will vary based on the blood samples available and individual student techniques.)

Name _____   Date _____

INSTRUCTIONS

1. Practice performing a manual platelet count following the step-by-step procedure.

2. Demonstrate the platelet count procedure satisfactorily for the instructor using the Student Performance Guide. Your instructor will explain the procedures for evaluating and grading your performance. Your performance may be given a number grade, letter grade, or satisfactory (S) or unsatisfactory (U) depending on course or institutional policy.

NOTE: The following is a procedure for performing a platelet count using the hemacytometer and the LeukoChek (Biomedical Polymers, Inc.) and/or Thrombo-TIC (bioanalytic GmbH) kits. Consult the package inserts for specific instructions.

MATERIALS AND EQUIPMENT

- gloves
- hand antiseptic
- full-face shield (or equivalent PPE)
- acrylic safety shield (optional)
- venous blood sample, anticoagulated with EDTA
- test-tube rack
- capillary puncture supplies (if EDTA blood not available)
- hemacytometer with coverglass (or disposable Neubauer-type hemacytometer)

- LeukoChek WBC/platelet kit including
  - reservoir containing 1.98 mL premeasured diluting fluid
  - pipet assembly (0.02 mL capillary pipet with shield)
  - kit instructions
- Thrombo-TIC kit for platelet count including
  - vial of diluting fluid (990 µL)
  - end-to-end 10-µL capillary
  - capillary holder
  - chamber-filling capillary (optional)
  - 10- to 20-µL micropipetter with tips
  - kit instructions
- microscope
- materials for moist chamber:
  - petri dish
  - moist cotton ball or moistened filter paper and wooden applicator sticks
- lens paper and lens cleaner
- ethanol (90% or 95%)
- timer
- laboratory tissue
- hand tally counter
- paper towels
- surface disinfectant (such as 10% chlorine bleach)
- biohazard container
- sharps container

© 2012 Delmar, Cengage Learning. Permission to reproduce for clinical use granted.

PROCEDURE

Record in the comment section any problems encountered while practicing the procedure (or have a fellow student or the instructor evaluate your performance).

S = Satisfactory
U = Unsatisfactory

You must:	S	U	Evaluation/Comments
1. Assemble equipment and materials			
2. Place a clean, dry hemacytometer coverglass over a clean hemacytometer			
3. Wash hands with antiseptic and put on gloves			
4. Put on face protection or work behind acrylic safety shield			
5. Perform blood dilution for platelet count following steps 6a through 6g using the LeukoChek system. If using the Thrombo-TIC system, skip to step 7			
6. For LeukoChek system: a. Puncture the reservoir cap diaphragm using the tip of the pipet shield b. Remove the pipet from the shield and fill the capillary pipet from a tube of well-mixed EDTA blood (preferred) or from a capillary puncture. The pipet will fill by capillary action and will stop filling automatically; be sure no air bubbles enter the capillary pipet c. Wipe excess blood from the outside of the capillary pipet with soft laboratory tissue NOTE: Do not allow tissue to touch pipet tip d. Squeeze the reservoir slightly, being careful not to expel any of the liquid. Maintain pressure on the reservoir, insert the capillary pipet into the reservoir, seating the pipet firmly in the neck of the reservoir. Do not expel any of the liquid e. Release the pressure on the reservoir, drawing the blood out of the capillary pipet into the diluent f. Squeeze the reservoir gently 3 or 4 times to rinse the remaining blood from the capillary pipet. NOTE: Do not allow the blood-diluent mixture to flow out the top of the reservoir g. Mix the contents of the reservoir thoroughly by gently swirling the reservoir or tilting it from side to side; remove the capillary pipet from the reservoir, and seat it in the neck of the reservoir in reverse position (the pipet tip should now project upward from the reservoir). Allow reservoir to stand at least 10 minutes but no longer than 3 hours. Skip to step 8 to continue			

© 2012 Delmar, Cengage Learning. Permission to reproduce for clinical use granted.

You must:	S	U	Evaluation/Comments

7. For the Thrombo-TIC procedure follow steps 7a through 7f:
   a. Attach a capillary holder to a 10-μL end-to-end capillary (open holder and attach to capillary about 2/3 of distance from end of capillary used to collect blood drop)
   b. Obtain blood from a tube of well-mixed venous EDTA anticoagulated blood or from capillary puncture; for capillary puncture, wipe away the first drop of blood
   c. Fill the end-to-end capillary; the capillary will fill by capillary action. Be sure no air bubbles enter the capillary
   NOTE: Hold capillary horizontal or at a slight (5 degrees) upward angle to avoid overfilling
   d. Wipe excess blood from the outside of the capillary with soft laboratory tissue, being careful not to remove any blood from the capillary
   NOTE: Do not allow tissue to touch capillary tip
   e. Drop the filled capillary into the vial of diluting fluid, close vial securely, and mix vial contents by inversion until all blood is removed from capillary
   f. Allow vial to stand at least 5 minutes for red blood cells to lyse			

8. Prepare a moist chamber using a petri dish and slightly moist cotton ball or moist filter paper and wooden applicator stick			

9. Load the hemacytometer using either the LeukoChek capillary pipet (step 9a) or a micropipetter for Thrombo-TIC method (step 9b)
   a. Mix the contents of the LeukoChek reservoir thoroughly; invert the reservoir and gently squeeze to discard 4 or 5 drops onto laboratory tissue; load both sides of the hemacytometer using the capillary pipet, using care not to overload
   b. Mix contents of Thrombo-TIC vial inverting several times; remove 10 to 20 μL immediately after mixing, using a chamber-filling capillary or a micropipetter with disposable tip; load both sides of the hemacytometer, using care not to overload			

10. Place the hemacytometer in the petri dish. If using a moist cotton ball, do not allow it to touch the hemacytometer; if using moist filter paper, support hemacytometer on wooden applicator sticks			
11. Place the cover on the petri dish and allow to remain undisturbed for 10 minutes to permit the platelets to settle in the hemacytometer NOTE: Do not wait longer than 20 minutes to begin the platelet count			
12. Place the hemacytometer on the microscope stage carefully and securely			

(Continues)

© 2012 Delmar, Cengage Learning. Permission to reproduce for clinical use granted.

You must:	S	U	Evaluation/Comments
13. Use the low-power (10×) objective to bring the ruled area into focus. Locate the large central square			
14. Rotate the high-power (40×) objective into position carefully and focus with the fine-adjustment knob until the ruled lines are in focus			
15. Adjust the condenser and reduce light intensity for best contrast. Platelets should appear as small round or oval particles that are refractile			
16. Count the platelets in the entire center square of the ruled area (all 25 small squares) using the left-to-right, right-to-left serpentine counting pattern and observing the boundary rule			
17. Record results			
18. Repeat the count on the other side of the hemacytometer			
19. Average the results from the two sides			
20. Calculate the platelet count: $$\text{platelets/}\mu L = \frac{\text{Avg} \times \text{DF}}{\text{A (mm}^2) \times \text{D (0.1 mm)}}$$ or $$\text{platelets/}\mu L = \text{average \# platelets} \times 1000$$			
21. Record the results			
22. Disinfect hemacytometer and coverglass with surface disinfectant and then wash and dry them			
23. Discard or store specimen as directed by instructor			
24. Discard sharps into sharps container			
25. Discard other contaminated materials into appropriate biohazard containers			
26. Clean microscope lenses, disinfect microscope stage, and return equipment to proper storage			
27. Clean work area with disinfectant			
28. Remove gloves and discard into biohazard container			
29. Wash hands with antiseptic			

Instructor/Evaluator Comments:

Instructor/Evaluator _____   Date _____

© 2012 Delmar, Cengage Learning. Permission to reproduce for clinical use granted.

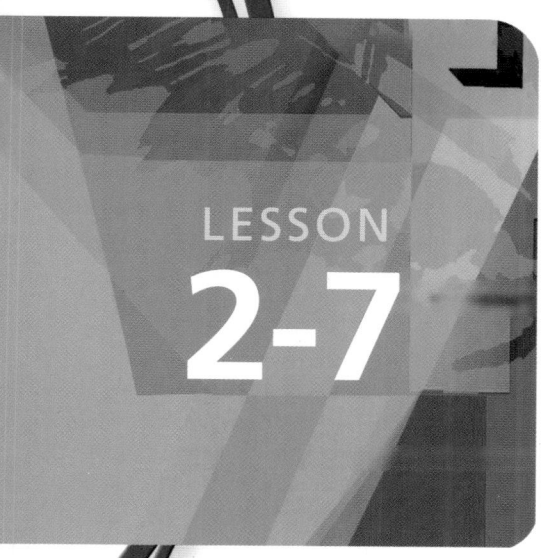

LESSON 2-7

Preparing and Staining a Blood Smear

LESSON OBJECTIVES

After studying this lesson, the student will:

- ⊙ Prepare a blood smear.
- ⊙ List five features of a properly prepared blood smear.
- ⊙ Preserve a blood smear.
- ⊙ Stain a blood smear.
- ⊙ Explain the purpose of staining blood smears.
- ⊙ Explain what information can be obtained from a stained blood smear.
- ⊙ List the blood components that can be observed in a stained blood smear.
- ⊙ List the safety precautions to observe when preparing and staining a blood smear.
- ⊙ Explain how techniques used in blood smear preparation and staining can affect the quality of blood smears.
- ⊙ Explain how the use of a blood sample containing EDTA can affect blood smear quality.
- ⊙ Define the glossary terms.

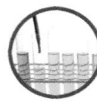

GLOSSARY

buffer / a solution that resists a sudden, marked change in pH when acid or base (alkali) is added

cytoplasm / the fluid portion of the cell surrounding the nucleus

eosin / a red-orange stain or dye

fixative / preservative; a chemical that prevents deterioration of cells or tissues

methylene blue / a blue stain or dye

morphology / the form and structure of cells, tissues, and organs

nucleus (pl. nuclei) / the central structure of a cell that contains DNA and controls cell growth and function

polychromatic / having many colors

Wright's stain / a combination of eosin and methylene blue in methanol; a polychromatic stain

INTRODUCTION

The examination of a stained blood smear is part of the complete blood count (CBC). Stains are applied to blood smears so that red blood cells (RBCs), white blood cells (WBCs), and platelets can be microscopically viewed, identified, and evaluated, as explained in the blood cell morphology and WBC differential count lessons (Lessons 2-8 and 2-9).

A well-made stained blood smear enables the technologist to view the cellular components of blood in as natural a state as possible. The **morphology**, or structure, of the cellular components can be studied. Examination of a well-prepared stained blood smear can provide valuable information to the physician for the detection of diseases in which changes to blood cell morphology occur. Examples of such diseases include infectious mononucleosis, leukemia, sickle cell anemia, and malaria.

Information gained during routine evaluation of blood smears can lead the physician to order special blood stains for further study. These special stains are used to identify specific components of cells such as iron granules or nucleic acids.

SAFETY AND QUALITY CONSIDERATIONS IN MAKING AND STAINING BLOOD SMEARS

Biological and chemical safety rules must be followed when preparing and staining blood smears. A high-quality stained blood smear is essential for successful microscopic examination.

Safety Precautions

Standard Precautions must be observed when preparing and staining blood smears. Gloves, full face protection, and a buttoned, fluid-resistant laboratory coat must be worn. Slides should be handled with care to prevent accidental cuts. The use of beveled-edge, rounded-corner slides reduces the chance of injury from slides. Because methanol is toxic, care should be taken to prevent skin contact or inhalation of fumes. After use, the slides must be discarded into sharps containers.

Quality Assessment

Slides used for blood smears must be free of oil, fingerprints, and dust. Slides can be purchased precleaned or can be washed with soap and water, rinsed thoroughly in warm water dipped in 95% ethanol, and polished with a clean, lint-free cloth. Clean slides can be stored in 95% ethanol and should be handled by the edges only. Slides with frosted ends are preferred because they are easily labeled.

Blood smears must be prepared in a manner that minimally alters the distribution and morphology of the cells. Capillary blood is preferred because no chemical is added to alter cell morphology. However, because platelets tend to clump rapidly in capillary blood, the anticoagulant ethylenediaminetetraacetic acid (ETDA) can be used, which minimally alters cell morphology and staining characteristics. No other anticoagulant can be used for blood smear. Anticoagulated blood can be used. Smears made from anticoagulated blood should be made within 2 hours of blood collection. All smears should be stained when dry or within 1 hour of being prepared. If smears cannot be stained within 1 hour of being prepared, they can be preserved by dipping into methanol for 30 to 60 seconds.

Exact staining times for the method being used must be followed. Stains should be kept tightly capped to prevent evaporation of stain or absorption of moisture; either situation can adversely affect staining results. Buffer pH should be checked frequently.

PREPARING A BLOOD SMEAR

Several factors must be considered when preparing a blood smear.

Collecting the Blood Specimen

The preferred specimen for blood smears is capillary blood that has no added anticoagulant. Capillary blood can be applied directly to the slide from the puncture site or can be collected in capillary tubes and then dispensed onto the slides. A satisfactory smear can also be made from venous blood that has the anticoagulant EDTA added to it, provided the smear is prepared within 2 hours of blood collection.

Making the Smear

Several techniques can result in good smears. Each technician must find the technique that is least awkward and provides good results. Tubes of anticoagulated blood must be mixed for at least 2 minutes by mechanical mixer or inverted gently 60 times immediately before the smear is made.

Two-Slide Method (Wedge Method)

The blood smear is prepared by placing a small drop of well-mixed blood about one-half to three-quarters of an inch from the right end (left end for left-handed) of a precleaned slide placed on a flat surface (Figure 2-43A). The end of a "spreader" slide is brought to rest at a 30- to 35-degree angle in front of the drop of blood and is then brought back into the drop of blood until the drop spreads along three-quarters of the edge of the spreader slide (Figure 2-43B). As soon as the blood spreads along the edge of the spreader, the spreader is lightly pushed to the left (right for left-handed) with a quick, steady motion (avoiding pressure on the slide) to spread the blood into a thin film (Figure 2-43C and D).

Each end of the spreader slide should be used only once, and then the slide should be discarded into a sharps container; or a slide can be used once to spread the smear and then used to have a smear applied to it. The smear is placed in a slide-drying rack and allowed to air-dry as quickly as possible. Slides must not be placed on a flat surface to dry. Dried slides are ready for staining or preserving.

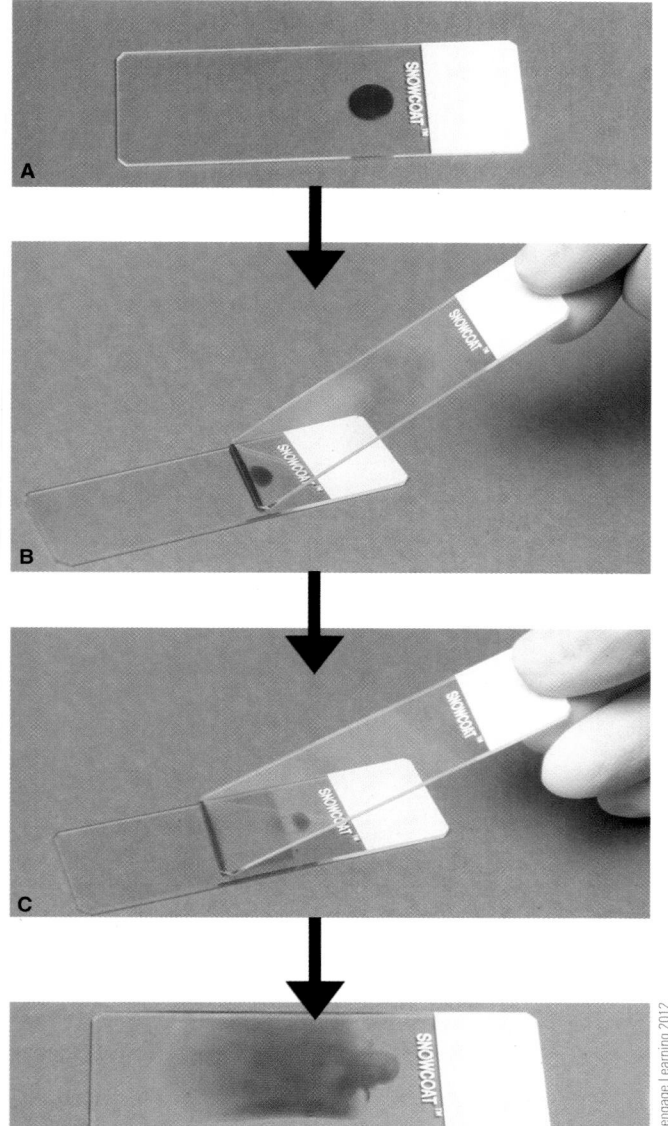

FIGURE 2-43 Making a blood smear: (A) dispense one drop of blood onto end of slide; (B) using a spreader slide, gently bring the back edge of the spreader slide into contact with the drop of blood; (C-D) quickly push the spreader slide forward to make the smear

© Cengage Learning 2012

Blood Drop Dispensers

Devices such as DIFF-SAFE (Alpha Scientific), Haemo-Diff (Sarstedt), and H-Pette Dispenser (Helena Laboratories) have cannulas that can penetrate the stoppers of blood collection tubes and deliver a drop of blood onto a slide. These devices eliminate the need to uncap the blood collection tube to make a blood smear. The procedure for dispensing blood using the DIFF-SAFE is shown in Figure 2-44. The H-Pette Dispenser and Haemo-Diff (shown in Figure 2-45) can be purchased fitted with paddles for spreading the blood drop to make the smear; these devices reduce the use of spreader slides and transfer-pipets as well as eliminating the hazard created by opening tubes of blood.

Preserving the Smear

If a dried smear cannot be stained immediately, it should be preserved by immersing in methanol for 30 to 60 seconds and then air-dried. The methanol is a **fixative**, or preservative, that prevents changes or deterioration of the cellular components. Slides preserved in this way can be stained at a later time.

Features of a Good Blood Smear

A well-prepared smear is illustrated in Figures 2-43D and 2-46A. The smear should cover about three-fourths of the slide and should show a gradual transition from thick to thin. It should have a smooth appearance, with no holes or ridges, and a feathered edge (about 1.5 cm long) at the thin end of the smear. When the smear is examined microscopically, the cells should be evenly distributed, with an area at the thin end of the smear where RBCs are not overlapping.

Factors Affecting Blood Smear Quality

Several factors can affect the quality of the blood smear (Table 2-11). The length and thickness of the smear are affected by:

- The size of the drop of blood
- The angle of the spreader slide
- The speed at which the smear is made

TABLE 2-11. Common problems in preparing blood smears and the possible causes

PROBLEM	POSSIBLE CAUSE(S)
Smear too thin or too long	Drop of blood too small
	Spreader slide at too low an angle
	Improper speed in making smear
Smear too thick or too short	Drop of blood too large
	Spreader slide at too high an angle
	Improper speed in making smear
Ridges or waves in smear	Uneven pressure on spreader slide
	Hesitation in pushing spreader slide
Holes in smear	Slides not clean
	Uneven or dirty edge of spreader slide
Uneven cell distribution	Uneven pressure during spread of blood
	Delay in spreading blood
	Uneven or dirty edge of spreader slide
Artifacts or unusual cell appearance	Smear dried too slowly
	Smear not fixed within 1 hour after preparation
	High humidity causing holes to appear in red cells

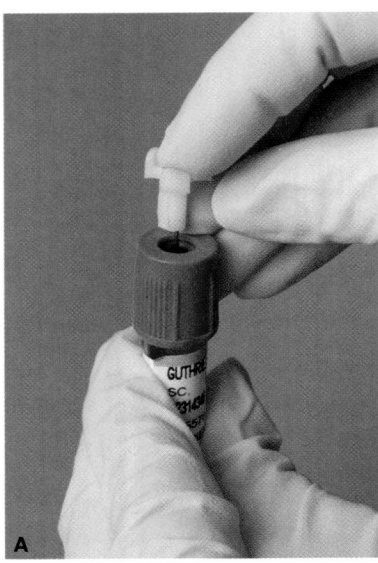
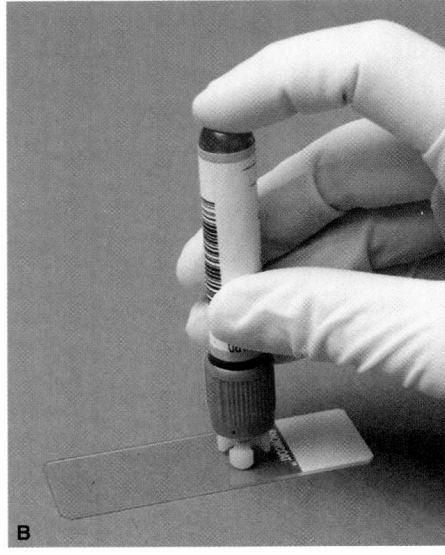
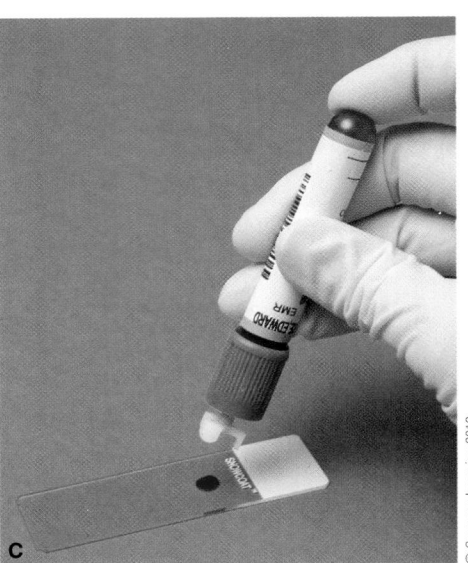

FIGURE 2-44 DIFF-SAFE blood dispensing device: (A) insert DIFF-SAFE cannula through rubber stopper; (B) invert tube and press against slide; (C) a drop of blood is dispensed onto slide

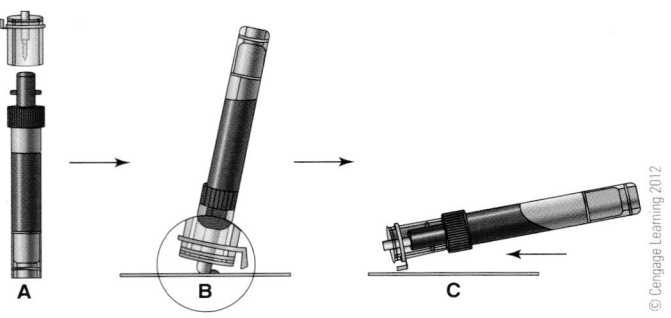

FIGURE 2-45 Haemo-Diff® blood drop dispenser: (A) Haemo-Diff is placed onto S-Monovette cap; (B) tube is inverted and a drop of blood is dispensed onto slide; (C) the spreader is used to make the blood smear

Thick, short smears occur when the angle of the spreader is too high or the drop of blood is too large. Thin smears occur when the blood drop is too small, the angle of the spreader slide is too low, or too much pressure is applied to the spreader. In the latter case, the smear can also be uneven. In general, the more rapid the spreading procedure is, the thinner the smear.

Applying too much pressure to the spreader slide can also push most of the WBCs to the end of the slide. This affects the distribution of the types of WBCs and decreases the number of WBCs seen in the rest of the smear.

The drying time of the smear can affect the appearance of the cellular elements. Smears dry slowly in a humid environment, causing abnormal cell appearance, such as RBCs that appear to have holes in them.

STAINING A BLOOD SMEAR

The **Wright's stain** used for the routine microscopic examination of blood is a **polychromatic** stain. It contains a combination of **methylene blue**, a basic dye that gives a blue color to stained

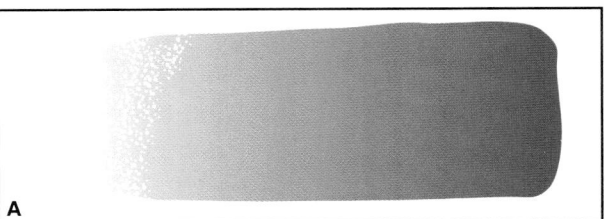

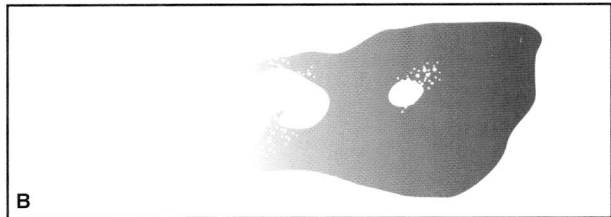

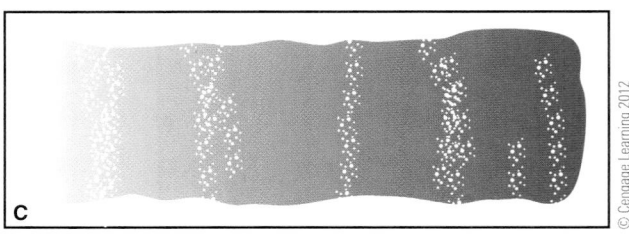

FIGURE 2-46 Properly prepared smear (A) versus improperly prepared smears (B and C)

structures **eosin**, an acid dye that gives a red-orange color to stained structures and methanol, a fixative.

Some structures, such as cell nuclei, attract the basic dyes and stain blue or purple. Other cell structures attract the acid dyes and stain pink-red. The cells and structures are thus more easily visualized and differentiated (hence the name differential count). Two commonly used blood stains are Wright's stain and Giemsa stain.

Procedure: Wright's Stain

Smears can be stained with Wright's stain by a quick stain method, two-step method, or an automatic stainer. A quick-stain is adequate for most routine work, but the two-step method (or automatic stainer) should be used to evaluate cell abnormalities and bone marrow cells.

Quick Stains

Quick stains are available in kits from several companies. These stains are modifications of Wright's stain. The kits contain three separate components: a fixative, a red dye such as eosin, and a blue dye such as methylene blue (Figure 2-47).

To perform a quick stain, the smear is is held with forceps and dipped sequentially into the staining solution(s) for a specified length of time and then rinsed and air-dried. The entire quick-stain method takes only 2 to 5 minutes. It can be easier for the inexperienced technician to obtain an adequate stain with quick methods, but experienced technicians can achieve superior results using the two-step method.

Two-Step Method

In a two-step method, a smear is placed on a staining rack and flooded with Wright's stain (Figure 2-48). The methanol in the stain acts a fixative in this step. After approximately 1 to 3 minutes, an equal volume of **buffer** is added dropwise to the stain, allowing the stain and buffer to mix. A buffer is a solution that resists marked change in the pH when acid or alkali is added. A green

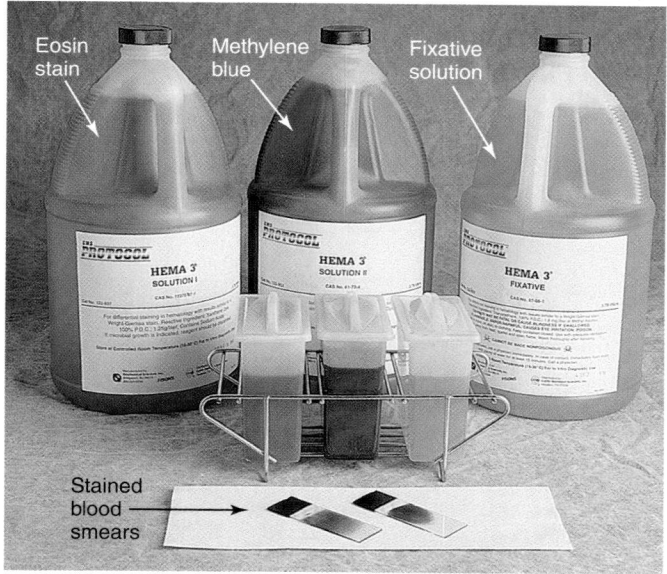

FIGURE 2-47 A quick stain kit for staining blood smears

metallic sheen appears when the solutions mix, usually within 2 to 4 minutes. The slide is held with forceps and rinsed gently with water, allowed to air-dry, and then examined using the microscope. The staining procedure, including stain and buffering times, will be included in the laboratory's procedure manual.

Automatic Stainers

There are two basic types of automatic slide stainers. In one type, the slides are placed on a moving belt, which carries them through the staining reagents (Figure 2-49). Another type of stainer is the "basket" or "batch" type, in which baskets of slides

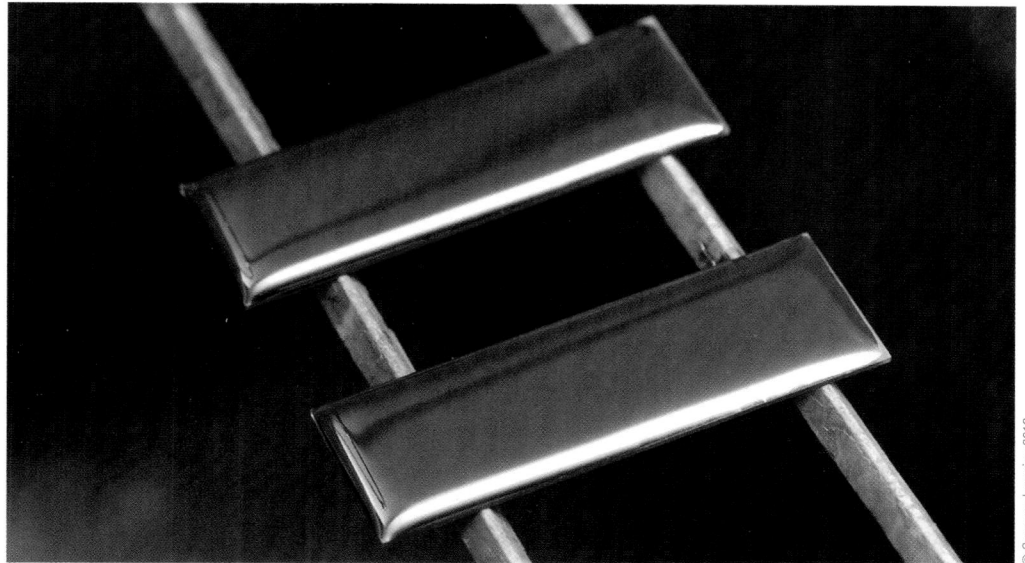

FIGURE 2-48 Staining blood smears on a simple slide-staining rack

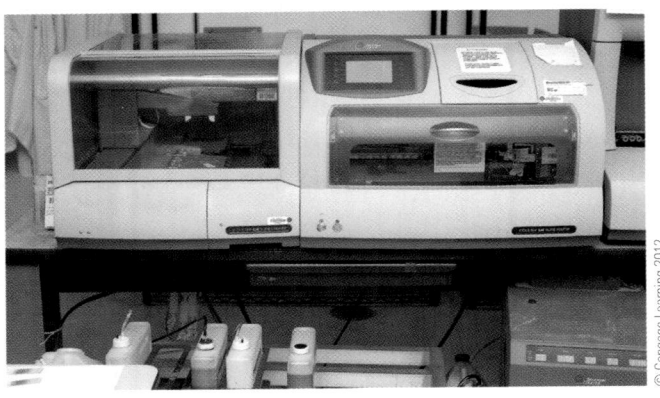

FIGURE 2-49 Automatic slide stainer

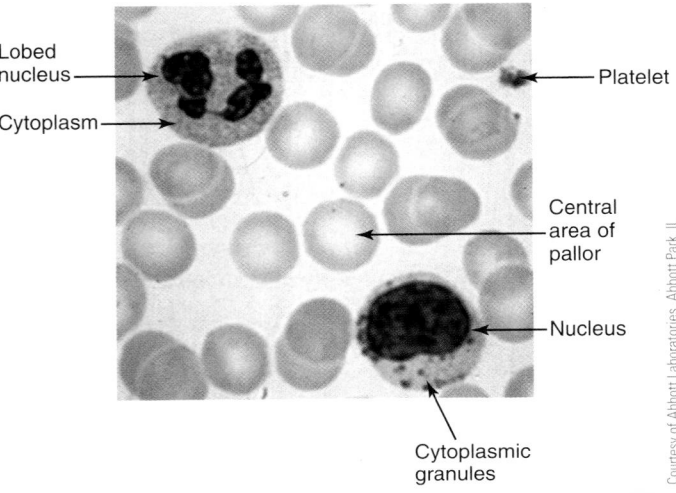

Lobed nucleus
Cytoplasm
Platelet
Central area of pallor
Nucleus
Cytoplasmic granules

FIGURE 2-50 Stained blood cells: neutrophil (top left), lymphocyte with azurophilic cytoplasmic granules (bottom right), red blood cells, and platelet (top right)

are taken stepwise through the staining process. One basket of slides is immersed in fixative, and then immersed into the stain solution, and so forth. This is continued throughout the complete staining process.

Automatic slide stainers are more efficient than manual staining when large numbers of slides must be stained or staining must be performed frequently during the workday. A disadvantage of automatic stainers is that if the stain solutions are not working properly, many slides can be processed before the technician becomes aware of the problem.

Evaluating Stain Quality

A properly stained smear should appear pinkish-blue to the naked eye. When viewed microscopically, the RBCs should appear pink-tan. The **nucleus**, or central structure, of the leukocytes should appear purple. The leukocyte **cytoplasm**, or area surrounding the nucleus, will vary from pink to blue or blue-gray, depending on the cell type (Figure 2-50). Inconsistencies in color or staining intensity can be caused by variations in pH, timing, or characteristics of the stain or buffer, and are best evaluated using the oil-immersion objective.

- Smears that are too pink can be caused by the stain time being too short, the wash time being too long, or the pH of the stain or buffer being too acidic.

- Smears that are too blue can be caused by overstaining, the wash or buffer time being too short, or the pH of the stain or buffer being too alkaline.

Storing Blood Smears

Stained smears and unstained preserved smears should be stored in a dust-free slide box or container with an opaque cover. If protected from light and moisture, stained smears will last for years, with little fading. Smears can be protected from scratches by covering the thin area of the smear(s) with a permanent coverglass. For routine work, however, this is not necessary.

SAFETY REMINDERS

- Review Safety Precautions section before beginning procedure.
- Observe Standard Precautions.
- Do not inhale methanol fumes or allow skin contact.
- Handle slides with forceps during staining.
- Use beveled-edge, rounded-corner slides.

PROCEDURAL REMINDERS

- Review Quality Assessment section before beginning procedure.
- Prepare smears from capillary blood immediately to avoid clotting.
- Preserve or stain smears within 1 hour after preparation.
- Use correct staining techniques.
- Store stains appropriately.

CASE STUDY 1

Vidya worked in the hematology laboratory of a small hospital. The laboratory's hematology procedure manual contained instructions for staining blood smears by the two-step method, and called for applying the stain for 2 minutes and the buffer for 2 minutes. Vidya stained three patient blood smears, but the smears appeared bluer than normal. When she examined the smears microscopically, the cells also appeared blue, making it difficult to identify them.

1. What can cause blood smears to stain too blue?
2. Discuss factors that could have affected the stain results.

CASE STUDY 2

Shana received a request to prepare smears from a tube of EDTA anticoagulated blood. The specimen was collected at 8 AM, and she prepared the smears at 8:30 AM. She allowed the smears to dry in the rack and processed several STAT specimens as well as routine tests. At 11:30 AM she stained the smears and observed one under the microscope. She was surprised by the appearance of the smears—the cells had bizarre morphology, and many of the red cells appeared moth-eaten.

1. Describe what could have happened in the process of preparing the stained smears.
2. What action could Shana have taken if she did not have time to stain the smears after they were made?

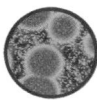

SUMMARY

Examination of a stained peripheral blood smear can contribute valuable information about a patient's condition. It is essential that the smear is made and stained correctly so that it presents an accurate representation of cells in the peripheral blood. It is essential that the smear is made and stained correctly. Blood smears can be made by a variety of methods, but the two-slide method is most frequently used. Capillary blood is the best specimen, but venous blood collected in EDTA can be used if the smear is made within 2 hours of blood collection. The most common blood stain is Wright's stain, a polychromatic stain composed of eosin and methylene blue in the fixative, methanol. Staining can be done manually or using an automatic slide stainer. Instructions for the particular stain being used must be followed exactly. Laboratory safety rules for handling blood, glass, and chemicals such as methanol must be followed.

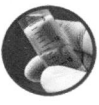

REVIEW QUESTIONS

1. What is the purpose of staining blood smears?
2. What specimen(s) can be used to prepare blood smears?

3. What blood components can be viewed on a stained smear?
4. Explain the two-slide method for making a blood smear.
5. What are five errors to avoid when making a blood smear?
6. Describe and diagram the appearance of a properly prepared blood smear.
7. How can unstained blood smears be preserved?
8. Explain what is meant by polychromatic stains.
9. Name two commonly used blood stains.
10. How should a properly stained smear appear?
11. In a correctly stained smear, what should be the color of the WBC nucleus?
12. What color is the cytoplasm of stained WBCs?
13. What is the proper method of storing preserved or stained smears?
14. Name three factors that can affect staining results.
15. How does the use of anticoagulated blood affect the quality of the smear?
16. Define buffer, cytoplasm, eosin, fixative, methylene blue, morphology, nucleus, polychromatic, and Wright's stain.

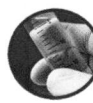

STUDENT ACTIVITIES

1. Complete the written examination for this lesson.

2. Practice preparing and staining blood smears by the two-step and/or quick-stain method as outlined in the Student Performance Guide.

3. Compare smears stained by the two-step and quick-stain methods. Which method produced the preferred results?

4. Experiment with variations in staining and buffering times using the two-step method. Explain the results.

WEB ACTIVITIES

1. Search the Internet for tutorials or videos demonstrating the preparation of blood smears.

2. Use the Internet to find an example of a material safety data sheet (MSDS) for Wright's stain. Determine if your laboratory is using appropriate safety measures when staining blood smears using Wright's stain.

LESSON 2-7
Preparing and Staining a Blood Smear

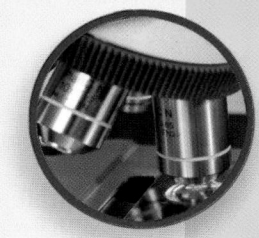

Name _____   Date _____

INSTRUCTIONS

1. Practice preparing and staining a blood smear following the step-by-step procedure.

2. Demonstrate the procedure for preparing and staining a blood smear satisfactorily for the instructor, using the Student Performance Guide. Your instructor will explain the procedures for evaluating and grading your performance. Your performance may be given a number grade, letter grade, or satisfactory (S) or unsatisfactory (U) depending on course on institutional policy.

NOTE: Stain characteristics can vary with stain lot. Follow manufacturer's instructions for best results.

MATERIALS AND EQUIPMENT

- gloves
- hand antiseptic
- full-face shield (or equivalent PPE)
- slide storage box
- pencil or diamond-tip etching pen
- 1 × 3 inch microscope slides (beveled-edge, rounded corners, frosted-end preferred)
- 95% ethanol
- laboratory tissue or gauze
- plastic or Mylar-sheathed capillary tubes (plain and heparinized)
- slide-drying rack
- through-the-stopper blood dispenser such as DIFF-SAFE or H-Pette Dispenser (optional)
- methanol in covered staining (Coplin) jar
- EDTA anticoagulated venous blood specimen
- test tube rack
- capillary puncture supplies
- blood stain reagents: Wright's stain and buffer, or commercial blood stain kit (quick stain)
- squirt bottle for rinsing slides (optional)
- transfer pipets
- staining rack
- immersion oil
- microscope
- lens paper
- lens cleaner
- forceps
- staining jars for quick stains
- timer
- paper towels
- surface disinfectant (such as 10% chlorine bleach)
- biohazard container
- sharps container

PROCEDURE

Record in the comment section any problems encountered while practicing the procedure (or have a fellow student or the instructor evaluate your performance).

S = Satisfactory
U = Unsatisfactory

You must:	S	U	Evaluation/Comments
1. Wash hands with antiseptic and put on gloves and face protection			
2. Assemble materials and equipment			

(Continues)

© 2012 Delmar, Cengage Learning. Permission to reproduce for clinical use granted.

You must:	S	U	Evaluation/Comments

3. Obtain several clean slides:
  a. Use precleaned slides, or
  b. Clean slides with 95% ethanol, and polish dry with lint-free laboratory tissue			

4. Prepare blood smears following steps 4a–4k:
  a. Place a clean slide on a flat surface, touching only the edges of the slide. Write patient identification on slide
  b. Obtain an anticoagulated blood sample
  c. Mix blood well and fill a plain capillary tube with blood or use through-stopper blood drop dispenser
  d. Dispense a small drop of blood onto the slide about one-half to three-quarters of an inch from the right end (if left-handed, reverse instructions)
  e. Rest the short end of a clean, polished, unchipped spreader slide in front of the drop of blood at a 30- to 35-degree angle; balance spreader slide lightly on fingertips
  f. Guide the spreader slide back into the drop of blood by sliding it gently along the slide until the blood spreads along three-fourths of the width of the spreader
  g. Push the spreader slide forward immediately with a quick steady motion, using the other hand to keep slide from moving while spreader is pushed
  h. Examine the smear to see if it is satisfactory
  i. Repeat steps 4a–4h until two satisfactory smears are obtained
  j. Perform a capillary puncture, wipe away the first drop of blood, and fill one or two capillary tubes
  k. Prepare two blood smears from capillary blood, following steps 4d–4i			

5. Allow the smear(s) to air-dry quickly by standing slides on end in slide-drying rack; do not dry flat			
6. Discard blood specimens appropriately or store for later use			
7. Preserve dried smears in absolute methanol for 30 to 60 seconds or skip to step 9 to stain the dried smears			
8. Remove preserved slides from methanol and allow smears to dry in slide-drying rack; store preserved slides for staining or proceed to step 9			
9. Stain blood smears by the two-step method (A) and/or quick stain method (B)			

A. Two-step method:
    (1) Place the dried smear on the staining rack, blood side up
    (2) Flood the smear with Wright's stain, but do not let stain overflow the sides of the slide
    (3) Leave stain on slide 1 to 3 minutes (obtain exact time from instructor)			

© 2012 Delmar, Cengage Learning. Permission to reproduce for clinical use granted.

You must:	S	U	Evaluation/Comments
(4) Add buffer drop by drop to the stain until buffer volume is about equal to that of the stain			
(5) Observe the stain surface for development of a green metallic sheen			
(6) Allow buffer to remain on slide for 2 to 4 minutes (do not allow mixture to run off slide); obtain exact time from instructor			
(7) Hold slide with forceps and rinse thoroughly and continuously with a *gentle* stream of water			
(8) Drain water from slide			
(9) Wipe the _back_ of the slide with a laboratory tissue or gauze to remove excess stain			
(10) Place smear in drying rack to dry			
B. Quick stain method:			
(1) Hold slide with forceps and dip slide into staining solutions as directed by manufacturer's instructions (do not allow slide to dry between solutions)			
(2) Rinse slide (if instructed to do so)			
(3) Remove excess stain from the _back_ of the slide with laboratory tissue			
(4) Place smear in drying rack to dry			
10. Observe stained smears microscopically:			
a. Be sure microscope objectives and eyepieces are clean. Place thoroughly dried slide on microscope stage, stain side up			
b. Focus with low-power (10×) objective			
c. Scan slide to find area where cells are barely touching each other (in feathered edge of smear)			
d. Place a drop of immersion oil on the slide			
e. Rotate oil-immersion lens carefully into position			
f. Focus with fine-adjustment knob only			
g. Observe red blood cells: color should be pink-tan			
h. Observe white blood cells nuclei should be purple; neutrophil granules should be pink-lavender, eosinophil granules should be orange; basophil granules should be dark blue; lymphocyte cytoplasm should be sky blue			
i. Observe platelets; they should appear blue-purple and granular			
11. Rotate the low-power (10×) objective into position			
12. Remove slide from microscope stage			
13. Clean oil objective thoroughly with lens paper and lens cleaner; clean oil from microscope stage if present			
14. Blot oil from slide gently with laboratory tissue			
15. Discard contaminated sharps into sharps container and other contaminated materials into biohazard container			
16. Discard stained smears as instructed or store in slide box for use in Lesson 2-8			

(Continues)

© 2012 Delmar, Cengage Learning. Permission to reproduce for clinical use granted.

You must:	S	U	Evaluation/Comments
17. Return all equipment and unused supplies to storage			
18. Wipe the work area with disinfectant			
19. Remove gloves and discard into biohazard container			
20. Wash hands with antiseptic			

Instructor/Evaluator Comments:

Instructor/Evaluator _____ Date _____

© 2012 Delmar, Cengage Learning. Permission to reproduce for clinical use granted.

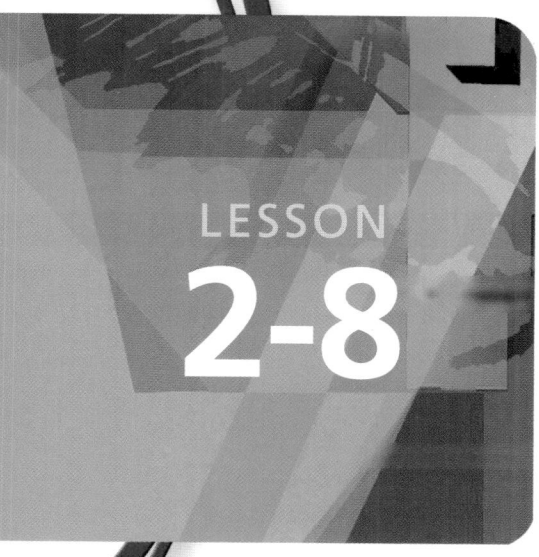

Normal Blood Cell Morphology

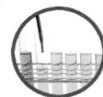

LESSON OBJECTIVES

After studying this lesson, the student will:

◉ State the importance of blood cell identification.

◉ List three morphological features of cells that are evaluated during blood cell identification.

◉ Name a unique morphological characteristic of each type of white blood cell.

◉ Use the microscope to identify five types of white blood cells from a stained smear of normal blood.

◉ Identify platelets microscopically.

◉ Identify red blood cells microscopically.

◉ Discuss safety precautions involved in the microscopic examination of blood smears.

◉ Explain how quality assessment affects the results of blood cell identification.

◉ Define the glossary terms.

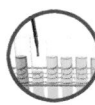

GLOSSARY

azurophilic / a term used to describe the reddis-purple staining characteristics of certain cells or cell structures; having an affinity for azure dyes

band cell / an immature granulocyte with a nonsegmented nucleus; a "stab cell"

basophil / a white blood cell containing basophilic-staining granules in the cytoplasm

basophilic / blue in color; having affinity for the basic stain

eosinophil / a white blood cell containing eosinophilic granules in the cytoplasm

erythrocyte / red blood cell; RBC

leukocyte / white blood cell; WBC

lymphocyte / a small basophilic-staining white blood cell having a round or oval nucleus and playing a vital role in the immune process

megakaryocyte / a large bone marrow cell from which platelets are derived

monocyte / a large white blood cell usually having a convoluted or horseshoe-shaped nucleus

neutrophil / a white blood cell containing neutral-staining cytoplasmic granules and a segmented nucleus; also called polymorphonuclear cell (PMN), poly, or seg

platelet / a formed element in circulating blood that plays an important role in blood coagulation; a small disk-shaped fragment of cytoplasm derived from a megakaryocyte; a thrombocyte

(continues)

red blood cell (RBC) / blood cell that transports oxygen (O_2) to tissues and carbon dioxide (CO_2) to the lungs; erythrocyte

vacuole / a membrane-bound compartment in cell cytoplasm

white blood cell (WBC) / blood cell that functions in immunity; leukocyte

INTRODUCTION

Much information can be gained from the observation and evaluation of the cellular components of the blood in a stained peripheral blood smear. The report on blood cell morphology combined with results from the red and white blood cell counts can often provide the physician the information needed to aid in diagnosis and treatment of the patient. Hematology technologists must be experienced in identifying normal blood cells and also in making the distinction between normal and abnormal blood cells. The examination of the stained blood smear, including the evaluation of cellular components, and the determination of the relative numbers of white blood cells (WBCs) is called the *white blood cell differential count*. The WBC differential count procedure is outlined in Lesson 2-9.

STUDYING BLOOD CELL MORPHOLOGY FROM A STAINED BLOOD SMEAR

Blood cell morphology is studied by microscopic examination of a Wright's-stained peripheral blood smear. The feathered edge (thin end) of the stained smear should be located using the low power (10×) objective of the microscope (Figure 2-51). In this area the cells are not overlapping, the RBCs are just touching each other, and the cells are slightly flattened, making cellular structures more easily seen. The feathered edge of the smear is then examined using the oil-immersion objective. The condenser of the microscope should be positioned so that it almost touches the bottom of the slide being examined. With the diaphragm open, the light should be bright enough to allow the features of the stained cells to be visible. WBCs and platelets should be evenly distributed throughout this portion of the smear.

Safety Precautions

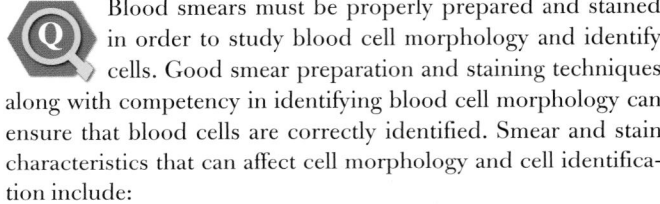

Stained dry blood smears are not a biological hazard. However, microscope slides present a physical hazard and must be handled carefully to prevent accidental cuts to hands or fingers. Used slides must be discarded into a sharps container. Electrical safety rules must be followed when operating the microscope.

Quality Assessment

Blood smears must be properly prepared and stained in order to study blood cell morphology and identify cells. Good smear preparation and staining techniques along with competency in identifying blood cell morphology can ensure that blood cells are correctly identified. Smear and stain characteristics that can affect cell morphology and cell identification include:

- The blood smear must be completely dry before the stain is applied to prevent distortion of cell morphology.

- The smear should be free of precipitate that could obscure cellular features and cause difficulty or confusion in identification.

- The smear must have a feathered edge, an area where the red cells are just touching each other. The cells in this area must be evenly distributed; they should not be in clumps or pushed to the smear edges.

Identification of Blood Cells in a Blood Smear

The formed elements of the blood seen in a stained blood smear include the **red blood cells (RBCs)**, also called **erythrocytes**, **white blood cells (WBCs)**, also called **leukocytes**, and **platelets** (Figure 2-52). Blood cell morphology can be learned through careful evaluation of the staining characteristics of the formed elements.

The cells seen in a normal peripheral blood smear are described in the following sections. The descriptions are for cells as they would appear in a Wright's-stained smear using the oil-immersion objective. A WBC identification guide with abbreviated descriptions is given in Figure 2-53.

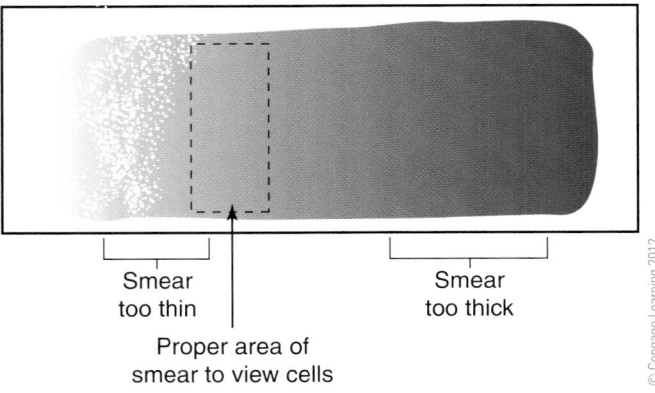

Smear too thin

Smear too thick

Proper area of smear to view cells

© Cengage Learning 2012

FIGURE 2-51 Proper area of the smear to view for microscopic identification of blood cells

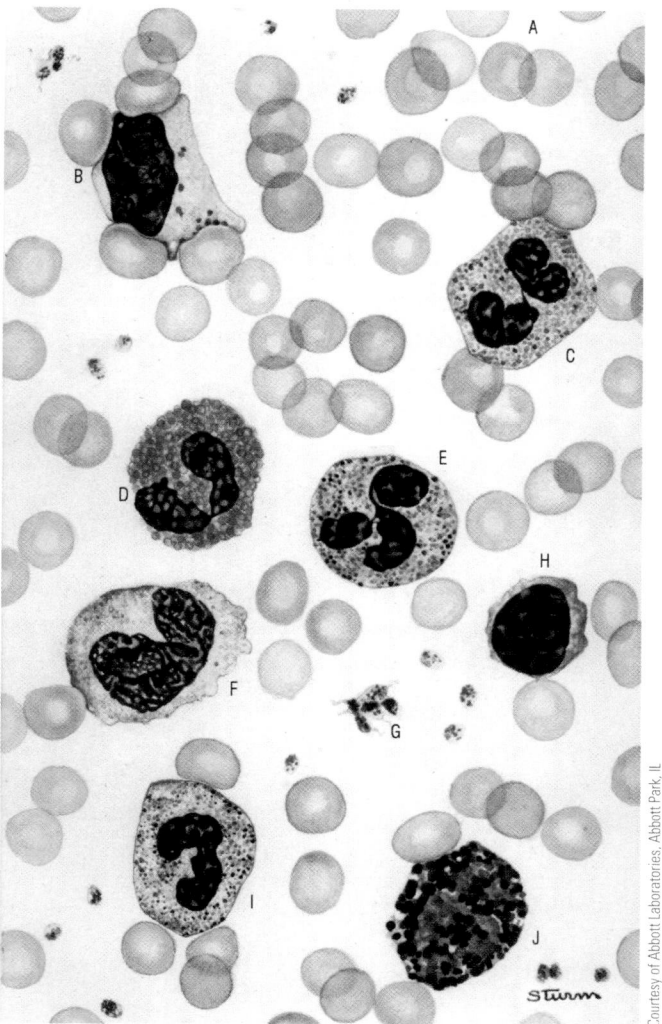

Courtesy of Abbott Laboratories, Abbott Park, IL.

FIGURE 2-52 Cells present in normal peripheral blood: (A) red blood cells; (B) large lymphocyte with azurophilic granules; (C) neutrophil; (D) eosinophil; (E) neutrophil; (F) monocyte; (G) platelets; (H) small lymphocyte; (I) band cell; (J) basophil

Features Evaluated in Cell Identification

RBCs and platelets are relatively easy to identify on a stained smear. However, the WBCs are more difficult to identify and classify. They can be classified by evaluating three features:

- Relative cell size
- Nuclear characteristics
- Cytoplasmic characteristics

The sizes of WBCs can be estimated by comparing them to the size of RBCs in the smear. The nucleus is observed for shape, size, structure, and color. The cytoplasm is evaluated by noting the color, amount, and type of granules. When the information from these three observations is combined, most normal WBCs can be easily identified (Figures 2-52 and 2-53).

Beginners will find it necessary to consciously consider each of the cell properties as they try to identify WBCs. As experience is gained, the process becomes almost automatic for normal cells. Much practice is required to be able to recognize and classify abnormal cells that are seen in various disease states.

Red Blood Cells

RBCs are the most numerous of the blood cells in the peripheral blood. Normally, an RBC loses its nucleus before it enters the peripheral blood, causing it to have a flattened, disk-like shape, often called a biconcave disk. Normal mature RBCs stain pink-tan, have no nucleus, and are 6 to 8 μm in diameter (Figures 2-52A and 2-54A). The pink-tan color is due to the staining of hemoglobin within the cells. Because RBCs are thin in the center, the centers of the cells stain lighter than the cell margins. This is called the "central area of pallor."

Platelets

Platelets, or thrombocytes, are the second most numerous of the formed blood elements in peripheral blood. They are also the smallest of the formed blood elements, being about 2 to 3 μm in diameter, or about one-third the diameter of a RBC. Platelets are not cells but are fragments of cytoplasm from a large bone marrow cell, the **megakaryocyte**. The platelet cytoplasm stains bluish and usually contains small reddish-purple granules (Figures 2-52G and 2-54A). Platelets can be round or oval or can have spiny projections. In a properly prepared smear, platelets are evenly distributed throughout the feathered edge of the smear and are not present in clumps.

White Blood Cells

WBCs are the largest of the normal peripheral blood components. Their sizes range from a diameter of approximately 8 μm to a diameter of 20 μm. Each of the five types of WBCs has a characteristic appearance (Figures 2-52 and 2-53). The granular WBCs—neutrophil, eosinophil, and basophil—contain numerous distinctive cytoplasmic granules, and each has a segmented nucleus. The lymphocyte and monocyte have few, if any, easily visible cytoplasmic granules, and each has a nonsegmented nucleus.

Neutrophil

The granular WBC with neutral-staining cytoplasmic granules is called a **neutrophil**. The neutrophil nucleus is usually segmented into two to five lobes, with each lobe connected by a nuclear strand or filament. The nucleus stains a dark purple and has a coarse, clumped appearance. The cytoplasm is pale pink to tan and contains fine pink or lilac granules. The neutrophil is about twice the diameter of an red blood cell and is the most numerous of the white blood cells in normal adult peripheral blood (Figures 2-52, 2-53, and 2-54B). Other names for the neutrophil are polymorphonuclear cell (*PMN*), *poly*, or *seg*.

A younger, or more immature, stage of the neutrophil called a **band cell** can occasionally be seen in normal peripheral blood.

	Neutrophilic Series		Eosinophil	Basophil	Lymphocyte	Monocyte
	Segmented (mature)	Band or Stab (immature)				
Cell Size (μm)	10–15	10–15	10–15	10–15	8–15	12–20
Nucleus						
Shape	2–5 lobes	Sausage or U-shaped	Bilobed	Segmented	Round, oval	Horseshoe
Structure	Coarse	Coarse	Coarse	Difficult to see	Smoothly stained, velvety	Folded, convoluted
Cytoplasm						
Amount	Abundant	Abundant	Abundant	Abundant	Scant	Abundant
Color	Pale pink-tan	Pale pink-tan	Pale pink-tan	Pale pink-tan	Blue	Gray-blue
Inclusions	Small, lilac granules	Small, lilac granules	Coarse, orange-red granules	Coarse, blue-black granules	Occasional red-purple granules	Ground-glass appearance

© Cengage Learning 2012

FIGURE 2-53 White blood cell identification guide

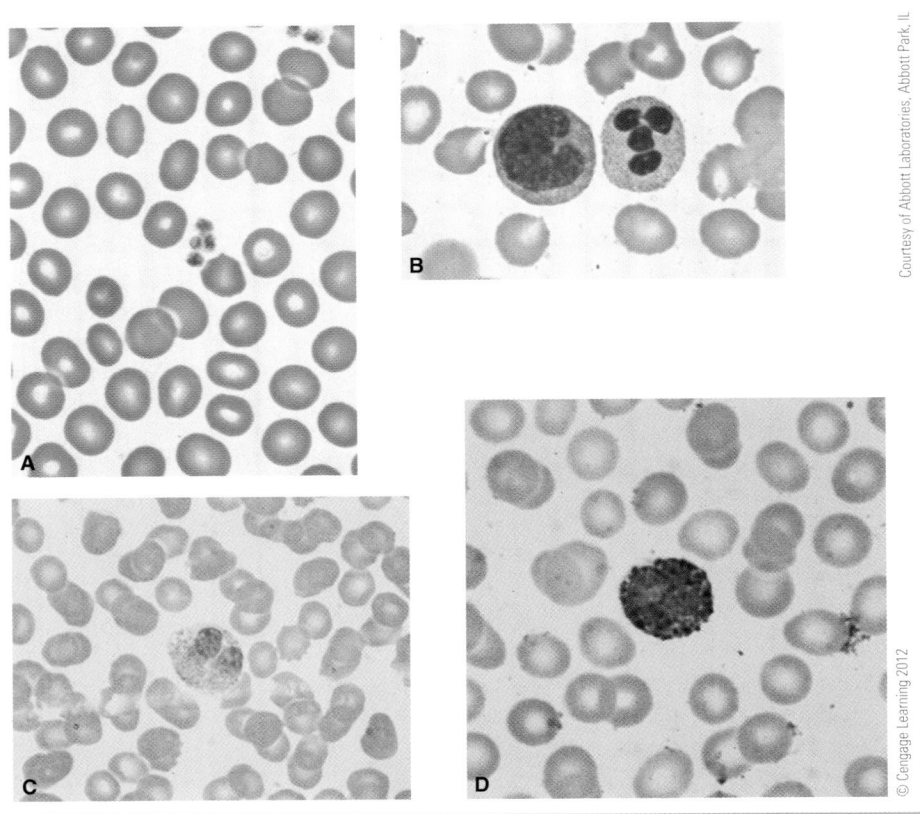

Courtesy of Abbott Laboratories, Abbott Park, IL

© Cengage Learning 2012

FIGURE 2-54 Photomicrographs of cells in peripheral blood: (A) normal red blood cells and platelets; (B) monocyte (left) and segmented neutrophil (right); (C) eosinophil; and (D) basophil

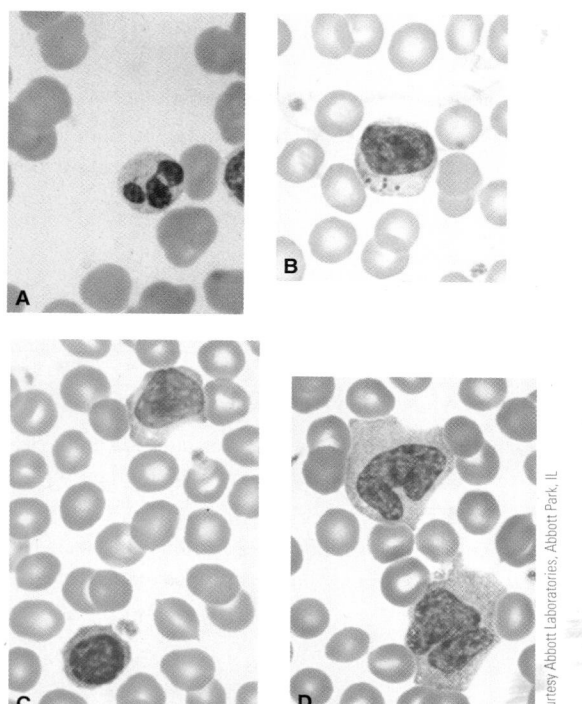

FIGURE 2-55 Photomicrographs of cells in peripheral blood: (A) segmented neutrophil; (B) lymphocyte with azurophilic granules; (C) intermediate lymphocyte and small lymphocyte; and (D) monocytes

The staining characteristics are similar to that of the neutrophil. However, the nucleus is not segmented but is shaped like a curved sausage (Figure 2-52I).

Eosinophil

The **eosinophil** is the WBC with granules that have an affinity for the eosin portion of the Wright's stain. The nucleus of the eosinophil is usually divided into two or three lobes and stains purple. The cytoplasm is pink-tan but is often difficult to see because it is filled with large red-orange (eosinophilic) granules (Figures 2-52, 2-53, and 2-54C). Eosinophils are approximately the same size as neutrophils but are much less numerous than neutrophils in the peripheral blood.

Basophil

The **basophil** is the WBC with granules that have an affinity for the basic portion of the Wright's stain. The basophil nucleus is segmented and stains light purple. However, the nuclear shape is often difficult to see because numerous large blue-black granules often obscure the nucleus and the cytoplasm (Figures 2-52, 2-53, and 2-54D). Basophils are only seen occasionally in smears from normal blood.

Lymphocyte

The **lymphocytes** are the smallest of the WBCs. The lymphocyte nucleus usually has a rather smooth appearance, a round or oval shape, and stains purple (Figures 2-52, 2-53, and 2-55B,C). The cytoplasm is **basophilic** (blue) and varies in amount.

Most lymphocytes are only slightly larger than a red blood cell and have a small rim of sky-blue cytoplasm visible around the large nucleus. However, some lymphocytes can be up to twice the diameter of an RBC and have a larger amount of cytoplasm—these are called *large lymphocytes* (Figure 2-52B). Occasionally, a few red-purple **azurophilic** granules are present in lymphocyte cytoplasm (Figures 2-52B and 2-55B).

Monocyte

The **monocyte** is the largest circulating WBC. The monocyte nucleus can be oval, indented, or horseshoe-shaped and can have brain-like convolutions or folds. The cytoplasm is gray-blue and often has an irregular margin. Very fine granules are distributed throughout the cytoplasm, giving it a dull, ground-glass appearance. **Vacuoles**, membrane-bound compartments in the cytoplasm, can also be present (Figures 2-52, 2-53, 2-54B, and 2-55D).

SAFETY REMINDERS

- Review Safety Precautions section before beginning procedure.
- Observe microscope safety.

PROCEDURAL REMINDERS

- Review Quality Assessment section before beginning procedure.
- Observe cells in an area of the smear where RBCs are just touching.
- Adjust microscope condenser and iris diaphragm to provide optimum light.

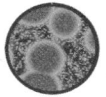 ## SUMMARY

The identification of cells in normal peripheral blood is an important task in the hematology laboratory. Much valuable information can be learned from the examination of a blood smear. Learning to identify the various types of blood cells and to recognize the differences between normal and abnormal cells is a necessary but also interesting and absorbing process. RBCs and platelets are relatively easy to identify, but identification of WBCs requires more practice. Because WBCs are nucleated, the characteristics that are considered in WBC identification are overall size of cell, size and shape of nucleus, amount of cytoplasm relative to nucleus, presence or absence of cytoplasmic granules, and staining characteristics of nucleus and cytoplasm.

Many blood cell atlases and visual aids are available to aid in blood cell identification. However, blood cell identification is best learned through examining numerous well-prepared stained blood smears and having the guidance of a laboratory scientist-proficient in blood cell morphology.

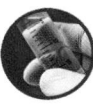 ## REVIEW QUESTIONS

1. Why is it important to identify blood cells?
2. What three features of cells are evaluated during cell identification?
3. List the five types of WBCs.
4. What is the source of platelets?
5. Describe the area of the smear used to identify blood cells.
6. What microscope adjustments or settings should be made to examine stained blood smears?
7. Describe the microscopic appearance of stained RBCs.
8. Describe the appearance of platelets in a stained blood smear.
9. What color granules are present in neutrophils? Eosinophils? Basophils?
10. How do small and large lymphocytes differ in appearance?
11. Define azurophilic, band cell, basophil, basophilic, eosinophil, erythrocyte, leukocyte, lymphocyte, megakaryocyte, monocyte, neutrophil, platelet, red blood cell, vacuole, and white blood cell.

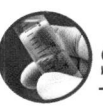 ## STUDENT ACTIVITIES

1. Complete the written examination for this lesson.
2. Practice blood cell identification as outlined in the Student Performance Guide, using the normal blood cell morphology worksheet.
3. Practice identifying blood cells on additional stained smears, from atlases, or from color illustrations of blood cells.

 ## WEB ACTIVITIES

1. Search the Internet for resources such as online blood cell atlases and other aids to help in learning normal blood cell identification. Look for online videos describing how to identify cells or showing WBCs in action.
2. Use the Internet to find images of stained peripheral blood cells. Make your own reference atlas of blood cells from online images. (Be sure that you do not violate any copyrights. Most web sites allow personal use of images.)
3. Search the Internet for free software applications, downloadable cell atlases, or blood cell identification tutorials such as CellAtlas.

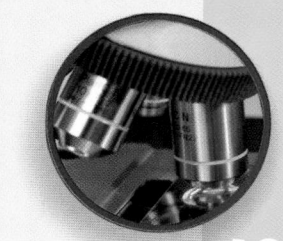

LESSON 2-8
Normal Blood Cell Morphology

(Results will vary based on the types of blood smears provided by the instructor.)

Name _____ Date _____

INSTRUCTIONS

1. Practice identification of RBCs, WBCs, and platelets from a stained smear.

2. Demonstrate blood cell identification satisfactorily for the instructor using the Student Performance Guide and the worksheet. Your instructor will explain the procedure for grading and evaluating your performance. Your performance may be given a number grade, a letter grade, or satisfactory (S) or unsatisfactory (U) depending on course or institutional policy.

MATERIALS AND EQUIPMENT

- hand antiseptic
- gloves (optional)
- stained normal blood smears
- microscope with oil-immersion objective
- immersion oil
- lens paper and lens cleaner
- laboratory tissue
- blood cell atlas; drawings or photographs and descriptions of stained blood cells
- worksheet
- colored pencils
- slide storage box
- sharps container
- paper towels
- surface disinfectant (such as 10% chlorine bleach)

PROCEDURE

Record in the comment section any problems encountered while practicing the procedure (or have a fellow student or the instructor evaluate your performance).

S = Satisfactory
U = Unsatisfactory

You must:	S	U	Evaluation/Comments
1. Wash hands with antiseptic; put on gloves (optional)			
2. Assemble materials and equipment; set up microscope and clean lenses			
3. Place stained blood smear on microscope stage and secure with clips			
4. Use the low-power (10×) objective to locate the feathered edge of the smear			
5. Bring the cells into focus using the coarse adjustment			
6. Scan the smear to find an area where the RBCs are barely touching			

(Continues)

© 2012 Delmar, Cengage Learning. Permission to reproduce for clinical use granted.

You must:	S	U	Evaluation/Comments
7. Place 1 drop of immersion oil on the smear			
8. Rotate the oil-immersion objective (97× or 100×) carefully into position			
9. Use only the fine adjustment knob to bring cells into clear focus			
10. Adjust the condenser and iris diaphragm to allow maximum light into the objective			
11. Scan the thin portion of the smear to observe the white blood cells			
12. Study the smear and find and identify all five types of WBCs. Use the worksheet to describe and sketch each cell type as it is found; label the nucleus and cytoplasm of each cell type			
13. Scan the smear to find platelets; sketch several platelets			
14. Scan the smear to observe RBCs; sketch several			
15. Repeat steps 11–14 until cell types can readily be identified			
16. Repeat steps 3–15 using a different smear			
17. Rotate the low-power (10×) objective into place			
18. Remove the slide from the stage			
19. Clean the oil-immersion objective thoroughly, using lens paper			
20. Check the microscope stage and condenser for oil and clean with lens paper			
21. Place the slide(s) in slide box and save for use in lesson 2-9 or discard into sharps container as instructed			
22. Clean remaining equipment and return it to storage			
23. Wipe work area with disinfectant			
24. Remove gloves (if used) and wash hands with antiseptic			

Instructor/Evaluator Comments:

Instructor/Evaluator _____ Date _____

© 2012 Delmar, Cengage Learning. Permission to reproduce for clinical use granted.

LESSON 2-8
Normal Blood Cell Morphology

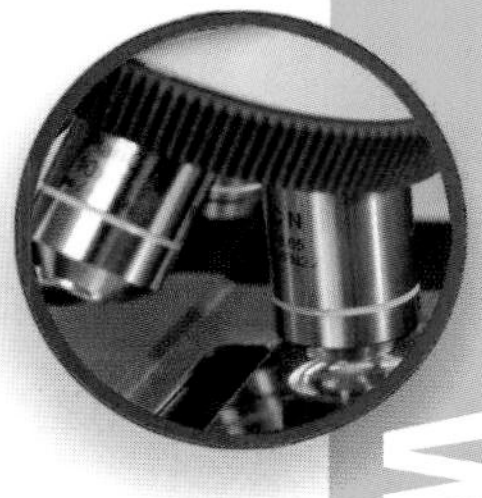

(Answers will vary based on the types of blood smears provided by the instructor.)

Name _____ Date _____

Specimen I.D. _____

Examine stained blood smears and identify the WBCs present. Draw two cells from each category below and describe their appearance, commenting on nuclear size and shape, cytoplasm color and inclusions, and relative cell size.

Segmented neutrophil:

Lymphocyte:

Monocyte:

Eosinophil:

Basophil:

Platelets:

Red blood cells:

Comments: _____

_____

_____

_____

© 2012 Delmar, Cengage Learning. Permission to reproduce for clinical use granted.

WORKSHEET

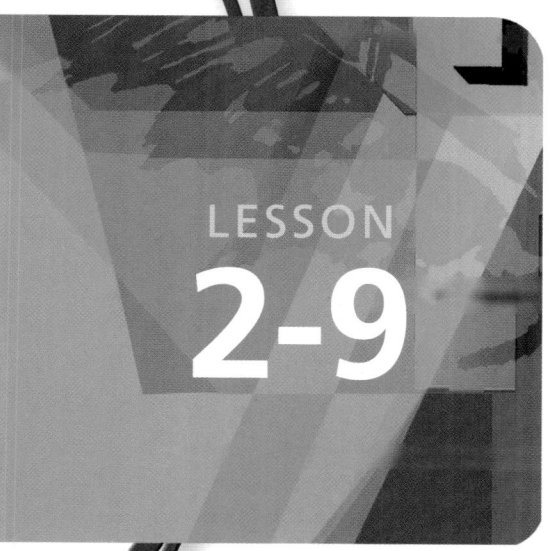

LESSON 2-9

White Blood Cell Differential Count

LESSON OBJECTIVES

After studying this lesson, the student will:

- ⊙ Explain the purpose of the white blood cell differential count.
- ⊙ State the importance of the white blood cell differential count.
- ⊙ List the reference ranges for the five types of white blood cells in a differential count.
- ⊙ Identify the five types of white blood cells microscopically on the stained smear.
- ⊙ Perform a white blood cell differential count and report the results.
- ⊙ Evaluate and report the morphology of red blood cells on a smear.
- ⊙ Observe the morphology of platelets and estimate the platelet count from a blood smear.
- ⊙ List the safety precautions to be observed when performing a differential count.
- ⊙ Discuss the role of quality assessment in performing a differential count.
- ⊙ Define the glossary terms.

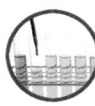

GLOSSARY

anisocytosis / marked variation in the sizes of erythrocytes

atypical lymphocyte / lymphocyte that occurs in response to viral infections and that is common in infectious mononucleosis; reactive lymphocyte

differential count / a determination of the relative numbers of each type of white blood cell when a specified number (usually 100) is counted; white blood cell differential count; leukocyte differential count

hypochromic / having reduced color or hemoglobin content

macrocytic / having a larger-than-normal cell size

microcytic / having a smaller-than-normal cell size

normochromic / having normal color

normocytic / having a normal cell size

phagocytosis / the engulfing of a foreign particle or cell by another cell

poikilocytosis / significant variation in the shape of red blood cells

reactive lymphocyte / see atypical lymphocyte

INTRODUCTION

The classification of white blood cells (WBCs) into different types and determination of their relative numbers is a **differential count**. The *diff*, as it is often called, is usually a part of a complete blood count (CBC). However, the *WBC count and diff* combination is also a frequent laboratory request. The procedure for the differential count involves counting 100 WBCs on a stained blood smear. During the differential count information is also obtained about the RBCs and platelets. The RBCs are evaluated for morphology and hemoglobin content. The platelets are evaluated for morphology, and platelet numbers are estimated.

The differential count can be used to diagnose and monitor the treatment of leukemias, anemias, and diseases and conditions that arise in other parts of the body. For example:

- The viral infection that causes infectious mononucleosis produces a characteristic WBC differential.
- In iron deficiency anemia, the characteristic RBC morphology with small RBCs that have a reduced amount of hemoglobin is seen.
- Infections in various areas of the body can cause increased WBC counts and changes in the percentages of types of WBCs.

Much useful information can be gained from the microscopic examination of a stained blood smear. By viewing a blood smear microscopically, the technologist can identify blood cells and evaluate any abnormalities present. The student must be proficient in identifying blood cells (Lesson 2-8) before performing differential counts.

ORIGIN AND FUNCTION OF WHITE BLOOD CELLS

The WBCs, RBCs, and platelets originate from hemopoietic stem cells. All WBCs are involved in the body's immune response in some way. Any condition or disease that damages or decreases the body's ability to produce normal functioning WBCs will also cause a compromised immune response.

The Granulocytes

The granulocytic (myeloid) blood cells—*neutrophils, eosinophils*, and *basophils*—develop in the bone marrow. They develop from a cell known as the colony-forming unit granulocyte-monocyte (CFU-GM), which arises from an earlier hematopoietic stem cell. The CFU-GM then can become a common precursor cell called a promyelocyte or progranulocyte. As a granulocyte matures, its nucleus changes from a round shape to a segmented shape. When granulocytic cells reach the stage in which the nucleus is either band-shaped or segmented, they migrate out of the bone marrow into the peripheral circulation. Mature granulocytes have a life span of only a few days.

The neutrophilic granulocytes are especially active in **phagocytosis**, the ingestion of foreign particles or cells, including bacteria. Normally in bacterial infections the number of neutrophilic granulocytes is increased. Eosinophils, and basophils to a lesser extent, are increased in allergic reactions.

The Monocytes

Monocytes also arise from CFU-GMs that develop from pluripotent hematopoietic stem cells in the bone marrow. These primitive cells are influenced by a growth factor called monocyte colony stimulating factor (M-CSF) to become monocytes instead of becoming neutrophils, eosinophils, or basophils. Mature monocytes often have vacuoles visible in their cytoplasm. Along with neutrophils, monocytes are a primary defense against invading pathogenic organisms. Phagocytosis and antigen-processing are two major roles of monocytes. Occasionally monocytes that have engulfed a cell or particle are seen in peripheral smears.

The Lymphocytes

Lymphocytes are derived from a pluripotent stem cell in the bone marrow, and mature in the bone marrow and lymphoid tissue. Lymphocytes play an important role in antibody production and in communicating with other cells in the immune system by producing messenger molecules called *cytokines*. These molecules help target cells such as tumor cells or virus-infected cells for destruction. Lymphocytes must be processed in the primary lymphoid organs (the thymus or the bone marrow) before they are fully functional in the immune responses. The lymphocytes known as T cells are processed in the thymus. The lymphocytes known as B cells develop in the bone marrow and in the secondary lymphoid tissue. B cells that are proficient in antibody production develop into *plasma cells*. Lymphocytes can have a life span ranging from a few days to months or years depending on the type.

PERFORMING THE DIFFERENTIAL COUNT

The purpose of a differential count is to determine the percentage of each type of WBC in peripheral blood, to make observations on RBC morphology, and to estimate platelet numbers. The WBC identification guide in Figure 2-56 shows examples of WBCs that are present in normal peripheral blood and lists characteristics important in cell identification.

Safety Precautions

Performing a WBC differential is a safe routine laboratory procedure when all safety policies are followed. Glass slides should be handled carefully to prevent cuts. The microscope cord and plug should be inspected for frayed or exposed wires. The microscope should be disconnected from the power supply before attempting repair or changing the bulb.

Quality Assessment

The written policy and procedure in each laboratory's standard operating procedure (SOP) manual must be followed when performing the WBC differential count. Because there are no controls for WBC differential counts, it

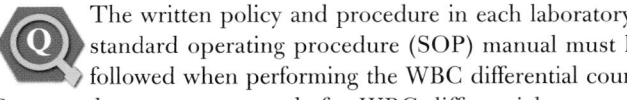

	Neutrophilic Series		Eosinophil	Basophil	Lymphocyte	Monocyte
	Segmented (mature)	Band or Stab (immature)				
Cell Size (μm)	10–15	10–15	10–15	10–15	8–15	12–20
Nucleus						
Shape	2–5 lobes	Sausage or U-shaped	Bilobed	Segmented	Round, oval	Horseshoe
Structure	Coarse	Coarse	Coarse	Difficult to see	Smoothly stained, velvety	Folded, convoluted
Cytoplasm						
Amount	Abundant	Abundant	Abundant	Abundant	Scant	Abundant
Color	Pale pink-tan	Pale pink-tan	Pale pink-tan	Pale pink-tan	Blue	Gray-blue
Inclusions	Small, lilac granules	Small, lilac granules	Coarse, orange-red granules	Coarse, blue-black granules	Occasional red-purple granules	Ground-glass appearance

© Cengage Learning 2012

FIGURE 2-56 White blood cell identification guide

is important that only qualified personnel perform differential counts and report the results. The count must be performed in an area of the smear where the RBCs are just touching, but not overlapping each other, when viewed microscopically. The edges of the smear and end of the smear should not be used for counting the cells; cells in these areas can be clumped, distorted, or unevenly distributed. The appropriate supervisor should always be consulted when abnormal cells are seen or when there is difficulty identifying cells.

The differential count report can give rise to a variety of actions, treatments, and further testing. Much repetition and practice are required to become proficient in performing the differential count. Cells do not always have a "textbook" appearance, therefore it is imperative that care and thoroughness are used when reporting the differential results.

Differential Count Procedure

The differential count is performed by counting and identifying 100 consecutive WBCs in a stained blood smear. The stained smear should always be examined using the oil-immersion objective (97× or 100×). The condenser of the microscope should be raised until it almost touches the bottom of the slide. The iris diaphragm should be adjusted, and the light should be bright enough so the stained cell features can be easily seen. The brightness of the light can be adjusted as necessary to examine details of the nucleus or cytoplasm of a cell.

Performing the WBC Differential Count

The area near the feathered edge of the smear is examined to locate a region where the RBCs are barely touching each other (Figure 2-57). Cells are easiest to identify in this area of the smear because of their slightly flattened shape, which allows better viewing of cell structures. When an area has been located in which the stain appears satisfactory and the cells are not crowded or distorted, 100 consecutive WBCs are counted. A definite pattern, such as the one shown in Figure 2-57, must be followed to avoid counting the same cells twice. As each type of WBC is seen, it is recorded using a differential counter that has keys designated for each cell type (Figures 2-58 and 2-59). Any cell abnormalities must be noted. The counting continues until 100 cells have been identified and recorded; the number of each cell type then represents a percentage of the 100 cells counted.

Red Blood Cell Observations

After the differential count has been completed, the RBCs are observed and evaluated for cell size and hemoglobin content. Normal RBCs are shown in Figure 2-60. Normal RBCs are round or slightly oval. With some experience, one can estimate the RBC size as **normocytic** (normal), **microcytic** (smaller than normal),

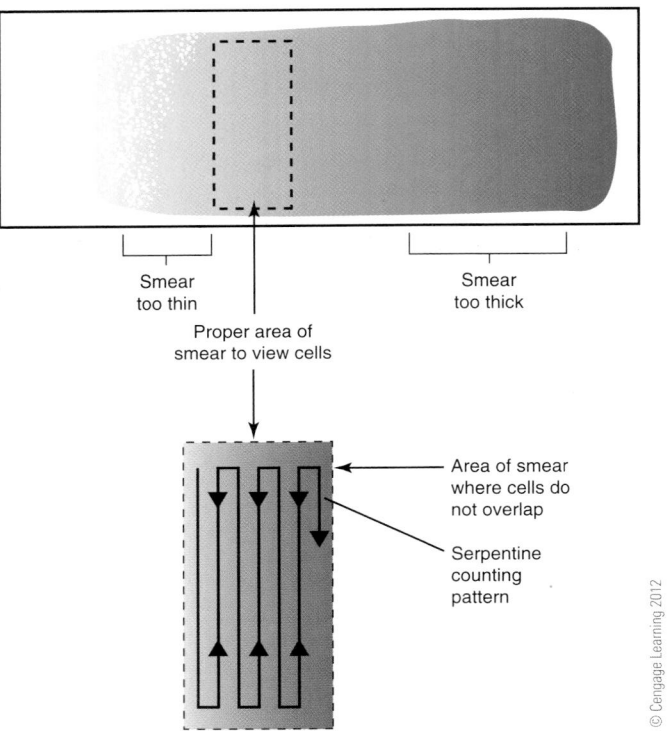

FIGURE 2-57 Proper area of a blood smear to view and illustration of counting pattern for the white blood cell differential count

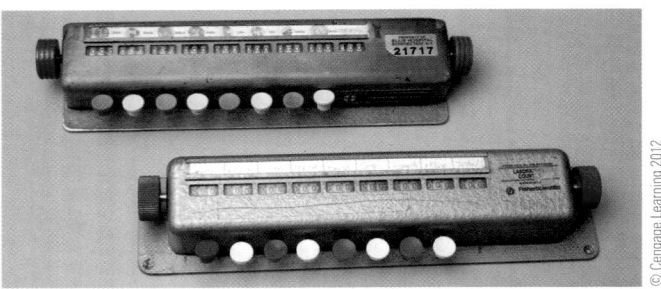

FIGURE 2-58 Manual differential cell counters

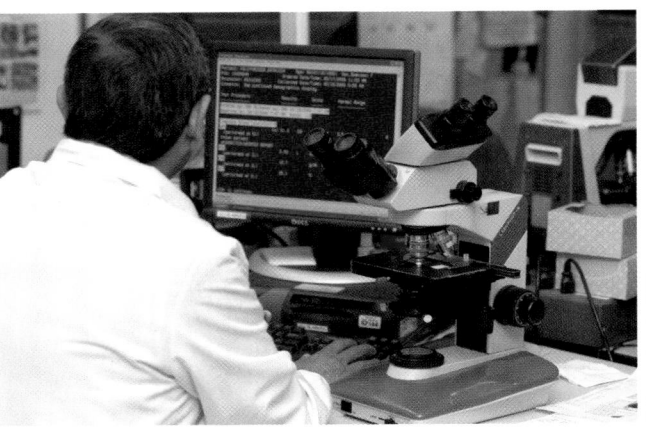

FIGURE 2-59 Reviewing differential count results using a computer

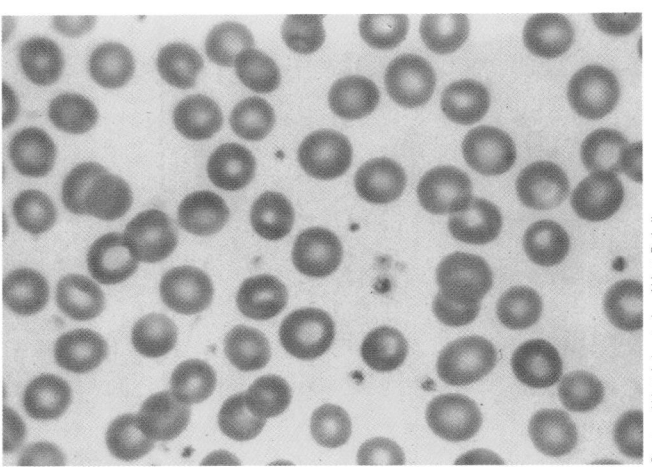

FIGURE 2-60 Photomicrograph of red blood cells and platelets in normal peripheral blood

or **macrocytic** (larger than normal). The condition in which markedly different sizes of RBCs are present is called **anisocytosis.** The presence of significant variation in the *shape* of RBCs is called **poikilocytosis.**

RBCs with the normal amount of hemoglobin are called **normochromic.** These cells stain evenly, with only a small pale area in the center of the cells. A **hypochromic** RBC has less than the normal amount of hemoglobin, with only a ring of hemoglobin around the cell's outer edge and a large central pale area.

Platelet Observations

Platelets are observed for any abnormalities in morphology, such as abnormally large size or absence of granules, and an estimate of platelet numbers is made. The total number of platelets counted in 10 oil-immersion fields is divided by 10 to give the average number per field. The presence of 7 to 20 platelets per oil-immersion field indicates a normal platelet count.

Reference Ranges for the White Blood Cell Differential Count

The reference ranges for the differential count vary with age. Normal values for adults and children are listed in Table 2-12. In a normal differential count, neutrophils and lymphocytes comprise 85% to 95% of cells, with monocytes, eosinophils, and basophils making up the remaining 5% to 15%. The percentage of lymphocytes is normally higher in children than in adults.

Absolute White Blood Cell Counts

It is often beneficial to the physician to be able to correlate the differential count with the WBC count. This is done by calculating the *absolute count,* the number of a particular WBC type per microliter (μL) or liter (L) of blood. The absolute counts are obtained by multiplying the WBC count by the differential

TABLE 2-12. Reference ranges for the white blood cell differential count and absolute white blood cell counts

| CELL TYPE | DIFFERENTIAL COUNT REFERENCE VALUES BY PERCENTAGE (%) | | | | ABSOLUTE COUNT REFERENCE VALUES (CELLS/μL) |
	1-MONTH-OLD	6-YEAR-OLD	12-YEAR-OLD	ADULT	ADULT
Neutrophil (seg)	15–35	45–50	45–50	50–65	2,250–7,150
Neutrophil (band)	7–13	0–7	6–8	0–7	0–770
Eosinophil	1–3	1–3	1–3	1–3	45–330
Basophil	0–1	0–1	0–1	0–1	0–110
Monocyte	5–8	4–8	3–8	3–9	135–990
Lymphocyte	40–70	40–45	35–40	25–40	1,125–4,400
Platelets	An average of 7–20 platelets per oil-immersion field is considered normal				

percentage (in decimals) of each cell type. For example, the absolute neutrophil count for a patient with a WBC count of 9,000/μL and 60% neutrophils is found by multiplying 9,000 × .60 to equal 5,400 neutrophils/μL. The adult reference ranges for absolute WBC counts are listed in Table 2-12.

Factors Affecting the White Blood Cell Percentages

Many disease states can change the percentages of the different types of WBCs (Table 2-13). Bacterial infections usually cause an increase in bands and segmented neutrophils. Viral infections can cause an increase in the number of lymphocytes; viral infections can also change lymphocyte morphology, causing them to appear atypical. The number of eosinophils is increased in parasitic infections and allergies. The number of monocytes is usually not affected by infections but occasionally will increase in tuberculosis. In leukemias, there is usually an increase and abnormality in one type of cell. The leukemia is named according to the predominant cell present. For example, an increased percentage of lymphocytes is found in lymphocytic leukemia.

Factors Affecting Red Blood Cell Morphology

Normal production and development of RBCs require certain factors such as vitamins and minerals. Iron deficiency is one cause of microcytic, hypochromic RBCs. Deficiencies of vitamins such as B_{12} and folic acid cause the cells to be macrocytic. Table 2-14 lists some conditions that affect RBC morphology.

TABLE 2-13. Examples of conditions affecting white blood cell percentages

CONDITION	EFFECT ON WHITE BLOOD CELLS
Bacterial infections	Increased total WBCs, increased percentage of neutrophils and bands
Viral infections	Decreased WBCs, increased percentage of lymphocytes
Infectious mononucleosis	Increased total WBCs, increased lymphocytes, increased atypical lymphocytes
Parasitic infections, allergic reactions	Increased eosinophils
Leukemias	Total WBCs usually increased, increase in type of leukocyte involved

TABLE 2-14. Examples of conditions that affect red blood cell morphology

CELL MORPHOLOGY	CONDITIONS
Size	
Normocytic	Normal
Microcytic	Iron deficiency anemia, thalassemias
Macrocytic	Vitamin B_{12} deficiency, folate deficiency
Shape	
Round, biconcave disk	Normal
Sickle	Sickle cell disease
Spherical	Hereditary spherocytosis
Hemoglobin Content	
Normochromic	Normal
Hypochromic	Iron deficiency anemia
Hyperchromic	Spherocytosis

Factors Affecting Platelets

The platelets can be affected by several factors. In some leukemias, the number of platelets is below normal. Exposure to chemicals, radiation, or drugs used in cancer therapy can also reduce platelets. If there is a delay in making a smear from a capillary puncture, clotting can begin, causing the platelet distribution to be uneven and the platelet estimate from a blood smear to be erroneous.

AUTOMATED DIFFERENTIAL COUNTS

Most hematology analyzers can perform some level of automated differential count. The automated differential can be either a three-part or five-part differential. In a three-part differential, the blood is subjected to a special reagent that shrinks the cytoplasm of each type of WBC in a specific way. The cells are then sorted by size and classified as lymphocytes, granulocytes, or mononuclear cells. In a five-part differential, neutrophils, lymphocytes, eosinophils, basophils, and monocytes are counted and classified.

The majority of hematology analyzers use impedance technology (electrical interruption) or a combination of impedance and light scatter to classify cells. Using hematology automation, several thousand cells can be scanned to obtain information for the automated differential count; however, abnormal cells are "flagged" and must still be verified by examination of the stained blood smear. Details about hematology automation are found in Lesson 2-10.

ABNORMAL OR ATYPICAL CELLS

Recognition and identification of atypical or abnormal WBCs requires much study and practice. Most laboratories require that abnormal cells be reviewed by the supervisor or pathologist before being reported. Exceptions to this are the reporting of **atypical** or **reactive lymphocytes** seen in infectious mononucleosis (Figure 2-61). Atypical lymphocytes are often characterized by a large nucleus and a large amount of blue cytoplasm easily indented by RBCs. The indentations cause the lymphocytes

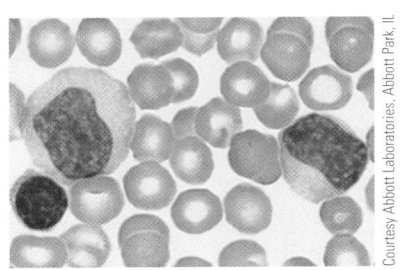

FIGURE 2-61 Photomicrograph showing two atypical (reactive) lymphocytes and one small lymphocyte (lower left)

to have a holly-leaf appearance. Lesson 2-11 contains more information on abnormal blood cell morphology.

When performing a differential count it is important to recognize what is normal so that it becomes easier to recognize the abnormal. If suspicious cells are seen, the differential can be repeated, counting 500 cells to increase the chances of finding more abnormal cells. When there is doubt about identification of a cell, more experienced personnel should be consulted.

SAFETY REMINDERS

- Review Safety Precautions section before beginning procedure.
- Handle slides with care.
- Observe microscope safety guidelines.

PROCEDURAL REMINDERS

- Review Quality Assessment section before beginning procedure.
- Follow procedure in facility SOP manual.
- Use the oil-immersion objective when counting cells.
- Adjust microscope for optimum light.

 ## CASE STUDY 1

Keisha is a technician in a physician office laboratory that has a cell counter for performing RBC and WBC counts. The physician ordered a WBC count and differential count on a patient who complained of pain and fever. Keisha performed the WBC count using the cell counter and prepared a stained blood smear to be sent to a reference laboratory for the differential count. The WBC count was 16×10^9/L. When checking the quality of the blood smear and stain before sending it to the reference laboratory, Keisha saw few WBCs on the smear.

1. Is the patient's WBC count obtained by the cell counter low, normal, or high?
2. Should Keisha have expected to see many WBCs on the smear?
3. Should either the WBC count or the smear be repeated?
4. Give your interpretation of this situation and state what you think Keisha's next step(s) should be.

CASE STUDY 2

Antonio, a technician who had completed school 3 weeks previously, was working alone in the laboratory when Dr. Moore ordered a WBC count and differential count. While examining the smear, Antonio noticed several blood cells he could not readily identify. The physician insisted on receiving a report on the WBC count and the differential count. Discuss the appropriate action(s) for Antonio to take.

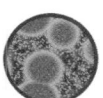

SUMMARY

The WBC differential count gives the relative numbers of each type of WBC in the peripheral blood. The reference ranges for the differential count vary according to age.

The technologist performing differential counts must have a thorough knowledge of blood cell morphology and be willing to ask a more experienced person for help in identifying cells that are difficult to categorize. In larger laboratories, WBC differential counts are routinely performed on hematology analyzers. These instruments flag abnormal results so an abnormality can be verified by a technologist. To ensure quality results that are helpful to the physician and to the patient, care must be exercised in all stages of the performance of the WBC differential count.

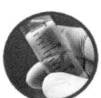

REVIEW QUESTIONS

1. What is the purpose of a WBC differential count?

2. Why is it important to correctly identify blood cells?

3. Describe the area of the smear in which the differential count should be performed.

4. What three characteristics of WBCs are evaluated in cell identification?

5. List the five types of WBCs, and state their reference ranges in percentages.

6. What are the functions of neutrophils? Of monocytes? Of lymphocytes?

7. How many platelets should be noted per oil-immersion field on a smear if the platelet count is normal?

8. What could cause the number of band cells to be increased above normal?

9. How is an absolute WBC count calculated?

10. What is the absolute lymphocyte count if 46% lymphocytes are counted in the differential count of a blood specimen with a total WBC count of $11.5 \times 10^3/\mu L$?

11. Describe the appearance of atypical lymphocytes and name one condition that causes them.

12. Contrast the appearance of normochromic RBCs and hypochromic RBCs.

13. What safety hazards are associated with performing the WBC differential count?

14. Why is it important that differential counts only be performed and reported by experienced, qualified personnel?

15. Define anisocytosis, atypical lymphocyte, differential count, hypochromic, macrocytic, microcytic, normochromic, normocytic, phagocytosis, poikilocytosis, and reactive lymphocyte.

STUDENT ACTIVITIES

1. Complete the written examination for this lesson.

2. Practice performing a differential count as outlined in the Student Performance Guide, using the worksheet or CBC report form for recording results.

3. Perform differential counts on additional smears provided by the instructor.

4. If an automated cell counter is available to perform differentials, compare the results of a manual differential count with the instrument result.

LESSON 2-9
White Blood Cell Differential Count

(Answers may vary based on the types of samples provided by the instructor and individual student results.)

Name _____ Date _____

INSTRUCTIONS

1. Practice identifying RBCs, WBCs, and platelets from a stained smear.

2. Practice the procedure for performing the WBC differential count following the step-by-step procedure

3. Demonstrate the WBC differential count procedure satisfactorily for the instructor, using the Student Performance Guide and the worksheet. Your instructor will explain the procedures for evaluating and grading your performance. Your performance may be given a number grade, a letter grade, or satisfactory (S) or unsatisfactory (U) depending on the course or institutional policy.

MATERIALS AND EQUIPMENT

- gloves (optional)
- hand antiseptic
- stained smears of normal peripheral blood
- microscope with oil-immersion objective
- immersion oil
- lens paper and lens cleaner
- laboratory tissue
- blood cell atlas; drawings, photographs and descriptions of stained blood cells
- differential counter
- slide storage box
- worksheet
- sharps container
- paper towels
- surface disinfectant (such as 10% chlorine bleach)
- Optional: tube of EDTA-venous blood (and test tube rack)
- supplies for making and staining blood smears
- supplies for performing WBC count, RBC count, Hgb determination and microhematocrit

PROCEDURE

Record in the comment section any problems encountered while practicing the procedure (or have a fellow student or the instructor evaluate your performance).

S = Satisfactory
U = Unsatisfactory

You must:	S	U	Evaluation/Comments
1. Wash hands with antiseptic and put on gloves (optional)			
2. Assemble materials and equipment; set up microscope and clean lenses			
3. Obtain blood smear for performing differential count: a. Obtain stained smear from instructor b. Prepare and stain a smear using venous-EDTA blood provided by instructor			

(Continues)

© 2012 Delmar, Cengage Learning. Permission to reproduce for clinical use granted.

You must:	S	U	Evaluation/Comments
4. Place stained blood smear on microscope stage and secure. Use the low-power (10×) objective to locate the feathered edge of the smear			
5. Bring the cells into focus using the 10× objective and coarse adjustment			
6. Scan the smear to find an area where the RBCs are barely touching			
7. Place 1 drop of immersion oil on the smear directly over the condenser			
8. Rotate the oil-immersion objective (97× or 100×) carefully into position so that the objective lens contacts the oil drop			
9. Use the fine adjustment to bring cells into focus			
10. Adjust the condenser and iris diaphragm to allow optimum light into the objective			
11. Locate the first WBC in the counting area and begin the count			
12. Use the differential counter to count 100 consecutive WBCs, moving the slide so that consecutive microscopic fields are viewed; use the counting pattern illustrated in Figure 2-57			
13. Record the numbers from the differential counter on the worksheet; check that the numbers of all the cell types add up to 100			
14. Observe the RBCs in at least 10 fields: Note the hemoglobin content; record as normochromic or hypochromic			
15. Observe the RBC size: Record as normocytic, microcytic, or macrocytic. If present, estimate the percentage of microcytic or macrocytic RBCs using a grading system of 1+ to 4+			
16. Observe platelets in at least 10 fields: a. Note platelet morphology b. Estimate the number of platelets per oil-immersion field: Count platelets in 10 fields and divide by 10 to obtain the average number per field c. Record as adequate, decreased, or increased, using the guide on the worksheet			
17. Rotate the low-power (10×) objective into place			
18. Remove the slide from the stage			
19. Clean the oil-immersion objective thoroughly using lens paper and lens cleaner, or following instructor's directions			

© 2012 Delmar, Cengage Learning. Permission to reproduce for clinical use granted.

You must:	S	U	Evaluation/Comments
20. Check the microscope stage and condenser for oil and clean with lens paper if necessary			
21. Discard slides as instructed or blot excess oil from the slides with laboratory tissue and place them in slide box			
22. Optional: Perform Hgb, microhematocrit, WBC count, and RBC count on the EDTA-venous blood used for the differential count; record results on CBC Report Form			
23. Clean remaining equipment, return it to storage, and wipe work area with disinfectant			
24. Remove gloves (if used) and discard into biohazard container			
25. Wash hands with antiseptic			

Instructor/Evaluator Comments:

Instructor/Evaluator_____ Date _____

© 2012 Delmar, Cengage Learning. Permission to reproduce for clinical use granted.

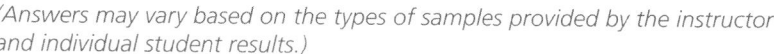

LESSON 2-9
White Blood Cell Differential Count

(Answers may vary based on the types of samples provided by the instructor and individual student results.)

Name _____ Date _____

Specimen I.D. _____

		REFERENCE VALUES (ADULT)
Segmented Neutrophils	_____ %	50%–65%
Lymphocytes	_____ %	25%–40%
Monocytes	_____ %	3%–9%
Eosinophils	_____ %	1%–3%
Basophils	_____ %	0%–1%
Bands	_____ %	0%–7%
Other	_____ %	

Platelet Estimate:

❑ Appear adequate

❑ Appear decreased
   (<7/ oil-immersion field)

❑ Appear increased
   (>20/oil-immersion field)

7–20/oil-immersion field

Red Blood Cell Morphology:

Cell size:

❑ Normocytic

❑ Microcytic

❑ Macrocytic

Normocytic (6–8 μm)

Cell color:

❑ Normochromic

❑ Hypochromic

Normochromic

Comments: _____

_____

_____

_____

© 2012 Delmar, Cengage Learning. Permission to reproduce for clinical use granted.

LESSON 2-9
White Blood Cell Differential Count

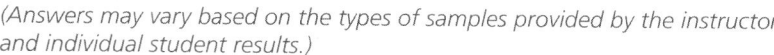

(Answers may vary based on the types of samples provided by the instructor and individual student results.)

Name _____ Date _____

Specimen I.D. _____

WBC/L   _____

RBC/L   _____

Platelets/L   _____

Hgb (g/L)   _____

Hct   _____

REFERENCE RANGES (ADULT)
$4.5–11.0 \times 10^9$/L ($4.5–11.0 \times 10^3$/µL)
Male: $4.5–6.0 \times 10^{12}$/L ($4.5–6.0 \times 10^6$/µL)
Female: $4.0–5.5 \times 10^{12}$/L ($4.0–5.5 \times 10^6$/µL)
$1.5–4.0 \times 10^{11}$/L ($1.5–4.0 \times 10^5$µL)
Male: 130–170 g/L (13–17 g/dL)
Female: 120–160 g/L (12–16 g/dL)
Male: 0.42–0.52 (or 42%–52%)
Female: 0.36–0.48 (or 36%–48%)

Differential Count:

_____%	Segmented neutrophils	50%–65%
_____%	Lymphocytes	25%–40%
_____%	Monocytes	3%–9%
_____%	Eosinophils	1%–3%
_____%	Basophils	0%–1%
_____%	Bands	0%–7%
_____%	Other	

Red Blood Cell Morphology:

Cell size:
- ❑ Normocytic
- ❑ Microcytic
- ❑ Macrocytic

Normocytic

Cell color:
- ❑ Normochromic
- ❑ Hypochromic

Normochromic

Platelet estimate:
- ❑ Appear adequate
- ❑ Appear decreased (<7/oil-immersion field)
- ❑ Appear increased (>20/oil-immersion field)

7–20/oil-immersion field

Comments: _____

_____

_____

© 2012 Delmar, Cengage Learning. Permission to reproduce for clinical use granted.

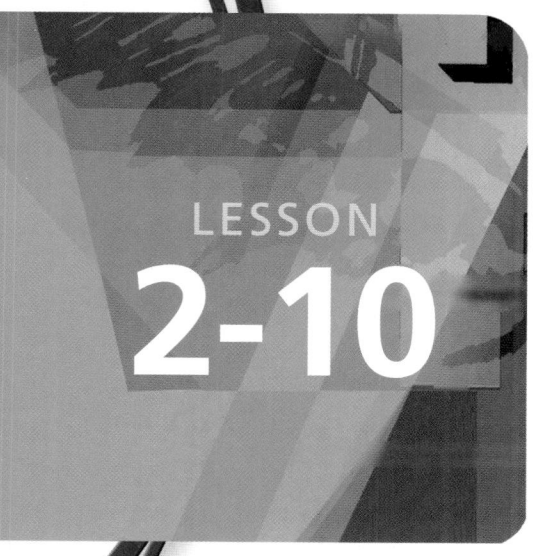

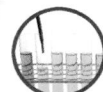

LESSON OBJECTIVES

After studying this lesson, the student will:

⊙ Describe the history of the counting of blood cells.

⊙ Compare the accuracy and precision of manual and automated blood cell counting methods.

⊙ Name two automated cell-counting technologies.

⊙ Give an example of an instrument that uses each type of counting technology.

⊙ Explain the principle of electrical impedance.

⊙ Explain the principle of light scatter.

⊙ Explain the principle of flow cytometry.

⊙ Explain the difference in the information obtained from 3-part and 5-part automated differential counts.

⊙ Discuss safety hazards associated with hematology instrumentation and precautions that should be followed when using hematology analyzers.

⊙ Discuss quality control and quality assessment procedures for automated hematology.

⊙ Define the glossary terms.

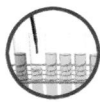

GLOSSARY

aperture / an opening

electrolyte solution / a solution that contains ions and conducts an electrical current

femtoliter (fL) / 10^{-15} liter

fluorescent / having the property of emitting light of one wavelength when exposed to light of another wavelength

histogram / a graph that illustrates the size and frequency of occurrence of articles being studied

impedance / resistance in an electrical circuit

index of refraction / the ratio of the velocity of light in one medium, such as air, to its velocity in another material

laser / a narrow, intense beam of light of only one wavelength going in only one direction

mean cell hemoglobin (MCH) / average red blood cell hemoglobin expressed in picograms (pg); mean corpuscular hemoglobin

mean cell hemoglobin concentration (MCHC) / comparison of the weight of hemoglobin in a red blood cell to the size of the red blood cell, expressed in percentage or grams per deciliter (g/dL); mean corpuscular hemoglobin concentration

(continues)

mean cell volume (MCV) / average red blood cell volume in a blood sample, expressed in femtoliters (fL) or cubic microns (μ^3); mean corpuscular volume

picogram / 10^{-12} gram

red blood cell indices / calculated values that compare the size and hemoglobin content of red blood cells in a blood sample to reference values; erythrocyte indices

INTRODUCTION

Humans have long been fascinated with blood, associating it with life in themselves and animals. In the 1600s, William Harvey recorded his observations of the direction of blood flow in the veins and put forth his theory of blood circulation.

In 1855, researchers devised the first counting chambers (hemacytometers) for viewing and counting cells using a microscope. Hemacytometers were gradually improved and standardized by changing the background color of the glass and adding some metal to the etched lines to make them brighter. By using special diluting pipets and these hemacytometers, blood cells in a specific volume of blood could be counted.

Blood cells were routinely counted manually until the late 1950s. In 1956, W. H. Coulter patented a device that counted blood cells using the method of *electrical impedance*, also known as *aperture impedance*. This invention made performance of blood cell counts faster, easier, and more available.

The first hematology instruments performed only the RBC and white blood cell (WBC) counts. Hemoglobin measurement was added later. Instruments are now available that provide direct or calculated values for 60 or more parameters. In these instruments, only the RBCs, WBCs, hemoglobin, platelets, and reticulocytes are counted or measured directly. The hematocrit, red cell indices, and other values are calculated from the RBC count and hemoglobin results.

The automated measurements are more accurate and precise than manual counts. Manual counts have a coefficient of variation (CV) of approximately ±10%, whereas reliable instrument counts have a CV of ±1% to 2%. Examples of the information available from various hematology analyzers are shown in Table 2-15.

TWO BASIC CELL-COUNTING TECHNOLOGIES

Electrical impedance was the only automated cell-counting method until the 1970s, when light-scatter cell-counting technology was developed. Today's cell counters are based on one of these two technologies.

Principle of Electrical-Impedance Cell Counting

Blood cells counted by electrical impedance are diluted in an **electrolyte solution** that conducts electricity. The electrical current flows in the electrolyte solution from one electrode to another across the opening, or **aperture** in the sampling probe (Figure 2-62).

TABLE 2-15. Examples of results available from hematology analyzers

RBC	MCHC	Atypical lymphocytes
WBC	MCV	Hypochromia
HGB	RDW*	RBC fragments
HCT	3-Part differential	Nucleated RBCs
PLT count	5-Part differential	Reticulocyte count
MPV†	Immature granulocytes	
MCH	Left shift	

* RDW: Red cell distribution width, a measure of RBC anisocytosis.
† MPV: Mean platelet volume, a measure of the average platelet volume.
Note: Instruments are available that perform other measurements of blood components; many measurements are only used for research purposes.

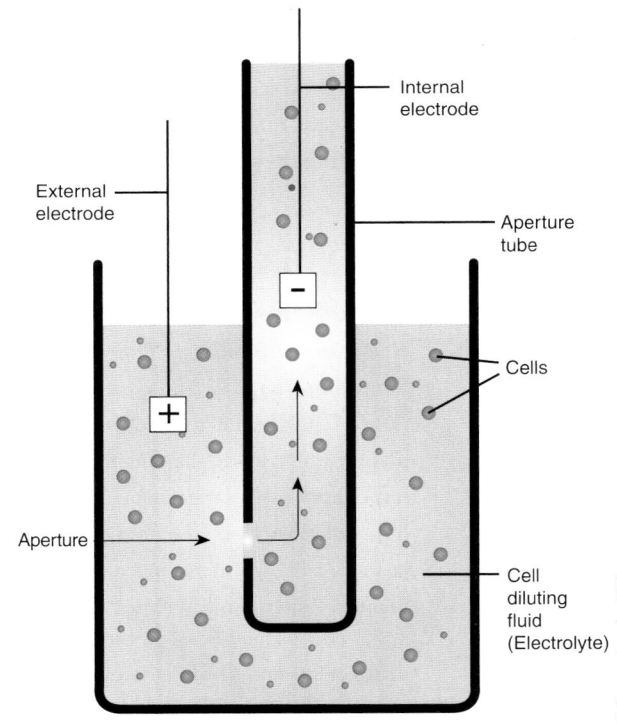

© Cengage Learning 2012

FIGURE 2-62 Illustration of electrical-impedance method of cell counting

Blood cells are poor conductors of electricity. As a cell suspended in the electrolyte solution passes through the aperture, the nonconducting cell causes an **impedance**, or interruption, of the electrical circuit. The impedance causes a pulse in the electrical circuit. These pulses are counted as cells. The size of the impedance is proportional to the size of the cell causing it. Therefore the instrument records not only how many cells pass through the aperture but also the size of each cell.

All electrical-impedance cell counters are based on Coulter's principles. The instruments using these principles have also been adapted for industrial use to count other types of particles in solutions.

Improvements in Electrical-Impedance Technology

The first electrical-impedance cell counters had some inherent problems. As cells passed through the aperture, cells not passing through the center of the aperture were measured as being larger than their real size. Also, cells that became trapped in the aperture were counted repeatedly, falsely increasing a count.

Accuracy and precision were improved by modifying cell counters so that the pulses were electronically edited and the flow was channeled to the center of the aperture. The information obtained was then more accurate for the purpose of sizing cells. Most cell counters display this sizing information on a screen in a graph called a **histogram**. The relative numbers of cells are plotted on the Y-axis and the relative cell sizes are plotted on the X-axis (Figure 2-63).

Examples of Electrical-Impedance Instruments

Several companies manufacture instruments that use electrical-impedance technology (Figure 2-64). Beckman Coulter, Inc., markets a variety of such instruments, including the Beckman Coulter Onyx for laboratories performing 10 to 100 complete

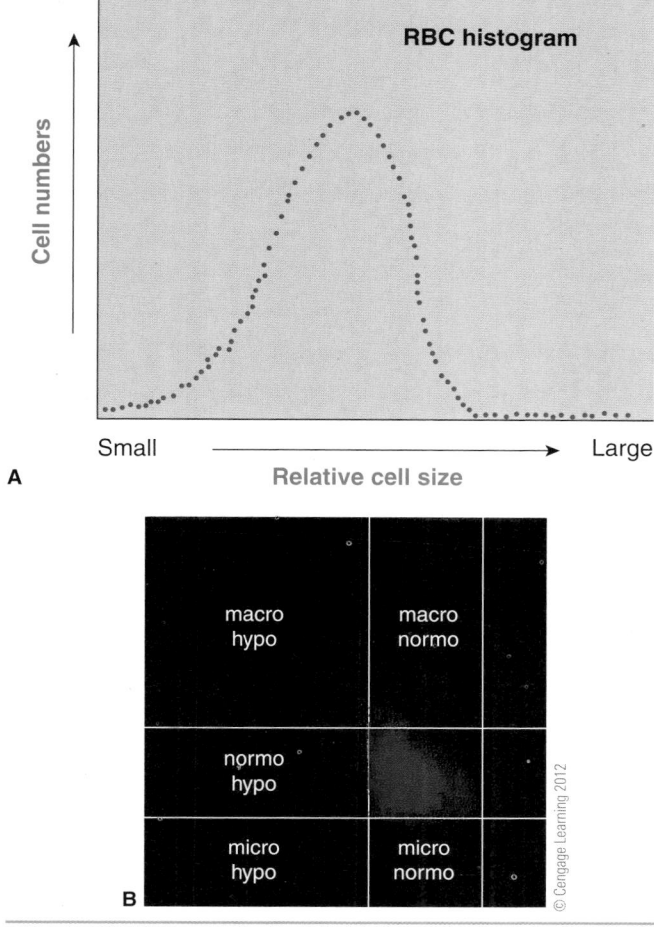

FIGURE 2-63 RBC histogram and cytogram: (A) RBC histogram showing relative red blood cell numbers plotted versus red blood cell size; (B) cytogram showing normal distribution of red blood cell sizes and hemoglobin content

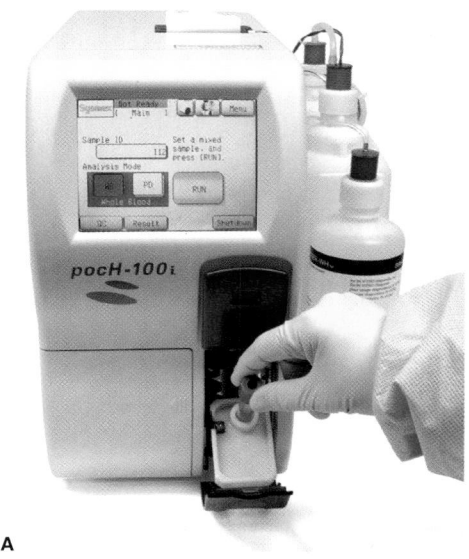

A

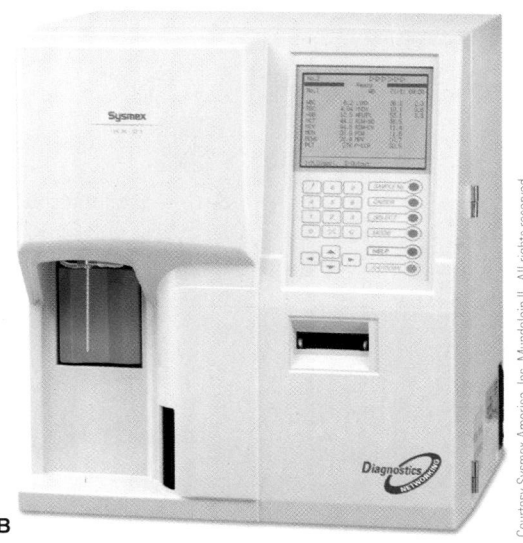

B

Courtesy Sysmex America, Inc. Mundelein IL. All rights reserved

FIGURE 2-64 Hematology cell counters: (A) pocH100i; (B) KX-21

blood counts (CBCs) per day and the Coulter Ac•T diff2 for laboratories such as physician office laboratories (POLs) that perform 1 to 50 CBCs per day. The Serono-Baker 7000, 8000, and 9000 series and the Horiba ABX Micros CRP 200 are all suitable for the workload in a small laboratory or a hematology or oncology practice. The Abbott Cell-Dyn 3500 uses electrical impedance coupled with an optical method. Many automatic cell counters perform 50 to 110 tests per hour, require small quantities of blood for testing, and have closed-tube sampling capability to reduce risk for exposure to blood.

Principle of Light-Scatter Cell Counting

In light-scatter cell counters, a **laser** beam or tungsten-halogen light beam is directed at a stream of blood cells passing through a narrow channel. The channel is extremely narrow to force the cells to pass through in single file. When the light beam strikes a cell, the beam is scattered at an angle. The speed and angle of scatter of the beam of light differ according to the cell type. This is called the **index of refraction** of the cell. The index of refraction is influenced by the shape and volume of the cell, although volume has the greater effect on the scatter. Sensors detect how much light is scattered and how much of the beam is absorbed by the cell (Figure 2-65A).

The laser light is monochromatic, which means it has only one wavelength and travels in only one direction. These two characteristics allow it to be more finely tuned than the tungsten-halogen light beam and enable it to produce scatter patterns more useful in diagnostic hematology. One disadvantage is that laser-beam instruments cannot be calibrated with the same materials as other cell counters. Only human blood cells can be used for calibrating the laser counters.

An important advantage added to light-scatter technology is *sheath-flow*, in which the cells are focused hydrodynamically (Figure 2-65B). Sheath flow improves performance and also helps avoid the cleaning and maintenance problems of electrical impedance models.

Light scatter is used in the Beckman Coulter GEN-S series, the LH 755, HMX, and MAXM. The GEN-S performs reticulocyte counts, makes a blood smear, and performs a 5-part differential for each sample (Table 2-16). The LH 755 and the Abbott SMS also make smears from each blood sample. The Sysmex XT

TABLE 2-16. Examples of hematology analyzers, the technology used, and the type of differential reported

TECHNOLOGY USED	INSTRUMENT	DIFFERENTIAL REPORTED
Electrical-impedance	Beckman Coulter Onyx	5 part
	Beckman Coulter Ac •T diff2	3 part
	Serono-Baker	3 part
Light-scatter	Beckman Coulter VCS, STKS, GEN-S, LH 755	5 part
	Sysmex XT 2000i	5 part
Combination of electrical impedance and light-scatter	Abbott Cell-Dyn 4000	5 part

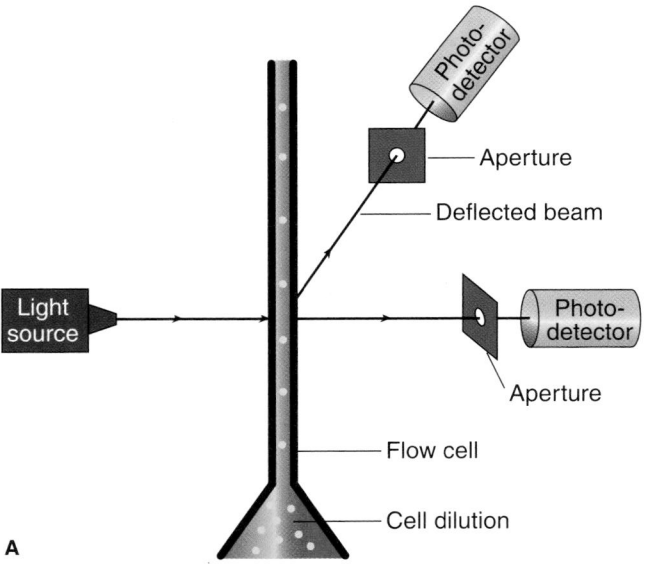

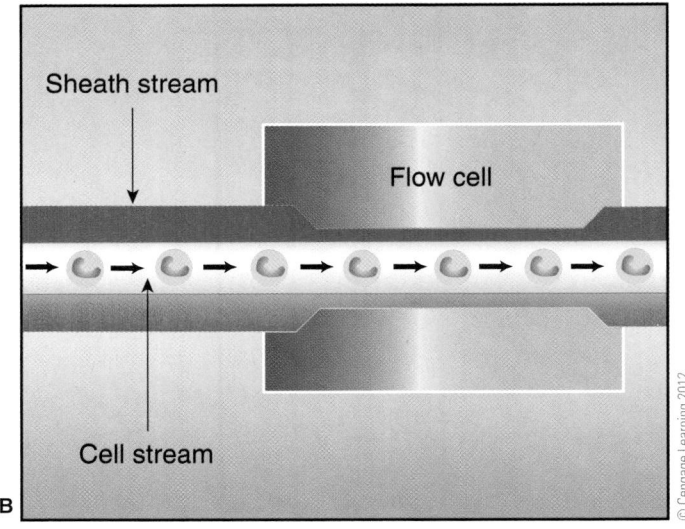

© Cengage Learning 2012

FIGURE 2-65 Light scatter technology: (A) schematic illustrating light-scatter method of cell counting; (B) schematic of sheath-flow, used to focus the cells hydrodynamically

2000i uses flow technology (see Current Topic) and performs a reticulocyte count, a 5-part differential and a fluorescent optical platelet count (Figure 2-66). The Abbott Cell-Dyn 4000 combines aperture impedance with light-scatter technology.

RED BLOOD CELL PARAMETERS

Automated hematology analyzers measure several RBC parameters in addition to counting the RBCs. The analyzers display cytograms or histograms showing the relative numbers of RBCs and degree of hypochromia. The red cell distribution width (RDW) is also shown, demonstrating the range of sizes of the RBCs in a population of cells.

Automated Calculation of Red Blood Cell Indices

Although estimates of size and hemoglobin content of RBCs can be made from microscopic examination of stained smears, the **red blood cell (RBC) indices** are calculated values that indicate the size and hemoglobin content of RBCs in a blood sample. The RBC indices provide a quantitative measurement of red cell volume and hemoglobin concentration that can be compared to

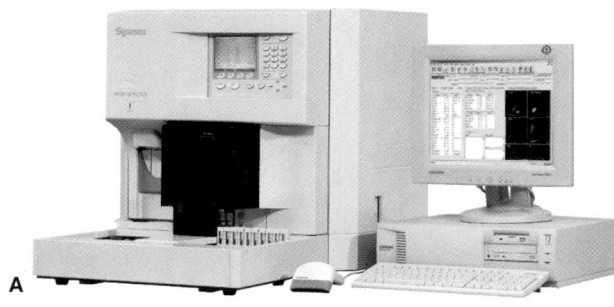

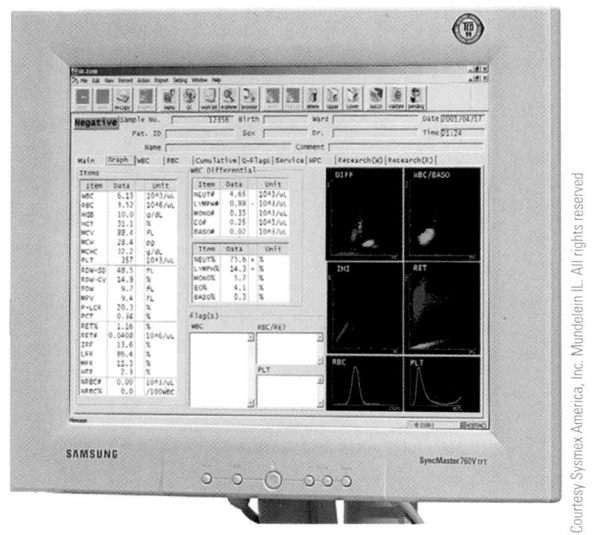

Courtesy Sysmex America, Inc. Mundelein IL. All rights reserved

FIGURE 2-66 Automated five-part differential: (A) Sysmex XT 2000i hematology analyzer with (B) five-part differential cytogram shown in right side of monitor

normal reference values. Laboratories with hematology analyzers rely on the instruments to automatically calculate the RBC indices. These calculations are made using the red blood cell count, hemoglobin concentration and the calculated hematocrit.

Manual Calculation of Red Blood Cell Indices

The three RBC indices are:

- Mean cell volume (MCV)
- Mean cell hemoglobin (MCH)
- Mean cell hemoglobin concentration (MCHC)

Manual calculations of the three RBC indices can be performed using the RBC count, hemoglobin concentration, and hematocrit and the formulas shown in Figures 2-67, 2-68, and 2-69.

$$MCV = \frac{\text{Hematocrit (percent)}}{\text{RBC}} \times 10$$

Using a hematocrit of 36% and an RBC of 4.0×10^{12}/L:

$$MCV = \frac{36}{4.0} \times 10$$

$$MCV = 90 \text{ fL (or } \mu^3)$$

© Cengage Learning 2012

FIGURE 2-67 Sample calculation of mean cell volume (MCV) from a blood specimen with hematocrit of 36% and RBC count of 4.0×10^{12}/L

$$MCH = \frac{\text{Hemoglobin (grams)}}{\text{RBC}} \times 10$$

Using a hemoglobin value of 15 g/dL and an RBC of 5.2×10^{12}/L:

$$MCH = \frac{15.0}{5.2} \times 10$$

$$MCH = 28.8 \text{ pg}$$

© Cengage Learning 2012

FIGURE 2-68 Sample calculation of mean cell hemoglobin (MCH) from a blood specimen with hemoglobin of 15 g/dL and RBC count of 5.2×10^{12}/L

$$MCHC = \frac{\text{Hemoglobin (grams)}}{\text{Hematocrit (percent)}} \times 100$$

Using a hemoglobin value of 15 g/dL and a hematocrit of 44%:

$$MCHC = \frac{15}{44} \times 100$$

$$MCHC = 34\%$$

© Cengage Learning 2012

FIGURE 2-69 Sample calculation of mean cell hemoglobin concentration (MCHC) from a blood specimen with hemoglobin of 15 g/dL and hematocrit of 44%

The indices can be used to classify anemias. The validity of the indices is dependent on the accuracy of the RBC count and the hemoglobin and hematocrit measurements.

Mean Cell Volume

The **mean cell volume (MCV)** is the volume of an average RBC in a blood sample. As shown in Figure 2-67, the MCV is calculated by dividing the hematocrit (%) by the RBC count (dropping the exponent) and is reported in **femtoliters (fL)**. The normal reference range for MCV is 80 to 98 fL (Table 2-17). An MCV above 98 fL indicates macrocytes; a value below 80 fL indicates microcytes. The red cell distribution width (RDW) provides a way to classify red cells by size. If the curve in the histogram is shifted to the left or right, it indicates that the sizes of the red cells in the sample are smaller or larger than normal cells (Figure 2-63).

Mean Cell Hemoglobin

The **mean cell hemoglobin (MCH)** estimates the average weight of hemoglobin in an RBC. The unit of weight is the **picogram (pg)**, which is equivalent to 10^{-12} g. The MCH is calculated by dividing the hemoglobin value in grams per deciliter by the RBC count (dropping the exponent) (Figure 2-68). The reference range for the MCH is 27 to 32 pg (Table 2-17).

Mean Cell Hemoglobin Concentration

The **mean cell hemoglobin concentration (MCHC)** expresses the concentration of hemoglobin in the RBCs in relation to their size and volume. The MCHC is calculated by dividing the hemoglobin (g/dL) by the hematocrit (%) (Figure 2-69). The result is expressed in percentage. Values within the reference range of 32% to 37% (Table 2-17) indicate *normochromia*, and values below 32% indicate *hypochromia*.

AUTOMATED DIFFERENTIAL COUNTING

Hematology cell counters and analyzers perform WBC differentials in addition to measuring or calculating several other cell parameters. Two types of differentials are produced. Electrical impedance instruments produce 3-part differentials; these are used as screening devices. The light-scatter instruments produce 5-part differentials.

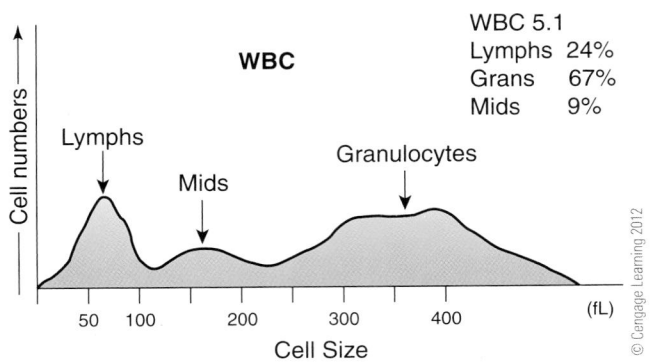

FIGURE 2-70 Histogram of 3-part differential illustrating normal white blood cell count and differential

The information from the blood cell count and differential count are shown on the instrument display screen in graphical form and can also be printed. The relative numbers of each type of cell are shown on the "Y" axis of the graph (Figure 2-70). The distribution of cell sizes in each category is shown on the "X" axis of the graph. These graphs are called histograms, cytograms, or *scattergrams* (Figure 2-66B). The histogram and cytogram are representations of the grouping of cell sizes around the mean cell size. The scattergram usually refers to the graph resulting from sample analysis using light-scatter technology.

Three-Part Differential

The analyzers that produce a 3-part differential subject the blood cells to a special reagent that shrinks the cytoplasm of each WBC type to a different degree, with the lymphocytes shrinking the most. This allows the cells to be sorted into 3 distinct size classifications: lymphocytes, mononuclear cells and granulocytes. WBCs of size range 35-99 fL are grouped as lymphocytes, cells in the range of 100-200 fL are grouped as mononuclear cells (or "mids"), and cells greater than 200 fL are called granulocytes (Figure 2-70). The 3-part differential does not separate the granulocytes into neutrophils, eosinophils, and basophils. The instrument alerts the operator to the presence of abnormal RBC or WBC counts, atypical lymphocytes, and giant platelets.

Beckman Coulter manufactures the Ac·T series and the "K" series of instruments that produce a 3-part differential. Serono-Baker has the Baker 9000 series analyzers that also report a 3-part differential.

Five-Part Differential

Several hematology analyzers provide 5-part differentials (Table 2-16). In the usual report, the WBCs are sorted into neutrophils, lymphocytes, monocytes, eosinophils, and basophils. Any variant lymphocytes or other immature cells are

TABLE 2-17. Reference ranges for the red blood cell indices		
	REFERENCE RANGE	**INTERPRETATION**
MCV	80–98 fL	<80 fL = microcytic
		>98 fL = macrocytic
MCH	27–32 pg	
MCHC	32%–37%	<32% = hypochromic

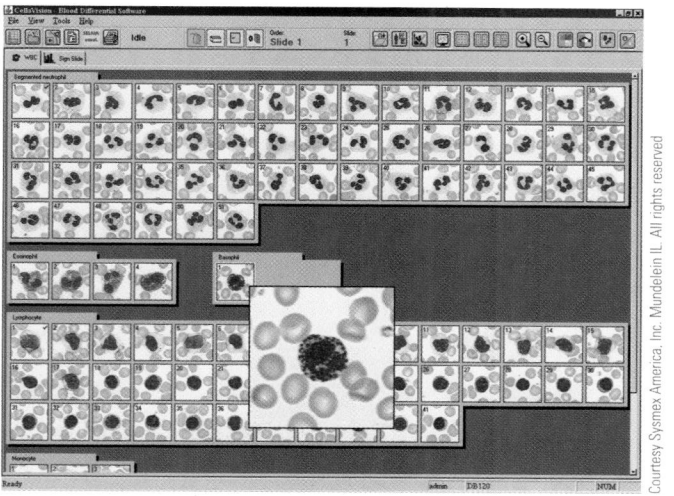

Courtesy Sysmex America, Inc. Mundelein IL. All rights reserved

FIGURE 2-71 Sysmex CellaVision DM96 screen showing image-recognition differential counting

included in an additional category called large unstained cells (LUCs). Instruments that perform a 5-part differential add chemicals or stains such as peroxidase and Alcian blue to the blood sample, subject the sample stream to a focused beam of light, and characterize each individual cell by its light-scatter pattern. The display of this information is called a cytogram or scattergram. The Sysmex XT2000i (Figure 2-66) and Technicon H series multichannel analyzers incorporate this technology.

Beckman Coulter has a variety of instruments that report a 5-part WBC differential. Their VCS (**V**olume, **C**onductivity and light **S**catter) technology allows the instrument to count and classify WBCs. These VCS modules are available on instruments such as the Coulter STKS, GEN-S, and MAXM. These instruments require as little as 100 μL of blood per sample and can process up to 75 samples per hour. The GEN-S system provides 33 the laboratory performing 100 to 1000 CBCs per day, parameters, including a 5-part differential and reticulocyte count. Abbott Diagnostics markets the Cell-Dyn series of analyzers that provide a 5-part differential using a system called multi-angle polarized light-scatter separation (MAPSS). Each cell is characterized by its light-scatter pattern measured from four specific angles.

IMAGE-PROCESSING INSTRUMENTS

Automated image-processing of differentials was first introduced in the 1980s. This technology was based on storing thousands of images of normal peripheral cells in the memory of the instrument's computer. The instrument scanned the blood smear and compared the cells in the smear with the images in its memory. The differential results were affected by some of the same disadvantages as the manual differential counting system—reliance on a well-made smear, good cell distribution, and proper staining technique. The early

CURRENT TOPICS

FLOW CYTOMETRY

Flow cytometers (*cyt* means cell, *meter* means measure) are analyzers used in both clinical and research applications. Flow cytometers combine the principles of light-scatter with light excitation and detection of the emission of **fluorescent** signals to classify and sort cells. Cells for flow cytometry analysis are stained with either a fluorescent dye or fluorescently labeled antibodies that can bind to specific cell surface markers. Clinical and research areas that use flow cytometry include:

- Hematology
- Immunology
- Urinalysis
- Tumor cell analysis
- Genetics
- Microbiology

In the flow cytometer, cells to be analyzed are hydrodynamically focused in a sheath of liquid. As cells approach the detector, they are focused into single file. This focused flow intercepts a laser light source that excites the fluorescent dye attached to the cells. A series of photodetectors collects the light emissions and converts the data to electrical signals. Flow cytometers can generate multiparameter data from particles and cells in the size range of 0.5 to 40 μm in diameter and can analyze up to 10,000 cells per second. A computer manages the data that are generated.

Cells for flow cytometry can be obtained from venipuncture, bone marrow aspirates, body fluids, or solid tissues such as tumors that have been disrupted to release the individual cells. One use of flow cytometry is to distinguish and quantitate subsets of lymphocytes. This is important in leukemias, lymphomas, human immunodeficiency virus (HIV) infections, and autoimmune diseases. The Beckman Coulter EPICS XL™ is a benchtop flow cytometer used in clinical and research laboratories. The Beckman-Coulter MoFlo XDP is a high-speed cell sorter for use in research.

instruments were almost too sensitive. Even though they could match a human technologist in cell recognition, they lacked the ability to correlate an abnormality in a particular cell with the morphology of the majority of a cell population. Therefore every abnormal cell had to be reviewed by a technologist.

Much-improved image-processing instruments are now available. Sysmex markets the CellaVision DM96 and the

DM1200, which display on a screen the cells that require reviewing so the technician does not have to find the particular smear and examine it microscopically (Figure 2-71). These instruments perform a preliminary differential on blood or body fluids, including preclassification of WBCs, preclassification of RBC morphology, and estimate of platelet numbers. The hematology technologist reviews and confirms the findings before the report is issued.

SAFETY PRECAUTIONS

   Automation substantially increases accuracy and reduces the time required to complete hematology testing. However, the use of instruments poses physical, chemical, and biological hazards. Standard Precautions must be followed and personal protective equipment (PPE) worn when using these instruments and performing maintenance and repairs, because the internal parts of the instrument can become contaminated with blood. Preparation of the blood sample for analysis and use of hematology controls and calibrators potentially expose technicians to bloodborne pathogens. Instruments with a through-the-cap sampler and that produce an automated differential greatly reduce this risk.

Safety rules to guard against physical and chemical hazards must be followed. Appropriate PPE must be worn and work practice controls used to prevent exposure to some of the chemicals used in the instruments. The material safety data sheets (MSDS) accompanying chemicals and reagents being used must be read and understood.

Routine maintenance or repair of an instrument can present hazards. Some instruments automatically perform routine maintenance procedures, but if the technician must do the procedures, the manufacturer's instructions must be closely followed. Removal of the outside instrument case and instrument repair should be performed only by qualified, trained personnel.

QUALITY ASSESSMENT

 Each laboratory will have a standard operating procedure (SOP) manual containing detailed instructions for the operation of hematology analyzers and the quality control measures that are required. Instrument manufacturers have responded the needs of laboratories for better quality assessment by designing instruments that can help the laboratory detect quality control (QC) problems, correct failures, and store and retrieve QC data. Subscription to a proficiency testing (PT) program is required; the PT test results allow a laboratory's performance to be compared to the performance of similar laboratories.

Many instruments record patient I.D. from bar codes on the sample tube, helping to reduce transcription errors. Some instruments can store up to 10,000 patient records at a time. A technologist can access a screen and compare a patient's results on one day with those from another day.

Manufacturers provide calibrators, controls, and specify the frequency of use. Some instruments also prepare Levey-Jennings charts for each run of control samples. In addition, as each control sample is run, any value not within the QC limits of the facility is flagged. The Levey-Jennings screen can be accessed and the results printed to see if a trend or shift might be developing. An inexpensive method of QC involves choosing 5 to 10 patient samples from a day's workload that have results within the reference ranges and reanalyzing them the next day on the same instrument. Statistical methods can then be used to determine if there is a significant change between the two sets of values.

 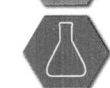

SAFETY REMINDERS

- Review Safety Precautions section before using an analyzer.
- Observe Standard Precautions.
- Wear appropriate PPE.
- Observe electrical safety when operating analyzers.
- Observe chemical safety when handling reagents.

PROCEDURAL REMINDERS

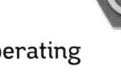

- Review Quality Assessment section before using an analyzer.
- Follow facility SOP manual when operating analyzers.
- Review control results to verify instrument performance.

CASE STUDY

Cheryl works the evening shift in an urgent care clinic. The first patient of the evening is a patient with a fever. Dr. McCloud ordered a WBC count and differential. The hematology analyzer in the clinic is one that performs cell counts and 3-part differentials. Cheryl collected the blood, but when she tried to use the analyzer, it malfunctioned, displaying the "Error 9!" message. When Cheryl consulted the instrument's operating manual to find the corrective action, she found that the Error 9 message indicated that the services of a certified repair technician were required.

1. Cheryl should:
   a. Tell the physician that it is impossible to perform the test
   b. Perform a manual WBC count and differential
   c. Tell the physician the test will be done after the instrument is repaired
   d. Send the test to a reference laboratory the next day
   e. Attempt to repair the analyzer because the test results are needed
2. Explain your answer.

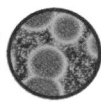

SUMMARY

The advent of the Coulter electrical-impedance counting technology revolutionized cell counting. For the first time it was possible to automate the process of cell counting which improved accuracy and precision of cell counts. Automated counts have a CV of ±1% to ±2% compared with ±10% for manual counts.

As cell counting technology advanced, analyzers and cell counters became more sophisticated. One improvement in cell-counting technology was to channel the flow through the aperture and edit the signals. Another improvement was sheath-flow, which reduced the need for frequent cleaning and maintenance of the aperture. Light-scatter technology was also introduced for cell counting. Today's instruments can perform cell counts, WBC differentials, reticulocyte counts, RBC indices, and several other parameters both directly measured and calculated. Flow cytometry has increased the ability of the laboratory to classify and sort cells into categories.

Hematology analyzers have simplified and somewhat reduced the hematology workload. At the same time, they have increased the laboratory's capacity and ability to perform a variety of hematology tests. When a laboratory maintains a good QC and quality assessment program and participates in a certified PT program, the physician can have confidence in the results.

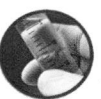

REVIEW QUESTIONS

1. Describe the history of blood cell counting.
2. Name two types of technology used to count blood cells and give an example of an instrument or analyzer that uses each type of technology.
3. How does the coefficient of variation for manual blood cell counts compare with that for automated counts?
4. Calculate the MCV for a blood sample with Hgb = 11 g/dL, Hct = 30%, and RBC = $3.8 \times 10^6/\mu L$. Classify the cells.
5. Discuss the importance of quality assessment and QC for automated instruments.
6. What is the difference between the technologies used in analyzers that perform 3-part differentials and those that perform 5-part differentials?
7. Explain the information illustrated by a histogram.
8. What is the importance of the RDW?
9. Define aperture, electrolyte solution, femtoliter, fluorescent, histogram, impedance, index of refraction, laser, mean cell hemoglobin (MCH), mean cell hemoglobin concentration (MCHC), mean cell volume (MCV), picogram, and RBC indices.

STUDENT ACTIVITIES

1. Complete the written examination for this lesson.
2. Interview a hematology laboratory employee and report on the types of hematology testing performed there. Ask for a copy of their CBC report form and list the parameters reported.
3. Practice calculating the red blood cell indices using the worksheet.
4. If a hematology cell counter is available, perform an automated CBC using a venous EDTA blood specimen provided by your instructor. Record your results on the CBC report form, page 123.

WEB ACTIVITY

Search the Internet for operating manuals or brochures describing two hematology analyzers that include automated differential counting. Report on the test capacity for each instrument. Estimate the time required to manually complete 50 CBCs with differential counts; compare this with the time required to complete 50 CBCs and differential counts using a hematology analyzer.

LESSON 2-10
Principles of Automated Hematology

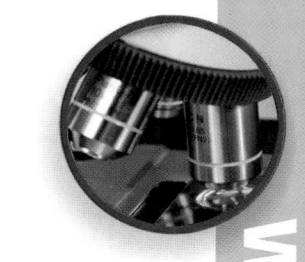

(Answers will vary based on the instruments available and blood specimens provided by the instructor.)

Name _____ Date _____

Specimen I.D. _____

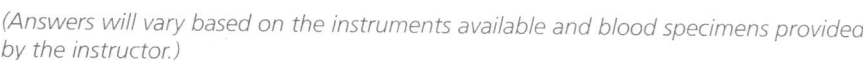

Calculating Red Blood Cell Indices

I. Depending on resources available, follow instructions in section A, B, or C to calculate the red blood cell indices.

A. If a hematology cell counter or analyzer is available, complete sections II and III. Determine the Hgb, Hct, and RBC count on a blood specimen and record the calculated indices. Then use the Hgb, Hct, and RBC values and the indices formulas to calculate your own set of indices. Compare your results with the calculated indices values.

B. If a cell counter is not available, complete sections II and III. Determine the Hgb, Hct, and RBC counts on a blood sample using available methods and calculate the indices.

C. Obtain Hbg, Hct, and RBC values from your instructor and calculate the indices, completing sections II and III.

II. Record values:

Hgb = _____ g/dL Hct = _____% RBC count = _____/μL

III. Calculate Indices:

1. Write the formula for the MCV: _____
    Calculate the MCV:

2. Write the formula for the MCH: _____
    Calculate the MCH:

3. Write the formula for the MCHC:_____
    Calculate the MCHC:

4. Compare your calculated indices values with the reference ranges in Table 2-17. Do the values fall within the reference ranges?_____

5. Compare your calculated indices values with the indices calculated by the cell counter. Do your values agree? _____

6. Classify the red blood cells according to hemoglobin content and cell size:

    a. The red blood cells are (circle one): normochromic / hypochromic
        Which one of the RBC indices did you use to classify hemoglobin content? _____

    b. The red blood cells are (circle one): normocytic / microcytic / macrocytic
        Which one of the RBC indices was used to classify cell size? _____

© 2012 Delmar, Cengage Learning. Permission to reproduce for clinical use granted.

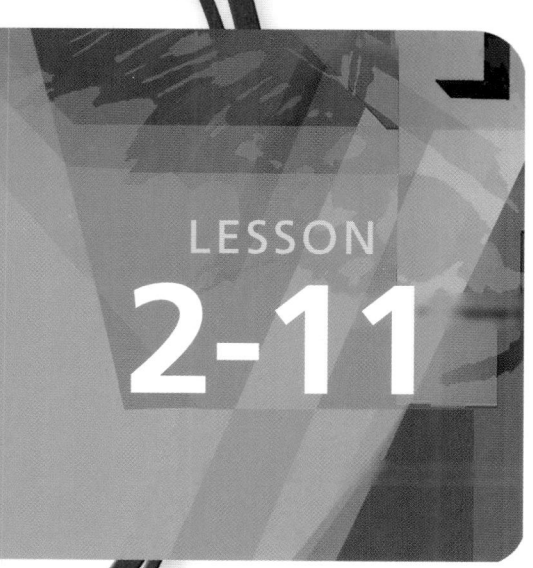

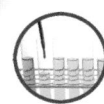

LESSON OBJECTIVES

After studying this lesson, the student will:

- State the importance of differentiating between normal and abnormal blood cells on a peripheral blood smear.
- List two conditions in which red blood cell anisocytosis is found.
- List two conditions in which red blood cell poikilocytosis is found.
- List two conditions in which red blood cell hypochromia can be found.
- Discuss the relationship of the red blood cell indices to red blood cell morphology.
- Discuss the significance of RBC inclusions.
- List two causes of leukopenia.
- List two causes of leukocytosis.
- Discuss neutrophilia and a shift to the left.
- Discuss the characteristics of leukemias.
- List conditions in which abnormal thrombocytes can be found.
- List safety precautions to be observed when examining a blood smear.
- Discuss the importance of quality assessment when examining blood smears that contain abnormal cells.
- Define the glossary terms.

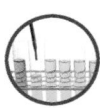

GLOSSARY

basophilia / abnormal increase in the number of basophils in the blood; basophilic leukocytosis; also, the affinity of cellular structures for basophilic dyes

basophilic stippling / remnants of RNA and other basophilic nuclear material remaining inside the red blood cell after the nucleus is lost from the cell; small purple granules in red blood cells stained with Wright's stain

blast cell / an immature blood cell normally found only in the bone marrow

codocyte / target cell

crenated cell / a shrunken red blood cell with scalloped or toothed margins

drepanocyte / sickle cell

elliptocyte / elongated, cigar-shaped red blood cell

eosinophilia / abnormal increase in the number of eosinophils in the blood

folic acid / a member of the B vitamin complex

(continues)

Howell-Jolly body / nuclear remnant remaining in red blood cells after the nucleus is lost and commonly seen in pernicious anemia and hemolytic anemias

keratocyte / a red blood cell deformed by mechanical trauma

leukemia / a cancer of white blood cells characterized by an abnormal increase of white blood cells and their precursors in bone marrow, tissue, and peripheral blood

neutrophilia / abnormal increase in the number of neutrophils in the blood

nucleated red blood cell (NRBC) / an immature red blood cell that has not yet lost its nucleus

red blood cell indices / calculated values that compare the size and hemoglobin content of red blood cells in a blood sample to reference values; erythrocyte indices

schizocyte / a fragmented red blood cell; formerly called schistocyte

shift to the left / the appearance of an increased number of immature neutrophil forms in the peripheral blood

sickle cell / crescent- or sickle-shaped red cell; drepanocyte

sickle cell disease / inherited blood disorder in which red blood cells can form a sickle shape because of the presence of hemoglobin S

stomatocyte / red blood cell with an elongated, mouth-shaped central area of pallor

target cell / abnormal red blood cell with target appearance; codocyte

thalassemia / a genetic disorder involving underproduction of the globin chains of hemoglobin and resulting in anemia

vitamin B$_{12}$ / a vitamin essential to the proper maturation of blood cells and other cells in the body

INTRODUCTION

The information gained from a complete blood count (CBC) with differential count can be valuable to the physician. The presence of abnormal red blood cells (RBCs) or white blood cells (WBCs) observed while performing a differential count can be a clue that disease or an abnormal condition is present.

Occasional abnormal RBCs and WBCs can be observed on a peripheral blood smear that is otherwise normal. This might be as simple as finding a few hypochromic red cells in the smear of a patient with mild iron deficiency anemia or observing a small number of atypical lymphocytes associated with a viral infection. Other times examination of a smear expected to be normal can yield unexpected results, such as the presence of immature WBCs. These abnormal cells could be few in number and might be recognized only by an experienced technologist, or they could be numerous but difficult to classify because of unusual characteristics in morphology.

Some conditions and diseases present very characteristic cellular changes in blood cells that can be observed on a Wright's-stained smear. Conditions such as iron deficiency anemia, **folic acid** deficiency, **vitamin B$_{12}$** deficiency, and **sickle cell disease** each produce characteristic changes in the red cell morphology. Abnormalities in the WBC count, percentages of WBCs, and WBC morphology can result from conditions such as viral or bacterial infections, hematological conditions and diseases, allergic reactions, stress, or recent exercise. Conditions such as exposure to radiation or chemotherapeutic drugs and diseases such as leukemia also cause abnormalities in platelet numbers and morphology.

Evaluation of RBC and WBC morphology is an important part of the WBC differential count. Becoming proficient in identifying abnormal cells comes only after much practice in identifying normal cells.

SAFETY PRECAUTIONS

   Standard Precautions must be observed and appropriate PPE must be worn during the preparation and staining of blood smears. Chemical and physical hazards are present when using stains, handling glass slides, and operating electrical equipment. The methanol used in the staining process is toxic; splashes onto the skin or into the eyes must be avoided. Glass slides should be handled carefully to avoid cuts. The microscope cord and plug should be inspected for damage before the microscope is connected to the power source.

QUALITY ASSESSMENT

 Personnel who perform and report WBC differential counts and evaluate WBC, RBC and platelet morphology must follow the policy contained in the facility's SOP manual. This will describe the area of the slide to be examined, the pattern of counting, and a standardized method of grading any abnormal morphology that is observed. The quality of the smear, the staining technique, and the method of examining the smear influence the quality of the results.

Technologists performing differential counts must be experienced and conscientious. A more experienced worker, laboratory supervisor, or pathologist must be consulted if any questions regarding cell identification arise.

ABNORMAL RED BLOOD CELL MORPHOLOGY

Disorders that affect the RBCs can cause variations in cell shape, variations in cell size, and hemoglobin content or RBC counts outside of the normal reference ranges.

Anisocytosis

RBCs of normal size, 6 to 8 μm in diameter, are said to be *normocytic*. RBCs that are smaller than 6 μm are *microcytic*; those that are larger than normal are *macrocytes*. *Anisocytosis* is the presence of varying sizes of red blood cells in a cell population. The mean cell volume (MCV) and the red cell distribution width (RDW) are calculated values that can be used to classify cells as normocytic, microcytic, or macrocytic (Table 2-18).

TABLE 2-18. Reference ranges for the red blood cell indices

	REFERENCE RANGE	INTERPRETATION
MCV	80–98 fL	<80 fL = microcytic
		>98 fL = macrocytic
MCH	27–32 pg	
MCHC	32%–37%	<32% = hypochromic

Patients with conditions such as iron deficiency anemia and inherited conditions such as **thalassemia** have microcytic RBCs. Thalassemias are caused by defects in the synthesis of the globin portion of the hemoglobin molecule. Iron deficiency anemia can be due to conditions such as inadequate intake of dietary iron, chronic blood loss, or an increased iron demand, such as that seen in pregnancy.

RBCs with a diameter greater than 8 μm are macrocytes, also called *megalocytes*. Macrocytes are produced in conditions such as deficiencies of vitamin B$_{12}$ or folic acid (folate) and in liver disease. Deficiency of folic acid or vitamin B$_{12}$ prevents proper maturation of blood cells in the bone marrow, causing the cells to remain larger than normal. Vitamin B$_{12}$ deficiency was formerly known as pernicious anemia because it was fatal until its cause was discovered in the mid-1950s.

Poikilocytosis

Poikilocytosis, variation in the shape of RBCs, can be inherited (have a genetic cause) or acquired

Sickle Cells: Drepanocytes

Sickle cell disease is an inherited condition in which Hb S causes the RBCs to have a characteristic *sickle* shape when oxygen levels are decreased (Figures 2-72B and 2-73A). Another name for a **sickle cell** is a **drepanocyte**. Because of their abnormal shape, sickle cells block blood flow in smaller vessels, cutting off oxygen to tissues in that area. The lowered oxygen level then causes more RBCs to change to the sickle shape. This can lead to a sickle cell

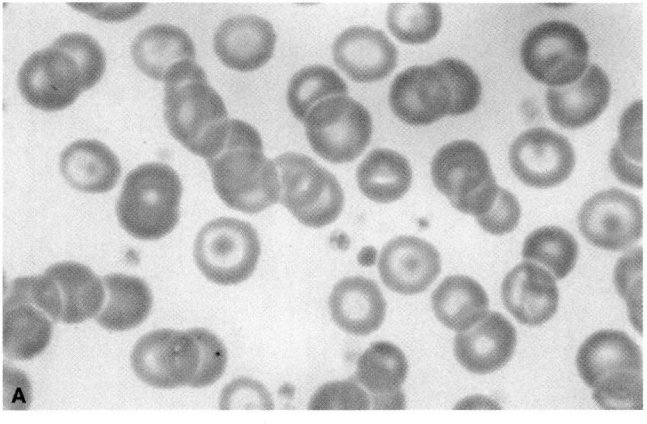
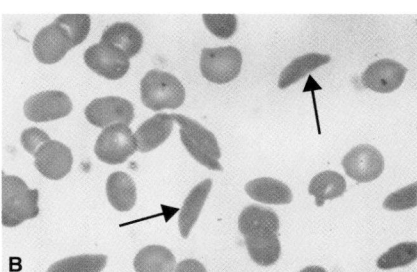
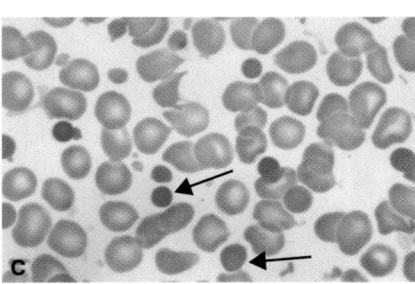
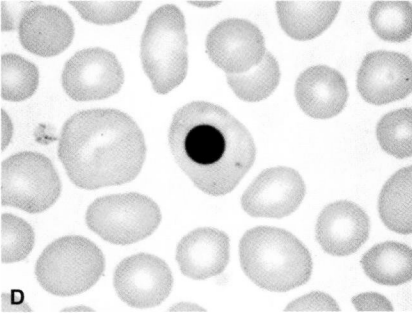

© Cengage Learning 2012

FIGURE 2-72 Abnormal red blood cell morphology: (A) target cells and hypochromic microcytes; (B) sickle-shaped cells in smear from patient with sickle cell anemia; (C) spherocytes and schizocytes in smear from burn patient; and (D) nucleated red blood cell

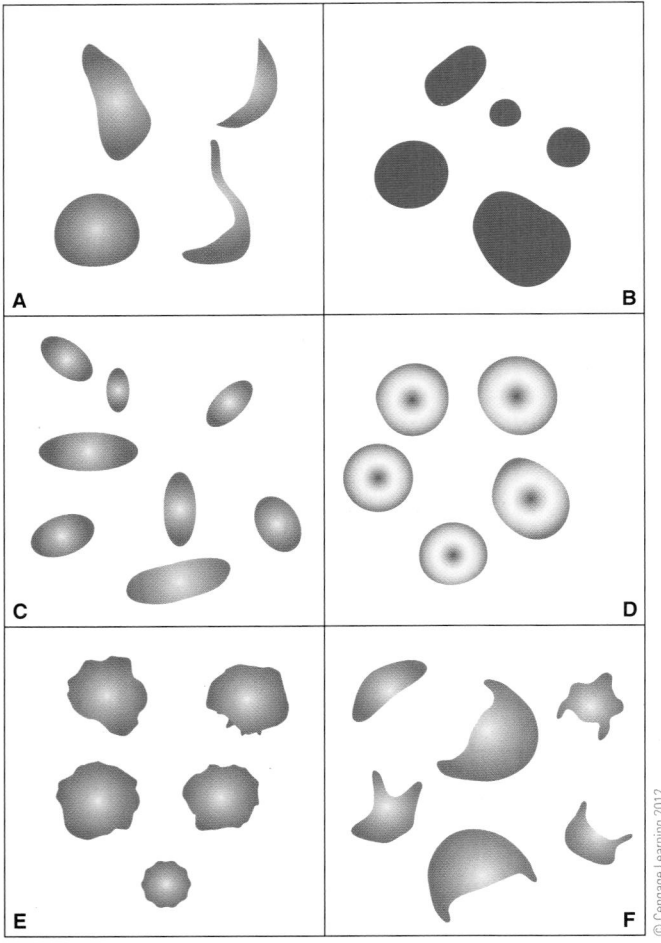

© Cengage Learning 2012

FIGURE 2-73 Morphology of selected abnormal red blood cells: (A) drepanocytes (sickle cells); (B) spherocytes; (C) elliptocytes; (D) codocytes (target cells); (E) crenated cells; and (F) keratocytes including helmet cells

Target Cells: Codocytes

Target cells are red blood cells that resemble a bull's eye target; they are also known as **codocytes**. Target cells can be seen in thalassemia, sickle cell disease, and other hemoglobin abnormalities (Figures 2-72A and 2-73D).

Keratocytes: Schizocytes

Fragmented RBCs are called either **keratocytes** or **schizocytes**. The keratocytes are RBCs that have been deformed by some mechanical trauma, such as passing through an artificial heart valve or being cut by a fibrin strand in a blood clot (Figures 2-72C and 2-73F). When cells are actually sheared into fragments, as can happen in patients with severe burns, they are called schizocytes.

Crenated Cells

Crenated RBCs have bumpy or spiny projections on the cell surface (Figure 2-73E). Crenated cells occur after prolonged exposure of the blood sample to anticoagulant or incorrect blood-to-anticoagulant ratio in the collection tube. These cells do not indicate a pathological condition. When using anticoagulated blood, it is important to make blood smears within 2 hours of blood collection to prevent alterations in blood cell morphology.

Variations in Hemoglobin Content

RBCs containing the correct amount of hemoglobin for their size are *normochromic*. A deficiency of hemoglobin resulting from lack of iron or another condition causes the RBCs to have a large central area of pallor with only a small outer rim of hemoglobin; these cells are *hypochromic* (Figure 2-74A). RBCs that appear to be completely filled with hemoglobin (have no central area of pallor) are called *hyperchromic*. The mean cell hemoglobin concentration (MCHC) is a calculated value that can be used to classify cells as normochromic or hypochromic (Table 2-18).

Red Blood Cell Inclusions

Red blood cell inclusions can indicate particular pathological conditions, such as toxic conditions, hemolytic anemias, or certain vitamin deficiencies.

Basophilic Stippling

Basophilic stippling is caused by the fine granular remnants of RNA and other basophilic substances remaining in the RBC after it loses its nucleus (Figure 2-74C). On a Wright's-stained smear, the RNA remnants cause cells to have a diffuse blue color (diffuse basophilia), orange and blue mottled appearance (polychromatophilia), or punctate fine and coarse granules (basophilic stippling). These RBCs are called reticulocytes when stained with a supravital stain such as new methylene blue stain (Lesson 2-12).

An occasional stippled cell or diffusely basophilic cell is normal. An increased number of stippled cells in the peripheral blood smear can indicate certain toxic conditions such as lead poisoning. An increase in stippled cells can also be seen

crisis, a serious and painful event for the patient because of damage to vital organs.

Spherocytes

Spherocytes are RBCs that are spherical instead of the normal biconcave shape (Figures 2-72C and 2-73B). Anemia develops because the spleen recognizes these cells as abnormal and destroys them prematurely.

Elliptocytes

Elliptocytes are elongated, cigar-shaped RBCs (Figure 2-73C). In hereditary elliptocytosis, the patient has large numbers of these abnormal cells. Anemia develops because the spleen destroys these RBCs and only a small number of normal RBCs remain.

Stomatocytes

RBCs with a linear area of pallor are called **stomatocytes** because the pale area is shaped like a mouth. These cells occur in the condition known as hereditary stomatocytosis.

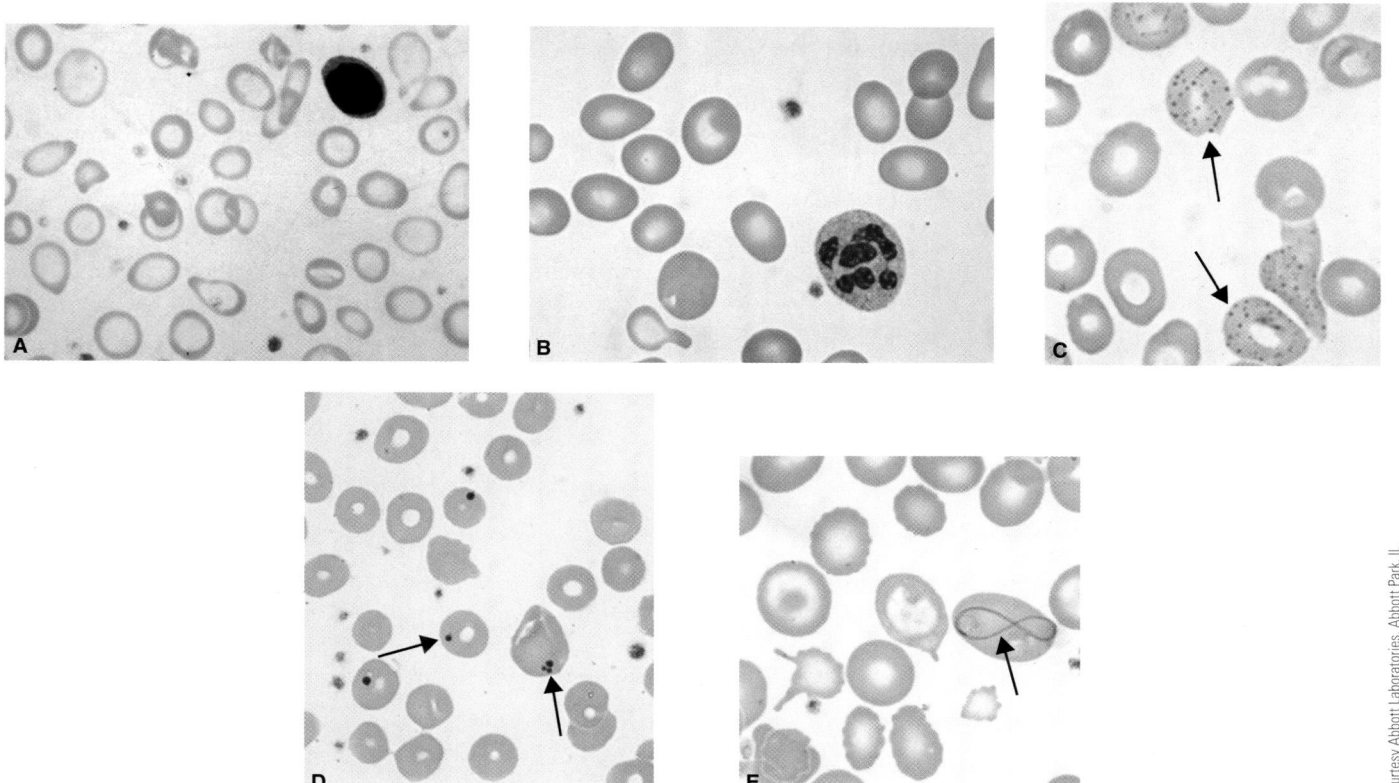

Courtesy Abbott Laboratories. Abbott Park. IL.

FIGURE 2-74 Photomicrographs of abnormal red blood cell morphology: (A) iron deficiency (microcytic) anemia; (B) megaloblastic anemia; (C) stippled cells; (D) Howell-Jolly bodies; and (E) Cabot ring

in response to increased RBC production resulting from acute hemorrhage or after treatment for iron, vitamin B_{12}, or folate deficiency.

Howell-Jolly Bodies

Howell-Jolly bodies are DNA remnants remaining in the RBC after the nucleus is lost. They appear on Wright's-stained smears as intense dark blue-purple bodies inside the cell and are common in pernicious anemia and hemolytic anemias (Figure 2-74D).

Cabot Rings

Cabot rings are found in RBCs in certain anemias and in lead poisoning. They appear as thin, dark blue-purple ring-like structures (Figure 2-74E).

Nucleated Red Blood Cells

Nucleated red blood cells (NRBCs), normally found only in bone marrow, can be seen in peripheral blood in severe anemia. The *metarubricyte* is the form most commonly seen (Figure 2-72D). Nucleated red blood cells are also present in small numbers in the peripheral blood of normal newborns.

Red Blood Cell Indices

The **red blood cell indices** are calculations that estimate the mean cell volume (MCV), mean cell hemoglobin (MCH), and mean cell hemoglobin concentration (MCHC). These calculations use the RBC count, hemoglobin, and hematocrit to define average cell size and concentration of hemoglobin within a population of red cells. Therefore the validity of the indices is dependent on the accuracy of the RBC count and the hemoglobin and hematocrit determinations. Laboratories with hematology analyzers rely on automation to calculate the indices. The formulas for arithmetically calculating the red cell indices are explained in Lesson 2-10.

Some information about RBC size and hemoglobin content can be obtained from microscopic examination of the stained smear. However, the RBC indices provide a quantitative measurement of average red cell volume and hemoglobin concentration that can be compared to normal reference values (Table 2-18). The two most useful indices are the MCV and the MCHC. RBCs can be classified as normocytic, microcytic, or macrocytic using the MCV. RBCs can be classified as normochromic or hypochromic using the MCHC value.

WHITE BLOOD CELL DISORDERS

Diseases or conditions affecting WBCs can be detected by finding abnormal WBCs on the peripheral blood smear or from the total WBC count (Table 2-19). A WBC count increased above the normal range is called *leukocytosis*; a count below the normal range is called *leukopenia*. The total WBC count and the types of cells present are often characteristic for a particular condition.

TABLE 2-19. Conditions that affect white blood cell counts and percentages

CONDITION	EFFECT ON WBC COUNTS
Bacterial infections	Increased total WBCs, increased percentage of neutrophils
Viral infections	Decreased total WBCs, increased percentage of lymphocytes
Infectious mononucleosis	Increased total WBCs, increased lymphocytes, increased atypical lymphocytes
Parasitic infections, allergic reactions	Increased eosinophils
Leukemias	WBC count usually increased, increase in one type of leukocyte

Leukopenia

Leukopenia occurs when the WBC count falls below the lower limit of the WBC reference range. A reduction in all WBC types is called *balanced leukopenia*; however, in most cases, only one WBC type is decreased.

Neutropenia, a reduced number of neutrophils, can be inherited or caused by certain infections, antibiotics, sulfa drugs, and chemotherapy treatments. *Lymphopenia*, a reduced number of lymphocytes, can be caused by exposure to radiation, steroid administration, and certain inherited or acquired immune disorders.

Leukocytosis

Several factors can cause an increase in circulating WBCs (leukocytosis). Bacterial infections, exercise, anxiety, or pain usually cause leukocytosis and neutrophilia. A *leukemoid reaction* is a transient excessive response in which the WBC count can reach 50×10^9/L or higher. The reason for the heightened response is infection or other condition, and the leukemoid reaction must be differentiated from leukemia, a malignancy. In leukemias, the total WBC count is increased, as well as an increase in the absolute count of one cell line, such as lymphocytes or granulocytes.

Neutrophilia

Neutrophilia is a type of leukocytosis that involves an abnormal increase in the number of the neutrophils. Bacterial infection is the most common cause of neutrophilia (Table 2-19). In acute infections, neutrophilia is accompanied by an increase in immature neutrophils in the peripheral blood. This is called a **shift to the left**, in which immature forms known as bands, *metamyelocytes* (juveniles), or *myelocytes* enter the peripheral blood prematurely to help fight the infection. In normal adult peripheral blood the presence of 1 to 5 band cells is normal; no metamyelocytes of myelocytes should be present (Table 2-20). In mild infections, usually only the neutrophils and band cells are increased. In more severe infections, the WBC count and the neutrophil count can increase, or more bands and metamyelocytes can appear in the peripheral blood. *Vacuoles* present in the cytoplasm of neutrophils can indicate a serious infection.

Eosinophilia

Eosinophilia is an abnormal increase in the percentage of eosinophils in the peripheral blood. Eosinophils increase in allergic conditions, parasitic infections, and certain skin diseases.

Basophilia

The number of basophils in the peripheral blood is usually constant and is not affected by physiological factors such as exercise or time of day. **Basophilia**, also called basophilic leukocytosis, is an abnormal increase in the number of basophils. It is usually associated with an increase in the other granulocytes and can be caused by conditions such as ulcerative colitis, chronic sinusitis, and viral infections such as smallpox and chickenpox. Increases in basophils are also seen in *chronic myelogenous leukemia* and *polycythemia vera*.

TABLE 2-20. Reference ranges for the white blood cell differential count and absolute white blood cell counts

CELL	DIFFERENTIAL COUNT REFERENCE VALUES BY PERCENTAGE (%)				ABSOLUTE COUNT REFERENCE VALUES (CELLS/µL)
	1-MONTH-OLD	6-YEAR-OLD	12-YEAR-OLD	ADULT	ADULT
Neutrophil (seg)	15–35	45–50	45–50	50–65	2,250–7,150
Neutrophil (band)	7–13	0–7	6–8	0–7	0–770
Eosinophil	1–3	1–3	1–3	1–3	45–330
Basophil	0–1	0–1	0–1	0–1	0–110
Monocyte	5–8	4–8	3–8	3–9	135–990
Lymphocyte	40–70	40–45	35–40	25–40	1,125–4,400
Platelets	An average of 7–20/oil immersion field is considered normal				

Monocytosis

Monocytosis, an increase in circulating monocytes, is rare but can occur in tuberculosis, subacute bacterial endocarditis, typhus, and rickettsial infections.

Lymphocytosis

The lymphocyte percentage is normally higher in infants and young children than in adults. In adolescents and adults, lymphocytosis can be due to acute viral infection, especially infectious mononucleosis. The predominant cell in infectious mononucleosis is the *atypical lymphocyte*, also called a reactive or variant lymphocyte. Most atypical lymphocytes are characterized by a large nucleus and large amount of intense blue cytoplasm easily indented by RBCs; the indentations can cause the lymphocytes to assume a holly-leaf shape (Figure 2-75).

Leukemias

Leukemias are distinguished by unrestrained production of leukocytes in the bone marrow, causing the production of red cells and platelets to be literally "crowded out" by the leukemic WBCs.

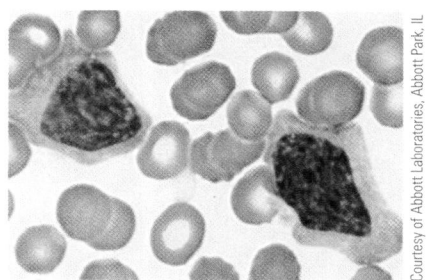

FIGURE 2-75 Photomicrograph showing two atypical lymphocytes

Usually the platelet count is decreased and anemia develops because leukemic cells inhibit the production of other cells in the bone marrow.

In acute leukemias, immature blood cells called **blast cells** and other immature forms of WBCs are the predominant cells in the peripheral circulation (Figures 2-76 and 2-77D).

CURRENT TOPICS

CHARACTERISTICS OF LEUKEMIAS

In earlier times leukemia was known as *blood cancer* or a condition in which the WBCs were crowding out the RBCs. Today leukemia, a type of cancer, is defined as an acute or chronic disease characterized by unrestrained growth of the WBCs and their precursors; the cause of the leukemia is often unknown.

Many of the symptoms of leukemia are related to the inability of the bone marrow to produce normal numbers of RBCs and platelets because of the large numbers of WBCs in the bone marrow. As a result, the patient develops anemia, fatigue, increased infections, and bleeding problems. In addition, the leukemic WBCs infiltrate the liver, spleen, lymph nodes, and nervous system, disrupting the normal functions of these organs. Blood flow in the smaller vessels such as capillaries can be slowed or blocked because of the large numbers of WBCs.

Classification of Leukemias

The leukemias are classified according to the severity of the disease and the dominant cell involved. *Chronic* leukemias worsen slowly. The total numbers of abnormal WBCs are relatively small, the abnormal cells can still function to some extent, and the bone marrow is not affected to a large degree.

Acute leukemias worsen rapidly and are characterized by abnormal immature cells that cannot carry out normal immune functions. Leukemias are further classified by the type of WBCs affected. Leukemia can arise from the *myeloid* line or the *lymphoid* line. Leukemia that arises from the myeloid cells is called *myelogenous*; when it arises from the lymphoid line it is called *lymphocytic*.

The four common types of leukemia are:

- *Chronic lymphocytic leukemia* (CLL): This type of leukemia primarily affects older adults, almost never affects children, and accounts for about 7,000 new cases each year.
- *Chronic myeloid leukemia* (CML): Also called chronic granulocytic leukemia, this type accounts for about 4,400 new cases each year and affects mainly adults.
- *Acute lymphocytic leukemia* (ALL): ALL is the most common leukemia in young children and accounts for about 3,800 new cases each year. Adults can also have ALL.
- *Acute myeloid leukemia* (AML): Also called acute nonlymphocytic leukemia, AML accounts for about 10,000 to 12,000 new cases each year and affects both children and adults. Other rarer types

(Continues)

CURRENT TOPICS (Continued)

of leukemia account for approximately 5,200 additional new cases each year.

Some causes of leukemia are known, such as the exposure to ionizing radiation that caused leukemia in many Japanese exposed to atomic bomb fallout at the end of World War II. Heredity has also been shown to play a part in developing leukemia; the siblings and twins of patients with leukemia have a greater chance of developing leukemia than the general population. However, other possible causes of leukemia have yet to be proven. Factors that have been identified as possible causes of leukemia include:

- Therapeutic radiation for treatment of another type of cancer
- Exposure to chemicals such as benzene or formaldehyde
- Drugs such as chloramphenicol, phenylbutazone, and certain chemotherapy agents
- Viruses, especially retroviruses

Treatment

New treatments for leukemia are constantly being developed. What works for one type of leukemia or one patient may not work for another. Treatment consists of four basic types:

- Chemotherapy is a mainstay of leukemia treatment. Chemotherapy agents kill leukemic cells but also damage or kill normal cells. Improvements in chemotherapy include *targeted therapy*, in which drugs target only the leukemic cells.
- Radiation therapy uses high-energy radiation directed at specific organs such as the spleen or brain to kill leukemic cells.

- Biological therapy is one of the newer forms of treatment in which monoclonal antibodies or interferon is used. Monoclonal antibodies are used against the abnormal cells in CLL; interferon has been found to be an effective treatment in CML.
- Stem cell transplants have been used for several years and have several variations. The patient is treated with high doses of drugs or radiation (or both), resulting in the destruction of both leukemic cells and normal cells in the bone marrow. The patient then receives a stem cell transplant from which new blood cells can develop. These stem cells can come from bone marrow transplantation, peripheral stem cell transplantation, or umbilical cord blood transplantation. Of the three, the public is probably most familiar with bone marrow transplants. The donated marrow usually comes from a donor whose tissue has been matched to the patient by tissue typing. In other cases, the patient's own blood cells can be harvested before the patient is subjected to whole body radiation. These harvested cells are treated to kill the leukemic cells, then frozen and stored until transfused back into the patient after radiation or chemotherapy is completed.

Although leukemia continues to cause many deaths each year, much progress has been made in the diagnosis, classification, and treatment of the disease. The hope is that, once specific causes are identified, new and improved treatments will result in leukemia becoming another curable disease.

Blast cells are the earliest identifiable blood cell precursors and are normally found only in the bone marrow. The total WBC count is usually, but not always, elevated in acute leukemia. Chronic leukemias are characterized by leukocytosis and can have WBC counts of 50,000 per microliter or greater. In the peripheral circulation, the predominant cells are mature cells along with some immature forms of the same cell type as well as some blast cells.

Diagnosing leukemias is a task for pathologists and hematology specialists. However, many cases are first noticed by a technologist performing a differential or because a hematology analyzer flags a sample as abnormal. It is critical for the

technologist to carefully perform every differential and to closely examine all the characteristics of any cells that appear unusual. Sometimes it is necessary to count 200 to 500 leukocytes to find more of the abnormal cells.

PLATELET DISORDERS

Platelets can be abnormal in number or in function. In *thrombocytopenia*, platelet numbers fall below the reference range. Many factors can cause decreased platelets, including radiation exposure, certain drugs, chronic alcoholism, destruction or

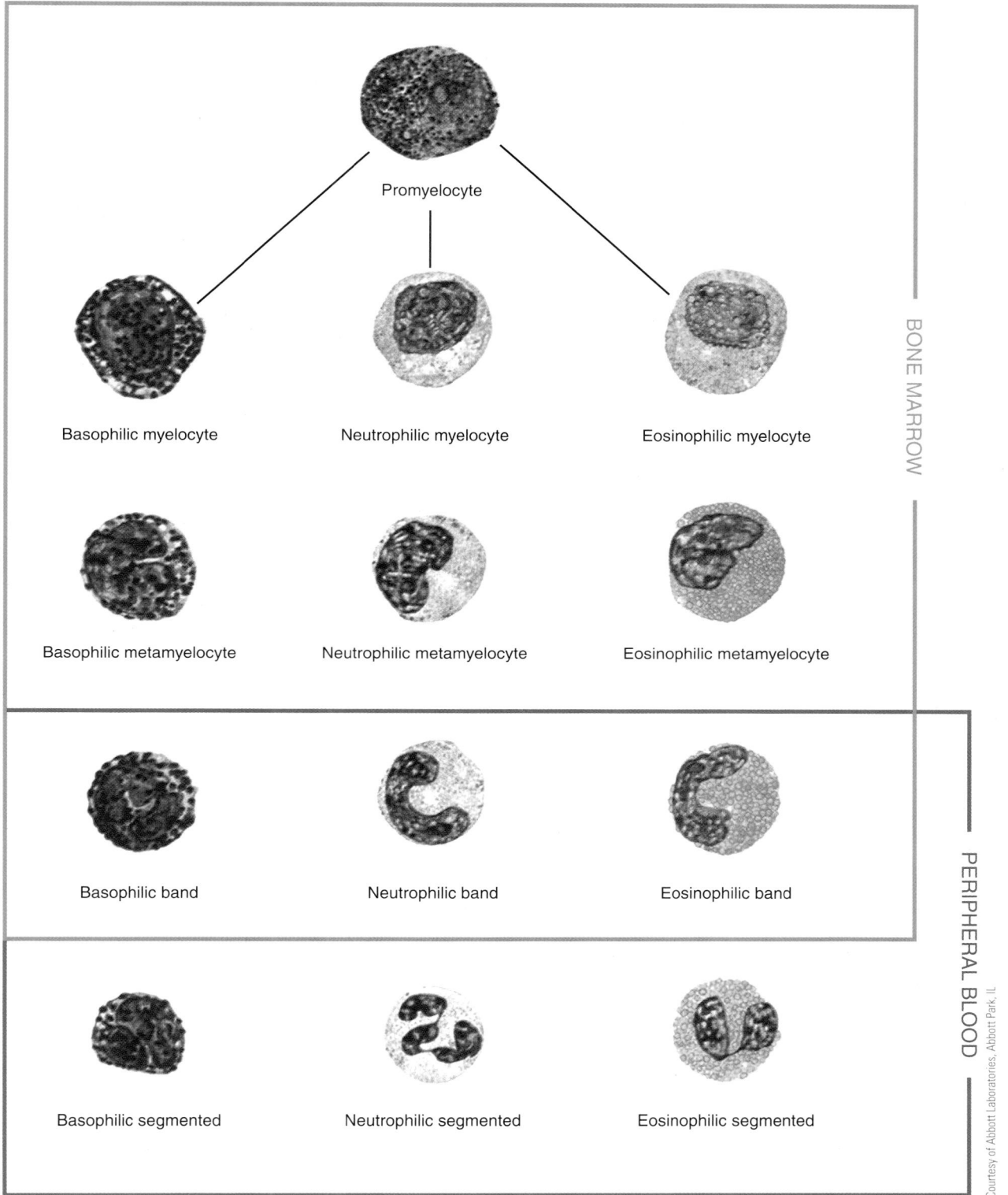

FIGURE 2-76 Origin and development of the granulocytic (myeloid) blood cells

sequestration by the spleen, and the effect of diseases such as leukemia on bone marrow.

Elevation of platelet numbers above the reference range is called *thrombocytosis*. Some causes of thrombocytosis include a reaction to inflammatory conditions, a secondary reaction to other blood disorders, and removal of the spleen. Platelet disorders are discussed in more depth in Lesson 3-2.

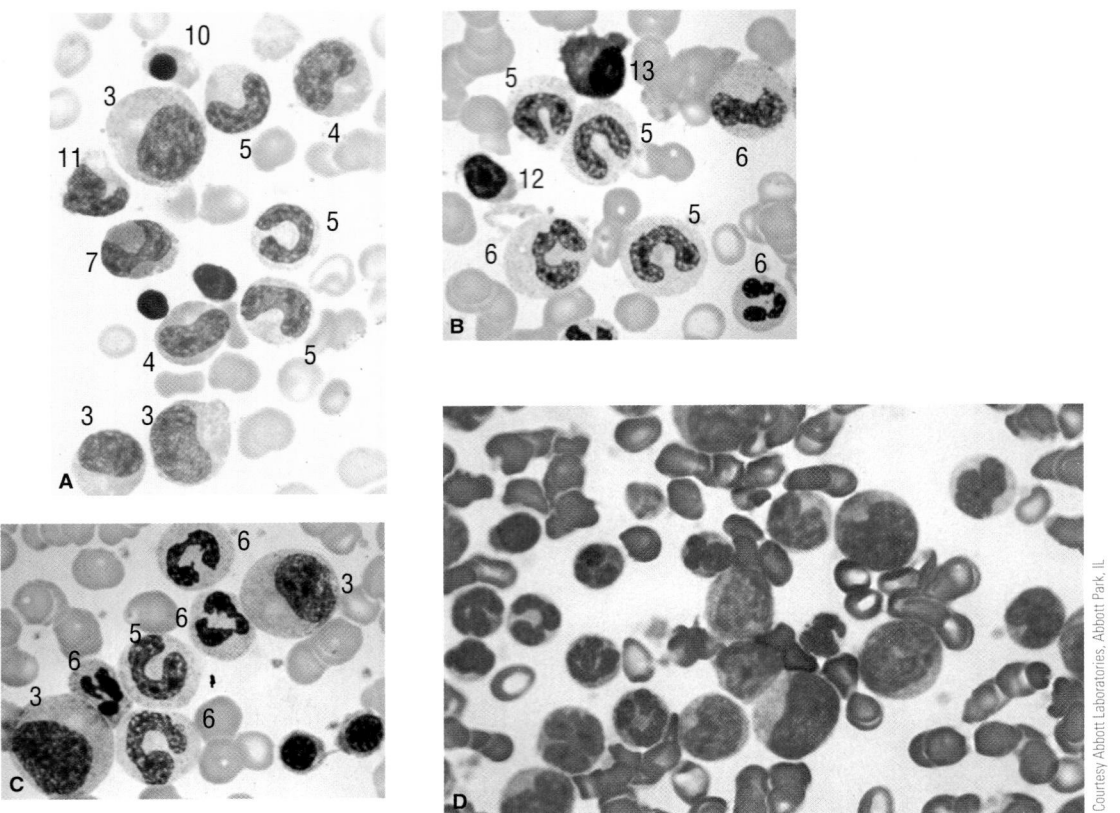

FIGURE 2-77 Photomicrographs of blood cells: (A-C) normal bone marrow cells and (D) peripheral blood cells of patient with chronic myelocytic leukemia. (Numbered key for A-C: 3, neutrophilic myelocyte; 4, metamyelocyte; 5, neutrophilic band; 6, segmented neutrophil; 7, eosinophilic metamyelocyte; 10, orthochromic erythroblast; 12, lymphocyte: and 13, plasma cell)

SAFETY REMINDERS

- Review Safety Precautions section before beginning procedure.
- Observe Standard Precautions,
- Follow electrical safety rules when using the microscope.

PROCEDURAL REMINDERS

- Review Quality Assessment section before beginning procedure.
- Follow the SOP manual for reporting abnormal cells.
- Have appropriate supervisor verify abnormal findings.

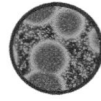

SUMMARY

Hematology technologists must remember that any smear being examined can contain abnormal blood cells even though the patient seems in good health. The technologist must be very familiar with normal and abnormal blood cell morphology to be able to accurately identify and evaluate the morphology of cells observed during the differential count. The peripheral blood smear must be properly prepared and stained to be of value for examination.

The supervisor, laboratory director, or the pathologist must be consulted before certain types of abnormal cells are reported. The policy of each institution regarding the reporting of abnormal cells will be outlined in the laboratory SOP manual.

This lesson is only an elementary introduction to the morphology of abnormal blood cells. It is not possible to adequately cover the subject in this space, but it is hoped that this lesson will stimulate students to desire to know more about disorders of the WBCs, RBCs, and platelets.

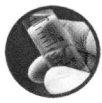

REVIEW QUESTIONS

1. Why is it important to recognize an abnormal blood cell?

2. List three conditions in which abnormal RBC morphology can be found.

3. Why is it important to report RBC inclusions?

4. How can RBC indices be used to classify anemias?

5. List three conditions in which abnormal WBC morphology can be found.

6. What is leukemia?

7. Discuss the differences between acute and chronic leukemias.

8. Why do leukemia patients develop anemia or bleeding problems?

9. List one cause of thrombocytosis and one cause of thrombocytopenia.

10. Define basophilia, basophilic stippling, blast cell, codocyte, crenated cell, drepanocyte, elliptocyte, eosinophilia, folic acid, Howell-Jolly body, keratocyte, leukemia, neutrophilia, nucleated red blood cell, red blood cell indices, schizocyte, shift to the left, sickle cell, sickle cell disease, stomatocyte, target cell, thalassemia, and vitamin B_{12}.

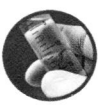

STUDENT ACTIVITIES

1. Complete the written examination for this lesson.

2. Practice recognizing and identifying abnormal blood cells as outlined in the Student Performance Guide.

WEB ACTIVITIES

1. Search the Internet for information on treatments for leukemia. Prepare a short report on the latest treatment regimen for one of the leukemias.

2. Use the Internet to find images of abnormal blood cells from peripheral blood and bone marrow. Make your own reference atlas of abnormal blood cell morphology from online images. (Be sure that you do not violate any copyrights. Most web sites allow personal use of images.)

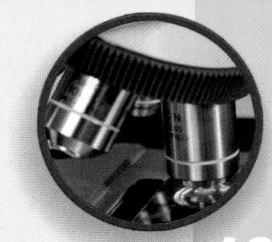

LESSON 2-11

Abnormalities in Blood Cell Morphology

Name _____ Date _____

INSTRUCTIONS

1. Practice identifying abnormal blood cells.

2. Demonstrate the recognition and identification of abnormal blood cells on peripheral smears or other visual learning aids using the Student Performance Guide. Your instructor will explain the procedure for evaluating and grading your performance. Your performance may receive a number grade, a letter grade, or satisfactory (S) or unsatisfactory (U) depending on the course or institutional policy.

MATERIALS AND EQUIPMENT

- hand antiseptic
- laboratory tissue
- microscope with oil-immersion objective
- microscope immersion oil
- microscope slides of various blood disorders such as iron deficiency anemia, B$_{12}$ or folate deficiency, infectious mononucleosis, leukocytosis, leukemias, and sickle cell disease
- blood cell atlas
- lens paper and lens cleaner
- slide storage box
- sharps container

PROCEDURE

Record in the comment section any problems encountered while practicing the procedure (or have a fellow student or the instructor evaluate your performance).

S = Satisfactory
U = Unsatisfactory

You must:	S	U	Evaluation/Comments
1. Wash hands with antiseptic			
2. Assemble appropriate equipment and materials to view blood smears using the microscope			
3. Observe the slide or visual aid of iron deficiency anemia. Look in several oil-immersion fields and identify microcytic red blood cells. Look for unusual cell shapes such as target cells			
4. Observe the slide or visual aid of B$_{12}$ or folate deficiency: a. Look in several oil-immersion fields and locate macrocytic RBCs b. Observe the WBCs and identify any that are larger than normal or have unusual nuclear characteristics			

(Continues)

STUDENT PERFORMANCE GUIDE

© 2012 Delmar, Cengage Learning. Permission to reproduce for clinical use granted.

You must:	S	U	Evaluation/Comments
5. Observe the slide or visual aid of infectious mononucleosis or other viral infection: a. Scan the differential counting area of the smear. Observe the WBCs for a relative increase in the number of lymphocytes b. Locate several reactive lymphocytes and note the characteristics of the cytoplasm and the nucleus			
6. Observe the slide or visual aid of sickle cell disease: a. Identify any sickled RBCs present b. Identify microcytic RBCs c. Examine several fields; identify target cells			
7. Observe the leukemia slide: a. Locate and identify the predominant white blood cell type present b. Observe the RBC morphology c. Observe the platelets for an increase or decrease in number			
8. Blot the immersion oil from the slides with laboratory tissue and replace slides in their storage containers or return visual aids to storage			
9. Clean the microscope objectives with lens paper and return the microscope to proper storage			
10. Wash hands with antiseptic			

Instructor/Evaluator Comments:

Instructor/Evaluator _____ Date _____

© 2012 Delmar, Cengage Learning. Permission to reproduce for clinical use granted.

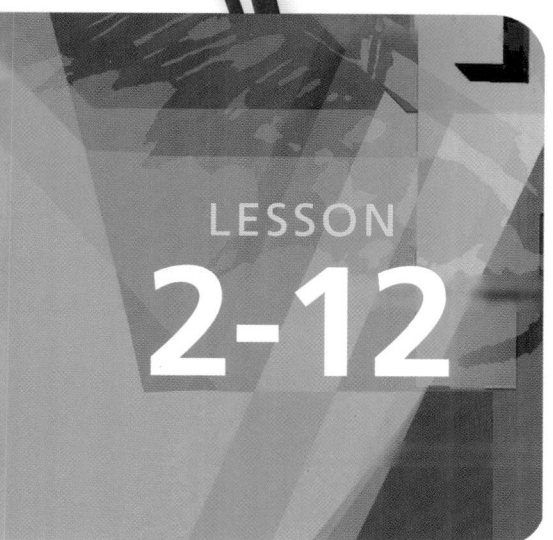

LESSON 2-12

Reticulocyte Count

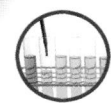

LESSON OBJECTIVES

After studying this lesson, the student will:

⊙ Explain the purpose of performing a reticulocyte count.
⊙ Name two dyes that can be used in the reticulocyte counting procedure.
⊙ Prepare smears for a reticulocyte count.
⊙ Perform a reticulocyte count.
⊙ Calculate a reticulocyte percentage.
⊙ Calculate an absolute reticulocyte count
⊙ Calculate a corrected reticulocyte count.
⊙ Explain the advantages of using the absolute or corrected count instead of the reticulocyte percentage.
⊙ List the normal reticulocyte reference ranges for adults and newborns.
⊙ Name two conditions in which the reticulocyte count would be low.
⊙ Name two conditions in which the reticulocyte count would be elevated.
⊙ Discuss the safety precautions to be observed when performing the reticulocyte count.
⊙ Discuss quality assessment guidelines that must be followed when performing the reticulocyte count.
⊙ Define the glossary terms.

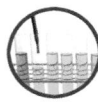

GLOSSARY

erythropoiesis / the production of red blood cells

Miller reticle / a reticle that imposes two squares over the field of view and that is used for reticulocyte counts

reticle / a glass circle etched with a pattern of calibrated grids, lines, or circles and inserted into a microscope eyepiece to allow the etched pattern to be imposed on the field of view

reticulocyte / an immature erythrocyte that still contains RNA remnants in the cytoplasm

reticulocytopenia / a decrease below the normal number of reticulocytes in the circulating blood

reticulocytosis / an increase above the normal number of reticulocytes in the circulating blood

reticulum / a filamentous network

ribonucleic acid (RNA) / the nucleic acid that is important in protein synthesis and that is found in all living cells

supravital stain / a nontoxic dye used to stain living cells or tissues

INTRODUCTION

The reticulocyte count estimates the number of immature red blood cells (RBCs) in the circulating blood; therefore, it is an indirect way of estimating the rate of **erythropoiesis**, RBC production. The test is used to help determine the cause of a low RBC count or anemia, to help classify the type of anemia, and to monitor the effectiveness of anemia treatment.

PRINCIPLE OF THE RETICULOCYTE COUNT

RBCs are produced in the bone marrow from hemopoietic stem cells. After a maturation process in which the RBCs lose their nucleus, the cells enter the peripheral blood circulation. For the first 24 hours in the circulation, RBCs still contain remnants of **ribonucleic acid (RNA)** in the cell cytoplasm. On a Wright's-stained blood smear, these immature cells stain bluish (polychromatophilia), appear slightly larger than other RBCs, and often do not have a distinct central area of pallor.

The reticulocyte staining technique identifies these immature RBCs in the peripheral blood. The reticulocyte stain is a **supravital stain**, a stain for living cells. Two common dyes used for reticulocyte staining are isotonic solutions of new methylene blue and brilliant cresyl blue.

When reticulocyte stain is applied to recently collected blood, the RNA in immature RBCs stains as granular aggregates or filaments called a **reticulum** (Figure 2-78). For this reason, these immature RBCs are called **reticulocytes** and represent the group of cells that have most recently entered the peripheral circulation. Reticulocytes appear as blue-tinged cells containing dark bluish-purple granules or reticulum and are slightly larger than mature RBCs (Figure 2-78). Mature RBCs appear bluish-green and contain no visible granules or other inclusions.

PERFORMING THE RETICULOCYTE COUNT

The manual reticulocyte count is performed by microscopically examining smears of freshly collected blood stained with new methylene blue stain.

Safety Precautions

  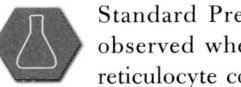 Standard Precautions must be observed when performing the reticulocyte count. In the reticulocyte procedure, cells are stained in the living state and no fixative is used. Therefore, the stained cells are still a biological hazard. Appropriate personal protective equipment (PPE) must be worn while obtaining the blood sample, staining the cells, making the smears, and performing the counts.

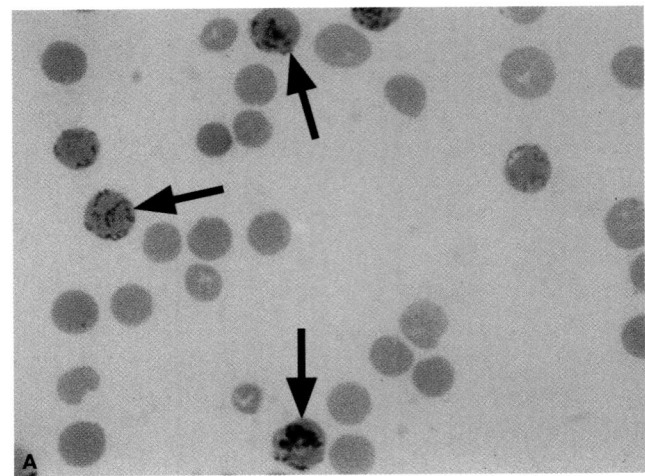

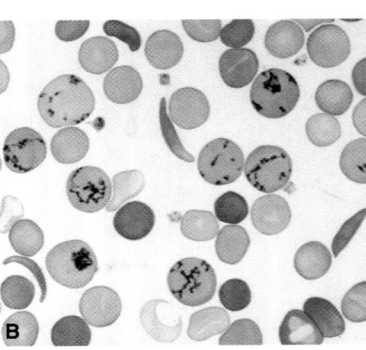

Courtesy Abbott laboratories, Abbott park IL.

FIGURE 2-78 Photomicrographs of reticulocytes stained with New Methylene Blue: (A) arrows indicate stained reticulum; (B) reticulocytes in blood of patient with sickle cell anemia

Quality Assessment

   The reticulocyte count must be performed following the method outlined in the laboratory's standard operating procedure (SOP) manual. The test must be performed within 4 hours of blood collection, because immature RBCs continue to mature as blood stands in a tube of anticoagulated blood. If the procedure is delayed, the reticulocyte count will be falsely decreased.

Stock stain must be stored at the recommended temperature and frequently filtered to eliminate debris and precipitate. The blood-stain mixture used to make reticulocyte smears is dilute; slides should be placed on a flat surface to dry to retain even distribution of cells and prevent pooling of the specimen at one end of the slide. Smears must be examined carefully, so that fine or faintly stained reticulum is not overlooked. When performing the reticulocyte count, the technician must be careful to distinguish reticulum from artifacts and debris.

A definite counting pattern must be used to avoid counting the same cells twice. Each laboratory must establish its own reference ranges, counting rules, and criteria regarding the designation of cells as reticulocytes. For instance, some laboratories specify that only cells

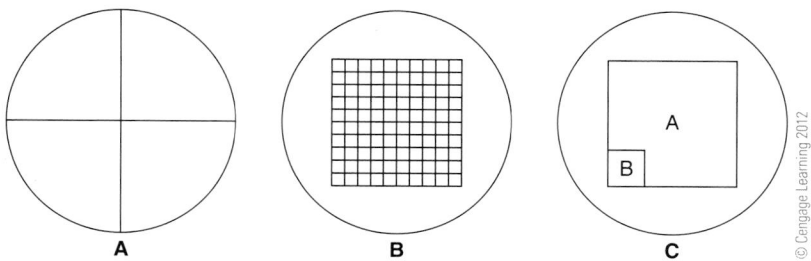

FIGURE 2-79 Reticles: (A) crosshair reticle; (B) grid reticle; and (C) Miller reticle

with more than one stained element (granule or filament) are counted as reticulocytes. Counting procedures must be followed uniformly by all technologists. Special eyepiece **reticles**, such as a **Miller reticle**, can be used to make cell counting easier (Figure 2-79). Reticulocyte controls are manufactured from human RBCs and are available for manual and automated counts.

Specimen Requirements

The reticulocyte procedure can be performed on capillary blood or venous ethylenediaminetetraacetic acid (EDTA)-anticoagulated blood and should be performed within 4 hours of blood collection.

Staining Procedure

A small volume of well-mixed blood (5 drops or 100 μL) is mixed with an equal volume of reticulocyte stain in a small vial. A stock solution of stain can be used or vials of premeasured reticulocyte stain can be purchased (Reti-TIC, bioanalytic GmbH). The blood-stain mixture is allowed to stand for 15 to 20 minutes to allow cells to take up the stain. The mixture is then used to prepare blood smears.

Smear Preparation

After the blood-stain mixture has incubated at room temperature for at least 15 minutes, the contents of the vial should be mixed gently. Two or three smears should be made from the well-mixed sample using a standard wedge blood smear technique such as that described in Lesson 2-7. Unlike blood smears for Wright's stain, reticulocyte smears should be placed on a flat surface to air dry.

Counting Procedure

The procedure used to count reticulocytes from the stained smears can vary slightly from laboratory to laboratory. Two counting methods described in this lesson are the standard method and the Miller reticle method.

Standard Counting Procedure

The dry smears are examined microscopically using the oil-immersion objective. A total of 1,000 RBCs are counted (500 per slide), and the number of reticulocytes observed per 1,000 RBCs is recorded. During the counting procedure, reticulocytes are counted twice—once as a reticulocyte and once as a red cell.

The use of an eyepiece reticle, if available, will make the counting process easier. A reticle seated in the microscope eyepiece allows the microscopist to view the cells through a lined measure that is imposed over the microscope image. Use of a quadrant or crosshair reticle (Figure 2-79A) or a grid reticle (Figure 2-79B) makes it easier for the microscopist to keep track of which cells in a field have been counted. Use of one of these types of reticles does not change the counting procedure.

Counting Procedure Using the Miller Reticle

A Miller reticle (Figure 2-79C) can be used for reticulocyte counts, however the standard reticulocyte counting procedure and calculation must be modified. The laboratory's SOP manual must be consulted for the exact counting method.

The Miller reticle imposes two squares—a large square (A) and a smaller inner square (B)—over the field of view. The small inner square of the reticle is one-ninth the size of the large outer square. For each field of view, the number of reticulocytes is counted in the entire large square (including the small square) and recorded; all red cells lying within the small square are counted, including reticulocytes, and that number is recorded as red cells. This is repeated for several fields until 100 to 200 red cells have been counted in the small squares and recorded.

Calculating the Reticulocyte Percentage

A reticulocyte count is reported as the *percentage* of RBCs that are reticulocytes. The calculations to find the percentage differ slightly depending on the counting procedure.

Calculations for the Standard Counting Method

For the standard method of counting reticulocytes, the percentage of reticulocytes is calculated using the following formula:

$$\frac{\text{\# Reticulocytes counted}}{\text{Total \# RBCs counted}} \times 100 = \% \text{ Reticulocytes}$$

or

$$\frac{\text{\# Reticulocytes}}{1000} \times 100 = \% \text{ Reticulocytes}$$

or

$$\frac{\text{\# Reticulocytes}}{10} = \% \text{ Reticulocytes}$$

This formula is only valid when 1,000 RBCs are counted during examination of the reticulocyte preparation. A sample calculation is shown in Figure 2-80A.

Calculations for the Miller Reticle Method

The reticulocyte count performed using the Miller reticle is also reported as the percentage of RBCs that are reticulocytes. However, the reticulocyte formula must be modified to take into account the different counting method.

When the Miller reticle is used to count cells, the reticulocyte percentage is calculated by dividing the total of number of reticulocytes counted (large square) by the total number of red cells counted (small square) multiplied by 9. The number obtained is then multiplied by 100 to obtain the percentage. Because the small square is one-ninth the area of the large square, the total count from the small squares must be multiplied by 9 before the percentage is calculated:

$$\frac{\text{\# Reticulocytes counted}}{(\text{Total \# RBCs counted}) \times 9} \times 100 = \% \text{ Reticulocytes}$$

A calculation of reticulocyte percentage from a count performed using the Miller reticle is shown in Figure 2-80B.

The advantage of this method is that a smaller number of RBCs can be counted. However, an additional calculation is required to obtain the reticulocyte percentage. Use of the Miller reticle also requires that blood cells are evenly distributed over a large portion of the blood smears.

Reference Ranges for Reticulocyte Counts

The normal reticulocyte percentage varies with age (Table 2-21). Newborn infants have high reticulocyte counts that decrease to adult levels by 2 weeks of age. In a healthy adult, the reticulocyte count is usually stable; approximately 1% of the RBCs will stain as reticulocytes when a supravital stain is applied to a blood sample.

Correcting the Reticulocyte Count for Anemia

For the reticulocyte percentage to give more meaningful information about RBC production, it should be correlated with the patient's RBC count or hematocrit. For example, the normal reticulocyte percentage is approximately 1%. A patient with an RBC count of $5 \times 10^6/\mu L$ and a reticulocyte percentage of 1% would have approximately 50,000 reticulocytes per microliter of blood. However, another patient with a reticulocyte percentage of 1% and an RBC count of $3 \times 10^6/\mu L$ would have only 30,000 reticulocytes per microliter.

Although the reticulocyte percentages are the same in these two individuals, the total numbers of reticulocytes are not. For this reason, reticulocyte percentages are often corrected for anemia to give the physician a more accurate reflection of the status of RBC production in the patient. The reticulocyte percentage can be correlated to the red cell count or hematocrit by calculating the *absolute reticulocyte count* or the *corrected reticulocyte count*.

TABLE 2-21. Reference ranges for reticulocyte counts

	REFERENCE RANGE (%)	UPPER LIMIT OF NORMAL (%)
Adults	0.5–1.5	3
Newborns	2.5–6.5	10

A. Perform a reticulocyte count using the Standard method:

I. Count the reticulocytes using two smears:

	Erythrocytes counted	Reticulocytes seen
Smear 1	500	7
Smear 2	500	5
Total	1000	12

II. Calculate the percentage of reticulocytes:

$$\% \text{ Retics} = \frac{\text{\# Reticulocytes counted}}{\text{\# RBC counted}} \times 100$$

$$\% \text{ Retics} = \frac{12}{1000} \times 100$$

$$\% \text{ Retics} = \frac{12}{10}$$

$$\% \text{ Retics} = 1.2$$

B. Perform a reticulocyte count using the Miller reticle:

I. Count the reticulocytes using two smears. Count all reticulocytes in the entire large square and count all red cells (including reticulocytes) in the small squares:

Smear 1	Smear 2
Retics counted = 18	Retics counted = 26
Red cells counted = 124	Red cells counted = 146

II. Compute the totals:
    Retics counted = 18 + 26 = 44
    Total red blood cells counted = 124 + 146 = 270

III. Calculate the percentage of reticulocytes:

$$\% \text{ reticulocytes} = \frac{\text{\# reticulocytes counted}}{(\text{Total \# RBCs counted}) \times 9} \times 100$$

$$\% \text{ Retics} = \frac{44}{270 \times 9} \times 100$$

$$\% \text{ Retics} = \frac{44}{2430} \times 100$$

$$\% \text{ Retics} = 1.8$$

© Cengage Learning 2012

FIGURE 2-80 Sample calculations of a reticulocyte percentage using the (A) standard counting method and (B) the Miller reticle counting method

CURRENT TOPICS

CLINICAL SIGNIFICANCE OF RETICULOCYTE COUNTS

The reticulocyte count alone cannot provide a specific diagnosis; it must be used with other factors to aid in diagnosis. Reticulocyte counts above 3% in an adult indicate that RBCs are being produced at an increased rate. **Reticulocytosis**, an increased number of reticulocytes, can occur in response to acute blood loss from hemorrhage, chronic blood loss such as from a bleeding ulcer, and response to treatment for anemia (Table 2-22). Increased reticulocyte percentages can also be seen in inherited and acquired hemolytic conditions. Examples of inherited conditions include certain hemoglobinopathies; examples of acquired conditions include trauma such as burns or artificial heart valve. If the cause of hemolysis is not corrected, the reticulocyte count will remain elevated. Thus a high reticulocyte count reflects a marrow that is responding to red cell destruction or loss by increasing red cell production.

Reticulocyte values below 0.5% indicate a decreased rate of RBC production. Low reticulocyte counts in the presence of anemia indicate a marrow unable to respond adequately to the need for red cells. A decrease in reticulocytes, **reticulocytopenia**, can occur in aplastic anemia. Anemias caused by iron, vitamin B_{12} or folate deficiencies can have normal to low reticulocyte counts (depending on severity), because the bone marrow lacks the hemoglobin building blocks necessary to increase red cell production (Table 2-22).

TABLE 2-22. Conditions causing increased or decreased reticulocyte counts

CONDITION	RETICULOCYTE COUNT
Aplastic anemia	Decreased
Vitamin B_{12} deficiency (untreated)	Normal to decreased
Iron deficiency anemia (untreated)	Normal to decreased
Bone marrow failure	Decreased
Hemolytic anemias	Increased
Hemorrhage	Increased
Factor deficiencies (folate, iron, B_{12}) following treatment	Increased
Living at high altitudes	Increased
Heavy smoking	Increased

Absolute Reticulocyte Count

The reticulocyte percentage simply estimates the percentage of RBCs that are reticulocytes. The *absolute reticulocyte count* is a calculation that estimates the number of reticulocytes per volume of blood by multiplying the reticulocyte percentage by the patient's RBC count.

For example, if a patient has 2% reticulocytes and an RBC count of $4 \times 10^6/\mu L$, the absolute reticulocyte count would be calculated as follows:

$$
\begin{aligned}
\text{Absolute reticulocyte count} &= \text{RBC count} \times \% \text{ Reticulocytes} \\
&= 4 \times 10^6/\mu L \times 2\% \\
&= 8 \times 10^4/\mu L \text{ or} \\
&= 80{,}000 \text{ reticulocytes}/\mu L
\end{aligned}
$$

Corrected Reticulocyte Count

Another way of correlating the reticulocyte percentage to anemia is to calculate the *corrected reticulocyte count*. This is done by dividing the patient's hematocrit by 45 (which represents a normal hematocrit) and then multiplying by the % reticulocytes. For example, if a patient has 3% reticulocytes and a hematocrit of 35%, the corrected reticulocyte count would be calculated as follows:

$$
\begin{aligned}
\text{Corrected retic count} &= \text{Retic count}(\%) \times \frac{\text{Patient Hct}}{45} \\
&= 3\% \times \frac{35}{45} \\
&= 2.3\%
\end{aligned}
$$

AUTOMATED RETICULOCYTE COUNTS

Automation makes it possible to count reticulocytes with more precision than is possible with manual counts. Most analyzers that perform reticulocyte counts use the principle of flow cytometry (see Lesson 2-10 for detailed discussion). These instruments use lasers and RNA-specific stains to identify reticulocytes in a blood sample as blood cells flow through a special counting chamber. Use of automated methods eliminates inconsistencies in counting techniques of different technicians and allows very large numbers of cells to be counted, which increases accuracy.

SAFETY REMINDERS

- Review Safety Precautions section before performing procedure.
- Observe Standard Precautions.
- Wear appropriate PPE.

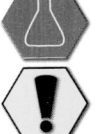

PROCEDURAL REMINDERS

- Review Quality Assessment section before performing procedure.
- Follow method in SOP manual.
- Examine cells carefully for reticulum.

CRITICAL THINKING

Mary Beth was preparing to perform a reticulocyte count on a blood specimen collected 3 hours earlier when she noticed sediment in the bottom of the stain bottle. However, Mary Beth decided not to use that stain.

1. What is the reason Mary Beth decided not to use the stain?
2. What should she do to make the stain usable?
3. Why was the time important?

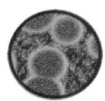

SUMMARY

Reticulocytes are immature RBCs in the peripheral blood circulation. They are identified by applying a supravital stain such as new methylene blue to red blood cells. The reticulocyte count is an important tool for assessing the bone marrow's ability to produce RBCs. The reticulocyte count is reported as a percentage of circulating RBCs. When the test is ordered with a RBC count an absolute reticulocyte count can be calculated.

The manual reticulocyte count is performed by microscopic examination of blood smears. Reticulocyte counts can also be performed using some hematology analyzers. The manual method is subject to more errors than the automated method, such as inadequate mixing of the blood before making the slides and incorrect or inconsistent counting procedures.

The reticulocyte count is useful in the diagnosis of certain anemias and to measure the response of anemia to treatment. The reticulocyte count gives the physician important information about red cell dynamics. A low reticulocyte count indicates decreased production of red cells by the bone marrow. A high reticulocyte count indicates an increased rate of blood loss which can be due to conditions such as blood loss from bleeding or from increased cell destruction.

REVIEW QUESTIONS

1. What is a reticulocyte?
2. What are two dyes (stains) used to stain reticulocytes?
3. Why would a reticulocyte count be ordered?
4. How is a standard reticulocyte count performed?
5. How is the Miller reticle used to perform a reticulocyte count?
6. What is the normal reticulocyte reference range for adults? For newborns?
7. What conditions can cause reticulocytosis?
8. Why must Standard Precautions be observed during the reticulocyte count?
9. What conditions can cause reticulocytopenia?
10. State the formula for calculating a standard reticulocyte count.
11. Calculate the absolute reticulocyte count and the corrected reticulocyte count from the following values: Hct = 32%; RBC = $3.8 \times 10^6/\mu L$; Reticulocyte count = 3%.
12. Define erythropoiesis, Miller reticle, reticle, reticulocyte, reticulocytopenia, reticulocytosis, reticulum, ribonucleic acid, and supravital stain.

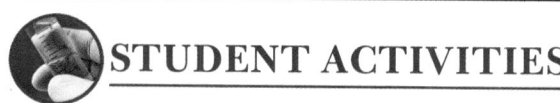

STUDENT ACTIVITIES

1. Complete the written examination for this lesson.

2. Practice performing reticulocyte counts and calculating reticulocyte percentages as outlined in the Student Performance Guide, using the worksheet.

3. Repeat a reticulocyte count on a specimen that has been stored at 4° C for 1 to 2 days after the initial reticulocyte count. Compare the two counts and discuss the results.

WEB ACTIVITIES

1. Use the Internet to find information about reticulocyte counts performed on hematology analyzers; report on the technology used to perform automated reticulocyte counts.

2. Use the Internet to find information and report on erythrocyte inclusions such as Heinz bodies, Howell-Jolly bodies, and Pappenheimer bodies. Discuss how the presence of any of these might affect the reticulocyte count.

3. Search the Internet for images of stained reticulocytes. Download these images and add them to your atlas of blood cell images. (Do not violate copyrights.)

LESSON 2-12
Reticulocyte Count

(Answers may vary based on the types of samples provided by the instructor and individual student results.)

Name _____   Date _____

INSTRUCTIONS

1. Practice the procedure for performing a reticulocyte count following the step-by-step procedure.

2. Demonstrate the procedure for the reticulocyte count satisfactorily for the instructor using the Student Performance Guide and the worksheet. Your instructor will explain the procedures for evaluating and grading your performance. Your performance may be given a number grade, letter grade, or satisfactory (S) or unsatisfactory (U) depending on course on institutional policy.

MATERIALS AND EQUIPMENT

- gloves
- hand antiseptic
- full-face shield (or equivalent PPE)
- acrylic safety shield (optional)
- microscope (optional: eyepiece with crosshair, grid, or Miller reticle)
- microscope slides
- lens paper and lens cleaner
- immersion oil
- laboratory tissue
- timer
- micropipetter (up to 100 µL capacity) with tips; plastic, disposable transfer pipets; or capillary (plain, blue-ring)
- freshly filtered new methylene blue stain or commercial reticulocyte kit
- Freshly collected EDTA–venous blood or capillary puncture supplies:
  - 70% alcohol or alcohol swabs
  - sterile cotton or gauze
  - sterile lancets
  - capillary tubes (heparinized, red-ring)
- disposable 1.5-mL vials with caps and vial rack
- test tube rack
- tally counters
- paper towels
- surface disinfectant (such as 10% chlorine bleach)
- biohazard container
- sharps container
- commercially prepared stained reticulocyte slides (optional)
- reticulocyte count worksheet

Optional:

- materials and equipment for RBC count and microhematocrit
- reticulocyte controls

PROCEDURE

    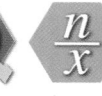

Record in the comment section any problems encountered while practicing the procedure (or have a fellow student or the instructor evaluate your performance).

S = Satisfactory
U = Unsatisfactory

You must:	S	U	Evaluation/Comments
1. Wash hands with antiseptic and put on gloves			
2. Assemble equipment and materials; set up microscope and clean lenses			

(Continues)

© 2012 Delmar, Cengage Learning. Permission to reproduce for clinical use granted.

You must:	S	U	Evaluation/Comments
3. Put on face protection or position acrylic safety shield on work area			

4. Set up test using freshly collected EDTA–anticoagulated blood following steps 4a–4e. If capillary blood is to be used, skip to step 5
  a. Pipet 100 µL reticulocyte stain into vial or obtain vial of premeasured reticulocyte stain
  b. Mix EDTA-anticoagulated blood well by inverting capped tube several times
  c. Pipet 100 µL of blood into the 100 µL of reticulocyte stain
  d. Cap vial and gently mix stain and blood
  e. Continue at step 6			

5. Perform a capillary puncture following steps 5a–5d
  a. Perform capillary puncture using standard technique
  b. Wipe away the first drop of blood with dry sterile cotton or gauze
  c. Fill one or two capillary tubes with capillary blood
  d. Dispense 3 to 5 drops of blood into the bottom of a small vial
  e. Add an equal amount of reticulocyte stain to the vial, cap vial, and gently mix contents			

6. Allow blood-stain mixture to stand for 15 to 20 minutes at room temperature			
7. Remix vial contents and use micropipetter or capillary to remove a small aliquot of the blood-stain mixture			
8. Prepare 2 or 3 blood smears from the blood-stain mixture and place smears on a flat surface to air dry. Discard used pipet tips or capillary tubes into sharps container			
9. Place one thoroughly-dry slide on the microscope stage and secure it			
10. Use the low-power (10×) objective to locate an area of the smear where cells do not overlap and are evenly spaced			
11. Place 1 drop of immersion oil on the slide and carefully rotate the oil-immersion (100×) objective into position			

12. Count all erythrocytes in one oil-immersion field and record the total number of red cells counted in the field as well as the number of reticulocytes in the field.
  a. If an eyepiece reticle with a grid is available, it can be used to help keep track of which cells have been counted.
  b. If a reticle is not available, mentally divide the field of view into four quadrants, and count the cells in each quadrant. A good area of the smear is one with about 80-100 cells per field of view
NOTE: Any reticulocytes seen are counted twice—once as a reticulocyte and once as an RBC			

© 2012 Delmar, Cengage Learning. Permission to reproduce for clinical use granted.

You must:	S	U	Evaluation/Comments
13. Move the slide to an adjacent microscopic field; count and record all erythrocytes in the (adjacent) field and record the number of reticulocytes in the field			
14. Continue steps 12 and 13 until 500 erythrocytes have been counted. Record counts on worksheet			
15. Repeat steps 9–14 using the second slide			
16. Add the counts from the two slides together			
17. Calculate the reticulocyte percentage using the worksheet and the formula: $$\frac{\#\ of\ retics\ counted}{1{,}000\ red\ blood\ cells} \times 100 = \%\ reticulocytes$$			
18. Record the results on the worksheet			

19. Repeat the reticulocyte count on the same blood smears using a Miller reticle if one is available. Refer to Figure 2-79 and follow steps 19a–19f. If the Miller reticle is not available, go to step 20
  a. Place a reticulocyte smear on the microscope stage, bring the cells into focus, put a drop of immersion oil on the slide, and rotate the oil-immersion lens into position
  b. Locate an area of the smear with 3 to 10 RBCs in the small square of the Miller reticle
  c. Count and record the *reticulocytes* within the entire large square including those that lie within the small square
  d. Count and record all RBCs in the smaller square (including reticulocytes)
  e. Move the slide to an adjacent field of view and continue counting all red cells in the small square and reticulocytes in the entire large square
  f. Continue counting cells in adjacent fields until 50 to 60 RBCs have been counted in the small square (usually 8 to 10 fields)
  g. Replace first smear with second reticulocyte smear and continue the counting process until approximately 100 to 120 red cells have been counted in the small squares. Calculate the reticulocyte percentage using the worksheet			

20. Clean the oil-immersion objective carefully and thoroughly with lens paper			
21. Clean any oil from the microscope stage with laboratory tissue and return microscope to storage			
22. Optional: If specimen used for reticulocyte count is from a tube of anticoagulated blood follow steps 22a – 22c. (If anticoagulated specimen is not available, go to step 23) a. Perform microhematocrit and RBC count on the same specimen			

(Continues)

© 2012 Delmar, Cengage Learning. Permission to reproduce for clinical use granted.

You must:	S	U	Evaluation/Comments
b. Record results on worksheet			
c. Use the worksheet to calculate the absolute reticulocyte count and the corrected reticulocyte count			
23. Return equipment to proper storage			
24. Store unused materials and discard used materials as instructed			
25. Discard sharps into sharps container			
26. Discard other contaminated materials into appropriate biohazard container			
27. Clean work area with disinfectant			
28. Remove gloves and discard into biohazard container			
29. Wash hands with antiseptic			

Instructor/Evaluator Comments:

Instructor/Evaluator _____   Date _____

© 2012 Delmar, Cengage Learning. Permission to reproduce for clinical use granted.

LESSON 2-12
Reticulocyte Count

(Answers may vary based on the types of samples provided by the instructor and individual student results.)

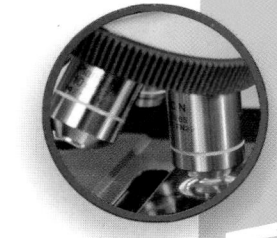

Name _____ Date _____

$\dfrac{n}{x}$ Specimen I.D. _____

I. Perform the reticulocyte count and record the results

A.   Red blood cells counted   Reticulocytes counted

    Slide 1   _____   _____

    Slide 2   _____   _____

    Total   _____   _____

B. Write the formula for the reticulocyte count:

C. Calculate the reticulocyte percentage: _____ = % reticulocytes

D. The reticulocyte percentage is (circle one): normal / increased / decreased

II. Optional: If available, perform RBC count and hematocrit on the same blood specimen used for the reticulocyte count, and record the results.

A. RBC/µL = _____ Hct (%) = _____

B. Absolute reticulocyte count: _____ .

    1. Write the formula for the absolute reticulocyte count:

       _____

    2. Calculate the absolute reticulocyte count: _____ .

C. Corrected reticulocyte count:

    1. Write the formula for the corrected reticulocyte count:

    2. Calculate the corrected reticulocyte count: _____ .

III. Optional: Reticulocyte count using Miller reticle

A. Record cell counts:

        Red blood cells counted (small square)   Reticulocytes counted (large square)

    Slide 1   _____   _____

    Slide 2   _____   _____

    Total   _____   _____

B. Calculate the reticulocyte percentage using the formula:

$$\% \text{ Reticulocytes} = \frac{(\text{Total reticulocytes counted in large square})}{(\text{Total RBCs counted in smaller square}) \times 9} \times 100$$

C. Reticulocyte percentage = _____ %

© 2012 Delmar, Cengage Learning. Permission to reproduce for clinical use granted.

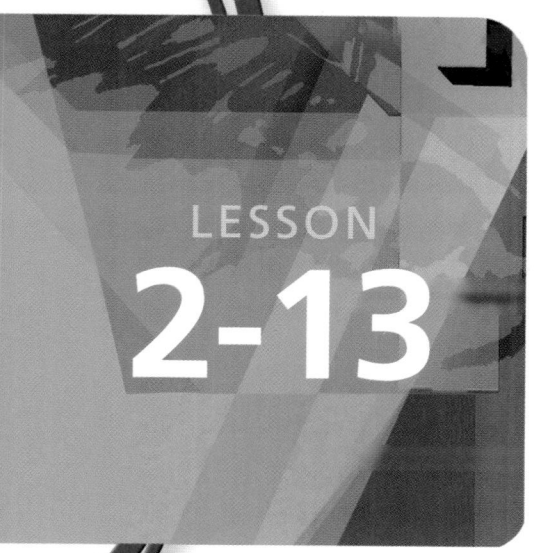

LESSON 2-13

Erythrocyte Sedimentation Rate

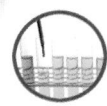

LESSON OBJECTIVES

After studying this lesson, the student will:

- ⊙ Explain the principle of erythrocyte sedimentation.
- ⊙ Explain the purpose of performing an erythrocyte sedimentation rate test.
- ⊙ Name four properties of blood that affect the erythrocyte sedimentation rate and explain how the rate is affected by each.
- ⊙ List five technical factors that can affect the erythrocyte sedimentation rate and explain how the rate is affected by each.
- ⊙ Discuss the relationship of the erythrocyte sedimentation rate to disease.
- ⊙ List five pathological conditions that affect the erythrocyte sedimentation rate.
- ⊙ State the reference ranges for three erythrocyte sedimentation rate methods.
- ⊙ Perform an erythrocyte sedimentation rate test.
- ⊙ Discuss automated erythrocyte sedimentation rate methods and compare to manual methods.
- ⊙ Discuss safety issues specific to the performance of the erythrocyte sedimentation rate.
- ⊙ List aspects of quality assessment especially relevant to the erythrocyte sedimentation rate.
- ⊙ Define the glossary terms.

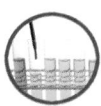

GLOSSARY

acute phase proteins / proteins that increase rapidly in plasma during acute infection and inflammation, or following tissue injury

aggregate / the total substances making up a mass; a cluster or clump of particles

inflammation / a nonspecific protective response to tissue injury that is initiated by the release of chemicals such as histamine and serotonin and the actions of phagocytic cells

polycythemia / an excess of red blood cells in the peripheral blood

rouleau(x) / group(s) of red blood cells arranged like a roll of coins

sedimentation / the process of solid particles settling to the bottom of a liquid

Westergren pipet / a slender pipet marked from 0 to 200 mm, used in the Westergren erythrocyte sedimentation rate method

Wintrobe tube / a slender, thick-walled tube used in the Wintrobe erythrocyte sedimentation rate

INTRODUCTION

The erythrocyte sedimentation rate (ESR), or *sed rate*, is a commonly performed hematology test. The ESR test measures the rate at which erythrocytes sediment in blood under standardized conditions. The ESR test is used to detect **inflammation**; it is elevated in acute and chronic inflammation and also in malignancies. The ESR can also be used to evaluate the treatment and course of certain inflammatory diseases.

The sedimentation of blood was one of the principles of ancient Greek medicine. In the more modern era of medicine, as early as 1836, it was noted that some factor in plasma increased the sinking rate of erythrocytes in whole blood. A procedure very similar to today's ESR test was first used in laboratory medicine around 1915 as a pregnancy test. Shortly after that, the ESR was used to screen for tuberculosis. Since the mid-1930s, the ESR test has been used as a test to detect inflammation and inflammatory disease.

PRINCIPLE OF THE ERYTHROCYTE SEDIMENTATION RATE TEST

The ESR test is based on the principle of **sedimentation**, the process of solid particles settling to the bottom of a liquid. In a sample of anticoagulated blood left undisturbed, the erythrocytes gradually separate from the plasma and settle to the bottom of the container. The rate at which the erythrocytes settle or fall under controlled laboratory conditions is the ESR.

To perform the manual ESR test, a calibrated tube of standard dimensions is filled with a sample of anticoagulated blood and placed in a rack in a vertical position for an exact time. At the end of the time, the distance the erythrocytes have fallen from the plasma meniscus (at the zero mark) is measured in millimeters (mm) and reported as the ESR (Figure 2-81).

In blood samples from most healthy persons, erythrocyte sedimentation occurs slowly; the erythrocyte-plasma suspension is fairly stable. In many diseases, particularly inflammatory diseases, the rate of sedimentation is rapid. In some cases, the rate is proportional to the severity of the disease.

FACTORS AFFECTING THE ERYTHROCYTE SEDIMENTATION RATE

Factors that affect the rate of erythrocyte sedimentation in a blood sample are: (1) properties of the plasma, (2) properties of the erythrocytes, and (3) technical factors.

Properties of Plasma

In normal blood, erythrocytes suspended in the plasma form few, if any, **aggregates** or clusters. Therefore the mass of the falling (settling) erythrocytes is small and the rate of sedimentation is slow.

In certain disease conditions, the erythrocytes sometimes form aggregates called **rouleaux**. This phenomenon is called rouleaux because the cells are arranged like rolls or stacks of coins (Figure 2-82), causing an increase in effective mass and an increased rate of sedimentation. (Clumps or clusters of cells are

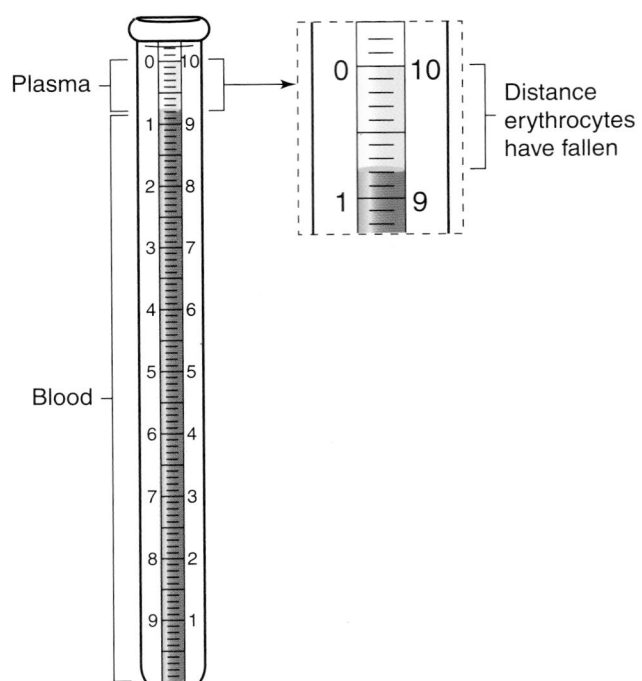

FIGURE 2-81 Illustration of sedimentation of cells in the erythrocyte sedimentation rate (ESR) test. Example shows Wintrobe ESR with sedimentation of 8 mm

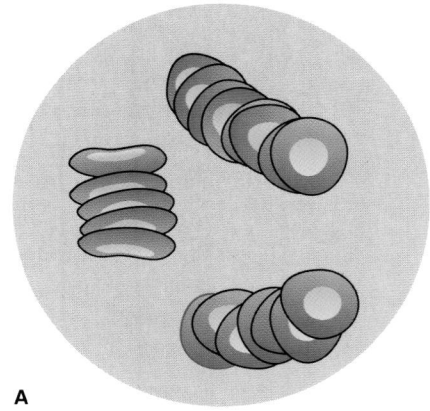

A

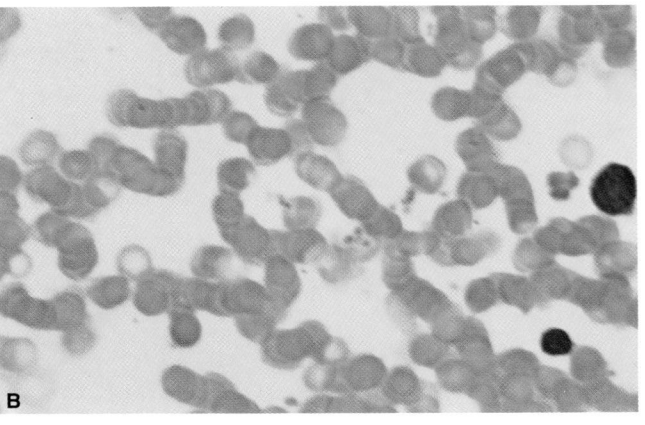

B

FIGURE 2-82 Rouleaux formation: (A) illustration of red blood cells forming "stacks of coins" (rouleaux); (B) rouleaux formation in a peripheral blood smear of a patient with multiple myeloma

heavier than single cells and will settle more rapidly.) Rouleaux formation is influenced by the amount and type of plasma proteins present in a blood sample. Increased levels of **acute phase proteins** or other plasma globulins enhance the tendency of RBCs to form rouleaux and therefore increase the sedimentation rate. Acute phase proteins include C-reactive protein (CRP), fibrinogen, alpha-1-antitrypsin, haptoglobin, ferritin, and complement components C3 and C4 (Table 2-23).

The ESR is an indirect measure of the amount of fibrinogen and other globulins in plasma; one or both of these protein groups are increased in many inflammatory or degenerative diseases, acute and chronic infections, and some tumors.

Properties of Erythrocytes

The ESR can also be affected by the size, shape, and number of red blood cells (RBCs).

Size

Macrocytic cells sediment more rapidly than microcytic cells because of their large size (increased mass).

Shape

The shape of the erythrocytes can also affect the ESR. For example, in sickle cell anemia the irregularly shaped erythrocytes cannot aggregate and the ESR is low or zero. Spherocytic cells also sediment at a slow rate.

Number

The ESR is affected by the RBC count. The sedimentation rate can be rapid in some anemias because the blood contains fewer erythrocytes. Therefore the hematocrit or RBC count should be checked on samples that have elevated ESRs to determine if the elevated rate is due to inflammation or to anemia. When the erythrocyte number is increased, as in **polycythemia**, the erythrocytes settle slowly and the ESR is low.

Technical Factors Affecting the Erythrocyte Sedimentation Rate

Several technical factors can affect the erythrocyte sedimentation rate. Temperature, timing, length and internal diameter of the sedimentation tube or pipet, pipetting technique, sample mixing, and

TABLE 2-23. Examples of acute phase proteins

C-reactive protein (CRP)
Alpha-1 acid glycoprotein
Alpha-1 antitrypsin
Haptoglobins
Ceruloplasmin
Serum amyloid A
Fibrinogen
Ferritin
Complement components C3, C4

TABLE 2-24. Technical errors that can cause a false increase or false decrease in the ESR

FALSE INCREASED RATE	FALSE DECREASED RATE
Tube not vertical	Air bubbles in tube
Incorrect timing (too long)	Incorrect timing (too short)
Test/Room temperature >25° C	Test/Room temperature >25° C
Incorrect mixing or sampling of blood	Incorrect mixing or sampling of blood
Vibration of tube during test	Blood specimen below room temperature

vibration during the test period will affect the sedimentation rate and are sources of error (Table 2-24). The precautions listed below must be followed to perform the test correctly.

- The sedimentation tube must be kept vertical during the test; even minor degrees of tilting can greatly increase the ESR.
- The test should be set up on a vibration-free counter. Vibrations, such as those occurring on a counter where a centrifuge is running, will cause a falsely increased ESR.
- The temperature in the testing area should be kept constant (20° to 25°C) while the test is being performed. Low temperatures cause erythrocytes to settle more slowly.
- The ESR test should be set up within 2 hours after the blood sample is collected or as specified in the laboratory's standard operating procedures (SOP) manual. Blood collected in ethylenediaminetetraacetic acid (EDTA) can be stored at 4° C for up to 6 hours for most ESR methods but must be brought to room temperature before the test is performed.
- The length and internal diameter (bore) of the sedimentation tube affect the rate of sedimentation. Therefore standardized tubes must be used in the test.
- Anticoagulated blood samples must be well mixed immediately before setting up the ESR test.
- Careful pipetting technique should be used when diluting blood samples and filling the sedimentation tube. Air bubbles in the tube will interfere with test accuracy.
- The test must be timed accurately. The ESR increases with time.

METHODS OF PERFORMING THE ERYTHROCYTE SEDIMENTATION RATE

Several methods of performing the ESR test are available, each with advantages, disadvantages, and different levels of sensitivity.

CURRENT TOPICS

RELATIONSHIP OF ERYTHROCYTE SEDIMENTATION RATE TO DISEASE

The erythrocyte sedimentation rate is a nonspecific test and is not diagnostic of any particular condition or disease. When the ESR is increased, it can be an indicator of inflammation somewhere in the body. Inflammation is a tissue response to injury or irritation that can be caused by a variety of conditions. The ESR and another test—the test for C-reactive protein (CRP)—are two inexpensive tests used to screen for inflammation. The CRP test, particularly the high sensitivity test (hs-CRP) is useful in detecting inflammation associated with coronary heart disease or cardiovascular disease. Results higher than the reference range for either the ESR or CRP test alerts the physician that more specific testing might be necessary. (The CRP test is also discussed in Lesson 6-1.)

The ESR is elevated in conditions that cause changes in plasma proteins, including inflammatory diseases such as rheumatic fever, rheumatoid arthritis, and lupus erythematosus. The ESR can also be increased in acute and chronic infections, tuberculosis, viral hepatitis, Hodgkin's and non-Hodgkin's lymphoma, and other cancers. Multiple myeloma, a malignant condition affecting B lymphocytes, causes an increased ESR because of the large amounts of immunoglobulins present in plasma.

Changes in shape, size, or number of RBCs can also affect the ESR. Patients with macrocytic anemia can have an increased ESR even though inflammation is not present. In sickle cell anemia, the ESR is low or sometimes zero, because sickle-shaped cells cannot form rouleaux. The ESR is also low in polycythemia.

The ESR can also be increased when disease is not present. For instance, pregnant woman often have an increased ESR because plasma fibrinogen usually increases during pregnancy. Table 2-25 lists conditions in which the ESR is increased and in which it is decreased.

Although the ESR is not used to make a specific diagnosis, the test can be used to follow the course of treatment of certain diseases, such as rheumatoid arthritis and lymphoma. An ESR that is elevated in the presence of active disease would be expected to decrease when treatment is successful. The ESR test also can be used to detect inflammation when white blood cell (WBC) counts are not elevated. For example, elderly patients can have normal WBC counts even in the presence of acute infection.

TABLE 2-25. Conditions in which the erythrocyte sedimentation rate can be increased or decreased

INCREASED SEDIMENTATION RATE	DECREASED SEDIMENTATION RATE
Pregnancy	Presence of sickle cells
Anemia	Polycythemia
Macrocytosis	Spherocytosis
Inflammatory diseases	Microcytosis
Cancer	
Acute and chronic infections	
Multiple myeloma	
Lymphoma	
Increased plasma fibrinogen	
Increased plasma globulins	
Tuberculosis	

Safety Precautions

  Standard Precautions must always be observed when performing the ESR test. Appropriate personal protective equipment (PPE) and engineering controls must be used. All sharps must be handled carefully and disposed of in sharps containers. The use of disposable ESR systems reduces the biohazard involved in disinfecting and cleaning reusable tubes.

Quality Assessment

   The ESR procedure in the facility's standard operating procedure (SOP) manual must be followed carefully, with special attention to technical factors that can affect the test, including test setup, specimen mixing, temperature, and timing. The procedure must include the use of approved commercial controls to help ensure that the ESR values reported by the laboratory are reliable. Control solutions for ESR tests are available from several suppliers. Some controls can

be used with both manual and automated methods; others are specific for particular methods.

Manual Erythrocyte Sedimentation Rate Methods

Manual methods described in this lesson are the Westergren (Modified) and the Wintrobe methods. Freshly collected EDTA-anticoagulated venous blood is used for both methods. Most procedures require that the test be set up within 2 hours after collection. Blood must be well mixed before setting up the test.

Westergren Method

The Westergren ESR method is performed using a **Westergren pipet** (or tube) graduated from 0 to 200 mm and a Westergren rack for holding the tubes. The Westergren test is more sensitive and slightly more complex to set up than the Wintrobe method. The Westergren method requires predilution of the blood with sodium citrate or saline before the pipet is filled. The test has been modified in recent years, and most laboratories now perform the modified Westergren method. The Westergren method is the ESR reference method of the Clinical and Laboratory Standards Institute (CLSI) and is the recommended standard method of the International Council for Standardization in Hematology.

Sediplast Erythrocyte Sedimentation Rate System

The Sediplast ESR System is a modified Westergren kit that uses a closed system consisting of a self-filling disposable pipet and sealed vial of premeasured diluent (Figure 2-83). Use of such a kit eliminates the biohazard risks present in the original Westergren method and also provides accurate filling of the pipet. The use of

the Sediplast ESR System is detailed in the Student Performance Guide at the end of this lesson and in Figure 2-84.

In the Sediplast ESR System, 0.8 mL of anticoagulated blood is mixed with 0.2 mL of premeasured 3.8% sodium citrate diluent in the sedivial (Figure 2-84A). The Westergren pipet is then inserted into the sealed vial with a twisting motion until the pipet reaches the bottom of the vial. The blood column will automatically zero itself, and any extra blood will overflow into the sealed reservoir (Figure 2-84B). The vial containing the pipet is placed in the sedimentation rack for 1 hour. At the end of the hour, the distance the erythrocytes have fallen is measured using the calibrated markings on the pipet (Figure 2-84C) and is reported in millimeters per hour. The nonautomated Sediplast ESR method is CLIA waived.

Wintrobe Method

The original Wintrobe ESR method is performed using a narrow-bore **Wintrobe tube** graduated from 0 to 100 mm (0 to 10 cm) and having a capacity of 1 mL of blood. The Wintrobe tube is placed in a special sedimentation rack on a level surface. Using a long-stemmed Pasteur-type pipet, the tube is filled with 1 mL of well-mixed anticoagulated blood. The tube is filled beginning at the bottom and filling to the top to prevent air bubbles in the tube. The meniscus must be adjusted to the "0" mark at the top of the tube. The rack holds the tube vertical.

At the end of 1 hour, the distance the erythrocytes have fallen in the blood sample is determined using the markings on the tube (reading from the "0" mark at the top of tube down to the top of red cells as shown in Figure 2-81). The ESR is recorded in mm/hour. The advantages of the Wintrobe method are its simplicity and the lack of expensive equipment. However, this method is not as sensitive as the Westergren ESR method and does not provide the safety of a closed system.

Self-filling Wintrobe kits are available, such as the Hypoguard Winpette system. These kits are similar to the Sediplast system—the plastic, disposable Winpette fills on contact with the accompanying reservoir and is self-zeroing. A difference is that the Winpette is 10 cm (100 mm) long, shorter than the 200 mm long Westergren pipet; this accounts for the lower sensitivity of the Wintrobe method.

Automated Methods

The SEDIMAT, Ves-Matic, ESR STAT-PLUS, and Zeta Sedimentation Ratio are four automated methods for performing the ESR. Most automated methods optically measure the change in opacity of blood as cells settle out of suspension. Automated ESR methods should only be adopted for use if they have high reproducibility, reliability and correlation with the Westergren reference method. Advantages of automated methods include:

- Save technician time
- Provide increased safety because the need for sample manipulation is decreased
- Interface with laboratory information systems (LIS)
- Use smaller sample volumes
- Provide more rapid results

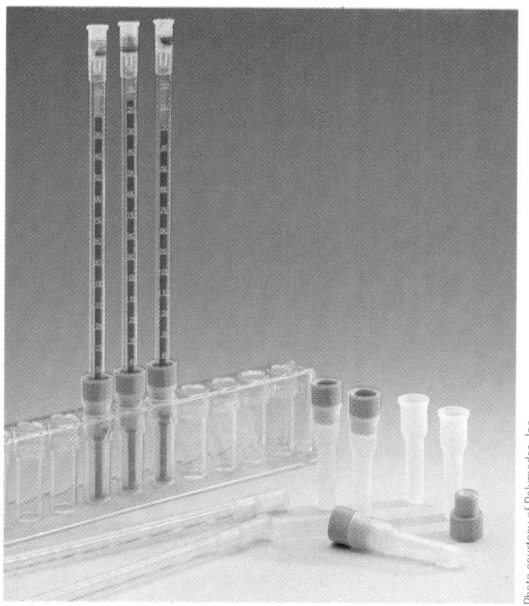

Photo courtesy of Polymedco, Inc.

FIGURE 2-83 Sediplast® ESR System showing three blood samples with different rates of sedimentation

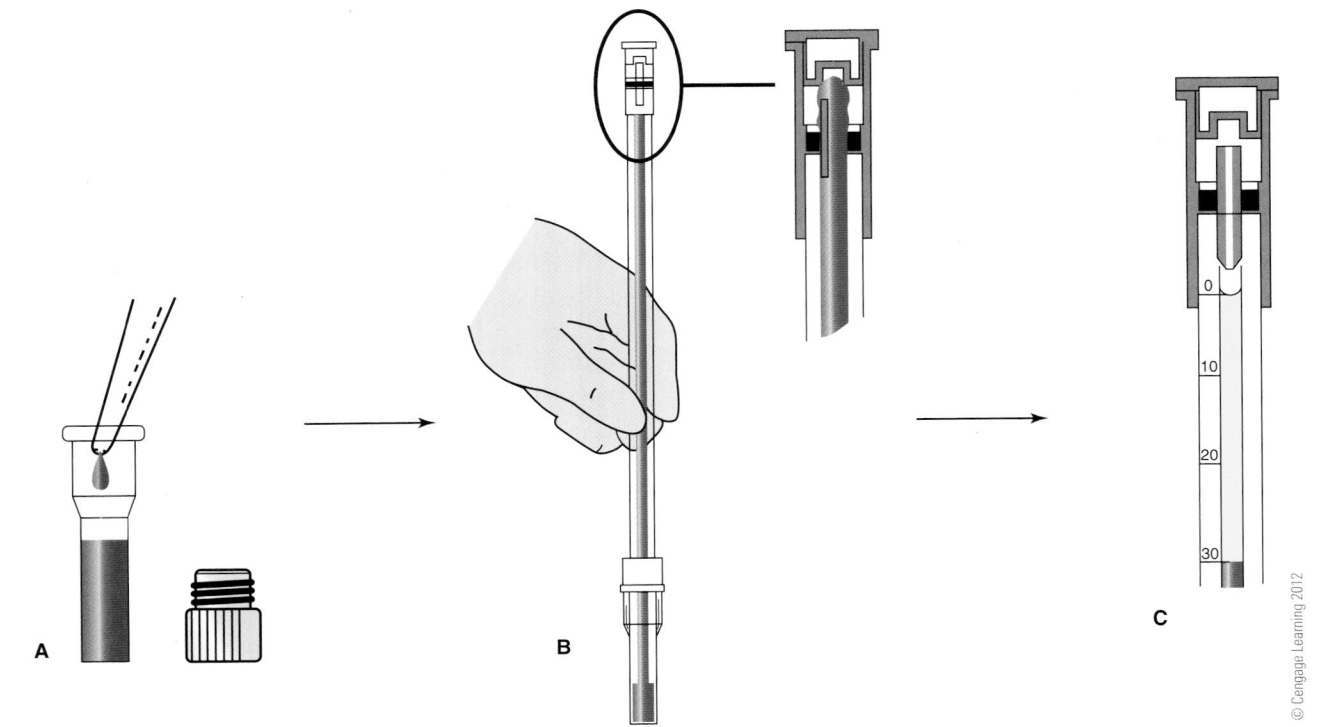

FIGURE 2-84 Steps for Sediplast® ESR test: (A) pipet blood into sedivial containing diluent, replace stopper, and mix; (B) insert pipet through piercable vial stopper, push down until pipet touches vial bottom, and allow tube to fill and autozero (inset); (C) read sedimentation distance from scale at top of pipet after one hour

SEDIMAT

The SEDIMAT 15 system (Polymedco) uses the principles, supplies, and setup procedures of the Sediplast system. The filled Sediplast Westergren pipet is placed into the SEDIMAT automated ESR reader, which accelerates sedimentation under controlled conditions. The reader displays the results of each sample on an LCD display after 15 minutes. The results are also stored in memory and can be printed out.

Ves-Matic

The Ves-Matic ESR system (Diesse) is an automated walkaway analyzer. A venipuncture is performed using a special vacuum tube that draws 1 mL of blood into a solution of sodium citrate. The tube is placed directly into the analyzer, the ESR is determined by infrared technology, and the results are available in approximately 22 minutes. An advantage is that the blood collection tube is also used as the sedimentation tube, eliminating the potential for exposure to blood during test setup

ESR STAT-PLUS

The ESR STAT PLUS analyzer (HemaTechnologies, Inc) is an automated sedimentation rate system that provides results in 5 minutes. Special EZ-SAFE Mylar-coated self-seal analysis tubes are filled with 25 µL of well-mixed EDTA blood. The tube is inserted into the analyzer, a centrifuge that uses infrared laser technology to track the plasma–erythrocyte interface. Readings from the laser measurements are used by software in the instrument to create a sedimentation curve. The sedimentation rate is calculated

and converted to millimeters per hour (mm/hour). The patient identification and test results are displayed on-screen at the end of the test period.

Zeta Sedimentation Ratio

The zeta sedimentation ratio (ZSR) is performed using a special, small-bore capillary tube that is filled with blood and spun for 3 to 4 minutes in a special centrifuge called the Zetafuge (Beckman Coulter). This centrifuge alternately compacts and disperses the RBCs under standardized centrifugal force. The tube is then read on a special reader to obtain a value called the zetacrit, which represents the percentage of sedimented erythrocytes. The zetacrit value is divided into the patient's hematocrit (also a percentage), and the result is the ZSR, expressed as a percentage. The ZSR's advantages are that it is rapid, corrects for anemia, and requires only a small blood sample, which is desirable for pediatric patients. However, a special centrifuge and reader are required to perform the test.

REFERENCE RANGES FOR THE ERYTHROCYTE SEDIMENTATION RATE

Each ESR method has its own set of reference values. Results must be compared with the appropriate reference ranges for the method used.

Reference values for the Sediplast ESR (Modified Westergren), Wintrobe ESR, and ZSR are given in Table 2-26. Sediplast and Wintrobe results are reported in millimeters per hour and have different reference ranges for males and females to account for differences in RBC counts in normal males and females. The reference values for the Wintrobe method are slightly lower than for the Sediplast, because blood is not diluted in the Wintrobe method.

The ZSR is calculated from the hematocrit and zetacrit and is reported as a percentage. Because the ZSR value is corrected for RBC volume, the reference range is the same for males and females of all ages.

TABLE 2-26. Reference ranges for Sediplast ESR (Modified Westergren), Wintrobe ESR, and Zeta Sedimentation Ratio (ZSR)

		SEDIPLAST ESR (mm/hr)	WINTROBE ESR (mm/hr)	ZSR PERCENTAGE (%) (ALL AGES)
Males:	<50 years	0–15	0–9	40–51 normal
	>50 years	0–20	0–9	51–54 borderline ≥55 elevated
Females:	<50 years	0–20	0–20	
	>50 years	0–30	0–20	
Newborns:		0–2		
Children (to puberty):		0–13		

SAFETY REMINDERS

- Review Safety Precautions section before beginning procedure.
- Observe Standard Precautions.
- Wear appropriate PPE.
- Use appropriate work practice controls.

PROCEDURAL REMINDERS

- Review Quality Assessment section before beginning procedure.
- Follow method in the SOP manual.
- Use reference ranges specific for the test method.

CASE STUDY

The laboratories at Community Hospital were being remodeled, and some equipment had to be moved temporarily from one laboratory room to another. On Friday the workmen had moved a tabletop centrifuge from the urinalysis station into one of the hematology laboratories. On Monday, Martha arrived at work in the hematology department. Her responsibility was to perform erythrocyte sedimentation rates (ESR) and to run the hematology cell counter. However, when Martha went to the ESR workstation, she noticed that the centrifuge had been moved onto the same counter. The technician from the urinalysis laboratory said he would be using the centrifuge most of the morning. Martha then told her supervisor that no ESR tests could be performed until the centrifuge was removed from that counter.

1. Why did Martha tell the supervisor no ESR tests could be performed? Was she simply upset because someone else was working in her laboratory? Explain your answer.
2. What technical factors can affect the Westergren ESR method?

CRITICAL THINKING

Howard, a hematology technologist in a small hospital, has been asked to investigate new ESR methods that give rapid results and require smaller blood volumes than the modified Westergren method currently used. He has found a method that meets the laboratory's budget and has listed five features of the test method:

1. Results available in 10 minutes
2. Capillary blood is collected into special microtubes that fit directly into instrument
3. Microtubes are plastic
4. Sample size is 20 µL
5. Method does not require transfer of blood from one tube to another

For each feature, note whether it is an advantage or disadvantage and explain why. Which feature has the biggest potential disadvantage, and why?

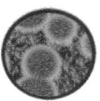

SUMMARY

The ESR is a nonspecific test. The results can be used to detect inflammation that might not be detected by other tests. The test can also be used to follow the progress of certain diseases or the response to treatment for diseases such as rheumatoid arthritis and other inflammatory diseases.

The ESR test is affected by many factors; the technician must follow the instructions for the specific method used and take care to eliminate environmental and technical factors that could cause erroneous test results. Several methods are available for measuring the ESR. The procedure for the particular method being used must be followed and the results must be compared to reference values for that method.

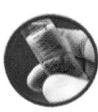

REVIEW QUESTIONS

1. Why would an ESR test be ordered?
2. What four properties of blood affect the ESR? Explain how the ESR is affected by each of these factors.
3. Name five conditions or diseases in which the ESR would be increased.
4. What two conditions usually have a low ESR?

5. How are the ESR and CRP test results used?
6. What are the reference values for the ESR using the Wintrobe method? Westergren method?
7. Name four technical factors that can affect the sed rate.
8. Name two automated methods for performing an ESR.
9. Name four advantages of automated ESR methods over manual methods.
10. Define acute phase proteins, aggregate, inflammation, polycythemia, rouleau(x), sedimentation, Westergren pipet, and Wintrobe tube.

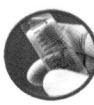

STUDENT ACTIVITIES

1. Complete the written examination for this lesson.
2. Practice performing the ESR as outlined on the Student Performance Guide.
3. Evaluate the effect of technical factors on the ESR: set up three ESR tests on the same blood sample. Follow the test procedure for one tube, place one tube in the refrigerator, and place one tube at an angle at room temperature. At the end of 1 hour, compare the results from the three tests and explain them.

WEB ACTIVITIES

1. Use the Internet to find information about two types of rapid, automated ESR tests not mentioned in this lesson. Report on the specimen required, technology incorporated, results time, and reliability of results compared to the Westergren reference method.
2. Search the Internet for tutorials or videos demonstrating the ESR procedure.

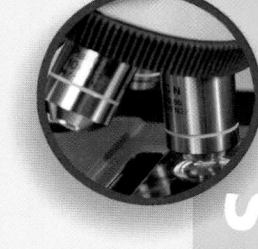

LESSON 2-13
Erythrocyte Sedimentation Rate

(Answers may vary based on the blood specimens provided by the instructor.)

Name _____ Date _____

INSTRUCTIONS

1. Practice performing the ESR test following the step-by-step procedure.

2. Demonstrate the ESR procedure satisfactorily for the instructor using the Student Performance Guide. Your instructor will explain the procedures for evaluating and grading your performance. Your performance may be given a number grade, letter grade, or satisfactory (S) or unsatisfactory (U) depending on course on institutional policy.

NOTE: Consult the manufacturer's package insert for specific instructions for the ESR kit being used.

MATERIALS AND EQUIPMENT

- gloves
- hand antiseptic
- full-face protection (or equivalent PPE)
- acrylic safety shield (optional)
- sample of venous blood collected in EDTA
- test tube rack
- Sediplast kit (or other ESR kit) with instructions for use:
  - Sedivial and rack
  - Sediplast autozeroing pipet
  - Micropipetter capable of delivering up to 1.0 mL
- timer
- paper towels
- laboratory tissue
- surface disinfectant (such as 10% chlorine bleach)
- biohazard container
- sharps container

PROCEDURE

Record in the comment section any problems encountered while practicing the procedure (or have a fellow student or the instructor evaluate your performance).

S = Satisfactory
U = Unsatisfactory

You must:	S	U	Evaluation/Comments
1. Wash hands with antiseptic and put on gloves			
2. Assemble equipment and materials for Sediplast ESR			
3. Put on face protection (or position acrylic safety shield)			
4. Mix blood sample gently for 2 minutes			
5. Remove stopper on sedivial and use micropipetter to fill vial to the indicated mark with 0.8 mL blood. Discard used pipet tip into sharps container. Replace stopper and invert vial several times to mix			
6. Place sedivial in Sediplast rack on a level surface			

(Continues)

You must:	S	U	Evaluation/Comments
7. Insert the disposable Sediplast autozeroing pipet gently through the pierceable stopper with a twisting motion and push pipet down until it rests on the bottom of the vial. The blood level will autozero in the pipet, and excess blood will flow into the sealed reservoir compartment			
8. Check to see that tube is vertical and set timer for 1 hour			
9. Return blood sample to storage. (If no laboratory work will be performed during the incubation, remove gloves, discard appropriately, and wash hands with antiseptic. Re-glove before handling test materials)			
10. Let the Sediplast pipet stand undisturbed for exactly 1 hour and then read the results of the ESR: Use the scale on the pipet to measure the distance from the plasma meniscus to the top of the RBC column			
11. Record the sedimentation rate as: ESR (Mod. Westergren, 1 hr) _____ mm			
12. Discard the Sediplast pipet and vial into a sharps container			
13. Discard other contaminated items into appropriate bio-hazard container			
14. Clean work area with disinfectant			
15. Remove gloves and discard into biohazard container			
16. Wash hands with antiseptic			

Instructor/Evaluator Comments:

Instructor/Evaluator _____ Date _____

© 2012 Delmar, Cengage Learning. Permission to reproduce for clinical use granted.

UNIT 3

Basic Hemostasis

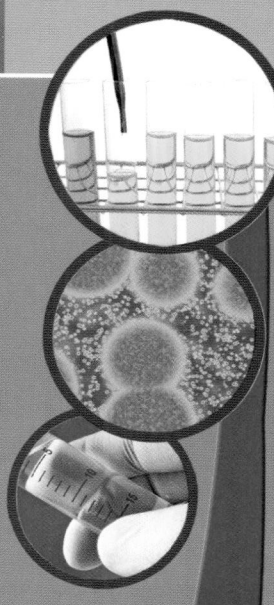

UNIT OBJECTIVES

After studying this unit, the student will:

- Explain the processes involved in hemostasis.
- Discuss acquired and inherited disorders of hemostasis.
- Discuss the use of instrumentation in coagulation testing.
- Discuss two principles of clot detection used in coagulation analyzers.
- Name five tests used to detect coagulation disorders and explain the purpose of each test.
- Explain how anticoagulant therapy is used and monitored.
- Perform an activated clotting time (ACT) test.
- Perform a prothrombin time test.
- Perform an activated partial thromboplastin time (APTT) test.
- Perform a D-dimer test.
- Correlate coagulation test results with hemostasis disorders.
- Discuss safety procedures that must be followed in coagulation testing.
- Discuss the importance of a comprehensive quality assessment program in coagulation testing.

UNIT OVERVIEW

Unit 3 is an introduction to the complex topic of hemostasis— the processes of stopping bleeding by the formation of clots— as well as fibrinolysis, the dissolving of clots. Lesson 3-1, Introduction to Hemostasis, describes the basic principles of hemostasis and the mechanisms that regulate blood clotting. Disorders of hemostasis, including inherited and acquired conditions of platelets and coagulation factors, are discussed in Lesson 3-2.

Coagulation testing methods and the technologies used in coagulation analyzers are discussed in Lesson 3-3. Also included is an explanation of the activated clotting time (ACT). The prothrombin time and the activated partial thromboplastin time (APTT), frequently ordered coagulation screening tests, are covered in Lessons 3-4 and 3-5. These tests illustrate and evaluate the ability of plasma proteins to form a fibrin clot. The tests are used to monitor anticoagulant therapy or to help identify coagulation factor deficiencies. Lesson 3-6 explains three coagulation problems that can create emergency situations and gives the principle and procedure for the D-dimer test—a rapid test useful in these situations.

Unit 3 covers selected clinical laboratory coagulation procedures that illustrate some basic principles of hemostasis and coagulation. However, these procedures represent only a few of the large variety of tests performed in the coagulation laboratory.

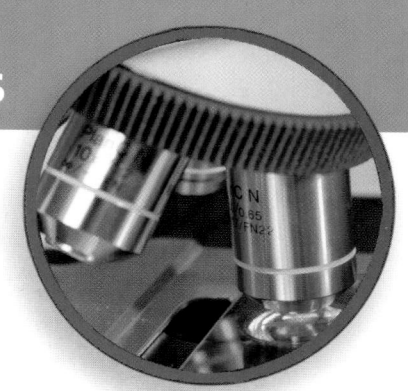

Garza, D. & Becan-McBride, K. (2009). *Phlebotomy handbook: blood specimen collection from basic to advanced.* (8th ed.). Upper Saddle River, NJ: Prentice Hall.

Goodnight, S. & Hathaway, W. E. (2001). *Disorders of hemostasis & thrombosis: A clinical guide.* (2nd ed.). Lancaster, PA: McGraw Hill.

Greer, J. P., et al. (Eds.). (2008). *Wintrobe's clinical hematology.* (12th ed.). Philadelphia: Lippincott Williams & Wilkins.

Harmening, D. M. (2008). *Clinical hematology and fundamentals of hemostasis.* (5th ed.). Philadelphia: F. A. Davis Co.

Hillman, R .S., et al. (2005). *Hematology in clinical practice.* (4th ed.). New York: McGraw-Hill Medical Publishing Division.

Hoeltke, L. B. (2006). *The complete textbook of phlebotomy.* (3rd ed.). Clifton Park, NY: Delmar Cengage Learning.

Jacobs, D. S., et al. (2004). *The laboratory test handbook.* (3rd ed.). Cleveland, OH: Lexi-Comp.

McClatchey, K. D. (Ed.). (2002). *Clinical laboratory medicine.* (2nd ed.) Baltimore: Lippincott Williams & Wilkins.

McPherson, R. A. & Pincus, M. R. (Eds.) (2006). *Henry's clinical diagnosis & management by laboratory methods.* (21st ed.). Philadelphia: Saunders Elsevier.

O'Shaughnessy, D., et al. (Eds.). (2005). *Practical hemostasis and thrombosis.* Ames, IA: Blackwell Publishers.

Rogers, G. M. (2001). *Case studies in hemostasis: laboratory diagnosis and management.* Chicago: American Society of Clinical Pathology.

Package Inserts

Clearview D-Dimer package insert. Distributed by Inverness Medical Professional Diagnostics, Princeton, NJ.

D-dimer Wellcotest package insert. Remel Inc., Lenexa, KS.

HEMOCHRON Jr. Package insert. ITC, Edison, NJ.

Web Sites of Interest

Lab Tests Online, www.labtestsonline.org

Medscape from WebMD, www.medscape.com

National Hemophilia Foundation, www.hemophilia.org

National Institutes of Health, www.nih.gov

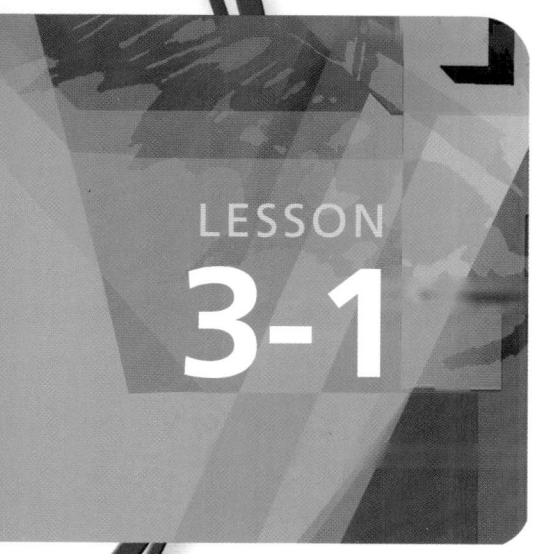

Introduction to Hemostasis

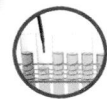

LESSON OBJECTIVES

After studying this lesson, the student will:

- ⊙ Explain the interaction of the blood vessels, platelets, and coagulation factors in hemostasis.
- ⊙ Describe the mechanisms of platelet adhesion and aggregation.
- ⊙ List the coagulation factors.
- ⊙ Name the coagulation factors produced in the liver.
- ⊙ Diagram the intrinsic pathway of hemostasis.
- ⊙ Diagram the extrinsic pathway of hemostasis.
- ⊙ Diagram the common pathway of hemostasis.
- ⊙ Explain how the three hemostasis pathways interact.
- ⊙ Explain the role of inhibitors in the hemostasis process.
- ⊙ Explain the process of fibrinolysis.
- ⊙ Describe the role of anticoagulant therapy in preventing and treating thrombus formation.
- ⊙ Define the glossary terms.

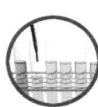

GLOSSARY

adhesion / the act of two parts or surfaces sticking together

aggregation / the collecting of separate objects into one mass

arteriosclerosis / abnormal thickening and hardening of the arterial walls, causing loss of elasticity and impaired blood circulation

atherosclerosis / a form of arteriosclerosis in which lipids, calcium, cholesterol, and other substances deposit on the inner walls of the arteries

coagulation / the process of forming a fibrin clot

coagulation factors / a group of plasma proteins (and the mineral calcium) involved in blood clotting

collagen / a protein connective tissue found in skin, bone, ligaments, and cartilage

Coumadin / an anticoagulant drug derived from coumarin that is administered orally to prevent blood clotting or to reduce the risk of clots; a trade name for warfarin

D-dimer / the smallest cross-linked fibrin degradation fragment formed from the breakdown of polymerized fibrin by plasmin

embolus (pl. emboli) / a mass (clot) of blood or foreign matter carried in the circulation

(continues)

endothelium / the layer of epithelial cells that lines blood vessels and the serous cavities of the body

FDPs / fibrinogen or fibrin monomer degradation products formed when plasmin cleaves fibrinogen or fibrin monomers into protein fragments; formerly called fibrin split products

fibrin / a protein formed from fibrinogen by the action of thrombin

fibrinogen / a plasma protein produced in the liver and converted to fibrin through the action of thrombin

fibrinolysis / enzymatic breakdown of a blood clot

glycoprotein/ a protein molecule having a carbohydrate component

hemorrhage / uncontrolled bleeding

hemostasis / the process of stopping bleeding, which includes clot formation and dissolution

heparin / an anticoagulant used therapeutically to prevent thrombosis; also used as an anticoagulant in certain laboratory procedures

inhibitor/ a substance that retards or stops a process or chemical reaction

intravascular / within the blood vessels

ionized calcium / in the body, a mineral that plays an important role in hemostasis

megakaryocyte / a large bone marrow cell from which platelets are derived

plasmin / an enzyme that binds to fibrin and initiates breakdown of the fibrin clot (fibrinolysis)

plasminogen / the inactive precursor of plasmin

prothrombin / the precursor of thrombin; factor II

sequestered/ isolated or set apart from the whole

thrombin / a protein formed from prothrombin by the action of thromboplastin and other factors in the presence of calcium ions; factor II_a

thromboplastin / a lipoprotein found in endothelium and other tissue; coagulation factor III; also called tissue factor

thrombus (pl. thrombi) / a blood clot that obstructs a blood vessel

vasoconstriction / narrowing of the diameter of a blood vessel

warfarin/ an anticoagulant drug taken to prevent blood clotting or to reduce the risk of clots

XDPs/ degradation products formed by plasmin action on cross-linked fibrin and containing the D-dimer fragment

INTRODUCTION

Blood normally circulates through the body in a liquid form via the arteries, veins, and capillaries. Problems arise when blood is lost from the vessels by bleeding, or when an **intravascular** clot obstructs a blood vessel.

    Hemostasis is the process of stopping the loss of blood from blood vessels. This process involves four interrelated and interdependent systems, as shown in Figure 3-1: the blood vessels, platelets, blood coagulation factors, and **fibrinolysis**, the enzymatic breakdown of a clot.

PRINCIPLES OF HEMOSTASIS

In the majority of patients, hemostasis functions normally; bleeding is stopped by clot formation, and unwanted or excessive clot formation is prevented by the body's circulating **inhibitors**. An inhibitor is a substance that retards or stops a process or chemical reaction.

    Congenital and acquired abnormalities can affect hemostasis. Problems can range from easy bruising to **hemorrhage**, which is uncontrolled bleeding. Conversely, undesirable clotting events

such formation of a **thrombus** or an **embolus** can occur. Both hemorrhage and excessive or pathological clotting can be life-threatening events.

The Role of Blood Vessels

The vascular phase of hemostasis includes a variety of responses that occur when a blood vessel is damaged. One reaction is **vasoconstriction**, the narrowing of the vessel to reduce blood flow to the damaged area. When a vessel is completely severed, the cut ends retract and are compressed by the contraction of skeletal muscle. Small capillary vessels seal themselves together if the damaged edges touch. **Collagen**, a protein connective tissue exposed when the **endothelium** lining the blood vessels is damaged, plays an important role in platelet activation.

The Role of Platelets

Platelets are cytoplasmic fragments of bone marrow cells called **megakaryocytes**. As platelets are released from the megakaryocyte, they enter the circulation (there is no bone platelet marrow

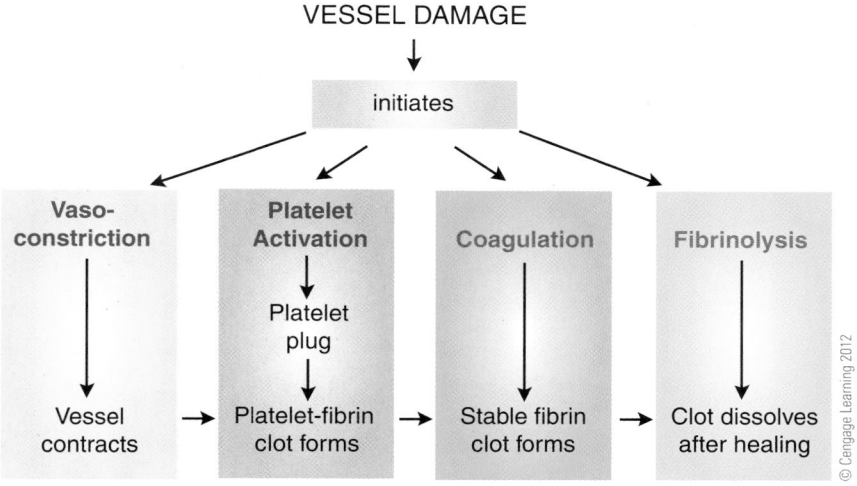

FIGURE 3-1 Interaction of the four processes involved in hemostasis

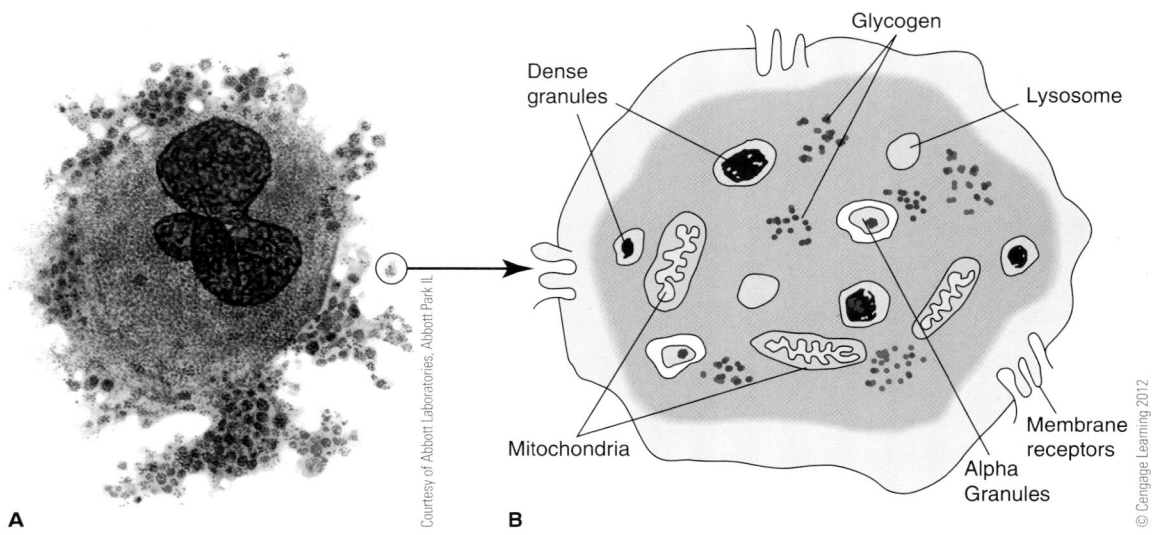

FIGURE 3-2 Megakaryocyte and platelets: (A) Illustration of megakaryocyte releasing platelets (circle with arrow); (B) enlarged diagram of the complex internal structure of a platelet, showing the various organelles

reserve). Eighty percent of platelets are circulating in the blood and the remaining 20% are **sequestered** in the spleen. The average life span of a platelet in circulation is 7 to 10 days.

Platelets do not have a nucleus and thus are not complete cells. However, platelets do contain mitochondria that act in metabolism and specific granules that are essential to **coagulation**, the formation of a fibrin clot (Figure 3-2B). Over 40 substances are secreted from platelet granules during the reactions that accompany adhesion and aggregation.

Platelets have a rounded disk-like shape while circulating in the bloodstream. However, platelets undergo a shape change when they come in contact with the exposed collagen in the wall of a damaged blood vessel. Platelet contact with collagen initiates platelet **adhesion**, the act of the individual platelets sticking to the damaged edge of the vessel (Figure 3-3). Normal adhesion requires von Willebrand's factor (vWF) and platelet **glycoprotein**.

As platelets adhere to the exposed endothelium, they become activated and release substances such as ionized calcium and the glycoprotein complex GP IIb/IIIa from their granules. The platelets then change from their normal disc-like shape into spheres with spiny projections forming over their surfaces. About 25% of the protein in platelets consists of the contractile proteins actin and myosin that are required for platelet shape change; this shape change is initiated by the release of ADP from the platelets and the exposed endothelium. These spiny platelets react with each other to form an aggregate (Figure 3-3). This **aggregation** reaction also requires sufficient ionized calcium and fibrinogen.

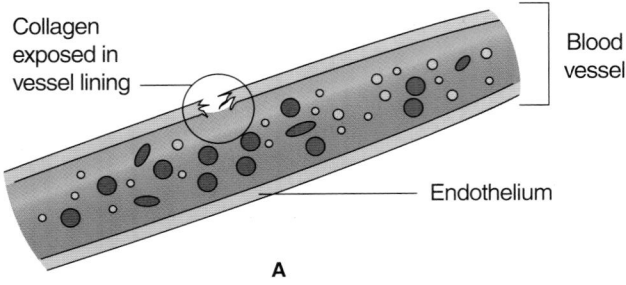

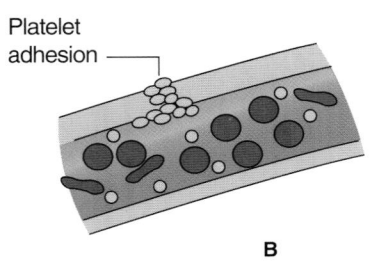

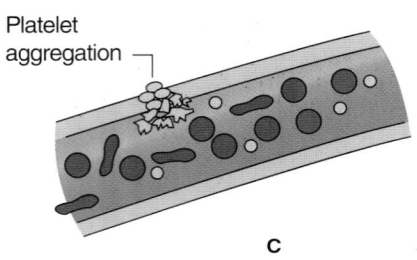

© Cengage Learning 2012

FIGURE 3-3 Illustration of platelet activation in a small wound: (A) collagen becomes exposed in vessel lining; (B) platelet adhesion occurs; followed by (C) platelet aggregation

Because of the large number of platelets present in circulating blood, a platelet plug forms within seconds to stop bleeding from a small wound, such as that caused by a capillary puncture (Figure 3-3). Platelets stabilize the clot and release factor V and platelet factor 3 (PF3) to accelerate the coagulation cascade. The result is stabilization of the platelet plug by strands of fibrin.

The Role of Coagulation Factors

The **coagulation factors** are plasma substances that participate in the formation of the fibrin clot. The coagulation factors are proteins except for **ionized calcium** (Ca^{++}), formerly called factor IV. Most of the protein coagulation factors are produced in the liver.

The coagulation factor numbers and names are listed in Table 3-1. The major coagulation factors are numbered I through XIII, in the order in which they were discovered, not in the order of their action. (The numbers IV and VI are no longer used.) Factors II, VII, IX, and X are vitamin K–dependent; sufficient vitamin K is required for these factors to be synthesized. In addition, two of the factors are named but have no number.

TABLE 3-1. The coagulation factor

FACTOR NUMBER	FACTOR NAME
Factor I	Fibrinogen
Factor II	Prothrombin
Factor III	Thromboplastin, tissue factor (TF)
[*formerly named Factor IV*]	Ionized calcium (Ca^{++})
Factor V	Prothrombin accelerator
Factor VII	Proconvertin
Factor VIII:C	Antihemophilic factor (AHF)
Factor IX	Christmas factor
Factor X	Stuart-Prower factor
Factor XI	Plasma thromboplastin antecedent (PTA)
Factor XII	Hageman factor (contact factor)
Factor XIII	Fibrin-stabilizing factor
[*no number assigned*]	Fitzgerald factor (high-molecular- weight kininogen)
[*no number assigned*]	Fletcher factor (prekallikrein)

Note: Some references use different names for the numbered factors.

The factors circulate in their inactive forms. When a vessel becomes damaged, a series of complex enzymatic reactions leads to the activation of the coagulation factors and formation of the fibrin clot. Platelets stabilize the clot and release factor V and platelet factor 3 (PF3) to accelerate the coagulation cascade by activating clotting factors. The result is stabilization of the platelet plug by strands of fibrin.

Coagulation factor interaction involves very complex reactions. However, the entire process can be summarized in two general reactions: (1) the conversion of **prothrombin** to **thrombin** in the presence of PF3, factor Va, and calcium ions and (2) the conversion of **fibrinogen** to **fibrin** as a result of the action of thrombin (Figure 3-4). The result is the production of a stable fibrin clot to stop the bleeding. Although many other factors, activators, and inhibitors have been discovered since this concept was first put forth, the basic concept developed in the early 1900s is still valid today.

Fibrinolysis

The fibrin clot serves as a temporary structure until the damaged area heals. The clot is then digested by the action of enzymes in a complex process called fibrinolysis (Figure 3-5). Two important components of the fibrinolytic system are **plasminogen** and **plasmin**. Plasminogen is the inactive form of plasmin

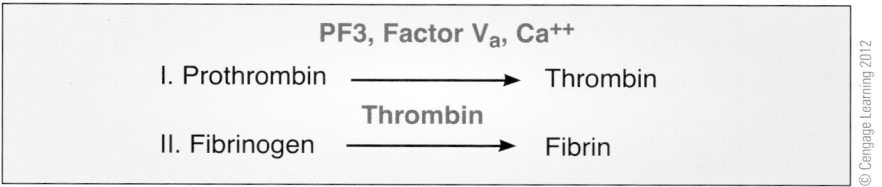

FIGURE 3-4 Simple illustration showing the conversion of prothrombin to fibrin

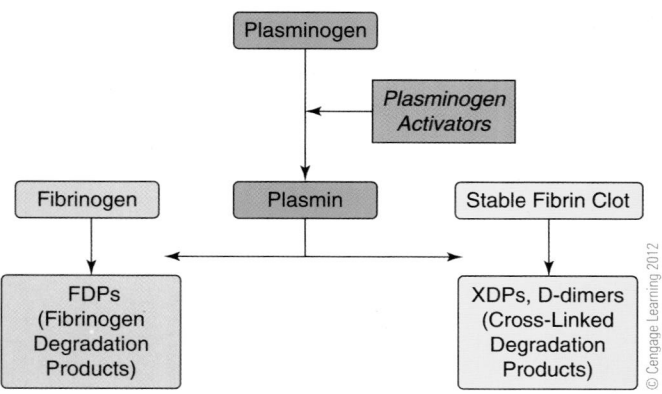

FIGURE 3-5 Diagram illustrating the mechanism of fibrinolysis

present in circulating blood. As blood flows past a fibrin clot, increasing amounts of plasminogen become bound to the clot. Endothelial cells around the injury site release *tissue plasminogen activator* (tPA), which converts the bound plasminogen to plasmin. Upon activation, plasmin acts enzymatically to break down fibrinogen and fibrin in the clot, creating fragments called fibrinogen and fibrin monomer degradation products (**FDPs**) and cross-linked fibrin degradation products (**XDPs**) which contain **D-dimers** (Figure 3-5). Undesired or excessive fibrinolysis is kept in check by inhibitors such as *alpha 2-antiplasmin* (α_2-antiplasmin) and *thrombin activatable fibrinolysis inhibitor* (TAFI).

THE COAGULATION PATHWAYS

The three coagulation pathways are the extrinsic, intrinsic, and common pathways. The coagulation process involves activation of the common pathway by either the extrinsic or the intrinsic pathway. Some interaction also occurs between the extrinsic and the intrinsic pathways. Figure 3-6 illustrates the interrelationship of the three pathways.

The Extrinsic Pathway

The extrinsic pathway is so named because one of the coagulation factors involved, factor III, is not present in circulating blood. Factor III, also called tissue factor or **thromboplastin**, is released when blood vessel endothelium is damaged. Factor III is a lipoprotein composed of protein and phospholipid and acts

as a cofactor in the activation of factor VII to VII$_a$. The calcium required for the reaction is released from platelet granules when the platelets adhere to the endothelial membrane. Activated factor VII (VII$_a$) then participates in the reaction converting X to X$_a$ (Figure 3-6).

The Intrinsic Pathway

All of the factors required to activate the intrinsic pathway are present in the circulating blood. This pathway is initiated when factor XII, contact factor, is activated by contact with certain surfaces to form XII$_a$. For instance, the intrinsic pathway is activated and clotting is initiated when blood contacts glass, such when blood is collected in a tube without anticoagulant.

The final reaction in the intrinsic pathway is the conversion of factor VIII to VIII$_a$. Platelet factor 3 (PF3), a phospholipid released from the platelet membranes, is also required in the activation of factor VIII to factor VIII$_a$ by IX$_a$. Factor IX can also be activated by factor III (tissue factor). Factor VIII$_a$ converts factor X to X$_a$ (Figure 3-6).

The Common Pathway

The extrinsic and intrinsic pathways both result in the conversion of factor X to activated factor X (X$_a$). The common pathway is a series of complex reactions initiated by X$_a$. The common pathway also includes activation of factor V in the presence of phospholipid and ionized calcium, resulting in the conversion of prothrombin to thrombin. Thrombin then acts as a catalyst in the conversion of fibrinogen to fibrin to form a fibrin clot (Figure 3-6). The fibrin clot is stabilized by factor XIII$_a$.

CONTROL MECHANISMS IN HEMOSTASIS

In normal circumstances, a clot forms only at the site of injury. Normal fibrinolytic mechanisms along with other regulating and inhibitor systems prevent an isolated injury from initiating the clotting mechanism throughout the body. Normal endothelium lining the blood vessels can also act as a regulator, preventing platelets from adhering and aggregating. In addition, certain plasma proteins can act as circulating coagulation inhibitors to prevent the formation of unwanted clots (Table 3-2). These proteins include protein C, protein S, and protein Z as well as antithrombin III and tissue factor pathway inhibitor (TFPI).

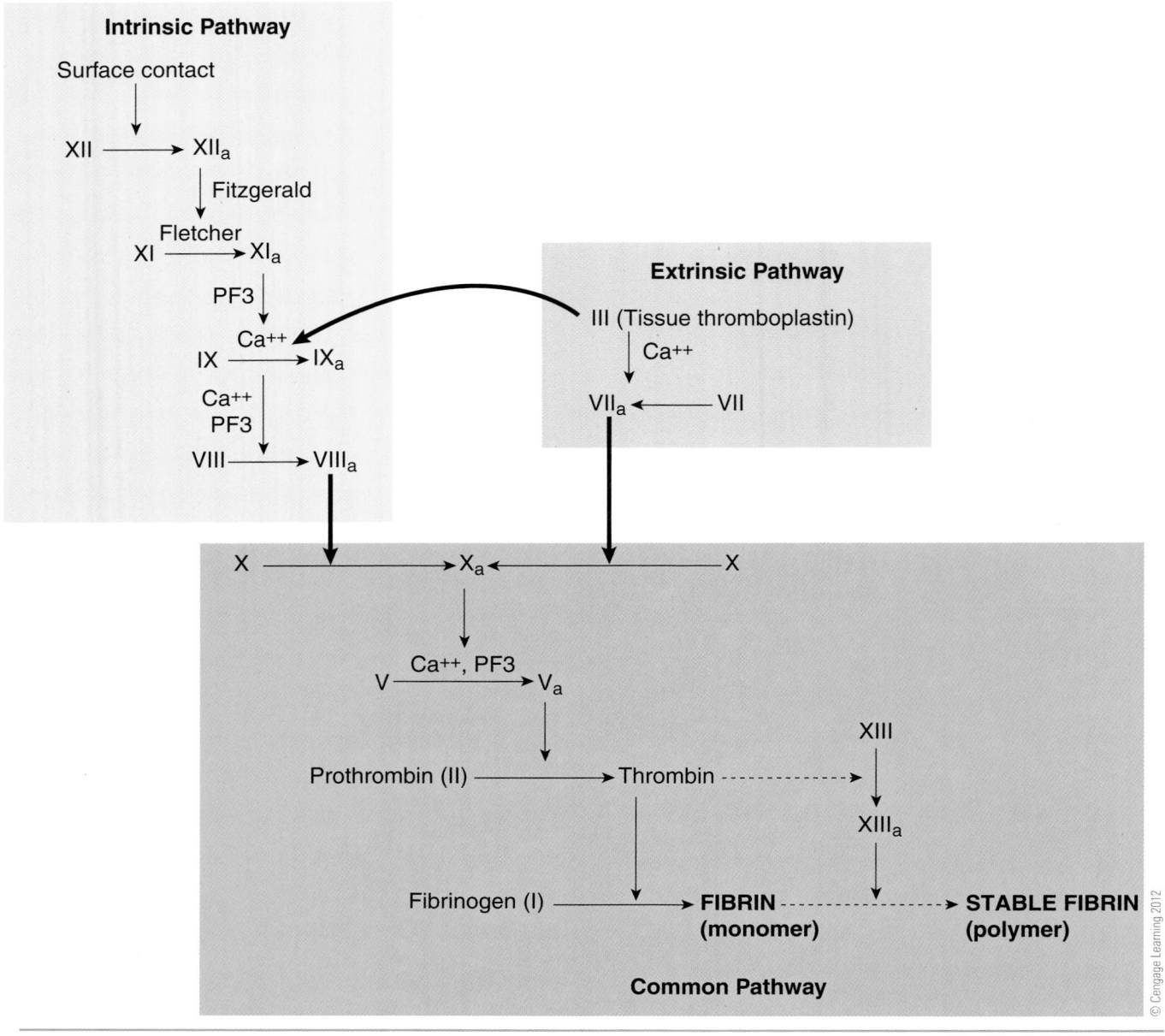

FIGURE 3-6 Schematic of the coagulation cascade showing the interractions of the intrinisic, extrinsic, and common coagulation pathways

TABLE 3-2. Naturally occurring coagulation inhibitors and their effects	
INHIBITOR	**EFFECT**
Antithrombin III	Inhibits thrombin
Protein C/S combination	Inactivates factors V_a and VIII_a
Tissue factor pathway inhibitor (TFPI)	Prevents activation of prothrombin by X_a
Protein Z	Inhibits factor X_a

CONDITIONS REQUIRING ANTICOAGULANT THERAPIES

Sometimes the hemostasis mechanism goes amiss and formation of intravascular blood clots becomes a problem. These situations can often be treated or managed by the use of anticoagulant drugs.

Thrombus and Embolus Formation

An example of a condition that can lead to intravascular blood clots is **atherosclerosis**, a form of **arteriosclerosis**.

In atherosclerosis, the endothelial lining of the blood vessel walls become rough and irregular. This can cause platelets to become activated and initiate the formation of clots within the blood vessels (intravascular clotting). A blood clot attached to a vessel wall is called a thrombus, but when it breaks off and travels through the circulatory system it is called an embolus. Emboli are especially dangerous because they can become lodged in small vessels in the brain, lungs, and other organs. This can cause serious damage and sometimes death unless the emboli are dissolved. In larger arteries, thrombus formation is not much of a problem because the velocity of blood flow quickly washes away and dilutes any initiator of such clots. Sluggish blood flow in smaller vessels caused by atherosclerosis or other conditions gives these thrombi a chance to form.

Anticoagulant Therapy

Patients who develop thrombi or have conditions that make them at risk for developing thrombi can be placed on anticoagulant therapy to reduce that risk. Examples are patients who have undergone major surgical procedures, such as heart valve replacement or joint replacement (hip or knee). Oral anticoagulants can also be prescribed for conditions such as atherosclerosis, phlebitis, or arterial stent implants.

Several drugs are available that can interfere with one or more parts of hemostasis. These drugs differ in mechanism of action, but the end result is the same—decreased tendency to form fibrin clots (Table 3-3).

Aspirin is a low-risk oral antiplatelet drug. Aspirin inhibits platelet aggregation, thereby decreasing the risk for clot formation caused by unwanted platelet activation. Clopidogrel (trade name Plavix) is another antiplatelet drug prescribed to prevent clot formation.

Other anticoagulant drugs work by inhibiting the activation of the plasma coagulation factors. Two anticoagulants in this category commonly used for prevention and treatment of thrombosis are **warfarin** (trade name **Coumadin**) and **heparin**. Warfarin is a vitamin K antagonist that interferes with production of the vitamin K–dependent coagulation factors. Heparin is a naturally occurring anticoagulant that inhibits the activation of thrombin and factor X. Heparin administered intravenously is effective immediately but is usually used only short-term. Both warfarin and heparin can be administered orally. Use of oral anticoagulants allows patients to return home and be treated as outpatients.

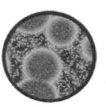

SUMMARY

Hemostasis, the process of stopping the loss of blood, is a delicate balance between coagulation and fibrinolysis. This balance is maintained through the interaction of the blood vessels, platelets, coagulation factors, and components of the fibrinolytic system. Abnormalities or deficiencies in any part of the hemostasis system can cause conditions of excessive clotting or excessive bleeding. These conditions can range from mild to life-threatening.

Blood vessels help control bleeding by vasoconstriction. Platelets help control bleeding by forming a plug at the site of vessel injury and releasing several chemicals that help initiate the coagulation process. Plasma coagulation factors undergo a series of chemical changes that result in the formation of a fibrin clot, providing a more stable way of inhibiting blood flow. The fibrin clot is then dissolved through a process of reactions called fibrinolysis. In certain conditions, regulation of the balance between clot formation and clot dissolution must be managed by drug therapy. Common drugs used are the anticoagulants heparin and warfarin and the antiplatelet drugs aspirin and clopidogrel; these drugs can prevent undesirable clot formation in patients at risk.

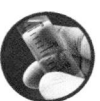

REVIEW QUESTIONS

1. List the four interrelated systems that have a role in hemostasis.
2. Describe the blood vessels' role in hemostasis.
3. Outline the role of platelets in clot formation.
4. Describe the role of the coagulation factors in hemostasis.
5. List the coagulation factors that are vitamin K dependent.
6. Explain how atherosclerosis can cause thrombus formation.
7. Name four naturally occurring inhibitors to coagulation.
8. What is the function of plasmin?
9. What products are formed as the result of plasmin activation?
10. Name the three pathways in the coagulation cascade and the factors involved in each.
11. How can vitamin K deficiency affect hemostasis?
12. Name two conditions for which anticoagulant (antithrombotic) therapy might be required.
13. Name three drugs commonly used for antithrombotic therapy.
14. Define adhesion, aggregation, arteriosclerosis, atherosclerosis, coagulation, coagulation factors, collagen, Coumadin, D-dimer, embolus, endothelium, FDPs, fibrin, fibrinogen, fibrinolysis, glycoprotein, hemorrhage, hemostasis, heparin, inhibitor, intravascular, ionized calcium, megakaryocyte, plasmin, plasminogen, prothrombin, sequestered, thrombin, thromboplastin, thrombus, vasoconstriction, warfarin, and XDPs.

TABLE 3-3. Antithrombotic drugs and their modes of action

DRUG	MECHANISM OF ACTION
Warfarin (Coumadin)	Inhibits vitamin K–dependent factors
Heparin	Inhibits thrombin and factor X
Clopidogrel (Plavix)	Inhibits platelet aggregation
Aspirin	Inhibits platelet aggregation and release of PF3

STUDENT ACTIVITIES

1. Complete the written examination for this lesson.

2. Research and report on laboratory tests of platelet function.

3. Interview a cardiac rehabilitation educator about causes and complications of atherosclerosis.

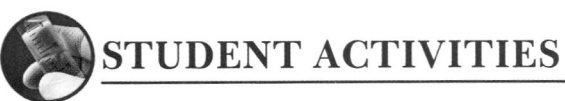

WEB ACTIVITIES

1. Use the Internet to find tutorials explaining components of hemostasis. Be sure to use only web sites from reliable sources such as the government, universities, professional organizations, or research foundations.

2. Use the Internet to find prescribing information from the manufacturer of either clopidogrel or oral heparin. Report on the drug's mechanism of action in clot prevention.

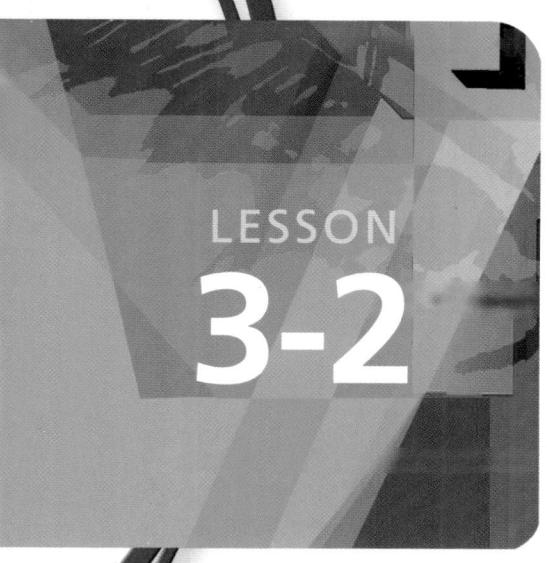

LESSON 3-2

Disorders of Hemostasis

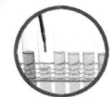

LESSON OBJECTIVES

After studying this lesson, the student will:

- ⊙ Discuss two inherited abnormalities of platelets.
- ⊙ Discuss two acquired abnormalities of platelets.
- ⊙ Discuss two inherited coagulation factor abnormalities.
- ⊙ Discuss two acquired coagulation factor abnormalities.
- ⊙ Explain the differences between hemophilia A and hemophilia B.
- ⊙ List the coagulation factors that are vitamin K dependent.
- ⊙ Explain the purpose of the bleeding time test.
- ⊙ Describe how the Ivy bleeding time test is performed.
- ⊙ Explain how disseminated intravascular coagulation (DIC) occurs.
- ⊙ Define the glossary terms.

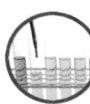

GLOSSARY

disseminated intravascular coagulation (DIC) / a bleeding disorder characterized by widespread thrombotic and secondary fibrinolytic reactions

epistaxis/ nosebleed

hemophilia / a bleeding disorder resulting from a hereditary coagulation factor deficiency or dysfunction

immune thrombocytopenic purpura (ITP) / a blood disorder characterized by purpura in skin and mucous membranes and low platelet count caused by the destruction of platelets by antiplatelet autoantibodies; also called idiopathic thrombocytopenic purpura

NSAIDs / acronym for nonsteroidal anti-inflammatory drugs

petechiae / small, purplish hemorrhagic spots on the skin; very small purpura

purpura / purple-colored areas that can occur in the skin, mucous membranes, or organs and that are caused when small blood vessels leak

recombinant / referring to molecules or cells created as a result of genetic engineering

thrombocytopathy / abnormal platelet function

(continues)

thrombotic thrombocytopenic purpura (TTP) / a blood disorder with varied causes and characterized by formation of clots in the small vessels, consumption of platelets, and skin purpura

von Willebrand's disease (vWD) / an inherited platelet disorder associated with decreased platelet adhesion and a bleeding tendency

INTRODUCTION

Hemostasis disorders have a variety of causes. A disorder can be inherited, such as classic hemophilia, or acquired such as factor abnormalities resulting from a vitamin K deficiency. Acquired disorders can also arise because of medications, such as the effect of aspirin on platelet aggregation. Other drugs or treatments can accelerate clot formation. These inherited and acquired disorders of hemostasis affect patients' lives and require a combination of clinical examination, laboratory tests, and investigation into family medical history for diagnosis.

HEREDITARY DISORDERS OF HEMOSTASIS

Inherited disorders of hemostasis cause lifelong problems with abnormal bleeding. Coagulation factors or platelets can be affected (Table 3-4).

TABLE 3-4. Examples of inherited and acquired disorders of hemostasis*

COAGULATION FACTOR DISORDERS	
ACQUIRED	**INHERITED**
Vitamin K deficiency	Hemophilia A
Anticoagulant therapy	Hemophilia B
Disseminated intravascular coagulation (DIC)	Deficiencies or dysfunction of coagulation factors
Autoantibodies to coagulation factor(s)	

PLATELET DISORDERS	
ACQUIRED	**INHERITED**
Aspirin ingestion	von Willebrand's disease (vWD)
Decreased megakaryocyte production	Bernard-Soulier syndrome
Immune thrombocytopenic purpura (ITP)	Glanzmann's thrombasthenia
Thrombotic thrombocytopenic purpura (TTP)	
Sequestration in spleen	

* This table lists only a few disorders and is not meant to be a comprehensive list.

Inherited Coagulation Factor Disorders

The **hemophilias** are inherited diseases in which a deficiency or functional disorder occurs in one or more of the coagulation factors (Table 3-4). Classic hemophilia, called *hemophilia A*, is caused by a functional deficiency of a portion of the coagulation factor VIII molecule, the VIII:C protein. Hemophilia B, also called Christmas disease, is named after the first patient in whom it was studied. The defect in Christmas disease is a functional deficiency of coagulation factor IX.

Hemophilias A and B are inherited as sex-linked recessive genes carried on the X chromosome. Because males inherit one X and one Y chromosome, if the inherited X chromosome carries the recessive hemophilia gene, the disease will be expressed. Females have two X chromosomes; those who carry the recessive hemophilia gene on one X chromosome will not manifest the disease because the normal gene on the other X chromosome will be dominant. These females are *carriers* and can pass the recessive gene to their offspring. Therefore, the diseases are limited almost exclusively to males, although there have been rare cases documented in females.

The clinical symptoms of hemophilia A and hemophilia B are identical. Affected infants do not have symptoms unless they undergo circumcision or other surgery. However, as the child grows and is subject to bumps and falls, large bruises appear. Abnormal bleeding occurs into the joints, causing swelling and pain. In addition, bleeding occurs in the mouth, muscles, renal tract, and gut, and after dental extractions.

Additional disorders caused by defects in the coagulation factors can also occur. The defect can be in the factor structure or function (qualitative defect) or the factor may be present in insufficient quantity to participate in a reaction (quantitative defect). These cases are rare, but the defective or absent factor can be identified by performing coagulation tests while substituting, one at a time, commercially available factors. The substituted factor that normalizes the patient's test result is the factor that is defective or missing in the patient.

Inherited Platelet Disorders

Several inherited disorders of platelets cause abnormal bleeding in the patient (Table 3-4). The most common inherited bleeding disorder is a platelet disorder called **von Willebrand's disease (vWD)**; the National Hemophilia Foundation estimates that over 2 million people in the United States have vWD. Von Willebrand's disease is not truly a disease, but is a hemostatic condition caused by a deficiency or functional abnormality of von Willebrand factor (vWF), a glycoprotein secreted by storage granules in platelets and by endothelial cells. If von Willebrand's factor is absent or deficient, the glycoprotein receptors Ib/IX on the platelet membrane cannot bind to the blood vessel endothelium. Platelet numbers are normal, but platelet adhesion is decreased or absent. Primary hemostasis is impaired because interaction between the platelets and the vessel wall is defective. Factor VIII also is affected because vWF binds and stabilizes it. Patients with vWD also have a decreased quantity of factor VIII. Most cases of von Willebrand's disease are mild and display symptoms such as **epistaxis** (nose bleeds), bleeding of the gums, and easy bruising. Unlike the classic hemophilias, von Willebrand's disease is inherited as an autosomal trait, and can occur in both males and females.

Two additional inherited conditions that have **thrombocytopathy**, or abnormal platelet function, are *Bernard-Soulier syndrome* and *Glanzmann's thrombasthenia*. Bernard-Soulier syndrome is a disorder in which the platelets are larger than normal and are present in normal or decreased numbers. The platelets' ability to adhere is decreased because of a defect in the platelet surface membrane. Affected patients develop small, purplish spots on the skin called **petechiae**. They also suffer gastrointestinal bleeding, nosebleeds, abnormal menstrual bleeding, or intracranial bleeding. The disease can be severe and even fatal.

In *Glanzmann's thrombasthenia*, the platelet count and platelet morphology are usually normal. The platelets have normal adhesion to collagen but do not have normal aggregation with other platelets. The surface membranes of platelets lack the glycoprotein complex GpIIb/IIIa necessary for the release mechanism that results in aggregation. In these patients, platelets do not form clumps when blood smears are made from blood collected without anticoagulant. The patient's bleeding problems are similar to those of the Bernard-Soulier patient.

ACQUIRED DISORDERS OF HEMOSTASIS

Acquired disorders of hemostasis can cause either abnormal bleeding or thrombus formation. The disorders can affect one or more of the coagulation factors or the platelets (Table 3-4).

Acquired Coagulation Factor Disorders

Examples of acquired factor disorders include:

- Vitamin K deficiency
- Disseminated intravascular coagulation (DIC)
- Circulating inhibitors to coagulation factors

Severe deficiency of vitamin K causes decreased production of the vitamin K–dependent coagulation factors, factors II, VII, IX, and X. The oral anticoagulant warfarin (Coumadin), often prescribed to reduce unwanted clotting, acts as a vitamin K antagonist, causing a decrease in the vitamin K–dependent factors. Other causes of vitamin K deficiency include insufficient vitamin K in diet (rare), malabsorption of vitamin K from the intestine, liver disease, and prolonged treatment with antibiotics.

Disseminated intravascular coagulation (DIC) is a serious condition in which trauma or a pathological process initiates coagulation and secondary fibrinolysis. Depending on the balance between the two systems, either thrombosis or bleeding can occur or a combination of the two. Some conditions that contribute to DIC are crushing injuries; certain bacterial, viral, or rickettsial infections; and drug reactions.

DIC occurs when intravascular coagulation is triggered. This causes fibrin deposition in blood vessels, which depletes the available supply of coagulation factors. Microthrombi form in vital organs, including the kidneys, lungs, heart, and brain. The fibrinolytic system is then activated, releasing fibrin fragments that can act as coagulation inhibitors.

Another cause of bleeding disorders is the development of circulating autoantibodies. These usually are directed at one or more of the clotting factors, causing the factor(s) to be removed from the blood and creating a factor deficiency.

Acquired Platelet Disorders

Acquired platelet disorders can arise from several sources (Table 3-4). *Acquired thrombocytopenia* can occur when the spleen enlarges, which can occur secondary to infection or a variety of diseases. The enlarged spleen traps (sequesters) many platelets inside the spleen, reducing the number of circulating platelets. Infection by certain viruses can decrease the bone marrow production of megakaryocytes, causing thrombocytopenia.

Immune thrombocytopenic purpura (ITP) occurs when the immune system produces antibodies against the patient's own platelets. ITP is characterized by low platelet count and the presence of **purpura**, purple-colored areas that can occur in the skin, mucous membranes, or organs caused when small blood vessels leak.

Thrombotic thrombocytopenic purpura (TTP) is a condition in which microthrombi are deposited in blood vessels. TTP can be acquired or congenital. The microthrombi block circulation, damaging various organs of the body. Many platelets are consumed in the formation of these microthrombi, causing the patient to become thrombocytopenic. Recent evidence has shown that in rare instances TTP can be caused by certain agents such as chemotherapeutic and immunosuppressant drugs.

Ingestion of aspirin affects the aggregation of platelets by inhibiting the platelet-release reaction. This inhibition begins within 45 minutes of aspirin ingestion. The effect on individual platelets is irreversible and continues for the life of the platelet (up to 8 to 10 days). Other nonsteroidal anti-inflammatory drugs (**NSAIDs**) such as ibuprofen and naproxen also affect platelets, but the effect is reversible within hours of discontinuing the drug.

TESTS OF HEMOSTATIC FUNCTION

Examination of hemostatic function can involve testing the platelets, the blood vessels, or the coagulation factors. Commonly performed tests include the prothrombin time, activated partial thromboplastin time (APTT), and platelet count. Less frequently performed coagulation tests include bleeding time, thrombin time, fibrinogen assay, and platelet function tests. Expected laboratory results for some disorders of hemostasis are shown in Table 3-5.

Tests of Vessel and Platelet Functions

Platelet Tests

The platelet count is a quantitative test for platelets. Even if the platelet count is in the normal reference range, a bleeding problem can still exist if the platelets do not function normally (Table 3-5). Platelet aggregation tests are tests of platelet function. (See Lesson 3-3 for more information on platelet aggregation.)

Bleeding Time

The *bleeding time* is a screening test for quantitative or qualitative abnormalities in the platelets and also for vascular integrity of the capillaries. The two methods of performing the bleeding time test are the Duke method and the Ivy method. However, the Duke method is rarely performed because of problems with standardization.

The Ivy method is performed on the patient's forearm in an area with no visible veins (Figure 3-7). The site is cleansed and

TABLE 3-5. Expected laboratory results for some disorders of hemostasis

CONDITION	TEST RESULTS			
	PROTHROMBIN TIME	ACTIVATED PARTIAL THROMBOPLASTIN TIME	BLEEDING TIME	PLATELET COUNT
Hemophilia A	Normal	Prolonged	Normal	Normal
Hemophilia B	Normal	Prolonged	Normal	Normal
von Willebrand's disease	Prolonged	Prolonged	Prolonged	Normal
Warfarin anticoagulant therapy	Prolonged	Prolonged	Normal	Normal
Glanzmann's thrombasthenia	Normal	Normal	Prolonged	Normal
ITP	Normal	Normal	Prolonged	Below normal

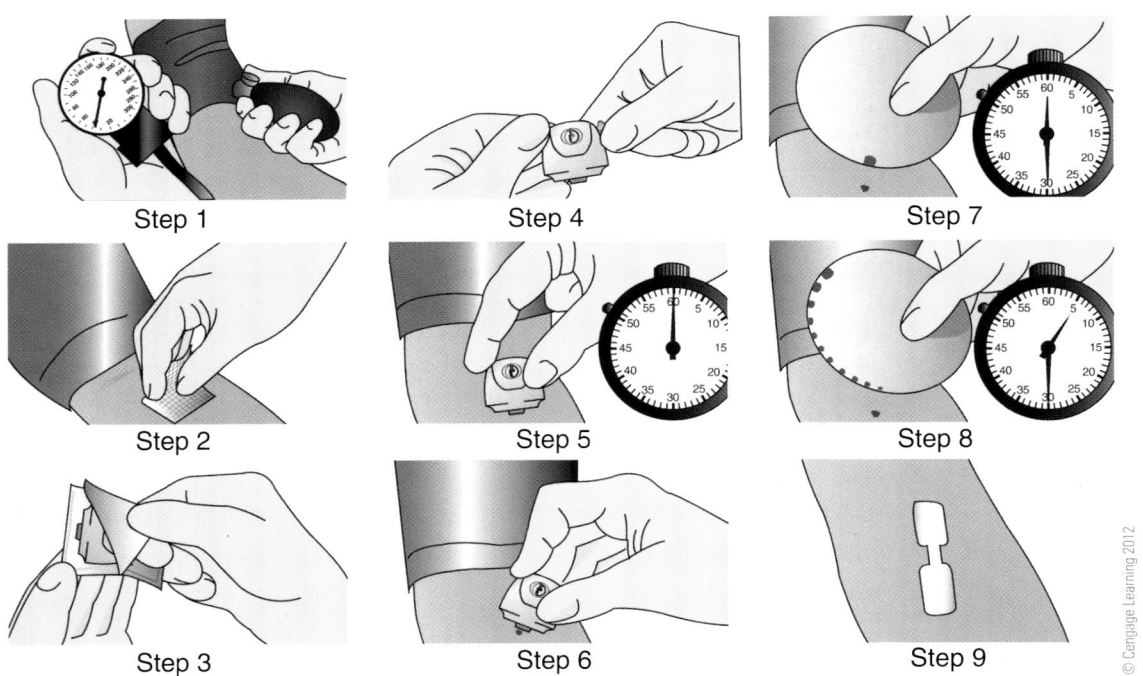

Step 1
Step 2
Step 3
Step 4
Step 5
Step 6
Step 7
Step 8
Step 9

© Cengage Learning 2012

FIGURE 3-7 Illustration of the Ivy bleeding time: (step 1) Blood pressure cuff is inflated to 40 mm Hg; (steps 5-6) incision is made on cleansed forearm; (steps 7-8) blood is wicked with filter paper every 30 seconds until blood flow stops

CURRENT TOPICS

HEMOPHILIA

Hemophilia, the oldest known inherited blood disorder, is caused by low levels or complete lack of a functional blood protein essential for clotting. Hemophilia A is caused by a deficiency in factor VIII; hemophilia B is caused by a lack of factor IX.

There are about 20,000 hemophiliacs in the United States; approximately 85% have hemophilia A, and 14% have hemophilia B (source: National Hemophilia Foundation Symposium, 2011). Each year about 400 infants are born with the disorder. The severity of the disease is related to the levels of functional coagulation factors in the blood. Approximately 70% of patients have less than 1% of the normal factor level and therefore have severe disease. However, when the factor level is increased to just 5% of normal, the patient usually has only a mild form of disease and bleeding events are rare except after injuries or surgery.

Treatment—Treatment of hemophilia has historically involved transfusion of plasma containing the needed factor. This traditionally has been *on-demand* therapy given only when bleeding symptoms appear. Usually by that time bleeding into the joints has already occurred. This repeated internal bleeding causes joint damage. In some European countries, treatments are given periodically to keep the factor level high enough to prevent bleeding, joint destruction, and hemorrhage. However, because these patients must have an indwelling venous catheter to have frequent access to the veins, there is an increased risk for infection.

The most serious challenges to successful treatment are:

- Maintaining safety of factor products
- Managing inhibitor formation
- Preventing irreversible joint damage
- Preventing life-threatening hemorrhage
- Making progress toward a cure

The Hemophilia Treatment Centers and National Institutes of Health (NIH) sponsor more than 100 hemophilia treatment centers around the United States. These organizations also coordinate treatment and offer grants for scientific research into improved treatment. For example, after hurricanes Katrina and Rita in 2005, they organized efforts to ensure that patients could receive treatments in Houston, Texas.

In the past, safety of blood products used for treatment of hemophilias has been a major concern. With improved testing methods and techniques to inactivate viruses, the risk for becoming infected with human immunodeficiency virus (HIV) or one of the hepatitis viruses is now mostly a thing of the past. However, there is still concern over the potential of these products to transmit emerging diseases such as variant Creutzfeldt-Jakob disease (vCJD)—the human form of "mad cow disease."

Research—Factor VIII can now be produced by biotechnology. **Recombinant** factor VIII is entirely free of blood components. Although the cost is higher for this form, it is clearly the choice for young children because it is free of viruses and plasma proteins that can cause allergic reactions and immunosuppression. Recombinant factor IX has also been produced. Research areas of special interest are the potential development of:

- Modified factor VIII or IX proteins with improved biological activity and/or increased functional half-life
- Drugs to improve the activity or biological availability of factors
- Novel hemostatic agents such as small molecules to promote hemostasis
- Ways to use immunosuppressive agents to prevent immune response to factor therapies

Although hemophilia remains a potentially life-threatening condition, progress is being made. Gene therapy is one area of current research. The prognosis should improve as more scientific research is applied to patient care.

a blood pressure cuff is placed on the upper arm and inflated to 40 mm Hg. A bleeding time device such as the Surgicutt is placed onto the site and the trigger is activated to release the blade, which makes a very small standardized incision. At the same time a timer is started. Filter paper is used to touch the blood (not the incision) at 30-second intervals, continuing until no blood appears on the paper. The timer is then stopped—this is the bleeding time. The normal reference range for the Ivy bleeding time is 2 to 9 minutes. When the bleeding time is prolonged, more definitive tests such as platelet adhesion and platelet aggregation must be performed (Table 3-5).

Tests of the Coagulation Pathways

Several tests of the coagulation pathways can be performed in the coagulation laboratory. These tests are discussed in general in Lesson 3-3. Two of the commonly performed tests, the prothrombin time and the APTT, are explained in Lessons 3-4 and 3-5. The prothrombin time is a measure of extrinsic coagulation pathway function; the APTT is a test of intrinsic coagulation pathway function. Instruments used in coagulation testing are discussed in Lessons 3-3 and 3-4.

CASE STUDY

Ms. Clark, a 63-year-old patient, had been taking an aspirin-containing over-the-counter medication daily for mild arthritic pain. She was scheduled for minor surgery, and her surgeon ordered an Ivy bleeding-time test after Ms. Clark reported that she had several bruises but did not remember injuring herself. The bleeding-time was 13 minutes; the surgeon postponed the surgery and told Ms. Clark to stop taking the medication.

1. When should the surgeon order another bleeding-time test?
   a. When the bruises are gone
   b. 8 to 10 days after the last dose of the pain reliever
   c. After results from other coagulation tests are received
   d. About 3 to 5 days after pain reliever is discontinued
2. Explain your answer.

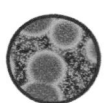

SUMMARY

Hemostasis disorders can result from abnormalities or deficiencies in platelets, blood vessels, coagulation factors, or a combination of these. Disorders can be inherited or acquired and can cause conditions ranging from mild to life-threatening. Hemophilia A and hemophilia B are examples of inherited disorders of hemostasis. Certain drugs and cancer treatments can cause an acquired thrombocytopenia. Acquired coagulation factor deficiencies can be occur because of anticoagulant therapy or conditions such as liver disease. Ongoing research in hemostasis disorders and improved treatments such as use of recombinant coagulation factors contribute to improved diagnosis and treatment of these disorders.

Coagulation testing is usually performed because a patient is receiving anticoagulant therapy, having an unwanted clotting or bleeding problem, or is scheduled for major surgery. Tests for hemostatic function can be as simple as a platelet count and prothrombin time or as complex as assays for factor deficiencies and platelet aggregation tests. Advances in knowledge about the hemostasis process and in instrument technologies have resulted in new and better tests available to aid in the diagnosis of hemostasis disorders.

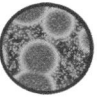

REVIEW QUESTIONS

1. Name two acquired platelet disorders and two inherited platelet disorders.
2. What is the effect of aspirin on platelets?
3. How do NSAIDs affect platelets?
4. List the vitamin K–dependent coagulation factors.
5. Name two hereditary coagulation factor disorders.
6. Describe the clinical symptoms of hemophilia A and hemophilia B.
7. Explain why hemophilia A and hemophilia B are almost exclusively limited to males.
8. What percent of hemophilia patients have hemophilia B?
9. Discuss treatments for hemophilia.
10. What is the purpose of the bleeding time test?
11. Explain the procedure for the Ivy bleeding time test.
12. Discuss conditions that contribute to DIC.
13. How does the defect in von Willebrand's disease affect platelets?

14. Define disseminated intravascular coagulation (DIC), epistaxis, hemophilia, immune thrombocytopenic purpura (ITP), NSAIDS, petechiae, purpura, recombinant, thrombocytopathy, thrombotic thrombocytopenic purpura (TTP), and von Willebrand's disease (vWD).

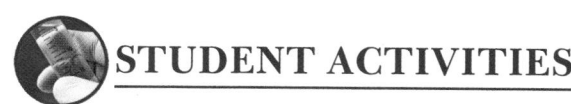

STUDENT ACTIVITIES

1. Complete the written examination for this lesson.
2. Research and report on a hemostasis disorder.

WEB ACTIVITIES

1. Find information about treatment(s) of hemophilias using the Internet and report on them. Use reliable sources such as the National Institutes of Health (NIH) or the National Hemophilia Foundation (www.hemophilia.org).

2. Use the Internet to find information on the genetics governing the inheritance of hemophilia B.

3. Find information about DIC using the Internet. Report on the clinical signs, treatments, and laboratory tests used to identify and evaluate the condition.

4. Use the Internet to research and report on the mechanisms by which nonsteroidal anti-inflammatory drugs (NSAIDs) such as aspirin and ibuprofen affect bleeding time. Find out if acetaminophen affects the bleeding time.

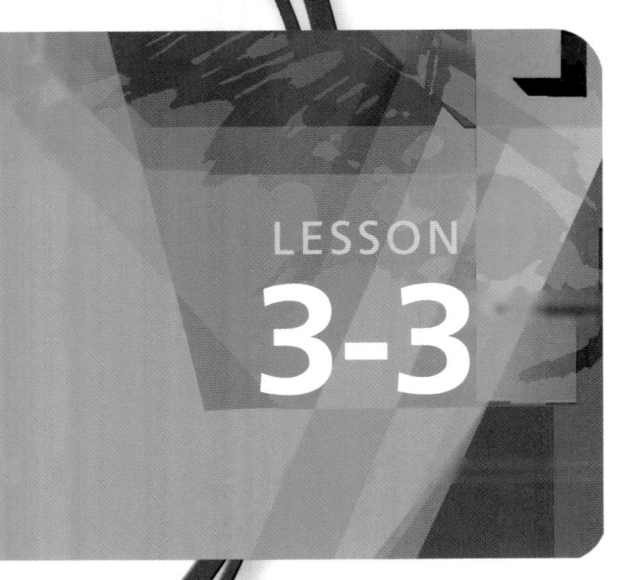

Principles of Coagulation Testing

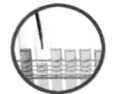

LESSON OBJECTIVES

After studying this lesson, the student will:

- ⊙ Discuss the history of coagulation testing.
- ⊙ Discuss manual and instrument methods of coagulation testing.
- ⊙ Discuss three types of technology used in coagulation analyzers.
- ⊙ List three instruments used in point-of-care coagulation testing.
- ⊙ Explain the significance of the development of the prothrombin time test.
- ⊙ Discuss the value of the activated clotting time (ACT) test.
- ⊙ Perform an activated clotting time (ACT) test.
- ⊙ List the safety precautions to be observed when performing coagulation tests.
- ⊙ Discuss quality assessment procedures to be followed when performing coagulation tests.
- ⊙ Define the glossary terms.

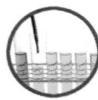

GLOSSARY

activated clotting time (ACT) / a test that assesses the effect of heparin on the ability of blood to clot

heparin / an anticoagulant used therapeutically to prevent thrombosis; also used as an anticoagulant in certain laboratory procedures

INTRODUCTION

Coagulation testing is now performed to determine the reasons for unwanted thrombosis and unexplained bleeding. However, this was not always the case. Until the twentieth century, research was concentrated on finding the reasons for thrombus and embolus formation. Physicians knew that these conditions caused the deaths of many patients. They also knew of the "free bleeders" (hemophiliacs) but were not as concerned with the cause(s) because thrombi and emboli were responsible for more deaths than excessive bleeding.

In the late nineteenth century Schimdt and Hammarsten presented the fundamental concepts of the conversion of

fibrinogen to fibrin by action of the enzyme thrombin (derived from prothrombin) and the requirement of calcium for clotting to occur. However, they were mistaken in their belief that the conversion of prothrombin to thrombin was a result of certain effects of white blood cells and tissues.

In 1905, Paul Morowitz proposed the basic scheme of coagulation in two operations: (1) the enzymatic conversion of prothrombin to thrombin in the presence of calcium and (2) the conversion of fibrinogen to fibrin by the enzyme thrombin. Although many additional coagulation factors and reactions have since been identified, these two reactions still represent the basics of hemostasis.

In the 1930s, Dr. A.J. Quick, a physician and researcher, proposed a test he called the prothrombin test, thinking that it measured only prothrombin. Even though it was later discovered that the test actually measures additional coagulation factors, the name of the test has remained prothrombin time or "protime." The 1930s are held to be the dividing line between the "old" and "new" ages of blood coagulation. Many tests of blood coagulation have been developed from this simple beginning. Some of these tests are used to monitor the therapeutic effects of the anticoagulants **heparin** and warfarin (Coumadin). Several tests have also been developed to detect the by-products of excess fibrinolysis such as occurs in disseminated intravascular coagulation (DIC), a potentially life-threatening condition.

COAGULATION INSTRUMENT TECHNOLOGY

Coagulation tests can be performed manually, one at a time using a point-of-care (POC) instrument, or in batches using semi-automated or completely automated technology (Table 3-6). Many types and sizes of instruments have been developed that can perform coagulation testing.

Most coagulation tests are based on detection of a fibrin clot. Clot detection in the various methods can be organized into the following categories:

- Visual
- Mechanical
- Optical
- Magnetic

Visual Clot Detection Methods

Manual methods for coagulation testing are "hands on." The technician places samples and reagents into a waterbath or heat-block to warm for a prescribed time. The reagents are then added by pipet to the patient sample and a timer started. The timer is stopped when a clot is *visually* observed in the test tube. For example, the prothrombin time can be performed manually by prewarming the patient's plasma and the prothrombin reagent in a water bath. The prothrombin reagent is then added to the pre-measured patient sample and the formation of a clot is viewed in a test tube that is being tilted back and forth by the technician.

TABLE 3-6. Clot detection technology used in coagulation instruments and examples of instruments or methods using the technology

DETECTION TECHNOLOGY	EXAMPLE OF METHOD OR INSTRUMENT
Visual	Manual prothrombin time
Mechanical/Optical	GEM PCL
Mechanical	FibroSystem
Mechanical/Magnetic	Trinity Biotech KCΔ series
LED optical	HEMOCHRON instruments

Fibrometer and Trinity KCΔ Technologies

For many years the standard method of performing a prothrombin time or activated partial thromboplastin time (APTT) was using a fibrometer, manufactured by BBL as the FibroSystem (Figure 3-8A). This test method mirrors the manual test except the heating unit is an integral part of the instrument and the pipetter used to dispense the reagents into the sample also starts the timer. The detection of the clot is *mechanical* (Table 3-6). The timer stops when the moving wire probes in the sample cup detect a clot. The time required for the clot to form, in seconds, is displayed on the fibrometer.

The Trinity Biotech KC1Δ and KC4Δ coagulation instruments are similar in function and ease of use to the FibroSystem (Figure 3-8B). These instruments can be used

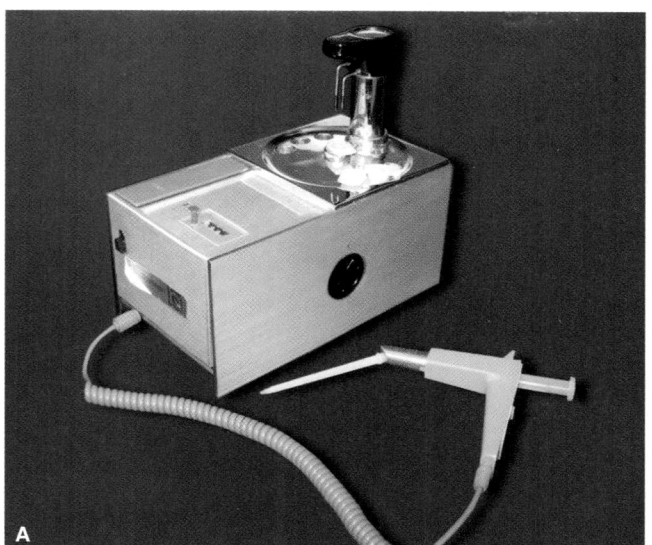

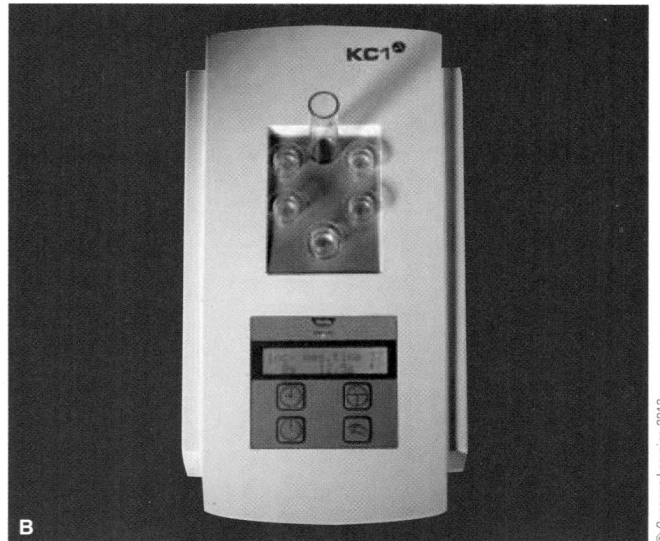

© Cengage Learning 2012

FIGURE 3-8 Coagulation Instruments: (A) FibroSystem; (B) Trinity KC1Δ™

to perform the prothrombin time (Lesson 3-4) and APTT described in Lesson 3-5. In the Trinity instruments, clot detection is by mechanical/magnetic method. The reaction cuvette contains a steel ball held in place by a magnet. The cuvette constantly rotates as reagents are added. The timer stops when the magnetic sensor can no longer hold the steel ball in place, indicating that a clot has formed.

Technologies in Point-of-Care Coagulation Instruments

Several small, handheld instruments are available for coagulation testing; tests performed with many of the instruments are CLIA-waived. These small instruments can be used for near-patient testing at the bedside and in physicians' offices, emergency departments, small clinic laboratories, and other Point-of-Care test sites. A few are approved for in-home testing by patients to monitor anticoagulant therapy (Figure 3-9).

In these POC instruments, the blood sample is introduced into a test cassette or test unit that is manually placed into the instrument. Mixing of the sample is achieved by movement of the reagents and sample within the test channels of the test cassette (within the instrument). When clot formation in the sample is detected, the result is reported digitally on a screen or printed out. Instrument functions available include automatically performing quality control checks, requiring operator identification, printing results, and in some cases storing results.

The HEMOCHRON microcoagulation series of analyzers (Figure 3-10A) and the ProTime analyzer, both from ITC, use *photo-optical* technology to detect the clot. In the HEMOCHRON, an array of LED optical detectors signals when

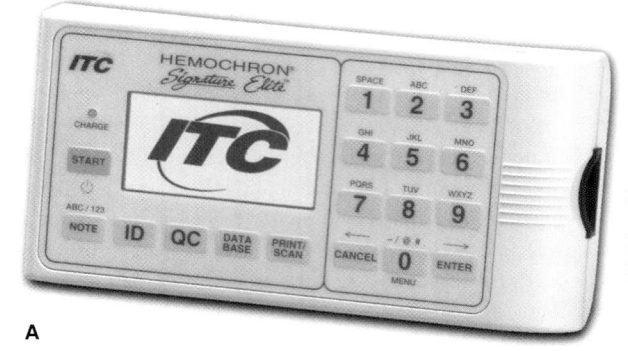

A

Courtesy of ITC, Edison, NJ

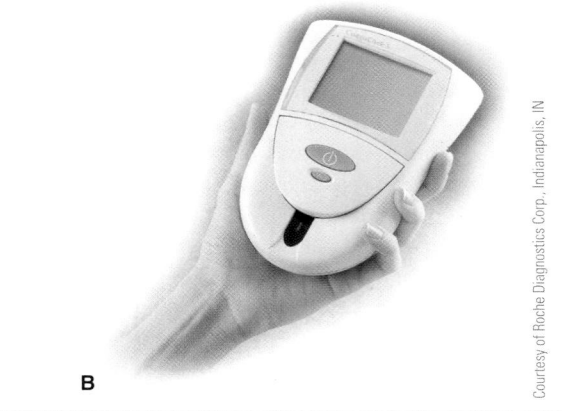

B

Courtesy of Roche Diagnostics Corp., Indianapolis, IN

FIGURE 3-10 Point-of-care coagulation analyzers: (A) Hemochron Jr. Signature Elite; (B) CoaguChek hand-held coagulation analyzer

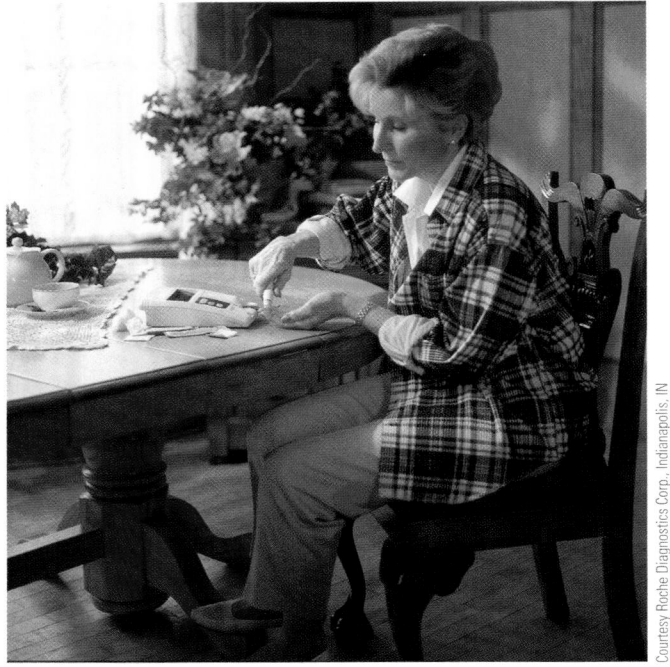

Courtesy Roche Diagnostics Corp., Indianapolis, IN

FIGURE 3-9 Patient performing at-home coagulation testing

movement ceases in the testing cuvette, indicating that a clot has formed. Citrated whole blood is used for the prothrombin time and APTT.

The GEM PCL PLUS from Instrumentation Laboratory (IL) uses a mechanical/optical method of detecting clot formation. The GEM PCL can perform the prothrombin time, the APTT, and the activated clotting time (ACT) using 50 microliters (μL) of whole blood for each. The CoaguChek S from Roche Diagnostics (Figure 3-10B) is CLIA-waived, making it suitable for testing in POLs and at POC. Clotting is detected optically in the COATRON M-1 from TECO, which performs a variety of coagulation tests.

Automated Methods for Coagulation Testing

Several automated instruments are available for use in laboratories performing larger volumes of coagulation tests or specialized testing. Most of these instruments use photometry and/or nephelometry; the ACL TOP$_{700}$ instrument from IL is an example of this type. It can be used for anticoagulant monitoring, but in addition can perform plasma assays for missing or deficient coagulation factors, antithrombin, protein C, protein S, and D-dimer (discussed in Lesson 3-6). This instrument is designed for use in a large hospital laboratory or regional laboratory. The Sysmex CA500 is an example of an instrument for use in a laboratory with a smaller volume or as a backup instrument in a large laboratory.

Platelet Studies

The evaluation of platelet function is important in the choice of therapies for several hemostasis disorders. Use of instruments such as platelet aggregometers makes these complex tests relatively simple to perform. The Bio/Data Platelet Aggregation Profiler Model PAP is a light transmission aggregometer (Figure 3-11). A variety of tests can be performed, including studies with antiplatelet drugs. Platelet aggregation tests are performed by measuring the rate of platelet aggregation when platelet-rich plasma is treated with known aggregating agents such as collagen, adenosine diphosphate (ADP), epinephrine, and ristocetin.

Safety Precautions in Coagulation Testing

  Standard Precautions must be observed while performing coagulation testing. Reagents and patient samples must be considered potential biohazards. Appropriate personal protective equipment (PPE) must be worn. When blood samples are collected, whether by capillary puncture or venipuncture, blood collection safety devices must be used, and contaminated materials and sharps disposed of in appropriate containers.

Centrifugation of blood and the transfer of plasma from blood collection tubes present potential hazards. Instruments that use whole blood and/or sample through the tube cap reduce the risk for exposure to biohazards.

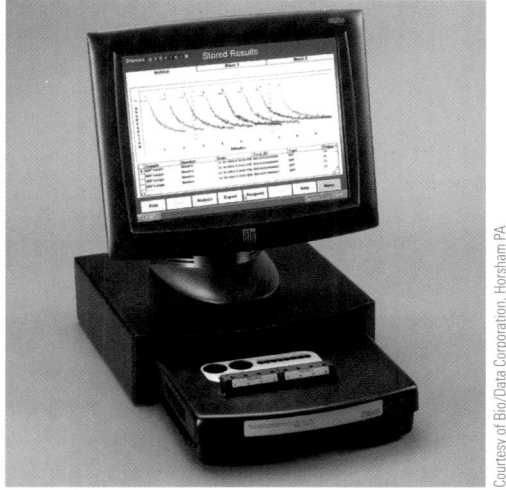

FIGURE 3-11 Platelet Aggregation Profiler Model PAP 8E showing aggregation graphs on screen display

Quality Assessment in Coagulation Testing

   Strict adherence to quality assessment (QA) procedures is essential in coagulation testing. Developing and following a QA protocol in coagulation testing contributes to overall quality management, reliable patient test results, and positive outcomes. The laboratory standard operating procedure (SOP) manual will contain details of test methods and QA procedures that must be followed. These include:

- Specimen collection techniques
- Order of draw
- Choice of anticoagulant and blood-to-anticoagulant ratio
- Specimen processing and storage
- Manufacturer's instructions for use of reagents and instruments
- Required quality control procedures

Specimen Collection

Specimen collection for hemostasis tests must be performed carefully. The venipuncture must be performed with minimal trauma. For capillary puncture, the first drop must be wiped away and excessive pressure at the puncture site must be avoided. Use of incorrect blood collection techniques can cause release of tissue thromboplastin into the blood sample, which can erroneously shorten the test result.

Anticoagulant and Order-of-Draw

The blood collecting tube must contain the correct type and amount of anticoagulant. Unless otherwise stated, the anticoagulant of choice for coagulation tests is 3.2% sodium citrate (in light blue–capped blood collection tubes). Plastic vacuum tubes are designed to draw 2.7 mL of blood into 0.3 mL of sodium citrate anticoagulant, creating a 9:1 blood-to-anticoagulant ratio.

Specimens for coagulation testing must be drawn using the CLSI criteria for order of draw. The sodium citrate tube is drawn first unless a blood culture is also being collected. Collecting the sodium citrate tube first prevents contamination of the sample by the clotting gels (agents) present in some of the red-topped tubes. If a winged collection system is used, a small plain discard tube is filled first and discarded, then the sodium citrate tube is filled. This prevents short draws caused by the air space in the winged collection tubing.

Specimen Processing

The anticoagulated specimen must be centrifuged using the time and speed guidelines in the facility's SOP manual for the coagulation test to be performed. Immediately following centrifugation, the top portion of plasma is removed to a clean tube, which is then capped to prevent evaporation. In general, plasmas can be stored for up to 4 hours before being tested. Temperature of storage is determined by the test procedure. For instance, plasma for APTT testing can be refrigerated at 4° C, but plasma for prothrombin time should not be refrigerated.

Test Reagents and Controls

Manufacturer's instructions must be followed for instrument use and preparation and use of reagents and controls. Controls are usually stored dehydrated and must be reconstituted according to manufacturer's directions. Appropriate controls must be run and the results recorded following the facility's SOP manual.

PERFORMING THE ACTIVATED CLOTTING TIME

The **activated clotting time (ACT)** is a test that assesses the effect of heparin on the ability of blood to clot. It is used to monitor patients receiving moderate- to high-dose heparin therapy while undergoing certain surgeries or procedures such as cardiac catheterization.

Safety Precautions

Standard Precautions must be observed while performing the activated clotting time. Safety needles and lancets should be used for collecting the blood specimen. All contaminated materials and used sharps must be discarded into the appropriate biohazard and sharps containers.

Quality Assessment

The laboratory's SOP manual will contain detailed instructions for the ACT test procedure, the use and maintenance of instruments, and the controls that must be run. Instructions for instrument care and maintenance can change, which makes it imperative to always read the package insert and operation manual accompanying an instrument and to incorporate all manufacturer's updates into the SOP manual. All time constraints of the test packets and blood collection procedures must be followed. Patient results must not be reported until the controls are within acceptable range.

Care and cleaning procedures can differ among instruments; the instructions included with the individual instrument must be followed. For example, the HEMOCHRON manufacturer issued a warning against the use of bleach to clean the instrument after it was found that excess liquid seeping into the instrument could cause falsely elevated ACT times. Instead, the HEMOCHRON should be cleaned with 90% ethanol.

ACT Test Procedure

The ACT test is a rapid test that measures how long it takes for blood to clot when the clotting mechanism is artificially activated. The ACT test measures the anticoagulant *effect* of heparin on the patient's clotting ability; the test does not measure the patient's blood heparin level. The ACT test is a modern version of the Lee-White clotting time, a test formerly used to estimate heparin effect, but which had the disadvantages of being lengthy, cumbersome, not easily standardized, and not very sensitive.

The ACT test is performed on fresh, non-anticoagulated whole blood collected by venipuncture using a plastic syringe. To perform the ACT test, a large drop of whole blood is added to an ACT cartridge containing a clotting activator such as kaolin, celite, silica, or glass particles. The timer starts when the cartridge is inserted into the instrument; the blood and reagent are mixed by internal tilting of the test cartridge. The timer stops when the instrument detects fibrin clot formation. The time required for the blood to clot is reported as the ACT. Laboratories must determine their own reference ranges based on the instrument and method used. The whole blood reference range for the ACT test performed on normal volunteers is 81 to 125 seconds, with the mean being 103 seconds.

The ACT PLUS by Medtronic, Inc. and the GEM PCL and HEMOCHRON (International Technidyne Corporation) are three POC instruments that can perform the ACT. The ACT PLUS is a dedicated ACT instrument. The GEM PCL and HEMOCHRON can perform several coagulation tests. In the HEMOCHRON ACT test, 0.2 mL of whole blood is added to a collection cup in the prewarmed cartridge. The START key is pressed, and the reactions take place in the cartridge inside the analyzer. Detection of a clot by the instrument's photometer determines the end-point. The ACT test result is automatically converted to a reference celite-ACT value reported in seconds.

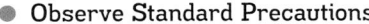

SAFETY REMINDERS

- Review Safety Precautions section before beginning procedure.
- Observe Standard Precautions.
- Wear appropriate PPE when handling control solutions.

PROCEDURAL REMINDERS

- Review Quality Assessment section before beginning procedure.
- Follow instructions in SOP manual.
- Collect correct blood specimen.
- Use the appropriate control solutions.

CASE STUDY

Josh, a newly hired technician, was taking a POC coagulation instrument to a patient's bedside to perform a coagulation test. The instrument was similar to one he had used at his previous employer's laboratory, so even though he had not been trained on the instrument at his new job, he was sure it operated just about the same. The instrument he had used previously accepted whole blood as a sample, so he took capillary puncture equipment with him. Evelyn, the section supervisor, came after him to bring him back to the laboratory.

What could be the reason(s) for Evelyn's action? Explain your answer.

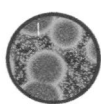

SUMMARY

Coagulation testing methods have evolved over the years. Automated and semi-automated instruments are available to perform coagulation tests. These instruments have simplified testing while improving laboratory efficiency. As new information is discovered about the hemostasis process, new methodologies are continually being developed to make it possible for laboratories to assay a patient's blood to help the physician diagnose and treat conditions more effectively.

Automated coagulation testing has greatly relieved the workload in the hemostasis laboratory. In the past, the technician had to separate the patient sample into aliquots for different instruments to assay. In automated methods, the specimen tube is placed in the instrument tray and the instrument reads the barcode on the tube's label and automatically performs the assays requested.

One of the most important developments in instrument technology is the availability of instruments for POC testing. Small, simple-to-operate instruments have made it possible to increase testing available in physician office laboratories and at POC. Many of these instruments are CLIA-waived, and a few are approved for in-home use by the patient. This is especially convenient for patients who must have the prothrombin time performed every week or two to monitor the therapeutic effect of warfarin.

Portable instruments used at POC require only a very small blood sample and provide results in a few minutes. The availability of POC hemostasis tests can be lifesaving in emergency situations. An example of this is the ability to perform the ACT test at POC in surgery or during heart procedures to evaluate the effect of moderate or high doses of heparin.

Coagulation testing must be performed using Standard Precautions and appropriate PPE. All quality controls, whether electronic or liquid, must be run as prescribed for each assay. The results of the controls must be within the assigned values. When the laboratory has good-quality assessment programs in place and participates in proficiency testing programs, the physician can have confidence in the results used for diagnosis, treatment, and management of hemostatic disorders.

REVIEW QUESTIONS

1. What is Dr. A. J. Quick's contribution to the field of coagulation testing?

2. When is the activated clotting time (ACT) test performed?

3. What is measured in the ACT test?

4. What reagent is used in the ACT test?

5. For tests that require citrated, anticoagulated plasma, state the correct blood-to-anticoagulant ratio.

6. Name three clot detection technologies used in coagulation testing.

7. List three advantages of portable coagulation analyzers.

8. Name an instrument that uses a magnetic sensor to detect clotting.

9. Name an instrument that uses mechanical means to detect the clot.

10. Name an instrument that utilizes photo-optics to detect clot formation.

11. What important error can occur while cleaning the HEMO-CHRON instrument?

12. Define activated clotting time (ACT) and heparin.

STUDENT ACTIVITIES

1. Complete the written examination for this lesson.

2. Practice performing the activated clotting time following the step-by-step procedure in the Student Performance Guide.

WEB ACTIVITIES

1. Use the Internet to find information on one of the following: fibrinogen assays, factor assays, or thrombin assays. Report on the assay and include method, instrument required, rationale for performing the test, and significance of test results.

2. Use the Internet to find information on an automated coagulation instrument that performs prothrombin time, APTT, and factor assays. Report the name of the instrument, the manufacturer, and at least five tests that can be performed using the instrument.

3. Search university or instrument manufacturers' web sites for tutorials explaining how to perform coagulation testing.

(Answers may vary based on the types of samples provided by the instructor and instrumentation available)

Name _____ Date _____

INSTRUCTIONS

1. Practice performing the activated clotting time following the step-by-step procedure.

2. Demonstrate the activated clotting time procedure satisfactorily for the instructor using the Student Performance Guide. Your instructor will explain the procedures for evaluating and grading your performance. Your performance may be given a number grade, a letter grade, or satisfactory (S) or unsatisfactory (U) depending on course or institutional policy.

NOTE: The instructions in this performance guide are for the HEMOCHRON instrument. Use the correct supplies and follow the manufacturer's instructions for the specific instrument being used.

MATERIALS AND EQUIPMENT

- gloves
- hand antiseptic
- full-face shield (or equivalent PPE)
- 1 to 3 mL plastic syringe and safety needle for venipuncture
- HEMOCHRON (or other instrument to perform the ACT)
- cuvettes, controls, package inserts, and operating manual for instrument being used
- paper towels
- laboratory tissue
- surface disinfectant (such as 10% chlorine bleach)
- biohazard container
- sharps container

PROCEDURE

  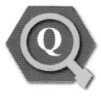

Record in the comment section any problems encountered while practicing the procedure (or have a fellow student or the instructor evaluate your performance).

S = Satisfactory
U = Unsatisfactory

You must:	S	U	Evaluation/Comments
1. Wash hands with antiseptic and put on gloves and face protection			
2. Assemble materials and equipment			
3. Perform the activated clotting time using the HEMOCHRON following steps 3a–3h. If another instrument is used skip to step 4 　a. Prepare whole blood controls for the HEMOCHRON 15 minutes before use, following manufacturer's instructions for rehydration and use 　b. Insert an ACT test cuvette into the slot to turn the instrument ON 　c. Wait for the ADD SAMPLE message to appear.			

(Continues)

© 2012 Delmar, Cengage Learning. Permission to reproduce for clinical use granted.

You must:	S	U	Evaluation/Comments
d. Apply whole blood control to the center of the cuvette well. Fill well, avoiding bubble or foam formation; allow excess sample to spill over into the outer well			
e. Depress the START button			
f. Wait for the result to be displayed, record the result, and compare with the acceptable range for the control level			
g. Repeat steps 3b–3f for a second control level (if available)			
h. Test patient sample following steps h1–h4:			
(1) Insert ACT test cuvette into instrument			
(2) Obtain 1.0 mL of whole blood by venipuncture using a plastic syringe			
(3) Add blood sample to the center of the cuvette well when ADD SAMPLE message appears. Fill well to the top, avoiding bubble or foam formation; allow excess sample to spill over into the outer well			
(4) Wait for the result to be displayed and record the test result			
4. Perform the ACT test using a different instrument, following the manufacturer's directions, or skip to step 5			
5. Discard all sharps into sharps container			
6. Discard other contaminated materials into biohazard container			
7. Clean and disinfect instrument(s) according to manufacturer's instructions and return to storage			
8. Wipe the work area with disinfectant			
9. Remove gloves and discard into biohazard container			
10. Wash hands with antiseptic			

Instructor/Evaluator Comments:

Instructor/Evaluator _____ Date _____

© 2012 Delmar, Cengage Learning. Permission to reproduce for clinical use granted.

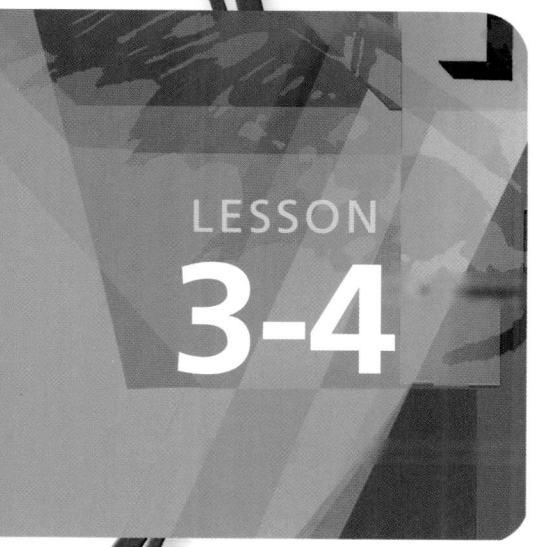

LESSON 3-4

Prothrombin Time

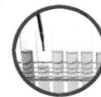

LESSON OBJECTIVES

After studying this lesson, the student will:

- ⊙ Discuss the role of prothrombin in blood coagulation.
- ⊙ Explain the major use of the prothrombin time test.
- ⊙ Perform a prothrombin time test.
- ⊙ State the reference values for the prothrombin time test.
- ⊙ Name three point-of-care (POC) testing instruments for prothrombin time.
- ⊙ Discuss the types of blood specimens used to perform the prothrombin time on POC instruments.
- ⊙ Explain the importance of and use of the international normalized ratio (INR).
- ⊙ Explain the reason for using the international sensitivity index (ISI).
- ⊙ Calculate the INR value.
- ⊙ Discuss how prothrombin time test results are used.
- ⊙ Discuss safety procedures that must be followed when performing the prothrombin time test.
- ⊙ Discuss quality assessment procedures for the prothrombin time test.
- ⊙ Define the glossary terms.

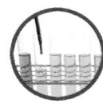

GLOSSARY

enzyme / a protein that causes or accelerates changes in other substances without being changed itself

hypercoagulation / a greater tendency than normal for blood to coagulate

international normalized ratio (INR) / a way of reporting a prothrombin time that takes into consideration the sensitivity of the prothrombin thromboplastin reagent used and the mean prothrombin time of a normal population

international sensitivity index (ISI) / a value assigned to each lot of prothrombin thromboplastin reagent to compensate for variations in sensitivities of thromboplastin from different sources

prothrombin ratio / a comparison of a patient's prothrombin time result with the mean prothrombin time of a normal population

prothrombin time test / a coagulation screening test used to monitor oral anticoagulant therapy

vitamin K / a vitamin essential for production of coagulation factors II, VII, IX, and X

INTRODUCTION

The prothrombin time test was an early coagulation test developed by Dr. A. J. Quick. He named the test prothrombin time because he thought it measured only prothrombin. Although it was subsequently recognized that the test was affected by several coagulation factors in addition to prothrombin, the name of the test has remained *prothrombin time*.

Prothrombin (factor II) is produced in the liver and is **vitamin K** dependent. A deficiency of vitamin K causes reduced production of prothrombin and can result in bleeding tendencies. Vitamin K deficiency can be caused by malabsorption of the vitamin from the intestine or prolonged antibiotic treatment; it is rare for it to occur as a result of a dietary deficiency.

The **prothrombin time** or *protime*, one of the most frequently performed coagulation tests, evaluates the function of the extrinsic and common pathways of hemostasis. The major use of the prothrombin time is to monitor warfarin (Coumadin) anticoagulant therapy; the test is also used as a presurgery coagulation screening test. Warfarin is a vitamin K antagonist, which means it blocks the action of vitamin K. The result is decreased production of prothrombin (factor II) and factors VII, IX, and X by the liver. Prothrombin times in factor deficiencies and other conditions are given in Table 3-7.

A therapeutic dose of warfarin can be prescribed for patients who have had an adverse clotting incident or who have risk factors for **hypercoagulation** (an increased tendency for blood clotting). The level of warfarin activity is indirectly measured by performing periodic prothrombin time tests on the patients' blood. The prothrombin time can be performed at the bedside, in a physician office laboratory (POL), an outpatient laboratory, a reference laboratory, or sometimes at home.

TABLE 3-7. Prothrombin time in factor deficiencies and other conditions

CONDITION	PROTHROMBIN TIME RESULTS
Factor Deficiencies	
VIII	Normal
XI	Normal
XII	Normal
II	Prolonged
V	Prolonged
VII	Prolonged
X	Prolonged
Other Conditions	
Warfarin therapy	Prolonged
Heparin therapy	Prolonged
Liver disease	Prolonged
Vitamin K deficiency	Prolonged

Prothrombin time results are used as a guide in regulating the patient's anticoagulant dosage.

PRINCIPLE OF THE PROTHROMBIN TIME TEST

The hemostasis pathway is activated when damage occurs to blood vessel endothelium or to tissue. The extrinsic pathway is activated by tissue thromboplastin (factor III) in the presence of calcium ions. Factor X, a proenzyme, is converted to the enzyme X_a, which in turn converts prothrombin to the enzyme thrombin (Figure 3-12). An **enzyme** is a protein that is able to cause or accelerate changes in other substances without being changed itself. Thrombin then acts on fibrinogen to form fibrin monomers that make up the initial clot.

The reagent used in the prothrombin test contains a commercial preparation of tissue thromboplastin and calcium chloride, substitutes for the tissue thromboplastin and calcium ions (Ca^{++}) that are coagulation activators of the extrinsic pathway. When anticoagulated normal patient plasma is combined with this reagent, the mechanism leading to formation of a fibrin clot is activated. The time required for the fibrin clot to form is the prothrombin time. If a coagulation factor deficiency exists within the extrinsic or common pathway, the prothrombin time will be prolonged (Table 3-7).

REFERENCE VALUES FOR PROTHROMBIN TIME

Depending on the thromboplastin reagent used, the typical prothrombin time reference range for tests performed using 3.2% citrated plasma is 10 to 13 seconds (Table 3-8). However, it is more useful to report the prothrombin time as either the **prothrombin ratio** or the (preferred) **international normalized ratio (INR)**.

The prothrombin ratio compares the patient's result with the mean of the prothrombin time from a normal population. The INR is a calculated value that allows standardization of prothrombin time reporting among different laboratories. Each lot or batch of thromboplastin reagent can have a different sensitivity in the prothrombin time test. An **international sensitivity index (ISI)** assigned by the manufacturer to each reagent lot is used with the prothrombin time to calculate the INR. Before the use of the INR, a patient could have a prothrombin time test performed on the same day by different laboratories and have different results even though the tests were performed correctly at each laboratory. The reference range for the INR is 1.0 to 1.4 (Table 3-8). Figure 3-13 shows an example of calculating the INR using the ISI.

PERFORMING THE PROTHROMBIN TIME TEST

The prothrombin time can be performed manually or using instruments such as the FibroSystem (Figure 3-14) or KCΔ series; small, handheld point-of-care (POC) instruments;

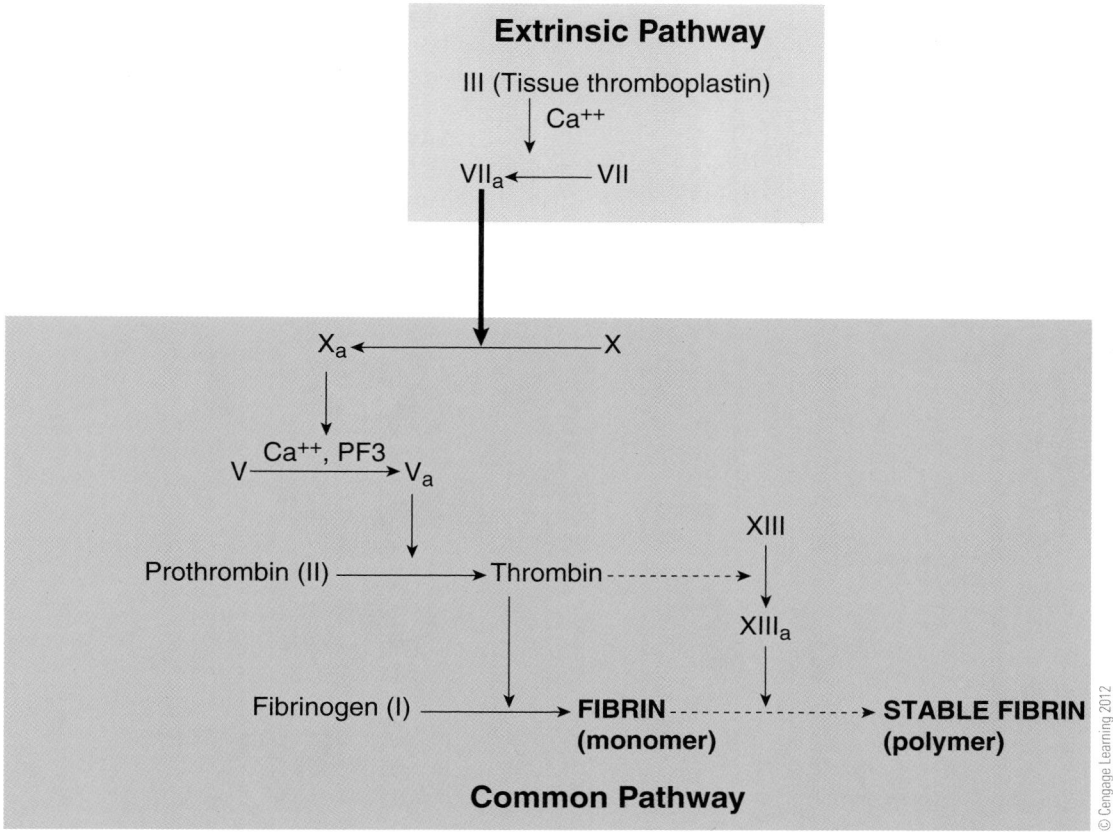

FIGURE 3-12 Diagram of the extrinsic and common coagulation pathways showing how factor X and prothrombin become activated

TABLE 3-8. Reference values for prothrombin time performed on citrated plasma		
	REFERENCE VALUES	
	MEAN	**RANGE (±2 SD)**
Plasma prothrombin time	11.5 seconds	10–13 seconds
INR	–	1.0–1.4

Calculate the International Normalized Ratio (INR) where:
   patient prothrombin time = 23 seconds
   mean normal protime of the facility = 10.5 seconds
   ISI = 1.2

$$INR = \left(\frac{\text{Patient result in seconds}}{\text{Mean normal of the facility in seconds}} \right)^{ISI}$$

$$INR = \left(\frac{23 \text{ sec}}{10.5 \text{ sec}} \right)^{1.2}$$

$$INR = (2.1)^{1.2}$$

$$INR = 2.52$$

FIGURE 3-13 Example of calculating the international normalized ratio (INR)

or coagulation analyzers that can perform several hemostasis tests on the same specimen. The manual method is rarely used, but it has the advantage of the clot being visible as it forms.

The FibroSystem has been used for performing the prothrombin time test for decades. A probe with moving wires detects the formation of the fibrin clot in the sample cup and stops the timer. Trinity Biotech's coagulation analyzers, which include the KC1Δ and the KC4Δ, can be used for prothrombin time tests as well. These instruments are similar to the Fibro-System in that they have a built-in heat block for warming the samples and reagents and a pipetter that starts the timer when the last reagent is added in the test.

Clot formation in the KC1Δ and KC4Δ is detected by a magnetic sensor. The test cuvette contains a steel ball held in place by a magnet; the cuvette rotates constantly during the test (Figure 3-15). When a clot forms, the steel ball becomes trapped in the fibrin clot and pulls away from the magnet, stopping the timer.

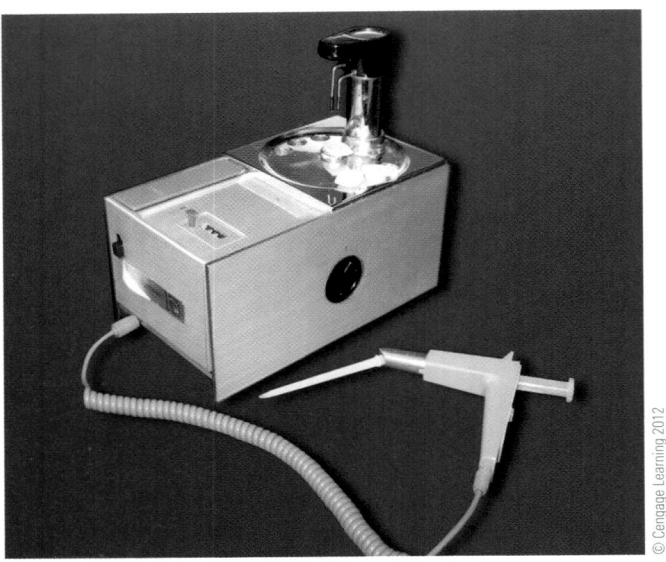

FIGURE 3-14 Fibrosystem

In higher volume laboratories, the prothrombin time test is performed on instruments that are capable of performing several different hemostasis tests on the same plasma sample. Most use photo-optical means to detect clot formation. The instruments for point-of-care (POC) are small, handheld devices that can perform several different coagulation tests, but one at a time.

Safety Precautions

  Standard Precautions must be observed to protect the worker from bloodborne pathogens. Performing the prothrombin time involves handling patient blood and control plasmas derived from human blood. In addition, the technician might also collect and process the blood specimen before testing it. Blood must be collected using safety needles or lancets. Used blood collecting devices must be discarded in appropriate sharps containers. Laboratory safety policies for use of the centrifuge must be followed. To reduce the chance of aerosol formation, tubes of blood must remain capped during centrifugation.

Quality Assessment

    The prothrombin time procedure is detailed in each laboratory's standard operating procedure (SOP) manual. Quality assessment (QA) programs for the prothrombin time test include all facets of the test from collecting and processing the specimen, analyzing control plasmas, and performing the test procedure, to reporting the results.

The venipuncture must be clean (performed without trauma), because trauma to the vein or surrounding tissues releases tissue thromboplastin into the specimen. The ratio of blood to citrate anticoagulant is critical; it must be 9 parts blood to 1 part anticoagulant. The blood collecting tube should be filled to the appropriate level, and must meet specimen acception criteria. The filled collection tube should immediately be gently inverted 4 or 5 times to mix the blood with citrate and avoid formation of microclots. Expired vacuum collection tubes should not be used; they can fail to draw the correct amount of blood because of loss of vacuum or evaporation of the anticoagulant.

Centrifugation time and speed will be specified in the SOP manual and must be adequate to create platelet-poor plasma. The top portion of plasma should be removed immediately after centrifugation and stored at room temperature in a capped tube if testing is going to be delayed. Plasma for prothrombin time should not be refrigerated.

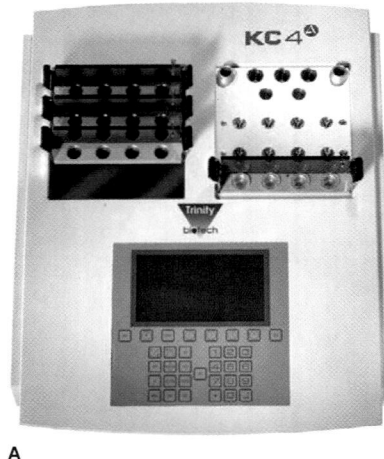 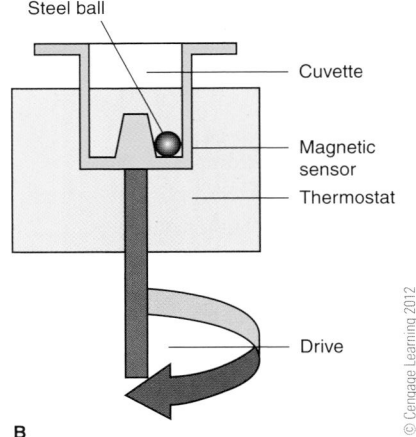

FIGURE 3-15 Coagulation analyzer with mechanical clot detection: (A) Trinity KC4Δ™ coagulation analyzer; (B) diagram of magnetic ball method of clot detection used in the KC1Δ™ and KC4Δ™ coagulation analyzers

Procedures requiring prewarming of the sample before testing will specify the maximum permitted warming time. This is usually 5 minutes at 37° C. All specimens, controls, and instruments must be at the proper temperature before the test is performed.

Collecting the Specimen

The specimen for the prothrombin time must be collected with minimal trauma to the vein and surrounding tissue. The blood is drawn into a vacuum tube (light blue top) that contains a 3.2% solution of sodium citrate. The 3-mL capacity blood collection tube is manufactured to draw 2.7 mL of blood into 0.3 mL of anticoagulant. Two-milliliter capacity tubes are also available.

Manual Prothrombin Time Procedure

In the manual method, the plasma and thromboplastin-$CaCl_2$ reagent are warmed in separate tubes in a heat block or waterbath. After warming, 0.1 mL of patient plasma is forcefully added to 0.2 mL of thromboplastin-$CaCl_2$ reagent while the tube is in the waterbath. A timer is started, and at the end of 10 seconds the tube is picked up, held horizontally in good light, and gently tilted back and forth until a thickening appears (Figure 3-16). This thickening is the fibrin clot, and the timer is stopped when it appears. The time for the clot to form is recorded in seconds. The manual test should be run in triplicate. Timing of the first test will be approximate, and the remaining two should agree with each other.

Prothrombin Time Using the FibroSystem

In the FibroSystem method, the plasma and premeasured thromboplastin-$CaCl_2$ reagent are pipetted into reagent cups and warmed in a heat block that is a part of the system (Figure 3-14). When the specimen and reagent are warm, the cup containing 0.2 mL of thromboplastin-$CaCl_2$ is placed into the center well of the instrument. The automatic pipetter attached to the instrument is used to draw up and then expel 0.1 mL of patient plasma into the reagent cup. This action simultaneously lowers the probe into the cup and starts the timer. Two moving wire probes detect the formation of the clot and stop the timer. The results are displayed in seconds. The tests are performed in duplicate and the results averaged. The average of the two times is used to calculate the INR. Abnormal and normal plasma controls are analyzed in the same manner as patient samples.

Prothrombin Time Using Trinity Biotech Coagulation Instruments

The KC1Δ and the KC4Δ are used similarly to the FibroSystem. The thromboplastin-$CaCl_2$ reagent is dispensed into a test cuvette and prewarmed in the heatblock. A tube containing patient plasma is also prewarmed. The timer is started when the prewarmed patient plasma is added to the cuvette containing prothrombin reagent. The test cuvette, which contains a steel ball, rotates constantly during the test while the ball is held in place with a magnet (Figure 3-15). When the fibrin clot forms, the steel ball is pulled away from the magnet, stopping the timer. The instrument displays the time in seconds and automatically calculates and displays the INR.

Automated and Semi-Automated Coagulation Analyzers

Several types of coagulation instruments are available for the high-volume laboratory. The plasma samples are prepared and placed into the instrument sample tray. The operator enters patient information and the test request information into the instrument. Many instruments identify patient samples and tests to be performed by reading and interpreting the barcode on the sample tube. Most automated analyzers detect clot formation by photo-optical density and print out a report or send the results directly to the laboratory information system (LIS).

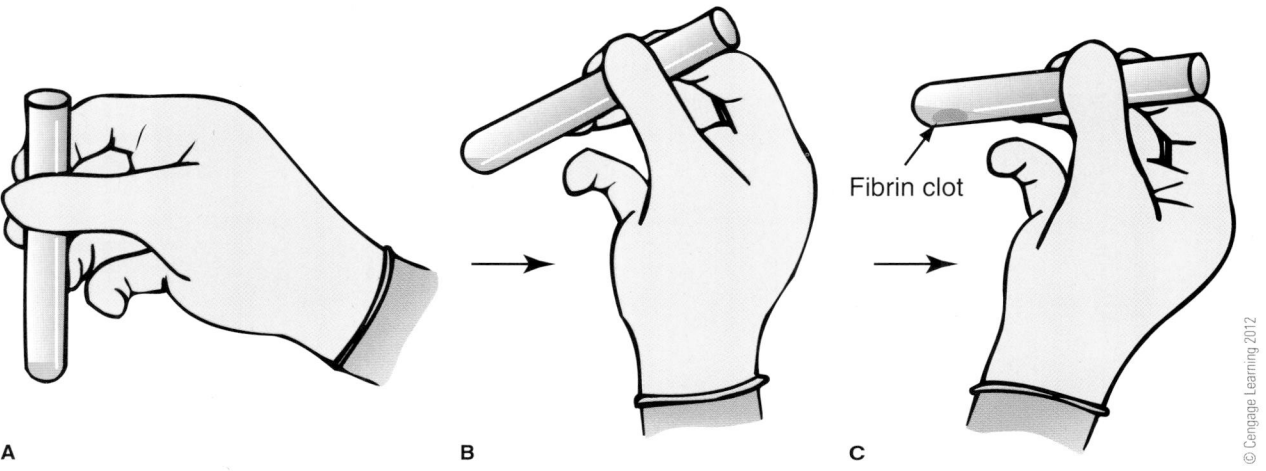

Fibrin clot

FIGURE 3-16 Illustration of the manual tilt-tube prothrombin time method: (A) lift tube out of waterbath; (B) tilt tube horizontally; (C) observe formation of fibrin clot

© Cengage Learning 2012

Point-of-Care Coagulation Analyzers

Many instruments are available for POC or near-patient coagulation testing. Examples include the HEMOCHRON Jr. Signature Elite (Figure 3-17) and the ProTime (Figure 3-18A), both from International Technidyne (ITC), and the CoaguChek S from Roche Diagnostics (Figure 3-18B). The CoaguChek S has a photo-optical system to detect the clot. The ProTime is marketed as a tool to monitor warfarin anticoagulant therapy. Prothrombin times performed on both the CoaguChek S and the ProTime are CLIA-waived, which makes them suitable for use in POLs and at POC.

The HEMOCHRON microcoagulation instruments use photo-optical technology to detect clot formation. Each individual test cuvette is contained in a foil packet that must be at room temperature before the test can be run (Figure 3-17B). When the test cuvette is inserted into the instrument, the instrument warm-up begins, which takes approximately 30 seconds. The specimen is citrated whole blood collected by venipuncture. When the instrument is ready, a tone alerts the operator and the screen alternately displays ADD SAMPLE and PRESS START. The operator then has 5 minutes to apply the blood sample to the cuvette. Two-hundred microliters (0.2 mL) of citrated whole blood are added to the cuvette sample well in the instrument and the START key is depressed. Inside the instrument, the blood and reagents in the cuvette are mixed as the blood moves back and forth in the test channel between two detectors. When cessation of movement is detected, the instrument signals the test is complete.

Whole blood is used in the HEMOCHRON test, but automated coagulation instruments typically use plasma for the test. To make results comparable between the plasma and whole blood methods, the HEMOCHRON automatically calculates the *plasma equivalent* from the whole blood prothrombin time result. The patient results are displayed as the plasma equivalent and as the INR. Whole blood prothrombin time reference values for the HEMOCHRON are given in Table 3-9.

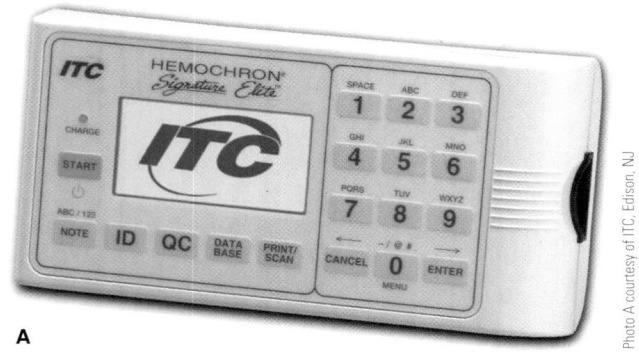

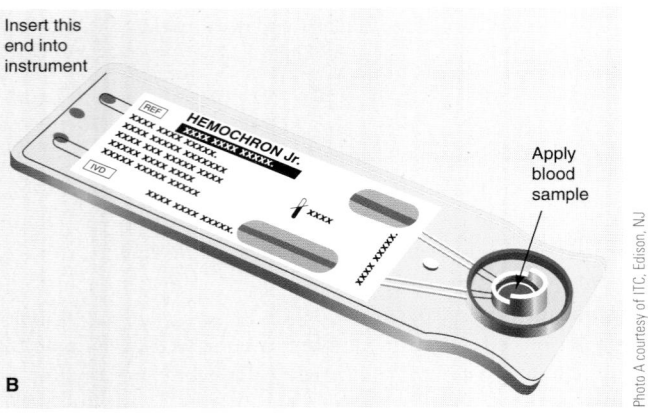

FIGURE 3-17 HEMOCHRON Whole Blood Microcoagulation System: (A) HEMOCHRON instrument for point-of-care testing; (B) diagram of test cuvette used in the HEMOCHRON Jr. System

Reporting and Using Prothrombin Time Results

The most common use of the prothrombin time test is monitoring the effectiveness of warfarin-type anticoagulant drugs. These drugs are prescribed for patients who are in danger of forming clots, such as those with artificial heart valves, arterial

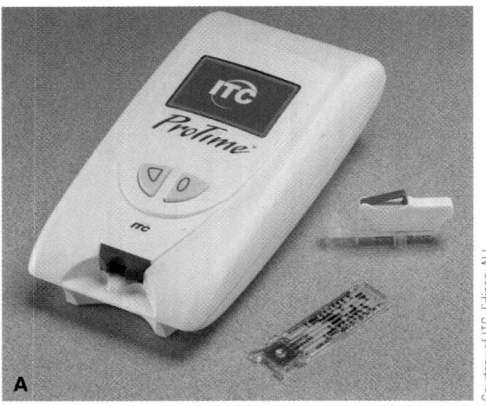

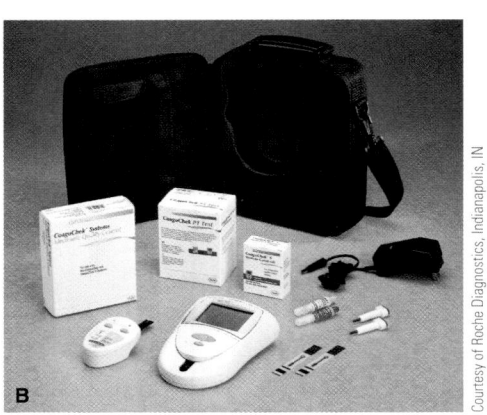

FIGURE 3-18 Point-of-care coagulation analyzers: (A) ProTime; (B) CoaguChek system

TABLE 3-9. Reference values for prothrombin time performed on 3.2% citrated whole blood using HEMOCHRON Jr. coagulation analyzer

REPORTING METHOD	MEAN	RANGE (±2 SD)
Whole Blood prothrombin time	23 sec	20–26 sec
Plasma Equivalent*	11 sec	8–15 sec
INR†	1.1	0.8–1.5

* Mathematically derived
† ISI = 1.0

SAFETY REMINDERS

- Review Safety Precautions section before beginning procedure.
- Observe Standard Precautions.
- Use safety devices when collecting blood.
- Follow centrifuge safety policies.

PROCEDURAL REMINDERS

- Review Quality Assessment section before beginning procedure.
- Follow method in SOP manual.
- Use correct blood collection technique, avoiding tissue trauma.
- Follow an established quality control program.

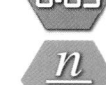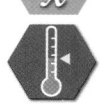

stents, or conditions such as phlebitis and other circulatory problems. The test is performed at regular intervals such as weekly, bi-weekly, or monthly. The physician uses the results to regulate the dose. It can take at least 2 weeks after beginning oral anticoagulant therapy for the prothrombin times to become stable.

Prothrombin times can be reported (1) in seconds, (2) as the prothrombin ratio, or (3) as the INR. The prothrombin ratio is obtained by dividing the patient's prothrombin time by the mean time of a normal population. The INR is calculated by using the patient's prothrombin time, the prothrombin time of the normal control plasma, and an index supplied by the manufacturer for each lot of prothrombin time reagent (Figure 3-13). The goal for most patients who are on warfarin anticoagulant therapy is to keep the anticoagulant dosage sufficient to maintain the INR between 1.5 and 2.5. When results are reported in seconds, the usual goal is to keep the patient's prothrombin time between 16 to 18 seconds, or 1.3 to 1.5 times the normal plasma control value.

CASE STUDY

A 54-year-old man had been injured in an industrial accident 10 years earlier. He had received two blood transfusions at the time of the accident, and in the intervening years, it was discovered that he had severe liver damage from a hepatitis C infection. He had a prothrombin time test performed along with other screening tests in preparation for him to have minor surgery.

1. What is a likely result?
   a. The prothrombin time was within the reference (normal) range.
   b. The prothrombin time was shorter than the reference range.
   c. The prothrombin time was longer than the reference (normal) range.
2. Explain your answer.

CRITICAL THINKING 1

How does severe liver disease affect the prothrombin time? Explain your answer.

CRITICAL THINKING 2

A physician prescribed Coumadin for his patient who had experienced a clotting incident. The patient's INR was 1.1 at the time the drug was prescribed. One week after beginning the oral medication, the patient's INR was 1.3 when the prothrombin test was performed. The physician wanted the patient's INR to stay between 1.5 and 2.0.

Should the patient's Coumadin dosage be increased? Discuss the correct use of the prothrombin time/INR results.

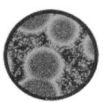

SUMMARY

The prothrombin time or protime, is one of the most frequently requested coagulation tests. It is used as a screening test to evaluate the function of the extrinsic and common pathways for coagulation abnormalities. It is also used to monitor the clotting times of patients receiving warfarin therapy. These patients are tested at regular intervals, sometimes as often as weekly.

The prothrombin time was formerly reported only in seconds. This has been replaced by the INR, which standardizes prothrombin time results among laboratories even if different instruments and brands of reagents are used. A sensitivity index, the ISI, assigned by the manufacturer to each lot of thromboplastin reagent, is used to calculate the INR.

Historically, the FibroSystem was used to perform the prothrombin time test, but several different technologies are now incorporated into coagulation instruments. The development of instruments that can use capillary blood have simplified prothrombin time testing; tests performed on some of these instruments are CLIA-waived. Although the prothrombin time test has been greatly simplified, the institution's safety guidelines and quality assessment procedures and policies must be followed to ensure worker safety and reliable patient test results.

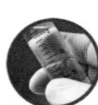

REVIEW QUESTIONS

1. What is the role of prothrombin in blood coagulation?
2. How does the physician use prothrombin time results?
3. Explain how a manual prothrombin time is performed.
4. Explain how to perform a prothrombin time using the FibroSystem.
5. What is the reference range for the prothrombin time test performed on citrated plasma? What is the INR reference range?
6. List three ways of reporting prothrombin times.

7. What is the preferred way of reporting the prothrombin time results? Explain why.
8. What is the desired range for the prothrombin time of a patient receiving warfarin anticoagulant therapy?
9. What type and concentration of anticoagulant is used to collect blood for a prothrombin time?
10. List four conditions in which the prothrombin time can be prolonged.
11. List two instruments that accept whole blood samples for the prothrombin time test.
12. How are prothrombin time results from a whole blood instrument correlated to results from an instrument that uses plasma?
13. Calculate the prothrombin ratio of a patient's plasma sample when the prothrombin time result = 21 seconds and the mean of normal = 12 seconds.
14. Calculate the INR when the ISI is 1.15, the patient's plasma prothrombin time is 20 seconds, and the mean of normal is 10 seconds. Is the INR value within the therapeutic range for Coumadin?
15. Explain why factor VIII deficiency does not affect prothrombin time results.
16. Define enzyme, hypercoagulation, international normalized ratio (INR), international sensitivity index (ISI), prothrombin ratio, prothrombin time test, and vitamin K.

STUDENT ACTIVITIES

1. Complete the written examination for this lesson.
2. Practice performing the prothrombin time as outlined in the Student Performance Guides.
3. If a second type of coagulation analyzer is available, perform the prothrombin time on the same sample tested using the first instrument and compare the results.

WEB ACTIVITIES

1. Locate the web site of a manufacturer of a point-of-care prothrombin time instrument mentioned in this lesson. Determine if other coagulation instruments are marketed by the company. Write a paragraph describing the instrument, procedure, sample size, etc.

2. Search the Internet for information about three different types of thromboplastin used in reagents for prothrombin tests. Report on differences and similarities.

3. Search the Internet for tutorials or videos describing or demonstrating how the prothrombin time test is performed.

LESSON 3-4

Prothrombin Time: Manual Method

(Answers may vary based on the types of samples provided by the instructor and individual student techniques.)

Name _____ Date _____

INSTRUCTIONS

1. Practice performing the manual prothrombin time test following the step-by-step procedure.

2. Demonstrate the manual prothrombin time test satisfactorily for the instructor, using the Student Performance Guide. Your instructor will explain the procedures for evaluating and grading your performance. Your performance may be given a number grade, a letter grade, or satisfactory (S) or unsatisfactory (U) depending on course or institutional policy.

NOTE: Follow manufacturer's directions for the reagents used.

MATERIALS AND EQUIPMENT

- gloves
- hand antiseptic
- full-face shield (or equivalent PPE)
- acrylic safety shield (optional)
- commercial thromboplastin reagent (thromboplastin-CaCl$_2$)
- reagent water or diluent for reconstituting reagents
- centrifuge for separating citrated plasma (if venipuncture is performed)
- citrated human plasma, recently collected, or venipuncture supplies including blue-top tubes
- coagulation plasma controls, normal and abnormal levels
- micropipetter and tips to transfer volumes from 0.1 to 1.0 mL (or pipets and pipetting aid)
- test tube rack
- test tubes (13 × 75 mm)
- waterbath at 37°C
- thermometer
- stopwatch or timer
- good light source
- laboratory tissue
- paper towels
- surface disinfectant (such as 10% chlorine bleach)
- biohazard container
- sharps container

PROCEDURE

  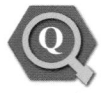

Record in the comment section any problems encountered while practicing the procedure (or have a fellow student or the instructor evaluate your performance).

S = Satisfactory
U = Unsatisfactory

You must:	S	U	Evaluation/Comments
1. Wash hands with antiseptic and put on gloves and face protection			
2. Assemble equipment and materials			
3. Obtain citrated plasma sample following step 3a or 3b: a. Collect venous blood into blue-top tube; centrifuge to obtain plasma; remove plasma to a separate tube, or b. Obtain citrated plasma sample from instructor			

(Continues)

© 2012 Delmar, Cengage Learning. Permission to reproduce for clinical use granted.

You must:	S	U	Evaluation/Comments

4. Perform a manual prothrombin time following steps 4a–4m:
  a. Check that waterbath temperature is 37° C
  b. Pipet 0.2 mL of thromboplastin-CaCl$_2$ reagent into seven labeled tubes (three for the patient, two for each normal and abnormal control)
  c. Place tubes in test tube rack in waterbath
  d. Label three tubes: patient, normal control, and abnormal control
  e. Pipet 0.4 to 0.5 mL each of patient plasma and control plasmas into labeled tubes (enough to perform each test in duplicate or triplicate)
  f. Place tubes in rack in waterbath
  g. Allow patient plasma, controls, and reagent to warm for the prescribed amount of time
  h. Draw up 0.1 mL warmed patient plasma and forcibly expel into a tube containing 0.2 mL warm thromboplastin-CaCl$_2$ reagent, starting timer simultaneously
  i. Allow tube to remain in waterbath about 10 seconds
  j. Work quickly—pick up the tube, dry the outside with tissue, and start tilting tube slowly back and forth in front of a good light source
  k. Stop the timer at the first sign of gelling or thickening (fibrin clot formation) in the moving liquid and record the time
  l. Repeat steps 4h–4k two times using patient plasma and another tube of warmed reagent each time (The first time observed is approximate; the second and third repeat tests should agree with each other)
  m. Perform steps 4h–4k in duplicate for each control plasma. Report results: report average of patient's second and third prothrombin times and record the average times for the controls			

5. Discard all sharps into sharps container and other contaminated materials into appropriate biohazard containers			
6. Clean equipment according to manufacturer's instructions and return all equipment to proper storage			
7. Wipe the work surface with disinfectant			
8. Remove gloves and discard into biohazard container			
9. Wash hands with antiseptic			

Instructor/Evaluator Comments

Instructor/Evaluator _____ Date _____

404

© 2012 Delmar, Cengage Learning. Permission to reproduce for clinical use granted.

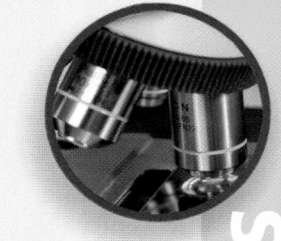

LESSON 3-4
Prothrombin Time: Semi-Automated Methods

(Answers may vary based on the types of samples provided by the instructor and instruments available.)

Name _____ Date _____

INSTRUCTIONS

1. Practice performing the prothrombin time test using instrumentation following the step-by-step procedure.

2. Demonstrate the prothrombin time test satisfactorily for the instructor, using the Student Performance Guide. Your instructor will explain the procedures for evaluating and grading your performance. Your performance may be given a number grade, a letter grade, or satisfactory (S) or unsatisfactory (U) depending on course or institutional policy.

NOTE: Follow manufacturer's directions for instruments and reagents used.

MATERIALS AND EQUIPMENT

- gloves
- hand antiseptic
- full-face shield (or equivalent PPE)
- acrylic safety shield (optional)
- calculator with exponential function
- paper and pen or pencil
- centrifuge for separating citrated plasma from cells
- commercial thromboplastin reagent (thromboplastin-CaCl$_2$)
- reagent water or diluent for reconstituting controls

- micropipetter and pipet tips capable of delivering 0.1 mL to 0.5 mL up to 1 mL
- coagulation instrument, such as FibroSystem or Trinity KCΔ series with automatic pipetters, pipet tips, and appropriate cups or cuvettes
- POC instrument such as HEMOCHRON Jr. and HEMOCHRON prothrombin time test cuvettes
- for FibroSystem or KCΔ series instruments:
  - venipuncture supplies including blue-top citrate tube, or citrated human plasma, recently collected
  - coagulation control plasmas, normal and abnormal levels
- for HEMOCHRON or other POC-type instrument:
  - citrated whole blood, or supplies for collecting citrated whole blood
  - whole blood coagulation controls (two levels) for the instrument in use
- test tube rack
- laboratory tissue
- paper towels
- surface disinfectant (such as 10% chlorine bleach)
- biohazard container
- sharps container

PROCEDURE

Record in the comment section any problems encountered while practicing the procedure (or have a fellow student or the instructor evaluate your performance).

S = Satisfactory
U = Unsatisfactory

You must:	S	U	Evaluation/Comments
1. Wash hands with antiseptic and put on gloves and face protection			

(Continues)

© 2012 Delmar, Cengage Learning. Permission to reproduce for clinical use granted.

You must:	S	U	Evaluation/Comments
2. Obtain citrated whole blood sample (if citrated plasma is provided, skip to step 5)			
3. Centrifuge the specimen as instructed			
4. Remove the plasma and transfer it to a clean test tube; label tube with sample ID			
5. Perform a prothrombin time following steps 5a–5r using the FibroSystem (If using a KCΔ series instrument, proceed to step 6; if using a POC instrument, proceed to step 7) a. Turn on instrument; reset timer to "0." If using the FibroSystem pipetter, be certain it is turned "OFF" b. Label desired number of sample cups and place in heat block (patient samples should be run in duplicate) c. Pipet 0.2 mL of thromboplastin-$CaCl_2$ into each cup, d. Pipet 0.4 mL patient plasma and controls into separate cups (enough to allow for duplicate testing of patient plasma and controls) e. Allow all components to warm the prescribed amount of time f. Place one sample cup with premeasured thromboplastin-$CaCl_2$ into center well of instrument g. Draw up 0.1 mL of warmed patient plasma with pipetter h. Turn pipetter "ON" i. Expel plasma into center cup containing 0.2 mL of thromboplastin-$CaCl_2$; the timer will start automatically when the plunger is depressed (if using the FibroSystem pipet) j. Wait for timer to stop, signaling the formation of a clot k. Record the time in seconds l. Lift probe and clean wire probes gently with laboratory tissue; reset timer between determinations m. Repeat steps 5f–5l using patient plasma n. Average the two times and record the results o. Repeat steps 5f–5l for the normal and abnormal controls p. Test each control in duplicate; average the two results of each control and record q. Turn off instrument r. Calculate the INR for the patient sample and the control plasmas and record			
6. Perform a prothrombin time following steps 6a–6p using a Trinity KCΔ instrument (Proceed to step 7 if using a POC instrument or to step 8 if testing is complete) a. Turn on instrument to warm up following manufacturer's instructions; connect pipet and cable to instrument b. Label desired number of test cuvettes and place in heat block as space permits (patient samples should be run in duplicate) c. Pipet 0.2 mL of thromboplastin-$CaCl_2$ into each test cuvette			

© 2012 Delmar, Cengage Learning. Permission to reproduce for clinical use granted.

You must:	S	U	Evaluation/Comments
d. Pipet 0.4 mL patient plasma and controls (amount sufficient to allow for duplicate testing of patient plasma and controls) into separate tubes and place into heat block as space permits e. Allow all components to warm the prescribed amount of time f. Place a cuvette with premeasured thromboplastin-$CaCl_2$ into the test position in instrument g. Draw up 0.1 mL of warmed patient plasma with pipetter h. Activate pipet automatic feature and expel plasma into the test position cuvette containing 0.2 mL of thromboplastin-$CaCl_2$; the timer will start automatically i. Wait for timer to stop, signaling the formation of a clot j. Record the prothrombin time in seconds and record the INR k. Repeat steps 6f–6j using patient plasma l. Average the two times and record the results m. Repeat steps 6f–6j for the normal and abnormal control plasmas o. Record the prothrombin times and INRs for the control plasmas p. Turn off instrument			
7. Perform a prothrombin time following steps 7a—7j using a POC-type instrument. If not available, proceed to step 8 NOTE: Instructions are given for HEMOCHRON using a venous citrated whole blood sample; follow the instructions for the instrument that is being used a. Allow test pack to come to room temperature and assemble all other supplies b. Collect venous blood in blue-top citrate tube c. Perform quality control checks if necessary; insert the cuvette into the instrument to initiate the prewarm/self-check mode (approximately 30 seconds) d. Observe the display screen for any error messages e. Wait for the audible signal indicating that the instrument is ready; the screen will alternately display ADD SAMPLE and PRESS START NOTE: The test must be run within 5 minutes or the instrument will go into timeout indicating that the test cuvette must be discarded and a new one obtained f. Dispense 1 drop (0.2 mL) of well-mixed citrated whole blood into the sample well of the test cuvette in the instrument. Fill the well flush to the top; if a large drop forms a dome, use the blood collection device to push it over into the outer sample well NOTE: Bubbles make the test invalid; do not force blood into the pin in the center of the sample well g. Depress the START key			

(Continues)

© 2012 Delmar, Cengage Learning. Permission to reproduce for clinical use granted.

You must:	S	U	Evaluation/Comments
h. Wait for the single beep that signals the completion of the test i. Record the results; they will be displayed for 120 seconds as the plasma equivalent value and the INR j. Repeat the test using whole blood controls as directed by instructor			
9. Discard all sharps into sharps container and other contaminated materials into appropriate biohazard containers			
10. Clean equipment or instruments according to manufacturer's instructions and return all equipment to proper storage. If Hemochron is used, clean with 90% ethanol			
11. Wipe the work surface with disinfectant			
12. Remove gloves and discard into biohazard container			
13. Wash hands with antiseptic			

Instructor/Evaluator Comments

Instructor/Evaluator _____ Date _____

© 2012 Delmar, Cengage Learning. Permission to reproduce for clinical use granted.

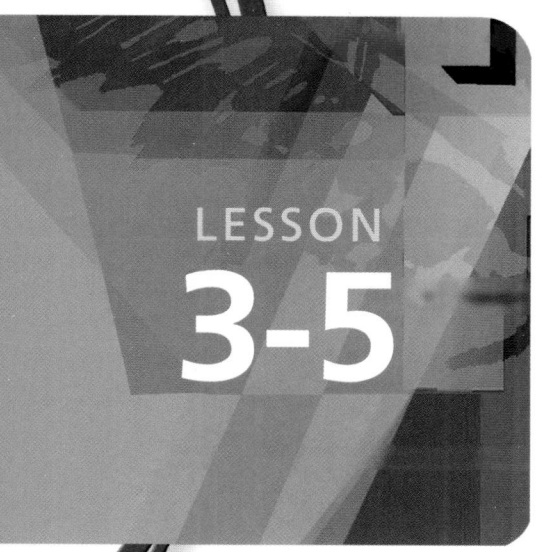

Activated Partial Thromboplastin Time

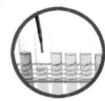

LESSON OBJECTIVES

After studying this lesson, the student will:

- ⊙ Explain the principle of the activated partial thromboplastin time (APTT).
- ⊙ Explain the reasons for performing an APTT.
- ⊙ Explain which coagulation pathway(s) is checked in the APTT.
- ⊙ List the coagulation factor deficiencies detected by the APTT.
- ⊙ Give the reference values for the APTT.
- ⊙ Explain how APTT results are used to monitor anticoagulant therapy.
- ⊙ List safety precautions to be observed when performing the APTT.
- ⊙ Discuss why quality assessment policies and procedures are important in the performance of the APTT.
- ⊙ Define the glossary terms.

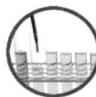

GLOSSARY

activated partial thromboplastin time (APTT) / the time required for a fibrin clot to form when $CaCl_2$ is added to citrated plasma that has been activated with partial thromboplastin reagent

partial thromboplastin / the lipid portion of thromboplastin, available as a commercial preparation; formerly called cephaloplastin

INTRODUCTION

The **activated partial thromboplastin time** (called APTT or aPTT) is a coagulation test used to monitor low-dose heparin therapy and to screen for function of the intrinsic and common pathways of hemostasis (Figure 3-19). **Partial thromboplastin**, the lipid portion of tissue thromboplastin, is the reagent used in performing the APTT. The partial thromboplastin reagent is manufactured from rabbit or bovine brain tissue as well as from vegetable sources such as soybeans. Partial thromboplastin performs the function of platelet factor 3 (PF3) in the APTT test. The APTT is so named because the partial

thromboplastin reagent used in the test contains activators such as kaolin or silica to activate the contact factors in the intrinsic pathway. Calcium chloride ($CaCl_2$) is the second reagent used in the test and is added to supply the ionized calcium required to activate prothrombin in the common pathway.

The APTT test will be normal only if factors in the intrinsic pathway (XII, XI, IX, and VIII) and in the common pathway (I, II, V, and X) are present in sufficient quantity and are functional (Table 3-10). The APTT test is sensitive to mild deficiencies of factors XII, XI, IX, and VIII and Fletcher and Fitzgerald factors. It is also useful for

409

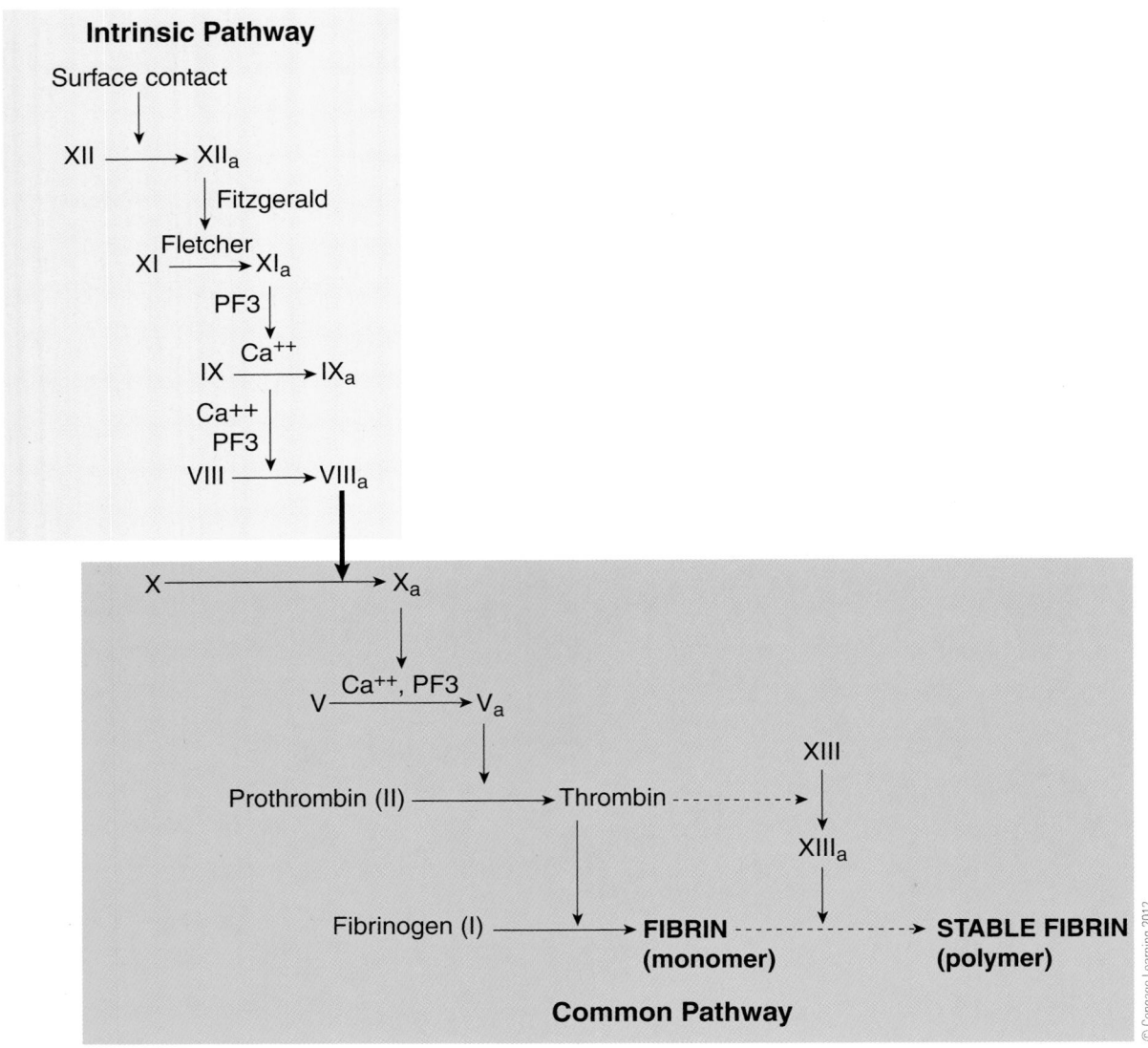

FIGURE 3-19 Diagram of fibrin formation via the intrinsic coagulation pathway

TABLE 3-10. Hemostasis pathways and coagulation factors tested by the activated partial thromboplastin time (APTT)

FACTORS OF INTRINSIC PATHWAY	FACTORS OF COMMON PATHWAY
XII	I
XI	II
IX	V
VIII	X
Fitzgerald factor	
Fletcher factor	

detecting deficiencies of factors X, V, II, and fibrinogen (I), although these factor deficiencies must be slightly more severe to cause a prolonged APTT. Factors VII, XIII, and platelet factor 3 (PF3) are not assayed in the APTT (Figure 3-19).

PRINCIPLE OF THE ACTIVATED PARTIAL THROMBOPLASTIN TIME

The APTT is performed by combining citrated patient plasma with two reagents—partial thromboplastin and calcium chloride ($CaCl_2$). The partial thromboplastin reagent differs from the thromboplastin reagent used in the prothrombin test. Prewarmed patient plasma is combined with partial thromboplastin and allowed to react. This begins activation of factors in the intrinsic pathway, activation that would be initiated by PF3 in vivo. $CaCl_2$

is then added to the plasma–partial thromboplastin mixture to allow the reactions necessary for forming the fibrin clot to be completed. The time required for the fibrin clot to form after addition of the $CaCl_2$ to the plasma-partial thromboplastin mixture is the activated partial thromboplastin time. The APTT can be performed using a variety of coagulation instruments.

PERFORMING THE ACTIVATED PARTIAL THROMBOPLASTIN TIME

The APTT can be performed on a FibroSystem, the KC1Δ, KC4Δ, a multisample coagulation analyzer, or small point-of-care (POC) analyzers. Semi-automated multisample analyzers are used in larger facilities and are now also designed for small laboratories. Small handheld analyzers can be used at point-of-care and in physician office laboratories (POLs).

Safety Precautions

 Standard Precautions must be observed to protect the worker from exposure to blood-borne pathogens. Appropriate personal protective equipment (PPE) must be used. Performing the APTT can expose the laboratory scientist to patient blood as well as blood-derived control plasmas. Blood collection safety devices must be used when performing venipuncture. Coagulation instruments that automatically pierce the tube cap and aspirate the sample lessen the potential for exposure. Contaminated materials must be discarded into biohazard containers and contaminated sharps into sharps containers. Centrifuge safety rules must be followed.

Quality Assessment

 The specimen collection and test procedures must be performed as outlined in the standard operating procedure (SOP) manual. The blood specimen must be collected with care; venipuncture must be performed with as little trauma as possible to avoid contaminating the sample. A difficult venipuncture can release excess tissue factor when the vein is punctured, which can activate clotting and falsely shorten the APTT time. When possible, the blood should be collected without using a tourniquet. If a tourniquet must be used, it should be left on *less* than 1 minute to prevent blood concentrating in that area. Hemoconcentration can activate some clotting factors and cause platelet release reactions, interfering with test results.

Blood should be collected into 3.2% sodium anticoagulant in a proportion of 9 parts blood to 1 part sodium citrate. Standard citrate tubes have a 3.0 mL capacity—the tubes contain 0.3 mL anticoagulant and draw 2.7 mL of blood; tubes are also available that contain 0.2 mL anticoagulant and draw 1.8 mL blood. The blood specimen should be centrifuged, and the platelet-poor plasma removed, placed into another tube, and stored in a capped tube at 4° C until tested. The APTT test should be run within 4 hours of collection. Controls must be run and be within assay limits before results are reported. Two or three levels of control plasmas can be used depending on the facility's protocol.

FibroSystem

The APTT procedure using the FibroSystem is similar to that for the prothrombin time. The patient plasma and the two APTT reagents—activated partial thromboplastin and $CaCl_2$—are prewarmed separately in the heatblock for the prescribed time, usually at least 3 minutes but no more than 10 minutes. The patient samples are prepared by combining 0.1 mL of the prewarmed patient plasma and 0.1 mL of warmed partial thromboplastin reagent into the patient sample cups. These are allowed to remain warm and activate for 3 minutes. To initiate the clotting reaction, 0.1 mL of prewarmed $CaCl_2$ is added using the FibroSystem automatic pipet, which simultaneously starts the timer and lowers the probes into the reaction cup. The two moving wire probes mix the sample until a clot is detected, which stops the timer. The number of seconds required for the clot to form is displayed on the instrument. Normal and abnormal controls must be run in the same manner as patient samples.

Trinity Biotech Instruments

The APTT test procedure using the Trinity Biotech KCΔ series instruments is similar to that for the prothrombin time test (Lesson 3-4). Reagents are the same as those used for the FibroSystem APTT. The instrument timer starts when the final reagent is added. The reaction cuvette containing a steel ball is constantly rotated during the test while the ball is held in place with a magnet. When the fibrin clot forms, the ball is pulled away from the magnet, stopping the timer. The time in seconds is displayed on the instrument.

Point-of-Care Instruments

Several small, handheld instruments are available to perform the APTT quickly and easily. These require only a small sample of whole blood for the assays. In International Technidyne's HEMOCHRON Jr. or HEMOCHRON Signature Elite, the individual test cuvettes containing all the needed reagents are enclosed in foil packets. The specimen required for the HEMOCHRON APTT test is whole venous blood collected in citrate anticoagulant.

The unopened test cuvette packet must be brought to room temperature before the cuvette is removed. The test cuvette is inserted into the instrument to begin the 30 second warm-up cycle. When the instrument is ready, an audible tone alerts the operator, and ADD SAMPLE is displayed on the screen. A large drop of citrated blood (0.2 mL) is added to the sample well in the center of the cuvette, and the START key is depressed to begin the assay. Inside the test cuvette, the blood is mixed with the cuvette reagents and the mixture is moved back and forth within the cuvette. When clotting occurs, LED photodetectors sense that movement of the blood within the cuvette has ceased and the timer stops automatically. The whole blood clotting time is converted to the plasma equivalent and displayed on the instrument screen.

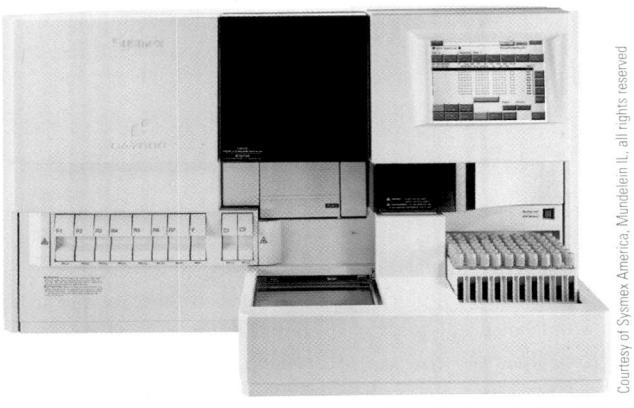

Courtesy of Sysmex America, Mundelein IL, all rights reserved

FIGURE 3-20 Sysmex CA-7000 automated coagulation analyzer

Automated Coagulation Analyzers

The APTT can be performed using automated and semi-automated analyzers that are capable of performing several different assays on a sample of citrated plasma (Figure 3-20). The technician loads the samples into the sample tray and enters the patient I.D., and tests to be run for each specimen. Many analyzers read the information on the barcode label of the tube and perform the test(s) requested for each sample. The analyzer performs the requested assays and then prints a report or sends the results directly to the laboratory information system (LIS).

Reference Values for the APTT

Reference ranges for the APTT vary according to test method, brands of reagents and controls used, instrument used, and technical procedure. Additionally, the ranges differ according to whether the test was performed on plasma or citrated whole blood. Each laboratory must establish its own reference range by periodically testing several specimens from the normal population. The technologists and healthcare providers must be familiar with and use the correct ranges established by the institution for the instrument and the method in use.

A typical mean normal reference value for the APTT performed on citrated plasma using a plasma instrument is 29 seconds, with a range of 24 to 34 seconds. For POC instruments that use citrated whole blood instead of the traditional citrated plasma sample, both the whole blood APTT result and the plasma equivalent, a mathematically derived value, are reported (Table 3-11).

As shown in Table 3-11 the reference range for the APTT performed by HEMOCHRON on citrated whole blood can be between 3 and 4 times longer than the plasma equivalent time. Failure to use the correct reference range could prove detrimental to the patient, so care must be taken to interpret and report test results correctly.

When the APTT is used to monitor heparin therapy, the usual goal is to keep the patient's APTT between 1.5 to 2.5 times the APTT of the normal plasma control. Table 3-12 lists examples of conditions that affect the APTT.

TABLE 3-11. Reference values for activated partial thromboplastin time (APTT) performed on 3.2% citrated whole blood using the HEMOCHRON Jr. coagulation analyzer

REPORTING METHOD	MEAN	RANGE (±2 SD)
Whole blood APTT	103 sec	93.2–116.8 sec
Plasma equivalent*	29.6 sec	20.6–38.6

* Mathematically derived

TABLE 3-12. Examples of conditions that affect the activated partial thromboplastin time (APTT)

CONDITION	EFFECT ON APTT
Factor deficiencies	
I, II, V, VIII, IX, X, XI, XII	Prolonged
VII, XIII	No effect
Other conditions	
Heparin therapy	Prolonged
Vitamin K deficiency	Prolonged

SAFETY REMINDERS

- Review Safety Precautions section before beginning procedure.
- Observe Standard Precautions.
- Treat control plasmas as if potentially infectious.
- Follow centrifuge safety rules.

PROCEDURAL REMINDERS

- Review Quality Assessment section before beginning procedure.
- Follow the manufacturer's instructions and the SOP manual.
- Collect blood specimen without trauma.
- Use correct reference values for test method.

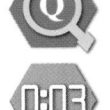

CASE STUDY

Alice Morrow came to the outpatient laboratory to have blood drawn for APTT. Usually Ms. Morrow did not have problems getting blood drawn. On that particular morning, the phlebotomist had difficulty, but he did finally obtain about 1.0 mL of blood in the light-blue capped blood collection tube that contained 0.3 mL of 3.2% sodium citrate. The phlebotomist labeled the tube with the date and a collection time of 8:45 AM. When the collection tube was received in the laboratory at 9:05 AM the technologist said the specimen was unacceptable and must be recollected.

1. Why was the specimen rejected?
   a. The APTT can only be performed on whole blood collected without anticoagulant.
   b. The phlebotomist waited too long to deliver the blood specimen to the laboratory.
   c. The ratio of blood-to-anticoagulant was incorrect.
   d. The blood was collected in the wrong anticoagulant.
2. Explain your answer and recommend a follow-up action.

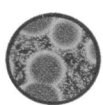

SUMMARY

The APTT is useful for monitoring patients on low-dose heparin anticoagulant therapy. In addition, it is used to screen for abnormalities in the intrinsic and common pathways. In the APTT test, a fibrin clot can form only if factors XII, XI, IX, and VIII in the intrinsic pathway and I, II, V, and X in the common pathway are functional and present in sufficient amounts. The APTT is not influenced by platelet numbers or function because the partial thromboplastin added in the test procedure performs the function of platelet factor 3 (PF3).

The APTT can be performed on multifunction coagulation instruments or on one of many handheld POC coagulation instruments. The instructions for each instrument must be followed carefully because some of the instruments use only plasma samples and others can use plasma or citrated whole blood. Standard Precautions must be observed while performing the test. In addition, all quality assessment procedures of the facility and the instrument manufacturer must be followed for test results to be valid.

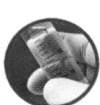

REVIEW QUESTIONS

1. Which hemostasis pathway is measured by the APTT?
2. What conditions could cause a prolonged APTT?
3. Name two uses of the APTT.

4. List two coagulation factors not measured by the APTT.
5. Why is the extrinsic pathway not measured by the APTT?
6. Why is $CaCl_2$ added in the APTT?
7. How would a traumatic venipuncture affect the activated partial thromboplastin time?
8. Why are activators added to the plasma during the APTT procedure?
9. What is the correct blood-to-anticoagulant ratio for specimens to be tested in the APTT?
10. Explain how the type of blood specimen tested affects the APTT reference values.
11. How does heparin anticoagulant therapy affect the APTT?
12. Define activated partial thromboplastin time (APTT) and partial thromboplastin.

STUDENT ACTIVITIES

1. Complete the written examination for this lesson.
2. Practice performing the APTT as outlined in the Student Performance Guide.
3. If available, use a coagulation analyzer to perform the APTT on the same sample tested using the FibroSystem or KC1Δ or KC4Δ. Compare the results obtained with the two instruments.

WEB ACTIVITIES

1. Use the Internet to find examples of two instruments that use whole blood to perform the APTT. Prepare a report comparing the sample type, sample size required, and time required to obtain test results for each of the two instruments. Discuss the advantages and disadvantages of using a whole blood sample for coagulation testing.

2. Search the Internet to find the explanation for "plasma equivalent" results. Report on how the plasma equivalent is determined in methods that perform the APTT on whole blood.

3. Search the Internet to find tutorials or self-tests for routine coagulation tests such as the APTT.

LESSON 3-5
Activated Partial Thromboplastin Time

(Answers may vary based on the types of samples provided by the instructor and type of instrument/analyzer used.)

Name _____   Date _____

INSTRUCTIONS

1. Practice performing the APTT following the step-by-step procedure.

2. Demonstrate the APTT procedure satisfactorily for the instructor, using the Student Performance Guide. Your instructor will explain the procedures for evaluating and grading your performance. Your performance may be given a number grade, a letter grade, or satisfactory (S) or unsatisfactory (U) depending on course or institutional policy.

NOTE: The instructions given are general instructions for the FibroSystem, KCΔ instruments, and HEMOCHRON. Follow manufacturers' instructions for the instrument and reagents being used.

MATERIALS AND EQUIPMENT

- gloves
- hand antiseptic
- full-face shield (or equivalent PPE)
- acrylic safety shield (optional)
- citrated plasma, citrated whole blood sample, or venipuncture materials required for obtaining citrated blood
- test tube rack
- clinical centrifuge
- Reagents for APTT:
  - commercial control plasmas, normal and abnormal levels
  - partial thromboplastin reagent
  - $CaCl_2$, 0.02 M
  - reagent grade water or diluent and pipets for reconstituting controls and reagents
- Manual clot detection system such as Fibro-System or KCΔ series:
  - For FibroSystem:
    - FibroSystem pipetter with cable and pipet tips
    - plastic reagent cups
    - 37° C heatblock with thermometer
    - manufacturer's instructions for FibroSystem
  - For KCΔ:
    - KC reaction cuvettes
    - KC pipetter with starter cable and pipet tips
    - manufacturer's instructions for KCΔ instrument
- HEMOCHRON or other POC coagulation analyzer with APTT test cuvettes and manufacturer's instructions
- laboratory tissue
- paper towels
- surface disinfectant (such as 10% chlorine bleach)
- biohazard container
- sharps container

PROCEDURE

Record in the comment section any problems encountered while practicing the procedure (or have a fellow student or the instructor evaluate your performance).

S = Satisfactory
U = Unsatisfactory

You must:	S	U	Evaluation/Comments
1. Wash hands with antiseptic and put on gloves and face protection			
2. Assemble materials and equipment			
3. Obtain citrated plasma from instructor and continue at step 4. If plasma is not available, use commercial plasma controls and continue at step 4 or obtain blood sample by venipuncture following steps 3a–3d: a. Collect venous blood in blue-top tube b. Centrifuge the blood sample for the specified time and speed to obtain platelet-poor plasma c. Remove plasma and place in a separate tube after centrifugation d. Label plasma tube			
4. Reconstitute the partial thromboplastin reagent according to manufacturer's instructions			
5. Select the clot detection system (FibroSystem or KCΔ). Follow instructions for the instrument being used			
6. Turn on the instrument; check to see that heat block is at 37° C before beginning			
7. Label 5 sample cups or tubes: normal control, abnormal control, patient ID, partial thromboplastin, and $CaCl_2$			
8. Pipet 0.4 to 0.5 mL of partial thromboplastin, $CaCl_2$, and plasmas into the separate labeled tubes and place tubes in heatblock to prewarm (following time specified in package inserts)			
9. For the FibroSystem, perform the APTT following steps 9a–9i: (for a Trinity KCΔ instrument go to step 10 or for a POC instrument go to step 11) a. Place a clean cup in the reaction well of the instrument and pipet 0.1 mL warmed partial thromboplastin into it using the FibroSystem pipet set to **OFF** b. Perform the APTT on a normal control plasma by pipetting 0.1 mL of the warmed control into the cup containing the 0.1 mL of prewarmed partial thromboplastin (in the reaction well) with pipet turned **OFF**			

© 2012 Delmar, Cengage Learning. Permission to reproduce for clinical use granted.

You must:	S	U	Evaluation/Comments
c. Let the mixture warm and activate for 3 minutes; **set instrument timer to "0"** d. Draw up 0.1 mL prewarmed CaCl$_2$, turn **ON** pipetter, and dispense CaCl$_2$ into the cup in the reaction well. The probe will lower into the cup; the timer will start automatically and will stop when a fibrin clot is detected e. Record the time from the instrument timer and **reset timer** f. Repeat steps 9a–9e using the normal control plasma g. Average the results from the duplicate samples and record the APTT normal control in seconds h. Perform the APTT in duplicate using the abnormal control plasma, following steps 9a–9e i. If all control values are within acceptable limits, repeat steps 9a–9e, using patient plasma			
10. For the Trinity KCΔ instruments, perform the APTT following steps 10a–10i: (if the instrument is not available, go to step 11 for POC instrument or to step 12 if no POC instrument is available) a. Place a cuvette in the test position of the instrument and pipet 0.1 mL warmed partial thromboplastin into it, following instructions with KC pipetter b. Perform the APTT on a normal control plasma by pipetting 0.1 mL of warmed normal control into the cuvette containing the 0.1 mL of prewarmed partial thromboplastin c. Let the mixture warm and activate for the specified time d. Pipet 0.1 mL prewarmed CaCl$_2$ into the cuvette in the test position; the KC pipetter will start the test automatically and the timer will stop when a fibrin clot is detected e. Record the results f. Repeat the test (steps 10a–10e) using the normal control plasma g. Average the results from the duplicate control samples; report the APTT normal control in seconds h. Perform the APTT in duplicate using the abnormal control plasma, following steps 10a–10e, averaging the results of the duplicate abnormal controls i. If all control values are within acceptable limits, repeat steps 10a–10e, using patient plasma. Test plasma in duplicate and average the results			
11. Perform APTT using a POC-type instrument following steps 11a–11j (Instructions given are for a HEMOCHRON type instrument using citrated whole sample; follow the instructions for the instrument that is being used) a. Allow test pack to come to room temperature and assemble all other supplies b. Obtain a citrated whole blood sample			

(Continues)

© 2012 Delmar, Cengage Learning. Permission to reproduce for clinical use granted.

You must:	S	U	Evaluation/Comments
c. Insert the cuvette into the instrument to initiate the prewarm/self-check mode (approximately 30 seconds)			
d. Observe the display screen for any error messages			
e. Wait for the audible signal that sounds when the instrument is ready; the screen display will alternate between ADD SAMPLE and PRESS START			
NOTE: If the test is not run within 5 minutes the instrument will go into timeout indicating that the test cuvette must be discarded and a new one obtained			
f. Dispense one drop (0.2 mL) of well-mixed citrated whole blood into the sample well of the cuvette. Fill the well flush to the top; if a large drop forms a dome, use the blood collecting device to push it over into the outer sample well			
NOTE: Bubbles make the test invalid; do not force blood into the pin in the center of the sample well			
g. Depress the START key			
h. Wait for the single beep that signals the completion of the test			
i. Record the results; they will be displayed as the time in seconds and the plasma equivalent value			
j. Repeat the test using whole blood controls as instructor directs			
12. Discard all sharps into sharps container and other contaminated articles into appropriate biohazard container			
13. Clean and disinfect equipment or instruments according to manufacturer's instructions and return all equipment to storage			
14. Wipe the work surface with disinfectant			
15. Remove gloves and discard into biohazard container			
16. Wash hands with antiseptic			

Instructor/Evaluator Comments

Instructor/Evaluator _____ Date _____

© 2012 Delmar, Cengage Learning. Permission to reproduce for clinical use granted.

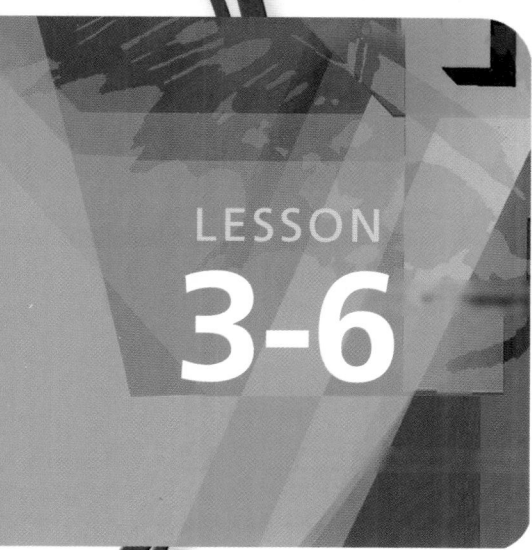

D-Dimers

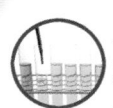

LESSON OBJECTIVES

After studying this lesson, the student will:

- ⊙ Explain the process of fibrinolysis.
- ⊙ Discuss the significance of D-dimers.
- ⊙ List three conditions for which D-dimer testing can be useful to the diagnosis.
- ⊙ Perform a test for D-dimers.
- ⊙ Explain two test methods for detecting D-dimers.
- ⊙ Discuss how the D-dimer test results help in the diagnosis of hemostasis emergencies.
- ⊙ Explain why it is important to be able to distinguish between FDPs and XDPs.
- ⊙ Discuss the interpretation of D-dimer test results.
- ⊙ Correlate D-dimer test results to the diagnosis of pulmonary embolism (PE), deep vein thrombosis (DVT), and disseminated intravascular coagulation (DIC).
- ⊙ Discuss safety precautions that must be observed when performing D-dimer tests.
- ⊙ Explain why it is important to follow quality assessment procedures when performing D-dimer tests.
- ⊙ Define the glossary terms.

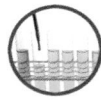

GLOSSARY

D-dimer / the smallest cross-linked fibrin degradation fragment formed from the breakdown of polymerized fibrin by plasmin

deep vein thrombosis (DVT) / occurrence of a thrombus within a deep vein, usually of the leg or pelvis

disseminated intravascular coagulation (DIC) / a hemostasis emergency characterized by widespread circulatory thrombotic events coexisting with fibrinolytic events

FDPs / fibrinogen or fibrin degradation products formed when plasmin cleaves fibrinogen or fibrin monomers into protein fragments; formerly called fibrin split products

pulmonary embolism (PE) / occlusion of a pulmonary artery or one of its branches, usually caused by an embolus that originated in a deep vein of the leg or pelvis

sepsis / the presence of microorganisms and/or their toxic products in the blood or other tissues

XDPs / degradation products formed by plasmin action on cross-linked fibrin and containing the D-dimer fragment

INTRODUCTION

Several medical emergency situations can require rapid hemostasis testing. These situations include circumstances in which the patient is suspected of having a condition such as deep vein thrombosis (DVT), pulmonary embolism (PE) or disseminated intravascular coagulation (DIC).

Two rapid hemostasis tests are the test for **FDPs** and the **D-dimer** test to detect **XDPs**, degradation products of cross-linked fibrin. The ability to distinguish between fibrinogen/fibrin monomer degradation products (FDP) and D-dimers is a helpful tool in differentiating among conditions with pathological clotting or fibrinolysis. The availability of rapid tests for D-dimers is an important aid in the diagnosis of these conditions. However, the D-dimer test results should never be used to diagnose DVT, PE, or DIC without taking into account other criteria, such as patient symptoms, other coagulation test results, and diagnostic imaging results.

Deep vein thrombosis (DVT) and **pulmonary embolism (PE)** are conditions that can be difficult to diagnose by clinical symptoms alone. DVT is the formation of a thrombus or thrombi caused by slow blood flow or stasis in the large veins (usually of the legs) resulting from long periods of inactivity.

Pulmonary embolism is a potentially lethal condition caused when a clot dislodges, is carried to the lungs, and blocks a pulmonary vessel. PE can be a complication of DVT. Rapid diagnosis and treatment are essential to recovery.

Disseminated intravascular coagulation (DIC) is a life-threatening condition in which widespread circulatory thrombosis and secondary hemorrhaging occur as a result of malfunctions in the mechanisms that maintain the balance between clotting and fibrinolysis, the process of dissolving clots. A patient can have hemorrhaging coexisting with the formation of microemboli. As clots are dissolved and new clots form, the circulating coagulation factors and platelets become depleted. DIC can be caused by conditions such as widespread inflammation, cancer, or **sepsis** resulting from systemic bacterial or fungal infections. Injuries that cause widespread damage to the vascular system, such as crushing injuries received in construction or automobile accidents, can also cause DIC. In disseminated intravascular coagulation, FDPs and XDPs are increased, platelet numbers are decreased, serum fibrinogen level is decreased, and both the prothrombin time and activated partial thromboplastin time (APTT) are prolonged (Table 3-13).

FIBRINOLYSIS AND FORMATION OF FDP AND XDP

The initial conversion of fibrinogen to fibrin results in the formation of fibrin monomers. The fibrin clot is stabilized when the fibrin monomers in a clot become cross-linked into polymers through the action of activated factor XIII, also denoted factor XIII$_a$.

Fibrinolysis

During fibrinolysis, both fibrinogen and fibrin are cleaved by plasmin, the major clot-lysing enzyme that is formed when clotting occurs. This cleaving yields fibrin degradation products called FDPs as shown in Figure 3-21. The action of plasmin on *cross-linked* fibrin polymers results in the formation of cross-linked fibrin degradation products (XDPs). The XDPs contain protein fragments called D-dimers, the terminal product formed when plasminogen cleaves cross-linked fibrin. It is important to distinguish between FDPs and XDPs because the presence of XDPs indicates a more serious condition. D-dimers are produced only as a result of lysis of the cross-linked fibrin and thus are a marker for pathological fibrinolysis.

Tests for FDP and XDP (D-Dimer)

Hemostasis tests used in the diagnosis of DVT, PE, and DIC include tests for fibrinogen and FDP and tests for D-dimers. Negative results from most D-dimer tests have a *negative* predictive value of 92% to 100% for pulmonary embolism and DVT. This means that a negative D-dimer result predicts with 92% to 100% certainty that pulmonary embolism is *not* present and predicts with 92% to 100% certainty that DVT is *not* present.

TABLE 3-13. Expected laboratory test results in disseminated intravascular coagulation (DIC)

TEST	RESULT IN DIC
Platelet count	Decreased
Serum fibrinogen	Decreased
PT	Prolonged
APTT	Prolonged
FDPs and XDPs	Increased

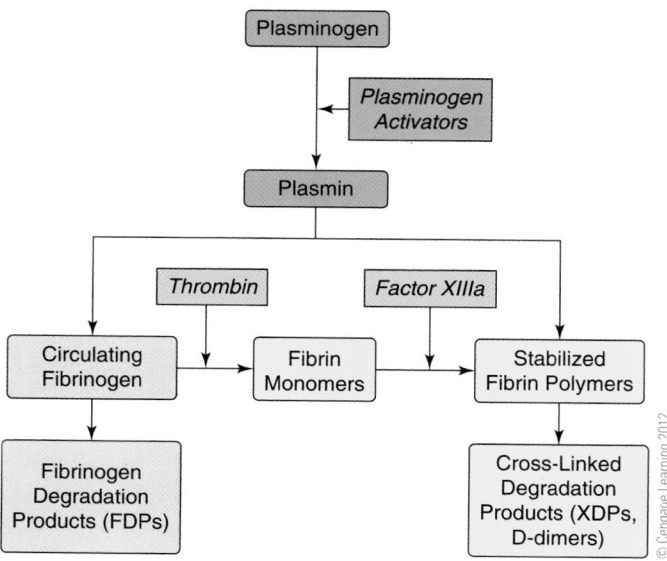

FIGURE 3-21 Illustration of the fibrinolytic pathway showing formation of D-dimers

Rapid Manual Tests

Several manual tests are available to detect D-dimer in serum or plasma. Some tests are based on the agglutination of latex particles; others are immunoassays. Results from both types of tests are available within minutes.

The D-dimer latex agglutination slide tests contain latex beads coated with a monoclonal antibody specific for the D-dimer. An example is the Remel D-Dimer test (Figure 3-22). When the patient sample is mixed with the latex reagent, any D-dimer present becomes bound to the antibody on the beads and visible agglutination forms.

The Clearview Simplify D-Dimer test is an example of a lateral flow immunoassay for D-dimer. The Clearview Simplify test uses an antibody specific for D-dimer incorporated into the test membrane to capture the D-dimer molecules in a patient sample. The end-point reaction is the formation of a colored line in the membrane.

D-Dimer Tests Using Point-of-Care Instruments

Small, portable coagulation analyzers are available that can be used at point of care (POC) to rapidly perform the D-dimer test. The Cardiac Reader (Roche Diagnostics) is a POC instrument that assays D-dimer as well as several cardiac markers using immunochemical assay technology (Figure 3-23). A photosensor detects and measures the reaction and provides a quantitative result directly from heparinized venous whole blood. The Triage D-Dimer Test is a fluorescent immunoassay test that is read on the Biosite Triage meter (Figure 3-24). Results are available within about 15 minutes.

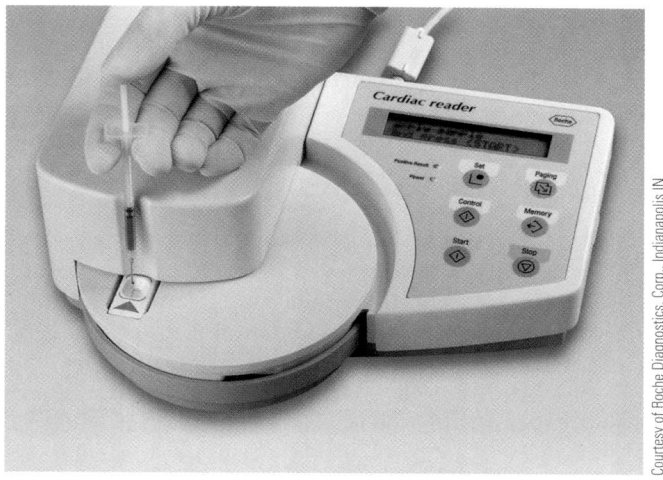

FIGURE 3-23 The Cardiac Reader®, a small analyzer that can measure D-dimers

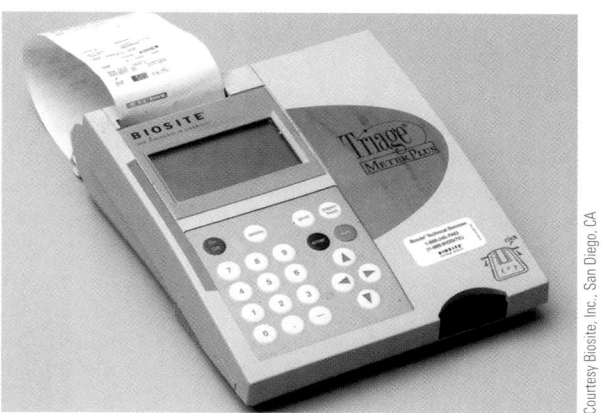

FIGURE 3-24 Triage® MeterPlus

Several POC instruments, such as FisherScientific's Di Stat, use latex-enhanced turbidimetric technology to measure the amount of D-dimer in the patient's sample. These systems report qualitative and quantitative results for the D fragments (D-dimers) in a plasma specimen. Latex particles coated with monoclonal antibody react with any D-dimers present in the patient plasma sample. The amount of agglutination that develops is proportional to the amount of D-dimers present. The DIMEX by TECO measures the amount of light transmitted through the test sample. As the D-dimer concentration increases (that is, as agglutination increases), the amount of transmitted light decreases. The concentration of D-dimer is calculated by the instrument and is reported in μg/L.

PERFORMING THE D-DIMER TEST

Manually performed assays for FDP and D-dimer have been used for several years to aid in diagnosis of DVT, PE, and DIC. The tests come as kits with a package insert containing instructions for use, the test device, pipettes for capillary and

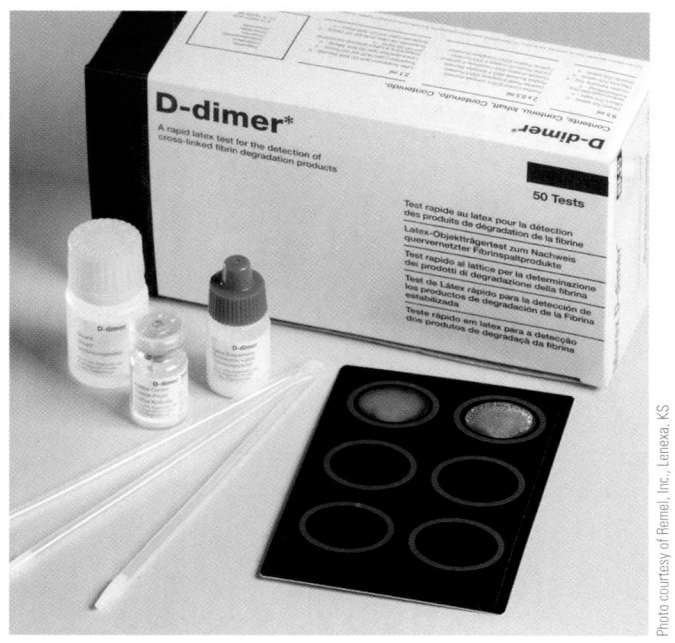

FIGURE 3-22 Rapid latex agglutination test for D-dimers showing negative (left) and positive (right) reactions

anticoagulated whole blood or plasma samples, plus other required reagents, such as control solutions and monoclonal antibodies. D-dimer tests are not CLIA-waived; they are classified as *moderately complex.*

Safety Precautions

Standard Precautions must be observed when handling patient specimens and control reagents. Appropriate personal protective equipment (PPE) must be worn when collecting the blood specimen and performing the test. The controls for rapid hemostasis tests are made from human blood and must be considered potentially infectious. Blood collection safety devices must be used when obtaining blood specimens. All used materials should be discarded into appropriate biohazard and sharps containers.

Quality Assessment

The D-dimer test methods and quality assessment procedures are detailed in each laboratory's standard operating procedure (SOP) manual. Specimen collection must be performed following manufacturers' instructions. The blood from a capillary puncture should be free-flowing. Venipuncture must be performed without trauma to avoid release of tissue thromboplastin into the specimen.

Some methods or instruments can analyze only one type of blood specimen. Other instruments can use more than one type of specimen, such as whole blood, ethylenediaminetetraacetic acid (EDTA) blood, heparinized blood, citrated whole blood, or citrated plasma. The technician must use the correct specimen for the particular instrument or method.

All reagents must be at the appropriate temperature before the tests are performed. For D-dimer latex agglutination tests,

pipetting must be precise; the tests must be read exactly at the specified time to avoid false-positive reactions caused by drying of the latex or other test materials.

Clearview Simplify D-Dimer Test

The Clearview Simplify D-dimer is a qualitative lateral flow immunoassay for the detection of D-dimer. The test is carried out on a membrane enclosed in a plastic case similar to tests for group A *Streptococcus*, human chorionic gonadotropin (hCG), and several other analytes. (See Lesson 4-1 for explanation of lateral flow immunoassays.) The Clearview Simplify test uses an antibody specific for D-dimer incorporated into the test membrane to capture the D-dimer molecules in a patient sample. The test can detect levels of D-dimer as low as 80 nanograms/milliliter (ng/mL).

The test is performed by adding a 35 microliter (μL) venous or capillary blood aliquot, or a 20 μL plasma aliquot, to the sample well in the device (Figure 3-25). A buffer is added to allow the reagents in the membrane to enter an aqueous phase. Any D-dimer molecules in the patient sample become bound to the anti–D-dimer antibody in the cartridge membrane. The antibody/D-dimer complexes migrate along the membrane until they are captured and immobilized by a second D-dimer specific dye-labeled antibody in the test (T) zone. This causes a pink-purple line to appear on the membrane. Unreacted patient sample and remaining unconjugated (unreacted) antibody continue to flow across the membrane to the procedural control zone. There the unreacted antibody becomes bound by a second antibody and immobilized in the membrane forming a pink/purple line. Results are available in 10 minutes (Figure 3-25 and Table 3-14).

The formation of the colored procedural control (PC) line indicates that the test procedure and the reagents were valid. If the PC line is not visible, the test is invalid. A positive test will have a purple/pink line visible in the test (T) area as well as in

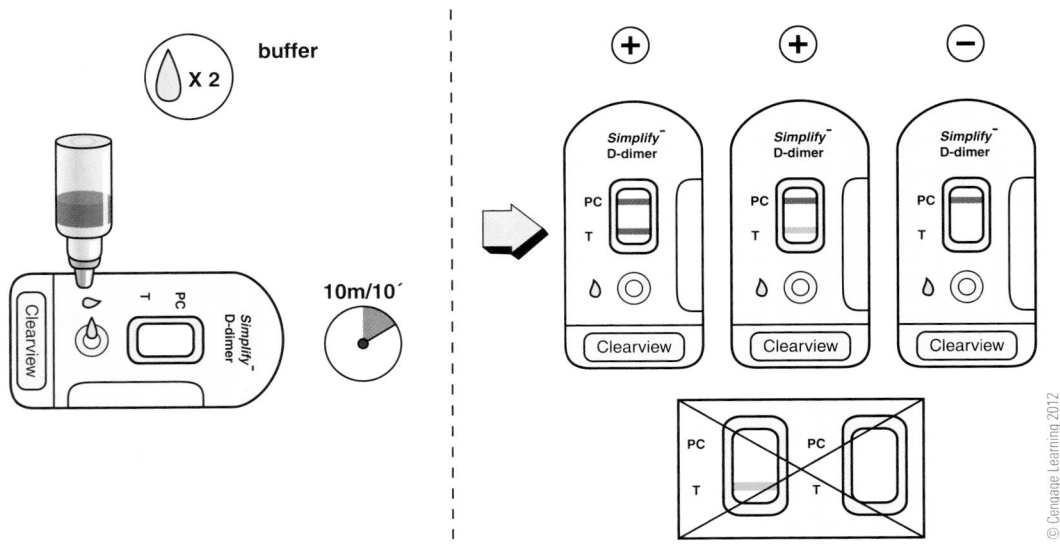

FIGURE 3-25 Diagram of Clearview Simplify D-dimer test procedure showing reactions

TABLE 3-14. Interpretation of results of the Clearview Simplify D-dimer test

VISIBLE RESULT	INTERPRETATION
Pink/purple line in test zone Pink/purple line in control zone	Positive for D-dimer
No line in the test zone Pink/purple line in control zone	Negative for D-dimer
No line in test zone No line in control zone	Invalid test*
Pink/purple line in test zone No line in control zone	Invalid test*

* Invalid test: Due to incorrect technique, defective reagents, or defective or damaged test cassette

in the patient reaction area (Figure 3-22). A semi-quantitative result can be obtained by preparing a doubling dilution series from 1:2 through 1:32 and testing 1 drop of each dilution separately. (See Lesson 1-8 for procedure for preparing doubling dilution series.) The detectable concentrations of D-dimers can range from 1 to 2 micrograms/mL (µg/mL) when positive only in the undiluted patient sample to greater than 32 µg/mL when the test is positive in the 1:32 dilution. The positive controls must give a positive reaction before results can be reported.

the PC area. The negative predictive value of the Clearview test is 100% for both PE and DVT (Figure 3-25).

Latex Agglutination Tests

The Remel D-dimer test is an example of a rapid slide agglutination assay for qualitative and semi-quantitative detection of XDP (cross-linked products). The Remel D-dimer test will detect only XDPs, not fibrinogen or fibrinogen degradation products (FDPs). The presence of these XDPs containing D-dimer is a marker for pathological fibrinolysis.

One drop of patient serum or plasma is mixed with one drop of latex suspension containing latex beads coated with antibodies to D-dimers. The slide is rocked gently by hand or mechanical rotator for 3 minutes. A positive test is indicated by agglutination

SAFETY REMINDERS

- Review Safety Precautions section before beginning procedure.
- Observe Standard Precautions.
- Discard used materials in appropriate biohazard containers.

PROCEDURAL REMINDERS

- Review Quality Assessment section before performing the procedure.
- Follow the procedures in the SOP manual.
- Run specified controls along with patient samples.
- Read test after specified time interval.

CASE STUDY 1

Jason had returned from Europe on a long transatlantic flight the previous day. During the flight, he had gotten chilled and developed a cough and some chest pain. Although the cough was uncomfortable, he was more concerned about the pain in his right calf. He called his physician, who instructed him to go to the emergency department. After hearing about his trip, the emergency department physician suspected DVT and ordered a rapid D-dimer test. The test result was negative; the test method performed had a negative predictive value of 100% for PE and 90% for DVT. The physician told Jason he did not have a PE but that he had not definitely ruled out the possibility of DVT.

1. Why did the physician order a D-dimer test?
2. Why is it important to use a type of D-dimer test that has a high negative predictive value?
3. What over-the-counter medication could possibly help prevent DVT?
4. Why might this help?

CASE STUDY 2

A farmer, Mr. Hawkins, was turning his tractor at the end of the row on a slight incline. The tractor flipped over. Mr. Hawkins could not jump clear and was pinned under the machine. Fortunately, a coworker was nearby and summoned help. In the emergency department his symptoms were pain and bleeding followed by signs of having blood clots. He continued to bleed.

1. What is a possible diagnosis?
2. What test(s) would you order?
3. Explain your answer.

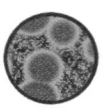

SUMMARY

D-dimers are produced when plasmin degrades stable fibrin clots, which are clots containing cross-linked fibrin. The presence of D-dimers in a patient's blood is an indicator of pathological fibrinolysis. The test for D-dimer is an important tool in the diagnosis of DVT, PE, and DIC.

A variety of manual and automated D-dimer test methods are available. All manufacturer's instructions and safety and quality assessment policies of the laboratory must be followed. Standard Precautions must be followed when handling patient specimens and controls. It is essential that the laboratory scientist follow the exact instructions for each brand of test, use the correct type of blood specimen, and use controls as prescribed by the package insert. The end-point of manually performed tests must be read at the exact timing specified, or the results are invalid. The D-dimer test can produce a valid result to aid in the diagnosis of hemostasis disorders.

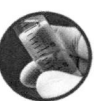

REVIEW QUESTIONS

1. What mechanisms occur in DIC that make it life-threatening?
2. What protein activates fibrinogen to begin clot formation?
3. The D-dimer test detects degradation products from the breakdown of which clotting proteins?
4. Name three conditions for which the D-dimer test can aid in evaluation and diagnosis.
5. Name three possible causes of DIC.
6. How do FDPs and XDPs differ? Detection of which indicates a more serious condition?
7. Describe two test methods for D-dimers.
8. Why is a quality assessment program important in a laboratory that performs D-dimer testing?
9. Explain what is meant when a test is said to have a negative predictive value?
10. What D-dimer test result would be expected in a patient who has DVT?
11. Explain why a bed-ridden patient might develop DVT or PE.
12. Define D-dimer, deep vein thrombosis (DVT), disseminated intravascular coagulation (DIC), FDPs, pulmonary embolism (PE), sepsis, and XDPs.

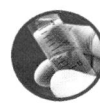

STUDENT ACTIVITIES

1. Complete the written examination for this lesson.
2. Practice performing a rapid test for D-dimers as outlined in the Student Performance Guide.

WEB ACTIVITIES

1. Use the Internet to gather information on DIC, DVT, or PE. For one of these conditions, report on the cause(s), symptoms, factors considered in diagnosis, laboratory tests that aid in diagnosis, and treatment.
2. Search the site of a scientific supplier for two tests for D-dimer not discussed in this lesson. List the names of the tests and types of specimens used (whole blood, plasma, etc.). Describe how the tests are performed (manual vs. automated, etc.)

D-Dimers

(Answers may vary based on the types of samples provided by the instructor and the type of test kit used.)

Name _____ Date _____

INSTRUCTIONS

1. Practice performing a rapid test for D-dimer following the step-by-step procedure.

2. Demonstrate the procedure for D-dimer satisfactorily for the instructor, using the Student Performance Guide. Your instructor will explain the procedures for evaluating and grading your performance. Your performance may be given a number grade, a letter grade, or satisfactory (S) or unsatisfactory (U) depending on the policy of the course or institution.

NOTE: The following is a general procedure for detecting D-dimer fragments using the Clearview Simplify D-Dimer test. The manufacturer's instructions for the specific method or instrument being used must be followed. If another kit is used, the procedure must be modified to fit the instructions accompanying that kit.

MATERIALS AND EQUIPMENT

- gloves
- hand antiseptic
- full-face shield (or equivalent PPE)
- marking pencil or pen
- timer
- test tube rack
- blood-collecting supplies:
  - for venous blood or plasma: citrate, heparin, or EDTA blood collection tube and venipuncture supplies
  - for capillary blood: capillary puncture materials
- commercial D-dimer kit (such as Clearview Simplify)
- optional: D-dimer control solutions
- disposable plastic transfer pipets
- micropipetter and tips capable of dispensing 20 μL
- paper towels
- laboratory tissue
- surface disinfectant (such as 10% chlorine bleach)
- biohazard container
- sharps container

PROCEDURE

Record in the comment section any problems encountered while practicing the procedure (or have a fellow student or the instructor evaluate your performance).

S = Satisfactory
U = Unsatisfactory

You must:	S	U	Evaluation/Comments
1. Wash hands with antiseptic and put on gloves and face protection			
2. Assemble equipment and materials			
3. Perform the manual test for D-dimer using the Clearview Simplify immunoassay (If this test kit is not available, carefully follow the instructions for the method being used)			

(Continues)

© 2012 Delmar, Cengage Learning. Permission to reproduce for clinical use granted.

You must:	S	U	Evaluation/Comments

4. Follow steps 4a–4i if using capillary blood; if using venous blood, go to step 5; if using control plasma, go to step 6
  a. Open the pouch containing the test components: *Use test within 10 minutes after opening*
  b. Perform a capillary puncture, wipe away the first drop, and collect the sample beginning with the second blood drop *using the capillary pipettes provided in the kit*
  c. Hold the filled capillary pipette in a vertical position above the round sample well of the device
  d. Squeeze the bulb and dispense all of the blood (35 μL) into the round sample well
  e. Allow the blood to completely penetrate the sample pad
  f. Hold the buffer bottle *vertically* and apply 2 drops of buffer to the sample well
  g. Leave the test device lying *flat* for the development time and discard sharps into sharps container
  h. Read the result after 10 minutes (see Table 3-14 and Figure 3-25)
  i. Go to step 5 if repeating the test using venous blood; if repeating the test using plasma, go to step 6; if not, skip to step 7			

5. Follow steps 5a–5g if using venous anticoagulated whole blood:
  a. Collect a venous blood sample using a collection tube containing trisodium citrate, heparin, or EDTA
  b. Open the pouch containing the test components: *Use test within 10 minutes after opening*
  c. Place test device on a flat horizontal surface.
  d. Use the *venous* pipettes included in the kit to deliver the blood specimen:
    (1) Squeeze the venous pipette near the sealed end and insert the open end into well-mixed venous anticoagulated sample
    (2) Release pressure to draw the sample into the pipette
    (3) Hold the pipette vertically and transfer 1 drop (35 μL) of whole blood to the round sample well
    (4) Discard pipette into sharps container
    (5) Allow the sample to completely penetrate the sample pad
  e. Hold the buffer bottle vertically and apply 2 drops of buffer to the well. *Do not disturb the device*
  f. Read the result after 10 minutes (see Table 3-14 and Figure 3-25)
  g. Go to step 6 if repeating the test using control plasma; if not, skip to step 7			

6. Follow steps 6a–6d if testing control plasma:
  a. Open the test pouch and place test unit on flat horizontal surface.
    NOTE: Test device must be used within 10 minutes after opening			

© 2012 Delmar, Cengage Learning. Permission to reproduce for clinical use granted.

You must:	S	U	Evaluation/Comments
b. Use a micropipetter to dispense 20 µL of control plasma into the sample well; allow plasma to completely penetrate the sample pad c. Hold the buffer bottle vertically and apply 2 drops of buffer to the sample well. Do not disturb the device d. Read the result after 10 minutes and record the result (see Table 3-14 and Figure 3-25)			
7. Discard all sharps into sharps container			
8. Discard other contaminated materials into appropriate biohazard container			
9. Clean the micropipetter with disinfectant following manufacturer's instructions			
10. Return unused supplies to storage			
11. Wipe the work area with disinfectant			
12. Remove gloves and discard into biohazard container			
13. Wash hands with antiseptic			

Instructor/Evaluator Comments:

Instructor/Evaluator _____ Date _____

© 2012 Delmar, Cengage Learning. Permission to reproduce for clinical use granted.

UNIT 4

Basic Immunology and Immunohematology

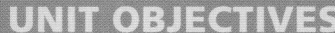

UNIT OBJECTIVES

After studying this unit, the student will:

- Discuss basic concepts of immunity and immune processes.
- Discuss how principles of immunology are used in the clinical laboratory.
- Explain the mechanisms of humoral and cell-mediated immunity.
- Compare the principles of tests based on agglutination and precipitation.
- Describe the principles and usefulness of labeled antibody techniques.
- Perform a rapid immunoassay for infectious mononucleosis.
- Perform a latex agglutination assay for rheumatoid factors.
- Perform a urine test for human chorionic gonadotropin (hCG).
- Discuss the functions of the immunohematology department.
- Explain guidelines for blood donation.
- Perform ABO grouping.
- Perform Rh typing.

UNIT OVERVIEW

Immunology is the study of the body's immune system and includes a variety of subdisciplines such as the study of immune diseases, tissue typing, blood banking, and organ transplantation. Even though most laboratories have a separate immunology department, every department in the clinical laboratory uses immunological principles and procedures in some way. Therefore, a basic knowledge of immunology is necessary to understand the principles of many laboratory tests.

Serology was the term first used for laboratory immunology because early immunological tests used serum for testing. Serological tests were designed around the *antigen-antibody* reaction. Today, *serological* procedures are more correctly called *immunological* procedures because they use serum, whole blood, urine, and other body fluids, as well as cells or tissues in a variety of test methods.

Many immunological tests are used in the clinical laboratory. These include:

- Antibody detection, identification, and measurement
- Identification of subsets of blood cells such as lymphocytes
- Detection of viral infections such as hepatitis, acquired immunodeficiency syndrome (AIDS), influenza, and infectious mononucleosis
- Identification of bacterial pathogens
- Clinical chemistry tests to identify analytes such as hormones or cardiac markers
- Toxicology tests to detect and measure drugs or monitor drug levels

A brief introduction to principles of immunology and basic techniques used in the immunology laboratory are described in Lesson 4-1. Medical laboratory scientists in all departments must have a good foundation and understanding of immunological principles.

Procedures for three commonly performed tests in the immunology laboratory are described in Lessons 4-2, 4-3, and 4-4. Lesson 4-2 explains the principle of immunochromatographic assays and describes how that technique is used in a rapid immunological test for diagnosing infectious mononucleosis, a viral disease. Lesson 4-3 explains a qualitative and semi-quantitative rapid agglutination assay to detect rheumatoid factors (RFs), one of the tests that can be used in the differential diagnosis of rheumatoid arthritis, an autoimmune disease. The urine test for human chorionic gonadatropin (hCG), commonly referred to as a pregnancy test, is discussed in Lesson 4-4. The test is based on immunological detection of the hCG hormone. Principles of the immunoassays presented in Lessons 4-2, 4-3, and 4-4 can be applied to many immunoassays performed in other departments of the laboratory.

Immunohematology, or blood banking, is the branch of immunology that uses immunological principles to identify and study the blood groups. Some blood banking procedures are relatively simple and easily interpreted, such as routine ABO grouping and Rh typing. Blood banking procedures such as compatibility testing for blood transfusion, antibody identification, and tissue typing are more complex and require knowledge and experience to perform and interpret.

Lessons 4-5, 4-6, and 4-7 introduce the student to immunohematology (blood banking) topics and basic blood typing procedures. Lesson 4-5 is an introduction to blood banking practices. Information and procedures for ABO grouping are discussed in Lesson 4-6. The Rh system and Rh typing procedures are presented in Lesson 4-7.

Delves, P.J. et al. (2006). *Roitt's essential immunology.* (11th ed.). Malden, MA: Blackwell Publishing Ltd.

Detrick, B. et al. (Eds.) (2006). *Manual of molecular and clinical laboratory immunology.* (7th ed.). Washington DC: American Society of Microbiology (ASM Press).

Engelkirk, P. G. & Duben-Engelkirk, J. (2010). *Burton's microbiology for the health sciences, North American edition.* (9th ed.). Baltimore, MD: Lippincott Williams & Wilkins.

Engelkirk, P. G. & Duben-Engelkirk, J. (2007). *Laboratory diagnosis of infectious diseases: Essentials of diagnostic microbiology.* Baltimore, MD: Lippincott Williams & Wilkins.

Flynn, J. C., Jr. & Kaszczuk, S. (Eds.). (1998). *Essentials of immunohematology.* Philadelphia: W. B. Saunders Co.

Forbes, B. A., et al. (2007). *Bailey & Scott's diagnostic microbiology.* (12th ed.). St. Louis: Mosby Year Book.

Harmening, D. (Ed.). (2005). *Modern blood banking and transfusion practices.* (5th ed.). Philadelphia: F. A. Davis Company.

Hilyer, C. D. et al. (2007). *Blood banking and transfusion medicine: Principles and practice.* (2nd ed.) Philadelphia, PA: Churchill Livingstone.

McPherson, R.A. & Pincus, M.R. (Eds.) (2007). *Henry's clinical diagnosis & management by laboratory methods.* (21st ed.). Philadelphia: Saunders Elsevier.

Paul, W. E. (Ed.). (2008). *Fundamental immunology.* (6th ed.). Philadelphia: Lippincott Williams & Wilkins.

Peakman, M. & Vergani, D. (2009). *Basic and clinical immunology.* (2nd ed.). London: Churchill Livingstone.

Quinley, E.D. (2010). *Immunohematology: Principles and practice.* (3rd ed.) Lippincott Williams & Wilkins.

Reid, M.E. & Lomas-Francis, C. (2004). *The blood group antigen facts book.* (2nd ed.). New York: Elsevier Academic Press.

Roback., J. et al. (2008). *Technical manual of the American Association of Blood Banks.* (16th ed.). Bethesda, MD: American Association of Blood Banks.

Rose, N. R., et al. (Eds.) (2002). *Manual of clinical laboratory immunology.* (6th ed.). Washington, D.C.: American Society for Microbiology (ASM Press).

Sacher, R. A. et al. (2000). *Widmann's clinical interpretation of laboratory tests.* (11th ed.). Philadelphia: F. A. Davis Company.

Shapiro, H. M. (2003). *Practical flow cytometry.* (4th ed.) Hoboken, NJ: John Wiley and Sons.

Sompayrac, L. M. (2008). *How the immune system works.* (3rd ed.). Oxford, UK: Blackwell Publishing.

Turgeon, M. L. (2003). *Fundamentals of immunohematology.* (2nd ed.). Baltimore: Lippincott Williams & Wilkins.

Turgeon, M. L. (2008). *Immunology and serology in laboratory medicine.* (4th ed.). St. Louis, MO: Mosby.

Whitlock, S. A. (2010). *Immunohematology for medical laboratory technicians.* Clifton Park, NY: Delmar Cengage Learning.

Package Inserts

Clearview Easy hCG. Package insert. Orlando, FL: Inverness Medical.

ICON II hCG. Package insert. Fullerton, CA: Beckman Coulter, Inc.

ICON 25 hCG. Package insert. Fullerton, CA: Beckman Coulter, Inc.

ICON Mono. Package insert. Fullerton, CA: Beckman Coulter, Inc.

QuickVue One-Step hCG Urine. Package insert. San Diego, CA: Quidel Corporation.

QuickVue+ Infectious Mononucleosis. Package insert. San Diego, CA: Quidel Corporation.

Remel Color Slide RF Test Kit. Package insert. Lenexa, KS: Remel, Part of Thermo Fisher Scientific.

Web Sites of Interest

American Association of Blood Banks, www.aabb.org
American Red Cross, www.redcross.org
American Society for Microbiology, www.asm.org
Centers for Disease Control and Prevention, www.cdc.org
National Institutes of Health, www.nih.org

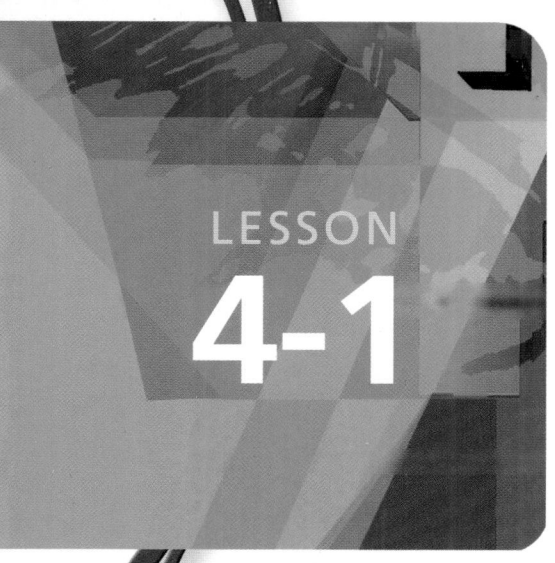

LESSON 4-1

Introduction to Immunology

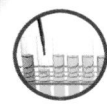

LESSON OBJECTIVES

After studying this lesson, the student will:

- ⊙ Explain the differences between natural resistance and acquired immunity.
- ⊙ Describe the process of inflammation.
- ⊙ State three characteristics of specific immunity.
- ⊙ Explain the differences between humoral and cell-mediated immunity.
- ⊙ Name the major cells that bring about specific immunity and describe their functions.
- ⊙ Diagram the structure of an immunoglobulin molecule.
- ⊙ Name the five immunoglobulin classes and give characteristics of each.
- ⊙ Explain the principle of agglutination and give an example of how it is used in the laboratory.
- ⊙ Explain the principle of precipitation and describe a precipitation technique.
- ⊙ Explain how nephelometry is used in immunological tests.
- ⊙ Explain the principles of labeled antibody tests and name three types of labels used.
- ⊙ Discuss the usefulness of flow cytometry in the immunology laboratory.
- ⊙ Define the glossary terms.

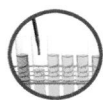

GLOSSARY

agglutination / the clumping or aggregation of particulate antigens resulting from reaction with specific antibody

allergy / a condition resulting from an exaggerated immune response; hypersensitivity

anamnestic response / rapid increase in blood immunoglobulins following a second exposure to an antigen; also called booster response or secondary response

antibody (Ab) / protein that is induced by, and reacts specifically with, a foreign substance (antigen); immunoglobulin

antigen (Ag) / foreign substance that induces an immune response by causing production of antibodies and/or sensitized lymphocytes that react specifically with that substance; immunogen

autoimmune disease / disease caused when the immune response is directed at one's own tissues (self-antigens)

B lymphocyte (B cell) / the type of lymphocyte primarily responsible for the humoral immune response

cell-mediated immunity / immunity provided by T lymphocytes and cytokines

(continues)

433

complement / a group of plasma proteins that can be activated in immune reactions, can cause cell lysis, and can help initiate the inflammatory response

cytokines / any of various nonantibody proteins secreted by cells of the immune system and that help regulate the immune response; lymphokines

dendritic cells / cells in lymphoid tissues that form a network to trap foreign antigens

enzyme immunoassay (EIA) / an assay that uses an enzyme-labeled antibody as a reactant

epitope / the portion of an antigen that reacts specifically with an antibody; antigenic determinant

humoral immunity / immunity provided by B lymphocytes and antibodies

immunocompetent / capable of producing a normal immune response

immunocompromised / having reduced ability or inability to produce a normal immune response

immunoglobulins (Ig) / antibodies; proteins that are induced by and react specifically with antigens (immunogens)

immunology / the branch of medicine encompassing the study of the immune processes and immunity

immunosuppression / suppression of the immune response by physical, chemical, or biological means

inflammation / a nonspecific protective response to tissue injury that is initiated primarily by the release of chemicals such as histamine and serotonin and by the actions of phagocytic cells

lymphokines / nonantibody proteins produced by lymphocytes in response to antigen stimulation and that play a role in regulating the immune response; cytokines

macrophages / long-lived phagocytic tissue cells that are derived from blood monocytes, function in destruction of foreign antigens, and serve as antigen-presenting cells

monoclonal antibody / antibody derived from a single cell line or clone

plasma cell / a differentiated B lymphocyte that produces antibodies

polyclonal antibodies / antibodies derived from more than one cell line

precipitation / formation of an insoluble antigen–antibody complex

primary lymphoid organs / organs in which B and T lymphocytes acquire their special characteristics; in humans, the bone marrow and thymus

secondary lymphoid tissue / tissues in which lymphocytes are concentrated, such as the spleen, lymph nodes, and tonsils

seroconversion / the appearance of antibody in the serum or plasma of an individual following exposure to an antigen

serology / the study of antibodies and antigens in serum or plasma using immunological methods

T lymphocyte (T cell) / the type of lymphocyte responsible for the cell-mediated immune response

thymus / a gland located in the upper chest that is the primary lymphoid tissue in which lymphocytes mature and acquire T cell characteristics

titer / in serology, the reciprocal of the highest dilution that gives the desired reaction; the concentration of a substance determined by titration

INTRODUCTION

Immunology had its beginnings in the study of infectious diseases and the development of vaccines to provide immunity. Early immunologists were physicians who worked to prevent infectious diseases through developing vaccines for bacterial and viral diseases such as smallpox, diphtheria, and tetanus. As advancements were made in knowledge about immunity, it became evident that the immune system was much more complex and had broader functions than just providing protection from invading microorganisms. The study of immunology now brings together a wide variety of disciplines, including segments of microbiology, oncology, allergy, laboratory science, genetics, and transplantation medicine to name a few.

It is now recognized that a healthy immune system is fundamental to overall good health. The immune system has an important role in protecting against tumors and toxins as well as microorganisms. The immune system can also be involved in the initiation of disease. For example, an **allergy** such as hay fever or a poison ivy rash is caused by an exaggerated immune response. **Autoimmune diseases** such as rheumatoid arthritis and lupus erythematosus result when components of the immune system react against one's own tissues. Deficiencies or malfunctions of the immune system can allow cancer cells to grow or allow the development of life-threatening infections by opportunistic organisms that are normally nonpathogenic.

A basic understanding of immunology is required to be able to generate, understand, and use much of the data in today's clinical laboratory. This lesson presents an overview of immunology and an introduction to principles of common immunological tests.

IMMUNOLOGY IN THE CLINICAL LABORATORY

Assays based on immunological principles are used in essentially all departments in the clinical laboratory where analytical tests are performed. These assays vary widely in design and purpose. Immunological assays are used to:

- Aid in the diagnosis of infectious diseases by detecting antibodies to bacteria, viruses, and parasites
- Detect or identify microorganisms using commercial antibodies
- Detect substances unrelated to the immune system, such as drugs or hormones, using antigen–antibody reactions
- Type blood and tissue
- Identify subsets of cells by detecting cell markers
- Evaluate patient immune function in cases of recurring infections, poor wound healing, or other symptoms indicating a possible problem with the immune response

THE IMMUNE SYSTEM

The immune system is a remarkably complex organization of tissues, cells, cell products, and biologically active chemicals, all of which interact to produce the *immune response*. The immune system provides specific defense mechanisms against a variety of foreign substances called **antigens (Ag)**. These antigens can be molecules, viruses, blood cells, tumor cells, bacteria, or fungi. For a substance to be strongly antigenic (capable of stimulating the immune response), it must contain protein or carbohydrate. However, only small portions of these molecules, called **epitopes**, are antigenic.

Natural Resistance

All of us have an innate *natural resistance* to harmful substances because of the presence of physical barriers, such as skin and mucous membranes, and protective secretions, such as mucus, stomach acid, and enzymes in tears. Also participating in this natural resistance are the actions of phagocytic cells, such as neutrophils and **macrophages**. These cells work together with certain naturally occurring biochemicals and proteins to initiate protective reactions such as **inflammation** (Figure 4-1 and Current Topic). These responses are nonspecific. This means that previous exposure to a foreign substance is not required for protective responses such as inflammation to be initiated, and that the body responds in the same way to a variety of substances and organisms.

Specific Immunity

The process of inflammation also helps initiate the *specific immune response* through interaction of macrophages and lymphocytes. Specific immunity is the type of immune response that recognizes and remembers different antigens. It is this response that most people think of as immunity.

Specific immunity is characterized by three properties:

- Recognition
- Specificity
- Memory

Recognition refers to the immune system's ability to recognize small differences in vast numbers of antigens in the environment and to distinguish them from self (one's own tissues).

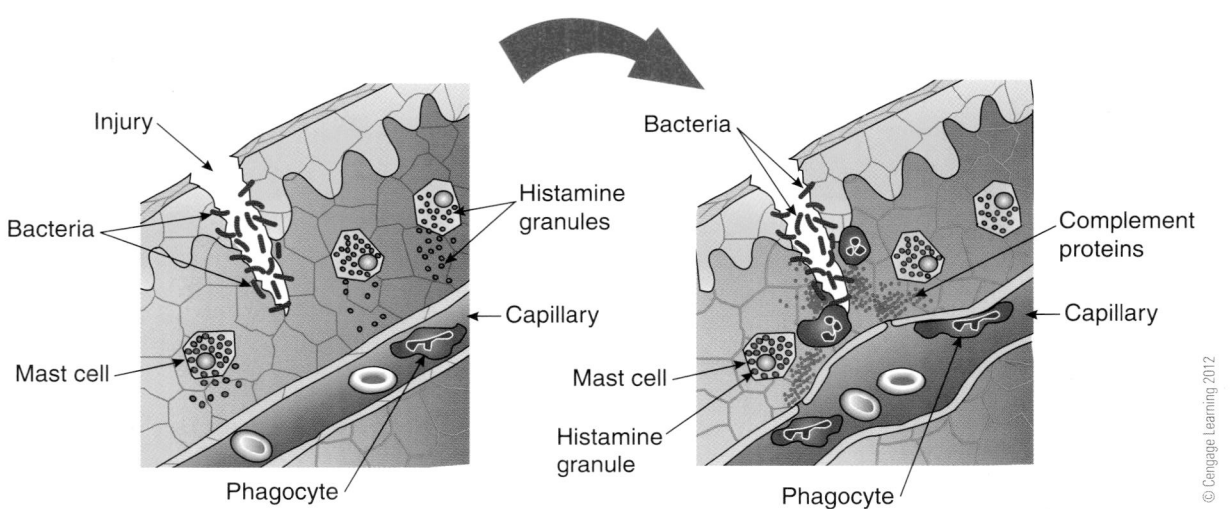

FIGURE 4-1 Inflammation: Left, tissue injury initiates a non-specific inflammatory response near the injured site and mast cells release histamine into tissue; right, histamine causes capillary dilation (redness) and plasma leaks into tissue causing swelling. Complement proteins and cytokines attract phagocytic cells which engulf and digest bacteria and tissue debris; on healing, histamine and complement signals cease, and tissue returns to normal

Specificity refers to the ability to direct a response toward a specific antigen without reacting with other similar antigens.

Memory refers to the immune system's ability to remember an antigen long after initial exposure. This ability, also called the **anamnestic response**, is the basis for immunizations. For example, a childhood immunization against the mumps virus will provide years of protection. The body's immune cells remember the viral antigens in the vaccine and will respond if they come in contact with the virus again, even years after the immunization.

Individuals normally have most contagious diseases only once because of the anamnestic response. After children have a disease such as measles, for instance, they usually develop lifelong immunity to the measles virus because of the memory response. Immunity to influenza viruses, however, is usually short-lived because influenza viruses have the ability to rapidly change their viral antigens.

Cells, Tissues, and Organs of the Immune System

Lymphocytes are important cells that help bring about the specific immune response. The two major types of lymphocytes are **T lymphocytes (T cells)** and **B lymphocytes (B cells)**, each having different functions in immunity. Lymphocytes circulate in the blood and in the lymph fluid and are also concentrated in lymphoid tissues throughout the body.

Lymphocytes are produced in the bone marrow and mature in the primary lymphoid organs. In mammals, the bone marrow and the **thymus** are the **primary lymphoid organs**. In humans, B cells mature and acquire their special characteristics in the bone marrow; T cells mature, proliferate and acquire T cell characteristics in the thymus. The spleen, lymph nodes, and tonsils are examples of **secondary lymphoid tissues** where lymphocytes can be found (Table 4-1).

Many cells in addition to lymphocytes contribute to and participate in immune responses and overall immunity through complex interactions. These include phagocytic cells such as granulocytes, monocytes, and **macrophages**, and **dendritic cells**, cells that form a network in lymphoid tissues to trap foreign antigens.

Two Types of Specific Immunity: Humoral and Cell-Mediated

The two types of specific immunity are **humoral immunity** and **cell-mediated** (cellular) **immunity** (Table 4-2). Both of these responses display recognition, specificity, and memory. The type of immunity predominating in an immune response to an antigen is primarily based on the type of lymphocyte that provides the major response to the antigen.

Humoral Immunity. B lymphocytes, or B cells, are responsible for humoral immunity. They provide primary protection against bacteria, toxins, and circulating antigens. B lymphocytes produce **antibodies (Ab)**, proteins that react specifically with antigens. B lymphocytes that have been converted to specialized and efficient antibody-producing cells are called **plasma cells** (Table 4-2).

Most vaccines stimulate humoral immunity. For instance, the DPT vaccine contains three antigens—killed *Corynebacterium diptheriae* (the bacterial species that causes diphtheria), killed *Bordetella pertussis* (the bacterium that causes whooping cough), and tetanus toxoid (an inactive toxin). After vaccination with these antigens, lymphocytes "learn" the antigens and produce specific antibodies against each antigen. If a child previously vaccinated with DPT vaccine is subsequently exposed to *B. pertussis*, the memory response will allow a rapid protective immune response.

Cell-Mediated Immunity. T lymphocytes, or T cells, help bring about cell-mediated immunity, providing protection against viruses, fungi, tumor cells, and intracellular organisms. Cell-mediated immunity is initiated by the interactions of T cells with foreign cells and antigens presented by macrophages and dendritic cells in secondary lymphoid tissue. T cells secrete **lymphokines**, also called **cytokines**, small molecules that communicate with other cells to help regulate the immune response (see Table 4-2 and Current Topic: Inflammation).

TABLE 4-1. Primary and secondary lymphoid organs and tissues

PRIMARY LYMPHOID ORGANS
- Thymus
- Bone marrow (bursa equivalent)

SECONDARY LYMPHOID ORGANS AND TISSUES
- Lymph nodes
- Spleen
- Gut-associated lymphoid tissue (GALT)
  - Peyer's patches
  - Appendix
  - Tonsils
- Bronchus-associated lymphoid tissue (BALT)

TABLE 4-2. Comparison of humoral and cell-mediated immunity

TYPE OF IMMUNITY	CELLS RESPONSIBLE	MEDIATED BY	PROVIDES PROTECTION AGAINST
Humoral	B cells (plasma cells)	Antibodies	Bacteria, toxins
Cell-mediated	T cells	Cells and lymphokines	Viruses, fungi, tumors

CURRENT TOPICS 1

INFLAMMATION

The inflammatory response is initiated by tissue injury from any trauma, mild or severe. The trauma can be internal or external and can be caused by burns, puncture wounds, toxins, bacteria, and other foreign substances, as well as by autoimmune disease. The four outward signs of inflammation are *redness*, *swelling*, *heat*, and *pain*. For example, when a superficial scratch becomes red, swollen, and tender, it is because of the inflammatory response, a nonspecific response.

The reactions that occur during the inflammatory response are directed at promoting healing of the injury. The typical inflammatory response is initiated when damaged tissue releases several different chemicals such as histamine, serotonin, and bradykinin. The immediate result of this chemical release is that capillary vessels become leaky, allowing fluid to move into the tissue, causing swelling and isolating any foreign substances from the rest of the body (Figure 4-1). The chemicals released are also *chemotactic*, which means they attract phagocytic cells to the site. The phagocytic cells engulf microorganisms that might have been introduced at the trauma site as well as damaged, dying, or dead cells. The phagocytes eventually die and accumulate at the site, forming what is commonly called *pus*. When the body senses that the foreign substance has been eliminated, the chemical releases subside and tissue returns to normal.

The inflammatory response just described is a greatly simplified version of the complex interactions that occur during inflammation. Also involved are the actions of complement proteins and many types of cytokines released by lymphocytes and macrophages. Complement proteins are a group of plasma proteins that can be activated in immune reactions, can cause cell lysis, and can help initiate the inflammatory response. Cytokines have far-reaching functions, which include recruiting cells such as neutrophils and *natural killer cells* to the site, causing fever by influencing the hypothalamus, and stimulating hematopoietic stem cells to produce more immune cells.

Acute inflammation is a natural part of the immune response. However, inflammation can occur inappropriately and lead to tissue destruction, such as occurs in autoimmune disorders, cardiovascular disease, and some degenerative disorders.

CURRENT TOPICS 2

T LYMPHOCYTE SUBSETS

T cells are the major players in cell-mediated immunity. The cell-mediated immune response is initiated when T cells encounter antigen processed and presented by cells such as macrophages and dendritic cells in the secondary lymphoid tissues. The pool of T cells consists of several subsets of cells, each with specific and different functions in the immune response. One way these subsets are identified is by the presence of *markers,* called CD markers, on the T cell membrane. Two T cell categories that are often measured in the immunology laboratory are *CD4 cells*, also called helper T cells, and *CD8 cells*, also called cytotoxic T cells. A CD4 cell has the CD4 marker on its membrane; a CD8 cell has the CD8 marker on its cell membrane.

CD4 cells cooperate with B cells to optimize antibody production. CD4 cells also contribute to regulation of the immune response by secreting cytokines, which influence the action of other cells of the immune system. CD8 cells are responsible for destroying tumor cells and virus-infected cells.

The human immunodeficiency virus (HIV) infects and destroys CD4 cells. Because CD4 cells are important to immune regulation and antibody production through their effects on B cells, this loss of CD4 cells produces a profound immunodeficiency in HIV-infected individuals. To monitor treatment or estimate immune suppression in HIV-positive patients, the patient's CD4 and CD8 cells are counted using flow cytometry (discussed later in this lesson). The results can be reported as the CD4/CD8 ratio, CD4 and CD8 percentages, or absolute CD4 and CD8 counts. The normal CD4/CD8 ratio ranges from approximately 0.8 to 3.0, and is usually ≥1.0. For example, a CD4/CD8 ratio of 2 indicates there are two CD4 cells for each CD8 cell. In HIV infection the ratio can fall to 0.1, meaning only 1 CD4 cell is present for each 10 CD8 cells.

IMMUNOGLOBULINS

Immunoglobulins (Ig), also called antibodies, are proteins produced by plasma cells and secreted into body fluids in response to antigen exposure. Immunoglobulins circulate in the blood and make up approximately 10% to 15% of serum protein.

Antibodies are named by placing the prefix *anti* before the antigen with which the antibody reacts. For example, one type of test for human immunodeficiency virus (HIV) infection detects the presence of *anti-HIV* (antibodies to HIV). In another example, the antibody specific for the A antigens on group A red blood cells is called *anti-A*.

An antigen entering the body triggers the production of immunoglobulins that can react specifically with epitopes found in that antigen. Epitopes are very small compared to the size of the antigen. In proteins, epitopes can consist of only five to six amino acids; in carbohydrates or polysaccharides an epitope might be only four to five sugar residues. The number of epitopes on a molecule is related to the size of the molecule. Smaller molecules contain only one or two epitope sites, meaning that an immunoglobulin would be able to bind to only one or two sites on the molecule.

The specific binding of epitope with immunoglobulin has been compared to fitting a key into a lock, with the epitope being the key and the immunoglobulin being the lock (Figure 4-2). The bonds holding the epitope to the antibody are noncovalent and are reversible. This interaction provides an important defense mechanism by targeting antigens for destruction.

Structure and Function of Immunoglobulins

The basic immunoglobulin (antibody) molecule consists of four polypeptide chains, two identical heavy (H) chains, and two identical light (L) chains. These four chains are linked together by interchain covalent bonds to form a shape similar to the letter **Y** (Figure 4-3). The region where the arms of the **Y** begin is called the hinge region because the molecule is flexible in this region (Figure 4-3).

Antibody monomers are bivalent; that is, each molecule contains two epitope-binding sites, one located at the end of each arm of the Y (Figures 4-3 and 4-4). These epitope-binding sites are composed of the variable (V) region and constant (C) region of one H chain and one L chain. These regions are named because of high variability in amino acid structure (V) or constancy (C) in amino acid structure. The epitope fits into a cleft formed by these portions of the chains; differences in amino acid structure in the variable regions of the H and L chains are responsible for the different specificities of antibodies.

Immunoglobulin Fragments

Much has been learned about the structure and function of immunoglobulin molecules by reacting immunoglobulin molecules with enzymes that can cut the protein chains into smaller segments. Two enzymes used early in these studies were papain (obtained from papaya) and pepsin (a digestive enzyme).

Papain treatment cleaves the immunoglobulin molecule at the hinge region of the Y, resulting in two identical fragments called *Fab fragments* and one fragment called the *Fc fragment* (Figure 4-4). Each Fab fragment contains one entire light chain and the portion of one heavy chain that contains the variable region. The fragments are named Fab because the fragments (F) contain the antigen binding (ab) sites of the Ig molecule. Each Fab fragment is monovalent (can bind to one epitope), but the intact immunoglobulin molecule is divalent (contains two antigen-binding sites).

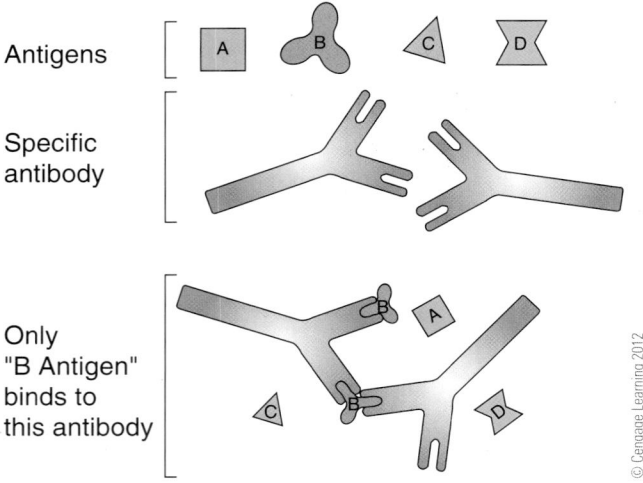

Antigens

Specific antibody

Only "B Antigen" binds to this antibody

© Cengage Learning 2012

FIGURE 4-2 Illustration of the lock-and-key concept of the antigen-antibody reaction: in the presence of 4 different antigens (A-D), only antibody molecules specific for the B antigens "recognize" and bind to antigen B

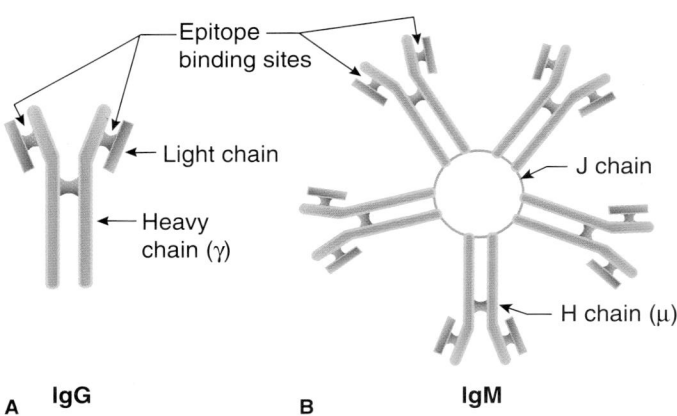

Epitope binding sites

Light chain

Heavy chain (γ)

J chain

H chain (μ)

A IgG   **B** IgM

FIGURE 4-3 Immunoglobulin structure: (A) IgG monomer is composed of 4 polypeptide chains, 2 heavy (H) chains and 2 light (L) chains all connected by disulfide bonds; (B) IgM pentamer is composed of 5 IgM monomers held together by a joining (J) chain. The heavy chain structure for each Ig class differs slightly, IgG having gamma (γ) chains, and IgM having mu (μ) chains. Each monomer has two epitope-binding sites; the IgM pentamer has 10 epitope-binding sites

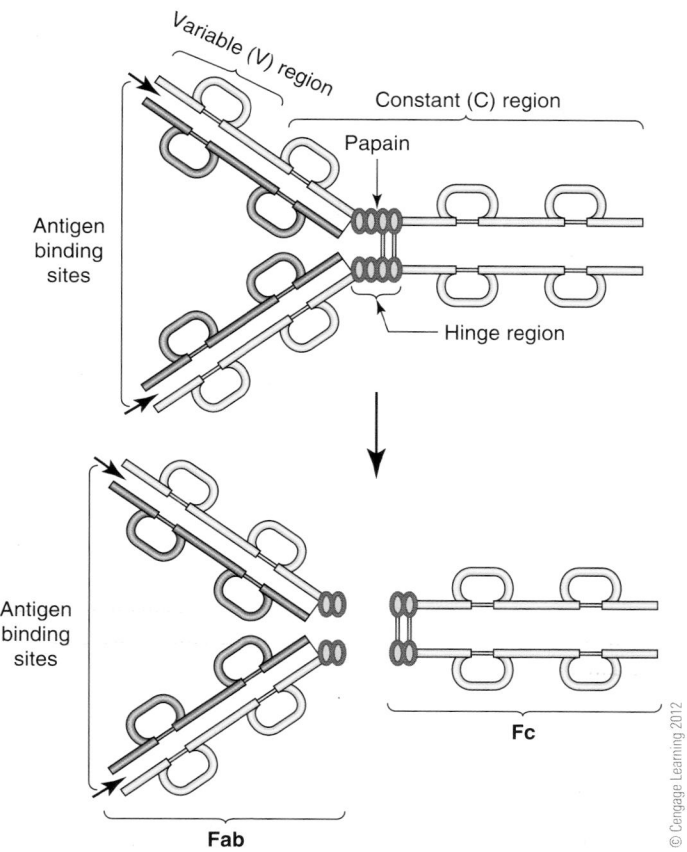

FIGURE 4-4 Immunoglobulin fragments: exposure of IgG to papain cleaves the Ig molecule into 3 fragments, 2 Fab fragments and 1 Fc fragment

The Fc fragment was named because it is easily crystallized (c). The Fc fragment of immunoglobulins has been shown to be responsible for binding to receptors on various cells—lymphocytes, mast cells, basophils, neutrophils, for example—leaving the epitope-binding "arms" of the molecule free to interact with epitopes/antigens (Figure 4-4). When immunoglobulins bind to cells through the Fc portion, the cells are often activated to perform a function.

Classes of Immunoglobulins

Several classes of immunoglobulins (Ig) exist, each with specific functions (Table 4-3). The Ig classes are structurally similar; a monomer of each class of Ig contains 2 H chains and 2 L chains. However, each Ig class has a unique H chain structure. That is, the H chains of one Ig class can be differentiated from the H chains of another Ig class by their chemical structure. The five classes of Ig in humans are:

- Immunoglobulin G (IgG)
- Immunoglobulin M (IgM)
- Immunoglobulin A (IgA)
- Immunoglobulin D (IgD)
- Immunoglobulin E (IgE)

TABLE 4-3. Characteristics and functions of immunoglobulin classes

IG CLASS	CHARACTERISTIC/FUNCTION
IgG	Long-lasting immunity, crosses placenta
IgM	First response antibody
IgA	Present in secretions
IgD	Function uncertain, present on B cell membrane
IgE	Allergic reactions

IgG

IgG is the antibody in highest concentration in blood. It is also called gamma globulin or immune globulin. IgG, once produced, remains in blood for a long time (has a long half-life) and provides long-lasting immunity. The Fc portion of IgG can bind to placental receptors, allowing transfer of the IgG across the placenta and providing immunity to the fetus and newborn. Therefore, newborns are born with humoral immunity that mirrors their mothers' IgG humoral immunity. This immunity lasts for several months after birth and is called *passive immunity* because the infant did not produce the antibodies. As the infant's level of maternal antibody decreases, the infant becomes susceptible to diseases. The infant's own immune system will be stimulated to produce antibodies when the infant is exposed to infectious agents or is vaccinated. This is called *active immunity* because the infant's immune cells are actively involved in producing the immune response.

IgM

IgM is the largest antibody, approximately five times larger than IgG. IgM is a pentamer, five IgM monomers bound together by a protein joining chain (J chain), leaving 10 epitope-binding sites free (Figure 4-3). IgM is the earliest antibody produced in response to an antigen but does not provide long-lasting immunity. IgM is also the first class of antibody to be produced by newborns after birth. Immunological tests based on detection of antibody in patient serum or plasma usually measure IgG or IgM. Because of its large size and many binding sites, IgM can be detected easily using laboratory tests based on agglutination principles. IgM is also effective in lysing cells because it can bind to multiple epitopes on a cell and can activate complement.

IgA

IgA is the second most abundant Ig in blood. It is called the secretory antibody because it is the predominant Ig in tears, saliva, breast milk, and secretions of the respiratory and intestinal tract. IgA provides protection against organisms that invade through these sites. IgA in breast milk provides passive immunity to newborns in addition to the passive immunity supplied by maternal IgG. Plasma or serum IgA is a monomer; secretory IgA is a dimer.

© Cengage Learning 2012

IgD

IgD is present in very small amounts in blood, and its function in blood is unclear. IgD is also found anchored in B cell membranes, where it can serve as a receptor.

IgE

IgE is the least common immunoglobulin in blood. IgE binds to eosinophils, basophils, and mast cells (tissue basophils) through its Fc region. IgE is involved in allergic reactions, such as hay fever and food allergies; IgE is increased in many parasitic infections. Immunoassays to detect IgE combine patient serum or plasma with specific allergens. These immunoassays are used to aid in diagnosis of allergies to food, pollen, chemicals, drugs, and various other substances.

Primary and Secondary Antibody Responses

The *primary antibody response* is the immune response occurring after the first exposure to an antigen. The first antibody detectable in plasma following initial antigen exposure is IgM, which usually is detectable in plasma or serum 3 to 4 days after antigen exposure. The IgM concentration quickly peaks and then drops rapidly over a few weeks (Figure 4-5). IgG is detectable in serum by 1 to 2 weeks after antigen exposure. The IgG level peaks within a few weeks and gradually decreases over a period of months (Figure 4-5).

Measurement or detection of IgM can provide information to aid in estimating when an individual was exposed to an organism or antigen. Because IgM is produced early and declines quickly, detection of IgM indicates acute disease (recent exposure). A rise in IgG concentration in blood samples collected 2 to 3 weeks apart also indicates recent exposure. **Seroconversion** is the term used when an antibody becomes detectable in the serum or plasma of a patient who previously tested negative for that antibody.

The anamnestic response, or *secondary antibody response*, is a rapid immune response seen after re-exposure to an antigen.

Antibody production increases rapidly and IgM and IgG levels rise quickly (within 2 to 3 days) following re-exposure to that antigen because immune cells remember the antigen. Booster vaccinations are based on the principle of the anamnestic response. IgG reaches higher levels in the anamnestic response than in the primary response, and the IgG remains detectable in the serum or plasma for months to years (Figure 4-5).

DISEASES INVOLVING THE IMMUNE SYSTEM

The immune system provides important protection from disease in **immunocompetent** individuals, individuals who have functioning immune responses. Any deficiency or damage to the immune system makes an individual more susceptible to disease, or **immunocompromised**.

Immune deficiencies can be mild or severe and can be acquired, congenital, or inherited. Most abnormalities of the immune system are acquired. Many drugs, especially corticosteroids and cancer chemotherapy agents, cause **immunosuppression** as an unwanted side effect. Infection with HIV results in interference with immune function, causing infected persons to become susceptible to opportunistic organisms such as *Pneumocystis*, an organism that causes no problems for healthy individuals. Other conditions that can cause abnormal or diminished immune responses include:

- Malignancies of the immune system, such as leukemia and lymphoma
- Diseases or abnormalities caused by overactive or misdirected immune system, as in allergies (hypersensitivities) or autoimmune diseases
- Inherited immunodeficiencies
- Congenital developmental abnormality in a fetus

Inherited immunodeficiencies and congenital developmental abnormalities affecting the immune system are uncommon.

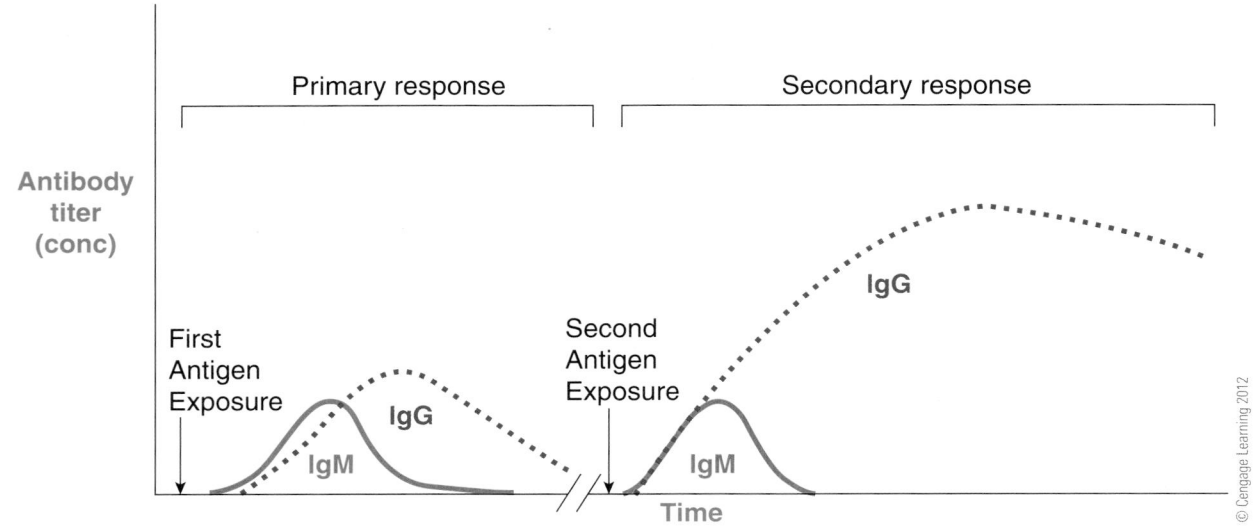

FIGURE 4-5 Comparison of IgM and IgG levels in the primary and secondary antibody responses

TABLE 4-4. Diseases and conditions associated with immune system abnormalities

DISEASE CATEGORY	EXAMPLES
Autoimmune diseases	Rheumatoid arthritis, lupus erythematosus, type 1 diabetes, myasthenia gravis
Hypersensitivities	Rhinitis, asthma, dermatitis
Malignancies	Lymphomas, leukemias, multiple myeloma
Acquired immunodeficiencies	Infections, systemic disease, malignancies, reactions to drugs, irradiation
Congenital immunodeficiencies	DiGeorge syndrome, agammaglobulinemia, severe combined immunodeficiency (SCID)

When they do occur, the effect is usually severe, causing a shortened life expectancy. Table 4-4 lists some diseases and conditions involving the immune system.

IMMUNOLOGICAL TESTS

Diagnostic tests based on immunological principles are diverse in design and are used in all departments in the clinical laboratory.

Tests of Immune Function

Many tests are designed to measure immune function or to detect immune deficiencies or irregularities. These include quantitating lymphocyte subsets such as CD4 and CD8 cells, quantitating immunoglobulin subgroups, tests of leukocyte function, allergy tests, and tests for specific complement proteins. Because of test complexity, most tests of immune function are performed in immunology laboratories located in large hospitals, transplant centers, reference laboratories, or medical schools.

Tests Based on Antigen-Antibody Reactions

Antibodies are incorporated into many clinical laboratory tests. They are useful because of their unique properties in recognizing and distinguishing among closely related antigens. Some tests aid in diagnosis of infections through the detection of antibodies to infectious agents in patient specimens; examples are the HIV, influenza, hepatitis, and rubella tests. These types of tests were commonly called **serology** tests because patient serum was the usual specimen. Some current serological methods can also use plasma or whole blood, as well as other body fluids.

Microbial antigens can be detected in patient specimens using commercial microbe-specific antibodies, as in tests to detect hepatitis viral antigens. Other laboratory tests use the antigen–antibody reaction to measure or detect a substance not a part of the immune system, such as using antibodies to measure drug or hormone levels or to identify a bacterial culture.

Monoclonal and Polyclonal Antibodies

Antibodies used in immunological tests can be monoclonal or polyclonal. **Monoclonal antibodies** are antibodies of one class and one specificity (react with only one epitope) and are derived from one (mono) clone, or cell line. Monoclonal antibodies are produced in laboratories and used as reagents in many immunodiagnostic kits.

Polyclonal antibodies are mixtures of antibodies produced by more than one (poly) cell line. We are constantly exposed to a broad array of antigens that stimulate our immune responses. For instance, one bacterial infection will stimulate many plasma cells (poly clones) to respond, each producing and secreting antibodies to a different bacterial epitope. This results in a mixture of antibodies in plasma that taken together can react with multiple antigens and reflect our history of antigen exposure.

Test Sensitivity and Specificity

Laboratories choose test methods based on the sensitivity and specificity of the method. *Sensitivity* refers to the lower limit of detection, or the lowest concentration capable of being detected by a test method (Table 4-5). Failure to detect small amounts of a substance in a test will result in a false-negative result.

Specificity refers to the ability to detect only the substance for which the test is designed. Reaction with other substances (cross-reactivity) decreases the specificity of the test and can cause false positive results.

Qualitative, Semi-quantitative and Quantitative Tests

Many immunological procedures are reported only as negative or positive; these are called qualitative tests. Other procedures are semi-quantitative or quantitative. Semi-quantitative procedures usually estimate concentrations of antibody or sometimes antigen. The antibody concentration can be estimated by making serial dilutions and determining the maximum dilution

TABLE 4-5. Immunological-based test methods in order of sensitivity (least sensitive methods are listed first; most sensitive methods are listed last)

Precipitation

Agglutination

Labeled antibody techniques

    Enzyme Immunoassay (EIA)

    Immunofluorescence (IF)

    Chemiluminescence

Flow cytometry

still capable of causing a visible reaction in the test procedure. Semi-quantitative estimates of antibody concentration can be expressed as a **titer**, the reciprocal of the highest dilution showing a reaction. (The procedure for serial dilutions is given in Lesson 1-8.) Quantitative immunological tests are less frequently performed. Examples of some quantitative tests are absolute T-cell counts, drug assays, and measurements of Ig subclass concentration expressed in units such as milligrams per liter (mg/L).

PRINCIPLES OF ANTIGEN-ANTIBODY TESTS

Examples of tests that incorporate the antigen–antibody reaction include:

- Agglutination tests
- Agar precipitation tests
- Nephelometric assays
- Immunofluorescence (IF) tests
- Enzyme immunoassays (EIAs)
- Chromatographic immunoassays
- Chemiluminescence immunoassays
- Flow cytometry techniques

Agglutination

Agglutination is the visible clumping or aggregation of cells or particles as a result of reaction with specific antibody (Figure 4-6). IgM is the antibody class that reacts best in agglutination reactions because of its large size and multivalent binding capacity. Antigen-coated cells or particles, such as red blood cells or latex beads, become linked together and form visible clumps when reacted with sufficient antibody. In most agglutination test designs, the presence of agglutination indicates a positive test. Blood typing (Lessons 4-6 and 4-7), bacterial identification, and the classic latex test for rheumatoid arthritis (described in Lesson 4-3) are tests based on the agglutination reaction. Agglutination tests can be qualitative or semi-quantitative.

Semi-quantitative tests can be performed on slides, in tubes, or in special microtiter plates having wells with rounded bottoms. Serial dilutions of serum are made and tested to determine the maximum dilution capable of causing agglutination, which is reported as a titer. When agglutination tests are performed in microtiter plates, a negative test is indicated by the presence of nonagglutinated particles concentrated in a small dot in the bottom of the well. A diffuse pattern of cells spread over the bottom of a round-bottomed well indicates a positive test (Figure 4-6B).

Precipitation

Precipitation is the formation of an insoluble complex when a specific antibody is reacted with a soluble antigen (Figure 4-7). IgG is the antibody class that reacts best in precipitation reactions. Agar or agarose, gelatin-like substances, provide a matrix for the reactions. The formation of a visible white precipitate in the agar is a positive reaction. Precipitation can occur only when antigen and antibody are in the correct proportions; excess of either reactant will inhibit formation of a visible precipitate. Radial immunodiffusion and rocket electrophoresis are examples of agar precipitation tests.

Radial Immunodiffusion (RID)

An example of a *radial immunodiffusion* (RID) test used in clinical laboratories is a test to estimate the concentration of IgG, IgM, or IgA in a patient's serum. Agar plates about the size of a microscope slide can be purchased that contain anti–human IgG (or anti–human IgA or IgM) diffused throughout the agar. The agar contains small wells. Each well is filled with patient serum

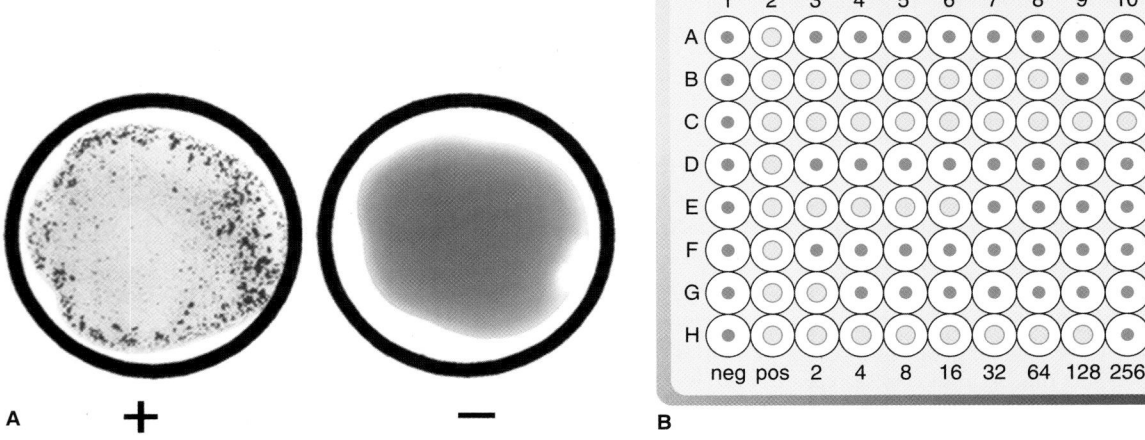

FIGURE 4-6 Agglutination: (A) slide agglutination showing positive (+) reaction in circle on left and negative (−) reaction in circle on right; (B) hemagglutination reactions in microtiter plate, small solid red dot is negative reaction, diffuse red circle is positive reaction; in row A all reactions are negative except well 2, which is positive

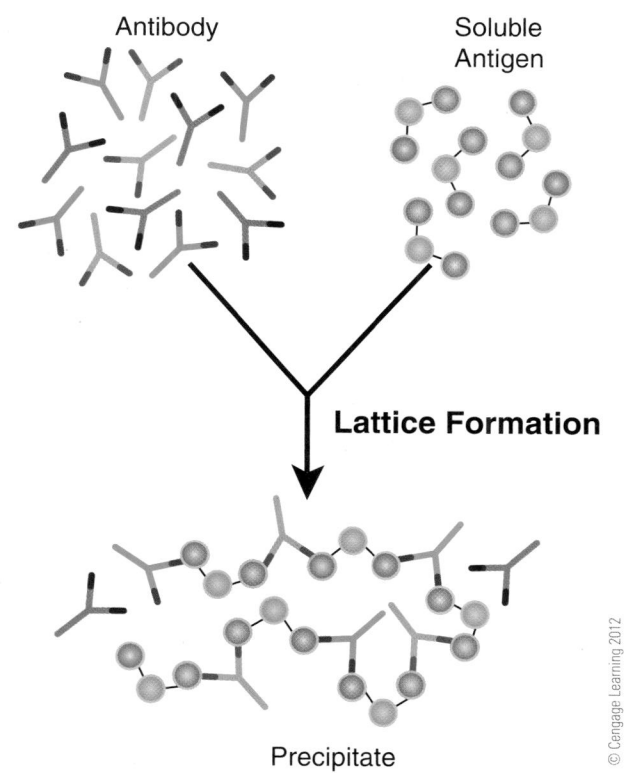

Lattice Formation

Precipitate

FIGURE 4-7 Precipitation: soluble antigen reacts only with specific antibody to form a lattice; when the size of the lattice complexes becomes large enough, the complexes fall out of solution and form a visible precipitate

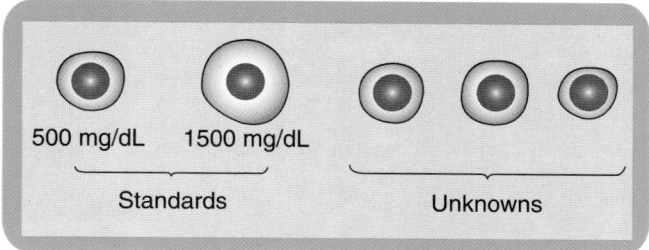

A **Radial Immunodiffusion**

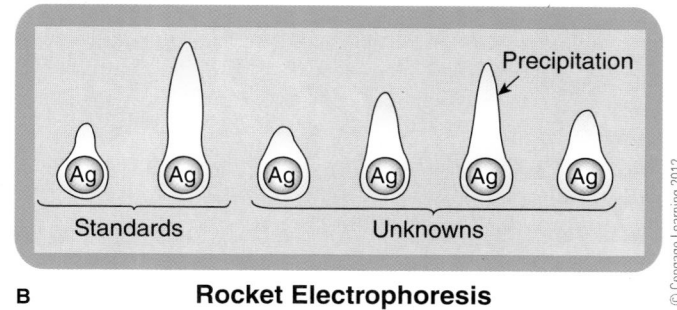

B **Rocket Electrophoresis**

FIGURE 4-8 Agar precipitation techniques: (A) in radial immunodiffusion, rings of precipitation form when serum diffuses into agar and reacts with specific antibody in agar; (B) in rocket electrophoresis, serum proteins diffuse out of wells under the influence of electric current and react with antibody in agar to form rocket-shaped precipitation patterns

(the test sample) or a standard (known amount of IgG), and the plate is incubated several hours. As the IgG in the serum or standard diffuses out of the well and into the agar, it reacts with the anti-IgG in the agar, forms immune complexes, and produces a visible white ring of precipitation around the well (Figure 4-8A). The diameter of the ring is proportional to the concentration of IgG in the sample. A standard curve is constructed using the diameters of the precipitation rings produced by the IgG standards and the concentrations of the IgG standards. The concentration of the unknown is determined by comparing the size of its precipitation ring with the standard curve.

Rocket Electrophoresis

Rocket electrophoresis is similar to radial immunodiffusion. A slide of antibody-containing agar is used. Standard-sized wells along one side of the slide are filled with standards or the serum that is being tested. An electric current is then applied to the agar to accelerate movement of the standards or samples out of the wells and into the agar. Movement of charged molecules in response to an electric current is called *electrophoresis*. If the antibody concentration in the agar is in the correct proportion to the antigen concentration in the samples applied to the wells (Figure 4-8B), precipitation will occur and a cone or *rocket*-shaped pattern will form. The area beneath the rocket is proportional to the concentration of the sample. A standard curve is constructed using the measurements of the

standards, and the concentration of the unknown is determined by comparison to the standard curve.

Nephelometry

Immunological tests based on precipitation methods can be automated using nephelometry. When specific antibody is reacted with soluble antigen, a suspension of very small particles forms that can be measured using an instrument called a nephelometer. Nephelometry is based on the principle that a suspension of small particles will scatter light when a beam is passed through it (Figure 4-9). The scattered light is collected electronically and measured. An increase in the concentration of the particle suspension causes the amount of light scatter to increase. In practice, antigen and antibody are combined in proportions to cause formation of small antigen–antibody complexes that remain suspended during measurement. A beam of light is passed through the suspension, and the degree of light scatter is compared to the light scatter from standards. The amount of unknown is determined from a standard curve.

Many tests that formerly were performed by agar precipitation techniques have been adapted to nephelometry, and several automated immunology analyzers operate on the principle of nephelometry. Tests for immunoglobulin subclasses and for specific plasma proteins such as haptoglobin, α-1 antitrypsin, rheumatoid factor, complement proteins, or C-reactive protein (CRP), can be performed quickly by nephelometry.

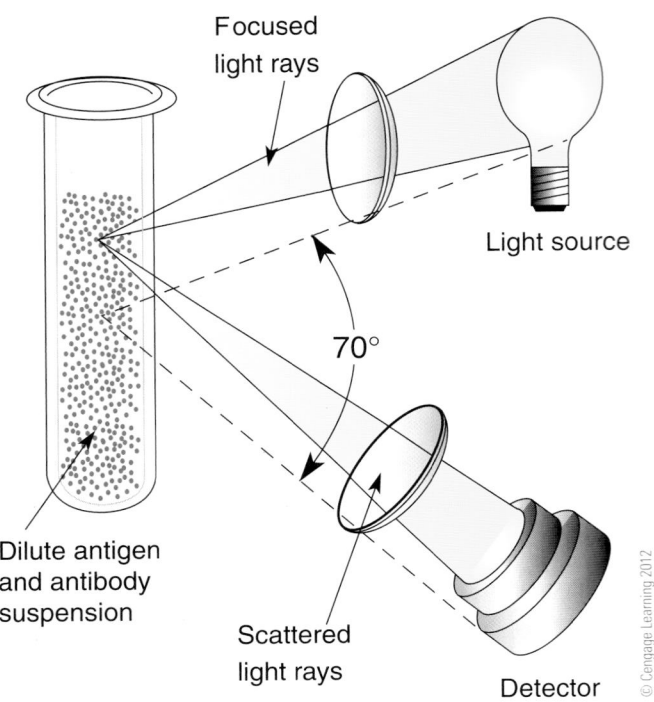

Focused
light rays

Light source

70°

Dilute antigen
and antibody
suspension

Scattered
light rays

Detector

© Cengage Learning 2012

FIGURE 4-9 Principle of nephelometry: light is deflected (scatters) when it interacts with small particles in solution, such as antigen-antibody (Ag-Ab) complexes; the measure of degree of scatter is proportional to the concentration of the Ag-Ab complexes

Labeled Antibody Techniques

Several types of immunological tests use *labeled* antibodies in the test design. Molecules (labels) such as dyes or enzymes are conjugated (attached) to the Fc portion of the antibodies (Figure 4-10). Attaching these labels to the immunoglobulins does not interfere with the immunoglobulins' ability to bind to antigens.

The first sensitive and reliable drug and hormone assays used antibodies labeled with radioisotopes, called *radioimmunoassays (RIAs)*. These early immunoassays required a radiation detector to measure the reaction. RIAs have been replaced by improved labeling techniques, eliminating the hazards of using radioactive materials.

Labeled antibody techniques are among the more sensitive immunoassays available (Table 4-5). Examples of labeled antibody techniques include:

- enzyme immunoassays
- membrane immunoassays using dyes or chemiluminescent labels
- immunofluorescence techniques
- protein immunoblotting
- flow cytometry

Enzyme Immunoassay

Enzyme immunoassays (EIAs) use enzyme-labeled antibodies to cause a visible reaction (Figure 4-10). The tests can be designed to detect either antibody in a patient specimen, or

antigen, such as viral antigen, in a patient specimen. Early EIAs were complex procedures, but many of today's tests, although sophisticated in internal design, are relatively simple to perform.

The following description of a test to measure rubella antibodies and determine immunity to rubella is an example of how an EIA works.

1. A reaction well or tube is coated with rubella viral antigen, patient serum is added, and the test is incubated to allow time for any anti-rubella antibody in the patient serum to bind to the viral antigen. The test well is then rinsed to remove nonspecific unbound antibody.

2. Anti-human IgG (antibody directed against human IgG) with an enzyme label attached to the Fc region is added to the well and allowed to incubate. (If anti-rubella was present in the patient serum and became bound to the viral antigen, the enzyme-labeled antibody will bind to the anti-rubella. If no anti-rubella was present in the serum, the enzyme-labeled antibody will not have anything to bind to.) The well is rinsed again to remove unbound enzyme-labeled antibody.

3. A colorless substrate specific for the enzyme is added to the well and allowed to react.

4. Test Interpretation: If no color forms after addition of the enzyme substrate, the test is negative—no enzyme remained to cause a color change in the substrate. If the enzyme substrate is converted to a colored form, the test is positive—indicating that enzyme-labeled secondary antibody was present.

Membrane, Lateral Flow, or Chromatographic Immunoassays

Numerous tests have been designed based on variations of the enzyme immunoassay. These are called by various names, such as *membrane immunoassays*, *lateral flow immunoassays*, or *immunochromatographic assays*.

In many immunoassays, most or all of the reagents are incorporated into an absorbent membrane enclosed in a plastic cassette. When a sample (serum, plasma, urine, or cell extract) is added followed by a buffer, molecules in the sample migrate across the membrane, reacting with the antibody and reagents in the membrane and forming a color or a reaction (Figure 4-11). Some tests are read and interpreted visually by the technologist; others are read using an instrument.

Most of these tests are simple to perform and interpret, even though the technology is complex. Examples of membrane immunoassays include over-the-counter urine pregnancy test kits, and tests for infectious agents such as for group A *Streptococcus*, influenza virus, *Helicobacter pylori* and *Trichomonas vaginalis*. Many membrane immunoassays are CLIA-waived.

Chemiluminescence immunoassays are recent modifications of enzyme assays that are increasing in use. Chemiluminescence is the generation of light by the release of energy from a chemical reaction. A familiar example of chemiluminescence is the light emitted by light stick toys. The light-emitting reactions of fireflies and certain marine organisms are similar to chemiluminescent reactions in that they are caused by chemical reactions; however, light emitted by organisms is called bioluminescence.

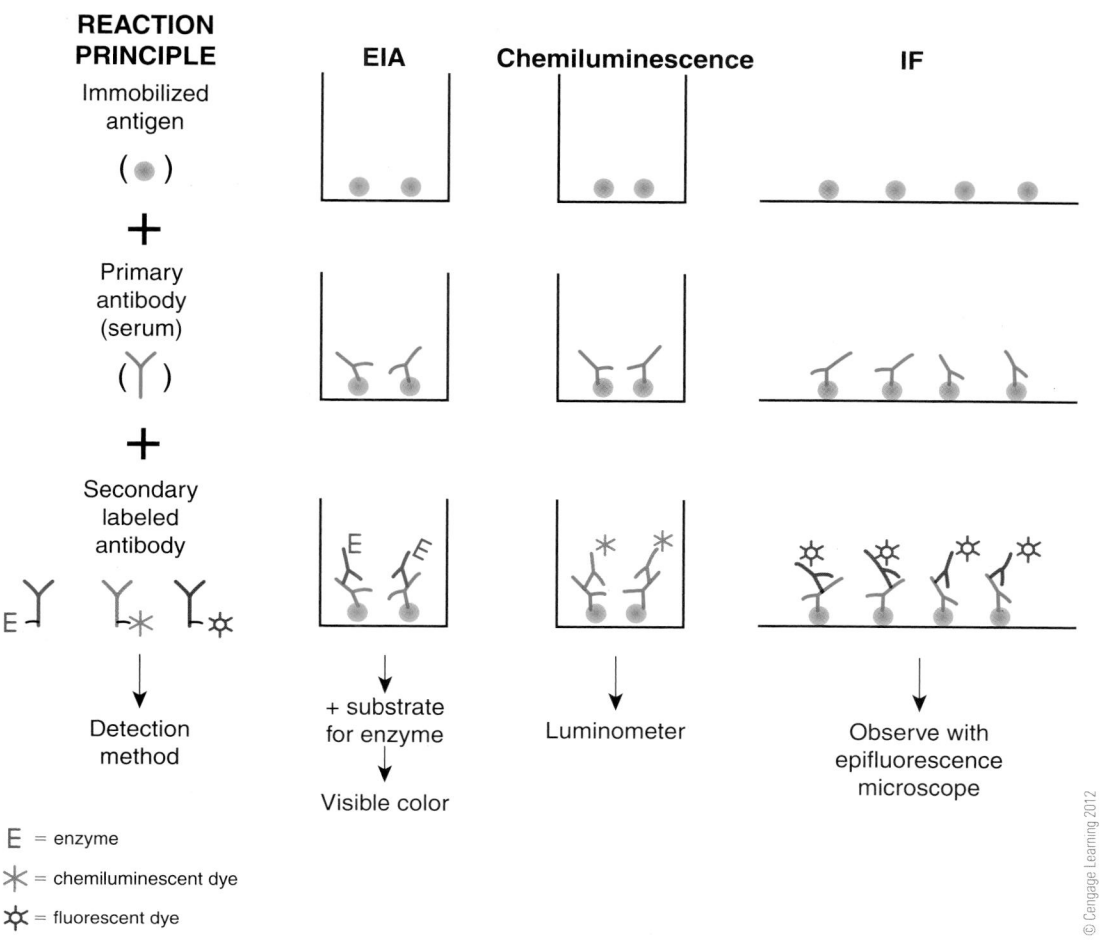

FIGURE 4-10 Comparison of labeled antibody techniques: (left) enzyme immunoassay (EIA); (center) chemiluminescence assay; (right) immunofluorescence assay (IF)

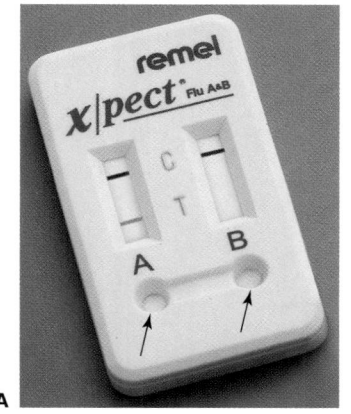

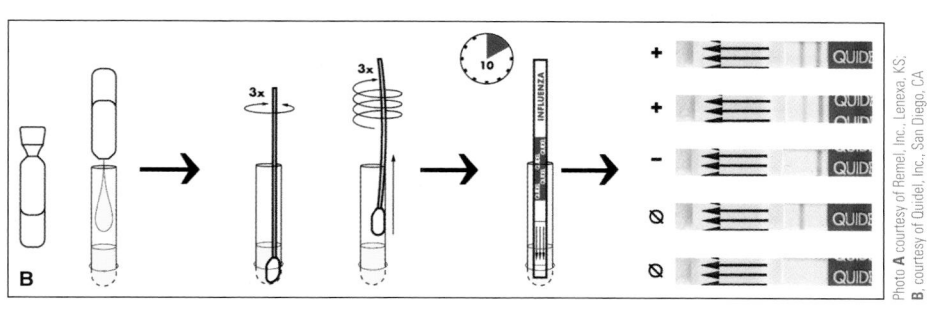

FIGURE 4-11 Two types of immunoassays for influenza: (A) in lateral flow immunochromatographic assay, patient serum was applied to wells A and B (arrows); after incubation the "C" lines appearing at the top of windows A and B indicate the internal controls are working properly; the blue "T" line in window A is a positive result for influenza A antibodies; absence of blue "T" line in window B is a negative result for influenza B antibodies. (B) Nasal swab is swirled in buffer to extract antigens; test strip is immersed in antigen extract; and formation of colored lines indicate control results and test results [+ = positive test; (−) = negative test; Ø indicates invalid test]

Immunofluorescence (IF) Techniques

Immunofluorescence (IF) techniques use antibodies labeled with a fluorescent dye to detect antigens or to detect antibodies. The fluorescent dyes emit a particular wavelength of light when excited by a beam of ultraviolet (UV) light. Epifluorescence microscopes are used to read and interpret reactions for tests performed using microscope slides (Figure 4-10 and Lesson 1-10). IF tests can also be performed in microtiter plates, and the reactions can be read using microplate readers.

Immunofluorescence tests can be direct or indirect. Direct tests use a labeled antibody that reacts directly with the antigen in question, such as identifying a viral antigen from a culture or from a patient specimen. Indirect tests use a labeled antibody to detect another antibody, creating a "sandwich" assay (Figure 4-10). Immunofluorescence tests are used in microbiology, parasitology, and immunology. Immunofluorescence techniques are often used to detect autoantibodies, such as those present in lupus erythematosus.

An example of an indirect immunofluorescence test is the classic test developed years ago for the diagnosis of *Treponema pallidum* infection (syphilis). This test is performed by incubating patient serum with a prepared slide of a laboratory strain of *Treponema*. The slide is rinsed to remove unbound, nonspecific antibody in the patient serum, and the specimen is then incubated with fluorescently-labeled anti-human globulin. The slide is rinsed again and examined microscopically. The presence of fluorescent spirochetes indicates that the patient serum was positive for anti-treponemal antibodies.

Pathogens such as mycobacteria, which include the bacteria causing tuberculosis, and *Cryptosporidium*, a pathogenic yeast, can also be identified using fluorescent antibodies. For these tests, a slide preparation prepared from a patient specimen is reacted with commercial microorganism-specific antibody. This first antibody can be fluorescently labeled (direct test) or, if not, is followed with a second labeled antibody (indirect test). The presence of fluorescing microorganisms of the correct morphology indicates that the patient is infected with the suspect microorganism. Indirect techniques are more sensitive than direct because more than one molecule of fluorescent-labeled second antibody can bind to the first antibody, increasing the amount of fluorescence.

Protein Immunoblotting Techniques

Protein *immunoblotting* techniques, sometimes called Western blots, combine electrophoresis with labeled antibody tests. The secondary antibodies used in immunoblotting can be labeled with enzymes, fluorescent dyes, or chemiluminescent molecules. These techniques are primarily performed in chemistry, reference, or research laboratories. One use of immunoblotting is to confirm positive results obtained with rapid screening tests for HIV infection. The immunoblotting procedure detects patient antibodies to the p24 antigen of HIV.

Flow Cytometry and Cell Sorting

Flow cytometry is a technique that is useful when cells in suspension need to be identified, categorized, or separated into groups. The term *flow cytometer* comes from cell (*cyto*) measurement (*meter*) as cells *flow* through a special narrow channel in single file. In clinical medicine, flow cytometry is used in immunology and hematology laboratories, as well as to identify urine sediment components.

To identify cells using flow cytometry, cell suspensions are treated with one or more fluorescent-labeled antibodies.

CASE STUDY

Ahmed, a 61-year-old man, came to see his physician because he had fever, headache, and fatigue for over a week and still was not feeling well. His physician ordered several tests for infectious diseases, including tests for influenza, toxoplasmosis, West Nile virus, and Epstein-Barr virus. These tests were performed by testing Ahmed's serum for the presence of both IgG and IgM antibody to the various infectious agents. The following results were reported:

Serum tested against:	IgG	IgM
Influenza A	Negative	Negative
Toxoplasma	Positive	Negative
West Nile virus	Negative	Positive
Epstein-Barr virus	Positive	Negative

1. What infectious agent(s) can be ruled out as the cause of Ahmed's illness? Why?
2. What is a possible cause of his illness? Explain your answer.

The labeled antibodies react with specific cell surface markers. The cell suspensions flow into a narrow channel and pass by a laser beam in single file. Cells passing through the beam are counted, cell or nuclear size is measured, or fluorescence pattern detected, and this information is stored in a database. A screen displays the information graphically showing percentages for each cell category or size distribution. Some analyzers can measure three different fluorescent colors, so three types of cells can be analyzed and sorted into groups simultaneously. Some cell sorting analyzers can separate cells by category and keep them alive for later use. Flow cytometry has many applications and is useful in separating stem cells or blood cells, such as subpopulations of lymphocytes. Specific applications of flow cytometry to hematology and urinalysis are discussed in Lessons 2-10 and 5-5.

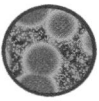

SUMMARY

This lesson is a brief introduction to the basic principles of immunology needed to understand procedures in the remaining lessons in this unit. Knowledge of the cells and organs of the immune system and the mechanisms of immune responses also aids the student in understanding how immunological tests work. This is important because tests based on immunological principles are performed in all laboratory departments.

Several test designs are based on the antigen–antibody reaction, so knowledge of the structure and functions of antibody subclasses is important. Antigen–antibody tests vary in sensitivity. Agglutination, agar precipitation techniques, and nephelometric assays are not as sensitive as labeled antibody techniques using enzymes, fluorescent dyes, or other chemical labels. Many immunological tests, such as membrane immunoassays, have been designed to be very easy to perform despite being based on complex principles. These tests often give rapid results and many are CLIA-waived. It is impossible to cover the complex topic of immunology in a single lesson, but it is hoped that the student will be stimulated to seek more information on this topic.

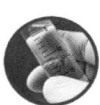

REVIEW QUESTIONS

1. What are the differences between specific immunity and natural resistance?

2. What are the differences between humoral and cell-mediated immunity?

3. What are the three characteristics of specific immunity?

4. What type of immunity most commonly develops from vaccinations?

5. Draw an IgG molecule. Show where the epitope binding sites are.

6. Name the five classes of immunoglobulins. Which is the most abundant in blood?

7. Which immunoglobulin class gives long-lasting immunity?

8. Which immunoglobulin class can increase in allergic reactions?

9. Which class of immunoglobulin can cross the human placenta? How does this affect the fetus and newborn?

10. Which class of immunoglobulin is called secretory antibody? Why?

11. Explain the principle of agglutination.

12. What tests are based on the principle of precipitation?

13. What instrument can be used to quantitate precipitation reactions?

14. What is meant by labeled antibody? What types of labels are used in immunological tests?

15. Explain the difference in test specificity and test sensitivity. How do these two characteristics affect test results?

16. How does the sensitivity of labeled antibody tests compare to that of precipitation and agglutination tests?

17. Explain the principle of flow cytometry and discuss how it is used in the clinical laboratory.

18. How do qualitative tests differ from quantitative or semi-quantitative tests?

19. Discuss how the inflammatory response stimulates healing.

20. How are lymphocyte markers used to follow the progress of HIV infection?

21. Why is the immunity present in newborns called passive immunity?

22. How do monoclonal antibodies differ from polyclonal antibodies?

23. Define agglutination, allergy, anamnestic response, antibody, antigen, autoimmune disease, B lymphocyte, cell-mediated immunity, complement, cytokines, dendritic cells, enzyme immunoassay, epitope, humoral immunity, immunocompetent, immunocompromised, immunoglobulins, immunology, immunosuppression, inflammation, lymphokines, macrophages, monoclonal antibody, plasma cell, polyclonal antibodies, precipitation, primary lymphoid organs, secondary lymphoid tissue, seroconversion, serology, T lymphocyte, thymus, and titer.

STUDENT ACTIVITIES

1. Complete the written examination for this lesson.

2. Look in magazines, newspapers, or other sources for information on the role of the immune system in allergies.

WEB ACTIVITIES

1. Use the Internet to find information on two brands of analyzers used for immunology testing. Compare the principle of operation of each and list tests that are included in the test menus.

2. Research an autoimmune disease or immune deficiency disease using reliable Internet sources. Report on the cause of the disease, symptoms, methods of diagnosis, and appropriate clinical laboratory tests.

3. Use the Internet to find information on C-reactive protein (CRP). Find three CRP tests that use at least two different technologies. Report on the test methods and the significance of CRP testing.

4. Search the Internet for tests that use chemiluminescence principles. Write a brief report explaining chemiluminescence and describing an example of how it is used in an assay design.

5. Search the Internet for tutorials on immunology topics such as inflammation, antibody structure and function, humoral and cell-mediated immunity.

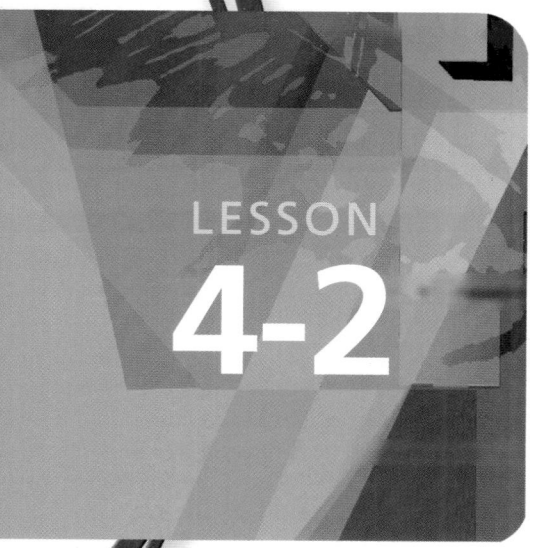

LESSON
4-2

Infectious Mononucleosis Tests

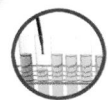

LESSON OBJECTIVES

After studying this lesson, the student will:

- ⊙ Name the cause of infectious mononucleosis (IM).
- ⊙ List five clinical symptoms of IM.
- ⊙ Explain how hematological and immunological findings are used in diagnosing IM.
- ⊙ Name two types of rapid tests used to diagnose IM.
- ⊙ Perform a rapid test for IM and interpret the results.
- ⊙ Discuss Epstein-Barr virus infections and explain how they relate to infectious mononucleosis.
- ⊙ Explain the safety precautions that must be observed when performing the test for IM.
- ⊙ Discuss procedures that must be followed to ensure the quality of results for the IM test.
- ⊙ Define the glossary terms.

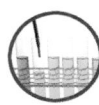

GLOSSARY

chronic fatigue syndrome (CFS) / a syndrome characterized by prolonged fatigue and other nonspecific symptoms, and for which the cause remains unknown

Epstein-Barr virus (EBV) / a virus that infects lymphocytes and is the cause of infectious mononucleosis

hepatosplenomegaly / enlargement of the liver and spleen

heterophile antibodies / a group of multispecific antibodies that are increased in infectious mononucleosis and that react with heterogeneous antigens *not* responsible for their production

incubation period / the time elapsed between exposure to an infectious agent and the appearance of symptoms

infectious mononucleosis (IM) / a contagious viral disease occurring in primarily the 15- to 25-year-old age-group and caused by infection with Epstein-Barr virus

latent / dormant; in an inactive or hidden phase

lymphadenopathy / a condition in which the lymph glands are enlarged or swollen

lymphocytosis / an increase above the normal number of lymphocytes in the blood

INTRODUCTION

Infectious mononucleosis (IM), also called *mono*, is a contagious viral disease that affects mostly the 15- to 25-year-old age-group. The disease is caused by infection of B lymphocytes with the **Epstein-Barr virus (EBV)**, a member of the herpes group of viruses and one of the most common human viruses. Individuals who are infected with EBV carry the virus in their throat and saliva. Transmission of the virus occurs when susceptible individuals have close contact with saliva from infected individuals, giving IM the common name of *kissing disease.*

EBV is found worldwide; by middle age, approximately 95% of adults have become infected with EBV. In developing countries EBV infection usually occurs in early childhood, before the age of 4 years. In the United States, peak infection is during adolescent years. When infection occurs in childhood, symptoms are either absent or so mild that treatment is not usually sought. However, when EBV infection occurs during the teenage years or young adulthood, the infection can cause IM in up to 50% of the cases.

Symptoms of IM are varied and nonspecific and can mimic symptoms present in other diseases. Early diagnosis of IM is usually based on laboratory test results combined with clinical symptoms and the age of the patient. The most common test for IM is a rapid immunological test that gives reliable results. Several test kits for IM are included in the list of CLIA-waived tests.

DIAGNOSIS OF INFECTIOUS MONONUCLEOSIS

Diagnosis of IM is based on clinical symptoms, hematological findings, and immunological test results.

Clinical Symptoms

Clinical symptoms of IM include fatigue, fever, sore throat, headache, and **lymphadenopathy**, or swollen lymph nodes. Patients can have some or all of these symptoms. During the acute phase, patients can also have **hepatosplenomegaly**, enlargement of the liver and spleen.

The **incubation period**, or the time between exposure to the virus and the appearance of symptoms, ranges from 4 to 6 weeks. Symptoms generally last for 1 to 4 weeks and seldom last for more than 4 months. When the symptoms last more than 6 months, other conditions associated with chronic symptoms or fatigue should be suspected, such as **chronic fatigue syndrome (CFS)**.

Hematological Findings

Infectious mononucleosis causes changes in circulating lymphocytes that can be detected by a white blood cell differential count and evaluation of white blood cell morphology from a stained blood smear. **Lymphocytosis**, an increase in lymphocytes, is usually present, and from 10% to more than 20% of the lymphocytes can be classified as *atypical* or *reactive* when viewed microscopically (See Figure 2-61 in Lesson 2-9).

Immunological Findings

Immunological tests for IM are designed to detect **heterophile antibodies** in the patient's blood. Heterophile antibodies are usually of the IgM class and react with structurally similar antigens found in bovine, horse, and sheep species. It is unclear why individuals produce these cross-reacting heterophile antibodies in cases of IM, but an increase in heterophile antibodies is associated specifically with IM, being present in 85% to 90% of IM cases. Laboratory diagnosis of IM based on detection of heterophile antibodies was one of the earliest immunological tests developed for clinical laboratory use.

Patients with IM begin producing heterophile antibodies early in the infection, and the immunological test for IM usually becomes positive after the first week of illness. The heterophile antibodies peak 2 to 4 weeks after symptoms begin and decline to low levels by 3 months. If the first immunological test is negative and clinical symptoms remain after a week, the patient should be retested. A positive test for heterophile antibodies combined with hematological and clinical findings provide the basis for diagnosing IM.

IMMUNOLOGICAL TESTS FOR INFECTIOUS MONONUCLEOSIS

Several commercial kits are available to test for the heterophile antibodies of IM. These tests provide results within a few minutes. The specimen used for the tests can be plasma, serum, or whole blood. Many of the kits are CLIA-waived when used with whole blood. If either serum or plasma is used, the tests are usually categorized as moderately complex. Test kits provide all necessary reagents, materials, and controls needed to perform the test.

Test kits for IM are adaptations of the Davidsohn differential test for heterophile antibodies, a time-consuming, cumbersome test that was developed in the mid-1900s to diagnose IM. Some IM kits are based on agglutination principles, with the end reaction being the presence or absence of agglutination. Other tests are immunochromatographic assays, which produce a color reaction. In some rapid tests for IM, the patient specimen is first pretreated to remove nonheterophile antibodies and then reacted with an antigen that binds only to heterophile antibodies. Because heterophile antibodies react with antigens found in several species, including bovine, sheep, and horse red blood cells, one or more of these are used as a source antigen in test kits.

Immunochromatographic Assays

In the past, many immunological tests were lengthy procedures, requiring special equipment and glassware, preparation and pipetting of several reagents, large sample volumes, and several complicated steps and incubations. Today, however, through the use of analyte-specific antibodies, complex test procedures have been miniaturized and simplified. Solid-phase immunochromatographic assays are now available for a multitude of analytes. In these assays, reagents and reactants are coated and immobilized on membranes enclosed in individual test units. In most cases, these assays require only that the technician add a drop or two of patient sample and perhaps one or two more reagents to the test cartridge. The test results are usually available in minutes.

By substituting the appropriate analyte-specific antibody into the test unit during manufacture, the same solid-phase technology can be adapted for the detection of several analytes. For this reason, many test cartridges made by a single company appear identical except for the label indicating which analyte can be detected using the test unit.

Principle of Immunochromatographic Assay for Infectious Mononucleosis

The procedure for detecting the heterophile antibodies of IM described in this lesson is the QuickVue+ Infectious Mononucleosis test (Quidel Corp.), an immunochromatographic assay (Figures 4-12 and 4-13). The methodology of this test is described in detail to illustrate the design of many such assays.

In the QuickVue+ Infectious Mononucleosis test, a membrane strip provides solid support for the assay. The membrane is housed in a plastic reaction unit containing three windows that expose three portions of the membrane. The membrane contains reagents in different zones. One end of the membrane lies under the sample well that contains an absorbent pad to promote an even flow of sample. Adjacent to the sample area, the membrane is coated with blue latex beads conjugated to goat anti–human IgM antibodies.

In the next membrane zone, which is exposed in the *read result* window, two reagents are immobilized. The first is blue latex beads immobilized in a pattern to provide a preprinted horizontal line. This line is visible when the test unit package is opened. The second reagent in this area is a bovine erythrocyte extract, which is immobilized in a vertical configuration, but is not visible before the test is begun.

The third zone of the membrane is exposed in the *test complete* window and contains an immobilized reagent in a

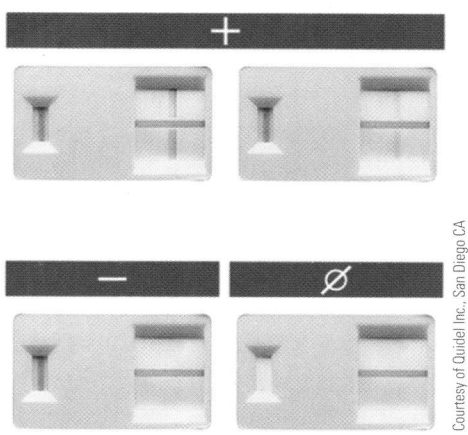

FIGURE 4-13 QuickVue+ Infectious Mononucleosis test results: (top row) reaction windows showing positive (+) tests; (bottom left) negative (−) test and (bottom right) invalid (Ø) test

vertical configuration. This reagent is capable of binding the antibody–blue latex conjugate to produce a visible vertical blue line. An absorbent pad is situated at the opposite end of the membrane from the sample end to promote fluid flow and retain fluid remaining after the reaction is completed.

Patient sample is added to the sample well, followed by a few drops of developer, which is simply an inert solution that provides enough liquid volume to promote capillary movement of the fluid sample through the membrane. As the sample flows through the membrane, the first reagent, anti–IgM–blue latex conjugate, is mobilized when it binds to IgM antibodies in the sample. This mixture is carried with the fluid sample along the membrane to the bovine erythrocyte zone.

If heterophile antibodies of IM are in the sample, they will bind to the immobilized bovine erythrocyte extract and be held in place. Because these IgM antibodies also have the goat–anti-IgM–blue latex bound to them, a visible blue vertical line will appear in the *read result* window forming a plus (+) sign (Figure 4-13 and Table 4-6). If no heterophile antibody is present in the sample,

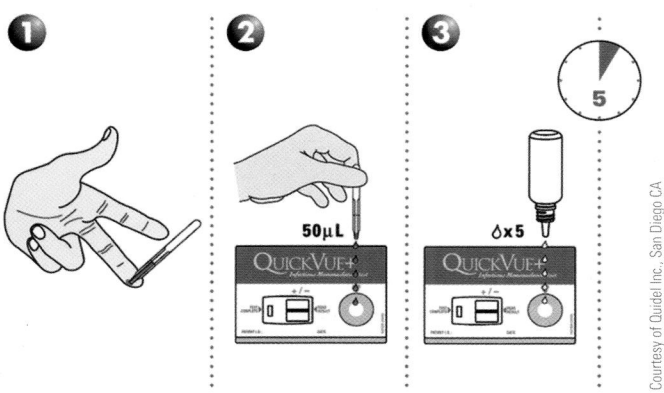

FIGURE 4-12 QuickVue+ Infectious Mononucleosis test: (1) collect blood sample; (2) add sample to well; (3) add developer and observe result after 5 minutes

TABLE 4-6. Interpretation of results with QuickVue+ Infectious Mononucleosis test	
Positive test	Any shade of blue vertical line forming a plus (+) sign in the *read result* window along with a vertical blue line in the *test complete* window
Negative test	No blue vertical line in *read result* window along with a vertical blue line in the *test complete* window
Invalid test	No line in *test complete* window after 10 minutes, OR Blue color fills *read result* window after 10 minutes

CURRENT TOPICS

CLINICAL SIGNIFICANCE OF EPSTEIN-BARR VIRUS INFECTION

Occurrence—The Epstein Barr virus (EBV) is a common virus found worldwide. Most people become infected with EBV by the age of 40. Because most adults have been infected with EBV, most newborns have some immunity to EBV at birth because of protection from maternal antibody. Once this passive protection subsides, infants become susceptible to EBV infection. Childhood infections with EBV are usually subclinical (asymptomatic) or have mild symptoms. However, approximately 50% of adolescents or young adults who become infected with EBV develop infectious mononucleosis (IM). Symptoms of IM usually last 1 to 2 months. EBV infection can cause more serious illness in severely immunosuppressed individuals, such as patients infected with human immunodeficiency virus (HIV) or those on immunosuppressant therapy following organ transplant.

EBV Persistence—EBV infections are lifelong. Once an individual becomes infected with EBV, the virus remains present in cells of the throat, blood, or immune system for the remainder of their life, but normally is in a dormant or latent state. Research has shown that periodically the virus can reactivate. If this happens, the virus is shed in saliva but the individual usually is asymptomatic and unaware of the virus reactivation.

Transmission of Epstein-Barr Virus—Transmission of EBV is almost impossible to prevent. Transmission of EBV does not normally occur by exposure to blood or aerosols (such as can be created by coughing or sneezing) but requires intimate contact with the saliva of an infected person. Healthy individuals can carry and spread the virus intermittently throughout their life and are usually the primary source for person-to-person transmission of the virus. However, most people who are exposed to an individual with IM have already been infected with EBV and so are not at risk for developing a new infection. Persons with active IM can spread the infection to others for a period of weeks. No special precautions or isolation procedures are recommended, because the virus is also frequently present in the saliva of healthy people.

Treatment for IM—There is no specific treatment for IM, other than treating the symptoms and recommending rest and a nutritional diet. Antiviral drugs are not used and vaccines are not available. If symptoms such as throat and tonsil swelling are a problem, the patient can be given a short course of corticosteroids to lessen symptoms. Because the spleen is often enlarged in cases of IM, vigorous activity is discouraged during the acute phase of IM.

Rapid Immunological Test for IM—The test for IM is *not* a test for EBV. Instead, patients are tested for heterophile antibody. In patients with clinical symptoms and other laboratory findings compatible with IM, a positive rapid test for heterophile antibodies is diagnostic, and no further testing is necessary.

False-positive rapid IM test results can occur in a few patients. False-negative results can occur in 10% to 15% of patients, primarily in young (preteen) children. If rapid IM tests or heterophile test results are negative, additional laboratory testing can differentiate EBV infections from IM-like illnesses caused by agents such as cytomegalovirus (CMV), adenovirus, or the parasite *Toxoplasma gondii*. This requires testing a patient's serum for antibodies to various EBV-associated antigens; these tests are expensive and more difficult and time-consuming than the rapid IM slide tests, so are not often done. Methods that detect EB virus in blood or tissue are used only as research tools and are not available for routine diagnosis.

EBV Link with Other Conditions—EBV infection during pregnancy has not been associated with miscarriage, nor has EBV been shown to cause birth defects. EBV infection was once suspected to be linked to chronic fatigue syndrome, but that link has never been proven. A rare event occurring in a very few EBV carriers is the development of either of two rare cancers not normally seen in the United States. These are *Burkitt's lymphoma* and *nasopharyngeal carcinoma*. These cancers seem to be closely associated with EBV, but EBV is not considered to be the sole cause.

this line will not form, leaving only the preprinted horizontal (–) blue line visible. The fluid sample will continue to move across the membrane carrying the antibody–blue latex conjugate until it contacts the binding agent in the *test complete* window. As the antibody–latex conjugate is bound, a vertical blue line will appear, indicating the test is complete.

PERFORMING A RAPID TEST FOR INFECTIOUS MONONUCLEOSIS

The manufacturer's instructions and the package insert provided with each kit must be strictly followed when performing and interpreting the test.

Safety Precautions

 Standard Precautions must be observed and gloves and other appropriate personal protective equipment (PPE) worn when performing immunological tests. Patient samples and controls made from human blood should be treated as if potentially infectious. Used test components must be discarded into appropriate biohazard containers.

Quality Assessment

 Manufacturer's instructions and information from the package insert for the kit being used will be incorporated into the standard operating procedure (SOP) manual and must be followed. Reagents must be stored and used appropriately and should not be used beyond the expiration dates. Positive and negative controls are provided with kits. These controls should be tested along with the patient specimen or following the schedule specified in the laboratory's SOP manual, to ensure that all reagents or kits are reacting correctly. Reagents from different kit manufacturers must not be interchanged. Reactions must be recorded and interpreted carefully, following the manufacturer's instructions and the laboratory's SOP manual.

Specimen Collection

The test can be performed using whole blood from capillary puncture or venous whole blood collected into either heparin anticoagulant or ethylenediaminetetraacetic acid (EDTA). The test can also be performed using serum, heparinized plasma, or EDTA-anticoagulated plasma.

Test Procedure

The reaction unit should be removed from its sealed pouch just before the test is to be run. A separate unit is used for each patient sample and each control. The reaction unit contains three areas: *add* well, to which reagents and specimen are added; *read result* window for reading and interpreting

reaction; and *test complete* window, which indicates if the test is working properly (Figure 4-13). The *read result* window should be observed before the unit is used to be sure a blue horizontal line is visible.

One drop (50 µL) of whole blood, serum, or plasma is introduced into the *add* well, using the pipette provided in the kit. If capillary blood is used, it should be drawn up to the line of the capillary tube included in the kit and the entire contents of the tube dispensed into the *add* well. Five drops of developer are then dispensed into the *add* well, the unit is allowed to remain undisturbed for the specified time, and the reaction is read.

Reading and Interpreting Results

Reactions that must be interpreted include the internal controls and patient results, as well as the reactions obtained with the positive and negative control solutions (external controls).

Internal Controls

Internal procedural controls are incorporated into immunochromatographic assays as one way of ensuring that the tests are set up correctly and the test units are working properly. The Quidel IM test includes both negative and positive internal controls. Failure of an internal control indicates either that the test was not performed correctly or the reagents were not working properly. The internal controls should be read and interpreted before reading patient results (Table 4-6 and Figure 4-13).

A clear *background* (other than the blue reaction lines) in the *read result* window at the end of the timed test is an internal negative control. If a blue color fills the *read result* window, the results are invalid.

A vertical blue line appearing in the *test complete* area is an internal positive control, indicating that the unit is performing correctly. If no blue line forms in the *test complete* window after 10 minutes, the results are invalid and patient results from the test cannot be reported.

External Controls

The positive control solution should cause a vertical line to form in the *read result* window, creating a plus (+) sign. When the negative control is tested, no vertical line should be seen in the *read result* window, leaving a minus (−) sign visible. A vertical blue line must form in the *test complete* window for the external control tests to be valid.

Patient Results

The *read result* window is observed for the test reaction. The presence of heterophile antibodies of IM (a positive result) is indicated by the formation of any shade of a blue vertical line forming a plus (+) in the *read result* window. The test is interpreted as negative if no vertical blue line appears in the *read result* window (Table 4-6 and Figure 4-13).

SAFETY REMINDERS

- Review Safety Precautions section before performing procedure.
- Observe Standard Precautions.
- Wear appropriate PPE when collecting blood samples and performing tests.

PROCEDURAL REMINDERS

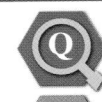

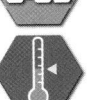

- Review Quality Assessment section before beginning procedure.
- Follow SOP manual and manufacturer's directions for the kit being used.
- Run positive and negative controls as specified in the SOP manual.
- Observe and interpret results carefully.

CASE STUDY

Josh, a college student, developed fever and sore throat a few days before spring break. He went to the university's health center, where the staff physician ordered a rapid immunological test for IM, and the results were negative. Josh went home for spring break, and his symptoms continued. After staying in bed for about a week, he went to see his hometown physician, who ordered another rapid immunological test for IM. The results were positive, and Josh began to improve within a few days.

Josh's mother called the university health center and complained that its testing was not reliable and she was unhappy with the level of health care her son was receiving.

1. Was her complaint valid?
2. Give your explanation for this scenario.

SUMMARY

Infectious mononucleosis (IM) is a contagious viral disease occurring primarily in teens and young adults. It is caused by infection with Epstein-Barr virus (EBV), a virus that is common worldwide. By middle age, most individuals have had an EBV infection, often subclinical (without noticeable symptoms). There is no specific treatment for IM, and in most cases the disease runs its course without complications.

Diagnosis of IM is made based on the combination of clinical symptoms, hematological findings, and immunological tests. Typical symptoms of IM include fatigue, fever, sore throat, and lymphadenopathy. Atypical lymphocytes are usually present in peripheral blood. Immunological tests for infectious mononucleosis detect the presence of heterophile antibodies in the patient's blood or serum, a characteristic finding in IM. Simple, rapid tests for IM can be performed at point of care. Some of these rapid IM tests are CLIA-waived.

3. What information can be gained from the hematological test for IM?

4. What substance is detected in the rapid immunological test for IM?

5. What safety precautions should be followed in performing a rapid test for IM?

6. What is the incubation period for IM?

7. How soon after IM begins will the immunological test usually be positive?

8. Describe the general principle of a rapid immunological test for IM.

9. Explain how internal and external controls are used with rapid tests for IM.

10. Define chronic fatigue syndrome, Epstein-Barr virus, hepatosplenomegaly, heterophile antibodies, incubation period, infectious mononucleosis, latent, lymphadenopathy, and lymphocytosis.

REVIEW QUESTIONS

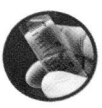

1. What is the cause of IM?
2. What are the clinical symptoms of IM?

STUDENT ACTIVITIES

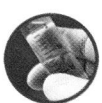

1. Complete the written examination for this lesson.
2. Practice performing the rapid test for IM as outlined in the Student Performance Guide.

WEB ACTIVITIES

1. Use the Internet to find information about a test kit for infectious mononucleosis other than the one described in this lesson. Download the package insert or manufacturer's information and explain the test design. Modify the steps in the Student Performance Guide for this lesson to fit the test instructions.

2. Using the Internet, look for information about chronic fatigue syndrome. Report on how it can be distinguished from infectious mononucleosis.

3. Use the Internet to find information about tests for Epstein-Barr viral antigens and antibodies to EBV. Write a brief report on your findings.

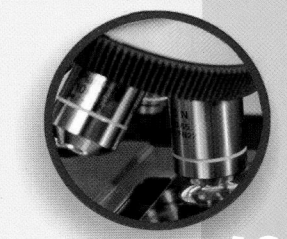

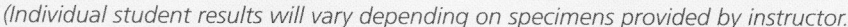

LESSON 4-2
Infectious Mononucleosis Tests

(Individual student results will vary depending on specimens provided by instructor.)

Name _____   Date _____

INSTRUCTIONS

1. Practice performing the rapid test for IM following the step-by-step procedure.

2. Demonstrate the rapid test for IM satisfactorily for the instructor, using the Student Performance Guide. Your instructor will explain the procedures for evaluating and grading your performance. Your performance may be given a number grade, letter grade, or satisfactory (S) or unsatisfactory (U) depending on course or institutional policy.

NOTE: Procedure given is for QuickVue+ Infectious Mononucleosis test by Quidel Corp. Instructions in package insert included with the kit should be followed. If another kit is used, the manufacturer's instructions for that kit must be followed.

MATERIALS AND EQUIPMENT

- gloves
- hand antiseptic
- full-face shield (or equivalent PPE)
- acrylic safety shield (optional)
- laboratory tissue
- paper towels
- test serum, plasma, or anticoagulated whole blood
- capillary puncture supplies (optional)
- test tube rack
- timer
- IM test kit including instructions, test units, dispensers, reagents, and positive and negative controls
- surface disinfectant (such as 10% chlorine bleach)
- biohazard container
- sharps container

PROCEDURE

Record in the comment section any problems encountered while practicing the procedure (or have a fellow student or the instructor evaluate your performance).

S = Satisfactory
U = Unsatisfactory

You must:	S	U	Evaluation/Comments
1. Wash hands with antiseptic and put on gloves			
2. Assemble equipment and materials			
3. Put on face protection (or set up acrylic safety shield)			
4. Remove test cartridge from sealed pouch and place it on a level, well-lit surface. Identify the *add* well, *read result* window, and *test complete* window. Check to see that *read result* window shows a preprinted blue horizontal line			
5. Dispense patient sample into the cartridge using method 5a, 5b, or 5c:			

(Continues)

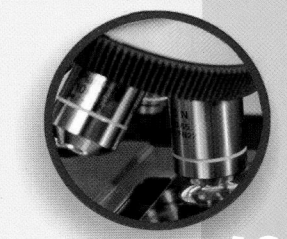

© 2012 Delmar, Cengage Learning. Permission to reproduce for clinical use granted.

You must:	S	U	Evaluation/Comments

a. For venous whole blood samples:
   1) Mix tube of blood well by inverting several times
   2) Draw blood into the pipet provided with the kit
   3) Dispense 1 drop into the *add* well and discard pipet into sharps container
b. For plasma or serum samples:
   1) Draw plasma or serum into the pipet provided with the kit
   2) Dispense 1 drop into the *add* well and discard pipet into sharps container
c. For capillary blood:
   1) Perform a routine capillary puncture and wipe away first drop of blood
   2) Fill the capillary tube provided with the kit to the line (50 µL)
   3) Dispense entire contents of tube into *add* well; discard tube and used lancet into sharps container			

6. Immediately dispense 5 drops of developer into the *add* well while holding the developer bottle vertically			
7. Start timer; do not pick up or move test cartridge			
8. Read test result when a blue color appears in the *test complete* window, approximately 5 minutes after test is set up. If blue *test complete* line is not visible by 10 minutes after test setup, the test is invalid and a result cannot be reported			

9. Interpret the results following instructions in package insert (refer also to guide in Table 4-6 and Figure 4-13):
a. Positive result—Formation of any blue vertical line forming a (+) sign in the *read result* window along with a vertical blue line in the *test complete* window
b. Negative result—A vertical blue line in the *test complete* window but no blue vertical line in the *read result* window
c. Invalid result—one or more of the following reactions:
   1) No vertical blue line in the *test complete* window after 10 minutes
   2) A blue color filling the *read result* window after 10 minutes			

10. Record results as positive or negative			
11. Repeat test procedure (steps 4–10) using positive and negative controls and record results			

© 2012 Delmar, Cengage Learning. Permission to reproduce for clinical use granted.

You must:	S	U	Evaluation/Comments
12. Discard used sharps into sharps container and other contaminated materials into appropriate biohazard container			
13. Store or dispose of specimen as instructed			
14. Clean work area with disinfectant			
15. Remove gloves and discard in biohazard container			
16. Wash hands with antiseptic			

Instructor/Evaluator Comments:

Instructor/Evaluator _____ Date _____

© 2012 Delmar, Cengage Learning. Permission to reproduce for clinical use granted.

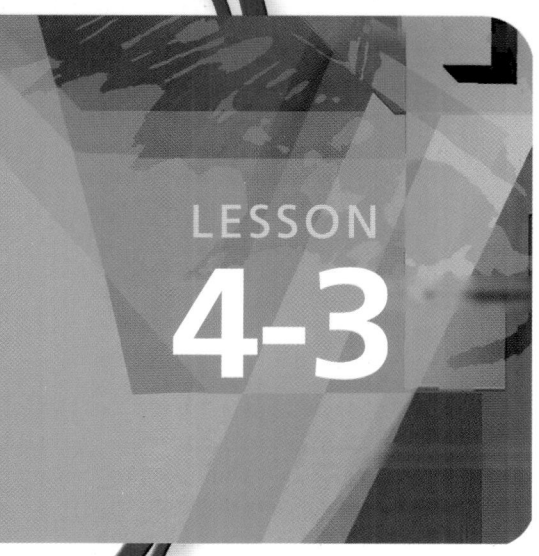

Test for Rheumatoid Factors

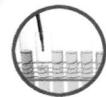

LESSON OBJECTIVES

After studying this lesson, the student will:

⊙ Explain the significance of rheumatoid factors.

⊙ Explain the reason(s) for performing the test for rheumatoid factors.

⊙ Explain the principle of latex agglutination tests.

⊙ Perform a qualitative latex agglutination test for rheumatoid factors and interpret the results.

⊙ Perform a semi-quantitative latex agglutination test for rheumatoid factors and interpret the results.

⊙ Discuss the clinical significance of a positive rheumatoid factor test and a negative rheumatoid factor test.

⊙ Discuss safety precautions that must be followed when performing the test for rheumatoid factors.

⊙ Discuss quality assessment practices used in performing the test for rheumatoid factors.

⊙ Define the glossary terms.

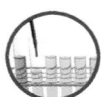

GLOSSARY

arthritis/ inflammation of the joints, due to several causes

autoantibody/ an antibody directed against self (one's own tissues)

reciprocal/ inverse; one of a pair of numbers (as 2/3 and 3/2) that has a product of one

rheumatoid arthritis (RA)/ an autoimmune disease characterized by pain, inflammation, and deformity of the joints

rheumatoid factors (RFs)/ autoantibodies directed against the Fc fragment of human immunoglobulin G (IgG) and often present in the serum of patients with rheumatoid arthritis

scleroderma / a systemic or localized autoimmune connective tissue disease characterized by a chronic hardening (*sclero*) of skin (*derma*) and connective tissue

Sjögren's syndrome / a systemic autoimmune disease affecting moisture-producing glands such as tear, sweat, and saliva glands but also affecting organs

synovial/ of, or relating to, the lubricating fluid of the joints

INTRODUCTION

Arthritis, an inflammation of the joints, can occur in several diseases. Among these are gout, rheumatic fever, osteoarthritis, and autoimmune diseases such as lupus erythematosus, **Sjögren's syndrome,** and **rheumatoid arthritis (RA).**

Rheumatoid factors (RFs) are **autoantibodies,** usually of the IgM class, directed against human immunoglobulin G (IgG). Rheumatoid factors are elevated in the blood and **synovial** fluid of 75% to 85% of people with RA; RFs are also elevated in a majority of patients with Sjögren's syndrome but are not typically elevated in osteoarthritis or gout. It is unclear what triggers the body to produce RFs.

In the early stages of disease, RA and other autoimmune diseases can be difficult to diagnose because symptoms of arthritis can be present in several diseases. No single test can confirm the diagnosis of most of these diseases.

The RF test is used with the physical examination, other laboratory tests, and sometimes radiological tests to aid in diagnosing RA and Sjögren's syndrome. The RF test is also used to follow the course of RA or Shögren's syndrome, or to help rule out these or other conditions as the cause of arthritis.

Immunological tests are used to detect and measure RFs in blood. Several tests for RFs are based on the detection of RFs in the patient's serum using a latex agglutination method. The rapid slide test for RFs is described in this lesson to demonstrate the principle of latex agglutination.

PRINCIPLE OF AGGLUTINATION TESTS FOR RHEUMATOID FACTORS

Several types of test kits are available to detect or measure RFs. Kits are designed using principles of enzyme immunoassay (EIA), nephelometry, or agglutination. Depending on the kit design, the specimen tested can be serum, plasma, or whole blood. Manual kits as well as kits for use with automated immunology instruments are available.

Most RF slide tests are modifications of a latex agglutination test developed by Singer and Plotz in 1956. In the RF test, small inert latex particles are coated with specially treated molecules of human IgG. When serum containing RFs is mixed with the IgG-coated latex particles, the RFs (which are autoantibodies) bind to the IgG and cause agglutination of the particles (Figure 4-14).

Commercial latex RF kits include the coated latex particles, positive and negative control sera, diluting buffer, and other materials necessary to perform the tests (Figure 4-15). Another type of slide agglutination test is a hemagglutination test that uses specially treated red blood cells to detect RF.

PERFORMING A QUALITATIVE TEST FOR RHEUMATOID FACTORS

The procedure described in this lesson provides general directions for performing a slide latex agglutination test to detect RF. When performing the test, the instructions in the package insert included with the test kit must be followed.

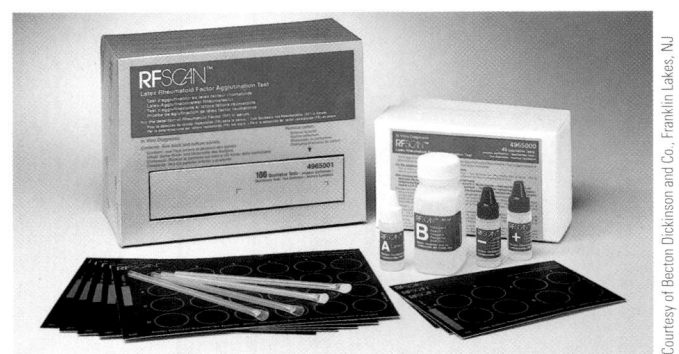

IgG Coated latex particles + Patient serum containing RF → Agglutination of latex

 = latex beads
▲ = human IgG
 = RF

FIGURE 4-14 Principle of latex agglutination test for rheumatoid factors: rheumatoid factors in serum react with IgG-coated latex particles to cause agglutination

FIGURE 4-15 Rheumatoid factor latex agglutination kit

Safety Precautions

Standard Precautions must be followed and appropriate personal protective equipment (PPE) worn when performing all immunological tests. Control solutions produced from human blood should be treated as if potentially infectious. All contaminated materials must be discarded into appropriate biohazard or sharps containers.

Quality Assessment

The laboratory's standard operating procedure (SOP) manual will contain the instructions for the particular kit being used; these instructions must be followed. Reagents from different manufacturers should not be interchanged. Storage recommendations must be followed, and reagents should not be used beyond the expiration dates.

Positive and negative control solutions provided with the kits must be run at the specified intervals and the results recorded. If controls do not give the expected reactions, patient specimens must not be tested until the problem has been identified and corrected. Dispensers, droppers, and stirrers must be used only once and discarded. Reactions must be timed carefully and results observed using good lighting.

CURRENT TOPICS

ARTHRITIS

Arthritis is a general term that means inflammation of the joints. Arthritis is usually a chronic condition involving pain, redness, and swelling of the joints. Arthritis can affect any joint in the body and has many causes. The three most common types of arthritis in adults are osteoarthritis, gout, and rheumatoid arthritis.

Osteoarthritis is the type of arthritis commonly seen as people age. It is sometimes called *wear and tear* arthritis. It usually affects joints of the hands, back, neck, hip, knee, or ankle. Cartilage, which cushions the ends of the bones in the joints, wears away, allowing bones to rub against each other. Osteoarthritis can begin in younger individuals, such as athletes who receive joint injury. Most individuals will have evidence of osteoarthritis in at least one joint by the time they become seniors. Although severe osteoarthritis can be debilitating and can severely affect mobility, it does not cause organ damage. There is currently no cure for osteoarthritis, but treatment includes exercise, joint care, anti-inflammatory drugs and drugs to relieve pain, and sometimes joint replacement surgery.

Another type of arthritis is associated with *gout*, a condition seen more commonly in middle-aged men. In this condition, sudden attacks of pain, redness, and swelling occur in the joints of the lower extremities such as the knees, ankles, heels, or toes. These attacks can be precipitated by stress, diet, or the presence of infection, and often occur in persons who have a family history of gout. The pain of gout is caused by a buildup of uric acid in the joint. Uric acid is a breakdown product of purines, which are found in many foods. The uric acid crystallizes in the joints, causing pain that usually subsides within a few days. Diagnosis of gout can be confirmed by finding uric acid crystals in microscopic examination of synovial (joint) fluid. Pain relief is often obtained with over-the-counter anti-inflammatory medications. Lifestyle changes, particularly dietary changes, can usually significantly reduce attacks or severity of symptoms.

Rheumatoid arthritis (RA) is an autoimmune disease that usually begins in young adulthood and is more common in women than men. When it begins in childhood, it is called juvenile RA. In the early stages of RA, small joints are usually affected first, such as wrists, hands, ankles, and feet. In RA, the symptoms are usually symmetrical; for example, both hands are usually affected rather than just one. RA can also affect other parts of the body, such as skin, lungs, vascular system, and eyes. Much is still unknown about RA, but it is thought that a combination of genetic factors, environmental factors, and hormones play a part in the disease. Some investigators have evidence that infections with certain viruses or bacteria can trigger onset of the disease in individuals with an inherited tendency to rheumatoid arthritis.

There is no one definitive test for rheumatoid arthritis, but the RF test is positive in a majority of cases. Depending on a patient's symptoms, other tests can be ordered at the same time as the rheumatoid factor (RF) test. Hematology tests that might be ordered include complete blood count (CBC) and erythrocyte sedimentation rate (ESR). Other immunological tests helpful in diagnosing or ruling out RA or other inflammatory diseases associated with arthritis include tests for antinuclear antibody (ANA), anticyclic citrullinated peptide (anti-CCP) antibodies, and C-reactive protein (CRP).

Diagnosis of the type of arthritis is made using a combination of family and personal medical history, physical examination, radiographs, and laboratory findings. Human leukocyte antigen (HLA) testing can be performed to identify cell markers associated with diseases that display arthritis-like symptoms. These include several autoimmune diseases such as ankylosing spondylitis, lupus erythematosus, Sjögren's syndrome, and scleroderma.

Treatments for arthritis are based on the severity of symptoms. Mild symptoms can be treated with exercise therapy and over-the-counter pain relievers or NSAIDs. More severe symptoms are treated with powerful medications such as corticosteroids, methotrexate (an antifolate drug) or adalimumab (tradename Humira), which blocks the action of tumor necrosis factor. In many cases, joint damage can be repaired by surgery.

Specimen Collection and Preparation

Serum is the usual specimen for latex agglutination tests. Blood is collected into a red-topped (or red/gray top) tube by venipuncture, the blood is allowed to clot, and the serum is separated from the cells by centrifugation. Many RF tests require that the serum be diluted 1:20 before testing, using a buffer included in the kit. This dilution is necessary because the sera of normal individuals can have low levels of RF. Testing diluted serum assures that only significant levels of RF will be detected in the test.

Test Procedure

To perform the test, 1 drop of positive control serum, negative control serum, and diluted patient serum are each placed in a separate test area on a slide included in the test kit. One drop of well-mixed latex reagent is dispensed into each test area. The latex reagent is then mixed with each serum using a clean stirrer or spreader for each. Each mixture is spread over the entire individual test area. The slide is then rocked or rotated for the specified time—usually 1 to 3 minutes—and immediately observed for agglutination under a bright light.

Interpreting the Results of a Rheumatoid Factor Test

The test area containing the positive control serum should show agglutination. Agglutination appears as small clumps against the background of the slide (Figure 4-16). The negative control serum should have no agglutination. A negative reaction will appear as a smooth solution with no clumping in the test area (Figure 4-16).

Absence of agglutination with the patient serum indicates the level of rheumatoid factors is within normal range and is reported as *negative*, *no agglutination seen*, or, if a 1:20 serum dilution was used, reported as *titer less than 20*.

The presence of agglutination with the patient serum is considered a positive test and indicates a significantly elevated level of RF. A semi-quantitative RF test should be performed on positive samples to determine the RF titer.

If undiluted serum is tested and shows agglutination, the serum should be diluted 1:20 or serially diluted and reassayed. Test kits differ in sensitivity. For most test kits, only serum that is positive at a 1:20 (or higher) dilution should be considered positive for RFs.

Significance of Rheumatoid Factor Test Results

Diagnosis of rheumatoid arthritis should not be based on the RF test alone because other conditions, particularly inflammatory diseases such as Sjögren's syndrome, can also cause a positive RF test.

Conversely, because only 75% to 85% of those with rheumatoid arthritis have increased levels of RF, *a diagnosis of rheumatoid arthritis cannot be ruled out solely on the basis of a negative RF test.*

Knowledge of the amount of RF present can be useful in monitoring the course of rheumatoid arthritis because RF levels tend to parallel the patient's condition and the effectiveness of treatment. Patients with active rheumatoid arthritis usually have higher RF levels than do patients with inactive disease.

PERFORMING A SEMI-QUANTITATIVE TEST FOR RHEUMATOID FACTORS

A semi-quantitative test for RF is performed by testing a series of dilutions of the patient's serum to determine the RF titer. The highest serum dilution showing agglutination (positive reaction) is recorded. The titer, which is the **reciprocal**, or inverse, of the highest dilution giving a positive result, is reported. For example, dilutions of 1:40, 1:80, and 1:160 were made from a serum that was positive in the qualitative test. When the dilutions were tested for RF, agglutination was observed in the 1:40 dilution, but the 1:80 and 1:160 dilutions were negative for agglutination. This serum would be reported to have an RF titer of 40 (the reciprocal of the 1:40 or 1/40 serum dilution). Some laboratories report the highest dilution showing a positive reaction instead of the titer; the laboratory's SOP manual will specify the policy for reporting results.

SAFETY REMINDERS

- Review Safety Precautions section before beginning procedure.
- Observe Standard Precautions.
- Handle controls and reagents as if potentially infectious.

PROCEDURAL REMINDERS

- Review Quality Assessment section before beginning procedure.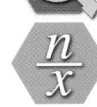
- Follow SOP manual and manufacturer's instructions for the kit used.
- Perform semi-quantitative test if initial test for RF is positive.
- Observe test reactions using good lighting.
- Run positive and negative controls each time a patient sample is tested.

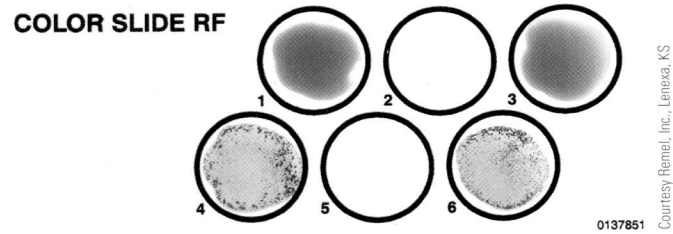

COLOR SLIDE RF

Courtesy Remel, Inc., Lenexa, KS

0137851

FIGURE 4-16 Illustration of agglutination in the rheumatoid factor latex test: wells 1 and 3 have no agglutination and are negative; wells 4 and 6 show agglutination and are positive

CASE STUDY 1

Ms. Jenkins, a 23-year-old woman, visited her physician and complained of joint pain and swelling. An RF test was ordered. The technician tested Ms. Jenkins' undiluted serum using a latex agglutination test for RF and observed agglutination. RF-positive and RF-negative serum controls performed as expected.

The technician should:

a. Report the test as negative

b. Report the test as positive

c. Report a titer of 20

d. Repeat the test using a 1:20 serum dilution or a dilution series

CASE STUDY 2

The following reactions were observed after performing a semi-quantitative RF latex agglutination test.

Serum Dilution	Agglutination Reaction
1:20	(+)
1:40	(+)
1:80	(+)
1:160	(−)
1:320	(−)

The RF titer is:

a. 1:80

b. 1:160

c. 80

d. 160

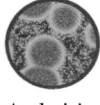

SUMMARY

Arthritis is a condition common in old age. Different types of arthritis occur, each with its distinct causes, symptoms, laboratory findings, and other disease associations. Arthritis associated with autoimmune disease, such as rheumatoid arthritis (RA), can occur at any age, and is typically more severe than other types of arthritis such as osteoarthritis or gout.

Rheumatoid factors (RFs) are autoantibodies that are increased in the serum of 75% to 85% of patients with rheumatoid arthritis and in the serum of a majority of patients with Sjögren's syndrome. The RF test is not specific for one disease. The RF test is one tool used in diagnosing or ruling out diseases associated with certain forms of arthritis, such as rheumatoid arthritis and Sjögren's syndrome.

RF tests can be manual or automated. Many manual RF tests are based on the principle of latex agglutination. Results of RF tests must be interpreted carefully. Because elevated levels of RFs are not detectable in all patients with rheumatoid arthritis, a negative RF test does not rule out rheumatoid arthritis. In addition, certain other inflammatory conditions can cause a positive RF test, so other clinical findings must be considered when interpreting the significance of a positive RF test.

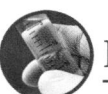

REVIEW QUESTIONS

1. What are rheumatoid factors (RFs)?

2. Name a disease associated with an elevated RF level.

3. Explain the principle of the latex agglutination test for RF.

4. Describe the appearance of a positive latex test and a negative latex test.

5. What is the difference between a qualitative and semi-quantitative agglutination test?

6. What is the significance of a positive RF slide agglutination test? Of a negative RF slide agglutination test?

7. Why is serum diluted before performing the RF test?

8. What is a titer?

9. Define arthritis, autoantibody, reciprocal, rheumatoid arthritis (RA), rheumatoid factors (RFs), scleroderma, Sjögren's syndrome, and synovial.

STUDENT ACTIVITIES

1. Complete the written examination for this lesson.

2. Practice performing qualitative and semi-quantitative slide agglutination tests for RF as outlined in the Student Performance Guide.

WEB ACTIVITY

1. Use the Internet to search for information on rheumatoid arthritis. Report on the pathology of the disease.

2. Use the Internet to find information about one of the following diseases that have symptoms similar to RA: lupus erythematosus, Sjögren's syndrome, ankylosing spondylitis, or scleroderma. Report on laboratory tests that are useful in diagnosis of the disease and give the expected results with the RF test. (Potential sources for information are medical research foundations for conditions such as arthritis, lupus, and Sjögren's syndrome.)

LESSON 4-3
TEST FOR RHEUMATOID FACTORS

(Individual student results will vary depending on specimens provided by instructor.)

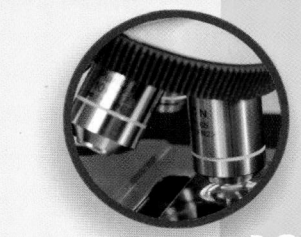

Name _____   Date _____

INSTRUCTIONS

1. Practice performing the latex slide test for RF following the step-by-step procedure.

2. Demonstrate the latex slide test for RF satisfactorily for the instructor, using the Student Performance Guide. Your instructor will explain the procedures for evaluating and grading your performance. Your performance may be given a number grade, letter grade, or satisfactory (S) or unsatisfactory (U) depending on course or institutional policy.

NOTE: Instructions given are general. The procedure should be modified to conform to the manufacturer's package insert provided with the kit being used.

MATERIALS AND EQUIPMENT

- gloves
- hand antiseptic
- full-face shield (or equivalent PPE)
- acrylic safety shield (optional)
- timer
- test tubes (13 × 75 mm)
- test tube rack
- serum samples
- micropipetters and appropriate pipet tips for delivering 0.05 mL (50 µL), 0.5 mL, 0.95 mL
- RF slide test kit that includes:
  - RF latex reagent
  - RF positive control
  - RF negative control
  - diluent
  - ringed test slides
  - dispensers/spreaders
- applicator sticks (if spreaders are not in kit)
- laboratory tissue
- paper towels
- surface disinfectant (such as 10% chlorine bleach)
- sharps container
- biohazard container

PROCEDURE

   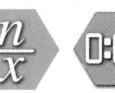

Record in the comment section any problems encountered while practicing the procedure (or have a fellow student or the instructor evaluate your performance).

S = Satisfactory
U = Unsatisfactory

You must:	S	U	Evaluation/Comments
1. Wash hands with antiseptic and put on gloves			
2. Assemble equipment and materials			
3. Allow all reagents to reach room temperature before performing test			
4. Put on face protection or position acrylic shield on work surface			

(Continues)

© 2012 Delmar, Cengage Learning. Permission to reproduce for clinical use granted.

You must:	S	U	Evaluation/Comments

5. Prepare a 1:20 dilution of the test serum:
  a. Pipet 0.05 mL (50 µL) of serum into a 13 × 75 tube
  b. Pipet 0.95 mL of diluent into the tube and mix well			

6. Label three test areas on slide: *positive control* (+), *negative control* (–), and *patient* (Pt)			
7. Add 1 drop of each control serum to appropriate labeled areas on the slide using a clean dispenser for each (pipet positive control serum into [+] ring and negative control serum into [–] ring)			
8. Use a clean dispenser to dispense one drop of diluted patient serum (from step 5) into ring on slide labeled *patient*			
9. Mix the RF latex reagent well by inverting several times			
10. Dispense 1 drop of well-mixed RF latex reagent into each ring that contains a control or test serum			
11. Use a separate spreader to thoroughly mix each serum with latex reagent, spreading the mixture over the entire surface of the ring NOTE: Be sure to use a clean spreader for each serum or control sample. An applicator stick can be used if no spreaders are included in the kit			
12. Start timer and rock the slide in a figure-eight motion for the appropriate time (usually 1 to 3 minutes)			
13. Observe the ringed areas for agglutination immediately at the end of the appropriate time period			
14. Record the results of the controls and patient serum (agglutination = positive; no agglutination = negative or titer less than 20)			
15. Perform the semi-quantitative test (steps 16–18) if the patient sample is positive for agglutination; if it is negative, go to step 20			

16. Prepare a two-fold serial dilution of patient serum (steps 16a-16h):
  a. Label five test tubes: **1** (1:40), **2** (1:80), **3** (1:160), **4** (1:320), and **5** (1:640)
  b. Pipet 0.5 mL of diluent into each tube
  c. Pipet 0.5 mL of the 1:20 dilution of patient serum (from qualitative test, step 5) into tube 1 (1:40) and mix contents of tube well
  d. Transfer 0.5 mL from tube 1 to tube 2 and mix well
  e. Transfer 0.5 mL from tube 2 to tube 3 and mix well
  f. Transfer 0.5 mL from tube 3 to tube 4 and mix well
  g. Transfer 0.5 mL from tube 4 to tube 5 and mix well
  h. Discard 0.5 mL from tube 5			

© 2012 Delmar, Cengage Learning. Permission to reproduce for clinical use granted.

You must:	S	U	Evaluation/Comments
17. Use each dilution (tubes 1 through 5) as a separate test specimen and perform the latex agglutination test as in steps 6–14			
18. Record the agglutination results for each tube			
19. Record the serum RF titer (the reciprocal of the highest dilution that shows agglutination)			
20. Discard specimens and used materials into appropriate sharps or biohazard containers			
21. Return all reagents and unused materials to proper storage			
22. Clean work area with disinfectant			
23. Remove gloves and discard into biohazard container			
24. Wash hands with antiseptic			

Instructor/Evaluator Comments:

Instructor/Evaluator _____ Date _____

© 2012 Delmar, Cengage Learning. Permission to reproduce for clinical use granted.

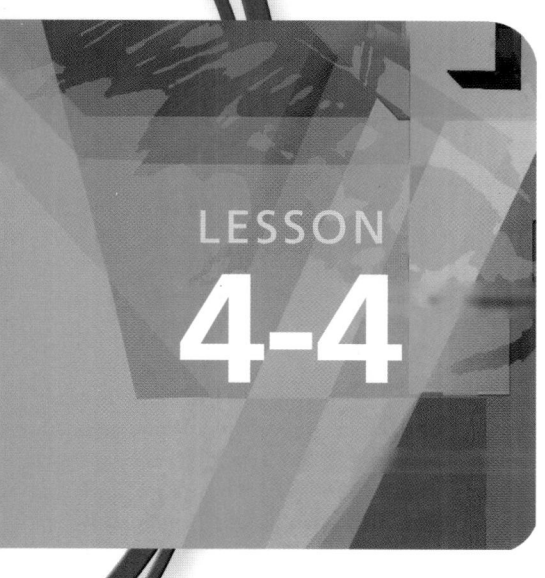

Tests for Human Chorionic Gonadotropin

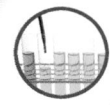

LESSON OBJECTIVES

After studying this lesson, the student will:

- ⊙ Explain why modern pregnancy tests are designed to detect human chorionic gonadotropin (hCG).
- ⊙ Discuss how solid-phase immunochromatographic assays are used to detect hCG.
- ⊙ Perform a test for urine hCG and report the results.
- ⊙ Discuss possible causes of false-positive and false-negative results in urine hCG tests.
- ⊙ Discuss factors that must be considered when interpreting hCG test results.
- ⊙ Explain the differences between internal and external controls in urine hCG tests.
- ⊙ List safety precautions to observe when performing urine hCG tests.
- ⊙ Explain the importance of quality assessment procedures in performing urine hCG tests.
- ⊙ Define the glossary terms.

GLOSSARY

agglutination inhibition / interference with, or prevention of, agglutination

ectopic pregnancy / development of fetus outside the uterus; extrauterine pregnancy

hemagglutination / the agglutination of red blood cells

human chorionic gonadotropin (hCG) / the hormone of pregnancy, produced by the placenta; also called uterine chorionic gonadotropin (uCG)

implantation / attachment of the early embryo to the uterus

teratogenic / relating to a substance or agent capable of leading to birth defects by causing change or harm to a fetus or embryo, or interfering with normal fetal development

trophoblastic / relating to embryonic nutritive tissue

INTRODUCTION

Pregnancy tests are based on the detection of the **human chorionic gonadotropin (hCG)** hormone. hCG is also called uterine chorionic gonadotropin (uCG). hCG is produced by the placenta shortly after fertilization and reaches detectable levels in urine and serum about 1 week after **implantation**, attachment of the early embryo to the uterine lining. Levels of hCG continue to rise during the first trimester of pregnancy, making it an excellent marker for pregnancy.

Tests for hCG are used when pregnancy is suspected and to rule out pregnancy before surgery or before prescribing birth control pills. Pregnancy should also be ruled out before prescribing therapies or procedures known to be **teratogenic**,

471

that is, capable of damaging a fetus or interfering with fetal development. These procedures include radiographic studies as well as administration of chemotherapy drugs and certain other medications and antibiotics.

Today's hCG tests are immunoassays and can be performed on urine or serum. Urine tests for hCG are designed to be sensitive, to be easy to perform and interpret, and to give rapid results. Many hCG kits are CLIA-waived if performed using urine. hCG tests performed on serum are in the moderately complex CLIA category. Principles of enzyme immunoassays (EIAs) and membrane or chromatographic immunoassays are also described in Lessons 4-1 and 4-2.

Some pregnancy test kits are intended for home use and can be purchased in pharmacies or drug stores. Whether kits are designed for home or clinical use, the tests use immunological methods to detect hCG. Positive results from home pregnancy tests should be confirmed by a physical examination and laboratory testing using appropriate controls, if warranted.

DEVELOPMENT OF PREGNANCY TESTS

Testing urine for pregnancy is one of the oldest documented tests. In Egyptian papyri over 3,000 years old a test for pregnancy is described: a woman's urine was placed on plant seeds, and if the seeds germinated or grew, the woman was predicted to be pregnant; if the seeds did not grow, she was declared not pregnant. In the Middle Ages and through later centuries, urine characteristics such as color and clarity, or the reaction of urine with wine, were used to predict pregnancy. It was not until the 1890s that scientists and physicians described the importance of certain internally secreted chemicals to the workings of the body, and named these chemicals *hormones*. However, even as the twentieth century began, physical symptoms such as morning sickness were still the most reliable predictors of pregnancy.

Early Pregnancy Tests

In the first half of the twentieth century, scientists began to unravel some of the mysteries of human reproduction. In the 1920s, it was recognized that a specific hormone was present only in pregnant women—the hormone we now know as hCG. The 1930s brought development of bioassays (assays using live animals) that required injection of a woman's urine into rabbits, frogs, or rats. The isolation of sex hormones in the late 1950s provided the foundation for development of the first nonanimal assay for pregnancy—a **hemagglutination** inhibition test that was an early type of immunoassay. Although the test was not very sensitive and many substances could cause false reactions, results were available within several hours rather than days. In the 1960s, research to understand antibodies, hormones, and other biochemicals continued, providing information used to improve test methods.

Beginning in the 1970s, increased attention was given to prenatal health care and early testing for pregnancy. A 2-hour test was developed that could detect hCG just a few days after a missed menstrual period. This test was an improvement of the original hemagglutination inhibition tube test, but false-positive reactions still occurred. Meanwhile researchers, primarily at the National Institutes of Health (NIH), discovered molecular characteristics of hCG and were able to develop specific antibodies against the antigenic hCG beta subunit.

Home Pregnancy Tests

In 1977, the e.p.t. (early pregnancy test) became available over-the-counter. Ads for e.p.t., as well as other home pregnancy tests also having Food and Drug Administration (FDA) approval, began appearing in women's magazines. These first home tests were based on the hemagglutination inhibition principle.

Rapid Tests for hCG

Through the 1970s and 1980s, women were encouraged to take an active role in their reproductive health and pregnancy tests continued to be improved.

Agglutination Inhibition

The rapid slide tests for hCG were developed, based on the principle of **agglutination inhibition** (Figure 4-17); these tests were sensitive, specific, and produced results in minutes. In a two-step reaction, urine was reacted with anti-hCG antibodies and then hCG-coated latex particles were added to the mixture. If hCG was in the urine, it would bind to the anti-hCG, thus preventing the anti-hCG from agglutinating the hCG-coated latex particles. Therefore, *absence of agglutination* was a positive result. If hCG was not present, agglutination occurred, and was reported as a negative result (Figure 4-17).

Enzyme Immunoassays

In the 1990s, pregnancy tests based on modified enzyme immunoassays (EIAs) were developed for both home and clinical use. These tests were called solid-phase EIAs, membrane immunoassays, or solid-phase chromatographic immunoassays and are the test methods currently used (Figure 4-18). To make results of home tests easier to interpret, in 2003 the Clear-Blue Easy Digital test was approved for over-the-counter sale. In this test, rather than colored lines or plus or minus signs, the results are displayed in word form—*pregnant* or *not pregnant.*

Most urine pregnancy tests use a plastic cassette or cartridge containing reactants such as specific antibodies, chromogens, and internal controls immobilized or coated on an absorbent membrane. The operator is only required to add urine to the cassette. When the urine containing hCG is applied, it migrates through the membrane, contacts the various reagents, and produces easy-to-read colored reactions in the *result* area of the test unit (Figure 4-18). The results are available within minutes and appear as colored lines, bars, or symbols such as "+" or "−". Siemens (formerly Bayer Corporation), a manufacturer of urine reagent strips, also makes the Clinitek hCG cassette, an hCG test that can be read on the Clinitek Status reagent strip reader. This test is CLIA-waived when performed using the strip reader.

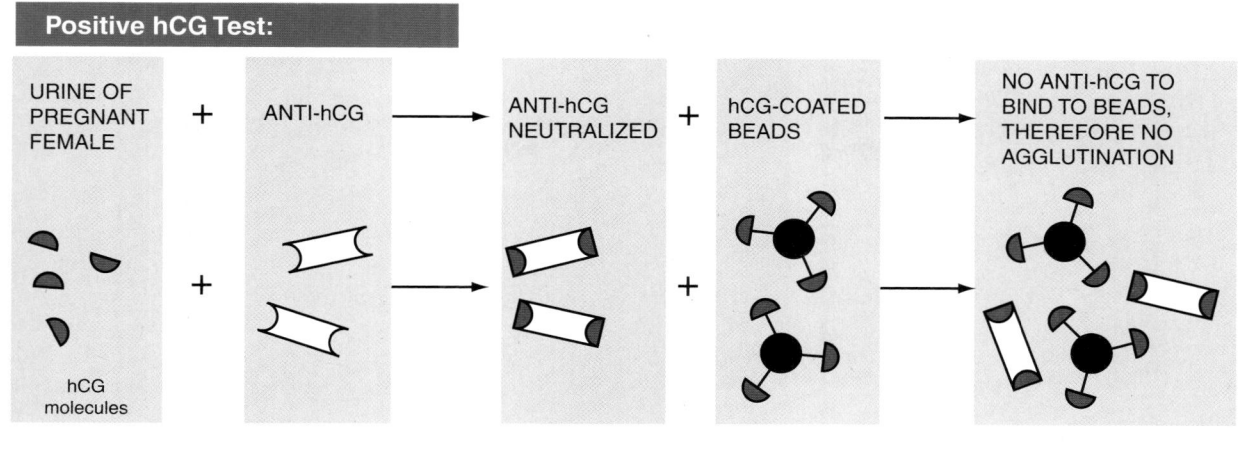

Positive hCG Test:

URINE OF PREGNANT FEMALE + ANTI-hCG → ANTI-hCG NEUTRALIZED + hCG-COATED BEADS → NO ANTI-hCG TO BIND TO BEADS, THEREFORE NO AGGLUTINATION

hCG molecules

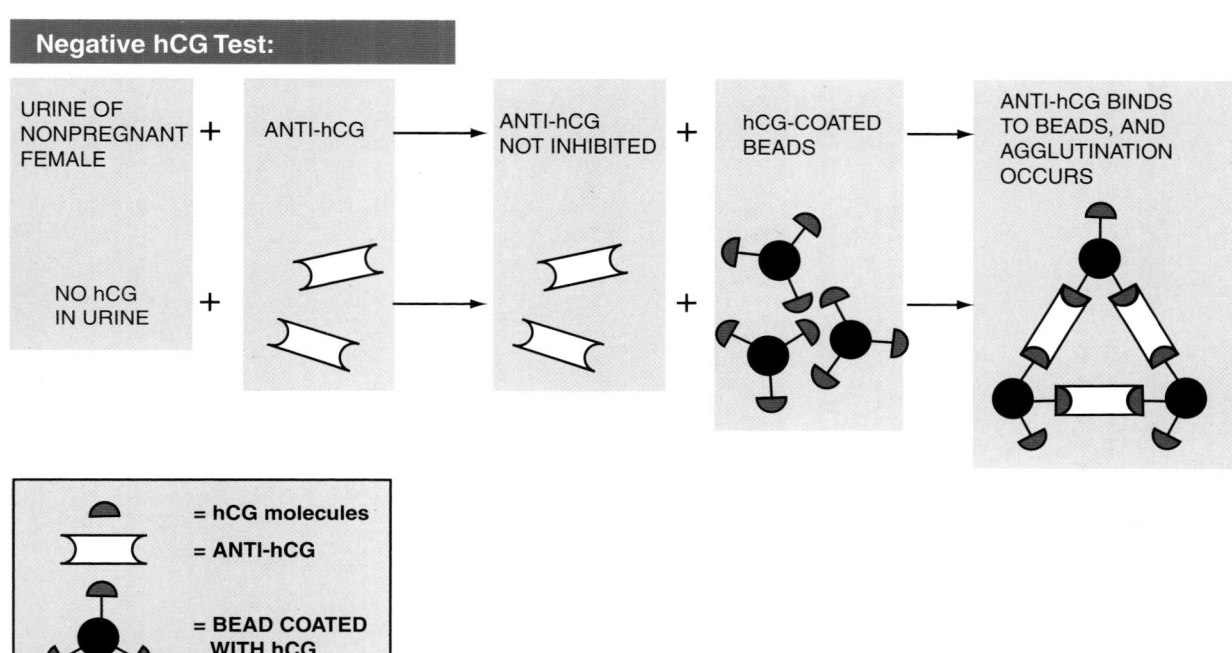

Negative hCG Test:

URINE OF NONPREGNANT FEMALE + ANTI-hCG → ANTI-hCG NOT INHIBITED + hCG-COATED BEADS → ANTI-hCG BINDS TO BEADS, AND AGGLUTINATION OCCURS

NO hCG IN URINE

= hCG molecules
= ANTI-hCG
= BEAD COATED WITH hCG

© Cengage Learning 2012

FIGURE 4-17 Principle of the agglutination inhibition test for hCG

PERFORMING A URINE HUMAN CHORIONIC GONADOTROPIN TEST

Several companies manufacture hCG tests for use in the clinical laboratory. Many test kits can be used with either serum or urine; other kits require only one or the other. Most quantitative tests must be performed using serum. The procedure described in this lesson is intended to present a general principle of hCG detection in urine.

Safety Precautions

  Standard Precautions must be observed and appropriate personal protective equipment (PPE) worn when performing urine hCG

tests. Exposure control methods should be used to avoid urine spills, splashes, or aerosol formation. If centrifugation of urine is required, centrifuge safety procedures must be followed. After testing, the used kit materials must be discarded into the appropriate sharps or biohazard container.

Quality Assessment

   The laboratory standard operating procedure (SOP) manual will contain instructions for specimen collection and preparation, urine hCG test procedure, reporting of results, and disposition of specimens. Specimen I.D. must be verified, and the institution's privacy policy and guidelines

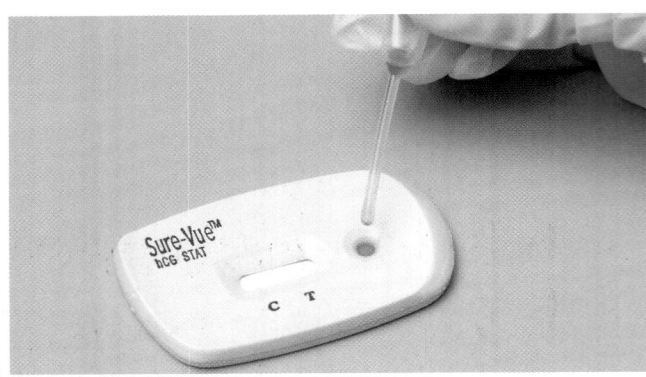

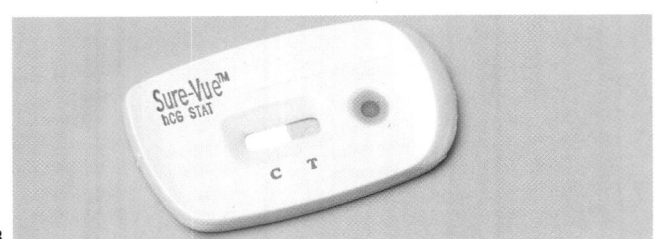

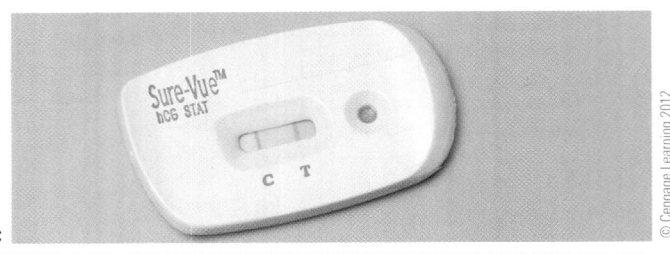

© Cengage Learning 2012

FIGURE 4-18 Chromatographic immunoassay for urine hCG: (A) urine is added to sample well; (B) development of pink background color in reaction window during incubation period indicates migration of sample through membrane; (C) positive reaction is indicated by presence of pink lines in control (C) and test (T) areas

for reporting hCG test results must be followed. The manufacturer's instructions must be rigorously followed for the kit in use, including:

- Specimens must be collected, stored, and used following manufacturer's directions
- Kits must be stored and used at manufacturer's recommended temperatures
- Urine must not be tested using a kit designed only for use with serum
- Kits must not be used after the expiration date
- Reagents must not be interchanged with other kits
- Reactions must be accurately timed, interpreted, and recorded

Most test kits contain an internal or procedural control that is positive when correct technique and sufficient sample volume are used. If the internal control is negative, the test is invalid. A positive hCG urine control (containing 25 to 250 mIU/mL) and negative hCG urine control (0 mIU/mL) must also be

run daily or as specified in the laboratory's SOP manual. Because hCG tests have different sensitivities, detection limits of the test in use must be considered when interpreting results.

Specimen Collection

Although any urine specimen can be used for most hCG tests, the first urine voided in the morning is the preferred specimen. This first morning specimen is the most concentrated urine specimen of the day, usually having a specific gravity of 1.020 or higher. This means that urine constituents, including any hCG present, will be concentrated in the early morning specimen. If the urine cannot be tested immediately, it can be stored for 24 to 48 hours; for some kits the urine can be stored frozen until testing. A clear aliquot must be used for testing. Visible precipitate should be removed by centrifugation or allowing it to settle.

ICON 25 hCG Procedure

The ICON 25 hCG is an example of a qualitative chromatographic immunoassay for hCG. In this test, anti-hCG antibodies are immobilized in a membrane enclosed in a test cartridge. The membrane contains a test region and an internal procedural control region. Three drops of urine are added to the sample well (S) of the cartridge. The urine migrates into the membrane by capillary attraction, and the test is read at 3 minutes. Any hCG in the urine binds to anti-hCG that is conjugated to a dye and immobilized in the test region. A colored line in the test (T) region indicates the specimen is positive for hCG and presumptive for pregnancy (Figure 4-19). Absence of a colored line in the test region is a negative test. A positive internal control is built in to the test and serves primarily to check technique. If the test has been performed properly, a colored line will always form in the control (C) region (Figure 4-19). Absence of a control line invalidates the test. Positive and negative external hCG controls must still be used with kits to ensure kit reliability.

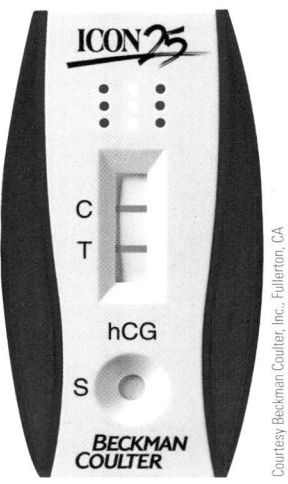

Courtesy Beckman Coulter, Inc., Fullerton, CA

FIGURE 4-19 Illustration of positive hCG result with ICON 25 hCG test

Reporting Human Chorionic Gonadotropin Results

The policy of the institution must be followed when reporting results of hCG tests, and patient privacy rights must be protected. The usual reporting method is to report the test as positive or negative for hCG, *not positive or negative for pregnancy*. Urine hCG tests are only presumptive for pregnancy, and positive hCG tests should be confirmed by physical examination and by ruling out other possible interfering conditions.

Significance of Human Chorionic Gonadotropin Test Results

Human chorionic gonadotropin appears in the urine and serum about 1 week after implantation, and the level rises during early pregnancy. By the first missed menstrual period, the hCG level can exceed 100 mIU/mL. By the 10th or 12th week of pregnancy, hCG levels are greater than 100,000 mIU/mL. The hCG level begins to decline about the third month of pregnancy and is not detectable within a few days after delivery.

Many tests are designed to detect hCG levels as low as 25 mIU/mL in urine and can often be positive before a menstrual period is missed. However, early in a pregnancy, urine hCG can be below test sensitivity levels, causing a (false) negative test result. Therefore, negative tests should be repeated on a first morning specimen after a few days to a week, if symptoms still warrant.

Conditions other than pregnancy can cause elevated hCG levels and positive reactions in hCG tests in the absence of pregnancy. These include **trophoblastic** disease, such as *choriocarcinoma*, and nontrophoblastic disease, such as breast, ovarian, and testicular tumors. Quantitative hCG tests performed on serum can be useful in diagnosing and following the course of these diseases as well as in diagnosing **ectopic pregnancy** (pregnancy outside the uterus) or suspected miscarriage (spontaneous abortion), which occurs in as high a rate as 25% to 50% of all pregnancies. Presence of hCG in urine should not be used to diagnose pregnancy unless other conditions have been ruled out and clinical findings support a pregnancy diagnosis.

SAFETY REMINDERS

- Review Safety Precautions section before beginning procedure.
- Observe Standard Precautions.
- Discard contaminated materials appropriately.

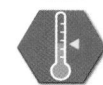

PROCEDURAL REMINDERS

- Review Quality Assessment section before beginning procedure.
- Follow SOP manual and manufacturer's instructions.
- Use appropriate control solutions to verify that kits are working properly.
- Interpret and report test results carefully, following institution's policy.

CRITICAL THINKING

A patient brought a urine specimen to the clinic for hCG testing. She reported that she had performed a home pregnancy test the previous evening on this same specimen and the results were negative, even though she felt sure that she was pregnant. The technician tested the specific gravity of the urine and found it to be 1.007.

1. What is the significance of a urine specimen with specific gravity of 1.007?
2. What advice should be given the patient? Explain your answer.

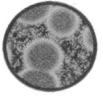

SUMMARY

Modern pregnancy tests are based on immunological detection of hCG in the urine or serum of pregnant females. The tests can detect hCG as early as a week or two after conception. Today's hCG tests give rapid results, and most are simple to perform. Many urine hCG test kits are CLIA-waived, and several are available over-the-counter for home use.

The laboratory's SOP manual will include manufacturer's directions, including specimen requirements, kit storage and use, test procedure, and interpretation of results. Positive and negative controls must be used to validate kit performance and procedural technique. The patient's right to privacy must be protected, and technicians must follow the institution's policy regarding the reporting of test results. Laboratory personnel must interpret urine hCG test results carefully, because the results reported will have certain consequences. For example, it is important that results are interpreted correctly and reported accurately when a patient is to receive a treatment that has the potential to cause damage to a fetus, such as radiography or drug therapy. Trophoblastic disease and certain types of cancers are sometimes associated with hCG production and can cause positive hCG tests.

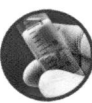 # REVIEW QUESTIONS

1. What hormone is detected in pregnancy tests? Where is the hormone produced?

2. What is the preferred specimen for urine hCG tests? Why?

3. What specimen is used for quantitative hCG tests?

4. What is the value of measuring the specific gravity of a urine specimen before performing the hCG test?

5. When does hCG first appear in pregnancy? When does it disappear?

6. Explain the principle of agglutination inhibition, which was used in the first rapid slide pregnancy tests.

7. Describe a general design of chromatographic immunoassays for hCG.

8. What safety precautions must be observed when performing hCG tests?

9. What is the purpose of an internal or procedural control?

10. Why are external controls required if internal controls are present?

11. What conditions other than pregnancy can cause a positive hCG test?

12. What action should be recommended to a woman who thinks she is pregnant but the urine hCG test is negative?

13. Define agglutination inhibition, ectopic pregnancy, hemagglutination, human chorionic gonadotropin, implantation, teratogenic, and trophoblastic.

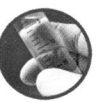 # STUDENT ACTIVITIES

1. Complete the written examination for this lesson.

2. Practice performing a urine test for hCG as outlined in the Student Performance Guide.

3. Survey over-the-counter pregnancy (hCG) test kits that are available; compare the major features of three kits.

 # WEB ACTIVITIES

1. Use the Internet to find the names and manufacturers of five CLIA-waived urine hCG test kits. Locate the manufacturers' web sites and look for package inserts or other descriptions of the principle and procedure for each kit. Make a table showing differences and similarities among the five kits, including principle of test design, endpoint reaction, types of internal controls, sensitivity level, specimen required, quantitative or qualitative, etc.

2. Download a package insert for a urine hCG test other than one discussed in this lesson. Use the package insert to write a procedure for performing the hCG test.

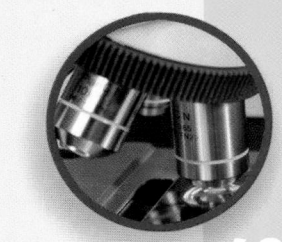

LESSON 4-4

Tests for Human Chorionic Gonadotropin

(Individual student results will vary depending on specimens provided by the instructor.)

Name _____ Date _____

INSTRUCTIONS

1. Practice performing a urine hCG test following the step-by-step procedure.

2. Demonstrate the urine hCG test procedure satisfactorily for the instructor, using the Student Performance Guide. Your instructor will explain the procedures for evaluating and grading your performance. Your performance may be given a number grade, letter grade, or satisfactory (S) or unsatisfactory (U) depending on course or institutional policy.

NOTE: Procedure given here is for the ICON 25 hCG test. Always follow the manufacturer's instructions and the package insert included with the kit being used.

MATERIALS AND EQUIPMENT

- gloves
- hand antiseptic
- full-face shield (or equivalent PPE)
- acrylic safety shield (optional)
- urine specimen
- timer
- ICON 25 hCG test kit or other rapid hCG test kit including:
  - kit instructions
  - test units
  - dispensers
  - hCG-positive and hCG-negative controls
- hCG-negative urine control (if not in kit)
- hCG-positive urine control (if not in kit)
- centrifuge and centrifuge tubes, with caps
- laboratory tissue
- paper towels
- surface disinfectant (such as 10% chlorine bleach)
- biohazard container
- sharps container

PROCEDURE

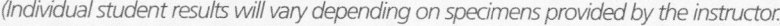

Record in the comment section any problems encountered while practicing the procedure (or have a fellow student or the instructor evaluate your performance).

S = Satisfactory
U = Unsatisfactory

You must:	S	U	Evaluation/Comments
1. Wash hands with antiseptic and put on gloves			
2. Put on face protection or position acrylic safety shield on work surface.			
3. Perform the ICON 25 hCG procedure following the steps 3a—3i (If a different hCG test kit is used go to step 4) a. Obtain test units, controls, timer, urine specimen, and test instructions b. Allow urine, test device, and controls to reach room temperature			
			(continues)

© 2012 Delmar, Cengage Learning. Permission to reproduce for clinical use granted.

You must:	S	U	Evaluation/Comments

c. Centrifuge urine to obtain clear supernatant if urine has visible precipitate
d. Open the pouch and place the test device on a level surface
e. Use the disposable dropper to dispense 3 drops of clear urine into the sample (S) well
f. Start the timer
g. Read the results in 3 minutes; the background of the test window should be white or light pink
h. Interpret and record the test results:
   1) A colored line appearing in the internal control (C) area indicates correct technique. Absence of the colored C line invalidates the test
   2) A colored line appearing in the test (T) area is a positive test for hCG
   3) Absence of a colored line in the test (T) area is a negative test for hCG
i. Repeat steps 3b–3h using both hCG-positive and hCG-negative urine controls			

4. Perform a urine hCG test following the manufacturer's instructions and steps 4a—4f: a. Obtain test units, controls, timer, urine specimen, and package insert for the test kit used b. Open test unit and place on level surface c. Apply specified volume of urine to the test unit and start timer d. Observe color development after specified time interval. Verify that internal control(s) displays correct reaction e. Record results, consulting manufacturer's pack-age insert to interpret test results f. Repeat steps 4b–4e using both hCG-positive and hCG-negative urine controls			
5. Discard used sharps into sharps container and other con-taminated disposable materials into biohazard container			
6. Dispose of specimen as instructed			
7. Clean work area with disinfectant			
8. Remove gloves and discard into biohazard container			
9. Wash hands with antiseptic			

Instructor/Evaluator Comments:

Instructor/Evaluator _____ Date _____

© 2012 Delmar, Cengage Learning. Permission to reproduce for clinical use granted.

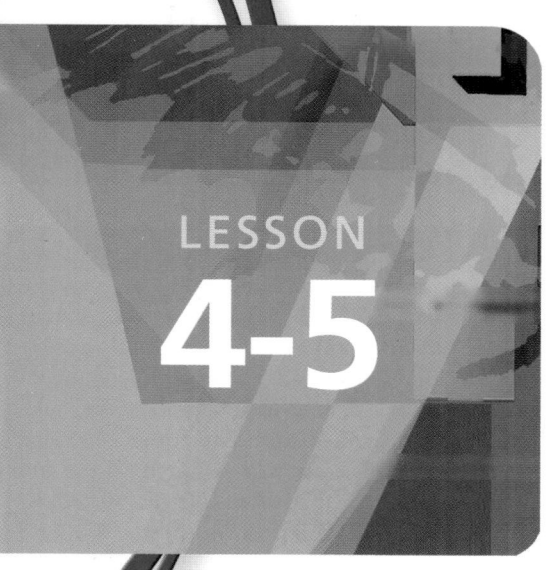

Introduction to Immunohematology

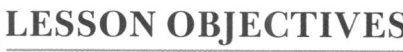

LESSON OBJECTIVES

After studying this lesson, the student will:

- ⊙ Discuss the functions of the immunohematology, or blood banking, department.
- ⊙ Name five procedures performed in the blood bank department.
- ⊙ Explain the process of blood donation.
- ⊙ Discuss requirements that must be met by blood donors.
- ⊙ Name eight tests that must be performed on donated blood before it can be transfused.
- ⊙ Name three blood components that can be obtained from a single unit of donated blood.
- ⊙ Discuss the safety procedures that must be followed in the blood bank.
- ⊙ Explain the importance of quality assessment policies to the operation of the blood bank.
- ⊙ Define the glossary terms.

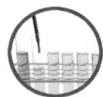

GLOSSARY

American Association of Blood Banks (AABB) / international association that sets blood bank standards, accredits blood banks, and promotes high standards of performance in the practice of transfusion medicine

apheresis / the process of removing a specific component, such as platelets, from donor blood, and returning the remaining blood components to donor circulation

blood bank / clinical laboratory department where blood components are tested and stored until needed for transfusion; also called immunohematology department or transfusion services; the refrigerated unit used for storing blood components

immunohematology / the study of the human blood groups; in the clinical laboratory, often called blood banking or transfusion services

transplant / living tissue placed into the body; the placing of living tissue into the body

INTRODUCTION

Immunohematology is the study of the human blood groups. In practice, immunohematology procedures are performed in the hospital blood bank or transfusion services department, by providers of blood components, and by immunology or histocompatibility laboratories. Examples of services performed can include:

- Evaluation of potential blood donors
- Collection and processing of donor blood
- Testing patient blood for blood group antigens

- Matching patient with compatible blood for transfusion
- Tissue typing
- Forensic studies
- Paternity tests
- Genetic studies

This lesson presents an introduction to the practice of immunohematology. Information is given about blood donation, collection and processing of donor blood, and the routine functions of the immunohematology department, also called the **blood bank** department. A discussion of ABO blood groups and procedures for ABO grouping are described in Lesson 4-6. The importance of the Rh blood group and procedures for Rh typing are given in Lesson 4-7.

HISTORY OF TRANSFUSION MEDICINE

The earliest recorded blood transfusion was attempted shortly after William Harvey reported his observations of blood circulation in 1628. For several decades following, crude blood transfusions were tried numerous times, sometimes transfusing blood from animals to humans, mostly with disastrous results. This eventually led to the prohibition of transfusion in the late 1600s.

In 1818, Dr. James Blundell, an English obstetrician, successfully transfused a woman suffering from postpartum hemorrhage using her husband's blood. He continued to experiment with transfusion, with some success, and also devised instruments for use in transfusion. In 1867, Joseph Lister proposed using antiseptic techniques during transfusions. In the late 1800s, U.S. physicians experimented with transfusing milk into patients, but because of adverse reactions, the physicians switched to saline. Throughout all of this time, some patients did well, some developed infections, and some suffered immediate severe reactions and died. Physicians had no way to anticipate which transfusions would be successful and which would fail.

In 1900, Karl Landsteiner discovered the ABO blood group and, in 1930, received the Nobel Prize for this discovery. Following this landmark discovery, in the first half of the twentieth century, physicians began developing ways to improve transfusion success. Some milestones were:

- The technique of crossmatching patient and donor blood was begun (patient blood is mixed with donor blood before transfusion and observed for a reaction)
- The discovery of the inheritance of blood groups
- Anticoagulants were developed that could preserve blood for longer periods
- The Rh blood group and other minor blood groups were discovered
- The first blood *depot* for storing donated blood was established during World War I
- The first hospital blood bank in the United States was established in 1937 in Chicago

- The U.S. government established a nationwide blood collection program in 1940 that was instrumental in saving lives during World War II

Beginning around 1950, and for the next three decades, improvements in blood banking were rapid and dramatic: sterile plastic blood bags were manufactured, improved blood preservation methods extended the shelf life of blood to 35 days, donor units were screened for hepatitis B, and hospital blood banks were established all over the country, even in small hospitals. Blood use increased dramatically as its value in trauma and major surgeries such as open heart surgery was recognized. Specialized treatments using components such as platelet concentrates, fresh frozen plasma, and anti–hemophilic factor (AHF) were used to treat bleeding disorders.

In the early 1980s, the discipline of *transfusion medicine* became a medical specialty. About this time the first cases of acquired immunodeficiency syndrome (AIDS) began to appear. In 1984, the cause of AIDs was proven to be the human immunodeficiency virus (HIV), and the virus was shown to be transmissible by blood. This immediately caused drastic changes in donor blood screening and intensified research into developing sensitive, reliable tests for HIV to prevent transmitting HIV from an infected donor to a patient. The need to guarantee a safe blood supply led not only to the development of sensitive tests to detect HIV but also to improved tests for other infectious agents. As new infectious diseases emerge, researchers act quickly to develop screening tests for the infectious agents. Blood donation requirements and screening tests are continually evaluated to ensure that procedures are in place to prevent potentially infected blood from entering the blood supply pool.

IMMUNOHEMATOLOGY OR BLOOD BANK DEPARTMENT

The application of immunohematology principles in the clinical laboratory is usually carried out in the blood bank, or *transfusion services*, department. The commonly used designation "blood bank" comes from the fact that blood units have traditionally been stored or *banked* in one location.

On a daily basis, scientists working in the blood bank are responsible for typing patient blood, testing blood for unexpected antibodies related to the blood groups, matching compatible blood units to patients for transfusion, and providing components such as red cells or platelets (Table 4-7). Because blood and blood components are administered intravenously, they are considered **transplants**; the operation of blood banks is regulated by the Food and Drug Administration (FDA). Depending on the size of the hospital, the blood bank department can perform blood group studies in paternity questions and work with transplant teams and tissue typing laboratories to ensure safe organ and tissue transplants (Table 4-7).

DONOR BLOOD

The **American Association of Blood Banks (AABB)** is an agency that accredits blood banks and also develops standards for blood banking practice. The AABB estimates that approximately

TABLE 4-7. Examples of tests performed in immunohematology laboratories

Identifying suitable blood donors
Collecting and processing donor blood
Routine blood typing
Providing compatible components for transfusion
Testing blood for unusual blood group antibodies
Tissue typing
Forensic studies
Paternity tests
Genetic studies

TABLE 4-8. Diseases and infectious agents capable of being transmitted by blood transfusion

VIRUSES	PARASITIC DISEASES	BACTERIAL DISEASES
Hepatitis A virus	Babesiosis	Syphilis*
Hepatitis B virus*	Chagas*	
Hepatitis C virus*	Malaria	
Cytomegalovirus†		
Human immunodeficiency virus (HIV)* types 1 and 2		
Human T-lymphotropic virus (HTLV)-I*		
Human T-lymphotropic virus (HTLV)-II*		
West Nile virus*		

*In the U.S., donor blood is routinely tested for this disease/agent
†Donor blood is screened only in selected cases

9.5 million donors donate 16 million units of blood in the United States each year. Donations are made at community blood donation centers as well as mobile blood donation centers at malls, schools, churches, and other areas participating in blood drives. Each year, these donations provide blood components for over 4 million patients, including trauma victims, surgical patients, and patients with bleeding disorders or diminished blood cell production.

Most hospitals acquire donor blood from blood donor processing centers, such as those operated by the American Red Cross (ARC) or other independent, nonprofit blood donation agencies. Blood donation centers strive to provide safe blood for transfusion, and this begins with accepting blood donation only from healthy donors. Volunteer donors provide the majority of donated blood in the United States and are highly recruited because the quality of volunteer donated blood is considered to be higher than that from paid donors.

Blood Donor Requirements

Several methods are used to eliminate unsafe blood from entering the blood supply—strict enforcement of donor eligibility standards, verification of donor I.D., donor medical screening, laboratory testing of donor blood, confidential exclusion of donors, and checks of donor records. Although donated blood is tested for several infectious agents, it is impossible to test for all possible agents (Table 4-8).

Before donating, prospective donors are provided educational materials explaining the requirements that must be met to be accepted as a donor, as well as diseases, conditions, or medical history that would cause a person to be excluded from donating. Potential donors who elect to continue with the process after reading the materials are given a brief physical examination and asked to answer extensive questions about their medical history. The questions are designed both to ensure that donation will not create a health risk to the donor and also to exclude donors whose blood might cause harm to the recipient if transfused. The safety of the blood supply depends on donor education and donor honesty in answering these questions. The privacy of prospective donors must be respected while obtaining medical history so that donors are not reluctant to provide honest answers.

The physical examination includes weight, temperature, blood pressure, pulse rate, blood hemoglobin level, and evaluation of general health and demeanor of donor (Table 4-9). The health questionnaire can contain as many as 100 questions, asking about date of last donation, current medications, recent immunizations, previous and existing diseases or medical conditions, and travel or residency outside of the United States. Behavioral history is also questioned, including questions about sexual behavior, illegal drug use, recent tattoos, body piercing, acupuncture, electrolysis, and other questions. Ultimately, the physician in charge of the donation center makes the final decision on whether to accept, defer, or exclude a donor. Deferrals can be temporary due to conditions such as fever, anemia, or high blood pressure. Permanent exclusions can be due to history of infectious disease,

TABLE 4-9. Examples of general health requirements for blood donors

PARAMETER	CRITERIA*
Age	At least 16 years old, conforming to state laws
Weight	110 pounds
Temperature	≤99.5° F (≤37.5° C)
Blood pressure	<180/<100 mm Hg
Hemoglobin	>11 g/dL (or >33% Hct)

*Requirements can differ slightly among blood collection agencies and according to state laws.

such as hepatitis or HIV infection, or lifestyle issues, such as history of use of intravenous drugs. Potential donors should be given the opportunity for confidential self-exclusion in a manner that avoids face-to-face interview. Potential donors should also be advised that all donated blood will be tested and the donor will be notified of any positive results.

Donor Blood Collection

All materials used to collect donor blood are sterile, so there is no danger of transmitting disease to the donor. Blood is collected by venipuncture from a large vein in the arm (usually the cephalic vein) after sterilizing the puncture site. Approximately 1 pint (about 450 mL) of whole blood is collected into a sterile closed bag containing anticoagulant and nutrients to prevent clot formation and keep blood cells viable for several weeks. A commonly used anticoagulant is a citrate-phosphate-dextrose-adenine (CPDA) solution that allows cells to be stored for up to 35 days. If mannitol and glucose are also added to the mixture, the shelf life of red blood cells can be extended to 6 weeks (42 days).

The donation process takes from 10 to 20 minutes. A small portion of the donor blood remains in sealed, segmented tubing external to the sterile unit (Figure 4-20). Each tubing segment is coded to match the code on the blood bag. The blood in these tubing segments is used for various tests so that unit sterility is maintained until it is transfused. At the time of donation, blood is also collected into vacuum tubes to be used for typing the blood and for other screening tests.

Adults average about 10 pints of blood in their circulation. The fluid lost from donation is replenished by the body within about 24 hours; the red blood cells are replaced in a few weeks. Blood donors must wait a minimum of 8 weeks (56 days) between donations of whole blood.

Processing and Testing Donor Blood

Donated blood is placed in "quarantine" immediately after the donation process. Technologists in donor processing centers determine the ABO group and Rh type of donor blood, screen the blood for unexpected antibodies to blood group antigens, and perform several other tests, most of which are designed to eliminate potentially infectious units from being transfused. Blood is tested for antibodies to hepatitis B and C viruses, HIV (HIV-1 and HIV-2), and human T-lymphotropic virus types I and II (HTLV-I, HTLV-II). Units are also tested for antigens of HIV, hepatitis B virus, hepatitis C virus and West Nile virus using very sensitive nucleic acid amplification tests (NATs) that detect viral genetic material. Additionally, blood is tested for evidence of syphilis and *T. cruzi* infections (Table 4-10).

Once all testing results are satisfactory, the blood component can receive its final labeling (Figure 4-20B). It is then removed from quarantine and becomes part of the available blood supply for distribution to healthcare facilities. Any unit that is confirmed positive for any test for infectious agents must be discarded, and the donor must be notified

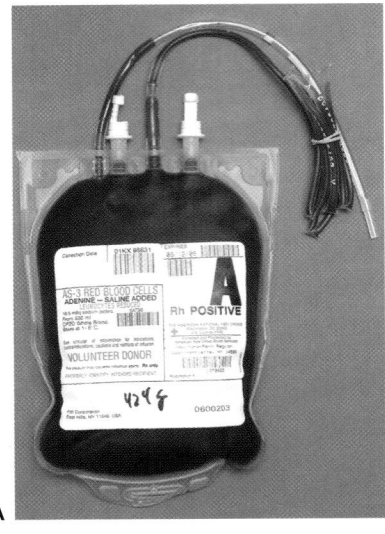

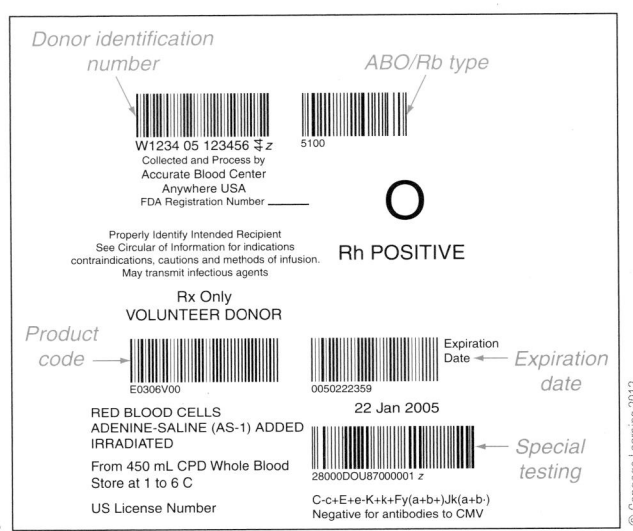

FIGURE 4-20 Blood component: (A) donor blood bag with attached segmented tubing and final labeling; (B) example of information provided on component label

and placed on a list prohibiting the person from giving blood. Table 4-10 lists the tests for infectious agents performed on donor blood in the United States in 2010. The list is constantly expanding as new infectious diseases emerge and tests become available.

Blood Components

Blood is collected as whole blood, which contains red and white blood cells and platelets suspended in plasma. Donated blood can then be separated into components, depending on the needs of the medical community in the region. In this way more than one patient can benefit from the donation of one unit of blood. Three components easily obtained from one donor unit are:

- Red blood cells
- Platelets
- Plasma (fresh frozen plasma [FFP])

TABLE 4-10. Tests for infectious diseases routinely performed on donated blood (as of June 2010)

ANTIBODY TESTS	ANTIGEN TESTS
Hepatitis B core antibody (anti-HBc)	Hepatitis B surface antigen (HBsAg)
Hepatitis C antibody (anti-HCV)	Nucleic acid amplification testing (NAT) for:
HIV-1 (anti-HIV-1)	HIV-1
HIV-2 (anti-HIV-2)	Hepatitis C virus
HTLV-I antibody (anti-HTLV-I)	West Nile virus (WNV)
HTLV-II antibody (anti-HTLV-II)	
Serologic test for syphilis	
Antibody test for *Trypanosoma cruzi*	

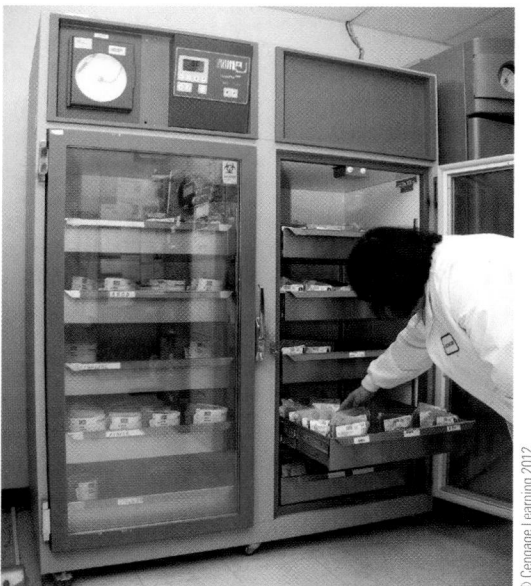

FIGURE 4-21 Refrigerated blood bank for storing blood components

Many other components can be prepared from donor blood but are used less frequently than red blood cells, platelets, and FFP. These components are usually prepared in a production facility other than the blood donation center and include cryoprecipitated antihemophilic factor (AHF), factor VIII concentrate, factor IX concentrate, and immune globulins, including Rh immune globulin. Emphasis is currently placed on producing certain components by recombinant DNA techniques to reduce or eliminate the risk for transmission of infective agents to patients.

Red blood cells are transfused into patients with low hemoglobin or hematocrit who need rapid improvement in the oxygen-carrying capacity of blood, usually because of hemorrhage. Plasma is a source of electrolytes and proteins such as albumin, globulins, fibrinogen, and other clotting proteins. If the plasma is frozen within hours after collection, it is designated as FFP and is useful in treating bleeding disorders caused by deficiency of clotting factors.

Platelet concentrates are prepared by centrifuging plasma to obtain platelet-rich plasma. Platelets are used to treat thrombocytopenia and other platelet or bleeding disorders.

DIC - TREATED BY FFD

Apheresis

Another type of donation is called **apheresis**, the process of removing one blood component and returning the remaining blood components to the donor's circulatory system. Apheresis can take 1 to 2 hours to complete and requires special cell-separating machines. This process can be used to donate red blood cells, plasma, platelets, and granulocytes. *Plateletpheresis* is the process of removing only platelets from a donor. Up to five times more platelets can be recoverd from one donor in a plateletpheresis session than are present in one unit of platelet concentrate prepared from a unit of whole blood.

Storage of Blood Components

Blood components are stored in temperature-controlled units such as blood bank refrigerators and freezers (Figure 4-21). The components must be stored within a very narrow temperature range. The temperature-controlled units are fitted with audible alarms that alert then the temperature falls above or below the set range, as well as backup power sources in case of power outages. Temperatures must be monitored and recorded as specified in the laboratory's standard operating procedure (SOP) manual.

PROCEDURES PERFORMED IN THE HOSPITAL BLOOD BANK

Blood banking is the common term referring to tests routinely performed in this department. Most routine blood banking procedures are based on the agglutination reaction. These procedures include:

- ABO grouping
- Rh typing
- Compatibility testing before blood transfusion
- Typing of donor blood
- Screening for and identification of unusual blood group antibodies
- Tests for hemolytic disease of the newborn

ABO is the major blood group. The Rh system of red cell antigens is second in importance. All donor blood and patients who might receive donor blood must have the ABO group and Rh type determined. These procedures are described in Lessons 4-6 and 4-7. Although donor units are labeled with ABO and Rh type before they are released from the processing center, hospital blood banks repeat the tests on all donor components.

CURRENT TOPICS

SYNTHETIC BLOOD AND BLOOD SUBSTITUTES

It is estimated that someone in the United States needs a blood transfusion every 2 to 3 seconds. During holidays or extreme winter weather, we often hear through the news media about blood shortages and pleas for volunteers to donate blood. Emergencies, natural disasters, and wars create immediate needs for increased donor units. Trauma victims needing blood must wait for a transfusion until they can reach a medical facility and laboratory testing can identify compatible blood.

Researchers have been searching for a safe blood substitute for years. Military-funded research began decades ago because of the need for a portable, stable product to transfuse into severely wounded personnel on the battlefield. HBO2-2-1 is one synthetic product developed by the military.

Research for blood substitutes continues today, using two main approaches: (1) use of liquid *perfluorochemicals*, synthetic chemicals related to Teflon, administered intravenously under high oxygen pressure and (2) use of *cell-free stable hemoglobin* derived from blood cells or genetically engineered. (The term *oxygen therapeutics* is often used in place of synthetic blood because it more closely describes the function of the products.) The ideal blood substitute would provide rapid oxygen delivery to the patient's tissues while eliminating the risk for transmission of infectious agents. It would also (1) reduce blood shortages, (2) have a long shelf life, (3) require no special storage conditions, and (4) be universally compatible. Each research approach has advantages and disadvantages, but neither has been able to overcome some of the major disadvantages, such as toxicity and short half-life of the product in plasma.

Clinical trials of several products have been conducted in animals, and some trials have been done in humans. Some hemoglobin products are already in limited use. Oxyglobin, a chemically stabilized hemoglobin, has been used successfully since 1998 to treat canine anemia. A stabilized bovine hemoglobin product is used in South Africa to treat severely anemic human adult patients. In the United States, blood substitutes have been tested in healthy volunteers and found to be safe in small amounts. As these products come into wider use, they will be useful at trauma sites to provide a means to stabilize patients who have sustained blood loss until they can receive donor blood.

The blood of patients requiring a transfusion must be matched to a compatible component. This test is called a *cross-match*, or *compatibility testing*. It involves combining patient plasma (or serum) with donor red blood cells and examining for an agglutination reaction. This is to be sure the patient has no antibody that could react with donor blood and cause an adverse reaction.

Safety in the Blood Bank

Standard Precautions must be followed when performing all blood bank procedures, whether at donor processing centers or hospital blood banks. Gloves and appropriate personal protective equipment (PPE) must be worn. Exposure control methods, such as working behind an acrylic safety shield (Figure 4-22), must be used to protect against exposure to blood and blood products. Because most reagents used in blood banking originate from human blood, all reagents must be handled as if potentially infectious. Disposable supplies should be used, and surfaces should be disinfected frequently. Safety rules must be followed when using electrical equipment and instruments with moving parts, such as centrifuges.

Quality Assessment

It is crucial to patient well-being that testing performed in the immunohematology department is of the highest quality and performed with the utmost attention to accuracy. Blood is a living tissue; a blood transfusion is a tissue transplant. The same precautions must be used with blood transfusions as with organ transplants. The methods and policies outlined in the facility's standard operating procedure (SOP) manual must be followed.

Donor blood must be collected and stored in a manner that maintains the sterility of the blood and the viability of the cells. Blood typing and crossmatching results are used to identify

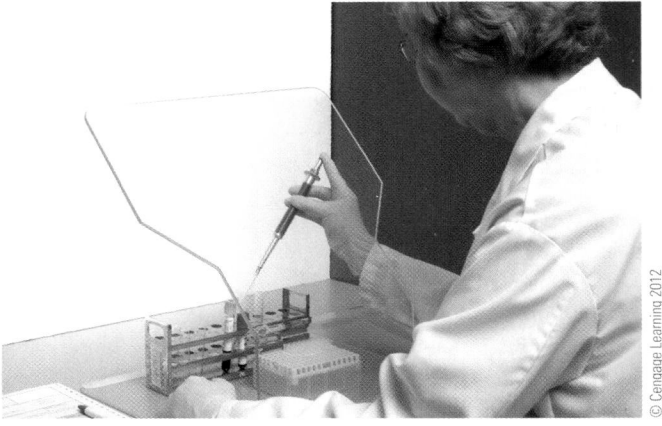

© Cengage Learning 2012

FIGURE 4-22 Exposure control method: use acrylic safety shield to prevent exposure to blood and blood products

donor blood compatible with the patient. Transfusion of the wrong blood into a patient can cause severe adverse reactions, such as kidney shutdown, or even death.

Strict quality assessment procedures must be followed in the blood bank department. Mandatory quality assessment guidelines include:

- Documenting proper working condition of refrigerators, freezers, water baths, centrifuges, and any other equipment used in preparing, testing, and storing blood components
- Monitoring temperatures at all times to ensure that components are constantly stored within acceptable temperature ranges
- Visually inspecting and testing reagents at designated intervals and recording control results
- Observing reagent expiration dates
- Using appropriate controls

Special attention must be paid to patient and donor blood identification. Special bar-coded armband systems can be used for inpatients and outpatients; matching bar-coded specimen labels are included with the system. Observation and interpretation of results must be carefully recorded.

CASE STUDY

Suri, a 31-year-old woman, heard about a need for blood donors in her area on the local television news broadcast. She went to the local blood donation center to volunteer to donate. Results of her physical examination and medical history included these findings:

Physical Exam:		Medications:		Travel in past year:	
Temperature	98.5°F	Antidepressant	Yes	Africa	No
Weight	115	Aspirin (last 8 days)	No	Europe	No
Hematocrit	31%	Birth control pills	Yes	Canada	Yes
Blood pressure	110/70				

Use information from the ARC or AABB web sites in addition to Table 4-9 to answer the following questions:

1. Are any of the Suri's findings reasons for deferring donation? If so, which one(s)?
2. Name three medications that can cause a donor to be permanently or indefinitely excluded from donating blood.

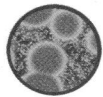

SUMMARY

Immunohematology covers several areas of study. These areas include research to ensure a safe blood supply, increase shelf life of donor blood, and develop synthetic blood. Transfusion practices are also continually evaluated to determine the best transfusion therapies for patients.

Blood donor collection and processing agencies provide a safe blood supply by screening donors through physical examinations and medical questionnaires. Laboratory tests are also used to screen donor blood for several infectious agents before it is approved and released to hospitals for use.

In the clinical laboratory, immunohematology procedures are performed in the blood bank or transfusion services department. Personnel type patient blood, confirm donor blood type, and provide compatible blood components for transfusion. The utmost care must be taken in all blood bank procedures

to ensure that patients receive transfusions that are life-saving, not life-threatening or otherwise detrimental to their health. Immunohematology is a challenging field, and requires dedicated, capable technologists working to provide the best possible patient care.

REVIEW QUESTIONS

1. What screening tests for viral diseases are performed on donated blood before the blood can be released to hospital blood banks?
2. What three components can be obtained from a single unit of donor blood?
3. Which governmental agency regulates blood banks?
4. What are the two major blood groups?

5. What is meant by synthetic blood? Why would it be beneficial?

6. What benefit could be gained by giving FFP to a patient?

7. What benefit is derived from transfusing red blood cells into a patient?

8. What important contribution was made to immunohematology by Karl Landsteiner? How did this change the practice of immunohematology?

9. Name five procedures performed in blood banks.

10. Explain the safety precautions that must be observed when performing blood bank procedures.

11. Why is it essential to have a comprehensive quality assessment program in place in blood banks?

12. Define American Association of Blood Banks, apheresis, blood bank, immunohematology, and transplant.

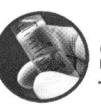

STUDENT ACTIVITIES

1. Complete the written examination for this lesson.

2. Visit a blood donation center. Ask for a copy of donor education information and donor questionnaire. Find out how donated blood is collected, tested, and processed for distribution. Find out what information is contained on the label attached to components of donor blood. Ask for information about how apheresis is performed.

WEB ACTIVITIES

1. Search web sites such as those of the ARC or AABB to find specific blood donor requirements. Print or download a donor medical questionnaire. List five conditions or criteria that would cause a potential donor to be deferred or excluded.

2. From reliable web sites such as those of the Centers for Disease Control and Prevention (CDC), ARC, or AABB, find out if the following diseases present a risk for transmission by blood transfusion: variant Creutzfeldt-Jakob disease (vCJD), Lyme disease, and smallpox.

3. Search the Internet for information on *autologous* blood donation. Write a report about it, including a definition, an explanation of how it differs from regular blood donation, and advantages and disadvantages.

4. Search the Internet for information about freezing blood cells for long-term storage. Describe how this process is performed and discuss advantages and disadvantages.

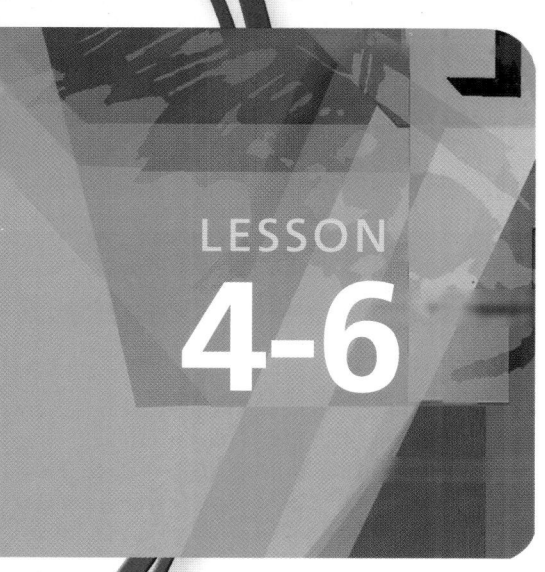

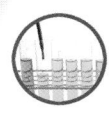

LESSON OBJECTIVES

After studying this lesson, the student will:

⊙ Name the four blood groups in the ABO system and state their frequencies in the United States.

⊙ Explain the inheritance of the ABO blood groups antigens.

⊙ Name the blood group antigens and antibodies in the ABO system.

⊙ Explain forward and reverse grouping.

⊙ Perform ABO slide grouping and interpret the results.

⊙ Perform ABO tube grouping and interpret the results.

⊙ Describe grading of agglutination in tube grouping.

⊙ Explain the use of gel typing in the blood bank.

⊙ Discuss safety precautions that must be observed when performing ABO grouping.

⊙ Discuss the importance of using controls and following quality assessment policies in the blood bank.

⊙ Define the glossary terms.

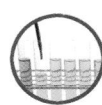

GLOSSARY

allele / one of two (or more) forms of a gene responsible for genetic variation

antiserum / serum that contains antibodies

blood bank / clinical laboratory department where blood components are tested and stored until needed for transfusion; also called immunohematology department or transfusion services; the refrigerated unit used for storing blood components

blood group antibody / a protein (immunoglobulin) that reacts specifically with a blood group antigen

blood group antigen / a substance or structure on the red blood cell membrane that stimulates antibody formation and reacts with that antibody

codominant / in genetics, a gene that is expressed in the heterozygous state, that is, in the presence of a different allelic gene

forward grouping / the use of known antisera (antibodies) to detect unknown antigens on a patient's cells; forward typing; direct grouping

genes / segments of DNA that code for specific proteins and that are the structural units of heredity

histocompatibility testing / assays to determine if donor and recipient tissue are compatible

human leukocyte antigen (HLA) / one of several antigens present on leukocytes and other body cells that are important in transplant rejection

(continues)

major histocompatibility complex (MHC) / the group of genes responsible for producing antigens such as HLA that are important in organ and tissue transplants

reverse grouping / the use of known cells (antigens) to identify unknown antibodies in the patient's serum or plasma

serological centrifuge / a centrifuge that spins small tubes such as those used in blood banking; serofuge

INTRODUCTION

The major blood group system is the ABO system; humans are grouped as one of four major types: A, B, AB, or O. ABO grouping tests are based on the principle of agglutination. The grouping tests can be performed by slide, tube, or gel methods. The slide method is quick and easy and requires no special equipment. However, the tube and gel methods are used in clinical laboratories because they are more sensitive than the slide test.

The ABO group of patient and donor blood must be determined before a blood transfusion can be given. Blood group determination must also be performed before organ transplants and in questions of paternity, forensic investigations, and genetic studies. This lesson presents information about the ABO blood group system and procedures for slide, tube, and gel methods of ABO grouping.

THE ABO SYSTEM

The ABO blood group system was discovered by Karl Landsteiner around 1900. All individuals can be placed into one of four major groups: A, B, AB, or O. According to the American Association of Blood Banks, in the United States, approximately 48% of the population is group O and 37% is group A. Only 11% of the population is B, and 4% is AB (Table 4-11). Distribution of the groups can differ regionally according to racial and ethnic populations.

Blood Group Antigens

ABO grouping is based on the presence or absence of two **blood group antigens** designated A and B. These antigens are found on the cell membranes of red blood cells, as well as platelets,

leukocytes, and most tissue cells. The blood group antigens are products of inherited allelic **genes**. Each individual inherits one blood group **allele** from each parent—the *A, B,* or *O* allele. *A* and *B* are **codominant** with respect to each other. Therefore, persons who inherit both an *A* and *B* allele will express both A and B antigens. A person who inherits one *O* allele and an *A* (or *B*) allele will express only A (or B) antigen. Individuals who inherit two *O* alleles have neither A nor B antigens.

Individuals are grouped according to the antigens present on their blood cells: a person who is group A has A antigen; a person who is group B has B antigen; a person who is group AB has A and B antigens; and a person who is group O has neither A nor B antigen (Table 4-12). The ABO grouping procedures are agglutination tests. A and B antigens on patient or donor red blood cells are detected by reacting the cells with known (commercial) antibodies in a procedure called **forward grouping**, or direct grouping.

Blood Group Antibodies

The discovery of the A and B antigens on blood cells was accompanied by the discovery of the corresponding ABO **blood group antibodies** in human blood. Blood group antibodies are named according to the antigen with which they react: an antibody that reacts with A antigen (A red blood cells) is called anti-A; an antibody that reacts with B antigen (B red blood cells) is called anti-B. The blood group O was so named because the red blood cells have neither A nor B antigen; therefore, there is no anti-O antibody.

ABO blood group antibodies occur naturally in blood and are of the immunoglobin M (IgM) class. If an antigen is missing from an individual's cells, the antibody specific for the missing antigen will be present. For example, group A individuals have anti-B antibody in their blood. An individual who is group O has

TABLE 4-11. ABO blood group frequencies in the United States*

ABO GROUP	PERCENTAGE (%) OF POPULATION
A	37
B	11
O	48
AB	4

*From AABB Website, 2010.

TABLE 4-12. Antigens and antibodies of the ABO system

ABO GROUP	ANTIGEN ON RED BLOOD CELLS	ANTIBODY IN BLOOD
A	A	Anti-B
B	B	Anti-A
AB	A and B	Neither anti-A nor anti-B
O	Neither A nor B	Both anti-A and anti-B

both anti-A and anti-B because O cells have neither A nor antigen (Table 4-12). Testing patient blood for the presence of the blood group antibodies is called **reverse grouping**, confirmatory grouping, or indirect grouping. It is performed by reacting patient serum or plasma with (commercial) red blood cells whose A and B antigens are known.

The blood group antigens are present on red blood cells of newborns; however, the blood group antibodies are not well developed at birth. Reverse grouping tests to detect the ABO antibodies are not reliable until the age of about 6 months. For this reason, only forward grouping is done in newborns and young infants.

Importance of ABO Grouping

The ABO group must be determined before procedures such as blood transfusion can be performed. An individual should be transfused with blood of the same ABO blood group. Because of the presence of the naturally occurring antibodies to A and B antigens, severe transfusion reactions can occur if blood is not matched properly.

The rule to follow in transfusing blood is to *avoid giving the patient an antigen he or she does not already have.* In an emergency, O blood can be used because it contains neither A nor B antigen. For this reason, people of blood group O are called *universal donors.*

Hospitals try to stick to same blood types

ABO GROUPING PROCEDURES

ABO grouping can be performed by slide, tube or gel techniques. The same safety and quality considerations apply to all blood typing techniques.

SAFETY PRECAUTIONS

  Standard Precautions must be followed when performing all **blood bank** procedures. Gloves and appropriate personal protective equipment (PPE) must be worn to protect against exposure to blood and blood products. Exposure control methods should be used to protect against accidental exposure to blood and blood typing reagents. Because most blood grouping reagents originate from human blood, all reagents must be handled as if potentially infectious. Disposable labware and supplies should be used and discarded into appropriate biohazard or sharps containers. Counter surfaces should be disinfected frequently with surface disinfectant. Safety rules must be followed to protect from physical and electrical hazards when using electrical equipment and instruments with moving parts, such as centrifuges.

QUALITY ASSESSMENT

   Quality assessment procedures and all test methods will be detailed in the blood bank standard operating procedure (SOP) manual. The manual will incorporate standards for good blood banking practice developed by the

American Association of Blood Banks (AABB), an agency that also accredits blood banks. The blood bank department must also follow Food and Drug Administration (FDA) guidelines and is subject to FDA inspections.

In immunohematology, the quality of laboratory testing can have a direct, immediate impact on the patient. A blood transfusion is a potentially lifesaving event. Errors or mistakes in identifying specimens, performing grouping tests, or interpreting grouping results can lead to serious consequences. Observations of test reactions must be carefully interpreted and recorded. Manufacturers' instructions must be followed for the particular reagents used. Technologists who work in the blood bank must be highly trained, conscientious, and vigilant.

Mandatory quality assessment guidelines include:

- Documenting proper working condition of refrigerators, freezers, water baths, centrifuges, and any other equipment used in preparing, testing, and storing blood components and reagents

- Monitoring temperatures at all times to ensure that components are constantly stored within acceptable temperature ranges

- Inspecting reagents visually, testing reagents at designated intervals, and maintaining records of results

- Observing reagent expiration dates

- Running appropriate controls and verifying reagent performance

The most important precaution in the blood bank department is to be sure that a patient requiring a transfusion receives a compatible blood component. Special bar-coded wristbands that come with matching bar-coded labels can be used. When blood is drawn for blood typing or compatibility testing, the wristband is placed on the patient and the matching bar-coded labels are placed on the tubes containing the patient's blood. Once compatible blood is identified for the patient, the units reserved for transfusion into that patient can be tagged with the matching bar-coded labels. Identification systems such as this provide a way of eliminating mistakes when a blood transfusion is required.

PRINCIPLE OF ABO SLIDE GROUPING

The slide test detects A or B antigens on red blood cells by combining the patient's blood cells with a known commercial **antiserum** on a slide and observing for agglutination. If the antigen present on the cells corresponds to the antibody in the antiserum, the antibody will bind to the antigen and cause clumping of the cells, or agglutination. If the antigen is not present on the cells, no agglutination will be observed.

Performing ABO Slide Grouping

ABO slide grouping is performed using commercial typing slides or microscope slides. One drop of commercial anti-A serum is added to one labeled slide, and one drop of anti-B serum is added to a separate labeled slide. A drop of well-mixed capillary or venous blood is placed adjacent to each drop of antiserum (Figure 4-23). The anti-A is mixed with the drop of blood using a disposable applicator stick, stirrer, or spreader. The procedure is repeated with the anti-B and the other drop of blood using a clean stirrer.

The slides are then rocked gently for 2 minutes and observed for agglutination using good lighting. Agglutination, a positive reaction, will appear as a clumping together of the red blood cells (Figure 4-24, top). Absence of agglutination is a negative reaction. The reactions with each antiserum should be recorded as positive (+) or negative (0).

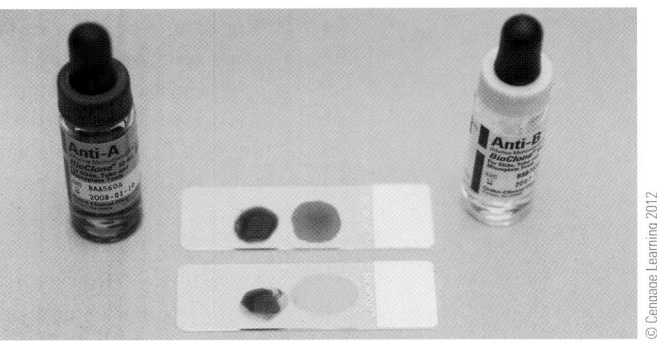

FIGURE 4-23 ABO slide grouping procedure: top slide contains one drop of blood and one drop of anti-A (blue); bottom slide contains one drop of blood and one drop of anti-B

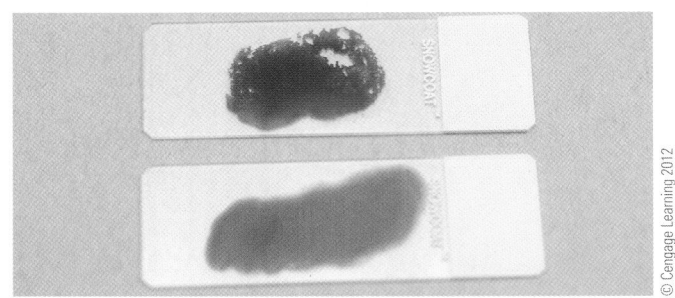

FIGURE 4-24 Blood group A typing results: agglutination of cells with anti-A (top slide) and absence of agglutination with anti-B (bottom slide) indicate that patient is blood group A

CURRENT TOPICS

ABO GROUPS AND ORGAN AND TISSUE TRANSPLANTS

Tissues or organs that are typically transplanted include kidney, liver, cornea, skin, pancreas, hemopoietic stem cell transplants (HSCT), bone marrow, heart, lung, intestine, and bone. Transplants that occur from one body site to another in the same individual are called *autologous transplants*, or *autografts*. An example of this would be skin grafts that are taken from one part of the body and transferred to a burned area. Because autologous transplants are of one's own tissue, the potential for tissue rejection is eliminated.

Transplants from a donor of the same species are called *allogeneic* or *allogenic transplants* (also called *allografts*). Allogeneic transplants can be from related individuals or unrelated individuals, such as a sister donating a kidney to her brother or a person receiving a heart transplant. According to the U.S. Department of Health and Human Services and the CDC, more than 30,000 people received solid organ transplants (SOT) in the United States in 2006, and more than 18,000 received HSCT. As many as 100,000 people are waiting to receive transplants at any one time.

Before an allogeneic transplant can be performed, the donor tissue or organ must be matched to the recipient (Figure 4-25). In the case of blood transfusions, which are tissue transplants, the ABO group and Rh type of the recipient is matched to the ABO group and Rh type of the donor blood. The ABO group must also be considered in other tissue and organ transplants because A and B antigens are present not only on red blood cells, platelets, and leukocytes, but also on many other cells in the body, particularly endothelial and epithelial cells.

After ABO matching, a second level of tissue matching involves histocompatibility testing, assays to determine whether donor and recipient share some tissue antigens. Important tissue antigens are coded for by the major histocompatibility complex (MHC), a complex of closely associated genes that code for highly variable antigens expressed on most cells of the body. These tissue antigens help distinguish one individual from another and are a major barrier to the ability to transplant tissues and organs from one individual to another.

Several antigens are produced by the MHC genes. Some of the most important are called human leukocyte antigens (HLA), named because they were first discovered on leukocytes. However, these antigens are present on many other types of body cells, and several different forms can be expressed

(Continues)

CURRENT TOPICS (Continued)

by the MHC, depending on which allelic genes are inherited. Therefore, family members are more likely to share some of the same antigens and be compatible donors. It is usually impossible to find a perfect HLA match because only identical twins have identical HLA antigens. However, when more HLA antigens are shared by donor and recipient, the chances of transplant rejection are lessened.

Transplant Rejection—The body's normal response to the introduction of foreign material is to mount an immune response and reject the foreign body.

This reaction occurs when allogeneic transplants are performed. Chances of rejection are minimized when donor histocompatibility antigens are matched to the transplant recipient. However, it is also necessary to use immunosuppressive drugs to further minimize the chances of rejection. Transplant rejection can be acute, chronic, or gradual, but can often be treated successfully with increased drug therapy. Individuals who receive allogeneic organ transplants usually must remain on immunosuppressive drugs for the remainder of their lives.

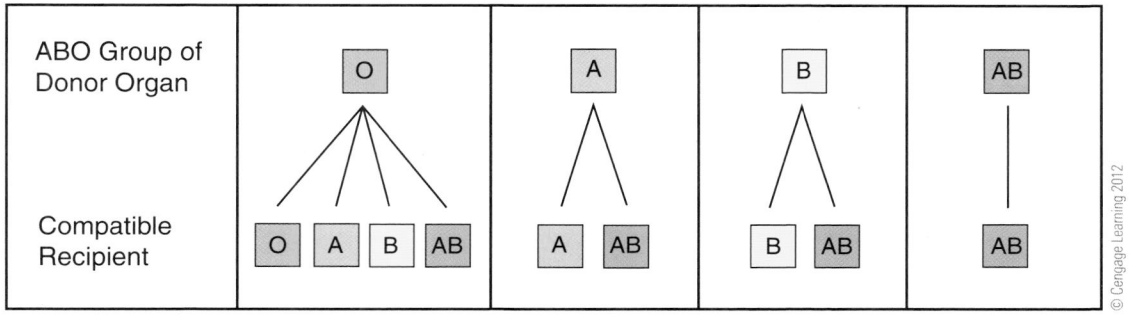

FIGURE 4-25 ABO compatibility chart for tissue and organ transplant

Interpretation of Slide Grouping Results

If only the A antigen is present on the red blood cells, the blood cells will agglutinate with anti-A but not with anti-B. If only B antigen is present, the blood cells will agglutinate with anti-B but not with anti-A. Group O blood cells will not agglutinate with either anti-A or anti-B. Group AB blood will agglutinate with both anti-A and anti-B (Table 4-13).

TABLE 4-13. Reactions of ABO groups with anti-A and anti-B sera

BLOOD	REACTIONS OF CELLS WITH: GROUP	
	ANTI-A	ANTI-B
A	+	0
B	0	+
AB	+	+
O	0	0

+ = agglutination
0 = no agglutination

PRINCIPLE OF ABO TUBE GROUPING

Tube testing is a more sensitive and reliable method of determining a patient's blood group than is slide testing. Tube testing is used in blood banks and in clinical laboratories; slide testing is more likely to be used in classrooms. ABO tube grouping consists of (1) direct or forward grouping, which identifies the antigens on the cells, and (2) reverse or confirmatory grouping, which identifies the blood group antibodies in patient plasma or serum.

Performing Forward Grouping

Forward or direct grouping identifies the antigens present on red blood cells by reacting a suspension of patient cells with commercial anti-A and anti-B sera and observing for agglutination after centrifugation. If a centrifuge is not available, the reactions can be observed after allowing the tubes to sit undisturbed at room temperature for 15 to 30 minutes.

A 2% to 5% red blood cell suspension of patient cells is made by combining 18 to 19 drops of saline with 1 drop of the patient's blood in a small (3 to 4 mL) test tube. Two tubes labeled *A* and *B* are set up: 1 drop of anti-A serum is placed in the *A* tube and 1 drop of anti-B serum is placed in the *B* tube.

One drop of the patient's 2% to 5% cell suspension is added to each tube, and the contents are mixed. The tubes are centrifuged for 15 to 30 seconds in a **serological centrifuge**, a specialized centrifuge that spins small test tubes, to speed up the reaction (Figure 4-26). (Centrifugation times can vary with the centrifuge. The centrifuges in each laboratory must be calibrated for optimum spin time.)

Interpretation of Forward Grouping

The tubes are tapped gently to loosen the cells from the bottom of the tube, and the cells are observed for agglutination. Clumping of the cells is a positive reaction indicating the antigen present on the cells corresponds to the antibody placed in the test tube (Tables 4-13 and 4-14). For example, based on the information in Table 4-14, a patient whose cells do not agglutinate with anti-A and do agglutinate with Anti-B is grouped as group B.

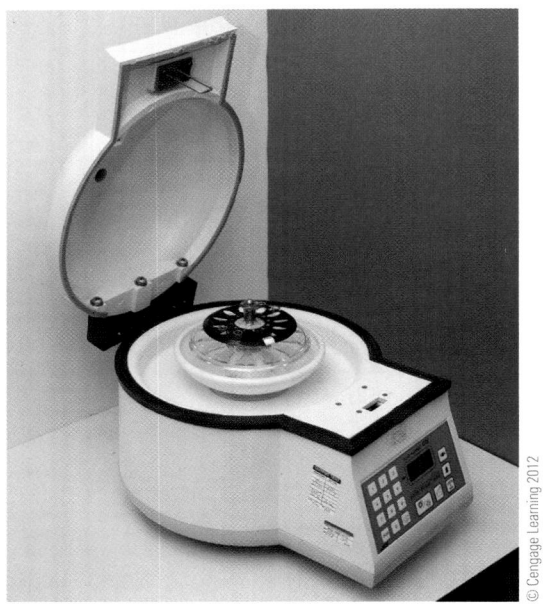

FIGURE 4-26 Serological centrifuge

Agglutination reactions should be graded using a plus system: neg or 0 (no agglutination); w+ (weak reaction); and 1+, 2+, 3+, and 4+ (strongest agglutination). Figure 4-27 gives an illustration and description of each grade of reaction.

Performing Reverse Grouping

Reverse (indirect or confirmatory) grouping identifies the antibodies present in a patient's serum or plasma by reacting the plasma with a commercial 2% to 5% suspension of group A cells and a commercial 2% to 5% suspension of group B cells and observing for agglutination.

Two drops of the patient's plasma are added to each of three tubes marked *a*, *b*, and *control*. One drop of the group A cell suspension is added to tube *a*, one drop of group B cell suspension is added to tube *b*, and one drop of a 2% to 5% suspension of patient cells is added to the *control* tube. The contents of the tubes are mixed, and the tubes are centrifuged for 15 to 30 seconds.

Interpretation of Reverse Grouping

After centrifugation or incubation, the tubes are tapped gently, the cells are observed for agglutination, and the reactions graded (Figure 4-27). A positive test, agglutination, indicates that the antibody present in the patient's plasma corresponds to the antigen on cells added to the tube. The control tube should always be negative for agglutination because it contains only the patient's plasma and cells. Reverse grouping results should confirm the results of forward grouping (Table 4-14).

PRINCIPLES OF GEL TYPING

Automated and semi-automated systems are available for blood grouping and crossmatching. Solid-phase and gel or column typing methods can be automated allowing some walkaway testing. This is particularly helpful when staffing is low and technologists must work in more than one department on their shift.

TABLE 4-14. ABO forward and reverse grouping results					
	FORWARD GROUPING		**REVERSE GROUPING**		
	REACTIONS OF CELLS WITH:		**REACTIONS OF PLASMA WITH:**		
ABO GROUP	**ANTI-A**	**ANTI-B**	**A CELLS**	**B CELLS**	**O CELLS**
O	0	0	+	+	0
A	+	0	0	+	0
B	0	+	+	0	0
AB	+	+	0	0	0
0 = no agglutination					
+ = agglutination					

Grading of Agglutination

The degree of red cell agglutination observed in any blood bank test procedure is significant and should be recorded. A system of grading is illustrated.

Description	Reaction	Grade
Button is one or two large clumps after being dislodged. Background is clear.		4+ (++++)
Button breaks into a few large clumps. Background is clear.		3+ (+++)
Button breaks into many medium-sized clumps. Background remains clear.		2+ (++)
Button breaks into numerous tiny clumps. Background becomes cloudy.		1+ (+)
A few small, very fine aggregates barely visible to the naked eye.		w+
No visible clumps or agglutinates.		0 (Neg)

FIGURE 4-27 Illustration of grading agglutination reactions in ABO tube typing

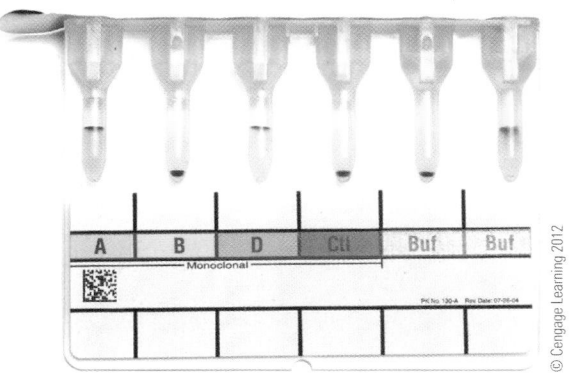

FIGURE 4-28 Gel typing card with columns (from left) for ABO forward typing, Rh D typing and control, and ABO reverse typing. Negative reactions (absence of agglutination) are indicated by the presence of cells at the bottom of the column; positive reactions (agglutination) are indicated by a cell layer at the top of the column. Patient specimen shown is "A positive"

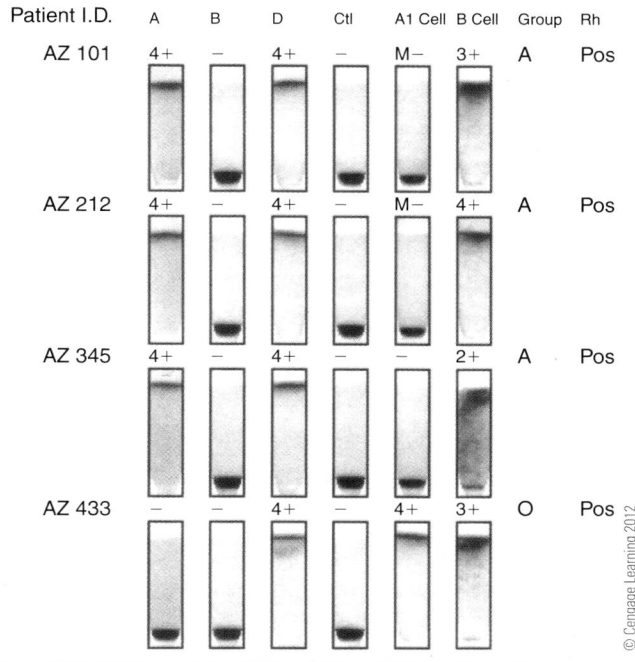

Patient I.D.	A	B	D	Ctl	A1 Cell	B Cell	Group	Rh
AZ 101	4+	−	4+	−	M−	3+	A	Pos
AZ 212	4+	−	4+	−	M−	4+	A	Pos
AZ 345	4+	−	4+	−		2+	A	Pos
AZ 433	−	−	4+	−	4+	3+	O	Pos

FIGURE 4-29 Gel typing report form: Shown are reports of ABO and Rh D typing for four patient specimens using the Ortho ProVue automated immunohematology testing system; from left are forward grouping (patient cells plus anti-A and anti-B), Rh D and control, and reverse grouping (A and B cells plus patient plasma)

Gel typing is sensitive and specific, and the procedure can be standardized, verified, and validated. Testing is performed in a card prefilled with gels mixed with the appropriate reagent (Figure 4-28). A dilution of patient cells is pipetted onto the gel column, and the card is incubated. The card is centrifuged and read. Agglutinated cells will not travel through the gel but remain at the top of the column, a positive reaction. Nonagglutinated cells travel through the gel to the bottom of the column, a negative reaction (Figures 4-28 and 4-29). Some gel typing reactions are stable for several hours, so tests can be retained and reread if necessary.

Gel typing techniques have several advantages over tube typing methods. Minimal handling of reagents and specimens increases biosafety. Endpoints are stable and well-defined, and interpretation of results is clear-cut and can be read manually or by instrumentation, eliminating technician subjectivity. The blood bank must continue to maintain strict standards and use the best available methods to guarantee patient safety and optimal patient outcome.

SAFETY REMINDERS

- Review Safety Precautions section before performing procedures.
- Observe Standard Precautions.
- Wear appropriate PPE.
- Observe centrifuge safety rules when operating the serofuge.

PROCEDURAL REMINDERS

- Review Quality Assessment section before performing procedures.
- Follow procedures in SOP manual.
- Store and use reagents according to manufacturer's instructions.
- Observe timing carefully when performing slide tests.
- Use good lighting to observe type typing reactions.
- Do not shake tubes too vigorously; weak agglutination reactions can be dispersed and misinterpreted.
- Record slide and tube typing results as soon as they are observed.

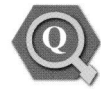

CRITICAL THINKING 1

Type O blood is considered the *universal* donor group. If a patient other than one in blood group O must receive a transfusion of group O blood, it is best to transfuse that patient with O packed or washed red cells rather than O whole blood.

Explain why this is so.

CRITICAL THINKING 2

A couple expecting their first child had ABO grouping performed. The husband was group AB and the wife was group O.

What are the possible ABO groups of the fetus?

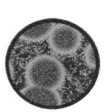

SUMMARY

The antigens and antibodies of the major blood group system, the ABO system, can be detected by agglutination tests performed by slide, tube, or gel methods. The gel methods have many advantages, such as stable reactions, well-defined endpoints, conservation of reagents and possibility of automation and walk-away technology.

Determination of ABO blood group is performed in hospital blood banks, blood donor centers, and other settings, such as forensic laboratories. Blood bank or immunohematology tests can often have life-changing consequences. These tests can lead to such outcomes as patients receiving transfusions of blood components, determination or ruling out of parentage, or evidence provided in forensic cases.

Blood banks, whether in hospitals or donor centers, are the only clinical laboratory service regulated by the FDA. Technologists who work in this department must be of the highest caliber and must adhere to strict quality assessment policies and procedures to ensure that a safe product is available for transfusion and that the patient receives the proper components.

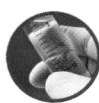

REVIEW QUESTIONS

1. Name the four groups in the ABO system.

2. What is the frequency of each ABO group in the United States?

3. What antigens present on red blood cells determine the ABO groups?

4. What antibody is present in the plasma of a person who is group B? Group O?

5. What is forward grouping?

6. What is reverse grouping?

7. What agglutination results would be observed when testing group A blood with anti-A and anti-B? When testing group AB blood?

8. How does ABO tube testing differ from ABO slide testing?

9. Why is timing important in slide testing?

10. How are the results of tube grouping tests interpreted? Explain the grading system for agglutination.

11. What safety precautions should be observed in ABO grouping?

12. Explain why adherence to quality assessment policies and procedures is important in the blood bank department.

13. Explain the principle of gel typing and list some of its advantages.

14. What is the MHC? How is it involved in tissue and organ transplants?

15. Define allele, antiserum, blood bank, blood group antibody, blood group antigen, codominant, forward grouping, genes, histocompatibility testing, human leukocyte antigen, major histocompatibility complex, reverse grouping, and serological centrifuge.

STUDENT ACTIVITIES

1. Complete the written examination for this lesson.

2. If possible, visit a hospital blood bank and find out how ABO testing is performed.

3. Practice performing ABO slide and tube groupings as outlined in the Student Performance Guides, using the worksheets.

4. Survey blood groups in your classroom. Make a chart showing the percentages of each ABO group. Do your percentages agree with published percentages?

WEB ACTIVITIES

1. Use the Internet to find two types of gel or solid-phase blood typing materials. Download or request package inserts. Read about instruments used to process and read the gel typing cards. Write a short report about one of the instruments, including information about how the gel card results are read, how many samples can be processed each hour, etc.

2. Search the Internet for tutorials or videos demonstrating ABO grouping test procedures.

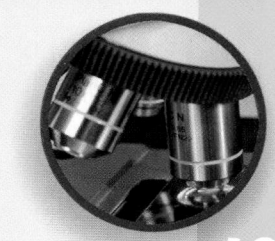

LESSON 4-6
ABO Grouping: Slide Method

(Individual student results will vary based on the specimens provided by the instructor.)

Name _____   Date _____

INSTRUCTIONS

1. Practice performing the slide method of ABO grouping following the step-by-step procedure.

2. Demonstrate the slide method of ABO grouping satisfactorily for the instructor, using the Student Performance Guide. Your instructor will explain the procedures for evaluating and grading your performance. Your performance may be given a number grade, letter grade, or satisfactory (S) or unsatisfactory (U) depending on course or institutional policy.

NOTE: Follow specific instructions in reagent package inserts.

MATERIALS AND EQUIPMENT

- gloves
- hand antiseptic
- full-face shield (or equivalent PPE)
- acrylic safety shield (optional)
- ethylenediaminetetraacetic acid (EDTA) anticoagulated blood specimens (pink-top or lavender-top tubes)
- test tube rack
- optional—capillary puncture materials: alcohol swabs, lancets, cotton balls or gauze, and capillary collection vials or tubes
- timer
- marker or wax pencil for labeling slides
- applicator sticks or stirrers
- disposable transfer pipets
- commercial anti-A
- commercial anti-B
- microscope slides or typing slides
- ABO Worksheet I
- laboratory tissue
- paper towels
- surface disinfectant (such as 10% chlorine bleach)
- biohazard container
- sharps container

PROCEDURE

Record in the comment section any problems encountered while practicing the procedure (or have a fellow student or the instructor evaluate your performance).

S = Satisfactory
U = Unsatisfactory

You must:	S	U	Evaluation/Comments
1. Assemble equipment and materials			
2. Wash hands with disinfectant and put on gloves			
3. Put on face protection or position acrylic safety shield on work area			
4. Perform slide grouping following steps 4a–4g a. Obtain two slides, label one A and one B			

(Continues)

© 2012 Delmar, Cengage Learning. Permission to reproduce for clinical use granted.

You must:	S	U	Evaluation/Comments
b. Place 1 drop of anti-A serum on the A slide and 1 drop of anti-B serum on the B slide. Do not allow dropper to touch the slide			
c. Dispense 1 drop of well-mixed venous blood or freshly collected capillary blood adjacent to the antiserum on each slide using a disposable pipet. Do not allow pipet to touch slide			
d. Use a disposable stirrer to mix the blood and antiserum on slide *A* into an area at least the size of a quarter. Repeat the procedure on the *B* slide, using a clean stirrer			
e. Rock the slides gently for 2 minutes and observe for agglutination using strong lighting			
f. Record agglutination results on ABO Worksheet I: agglutination = +; no agglutination = 0			
g. Determine the blood group and record			
5. Repeat steps 4a–4g using additional blood samples			
6. Discard all specimens appropriately or return them to storage as directed by instructor			
7. Discard sharps into sharps container and other contaminated materials into appropriate biohazard container			
8. Return reagents and equipment to proper storage			
9. Clean work area with surface disinfectant			
10. Remove gloves and discard into biohazard container			
11. Wash hands with antiseptic			

Instructor/Evaluator Comments:

Instructor/Evaluator _____ Date _____

© 2012 Delmar, Cengage Learning. Permission to reproduce for clinical use granted.

LESSON 4-6
ABO Grouping—Slide Method

(Individual student results will vary based on the specimens provided by the instructor.)

Name _____ Date _____

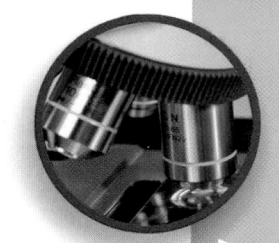

| Specimen I.D. | AGGLUTINATION RESULTS* | | INTERPRETATION |
	Anti-A	Anti-B	ABO Group
_____	_____	_____	_____
_____	_____	_____	_____
_____	_____	_____	_____
_____	_____	_____	_____
_____	_____	_____	_____

*Record results as:
0 = no agglutination
+ = agglutination

© 2012 Delmar, Cengage Learning. Permission to reproduce for clinical use granted.

LESSON 4-6
ABO Grouping: Tube Method

(Individual student results will vary based on the specimens provided by the instructor.)

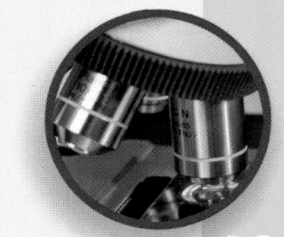

Name _____ Date _____

INSTRUCTIONS

1. Practice performing ABO grouping by the tube method following the step-by-step procedure.

2. Demonstrate the tube method for ABO grouping satisfactorily for the instructor, using the Student Performance Guide. Your instructor will explain the procedures for evaluating and grading your performance. Your performance may be given a number grade, letter grade, or satisfactory (S) or unsatisfactory (U) depending on course or institutional policy.

NOTE: Follow specific instructions in reagent package inserts.

MATERIALS AND EQUIPMENT

- gloves
- hand antiseptic
- full-face shield (or equivalent PPE)
- acrylic safety shield (optional)
- EDTA anticoagulated blood specimens (pink-top or lavender-top tubes)
- marker or wax pencil for labeling tubes
- blood bank saline (physiological saline)
- plastic, disposable transfer pipets
- commercial anti-A
- commercial anti-B
- commercial A cells (2% to 5% suspension)
- commercial B cells (2% to 5% suspension)
- disposable test tubes, 13 × 75 mm
- test tube rack
- timer
- optional: serological centrifuge capable of spinning 13 × 75 mm tubes at 2000 to 2500 rpm
- ABO Worksheet II
- paper towels
- laboratory tissue
- surface disinfectant
- biohazard container
- sharps container

PROCEDURE

  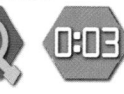

Record in the comment section any problems encountered while practicing the procedure (or have a fellow student or the instructor evaluate your performance).

S = Satisfactory
U = Unsatisfactory

You must:	S	U	Evaluation/Comments
1. Assemble equipment and materials.			
2. Wash hands with disinfectant and put on gloves			
3. Put on face protection or position acrylic safety shield on work area			
4. Perform ABO forward tube grouping following steps 4a–4i			

(Continues)

STUDENT PERFORMANCE GUIDE

© 2012 Delmar, Cengage Learning. Permission to reproduce for clinical use granted.

You must:	S	U	Evaluation/Comments
a. Prepare a 2% to 5% suspension of patient cells by placing 1 drop of well-mixed EDTA-anticoagulated blood into a test tube and adding 18 to 19 drops of saline. Label the tube *patient cells* b. Label two test tubes *A* and *B* c. Place 1 drop of anti-A in tube *A* and 1 drop of anti-B in tube *B* d. Place 1 drop of the 2% to 5% patient cell suspension into each tube and mix gently e. Place tubes in serological centrifuge and spin 15 to 30 seconds (as directed by instructor) NOTE: Balance the centrifuge by placing tubes opposite each other. (If no centrifuge is available, allow tubes to stand at room temperature for 15 to 30 minutes and go to step 4g) f. Allow the centrifuge to come to a complete stop and remove the tubes g. Tap each tube gently to loosen cells from the bottom of the tube and observe cells for agglutination using good lighting. Grade agglutination using the guide in Figure 4-27 h. Record results from each tube on Worksheet II i. Determine the blood group of the sample and record			
5. Perform ABO reverse grouping on the blood sample following steps 5a–5k a. Centrifuge the EDTA-anticoagulated blood specimen, remove 0.5 to 1.0 mL of plasma from the sample, and place it in a clean test tube b. Label three test tubes *a, b,* and *control* c. Place 2 drops of patient plasma into each of these tubes d. Place 1 drop of a 2% to 5% commercial suspension of A cells into tube *a* and mix e. Place 1 drop of a 2% to 5% commercial suspension of B cells into tube *b* and mix f. Place 1 drop of the patient's 2% to 5% cell suspension into *control* tube and mix g. Place tubes in serological centrifuge (be sure to balance tubes in rotor) and spin 15 to 30 seconds (or allow tubes to sit at room temperature 15 to 30 minutes and go to step 5i) h. Remove the tubes from the centrifuge after it stops completely i. Tap each tube gently, observe cells for agglutination, and grade agglutination using guide in Figure 4-27 j. Record the results from each tube on ABO Worksheet II k. Determine the blood group of the sample and record			
6. Compare results of forward grouping with results of reverse grouping of the same sample. Reverse grouping should agree with results of forward grouping			

© 2012 Delmar, Cengage Learning. Permission to reproduce for clinical use granted.

You must:	S	U	Evaluation/Comments
7. Repeat forward and reverse grouping (steps 4 and 5) on additional blood specimens if available			
8. Discard all specimens appropriately or store specimens as directed by instructor			
9. Discard disposable labware into appropriate sharps or biohazard container			
10. Return all equipment and reagents to proper storage			
11. Clean work area with disinfectant			
12. Remove gloves and discard in biohazard container			
13. Wash hands with antiseptic			

Instructor/Evaluator Comments:

Instructor/Evaluator _____ Date _____

© 2012 Delmar, Cengage Learning. Permission to reproduce for clinical use granted.

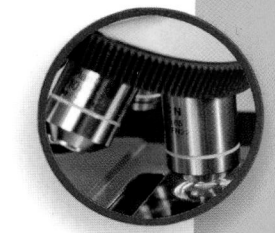

LESSON 4-6
ABO Grouping—Tube Method

(Individual student results will vary based on the specimens provided by the instructor.)

Name _____ Date _____

	DIRECT (FORWARD) GROUPING*		INTERPRETATION	INDIRECT (REVERSE) GROUPING*			INTERPRETATION
Specimen I.D.	Anti-A	Anti-B	ABO Group	A Cells	B Cells	Control	ABO Group

*Record results as:

0 = no agglutination

w+ = fine agglutinates, most cells not agglutinated

1+ = numerous tiny clumps, cloudy background

2+ = several small to medium clumps, clear background

3+ = a few large clumps, clear background

4+ = two to three large clumps, clear background

© 2012 Delmar, Cengage Learning. Permission to reproduce for clinical use granted.

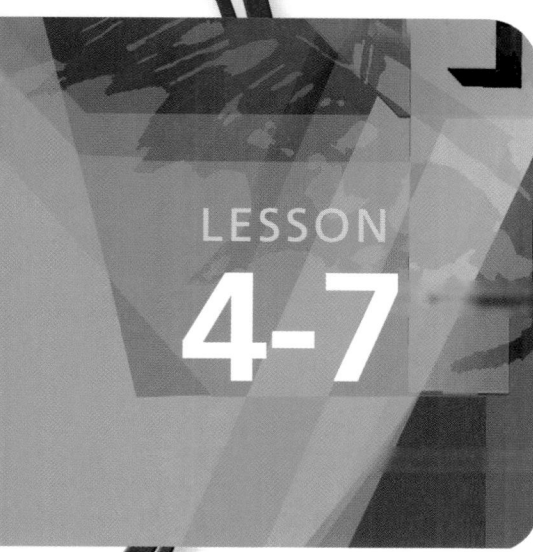

Rh Typing

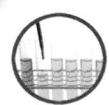

LESSON OBJECTIVES

After studying this lesson, the student will:

⊙ Explain the importance of the Rh blood group system.

⊙ Discuss the antigens of the Rh system and explain how they are inherited.

⊙ Name two ways in which immunization to the Rh D antigen can occur.

⊙ Name two problems that can occur as a result of immunization to the D antigen.

⊙ Explain why Rh D immune globulin (RhIG) is used.

⊙ Perform Rh D slide typing.

⊙ Interpret the results of Rh D typing.

⊙ Explain the significance of the weak D antigen.

⊙ Describe safety precautions that should be observed while performing Rh D typing.

⊙ Discuss quality assessment policies and procedures that must be followed to ensure reliable Rh typing results.

⊙ Define the glossary terms.

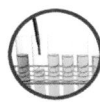

GLOSSARY

allele / one of two (or more) forms of a gene responsible for genetic variation

anti-human globulin test / a sensitive test that uses a commercial anti-human globulin reagent to detect human globulin coated on red blood cells; antiglobulin test; Coombs' test

feto-maternal hemorrhage (FMH) / the occurrence of fetal blood cells entering into the maternal circulation before or during delivery

genotype / the genetic makeup of a cell or organism

hemolytic disease of the newborn (HDN) / a condition in which maternal antibody targets fetal red blood cells for destruction

phenotype / the observable characteristics in a cell or organism as determined both by genetic makeup and environmental factors

Rh D immune globulin (RhIG) / a concentrated, purified solution of human anti-D antibody used for injection

INTRODUCTION

The Rh blood group was discovered in the 1940s. It is the second most important human blood group system. The Rh blood group received its name because rhesus monkeys were being used in the experiments when it was discovered.

The complexity of the Rh antigen system has only been fully realized in recent years, once researchers could study the system using molecular techniques. Over 50 Rh antigens have been identified in the Rh system; the Rh D antigen is the most clinically significant of the Rh antigens.

The Rh antigens are highly immunogenic. Individuals whose red blood cells do not have a particular Rh antigen can produce an immune response when exposed to that antigen. For this reason, Rh D typing must be performed on all donor blood and on patient blood before a blood transfusion can be given. Rh typing is also a routine part of the prenatal workup. Rh typing can be performed by slide, tube, or gel methods. Both tube and gel methods are used in blood banks.

THE Rh BLOOD GROUP SYSTEM

The first antigen of the Rh system recognized was the D antigen. It remains the most important antigen in the system because it is the most antigenic and the only one for which blood is routinely tested. Like the antigens of the ABO system, Rh antigens are products of inherited genes and are present on the surface of red blood cells. Unlike the ABO antigens, the Rh antigens are proteins and only red blood cells express the Rh antigen—other blood and tissue cells do not have Rh antigens. Also unlike the ABO system, antibodies to Rh antigens do not occur naturally (Table 4-15).

The functions of the Rh antigens are not entirely understood. However, by studying some of the rare Rh antigen variants, scientists have gained a better understanding of the function of the Rh antigens. One extremely rare Rh type is called Rh null (written as Rh$_{null}$); red cells designated as Rh$_{null}$ lack *all* known Rh antigens. Rh$_{null}$ cells have abnormal shape and decreased life span. Studies of these cells show that Rh antigens play a structural role in maintaining the red cell membrane and also allow transport of some molecules across the cell membrane.

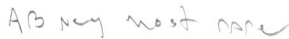

Occurrence of Rh D Antigen

The major antigen in the Rh system is the D antigen. Red blood cells that possess the D antigen are called Rh D positive. Cells that lack the D antigen are called Rh D negative. It has become common to refer to the Rh D antigen simply as D antigen, and Rh D-positive blood as D-positive blood or Rh-positive blood. Donor blood, in addition to being labeled with the ABO group, must be labeled as Rh positive or Rh negative (Figure 4-30), referring to the presence or absence of the Rh D antigen.

The D antigen occurs in the large majority of the population, but the incidence differs according to ethnic or racial group (Table 4-16). In the United States, according to 2011 AABB statistics (www.aabb.org), approximately 82% of the population are D positive and 18% are D negative.

Detection of Rh D Antigen

The Rh D antigen is detected using agglutination techniques similar to those used for ABO typing. A drop of blood is mixed with Anti-D, a commercial antibody directed against the D antigen.

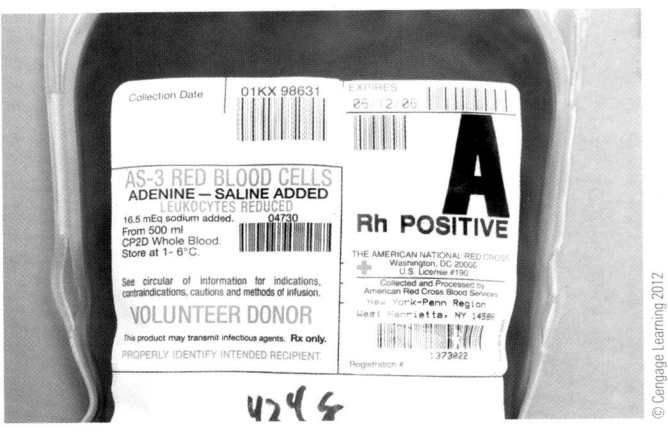

FIGURE 4-30 Donor bag containing group A, Rh positive blood

TABLE 4-15. Comparison of ABO and Rh blood group antigens and antibodies

CHARACTERISTIC	ABO GROUP	Rh GROUP
Antigen structure	Carbohydrate	Protein
Antigen location	Surfaces of all cells and tissues	Surfaces of red blood cells only
Naturally occurring antibodies	Yes	No
Antibody class	IgM	IgG

TABLE 4-16. Frequency of Rh D-positive and D-negative blood among different ethnic populations

ETHNIC GROUP	D POSITIVE (%)	D NEGATIVE (%)
Caucasian	85	15
African-American	93	7
African	99	1
Asian	99	1
Western European (Basque)	65	35
Native American Indian	99	1

If the red cells contain D antigen on their membranes, the cells will agglutinate in the presence of the antibody, and the cells are designated D positive.

Weak D Antigen

Less than 1% of the general population has a form of the D antigen that reacts weakly or gives a negative result in the Rh D typing procedure. These cells are called *weak D* and are considered D positive. The test for *weak D* must be performed before the Rh D type can be reported. Donor blood can only be labeled D negative after the weak D test confirms that no D antigen is detectable.

The Anti-Human Globulin Test

The test for detection of weak D uses the principles of the **anti-human globulin (AHG) test**, a sensitive method of detecting antibody bound to red blood cells by using a commercial anti-human immunoglobulin G (AHG) reagent. Red blood cells incubated with commercial anti-D of the IgG class and initially showing no agglutination reaction are tested further by the AHG test (also called the indirect antiglobulin test [IAT]). The red blood cells that were exposed to anti-D in the initial test are further incubated, then rinsed several times to remove any unbound anti-D. A drop or two of AHG reagent is then added to the cells; this anti-IgG will react with any anti-D antibodies that became bound to the red blood cells during the initial typing test. The tube is centrifuged, and cells are observed for agglutination. Only units of donor blood that are negative in the weak D test (AHG test) can be labeled D negative.

Rh Antigens Other Than D

Dozens of antigens have now been identified in the Rh system. Most of these antigens occur only rarely. However, four Rh antigens rank next in importance behind D. The most common name for these antigens are C (called "big C"), c (called "little c"), E ("big E"), and e ("little e"). The methods for naming the Rh antigens are listed in Table 4-17 and explained in the Current Topic, Nomenclature and Inheritance of the Rh System.

In certain cases, blood must be typed for the C, c, E, and e Rh antigens in addition to being typed for the D antigen. Rh typing to identify the Rh antigens present on red cells reveals the individual's Rh **phenotype**. Infrequently, an individual negative for one of these antigens (C, c, E, e) will produce antibodies against the antigen if they are exposed to blood containing the antigen.

Rh Antibodies

Although antibodies to Rh antigens do not occur naturally in the blood, antibody to D antigen (anti-D) can be produced by a D-negative individual who becomes sensitized or immunized to the D antigen. This can occur following blood transfusion with D-positive blood or during pregnancy (see Current Topic on hemolytic disease of the newborn). Anti-D, when produced, is primarily of the immunoglobin G (IgG) class.

TABLE 4-17. Comparison of Fisher-Race, Wiener, and Rosenfield et al. methods of naming Rh antigens

FISHER-RACE METHOD	WEINER METHOD	ROSENFIELD et al. METHOD
D	Rh_o	Rh 1
C	rh′	Rh 2
E	rh″	Rh 3
d*	Hr_o	—
c	hr′	Rh 4
e	hr″	Rh 5

*No d antigen has been found; d denotes absence of D antigen

Importance of Rh Typing

It is important to test for the D antigen in all patients who are to receive transfusions so that the correct type of blood will be given. Rh D–negative patients should only be transfused with Rh D-negative blood. On the other hand, blood that has the D antigen in any form, even the weak D form, must be considered Rh positive and must not be transfused into a D-negative person.

Testing for the D antigen is also used to identify females at risk for giving birth to an infant with **hemolytic disease of the newborn (HDN)**, in family genetic studies, and in legal cases to establish parentage.

Rh TYPING PROCEDURES

The Rh D antigen is identified using agglutination techniques. Venous anticoagulated blood is the preferred specimen, but capillary blood can also be used for some procedures.

Safety Precautions

  Standard Precautions must be followed when collecting blood specimens and when performing typing procedures. Gloves and other appropriate personal protective equipment (PPE) must be worn. All reagents must be treated as if potentially infectious because many are derived from human blood. Used slides or tubes must be discarded into a sharps container. Centrifuge safety rules must be followed, including always balancing tubes in the rotor and allowing the centrifuge to come to a complete stop before opening the lid.

Quality Assessment

   Accuracy in Rh typing and reporting results is critical to a patient's well-being. To reduce the chance of errors, quality assessment policies must be followed. Detailed

CURRENT TOPICS 1

NOMENCLATURE AND INHERITANCE OF THE Rh SYSTEM

Over the history of the Rh system, three nomenclatures (naming systems) have been suggested by different researchers. The three naming systems are those of Fisher and Race, Weiner, and Rosenfield et al. Manufacturers of blood bank reagents use one or more of these naming systems on their products (Table 4-17). In practice, the Fisher-Race nomenclature is used most frequently in naming the Rh antigens because of its simplicity.

The inheritance of the genes responsible for the Rh system is complex and still not fully explained. The genes coding for the Rh antigens are positioned very close to each other on chromosome 1, causing the Rh genes on each chromosome to normally be inherited together. An individual's Rh genotype is determined by the allelic genes of the Rh system inherited from each parent.

In the simplest explanation, allelic genes at two closely linked loci on the chromosome code for the five most important Rh antigens. The D antigen is coded for by the allelic gene *RHD*. (Italics are used to denote genes; antigens are non-italicized.) Individuals who are D positive have inherited at least one *RHD* allele; individuals who are Rh D negative have no *RHD* alleles—the *RHD* alleles have been deleted from both copies of chromosome 1. This is the reason that there is no corresponding "d" (little d) antigen.

Alleles of another gene, the *RHCE* gene, code for the C, c, E, and e antigens. The *RHCE* gene has four possible alleles: *RHCE*, *RHCe*, *RHcE*, and *RHce*. These genes are codominant. This means that if a person inherits one *RHCe* allele and one *RHcE* allele, all four antigens (CcEe) will be expressed on the person's red blood cells. The genes coding for CcEe antigens are located near the *RHD* gene locus (Table 4-18).

TABLE 4-18. Rh gene complexes, antigens encoded, and observed red cell phenotypes

POSSIBLE ALLELIC GENES PRESENT[†] (ON A CHROMOSOME)	ANTIGENS ENCODED	RED CELL PHENOTYPE
RHD, RHCe	D, C, e	D+, C+, e+
RHD, RHcE	D, c, E	D+, c+, E+
RHD, RHce	D, c, e	D+, c+, e+
RHD, RHCE	D, C, E	D+, C+, E+
—, *RHCe**	C, e	C+, e+
—, *RHcE**	c, E	c+, E+
—, *RHce**	c, e	c+, e+
—, *RHCE**	C, E	C+, E+

[†]This list represents possible combinations of allelic genes present on one chromosome; each individual inherits two chromosomes, each containing two allelic genes
RHD gene is absent

- Testing commercial reagents with controls at designated intervals
- Using and storing reagents according to manufacturer's directions and observing expiration dates
- Observing strict test conditions for typing tests
- Carefully interpreting and recording results

Rh Slide Typing

To perform Rh D slide typing, a drop of commercial anti-D antiserum is added to a labeled microscope slide. Two drops of well-mixed blood are added to the slide. The blood and antiserum are mixed with a stirrer and spread over at least half of the slide. The slide is placed on a heated, lighted viewbox to heat the slide to 37° C. The box is rocked back and forth for 2 minutes while the mixture is observed for agglutination (Figure 4-31). The presence or absence of agglutination is recorded.

It is usual to also prepare a control slide that is tested in the same manner as the patient sample if high-protein anti-D antisera is used for slide typing. A drop of commercial protein control solution (identical to the anti-D reagent except that the control does not contain antibody) is placed on a slide and two drops of well-mixed blood are added. The blood and control solution are mixed on the slide, the slide is heated on the viewbox, and observed for agglutination. The control slide should not show agglutination.

Several types of commercial anti-D are available for Rh slide typing, including high-protein anti-D, chemically modified anti-D, monoclonal anti-D, and saline anti-D. Control procedures and instructions for use can differ for each type of antiserum. Recommendations in package insert(s) for the reagents being used must be followed.

instructions of all test methods and QA procedures will be outlined in the blood bank's standard operating procedures (SOP) manual. Examples of required QA practices include:

- Identifying patient, patient specimen, reagents, and test vessels with accuracy
- Visually inspecting typing reagents for contamination

CURRENT TOPICS 2

HEMOLYTIC DISEASE OF THE NEWBORN

Hemolytic disease of the newborn (HDN) is a condition in which antibody from the mother enters the fetal circulation and attacks or destroys the fetal red blood cells. (An older term for HDN is *erythroblastosis fetalis*; HDN is also called HDFN, hemolytic disease of the fetus and newborn.)

In the past, HDN was caused primarily by maternal anti-D reacting with D antigen on the fetal red cells. However, through prenatal testing and aggressive use of methods to prevent HDN caused by D antigen, non-D Rh antigens (such as C, c, E, or e) are now responsible for the largest proportion of HDN cases.

HDN can occur when an antigen-negative mother becomes pregnant with an antigen-positive fetus. For example, in a case of HDN caused by anti-D, during pregnancy or at birth, some of the fetus's D-positive blood cells can leak into the mother's circulatory system. Bleeding of fetal blood into the mother's circulation is called feto-maternal hemorrhage (FMH). Exposure to the fetal cells stimulates the mother's immune system to produce antibodies—essentially she becomes immunized to D-positive cells. This antibody (anti-D) is of the IgG class, which can cross the placenta and enter the fetal circulation. Situations that can cause feto-maternal hemorrhage include:

- Amniocentesis or other invasive procedure
- Miscarriage or abortion
- Ectopic pregnancy
- Heavy bleeding during pregnancy
- The birth process

In most cases, women are not exposed to fetal blood until the time of birth, which means that the first baby usually will not have HDN. However, large amounts of newborn blood often leak into the mother's circulation during delivery. If a D-negative woman is exposed to D-positive blood and produces anti-D antibodies, these can cross the placenta in subsequent pregnancies. If a subsequent fetus also has D-positive red cells, the anti-D will destroy (cause hemolysis of) the fetus's red blood cells—thus the name *hemolytic* disease of the newborn.

SYMPTOMS AND CONSEQUENCES OF HDN

The mother of a fetus with HDN usually experiences no symptoms during pregnancy unless the HDN is very severe. For this reason it is very important that at-risk expectant mothers have prenatal screenings in their first trimester to determine their Rh D type and to test for any antibodies that are already present. At-risk mothers will usually have frequent fetal monitoring so that any signs of fetal stress will be detected early. The father can also be typed—there is no risk for Rh D HDN when both parents are D negative.

HDN can be mild to severe; the degree of severity is usually related to the mother's antibody level and the length of time during the pregnancy that she produced antibodies. In mild cases, signs of HDN may not be detected until birth and can include anemia, jaundice, or breathing problems. In very severe cases, heart failure or brain damage can occur or even stillbirth or miscarriage.

PREVENTION OF Rh D HEMOLYTIC DISEASE OF THE NEWBORN

Since 1968, it has been possible to prevent almost all cases of HDN caused by the D antigen by administering injectable Rh (D) immune globulin (RhIG) to the D-negative mother. Development of this treatment was a significant breakthrough in obstetrics and is estimated to have saved the lives of approximately 10,000 infants each year. RhIG is a concentrated solution of anti-D purified from human plasma. When RhIG is administered at the appropriate times, it will prevent the mother from producing her own antibody to D cells. The injected anti-D will bind to any red blood cells from the fetus that have entered maternal blood, causing them to be eliminated from circulation before the mother's own immune system becomes stimulated. Current treatment regimen is to administer Rh-immune globulin to D-negative expectant mothers at 28 weeks of pregnancy and within 72 hours after birth of a D-positive baby. RhIG is also administered following events such as miscarriage, abortion, or amniocentesis. By receiving the injection at 28 weeks and after delivery, sensitization will be prevented and Rh D incompatibility should not be a problem during the next pregnancy. This treatment must be repeated with every pregnancy unless it is positively known that the fetus/baby is D negative. This treatment is only successful with D antigen incompatibilities.

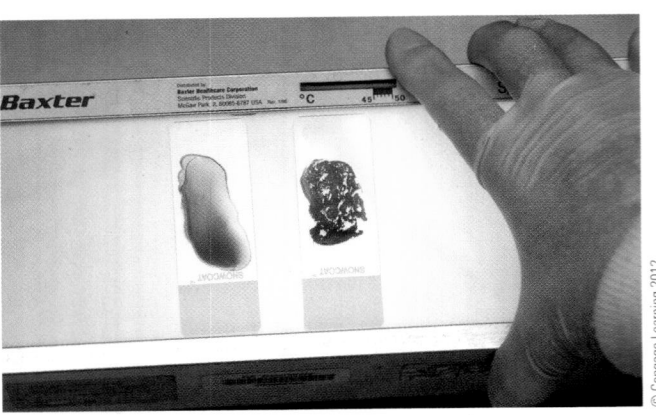

FIGURE 4-31 A heated, lighted viewbox is used for Rh slide typing: specimen on the right slide is D positive

Interpreting Rh Slide Typing Results

Agglutination with anti-D and absence of agglutination with the control reagent constitutes a valid positive test; the cells are D positive (Table 4-19). Absence of agglutination with both anti-D and control reagent *suggests* that the cells are D negative, but the cells must be tested further (for weak D) using a tube test or the AHG procedure before the blood can be designated as Rh D negative.

The control slide should always be negative for agglutination. If the control is positive, the test is invalid and must be repeated using a different method or different reagents. Positive control results can be due to contaminated control serum or abnormalities in the patient blood sample.

Rh Tube Typing

Rh tube typing is more sensitive than slide typing. Rh D tube typing is performed in the same manner as ABO grouping. A 2% to 5% suspension is made from the patient's cells using physiological or blood bank saline. One drop of this suspension is mixed with one drop of anti-D and the tube is centrifuged. The cell pellet is gently dislodged and observed for agglutination, and the reaction is graded. The patient plasma normally contains no natural anti-D antibody, so reverse (confirmatory) typing is not performed. Many laboratories routinely type each specimen with two different types of anti-D to increase the chances of detecting weak D antigen.

Commercial anti-D for tube typing is available as monoclonal antisera, polyclonal antisera, purified IgG antisera, purified IgM antisera, combinations of IgG and IgM, and chemically modified antisera. The antisera manufacturer's package insert will give instructions for performing the control test if one is needed.

Interpreting Results of Rh Tube Typing

If a patient has Rh D–positive blood, the patient's cells will agglutinate when reacted with anti-D. If the patient has Rh D–negative blood, no agglutination will be present (Table 4-19). Negative Rh D typing results must be confirmed according to laboratory policy before being reported.

Laboratories must have a clear written procedure regarding D typing and interpretation. It is particularly vital that weak D-positive donor blood not be misidentified as D-negative blood. If that were to happen, a D-negative person could be given blood containing D antigen. Some laboratories have a policy of transfusing a weak D patient with D-negative blood. However, blood from weak D donors is labeled D positive and is only transfused into patients with D-positive blood.

Gel Typing for Rh D

Gel cards used for ABO typing also contain columns for D typing (see Lesson 4-6). The tests are performed and interpreted as for the ABO forward and reverse grouping. Dilute red cell suspensions are added to the columns that contain antiserum or control reagent in a gel matrix. Under controlled centrifugation, the cells are forced into the gel matrix, where they contact anti-D or control reagent. If D antigen is not present on the red cells, the cells will fall to the bottom of the column without reacting with the antisera. Anti-D in the gel will bind to D-positive cells, causing agglutination and preventing the cells from traveling through the gel. A cell layer remaining at the top of the column is a positive result.

TABLE 4-19. Interpretation of results of Rh D slide typing

REACTIONS OF RED CELLS WITH:

ANTI-D	CONTROL	INTERPRETATION
+	0	D positive
0	0	Presumptive Rh D negative; confirm with additional testing before reporting results
+	+	Invalid test; repeat test using another method
0	+	Invalid test, repeat test using another method

+ = agglutination.
0 = no agglutination.

SAFETY REMINDERS

- Review Safety Precautions section before beginning procedure.
- Observe Standard Precautions.
- Wear appropriate PPE.
- Avoid spills, splashes, or creation of aerosols.

PROCEDURAL REMINDERS

- Review Quality Assessment section before performing procedure.
- Follow SOP manual and reagent manufacturers' instructions.
- Identify patient and patient specimens correctly.
- Label reaction vessels accurately.
- Perform Rh D slide typing using a lighted, heated viewbox.
- Observe Rh slide typing reactions within 2 minutes.
- Confirm negative Rh D slide typing according to laboratory policy.

CASE STUDY 1

Mr. Morris came into the blood donation center to donate blood. When the processing center performed initial ABO and Rh D typing of his blood, the results indicated that Mr. Morris was A negative. The ABO grouping was done by tube typing, and the Rh D typing was done by the slide method.

The next step for the processing center should be:

a. Label the blood A negative

b. Repeat the ABO grouping by the slide test that is more reliable

c. Perform further typing to test for weak D before labeling unit

CASE STUDY 2

Mrs. Rodriguez, who had been typed as B negative, needed a transfusion. The only blood components available were B positive and O negative.

Which blood type should she receive? Explain your answer.

CASE STUDY 3

Mr. Gupta, whose Rh phenotype was DCe, was transfused with D-negative blood.

Which of the following could occur?

a. He could produce anti-d

b. He could produce anti-c

c. He could produce anti-D

d. He could produce anti-e

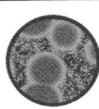

SUMMARY

The Rh blood group system is composed of red blood cell antigens that are products of inherited genes. The D antigen is the major antigen in the system, but other lesser antigens, including C, c, E, and e, are also important in blood banking. Donor blood units and potential transfusion recipients are routinely typed for D antigen. Rh typing can be performed by slide, tube, or gel methods. D negative typing results must be confirmed according to laboratory policy.

Determining the Rh D type is especially important in transfusion medicine and in obstetrics. Persons who are typed as D negative should only be transfused with blood that is also D negative. Rh D negative expectant mothers must be monitored and treated with Rh immune globulin to prevent the possibility of the fetus developing HDN. Testing for the Rh D antigen must be performed, interpreted, and reported only by qualified personnel and following the policy and procedures of the laboratory SOP manual.

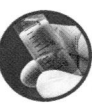

REVIEW QUESTIONS

1. What is the major antigen in the Rh system?
2. What circumstances must exist before anti-D antibody is produced by an individual?
3. What is the weak D antigen?
4. Explain how HDN occurs.
5. Why is Rh D typing performed?
6. Why must D-positive blood not be transfused into a D-negative patient?
7. Which is more sensitive, slide or tube typing?
8. Why is reverse typing not done for the Rh system?
9. How are the major Rh antigens inherited?
10. Define allele, anti–human globulin test, feto-maternal hemorrhage, genotype, hemolytic disease of the newborn, phenotype, and Rh D immune globulin.

STUDENT ACTIVITIES

1. Complete the written examination for this lesson.
2. Practice performing Rh D typing on several blood samples as outlined in the Student Performance Guide, using the worksheet.
3. Survey the Rh D types among your classmates. Compare your findings with the distribution of D antigen in the United States.

WEB ACTIVITIES

1. Use the Internet to find information about transfusion reactions. Write a one-page report describing causes, symptoms, and treatment.
2. Find information about different types of Rh typing sera using the Internet; list three types and explain the differences in the three.

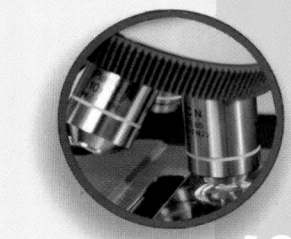

LESSON 4-7
Rh Typing

(Individual student results will vary based on the specimens provided by the instructor.)

Name _____   Date _____

INSTRUCTIONS

1. Practice performing Rh D typing following the step-by-step procedure.

2. Demonstrate Rh D typing satisfactorily for the instructor, using the Student Performance Guide. Your instructor will explain the procedure for evaluating and grading your performance. Your performance may be given a number grade, a letter grade or satisfactory (S) or unsatisfactory (U) depending on course or institutional policy.

NOTE: Several types of anti-D typing sera are available; instructions for correct use and level of test sensitivity can differ among typing sera. Follow instructions in the package insert included with the particular typing reagent(s) being used.

MATERIALS AND EQUIPMENT

- gloves
- hand antiseptic
- full-face shield (or equivalent PPE)
- acrylic safety shield (optional)
- serological centrifuge
- test tube rack
- serological tubes, 13 × 75 mm
- disposable transfer pipets
- microscope slides
- applicator sticks or stirrers
- blood bank saline (physiological saline)
- anti-D typing serum (for tube typing)
- Rh protein control solution
- anti-human globulin serum (optional, for use in weak D test)
- EDTA blood specimens (pink-top or purple-top tubes)
- lighted, heated viewbox for Rh typing
- Rh worksheet
- wax pencil or sharpie
- timer
- laboratory tissue
- paper towels
- surface disinfectant
- biohazard container
- sharps container

PROCEDURE

  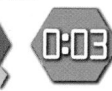 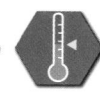

Record in the comment section any problems encountered while practicing the procedure (or have a fellow student or the instructor evaluate your performance).

S = Satisfactory
U = Unsatisfactory

You must:	S	U	Evaluation/Comments
1. Assemble equipment and materials			
2. Wash hands with antiseptic and put on gloves			
3. Put on face protection or position acrylic safety shield in work area			
4. Perform Rh D slide typing following steps 4a–4k:			

(Continues)

© 2012 Delmar, Cengage Learning. Permission to reproduce for clinical use granted.

You must:	S	U	Evaluation/Comments
a. Turn on viewbox. Label two microscope slides *D* and *C* (control) b. Place 1 drop of anti-D serum on the *D* slide c. Place 1 drop of Rh control solution on the *C* slide d. Place 2 drops (or 1 large drop) of patient's well-mixed whole blood on each slide e. Mix blood and anti-D with an applicator stick, spreading the mixture over at least half of the slide f. Repeat procedure for the control slide using a clean applicator stick g. Place slides on the lighted viewbox and start timer h. Tilt the viewbox slowly back and forth for 2 minutes i. Observe the slides for agglutination at the end of 2 minutes j. Record results on Rh Worksheet: agglutination = +; no agglutination = 0 k. Determine the Rh type and record on Rh Worksheet			
5. Repeat steps 4a–4k on other blood samples, as directed by instructor			
6. Perform Rh D tube typing on a specimen following steps 6a–6i (or go to step 7); use anti-D specified for use in tube typing; commercial control solution is not required but patient plasma can be used for control a. Prepare a 2% to 5% suspension of the patient blood specimen by adding 18 or 19 drops of saline to 1 drop of well-mixed anticoagulated whole blood b. Centrifuge patient whole blood specimen, remove a small portion of plasma, and place in tube labeled patient plasma c. Label one tube *patient* and one tube *patient control* d. Add 1 drop of anti-D to *patient* tube; add 1 drop of patient plasma to the *patient control* tube e. Add 1 drop of patient cell suspension to the *patient* tube and 1 drop to the *patient control* tube f. Mix contents of tubes and centrifuge for 15 to 30 seconds (as directed by instructor) g. Gently tap tubes to loosen cell pellets and observe for agglutination h. Grade the reactions and record results on Rh Worksheet. NOTE: Absence of agglutination in patient tube is a presumptive D negative reaction and requires a test for weak D before the patient can be definitively typed as D negative i. Optional: perform weak D test on presumptive D negative blood as directed by instructor or go to step 7			
7. Discard specimens, tubes, and slides into appropriate sharps container			
8. Discard other contaminated materials into appropriate biohazard container			

© 2012 Delmar, Cengage Learning. Permission to reproduce for clinical use granted.

You must:	S	U	Evaluation/Comments
9. Clean and disinfect equipment and return to proper storage			
10. Clean work area with disinfectant			
11. Remove gloves and discard into biohazard container			
12. Wash hands with antiseptic			

Instructor/Evaluator Comments:

Instructor/Evaluator _____ Date _____

© 2012 Delmar, Cengage Learning. Permission to reproduce for clinical use granted.

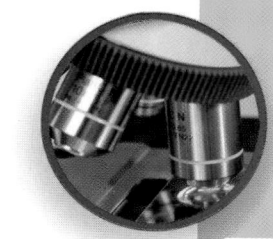
LESSON 4-7
Rh Typing

(Individual student results will vary based on the specimens provided by the instructor.)

Name _____ Date _____

| Specimen I.D. | AGGLUTINATION RESULTS* | | INTERPRETATION† |
	Anti-D	Control	Rh Type
_____	_____	_____	_____
_____	_____	_____	_____
_____	_____	_____	_____
_____	_____	_____	_____
_____	_____	_____	_____

*Record tube typing results as:

0   = no agglutination
w+ = fine agglutinates, most cells not agglutinated
1+ = numerous tiny clumps, cloudy background
2+ = several small to medium clumps, clear background
3+ = few large clumps, clear background
4+ = two to three large clumps, clear background

†Record interpretation as:
Rh D positive or presumptive Rh D negative

UNIT 5

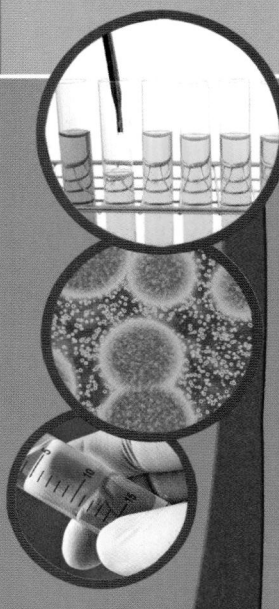

Urinalysis

UNIT OBJECTIVES

After studying this unit, the student will:

- Identify the organs of the urinary system.
- Identify the parts of the kidney and state the function of each part.
- Explain how urine is formed.
- Discuss diseases that affect kidney function.
- Describe urine collection and preservation methods.
- Perform a physical examination of urine.
- Perform a chemical examination of urine.
- Perform a microscopic examination of urine sediment.
- State the reference values for the tests included in the routine urinalysis.
- Correlate results of urine physical, chemical, and microscopic examinations with physiological and disease states.
- Explain how urinalysis results can give important information about the status of a patient's health.

Urine has long been used as an indicator of a person's health. References to testing urine date back to ancient Egyptian hieroglyphics and are found in the writings of Hippocrates. By the Middle Ages, early physicians often examined urine, sometimes without ever seeing the patient. Although these physicians did not have the sophisticated tests that we have now, they did examine the color, odor, volume, viscosity, and even sweetness of urine. With the invention of the microscope, urine could be examined microscopically.

In 1850, a French chemist developed the first crude urine "test strip" to detect urine sugar. It took decades for anyone to take an interest in further developing the strip technology. By the beginning of the twentieth century, a few filter paper tests were available for performing spot tests on urine.

In the first half of the 1900s, when laboratory medicine was in its infancy, many chemical tests were developed for urine. For the most part these tests were complex and time-consuming, causing urine testing to be rather impractical and infrequently done. With the commercial production of urine reagent strip tests around the middle of the twentieth century, urinalysis became an important part of the routine physical examination. Since that time the appearance of reagent strips has changed little, but the technology incorporated into the tests on the reagent strips has changed significantly. Routine physical examinations often include a routine urinalysis in which several tests are performed on one urine sample.

Modern urinalysis has several major advantages: (1) the urine specimen is easily obtained; (2) the reagent strip tests are rapid, simple, reliable and inexpensive; and (3) the tests provide much information about the body's metabolism. Changes occur in urine when kidney disease or certain other diseases are present. Urinalysis can be performed to detect physical, chemical, and microscopic characteristics that indicate disease of, or damage to, the urinary system. Urine tests can also detect metabolic end products that indicate particular diseases unrelated to the urinary system. Urinalysis results can give the physician valuable information about a patient's health and information useful in diagnosing disease or following the course of treatment.

This unit presents basic information about the urinary system, collection of urine specimens, and the procedures included in the routine urinalysis, one of the most frequently performed laboratory procedures. Lesson 5-1 contains fundamental information about the anatomy of the urinary system, kidney structure and function, urine formation and composition, and diseases that affect the urinary system. This information provides a foundation for understanding the importance of urine testing and test results.

Lesson 5-2 describes routine and special urine collection procedures. Lessons 5-3, 5-4, and 5-5 describe the three parts of the routine urinalysis—the physical, chemical, and microscopic examinations of urine. The lesson explaining the test for human chorionic gonadotropin (hCG), commonly called the pregnancy test, is included in Unit 4, Basic Immunology and Immunohematology.

READINGS, REFERENCES, AND RESOURCES

Brunzel, N. A. (2004). *Fundamentals of urine and body fluid analysis.* (2nd ed.) Philadelphia: W. B. Saunders Company.

Brunzel, N. A. (2010). *Urinalysis and body fluid basics: A text and atlas.* Philadelphia: W. B. Saunders Company.

Burtis, C. A., et al. (Eds.) (2008). *Tietz fundamentals of clinical chemistry* (6th ed.). Philadelphia: W. B. Saunders Company.

Haber, M. H. (1991). *A primer of microscopic urinalysis.* (2nd ed.) Garden Grove, CA: Hycor Biomedical, Inc.

Hohenberger, E. F & Kimling, H. (2008). *Compendium urinalysis: Urinalysis with test strips.* Mannheim, Germany: Roche Diagnostics Company Brochure.

KOVA System for Standardized Urinalysis. Package insert. Garden Grove, CA: HYCOR Biomedical Corporation.

McBride, L. J. (1998). *Textbook of urinalysis and body fluids: A clinical approach.* Philadelphia: Lippincott-Raven.

McPherson, R. A. & Pincus, M. R. (Eds.) (2007). *Henry's clinical diagnosis and management by laboratory methods.* (21st ed.). Philadelphia: Saunders Elsevier.

Mundt, L. A. and Shanahan, K. (2010). *Graff's textbook of urinalysis and body fluids.* (2nd ed.). Philadelphia, PA: Lippincott Williams & Wilkins.

Ringsrud, K. M. & Linne, J. J. (1995). *Urinalysis and body fluids: A color text and atlas.* St. Louis: Mosby Yearbook.

Rizzo, D. C. (2009). *Fundamentals of anatomy and physiology.* Clifton Park, NY: Delmar Cengage Learning.

Saladin, K. S. (2009). *Anatomy and physiology: The unity of form and function.* (5th ed.). Columbus, OH: McGraw-Hill.

Scanlon, V. C. & Sanders, T. (2006). *Essentials of anatomy and physiology.* (5th ed.). Philadelphia, PA: F. A. Davis Company.

Siemens Healthcare Diagnostics' Modern Urine Chemistry Series. (2008). *Siemens encyclopedia of urinalysis: CD-ROM.* Deerfield, IL: Siemens Healthcare Diagnostics.

Siemens Healthcare Diagnostics' Modern Urine Chemistry Series. (2008). *Application of urine chemistry and microscopic examination in health and disease.* Deerfield, IL: Siemens Healthcare Diagnostics.

Strasinger, S. K. & Di Lorenzo, M. S. (2008). *Urinalysis and body fluids.* (5th ed.) Philadelphia: F. A. Davis Company.

Web Sites of Interest

American Diabetes Association, www.diabetes.org
National Institutes of Health, www.kidney.niddk.nih.gov
National Kidney Foundation, www.kidney.org

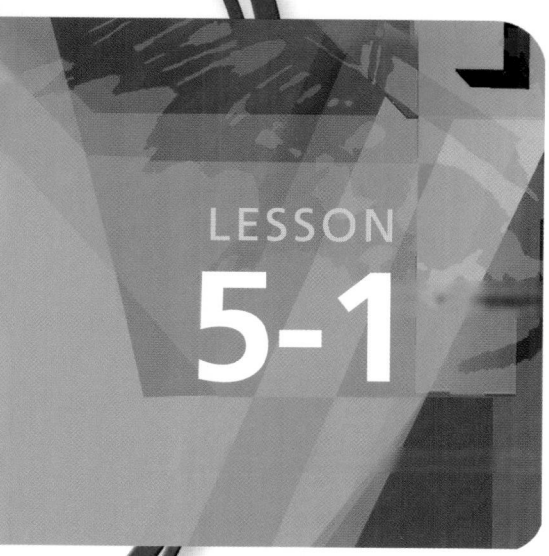

LESSON 5-1 Introduction to Urinalysis

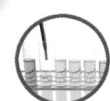

LESSON OBJECTIVES

After studying this lesson, the student will:

- ⊙ Identify the organs of the urinary system.
- ⊙ List four major functions of the kidney.
- ⊙ Explain the importance of the kidneys to overall health.
- ⊙ Identify the parts of the kidney.
- ⊙ Describe the anatomy of a nephron and discuss the functions of its parts.
- ⊙ Explain how urine is formed.
- ⊙ Describe the composition of urine.
- ⊙ List five factors that affect urine volume.
- ⊙ List the three parts of a routine urinalysis.
- ⊙ Explain the value of performing a routine urinalysis.
- ⊙ Name three hormones that are produced in the kidneys and give the function of each.
- ⊙ Name three hormones that influence kidney function and give the function of each.
- ⊙ Discuss the differences between hemodialysis and peritoneal dialysis.
- ⊙ Describe three kidney diseases that can cause abnormal urinalysis results.
- ⊙ List three systemic diseases that can cause abnormal urinalysis results.
- ⊙ Define the glossary terms.

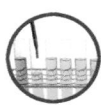

GLOSSARY

Bowman's capsule / the portion of the nephron that receives the glomerular filtrate

cortex / the outer layer or portion of an organ

cystitis / inflammation of the urinary bladder, usually caused by an infection

dialysate / in kidney dialysis, a solution used to draw waste products and excess fluid from the body

distal convoluted tubule / the portion of a renal tubule that empties into the collecting tubule

glomerular filtrate / the acellular, low-protein ultrafiltrate of plasma that passes from the glomerular capillary to the space of Bowman's capsule and from which urine is formed

glomerulonephritis / inflammation of the glomeruli

glomerulus (pl. glomeruli) / a small bundle of capillaries that is the filtering portion of the nephron

kidney / the organ in which urine is formed

(continues)

loop of Henle / the U-shaped portion of a renal tubule between its proximal and distal portions

medulla / the inner or central portion of an organ

nephron / the structural and functional unit of the kidney composed of a glomerulus, Bowman's capsule, and its associated renal tubule

nephropathy / general term for kidney disease

nephrotoxic / toxic or destructive to kidney cells

peritoneum / a membrane lining the abdominal cavity and containing a fluid that keeps abdominal organs from adhering to the abdominal wall; parietal peritoneum

proximal convoluted tubule / the portion of a renal tubule that collects the filtrate from Bowman's capsule

pyelitis / inflammation of the renal pelvis, usually caused by an infection

pyelonephritis / inflammation of the kidney and the renal pelvis, usually caused by an infection

renal hilus / the concavity in the kidney where nerves and vessels enter or exit

renal pelvis / the funnel-shaped expansion of the upper portion of the ureter that receives urine from the renal tubules

renal threshold / the blood concentration above which a substance not normally excreted by the kidneys appears in urine

renal tubule / a small tube of the nephron that collects and concentrates urine

tubular necrosis / death of the tissue comprising the renal tubules

ureter / the tube carrying urine from the kidney to the urinary bladder

urethra / the canal through which urine is discharged from the urinary bladder

urinary bladder / an organ for the temporary storage of urine

urinary tract infection (UTI) / an infection of the urinary tract, usually of the urethra

urine / excretory fluid produced by the kidneys

INTRODUCTION

The urinary system has a vital role in regulating many bodily processes. The kidneys are the primary functional organs of the urinary system. The major functions of the kidneys include:

- Elimination of metabolic and toxic waste products from the body
- Regulation of acid–base balance (pH)
- Regulation of the composition and volume of body fluids
- Production of hormones necessary for proper function of body tissues and organs
- Production and excretion of urine

The kidneys function as biological purification factories, filtering and cleansing the blood of harmful metabolic wastes, and excess ions. These waste products then leave the body in the urine. If waste products are not removed from the body, they can rapidly reach toxic levels and cause death within a few days.

The urinary system also regulates blood volume, blood chemistry, pH, and electrolyte concentrations through a complex process of excretion and reabsorption. Hormones produced in organs of the urinary system are integral to red blood cell production, blood pressure regulation, and bone calcium absorption.

This lesson presents introductory material about the anatomy and functions of the urinary system, basic knowledge that is necessary to understand the relationship between the urinary system and health. Later lessons in this unit explain the routine urinalysis procedure and show how urinalysis test results can give important information about the state of a patient's health.

THE URINARY SYSTEM

The urinary system is an excretory system consisting of two kidneys, two ureters, the urinary bladder, and the urethra. The **kidneys** are the organs in which **urine** is formed. Humans have two kidneys, bean-shaped organs that lie behind the abdominal **peritoneum**, one on each side of the vertebral column. Connected to each kidney is a **ureter**, a funnel-shaped tube that carries urine from the kidney to the **urinary bladder**, where it is temporarily stored. The **urethra** is the canal through which urine is carried from the urinary bladder to the outside. Figure 5-1 is a diagram of the urinary system, showing the kidneys, ureters, urinary bladder, and urethra.

Anatomy of the Kidneys

Each kidney is surrounded by a fibrous protective capsule. The **renal hilus** is the concave region of the kidney where blood vessels, lymphatic vessels, nerves, and the ureter enter or exit the kidney (Figure 5-1). Internally, the kidney has three major regions: the cortex, the medulla, and the renal pelvis (Figures 5-1 and 5-2). The **cortex** is the outermost layer of

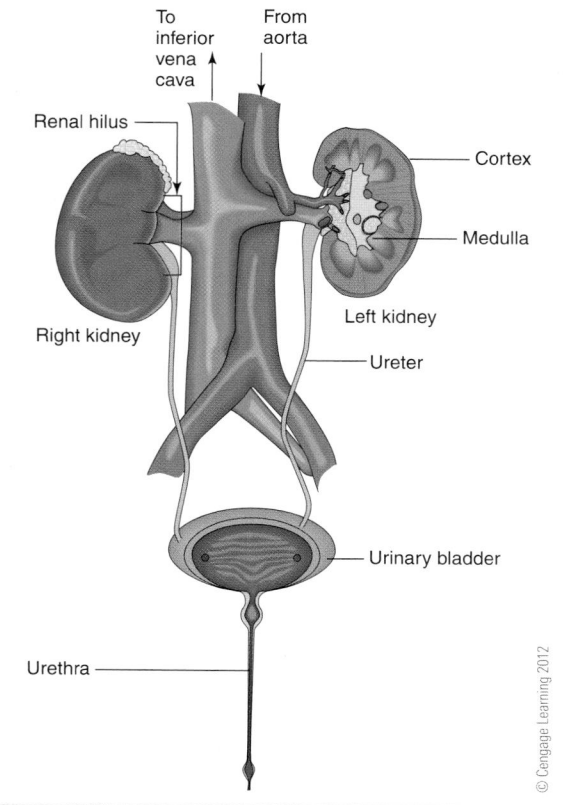

FIGURE 5-1 Organs of the urinary system

tissue, lying beneath the capsule. The **medulla** lies beneath the cortex and contains the renal pyramids, cone-shaped tissue masses. The renal columns are extensions of the renal cortex that separate the renal pyramids. Each pyramid and its associated cortical region make up a kidney lobe. The **renal pelvis** is the funnel-shaped expansion of the upper (proximal) portion of the ureter.

The Nephron

The functional unit in the kidneys is the **nephron** (Figure 5-3). Each kidney has approximately 1 million nephrons, which are located in the kidney cortex. Each nephron is composed of a *glomerulus, Bowman's capsule,* and its associated *renal tubule.*

The Glomerulus

The **glomerulus**, the filtering unit of the kidney, is a bundle of blood capillaries (Figure 5-3). Surrounding each glomerulus is a layer of cells called **Bowman's capsule**. In the glomerulus, water and other small molecules such as glucose, salt, and urea are filtered from the blood (leave the circulatory system) and pass into Bowman's capsule, while blood cells and larger molecules such as proteins remain in the blood. This filtered fluid is called the **glomerular filtrate** and is funneled by Bowman's capsule into the renal tubule (Figures 5-3 and 5-4).

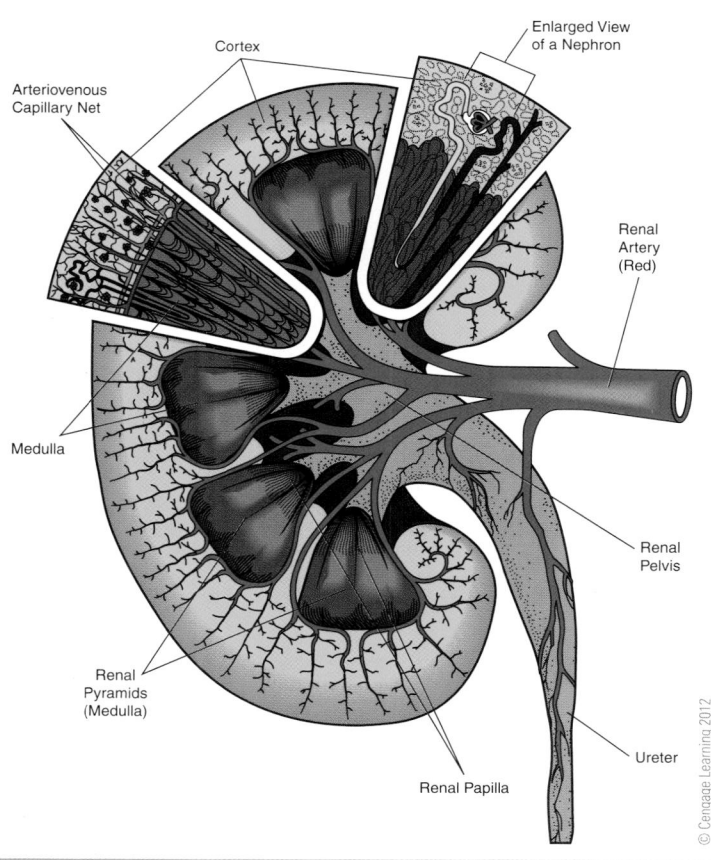

FIGURE 5-2 Diagram of longitudinal cross-section of a kidney. Enlarged insets show position of nephrons spanning renal cortex and medulla (red indicates arterial blood, blue indicates venous blood)

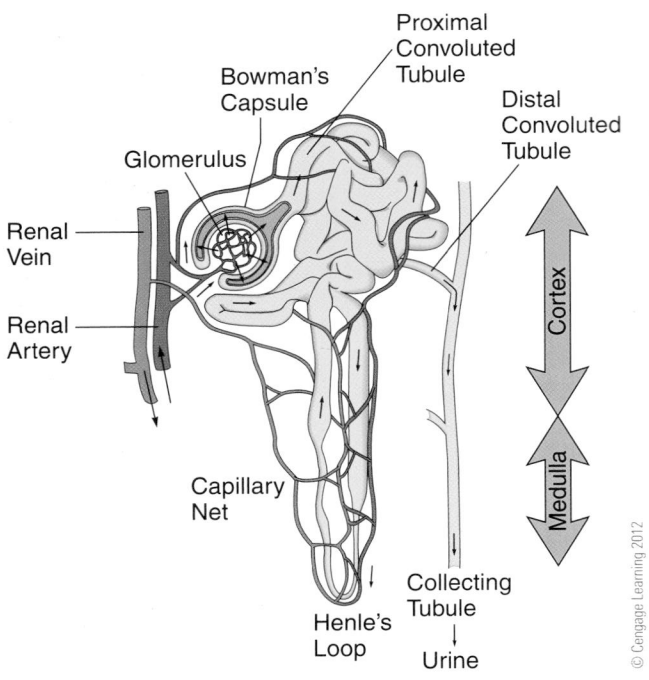

FIGURE 5-3 The nephron: shown are the glomerulus, Bowman's capsule (orange), renal tubule (tan) and nephron blood supply (small arrows indicate direction of blood flow in renal artery and renal vein)

The Renal Tubule

Each glomerulus has an associated **renal tubule**. The three parts of a renal tubule are (1) the **proximal convoluted tubule**, (2) the **loop of Henle**, and (3) the **distal convoluted tubule**, which empties into a collecting tubule (Figure 5-3). The renal tubule is surrounded by blood capillaries (peritubular capillaries), and portions of the tubule can extend into the medulla of the kidney (Figure 5-3).

Urine Formation

Urine is formed by concentration and acidification of the glomerular filtrate as it passes through the renal tubules. Substances such as vitamins, electrolytes, amino acids, and glucose are selectively reabsorbed from the filtrate by cells lining the renal tubules (Figure 5-4). Most of the water in the filtrate is also reabsorbed, producing a concentrated fluid. Water reabsorption takes place in the proximal and distal tubules; glucose reabsorption takes place in the proximal tubules. In addition, some molecules, such as potassium and hydrogen ions, are secreted into the filtrate by tubular cells. The resulting concentrated fluid is urine, which passes into the collecting tubules, collects in the renal pelvis, and flows through the ureters into the urinary bladder.

The kidneys have an extremely high rate of blood flow—approximately 1,200 mL of blood are cleansed of waste products

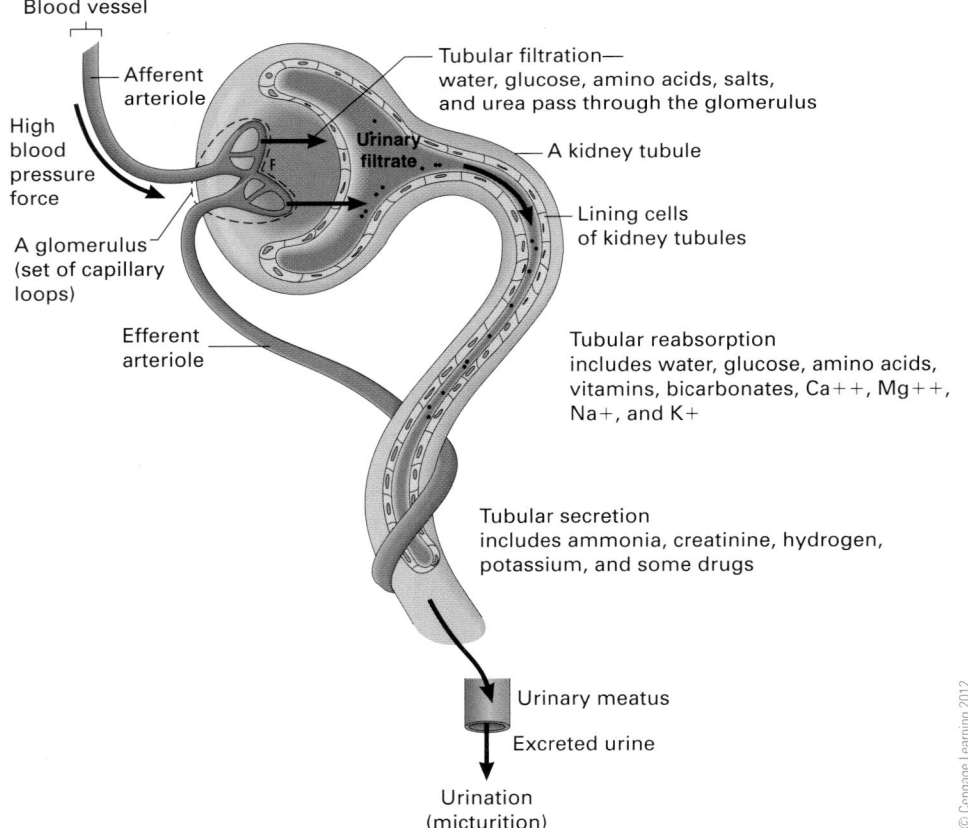

FIGURE 5-4 Diagram of glomerular filtration and tubular reabsorption and secretion (loop of Henle and convoluted and distal tubules not shown)

each minute. As a result, the glomeruli form approximately 180 liters (L)—about 45 gallons!—of filtrate each day. After concentration in the tubules, this volume is reduced to between 750 mL and 2 liters (L) of urine produced daily in a healthy adult.

Urine Composition

Approximately 95% of urine is water, and the other 5% is solutes (dissolved substances). Urea, a breakdown product of amino acids, is the solute in highest concentration, followed by sodium and chloride. Other urine solutes include creatinine, uric acid, potassium, phosphate and sulfate ions, as well as small amounts of bile pigments and calcium, magnesium, and bicarbonate ions (Table 5-1). One way to determine if an unknown fluid is urine is to measure the urea, creatinine, sodium, and chloride levels—the concentration of these is higher in urine than in other body fluids.

The composition of urine can change depending on factors such as the time of day (diurnal change) and the physical state, diet, and health of the individual. In some diseases, substances such as glucose, blood cells, protein, or bile pigments can be present in the urine.

Hormones and the Urinary System

Kidney function is under the influence of several hormones. In addition, the kidneys produce hormones that affect other body processes and organ systems (Tables 5-2 and 5-3).

Hormones That Affect Kidney Function

Hormones that influence kidney function include:

- Parathyroid hormone (PTH)
- Calcitonin
- Aldosterone
- Antidiuretic hormone (ADH)
- Atrial natriuretic peptide (ANP)

Parathyroid hormone (PTH) is produced in the parathyroid glands. PTH influences calcium reabsorption in the kidney tubules and works with vitamin D_3 to regulate bone calcium. *Calcitonin* is produced in the thyroid and inhibits reabsorption of calcium by kidney tubules, leading to increased calcium loss

TABLE 5-2. Hormones that influence kidney function

HORMONE	SITE OF PRODUCTION	FUNCTION
Aldosterone	Adrenal cortex	Regulates electrolytes, especially sodium and potassium
Antidiuretic hormone	Hypothalamus	Regulates water reabsorption
Atrial natriuretic peptide	Heart	Influences sodium excretion
Parathyroid hormone	Parathyroid	Regulates calcium reabsorption
Calcitonin	Thyroid	Inhibits calcium reabsorption

TABLE 5-3. Hormones produced by the kidneys

HORMONE	FUNCTION
Erythropoietin	Stimulates red blood cell synthesis
Renin	Influences blood pressure
Active vitamin D_3	Influences bone calcium levels

TABLE 5-1. Some solutes found in normal urine

Urea	Magnesium	Vitamins
Sodium ions	Potassium ions	Bile pigments
Chloride	Amino acids	Calcium ions
Creatinine	Uric acid	Phosphate ions
Sulfate ions	Bicarbonate ions	

in urine. *Aldosterone* is a mineralocorticoid hormone produced in the adrenal cortex; it helps regulate electrolytes by promoting excretion of potassium and retention (reabsorption) of sodium from the glomerular filtrate. *Antidiuretic hormone (ADH)*, also called *vasopressin*, is produced in the hypothalamus and is then transported to and released by the pituitary gland. ADH regulates water reabsorption by the kidney tubules. *Atrial natriuretic peptide* is produced by heart cells. It helps reduce plasma volume by increasing sodium excretion in the kidneys (Table 5-2).

Hormones Produced by the Kidneys

Although kidney function is influenced by hormones such as ADH that are produced in other organs, the kidneys also produce hormones that influence physiological processes in other parts of the body (Table 5-3). Three hormones produced by the kidneys are:

- Erythropoietin
- Renin
- Active vitamin D_3

Erythropoietin stimulates red blood cell production in the bone marrow. *Renin* indirectly influences blood pressure. *Vitamin D_3*, which is actually a hormone rather than a vitamin, helps regulate bone calcium and phosphorus by increasing absorption of dietary calcium and phosphorus.

Urine Volume

The amount of urine formed daily depends on age, fluid intake, metabolism, blood pressure, diet, hormone balance, and many other factors. Healthy adults excrete between 750 mL and 2 liters of urine per day. *Diuretics* (substances that promote the formation of urine) increase urinary output and therefore dilute the urine. Caffeine and some hypertension medications act as diuretics. *Antidiuretic hormone* stimulates water reabsorption by the kidneys, thus creating concentrated urine and decreasing urine volume.

Renal Threshold

Most components present in urine are also present in blood, but in different amounts and proportions. Many small molecules that enter the glomerular filtrate become reabsorbed into the blood as the filtrate passes through the tubules of the nephron. When the blood level of a substance becomes high enough to exceed the tubular reabsorption capacity, then the substance will be excreted in the urine. In those cases, the blood concentration is said to have exceeded the **renal threshold**. For example, the renal threshold of glucose ranges from 160 to 180 mg/dL. At blood glucose levels below this range, glucose is reabsorbed from the filtrate by the tubules. When blood glucose levels exceed this threshold, glucose will be excreted in the urine.

TESTS OF RENAL FUNCTION

Several tests can be performed on urine. Some are simple and rapid, such as the tests included in the routine urinalysis. The routine urinalysis procedure has three parts: the physical and chemical examinations of urine, described in Lessons 5-3 and 5-4, and the microscopic examination of urine sediment described in Lesson 5-5.

Abnormalities discovered during a routine urinalysis can lead the physician to request more specific tests of renal function. Serum tests for metabolites such as creatinine and blood urea nitrogen (BUN) are important in monitoring kidney function. Other tests used to assess renal function can be performed on 24-hour urine specimens, such as the creatinine clearance test, and tests for certain hormones or metabolites. These tests can be complex and time-consuming. Although the procedures for tests on 24-hour urines are beyond the scope of this text, the procedure for collecting 24-hour urine specimens is covered in Lesson 5-2.

CURRENT TOPICS

RENAL DIALYSIS

The kidneys cleanse the blood and remove excess fluid, minerals, and waste products; they also produce hormones necessary for strong bones and blood cell production, all vital functions. There are several causes of kidney failure, but whatever the reason, the consequences are the same—harmful wastes build up in the body, blood pressure rises, excess fluid is retained, and red cell production decreases. Acute kidney failure can cause death in only a few days if untreated. In some cases acute kidney failure responds to treatment, and kidney function is regained. Chronic kidney failure, also called *chronic renal insufficiency*, leads to kidney failure more slowly. When a patient reaches the point at which 85% to 90% of kidney function has been lost, treatment is required.

The two major treatments for kidney failure (end-stage kidney disease) are dialysis and kidney transplant. Dialysis is used to treat acute kidney failure and to treat patients with chronic kidney failure until they can receive a kidney transplant. In many cases, patients never receive a transplant but remain on dialysis for years.

Dialysis attempts to replace the function of the failed kidneys by using artificial means to remove harmful wastes, salts, and excess fluid. Two types of

dialysis are used, *hemodialysis* and *peritoneal dialysis*. Hemodialysis is used to treat acute kidney failure; chronic kidney failure can be treated with hemodialysis or peritoneal dialysis. With both types of dialysis, the patient's condition must be closely monitored by frequent physical examinations and laboratory tests. Dialysis patients must follow a precise, restricted

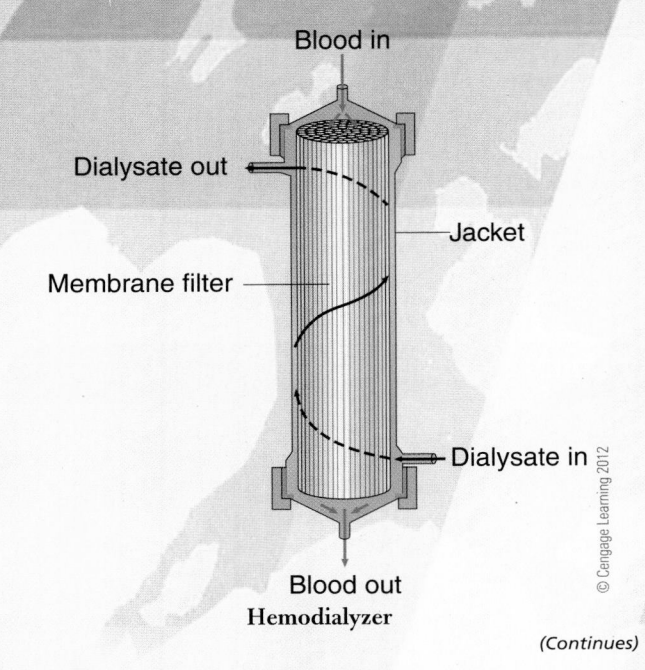

Blood in

Dialysate out

Jacket

Membrane filter

Dialysate in

Blood out

Hemodialyzer

© Cengage Learning 2012

(Continues)

CURRENT TOPICS (Continued)

diet low in sodium, phosphorus, potassium, and fluid intake. Vitamin and mineral supplements are required because of diet limitations and loss of vitamins and minerals during dialysis.

Hemodialysis

In hemodialysis, blood from a patient's vein is slowly passed through a *dialyzer* that removes wastes and extra fluid. The dialyzer, also called an artificial kidney, is a canister containing special membrane filters (Diagram 1). A permanent *fistula* or graft connecting a vein to an artery is surgically created beneath the patient's skin. A dialysis machine pumps blood from this fistula or graft to the dialyzer (Diagrams 1 and 2). Blood remains on one side of the membrane filters, and a fluid called a dialysate is constantly pumped around the other side of the dialyzer membranes, drawing wastes and excess fluid from the blood across the membranes into the dialysate. The wastes and excess fluid are carried away as the dialysate leaves the dialyzer, and the cleansed blood is returned to the body. Hemodialysis is a slow process, taking 4 to 5 hours, and must be done three to four times a week. Most patients go to a dialysis center for treatment; some patients are trained to perform hemodialysis at home.

Peritoneal Dialysis

The peritoneum is the membrane that lines the walls of the abdominal cavity, creating a peritoneal space or cavity. In peritoneal dialysis, the peritoneal cavity is used as the exchange container and the peritoneal membrane acts as a filter. The patient's abdomen is filled with a dialysate (usually containing dextrose) using a soft tube called a catheter (Diagram 3). The dialysate pulls wastes and extra fluid from the blood into the peritoneal cavity by diffusion. After a few

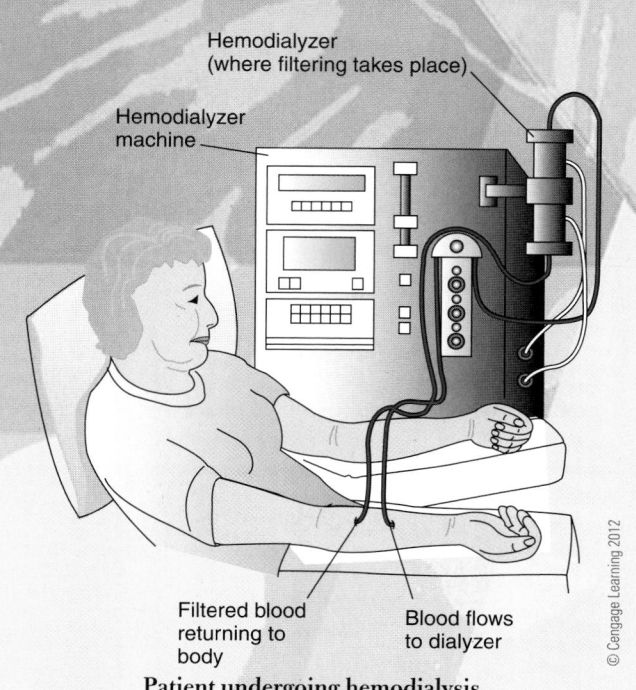

Patient undergoing hemodialysis

hours, the dialysate fluid containing this waste and excess fluid is drained and discarded. More dialysate fluid is then pumped into the cavity to begin another exchange. A typical schedule calls for four exchanges a day, each with a dwell time (time the dialysate is in the peritoneal cavity) of 4 to 6 hours. Peritoneal dialysis can be the *ambulatory* type that does not require a machine and allows the patient to remain mobile. In other cases, a cycler machine fills and drains the abdomen while the patient sleeps. Both types require that a catheter be permanently placed in the abdomen to carry the dialysis solution into and out of the abdomen. Peritoneal dialysis gives the patient more freedom and independence than renal dialysis.

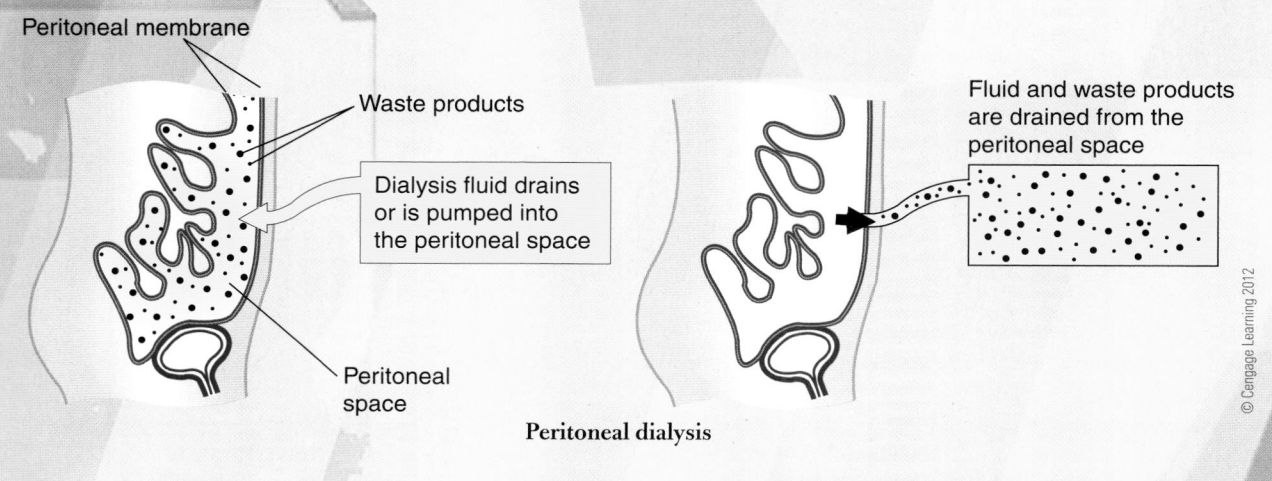

Peritoneal dialysis

CONDITIONS AND DISEASES AFFECTING URINALYSIS RESULTS

Abnormal urinalysis results can be seen in disorders or diseases of the urinary tract or in situations in which disease in other parts of the body affects kidney function or urine composition. Disease can cause changes in the:

- Urine volume
- Urine color
- Urine transparency or clarity
- Urine odor
- Cells present in urine
- Chemical constituents of urine

Urinary Tract Infections

Urine stored in the urinary bladder is normally sterile. **Urinary tract infections (UTIs)** most commonly occur in the urethra and can be caused by bacteria, yeasts (fungi), or protozoan parasites. Untreated UTIs can spread to the urinary bladder, causing **cystitis**. In severe cases, the kidney can become involved, resulting in **pyelitis**, an inflammation or infection of the renal pelvis, or **pyelonephritis**, an inflammation or infection of the renal pelvis and the kidney.

Diseases of the Kidneys

Kidney disease can be mild or severe and acute or chronic. Chronic kidney disease is often far advanced by the time it is discovered because kidney failure does not occur until a large percentage of the nephrons are nonfunctional. When kidney function decreases, toxic products such as urea, uric acid, and creatinine accumulate in the blood. Kidney failure can be treated by dialysis (see Current Topics) or kidney transplant. Some examples of diseases of the kidneys include glomerulonephritis, polycystic kidney disease, and tubular necrosis (Table 5-4).

Glomerulonephritis

Glomerulonephritis (GN) is an inflammation of the glomeruli, usually caused by deposition of antibodies or immune complexes in the glomeruli, causing glomerular damage. Glomerulonephritis can develop as a result of infection somewhere in the body, autoimmune diseases, or systemic diseases in which capillary damage occurs (because the glomeruli are made of capillaries). Damage to glomerular capillaries results in inefficient filtering; protein and blood cells can be present in urine, and excess body fluid accumulates, causing edema and hypertension.

Poststreptococcal GN is a well-known but infrequently occurring type of glomerulonephritis. It is a complication of untreated or incompletely treated group A *Streptococcus* throat or skin infection. The glomerular damage in poststreptococcal GN is caused when immune complexes that form in response to the infection are deposited in the glomeruli, causing inflammation and interfering with glomerular function. All group

A streptococcal infections should be treated promptly with antibiotics to avoid the possibility of complications. When symptoms associated with poststreptococcal GN are treated, the condition often subsides after a few months. However, in some cases the condition can progress to chronic renal failure.

Polycystic Kidney Disease

Polycystic kidney disease is an inherited condition in which glomerular function is lost because of formation of multiple cysts in the kidneys. Patients with polycystic kidney disease in time usually become candidates for kidney dialysis or kidney transplant.

Tubular Necrosis

Tubular necrosis can occur when the blood supply to the kidney is diminished, or upon exposure to, or ingestion of, substances that are **nephrotoxic** (toxic to kidney cells). The capacity of the tubules to concentrate urine is affected in this condition.

Systemic Diseases Affecting Urinalysis Results

Several systemic diseases can cause **nephropathy**, a general term referring to kidney disease. Diseases that can cause abnormal urinalysis results include diabetes mellitus, hypertension, atherosclerosis, autoimmune diseases, nephrotic syndrome, and malignancies (Table 5-4). Uncontrolled diabetes, prolonged hypertension, and autoimmune diseases such as lupus erythematosus can cause glomerular damage. Nephrotic syndrome is a complex condition associated with circulatory disorders and is characterized by tissue edema and protein in the urine. Malignancies developing in the urinary system can cause obstruction, abnormal urinalysis results, or the appearance of malignant cells in the urine.

TABLE 5-4. Examples of conditions and diseases that can affect urinalysis results

KIDNEY DISEASES

Glomerulonephritis
Polycystic kidney disease
Tubular necrosis

SYSTEMIC DISEASES AFFECTING KIDNEY FUNCTION

Diabetes mellitus
Hypertension
Atherosclerosis
Autoimmune diseases
Nephrotic syndrome
Malignancies

OTHER CONDITIONS

Urinary tract infections

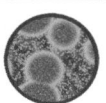

SUMMARY

A normal functioning urinary system is necessary for good health. The kidneys are responsible for the formation and excretion of urine, the principal way the body eliminates waste products and excess fluid. Urine excretion provides a means of regulating the body's state of hydration and the blood concentration of ions such as sodium, potassium, and other small molecules. Three processes are involved in urine formation:

- *Filtration* of waste products, salts, and excess fluid from the blood by glomeruli
- Tubular *reabsorption* of water and solutes from the glomerular filtrate
- Tubular *secretion* of ions and molecules into the urine

Although urine production is a primary function of the kidneys, the kidneys also have other functions, such as the production of hormones necessary for strong bones, blood pressure control, and red blood cell production.

Diseases or conditions that interfere with normal kidney function allow buildup of toxic waste products in the body. This condition can be life-threatening and must be treated promptly. Cases of irreversible kidney failure can be treated by dialysis or kidney transplant.

Tests such as those performed in the routine urinalysis provide an indication of an individual's metabolism and general state of health. An understanding of kidney function and urine composition helps laboratory personnel understand and interpret routine urinalysis results.

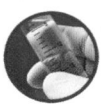

REVIEW QUESTIONS

1. Name the organs of the urinary system.
2. Draw a kidney and label the parts.
3. What are four major functions of the kidneys?
4. Draw a nephron and label the parts; state the function associated with each part.
5. Explain how urine is formed.

6. What components are in urine?
7. What is the normal daily urine volume of an adult?
8. Name four factors that can influence urine volume.
9. What is the function of a diuretic?
10. What are the three parts of a routine urinalysis?
11. List three hormones produced by the kidneys, and give the function of each.
12. List three hormones that influence kidney function, name the sites of production, and explain their function.
13. Name three conditions or diseases of the urinary system that can affect urinalysis results.
14. Name three systemic diseases that can affect urinalysis results.
15. Why is dialysis useful as a treatment for kidney disease?
16. Explain peritoneal dialysis.
17. Explain hemodialysis.
18. Define Bowman's capsule, cortex, cystitis, dialysate, distal convoluted tubule, glomerular filtrate, glomerulonephritis, glomerulus, kidney, loop of Henle, medulla, nephron, nephropathy, nephrotoxic, peritoneum, proximal convoluted tubule, pyelitis, pyelonephritis, renal hilus, renal pelvis, renal threshold, renal tubule, tubular necrosis, ureter, urethra, urinary bladder, urinary tract infection (UTI), and urine.

STUDENT ACTIVITIES

1. Complete the written examination for this lesson.
2. Select five urine solutes listed in Table 5-1. Consult an anatomy/physiology text and find out how the urine concentration of each solute is influenced. That is, is the solute secreted from a portion of a renal tubule, filtered by the glomerulus, or partially reabsorbed in a portion of the renal tubule?
3. If possible, tour a dialysis center.

WEB ACTIVITIES

1. Use the Internet to search for general information on kidney disease, using reliable sources such as medical school web sites, research institutes such as the National Institutes of Health, or nonprofit kidney disease associations or foundations.
2. Select a disease from Table 5-4 and use the Internet to find information about the disease. Prepare a one-page report on the disease. Include information about the cause(s) of the disease, how kidney function is affected, and types of treatment available.
3. Use the Internet to search for information about kidney transplantation. Report on why it would be performed, how donor kidneys are obtained, and what criteria must be met for the patient and the donor.

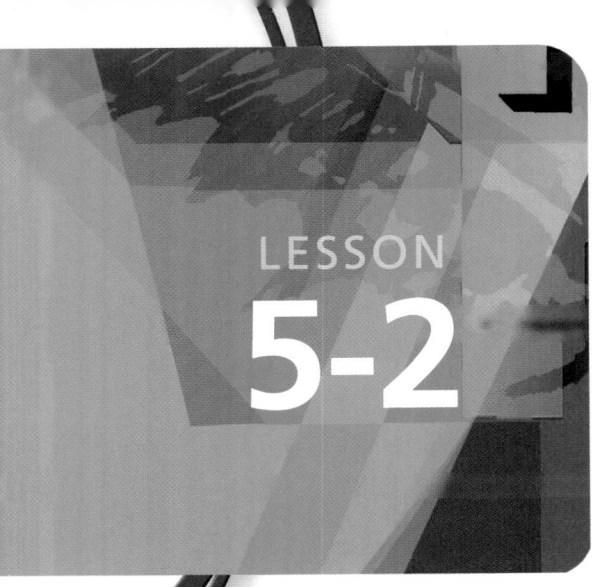

Urine Collection and Processing

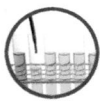

LESSON OBJECTIVES

After studying this lesson, the student will:

⊙ Explain the importance of the proper collection of urine specimens.

⊙ List four types of urine specimens and explain when each might be required.

⊙ State the normal 24-hour urine volumes for adults, children, and newborns.

⊙ Discuss why a preservative is required for some urine specimens.

⊙ Explain how to collect a midstream urine specimen.

⊙ Explain how to collect a clean-catch urine specimen.

⊙ Explain how to collect a 24-hour urine specimen.

⊙ Explain how collection of urine specimens for drug screens differs from collection for routine urinalysis.

⊙ Explain safety precautions that must be observed when handling urine specimens.

⊙ Discuss the importance of quality assessment in urine collection and processing.

⊙ Define the glossary terms.

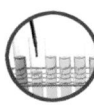

GLOSSARY

anuria / absence of urine production; failure of kidney function and suppression of urine production

clean-catch urine / a midstream urine sample collected after the urethral opening and surrounding tissues have been cleansed

midstream urine / a urine sample collected from the mid-portion of a urine stream

nocturia / excessive urination at night

oliguria / decreased production of urine

polyuria / excessive production of urine

random urine specimen / a urine specimen collected at any time, without regard to diet or time of day

INTRODUCTION

The proper collection and processing of urine specimens are the first steps leading to reliable urine test results. The type of specimen required for a urine test depends on the nature of the test that is ordered. For example, quantitative chemical tests, such as

measurement of urine calcium, require a different type of specimen than is required for a routine urinalysis. Because urine specimens are usually collected by the patient, it is important that the patient be given specific instructions about how to collect the urine specimen.

Urine specimens must sometimes be transported to a laboratory for testing, so it is also important that personnel at the collection site, transport service, and receiving laboratory all understand transport requirements and limitations. This lesson explains the various types of urine specimens that are used for urine tests and describes the urine collection and handling procedures for each.

TYPES OF URINE SPECIMENS

Common types of urine specimens submitted for laboratory analysis are:

- Random urine specimen
- Fasting or first morning urine specimen
- Clean-catch urine specimen
- Timed specimen, such as 24-hour urine specimen

All urine specimens except 24-hour urine specimens, should be collected by the midstream procedure. A **midstream urine** specimen is one in which the patient collects only the middle portion of the urine flow.

Specimens for Routine Urinalysis

The preferred specimen for routine urinalysis is the *first morning specimen*, obtained immediately on arising. This specimen is normally more concentrated than a random specimen and usually has an acid pH that helps preserve any cells present. The first morning specimen can be designated as a *fasting* specimen if it is collected before the patient has eaten. Most specimens received for routine urinalysis, however, are **random urine specimens**—specimens obtained at any time of day and without regard to food intake.

Clean-Catch Urine Specimens

A **clean-catch urine** specimen is required when urine is to be cultured for microorganisms. The clean-catch procedure requires cleansing of the urethral opening before the urine is collected. The detailed procedure for collecting clean-catch urine is described in this lesson; the urine culture procedure is explained in Lesson 7-6.

Timed Specimens: Twenty-Four–Hour Urine Specimens

Most quantitative urine tests require a *24-hour urine specimen*; 8-hour urine specimens can also be used for certain tests. Analyses of timed specimens are usually performed in large hospital or reference laboratories. Collection procedures for timed specimens must be followed carefully to ensure that the laboratory has a complete specimen to examine. Protein, creatinine, urobilinogen, calcium, hormones, amino acids, metabolic products, heavy metals, and drugs are just a few examples of analytes that can be measured in 24-hour urine specimens. Results are expressed as analyte units per 24 hours. Instructions for collecting 24-hour urine specimens are given in this lesson.

Collection of Urine by Catheter

Occasionally, urine for culture or routine analysis must be collected by catheterization, a procedure normally performed by nursing service personnel. Catheterization is required when a patient is unable to urinate independently. A catheter is inserted into the bladder through the urethra and the urine is collected directly into the appropriate collection container.

Pediatric Urine Specimens

When a urine specimen is needed from infants or small children who cannot urinate on demand, a special urine collection bag is fitted to the skin surrounding the urethra. Once sufficient urine is obtained, the collection bag is removed and the urine is transferred into a urine container.

HANDLING AND PRESERVING URINE SPECIMENS

Specific guidelines for the collection, transport, preservation, and storage of urine will be included in the laboratory's standard operating procedure (SOP) manual.

Urine Containers

Several sizes and shapes of containers are available for collecting urine specimens. Random and first morning specimens should be collected in lidded, disposable containers with at least a 50-mL capacity. (Table 5-5 lists criteria for urine collection containers.) For clean-catch specimens, urine containers must be sterile (Figure 5-5, Table 5-5). Large, amber, opaque containers capable of holding at least 3 to 4 liters (L) are provided to patients for collecting 24-hour urine specimens (Figure 5-6, Table 5-5). These containers often contain preservatives.

Labeling Urine Specimens

Urine specimens must be labeled clearly with the patient's name, as well as the date and time of collection. Labels must be placed on the container, not on the lid. For timed specimens,

TABLE 5-5. Criteria for urine collection containers	
CRITERIA FOR ALL URINE CONTAINERS	**ADDITIONAL SPECIAL CONTAINER REQUIREMENTS**
50-mL minimum capacity	Amber color for light sensitive analytes
Break-resistant plastic, leach-resistant	Sterile container for urine culture
Clean, chemical free	3–4 liter capacity for 24-hour urines
Wide mouth, wide stable base	
Secure, leak-resistant lid or closure	
Single-use, disposable	

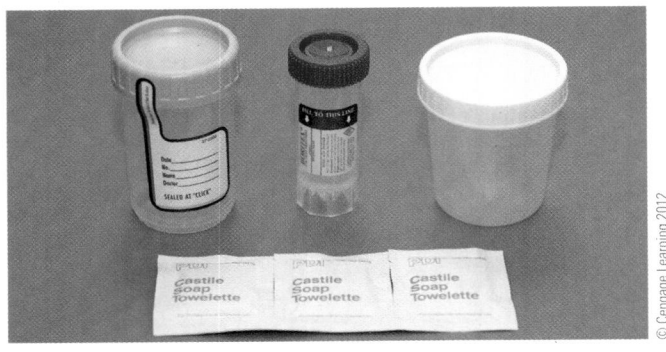

© Cengage Learning 2012

FIGURE 5-5 Clean-catch urine collection kits

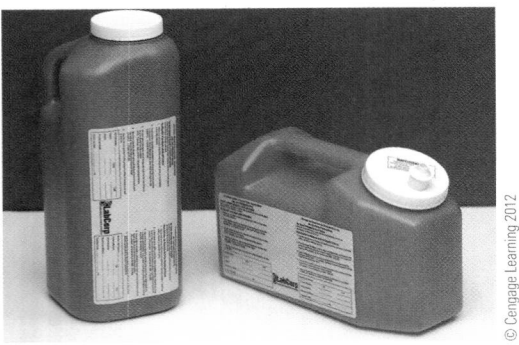

© Cengage Learning 2012

FIGURE 5-6 Twenty-four-hour urine specimen containers

the start and stop times should be included on the label or requisition form.

Specimen Log-In

The time the specimen is received by the testing site should be recorded on the laboratory log, requisition form, or specimen label. The requisition form should be checked to be sure the specimen collection meets the criteria for the type of test to be performed. The specimen volume should be observed to be sure it is sufficient for testing, usually a minimum of 15 mL. The guidelines in the SOP manual should be followed when urine volume is less than specified for the test procedure.

Storage of Urine Specimens

For all tests except 24-hour tests, urine specimens should be examined within 1 to 2 hours of collection. If this is not possible, deterioration of the specimen can be prevented by refrigerating the urine at 4° to 6°C for up to 4 hours in the dark in a lidded container or, less commonly, by adding a preservative.

Test results are affected by the way urine specimens are handled after collection. When urine remains at room temperature for an extended time, any bacteria present will multiply rapidly, increasing the urine pH and causing an unpleasant, ammonia-like odor to develop. Refrigeration of urine can slow bacterial growth, but it does not preserve urine sediment components such as casts

and cells. Refrigeration also protects labile urine components such as ketones, bilirubin, and urobilinogen, which deteriorate more rapidly at room temperature.

Preservation of Urine

Preservatives are used to prevent bacterial growth and to preserve certain chemical or microscopic components of urine. The simplest method of temporarily preserving urine quality is to refrigerate specimens. Chemical preservatives can be added to urine specimens that must be mailed or otherwise transported. Refrigeration slows bacterial growth, whereas the addition of a chemical preservative both retards the growth of bacteria and slows the destruction or decomposition of other urine components. For some chemical tests, urine can be frozen until testing.

All chemical preservatives should be environmentally safe and mercury-free. The preservative must not interfere with the tests that have been ordered and should be used in the correct preservative-to-urine ratio. Some commonly used chemical preservatives are HCl, acetic acid, NaOH, sodium carbonate, and boric acid (Table 5-6). When urine is to be cultured, buffered boric acid can be added to prevent further growth of any bacteria present. Containers for 24-hour urine specimens usually have preservatives added before the urine is collected.

Urine for Culture

When infection of the urinary tract is suspected, a test for urine *culture and sensitivity* (C & S) is ordered. Urine to be cultured for the presence of microorganisms must be collected, processed, and transported in a manner that prevents contamination. If both culture and routine urinalysis are to be performed on the same specimen, the urine must be sent to the microbiology department first for culture, because aseptic techniques are not used in routine urinalysis procedures. When urine to be cultured must be transported over a distance, a kit containing a vacuum tube and sterile straw (Figure 5-7A, B) can be used. These kits work similar to vacuum blood collecting systems. An aliquot of clean-catch urine is drawn into a sterile vacuum tube containing a preservative that is not toxic to microorganisms in the specimen (Figure 5-7C).

TABLE 5-6. Common urine preservatives and their uses

PRESERVATIVE	PRESERVES FOR ANALYSIS OF
Hydrochloric acid (HCl)	Genetic metabolic screens, ketoacids, mucopolysaccharides
Sodium carbonate	Porphyrins, urobilinogen
Sodium hydroxide (NaOH)	Uric acid, myoglobin
Boric acid	Uric acid, citrate, cortisol
Acetic acid	Ketosteroids, aldosterone
Refrigeration or freezing	Protein, potassium, iron, sodium, amylase, creatinine, drug screen, heavy metals screen

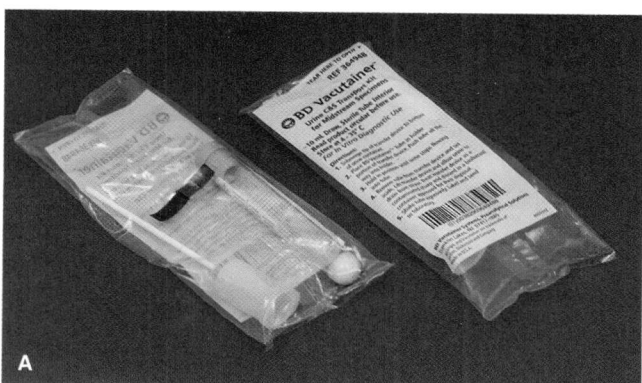
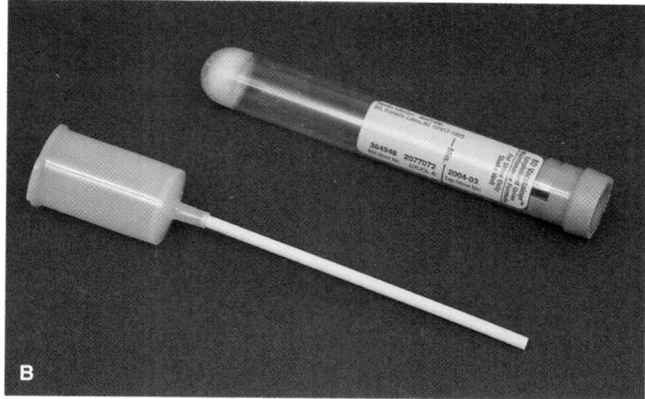
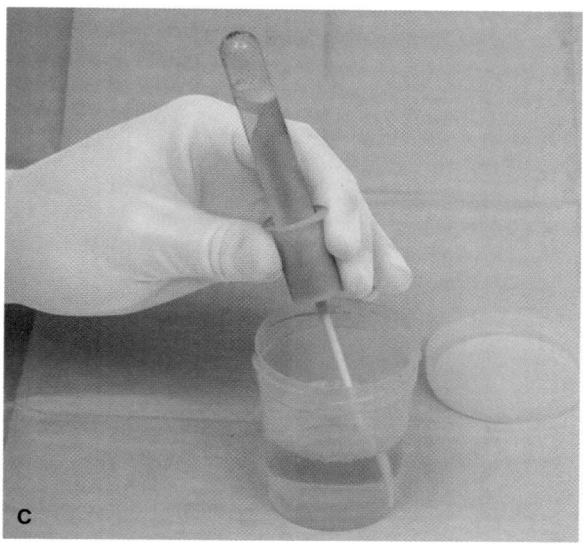

FIGURE 5-7 Method for transport of urine for culture and sensitivity: (A) kit contains (B) sterile vacuum tube containing preservative and sterile collecting straw; (C) urine is aseptically collected into vacuum tube using collecting straw

© Cengage Learning 2012

PROCEDURES FOR COLLECTING URINE SPECIMENS

Urine collection procedures differ slightly depending on the the test ordered. Instructions for urine collection, including procedures for midstream collection, clean-catch collection, 24-hour urine collection, and collection for drug screens will be specified in the SOP manual.

Safety Precautions

Standard Precautions must be observed by all personnel. Personal protective equipment (PPE) such as gloves, face protection, and a buttoned, fluid-resistant laboratory coat should be worn when working with specimens. To protect healthcare personnel as well as specimen integrity, leak-resistant urine containers must be used. Specimens submitted in leaking containers should not be accepted for testing.

Splashes or the creation of aerosols must be avoided when pouring or discarding urine. Urine can be discarded in sinks, followed by rinsing the sink with water and then surface disinfectant. Spills of urine must be wiped up with disinfectant. Patients who must collect 24-hour urine specimens should be given the material safety data sheet (MSDS) information or written instructions for safe handling of any preservative in the collection container.

Quality Assessment

Detailed instructions must be given to patients so they understand how to correctly collect the specimen. Written instructions must be understandable to all patients and should be available in non-English versions.

Specimen labeling must be accurate and complete. Containers (not lids) should be labeled with the patient's name, date, time, and method of collection. Specimens must be delivered to the testing site as soon as possible after collection and logged in with time received, so that testing can be performed within the accepted time limits. Specimens that cannot be tested within 1 to 2 hours of collection should be stored in the dark with lid on at 4° to 6° C until tested.

Collecting Midstream Urine Samples

The midstream collection method is used for all first morning, random, and clean-catch specimens. The patient should be instructed to begin voiding into the toilet and then to interrupt the urine stream to collect only the middle portion of the urine stream in the specimen container. This is to prevent contaminating the specimen with epithelial cells, microorganisms, or mucus from the urethra.

Collecting Clean-Catch Urine Samples

A clean-catch urine specimen is required if urine is to be cultured. Hospitals and physician offices will provide the patient with a kit containing towelettes and a sterile urine container (Figure 5-5). Patients should be instructed to cleanse the urethral opening, carefully collect the urine specimen using the midstream collection method, and avoid touching the inside of the sterile container. Written or pictorial instructions that are understandable to all patients should be available and should also be posted in the restroom near the toilet.

Instructions to the Male Patient

The patient should wash his hands with soap and water and retract the penis foreskin (if not circumcised), using a towelette. A second towelette should be used to cleanse the urethral opening with a single stroke directed from the tip of the penis toward the ring of the glans. The towelette should then be discarded and the cleansing procedure repeated using two more towelettes.

The patient should begin to void into the toilet. The urine stream should be interrupted to collect only the middle portion of the urine flow in the supplied container. After the specimen has been collected, the lid should be placed securely on the container, avoiding touching the inside of the container or lid. The information on the label should be completed and attached to the specimen container.

Instructions to the Female Patient

The patient should wash her hands with soap and water, position herself comfortably on the toilet seat, and swing one knee to the side as far as possible. She should spread the outer vulval folds (labia majora) using a towelette and wipe the inner side of one inner fold (labium minora) with a towelette, using a single stroke from front to back. The towelette should then be discarded and a second towelette used to repeat the procedure on the opposite side. A third towelette should be used to cleanse the urethral opening with a single front-to-back stroke.

The patient should then begin to void into the toilet. The urine stream should be interrupted to collect only the middle portion of the urine flow in a container. Touching only the outside of the container and the lid, the patient should close the container securely, complete the label, and attach it to the container. If the patient has vaginal discharge, a clean tampon should be inserted before urine collection to decrease the possibility of specimen contamination.

Collecting Urine for Drug Screens

Urine drug screens can be required in a number of situations, such as participation in athletic events, job applications, or cases of suspected drug abuse. Although a random urine specimen is used for drug screens, much documentation is required to guarantee the reliability of the collection procedure and the identity of the person submitting the specimen. Each laboratory that handles specimens for drug screening must follow the written protocol in the laboratory's SOP manual. Chain-of-custody of the specimen must be documented to safeguard against possible tampering and to guarantee the specimen's integrity (Figure 5-8). Some requirements usually included in a protocol for urine drug-screen collection are:

- Photo identification
- Signed consent of patient/donor
- Use of special collection kits provided to the patient by the laboratory
- Inspection of bathroom before and after collection, with a monitor stationed outside during collection
- Urine temperature measured and recorded immediately after collection
- Specimen labeled in presence of donor, sealed in outer container, and secured until transported to testing agency.

Collecting Twenty-Four–Hour Urine Specimens

The collection procedure for a 24-hour urine specimen must be followed carefully. The laboratory will provide the patient a collection container and verbal and written instructions describing how to collect the specimen (Figure 5-9).

Specimen Containers

Specimen containers for 24-hour urine collection must have a 3- to 4-L capacity and should be opaque to protect light-sensitive urine components. Laboratory personnel should consult the SOP manual for a list of tests that can be performed on 24-hour urines, the preservative (if any) required for each, and the temperature at which the specimen should be stored during the 24-hour collection period. Most procedures require the specimen to be stored at 4° to 6° C (refrigerated) during the collection period. Any preservative needed will be added to the container before collection or upon receipt of the 24-hour specimen, depending on the test to be performed. If a preservative is used, the patient should be provided written safety information, such as the MSDS, explaining any hazards associated with exposure to the preservative. Patients should be cautioned against accidentally splashing the preservative on their skin or in their eyes.

Patient Collection Instructions

Twenty-four–hour urine specimens must contain all of the urine excreted by the patient in a 24-hour period. Collection usually begins at a designated morning hour, for example, 8 AM. The patient should be instructed to completely empty the bladder by voiding into the toilet at 8 AM on the day collection begins.

This urine is not included in the 24-hour collection. The patient should then collect ALL urine produced until 8 AM the following morning. Urine should be collected in a small container and then carefully transferred to the large 24-hour urine container. At 8 AM on the day after collection began (24 hours later), the patient should empty the bladder and add this urine to the 24-hour container. The container should then be delivered to the laboratory. An example of patient instructions for collecting a 24-hour urine is shown in Figure 5-9.

USA LABS
ID#

Referred by

Health Care Provider
Address
Phone

DO NOT WRITE
IN THIS AREA

CHAIN OF CUSTODY

STEP 1 — TO BE COMPLETED BY EMPLOYER/COLLECTOR.
DONOR IDENTIFICATION—PLEASE PRINT

LAST NAME

FIRST NAME   M.I.

SOC. SEC. NO. _____ — _____ — _____

EMPLOYEE NO. _____

DONOR I.D. VERIFIED   ☐ PHOTO I.D.
                         ☐ EMPLOYER REPRESENTATIVE

_____
SIGNATURE OF EMPLOYER REP.
REASON FOR TEST (CHECK ONE)
☐ (1) PRE-EMPLOYMENT ☐ (2) POST ACCIDENT ☐ (3) RANDOM
☐ (4) PERIODIC ☐ (5) REASONABLE SUSPICION/CAUSE
☐ (6) RETURN TO DUTY
☐ (99) OTHER (SPECIFY)

TESTS REQUESTED: TOTAL TESTS ORDERED ☐

SPECIMEN   ☐ Urine   ☐ Blood   (SUBMIT ONLY ONE SPECIMEN WITH EACH REQUISITION)

STEP 2—COLLECTOR, FOR URINE SPECIMENS, READ TEMPERATURE WITHIN FOUR MINUTES OF COLLECTION.
CHECK THE BOX IF TEMPERATURE IS WITHIN THE SPECIFIED RANGE ☐90°–100°F / 32°–38°C

OR RECORD ACTUAL TEMPERATURE HERE: _____

STEP 3—TO BE COMPLETED BY COLLECTOR.   COLLECTION SITE

COLLECTION DATE _____ TIME _____ ☐ AM PM
                                           ADDRESS
REMARKS _____
                                           CITY   STATE   ZIP
_____   ( )
                                           PHONE

I certify that the specimen identified on this form is the specimen presented to me by the employee identified in Step 1 above, and was collected, labeled and sealed in the donor's presence.

COLLECTOR'S NAME PRINT (FIRST, M.I., LAST)   SIGNATUE OF COLLECTOR

STEP 4—TO BE INITIATED BY THE DONOR AND COMPLETED AS NECESSARY THEREAFTER.

PURPOSE OF CHANGE	RELEASED BY SIGNATURE	RECEIVED BY SIGNATURE	DATE
A. PROVIDE SPECIMEN FOR TESTING			
B. SHIPMENT TO LABORATORY			
C.			

COMMENTS:

Self-stick   identification
Labels for sealing specimen:

(123) (123) (123) (123)

SPECIMEN PACKAGE INTEGRITY WAS ☐ACCEPTABLE ☐UNACCEPTABLE WHEN RECEIVED IN LAB.

RECEIVER'S INITIALS

FOR OFFICE USE

© Cengage Learning 2012

FIGURE 5-8 Sample chain of custody form

Patient Instructions for 24-Hour Urine Collection

(Shaded area to be completed by laboratory)

Patient Name _____ Date _____

Test to be Performed _____

Preservative Added _____

Safety Precautions _____

_____

Once urine collection begins, store the 24-hour urine container:

☐ at room temperature   ☐ in the refrigerator

- -

Your physician has ordered a 24-hour urine test. It is important that you carefully follow these instructions:

For this test, urine is usually collected from the morning of one day until the same time the following day (for example, from 8 AM one day to 8 AM the following day).

1. To begin the collection void into the toilet as usual. DO NOT SAVE THIS URINE. Record the time and date on the collection container label as "START" time and date.

2. Collect ALL urine the next time you void, and ALL urine voided for the next 24 hours. Each time you urinate, collect the urine into a specimen container and then transfer the entire amount to the 24-hour urine container given to you.

3. At 24 hours from the time you began the test (the morning of the second day), empty your bladder and add ALL of this urine to the 24-hour container. Record the STOP date and time on the container label and bring all the urine in the collection container to the laboratory.

Additional Instructions:
- Read and follow the safety information given you for this test
- Time the test to end on a day when the laboratory is open to receive the specimen
- Keep the 24-hour urine container tightly capped during the collection period

If you have any questions about this procedure, please contact the laboratory at 555-1234.

© Cengage Learning 2012

FIGURE 5-9 Example of patient instructions for collecting a 24-hour urine specimen

Measuring Urine Volume

When a routine urinalysis is performed, the volume of the specimen is usually not recorded. However, the volume of a 24-hour urine specimen must be measured and recorded because the volume measurement is used in calculating the test results. Urine volume is measured using a large graduated cylinder, the urine is returned to its container, and the total volume is recorded on the specimen label and the accompanying requisition form.

If the 24-hour volume is unexpectedly low, the laboratory can measure the creatinine level of the urine specimen and correlate it with the urine volume. At least 1 g of creatinine should be excreted in a 24-hour period; a value less than this suggests incomplete collection.

Reference Ranges for 24-Hour Urine Volumes

The volume of urine normally excreted in 24 hours varies according to age (Table 5-7). Newborns produce between 20 and 350 mL of urine in 24 hours. By the age of 1 year, 300 to 600 mL/24 hours is normal. For 10-year-olds, the 24-hour urine volume can range from 750 to 1,500 mL. Adults produce from 750 to 2,000 mL in 24 hours, with 1200–1500 mL per day being the average.

Several factors influence urine volume. These include fluid intake, diet, time of day, fluid lost in exhalation and perspiration, hormone levels, and the status of renal and cardiac functions. Urine excretion during the day is usually three times the volume excreted at night. Excessive production of urine (over 2000 mL/24 hours) is called **polyuria**. **Oliguria** is insufficient production of urine (less than 500 mL/24 hours), and **anuria** is absence of urine production. The term **nocturia** refers to excessive production of urine at night.

TABLE 5-7. Reference ranges for 24-hour urine volumes

AGE	VOLUME (mL/24 HOURS)
Newborn	20–350
1 year	300–600
10 years	750–1,500
Adult	750–2,000

SAFETY REMINDERS

- Review Safety Precautions section.
- Observe Standard Precautions when handling urine specimens.
- Wear appropriate PPE.
- Handle preservatives with care.
- Avoid creating splashes or aerosols.

PROCEDURAL REMINDERS

- Review Quality Assessment section.
- Follow SOP manual.
- Refrigerate specimens that cannot be tested within 1 to 2 hours.
- Instruct patients in urine collection procedures.

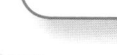

CASE STUDY 1

A hospital laboratory employee working in urinalysis received an unrefrigerated specimen for routine urinalysis at 2 PM. The collection time on the specimen label was 8:30 AM the same day.

1. What would be the appropriate action for the laboratory employee?
2. Explain your answer.

CASE STUDY 2

On Thursday morning, Mr. Strickland, a healthy-appearing 62-year-old patient, brought a 24-hour urine specimen to the laboratory. He said that he had begun the collection on Wednesday morning and had just completed collection that morning. Alice, the laboratory technician, measured the urine volume and found it to be 550 mL.

1. This 24-hour urine volume is:
   a. Within the reference range
   b. Greater than the reference range
   c. Less than the reference range
2. The correct procedure for Alice to follow is:
   a. The urine volume is acceptable; Alice should forward the urine to the chemistry department for the 24-hour test to be performed.
   b. The urine volume is suspect; Alice should question Mr. Strickland about how he collected the specimen.
   c. Alice must follow the facility's SOP manual concerning acceptance criteria for 24-hour urines.
   d. Both b and c are correct

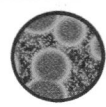

SUMMARY

The examination of a patient's urine can yield many helpful results. The quality of the test results is influenced by specimen collection, handling, transport and processing methods. Urine collection procedures can differ slightly, depending on the test to be performed. The first morning specimen is the preferred specimen for routine urinalysis. First morning, random, and clean-catch specimens should all be collected midstream; this minimizes introducing urethral and external skin contaminants into the specimen. When bacterial culture is to be performed, the urine specimen must be a clean-catch specimen. Urine for timed tests, such as the 24-hour collections required for some quantitative chemical tests, are not collected midstream.

Standard Precautions must be followed when handling urine, as with all other body fluids. Collection procedures for all urine tests are detailed in each laboratory's SOP manual and must be strictly followed. Adherence to quality assessment guidelines for specimen collection, labeling, handling, transport, and storage ensures that the laboratory receives an acceptable specimen.

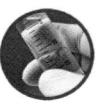

REVIEW QUESTIONS

1. Why is proper urine collection important?

2. How is a clean-catch urine collected?

3. When is a clean-catch urine required?

4. What is a midstream urine specimen? When is it the preferred specimen?

5. Describe the procedure for collecting a 24-hour urine specimen.

6. What is a nonchemical method of preserving urine?

7. Name three chemicals used to preserve urine specimens.

8. In what circumstances should urine be refrigerated? Name two advantages of refrigerating urine.

9. What is the normal 24-hour urine volume for newborns? One-year-olds? Adults?

10. How can incorrect collection of urine affect urinalysis test results?

11. Why is the first morning specimen preferred for routine urinalysis?

12. How does urine collection for drug screening differ from urine collection for routine urinalysis?

13. What PPE should be worn when handling urine specimens?

14. What is the correct method of urine specimen disposal?

15. Why might a 24-hour urine test be ordered?

16. Define anuria, clean-catch urine, midstream urine, nocturia, oliguria, polyuria, and random urine specimen.

STUDENT ACTIVITIES

1. Complete the written examination for this lesson.

2. Design cards that instruct male and female patients how to collect clean-catch urine specimens. Practice giving instructions to male and female patients for collecting clean-catch urine samples, using the patient instruction cards.

3. Practice instructing a patient in the collection of a 24-hour urine specimen.

WEB ACTIVITIES

1. Use the Internet to find information about 24-hour urine tests from web sites of hospitals or reference laboratories. Make a list of urine tests that require the following preservatives: sodium hydroxide, hydrochloric acid, sodium carbonate, and boric acid.

2. Find MSDS information for three preservatives listed in Web Activity 1. For each preservative, list the safety information that should be given to patients provided with 24-hour urine containers with these preservatives.

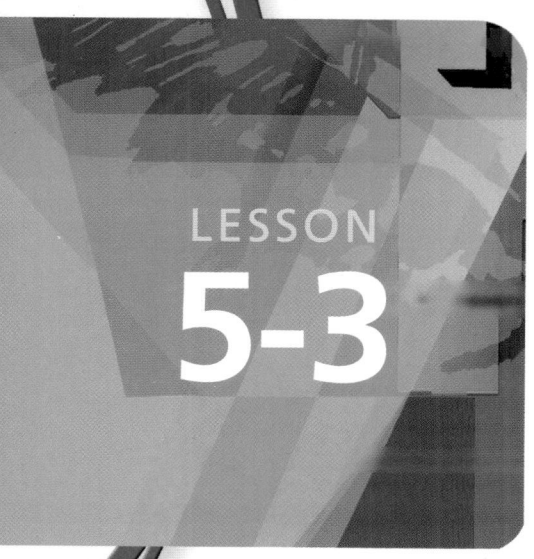

LESSON 5-3

Physical Examination of Urine

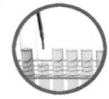

LESSON OBJECTIVES

After studying this lesson, the student will:

⊙ Name the physical characteristics of urine evaluated during a routine urinalysis.

⊙ List three causes of abnormal urine odor.

⊙ Explain why normal urine is yellow.

⊙ List three abnormal urine colors and give a cause for each.

⊙ Name two conditions that can affect the appearance or transparency of urine.

⊙ Explain factor(s) that influence urine specific gravity.

⊙ Demonstrate the use of the urinometer and refractometer.

⊙ Perform a physical examination of urine and report the results.

⊙ Discuss the safety precautions that must be observed when performing the physical examination of urine.

⊙ Explain the importance of quality assessment in the physical examination of urine.

⊙ Define the glossary terms.

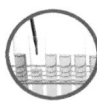

GLOSSARY

amorphous / without definite shape

amorphous phosphates / granular crystals without uniform shape that can form in alkaline urine, give urine sediment a whitish appearance after centrifugation, and appear clear microscopically

amorphous urates / granular crystals without uniform shape that can form in acid urine, can give urine sediment a pink appearance after centrifugation and appear yellowish microscopically

hematuria / the presence of blood in the urine

hemoglobinuria / the presence of hemoglobin in the urine

ketones / a group of chemical substances produced during increased fat metabolism; ketone bodies

maple syrup urine disease (MSUD) / a rare metabolic condition in which the amino acids leucine, isoleucine, and valine are not metabolized, causing the urine to have the odor of maple syrup

melanin / a dark pigment of skin, hair, and certain tumors

mucus / a substance secreted by cells lining the urethra and vagina and that can be present in urine

myoglobin / a pigmented, oxygen-carrying protein found in muscle tissue

opalescent / having a milky iridescence

(continues)

phenylketonuria (PKU) / an inherited condition in which the amino acid phenylalanine is not metabolized, but is excreted into the urine and causes urine to have a mousy or musty odor

porphyrins / a group of light-sensitive, pigmented, ringed chemical structures that are required for the synthesis of hemoglobin

refractive index / the ratio of the speed of light in air to the speed of light in a solution

refractometer / an instrument for measuring the refractive index of a substance; also called a total solids meter

specific gravity (sp. gr.) / the ratio of the weight of a solution to the weight of an equal volume of distilled water; a measurement of density

turbid / having a cloudy appearance

urinometer / a float with a calibrated stem used for measuring specific gravity of urine; hydrometer

urochrome / the yellow pigment that gives urine its color

INTRODUCTION

A routine urinalysis consists of three parts—the physical, chemical, and microscopic examinations. This lesson covers the physical examination; the chemical and microscopic examinations are covered in Lessons 5-4 and 5-5. An example of a laboratory requisition and report form for a routine urinalysis is shown in Figure 5-10.

The physical examination is the first part of the urinalysis performed and includes observing and reporting urine color, transparency, and specific gravity. The physical examination of urine is the first part of the routine urinalysis and can be performed while the urine specimen is being prepared for the rest of the urinalysis procedure.

PHYSICAL CHARACTERISTICS OF URINE

The physical characteristics of urine evaluated and recorded during urinalysis are color, transparency or clarity, and specific gravity. Urine odor is not typically reported. However, unusual urine odors can lead the technician to investigate the reason for the odor.

Urine Color

The normal color of urine ranges from pale yellow to amber (Table 5-8). The pigment that produces the normal yellow-to-amber color of urine is **urochrome**. As the urine concentration varies, the color intensity will change. Dilute urine samples are almost colorless, pale yellow, or straw-colored; more concentrated urine samples are darker yellow or amber. Variations in urine color can also be caused by diet, medications, physical activity, and disease (Table 5-9). Urine color can sometimes provide a clue to certain diseases or conditions.

Dark Amber Urine

Dark amber urine can be due to several causes. Urine of high specific gravity is often a dark amber color. Other causes of dark amber urine include the presence of bilirubin, certain drugs such as nitrofurantoin, and supplements such as large doses of vitamin A.

Red Urine

The abnormal color seen most frequently in urine is red or red-brown. **Hematuria**, the presence of blood, can cause urine to be cloudy red, sometimes described as "smoky." Clear red urine can be due to **hemoglobinuria**, the presence of hemoglobin from lysed red blood cells. The presence of **myoglobin**, a pigmented oxygen-carrying protein found in muscle tissue, can also cause urine to appear red. Acidic urine causes hemoglobin and myoglobin to form a red-brown color. **Porphyrins**, molecules that are building blocks of the heme portion of hemoglobin, can cause the urine to be red or wine-red, sometimes called port-wine colored.

Brown or Black Urine

Brown-black urine can be caused by the presence of hemoglobin that has become oxidized to form methemoglobin in acidic urine that has been standing. The presence of **melanin**, a dark pigment, will also cause urine to become dark or black on standing. Melanin can be present in the urine of patients with advanced metastatic melanoma, a tumor of melanin-producing cells. Homogentisic acid can also cause a brown-black color to form in urine that has been standing. Homogentisic acid is present in urine in *alkaptonuria*, an inborn error of metabolism in which the body cannot metabolize certain amino acids, causing homogentisic acid to accumulate in the blood, tissue, and urine.

Yellow-Brown or Green-Brown Urine

Bilirubin, biliverdin, or other bile pigments can cause urine to be dark yellow-brown or yellow-green. Urine specimens containing these substances can form a yellow-green foam when shaken. Bilirubin can be present in the urine of patients with hepatitis or certain other liver disorders.

Urine Transparency (Clarity)

Normal urine is usually clear or transparent immediately after voiding (Table 5-8). Clear urine usually has normal microscopic results; abnormalities in a clear specimen are usually detected in the chemical examination.

Urine that is **turbid** or cloudy can be due to normal or abnormal conditions (Table 5-10). The cause of a cloudy or turbid urine specimen usually becomes evident during the microscopic examination. As normal, recently voided urine reaches room temperature, or after refrigeration, it can become cloudy. Depending on the urine pH, this cloudiness can be due to **amorphous urate** or **amorphous phosphate** crystals. The presence of **mucus**, secretions from the genitourinary tract, can also cause urine to have a cloudy or hazy appearance. Amorphous crystals or mucus in urine are common findings with no clinical significance and can be confirmed as a cause of cloudy urine when the microscopic examination is performed.

Tri-Cities Family Health Clinic
Urinalysis Laboratory Request Form

Patient _____ Date_____

Age_____   Gender: M ____ F ____

Ordering Physician_____

☐ Routine Urinalysis with Microscopic
☐ Dipstick Urinalysis
☐ Urine Culture and Sensitivity
☐ Other _____

Specimen Collection Time _____   ☐ a.m.   ☐ p.m.
Laboratory Log-in Time   _____   ☐ a.m.   ☐ p.m.

Results		**Reference**
Color	_____	yellow to amber
Transparency	_____	clear
Specific Gravity	_____	1.010-1.025

Dipstick:

Glucose	_____	negative
Bilirubin	_____	negative
Ketone	_____	negative
Blood	_____	negative
pH	_____	5.0-8.0
Protein	_____	negative-trace
Urobilinogen	_____	0-1.0 mg/dL
Nitrite	_____	negative
Leukocyte	_____	negative

Microscopic:

WBC/HPF	_____	
RBC/HPF	_____	0-4
Epith. Cells	_____	occas, squamous
Casts	_____	occas, hyaline
Bacteria	_____	none
Mucus	_____	0 to 2+
Amorphous Sediment	_____	
Crystals	_____	
Type	_____	
Other	_____	

Tech: _____
Date: _____
Time: _____

© Cengage Learning 2012

FIGURE 5-10 Example of a urinalysis request and report form

TABLE 5-8. Physical characteristics of normal adult urine

PHYSICAL CHARACTERISTIC	REFERENCE VALUE
Transparency	Clear
Color	Pale yellow to amber
Specific gravity	1.010 to 1.025 (adult)

TABLE 5-9. Abnormal urine colors and their cause

COLORS CAUSED BY DIET OR MEDICATIONS

COLOR	CAUSE
Red	Beets, rhubarb (in alkaline urine)
Yellow-orange	Carrots, vitamins, some antibiotics
Green, blue-green	Drugs such as amitriptyline
Brown-black	Methyldopa, metronidazole

COLORS CAUSED BY DISEASE STATES

COLOR	CAUSE
Red, red-brown	Red blood cells, hemoglobin, myoglobin
Wine-red	Porphyrins
Brown-black	Melanin, homogentisic acid, hemoglobin (in acid urine)
Dark yellow-brown or green-brown	Bilirubin, bile pigments

TABLE 5-10. Conditions affecting the transparency of urine

NORMAL URINES

TRANSPARENCY	CAUSES
Hazy	Mucus (females), talcum powder, squamous epithelial cells
Cloudy	Amorphous phosphates, amorphous urates

ABNORMAL URINES

TRANSPARENCY	CAUSES
Cloudy-red	Red blood cells
Turbid or cloudy	White blood cells, bacteria, yeasts, renal epithelial cells, lipids
Opalescent, milky	Excess lipids (fats)

Turbidity in a fresh urine sample can be an indication of disease. Common causes of turbidity in recently voided urine are increased numbers of white blood cells, red blood cells, epithelial cells, or bacteria. If a significant amount of red blood cells is present, the urine can appear cloudy and red. Excess fats or lipids can cause urine to appear **opalescent** (milky).

Specific Gravity

The **specific gravity (sp. gr.)** of a solution is the ratio of the weight of the solution compared to the weight of an equal volume of distilled water at the same temperature. Stated another way, the specific gravity is the density of a solution compared to the density of distilled water, which is 1.000.

The range of specific gravity for normal urine is 1.010 to 1.025 (Table 5-8). Specific gravity is highest in the first morning specimen, which usually has a specific gravity greater than 1.020. The specific gravity of urine estimates the concentration of solutes such as urea, phosphates, chlorides, proteins, and sugars in the urine. Specific gravity is an indicator of renal tubular function; it is used to assess the ability of the kidneys to reabsorb essential chemicals and water from the glomerular filtrate.

More concentrated urines, those with higher specific gravities, are usually darker in color than urines with low specific gravity. Patients who become dehydrated as a result of excessive sweating, diarrhea, or vomiting can have concentrated urine with high specific gravity. High urine specific gravity can also be caused by decreased blood flow to the kidneys, such as in heart failure.

Urines from healthy infants have low specific gravity because the kidneys have not matured sufficiently to concentrate urine. Neonate urine should have a specific gravity of about 1.003.

Urine Odor

Normal, recently voided urine has a characteristic aromatic and not unpleasant odor. Changes in urine odor can be due to disease, diet, or the presence of microorganisms. Although urine odor is not reported on the urinalysis form, it is a noticeable property that can give valuable information and alert the technologist to possible abnormalities or improper handling of the urine specimen.

The odor of urine from a person with uncontrolled diabetes is described as fruity. This is due to the presence of **ketones**, products of fat metabolism. This fruity odor can also be present in urine from an individual following a strict high-protein diet.

Metabolic diseases other than diabetes can also cause an unusual urine odor. **Phenylketonuria (PKU)**, an inherited condition in which the amino acid phenylalanine is not metabolized, causes urine to have a mousy or musty odor. All newborns are tested for PKU because mental retardation will result if the condition is allowed to go untreated. **Maple syrup urine disease (MSUD)** is a rare metabolic condition in which the amino acids leucine, isoleucine, and valine are not metabolized. The condition is named because urine has the odor of maple syrup. This condition is evident in the first weeks of life in affected infants.

If urine is allowed to remain unrefrigerated for a few hours, any bacteria present can multiply and break down urea to form ammonia; the resulting urine odor is similar to ammonia.

A recently voided sample of urine with a foul, pungent odor suggests urinary tract infection.

Foods such as garlic and asparagus can also produce an abnormal urine odor. Although urine odor can be striking in certain instances, odor alone is not a reliable enough characteristic to use in making a diagnosis.

Reference Values

Freshly voided urine is normally clear, pale yellow to amber in color, and has a specific gravity between 1.010 and 1.025. Some laboratories have a policy of not performing the microscopic examination of urine when a urine sample is yellow, clear, and the specific gravity and chemical results are normal. Table 5-8 lists the physical characteristics of normal adult urine.

PERFORMING A PHYSICAL EXAMINATION OF URINE

The laboratory's standard operating procedure (SOP) manual will contain instructions for the routine urinalysis procedure, including quality assessment (QA) methods, specimen collection, handling and processing, testing, and reporting results.

Safety Precautions

 Standard Precautions must be observed when handling urine and all other body fluids. Appropriate personal protective equipment (PPE) must be worn. Infectious agents such as the hepatitis virus can be present in urine, so all urine specimens must be handled with caution to prevent possible exposure of laboratory personnel. Urine specimens often require more handling than other laboratory specimens, such as swirling to mix and pouring. If a face shield is not available, the technician should work behind an acrylic safety shield to prevent splashes to the eyes or other mucus membranes.

Specimens can be discarded in a sink, followed by rinsing with water and disinfectant, but the creation of aerosols or splashes must be avoided. Reusable equipment must be disinfected with surface disinfectant and then washed after each use. Refractometers should be disinfected by placing a drop or two of surface disinfectant on the surfaces of the glass plate and cover, rinsing with a drop of water, and wiping dry. The work area should be disinfected frequently.

Quality Assessment

   Adherence to a comprehensive QA program ensures that the results from urine tests are reliable. Only specimens meeting the specimen acceptance criteria in the SOP manual should be accepted for testing. Specimens that cannot be tested within 1 to 2 hours after collection can be refrigerated for up to 4 hours. Before testing, urine samples should be allowed to reach ambient temperature (21° to 25°C) and should be mixed well by gentle swirling.

Refractometers and urinometers must be checked at specified intervals with distilled water (specific gravity, 1.000) and control solutions, and the results should be documented. If the specific gravity of distilled water does not read 1.000, the refractometer should be adjusted using the adjustable set screw. Refractometer accuracy must also be checked at specified intervals with solutions of known specific gravity such as 5% NaCl (1.022), and urine control solutions (such as KOVA-Refractrol SP), and the results documented.

Specimen Requirements

The preferred specimen for routine urinalysis is a recently voided, first morning midstream specimen. Random specimens are also acceptable. Physical characteristics are best observed by examining a urine sample immediately after voiding before the sample is refrigerated. Because some urine components are volatile, labile, or light-sensitive, specimens should remain tightly covered and in the dark until tested.

Procedure

The room temperature urine specimen is mixed well by gentle swirling, a portion is poured into a clear tube, and the urine color and transparency are observed and recorded. The specific gravity of the urine is measured, and the urine is then prepared for chemical and microscopic examination.

Color and Transparency

Urine color is observed and recorded. The urine should be observed for transparency (clarity) using good light. Transparency is usually reported as clear, hazy (slightly cloudy), cloudy (turbid), or milky (opalescent).

Specific Gravity

Specific gravity can be measured with a urinometer (Figure 5-11), refractometer (Figure 5-12), or reagent strip. The urinometer method requires 20 to 50 mL of urine, depending on the size of the urinometer. The refractometer method uses only a drop of urine. The procedure for measurement of specific gravity with a reagent strip is included in Lesson 5-4, Chemical Examination of Urine.

Urinometer Method. Well-mixed urine is poured into a special glass cylinder, and the **urinometer**, a weighted float with a calibrated stem, is placed into the urine with a slight spinning motion. The specific gravity is read at the urine's meniscus on the float's stem (Figure 5-11). The urinometer will float high in a concentrated sample (high sp. gr.) and will sink lower in a dilute sample (low sp. gr.). Disadvantages of this method are the large urine volume required and the need to disinfect, wash, and dry the cylinder and urinometer after each use.

Refractometer Method. A **refractometer**, also called a *total solids meter* (TS meter), measures specific gravity optically by measuring the **refractive index** of the urine. The refractive index is the ratio of the speed of light in air to the speed of light in a solution. To use the refractometer, 1 drop of well-mixed urine is placed on the glass plate and the cover is gently closed (Figure 5-13). While looking through the ocular, the specific gravity is read directly from a scale that converts refraction to specific gravity (Figure 5-14).

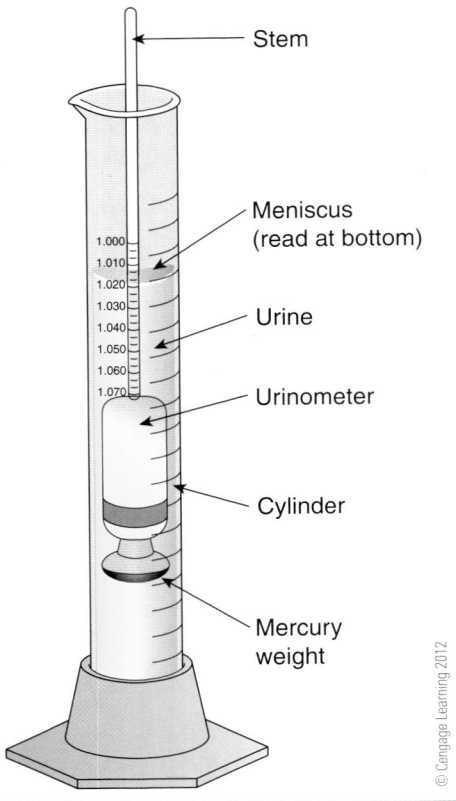

FIGURE 5-11 Urinometer used for specific gravity measurement

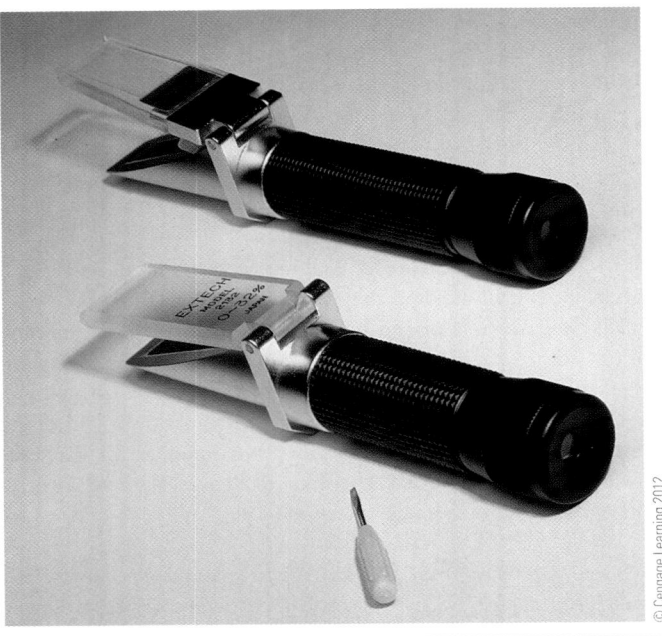

FIGURE 5-12 Refractometers and calibration tool

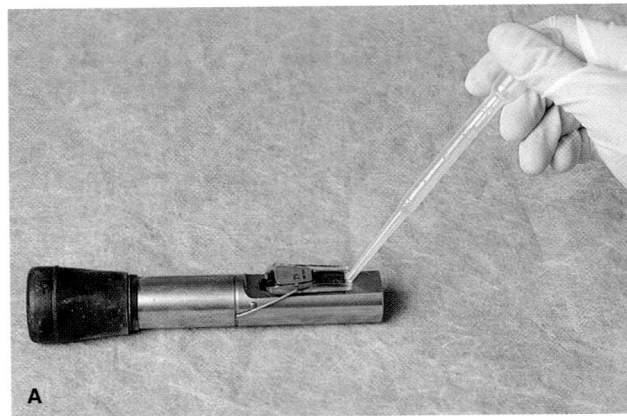

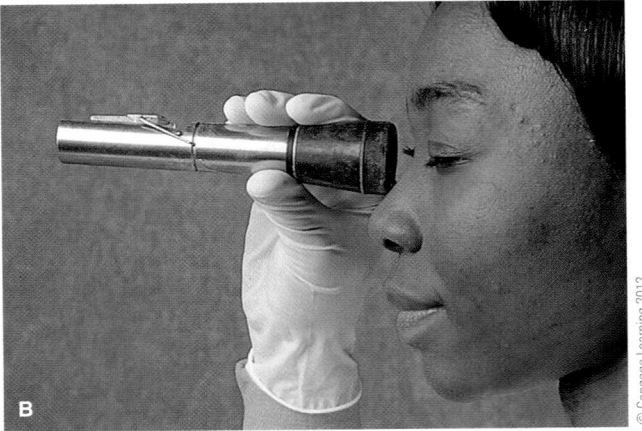

FIGURE 5-13 Measuring specific gravity using the refractometer: (A) a drop of urine is placed on the glass plate; (B) the technician looks through the eyepiece to view the scale

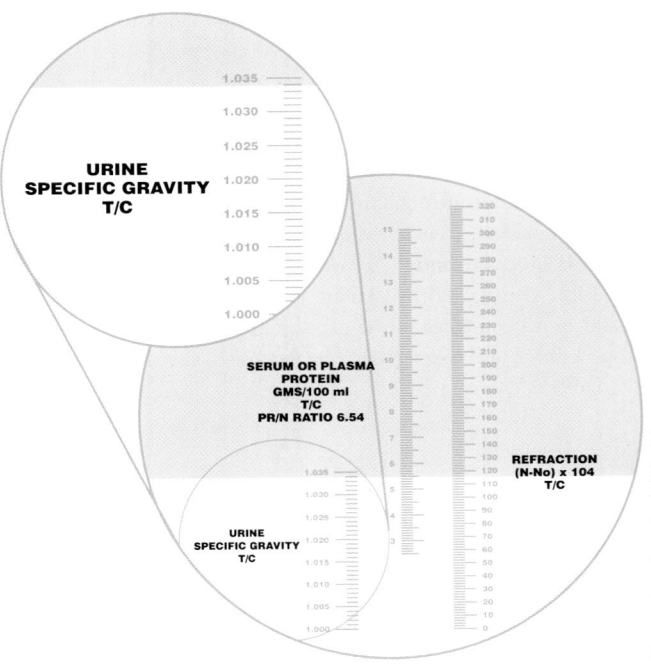

FIGURE 5-14 Refractometer scale showing a specific gravity reading of 1.034. The small scale (lower left and shown enlarged at upper left) is used to read urine specific gravity

SAFETY REMINDERS

- Review Safety Precautions section before beginning procedure.
- Observe Standard Precautions.
- Wear appropriate PPE.
- Disinfect equipment and work area.
- Avoid creating splashes or aerosols.

PROCEDURAL REMINDERS

- Review Quality Assessment section before beginning procedure.
- Follow instructions in SOP manual.
- Mix urine before testing.
- Test urines at room temperature.
- Test refractometer daily with distilled water and urine controls.

CASE STUDY 1

A urine specimen from a 48-year-old woman was received in the urinalysis laboratory at 9 AM. The specimen label indicated the urine was collected that morning at 8:30 AM, and the laboratory log-in time was 8:46 AM. While preparing the specimen for urinalysis, the technician noticed that the urine had a strong, unpleasant odor and was very cloudy.

1. Discuss the possible cause(s) of this finding.
2. What is the appropriate action of the laboratory technician?

CASE STUDY 2

A urine specimen submitted from a patient suffering from severe vomiting and diarrhea was a dark amber color.

1. This color is most likely due to:
   a. Myoglobin in the urine
   b. Bilirubin in the urine
   c. High specific gravity of the urine
   d. White blood cells in the urine
2. Explain your answer.

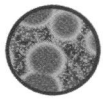

SUMMARY

The physical examination of urine includes reporting the color, transparency, and specific gravity of urine. The results of the physical examination of urine often confirm or explain chemical or microscopic results. Although abnormalities in the physical characteristics of urine can provide significant clues to renal or metabolic disease, variations in characteristics such as color or transparency do not always reflect pathological changes. Sometimes variations seen in normal urine can be caused by incorrect handling of the specimen, such as improper storage temperature or delay in examination. Standard Precautions must be observed when performing the physical examinations of urine. Quality assessment procedures must be performed as specified in the SOP manual.

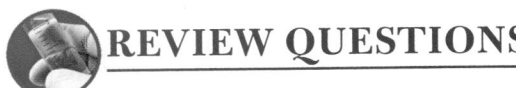

REVIEW QUESTIONS

1. What observations are included in the physical examination of urine?

2. Name three metabolic conditions in which abnormal urine odor can occur.

3. If a urine specimen smells like ammonia, what should be suspected?

4. What gives urine its normal color?

5. Name four abnormal urine colors and list a possible cause for each.

6. What is the normal transparency of urine?

7. What are three causes of cloudy urine?

8. What is the normal specific gravity of urine?

9. What kidney function is reflected by urine specific gravity?

10. Which physical characteristic of urine is not usually reported on the urinalysis report form?

11. What type of urine specimen is preferred for examining physical characteristics?

12. How can handling and storage of urine specimens influence the results of physical tests?

13. What two things should be done before testing a specimen that has been refrigerated?

14. What safety precautions should be observed when performing urine tests?

15. Define amorphous, amorphous phosphates, amorphous urates, hematuria, hemoglobinuria, ketones, maple syrup urine disease, melanin, mucus, myoglobin, opalescent, phenylketonuria, porphyrins, refractive index, refractometer, specific gravity, turbid, urinometer, and urochrome.

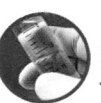

STUDENT ACTIVITIES

1. Complete the written examination for this lesson.

2. Practice performing physical examinations of several urine specimens as outlined in the Student Performance Guide, using the worksheet.

3. Obtain several urine specimens. Compare the specific gravities of lighter-colored urines with those of darker-colored urines.

4. Divide a urine sample. Put one part in the refrigerator; place the other part on the counter at room temperature. Observe each for transparency changes and odor changes at the end of 1 hour, 2 hours, 4 hours, or more.

WEB ACTIVITY

Use the Internet to find information on hyposthenuria, isosthenuria, and diabetes insipidus. Explain the cause of each of the conditions and report on the expected urine specific gravity in each of the conditions.

(Individual student results will differ depending on specimens provided by instructor.)

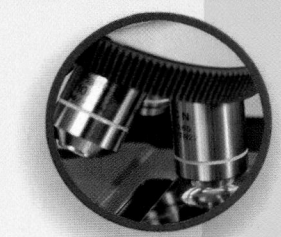

Name _____   Date _____

INSTRUCTIONS

1. Practice performing the physical examination of urine following the step-by-step procedure and using the worksheet.

2. Demonstrate the procedure for the physical examination of urine satisfactorily for the instructor, using the Student Performance Guide. Your instructor will explain the procedures for evaluating and grading your performance. Your performance may be given a number grade, letter grade, or satisfactory (S) or unsatisfactory (U) depending on course or institutional policy.

NOTE: Consult manufacturers' directions before using instruments or performing tests.

MATERIALS AND EQUIPMENT

- gloves
- hand antiseptic
- full-face shield (or equivalent PPE)
- acrylic safety shield (optional)
- clear plastic conical centrifuge tubes with caps, 15 mL capacity
- test tube rack
- recently collected urine specimens
- disposable transfer pipets
- refractometer and/or urinometer
- distilled water for calibrating refractometer
- reagent grade water for reconstituting controls
- urine controls, normal and abnormal levels
- pipets, or micropipetter with disposable tips (for reconstituting controls)
- worksheet
- laboratory tissue
- paper towels
- surface disinfectant (such as 10% chlorine bleach)
- biohazard container
- sharps container

PROCEDURE

Record in the comment section any problems encountered while practicing the procedure (or have a fellow student or the instructor evaluate your performance).

S = Satisfactory
U = Unsatisfactory

You must:	S	U	Evaluation/Comments
1. Wash hands with antiseptic and put on gloves and face protection (if not wearing face protection, work behind acrylic safety shield)			
2. Assemble equipment and materials			
3. Obtain a recently collected urine specimen. If specimen has been refrigerated, allow it to reach room temperature before proceeding			
4. Record specimen ID on the worksheet			

(Continues)

© 2012 Delmar, Cengage Learning. Permission to reproduce for clinical use granted.

You must:	S	U	Evaluation/Comments
5. Mix urine by gentle swirling and pour approximately 10 mL into a clear, conical centrifuge tube			
6. Observe the color of the urine and record on the worksheet			
7. Observe and record the transparency of the urine			
8. Note the odor of the urine; if unusual, record in the comment section of the worksheet			
9. Measure specific gravity using the refractometer:			

a. Place 1 drop of distilled water on the glass plate of the refractometer and close gently
   b. Look through the ocular and read the specific gravity from the scale. For water, the specific gravity should read 1.000; if it does not, calibrate the refractometer with the screwdriver provided
   c. Disinfect the refractometer glass plate and cover, rinse with 1 or 2 drops of water, and dry with laboratory tissue
   d. Place 1 drop of normal urine control solution on the plate and close gently
   e. Look through the ocular and read the specific gravity from the scale
   f. Record the control value on the worksheet and compare the result with the accepted range for the urine control
   g. Repeat steps 9c-9f using the abnormal urine control
   h. Test patient urine following steps 9c-9e and record the results on the worksheet
   i. Clean the glass plate with surface disinfectant, rinse, and dry with a laboratory tissue			

10. Repeat physical examination of additional urine specimens, if available, following steps 4-9			

11. Measure specific gravity using the urinometer (if urinometer is not available, go to step 11):
   a. Fill urinometer cylinder approximately three-fourths full with distilled water
   b. Insert urinometer with gentle spinning motion
   c. Read the specific gravity at the meniscus on the stem of the urinometer when it stops spinning and record (specific gravity of water should be 1.000)
   d. Rinse and dry equipment with laboratory tissue; repeat steps 10a–10c using a urine specimen and record the result
   e. Disinfect, rinse and dry urinometer and cylinder			

12. Discard urine specimen(s) as instructed			
13. Disinfect and clean all equipment and return to proper storage			

© 2012 Delmar, Cengage Learning. Permission to reproduce for clinical use granted.

You must:	S	U	Evaluation/Comments
14. Discard contaminated materials into appropriate sharps or biohazard container			
15. Clean work area with disinfectant			
16. Remove gloves and discard into biohazard container			
17. Wash hands with antiseptic			

Instructor/Evaluator Comments:

Instructor/Evaluator _____ Date _____

© 2012 Delmar, Cengage Learning. Permission to reproduce for clinical use granted.

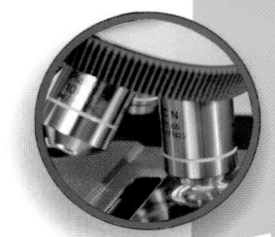

LESSON 5-3
Physical Examination of Urine

(Individual student results will differ depending on the specimens provided by the instructor.)

   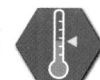

Name _____   Date _____

Specimen I.D. _____

OBSERVATION	PATIENT RESULTS	NORMAL CONTROL	ABNORMAL CONTROL	REFERENCE VALUES
Transparency (appearance)				
clear	_____	_____	_____	clear
hazy (slightly cloudy)	_____	_____	_____	
cloudy (turbid)	_____	_____	_____	
milky (opalescent)	_____	_____	_____	
other	_____	_____	_____	
Color:	_____	_____	_____	pale yellow to amber
Specific gravity:	_____	_____	_____	1.010–1.025

Comments: _____

_____

Date _____	**Normal Control**	**Abnormal Control**
Time _____	**Lot No.** _____	**Lot No.** _____
	Exp. Date _____	**Exp. Date** _____

© 2012 Delmar, Cengage Learning. Permission to reproduce for clinical use granted.

WORKSHEET

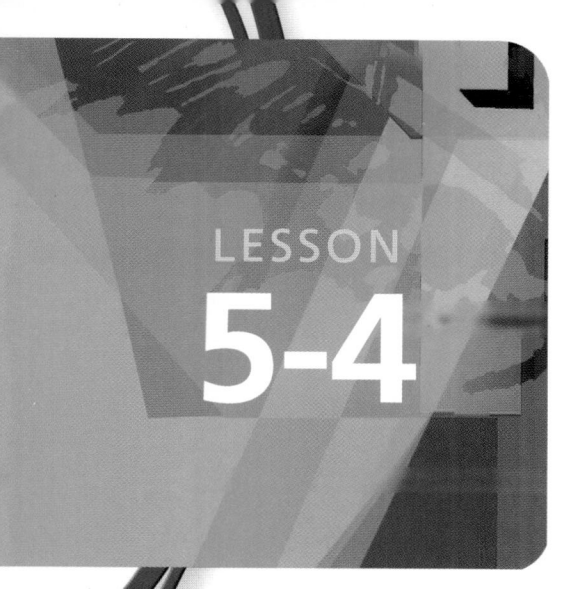

Chemical Examination of Urine

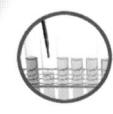

LESSON OBJECTIVES

After studying this lesson, the student will:

- ⊙ Explain the specimen requirement for the chemical examination of urine.
- ⊙ List 10 urine chemical tests routinely performed by reagent strip, explain the principle of each, and give the reference values for each.
- ⊙ Name a condition that can cause an abnormal result for each of the chemical tests routinely performed on urine.
- ⊙ Perform a chemical examination of urine using a reagent strip and report the results.
- ⊙ Perform the copper reduction test on urine.
- ⊙ Perform confirmatory tests for protein, ketones, and bilirubin in urine.
- ⊙ Correlate results of the physical examination of urine with those of the chemical examination.
- ⊙ Discuss the safety precautions that must be observed when performing chemical testing of urine.
- ⊙ Explain the importance of quality assessment in the chemical examination of urine.
- ⊙ Define the glossary terms.

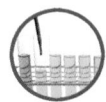

GLOSSARY

albumin / the most abundant protein in normal plasma; a homogeneous group of plasma proteins that are made in the liver and help maintain osmotic balance

bilirubin / a product formed in the liver from the breakdown of hemoglobin

chromogen / a substance that becomes colored when it undergoes a chemical change

galactosuria / the presence of galactose in the urine; the condition in which galactose is excreted into the urine

globulins / a heterogeneous group of serum proteins with varied functions

glycosuria / glucose in the urine; glucosuria

hematuria / the presence of blood in the urine

hemoglobinuria / the presence of hemoglobin in urine

ketones / a group of chemical substances produced during increased fat metabolism; ketone bodies

ketonuria / ketones in the urine

microalbumin / a small amount of albumin in urine that is not detectable by routine reagent strip

microalbuminuria / condition in which small amounts of albumin are present in the urine but are not detectable by routine reagent strip

proteinuria / protein in the urine, usually albumin

(continues)

specific gravity (sp. gr.) / the ratio of the weight of a solution to the weight of an equal volume of distilled water; a measurement of density

urobilinogen / breakdown product of bilirubin formed by the action of intestinal bacteria

INTRODUCTION

The chemical examination of urine can be performed using reagent strips, single-use narrow plastic strips with several reagent pads attached. Reagent strip analysis is also called biochemical, analyte, or "dipstick" analysis of urine. Before the development of reagent strip technology, these chemical tests had to be performed individually using time-consuming manual methods.

A single reagent strip can test for as many as 10 different substances; other types of test for only one or two substances or analytes. Strips used in routine urinalysis usually include tests for acid–base balance (pH), protein, bilirubin, blood, nitrite, ketones, urobilinogen, glucose, leukocyte esterase, and specific gravity.

Chemical testing by reagent strip is part of a routine urinalysis but can also be ordered separately, without the urine physical and microscopic examinations. Chemical analysis of urine by reagent strip method is a CLIA-waived procedure. The urine chemical test results can be an aid to diagnosis. The results of chemical analysis of urine provide information on the patient's carbohydrate metabolism, kidney and liver function, and pH balance.

This lesson presents the principles and methods of chemical analysis of urine using reagent strips. Procedures for performing the test for reducing sugars and confirmatory tests for protein, ketones, and bilirubin are also given. The urine microscopic examination is covered in Lesson 5-5.

PRINCIPLES OF URINE CHEMICAL TESTS

Each reagent pad on a reagent strip contains the chemicals required for a specific chemical reaction. Reagent strips are available in a variety of types. Two common brands of urine reagent strips are the Multistix line (Siemens Medical, formerly Bayer Corp.) and Chemstrip line (Roche Diagnostics Corp.), shown in Figure 5-15.

Reagent strips are used by dipping the strip into urine and observing chemical reactions on each reagent pad within a specified time. The chemicals within the reagent pads react rapidly with substances in the urine causing color changes in the pads. Color and timing guides for interpreting results are specific for each brand or type of strip and are provided by each reagent strip manufacturer (Figure 5-16).

In routine urinalysis, the reagent strips commonly used test 10 parameters:

- Glucose
- Bilirubin
- Ketones
- Blood

- pH
- Protein
- Urobilinogen
- Nitrite
- Leukocyte esterase
- Specific gravity

Basic principles of the biochemical reactions involved in each of these 10 tests are discussed briefly in this section. However, because reagent strip manufacturers can use different biochemical detection methods in their strips, the manufacturer's instructions must be consulted for specific chemical principles, correct procedure, and possible interferences for the test strip being used.

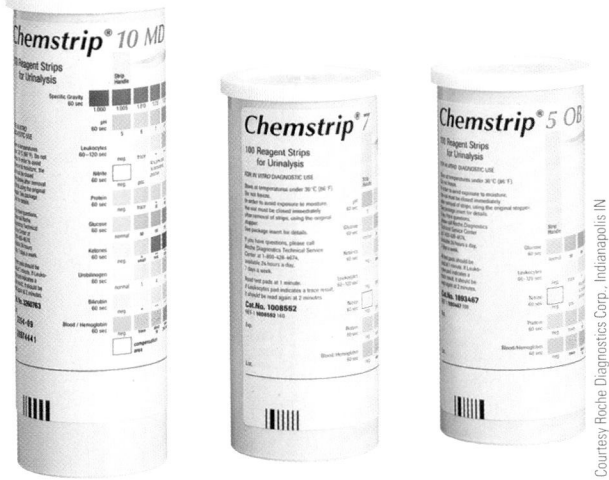

FIGURE 5-15 Chemstrip urine reagent strip vials showing color charts

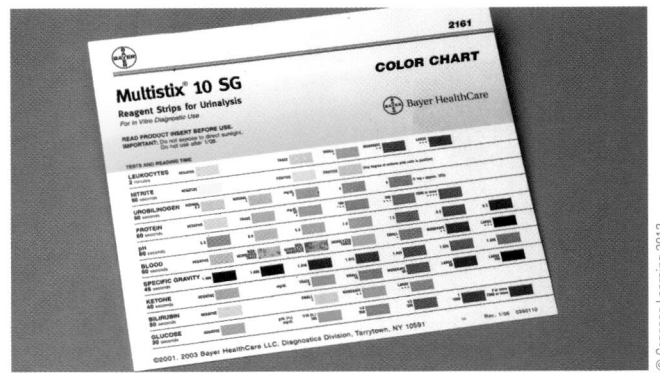

FIGURE 5-16 Bayer Multistix 10 SG reagent strip color chart

Glucose

The presence of detectable glucose in urine is called glycosuria and indicates that the blood glucose level has exceeded the renal threshold for glucose (160 to 180 mg/dL). This condition can occur in diabetes mellitus and gestational diabetes. The presence of glucose in urine can be an indication that diabetes is not being well controlled.

The reagent strip is specific for glucose and will not react with other sugars. The glucose reagent pad contains the enzymes glucose oxidase and peroxidase plus a **chromogen**, a substance that produces a color in the chemical reaction. The enzymes react with glucose in the urine to change the color of the reagent pad. The intensity of the color formed is proportional to the glucose concentration. Normal urine is negative for glucose by the reagent strip method.

Bilirubin

TURNS URINE DARK COLOR

Bilirubin is the primary bile pigment. Bilirubin is a hemoglobin breakdown product formed in the liver from senescent (old) red blood cells. When bilirubin is present in urine, it can indicate liver disease, bile duct obstruction, or hepatitis. The test for bilirubin is based on coupling bilirubin with a diazonium salt in the reagent pad to form a purple-brown color. Direct light causes decomposition of bilirubin, so specimens should be protected from light until testing is completed to prevent false-negative results. A positive reagent strip bilirubin test should be followed by the Ictotest, which is more sensitive and has fewer interferences. Normal urine contains no detectable bilirubin by the reagent strip method.

Ketones

When the body burns fat rather than sugar for energy, a group of molecules collectively called **ketones are produced**. Ketones are a mixture of acetone, acetoacetic acid (also called diacetic acid), and beta-hydroxybutyric acid. In uncontrolled diabetes, starvation, or prolonged dieting or fasting, ketones are excreted into the urine, a condition called **ketonuria**. The ketones reagent strip pad is more sensitive for acetoacetic acid than acetone; beta-hydroxybutyric acid is not detected.

The ketone test is based on the reaction of ketones with sodium nitroprusside in the ketone reagent pad, causing a dark pink to maroon color to form. Because ketones evaporate at room temperature, urine should be kept tightly capped and refrigerated if it cannot be tested promptly. Normal urine is negative for ketones when tested by reagent strip.

Blood

CAN BE WHOLE OR Hemoglobin

The presence of blood in the urine is called **hematuria**. **Hemoglobinuria** is a more specific term referring to the presence in urine of hemoglobin from lysed red blood cells. Hematuria can occur in conditions such as infection, bleeding in the kidneys, glomerular damage, tumor in the urinary tract, or trauma to the urinary tract from surgery or catheter insertion. Blood cells can also contaminate urine as a result of menstruation.

The blood reagent pad detects both intact red blood cells and free hemoglobin from lysed red cells. Myoglobin will also cause a positive reaction. In the presence of blood, a color forms because of the peroxidase-like action of hemoglobin in the red blood cells reacting with chromogen and peroxide in the reagent pad. The resulting color ranges from orange through green to dark blue and the degree of color change is proportional to the amount of blood present. Intact red blood cells can cause a spotty appearance on the reagent pad. Normal urine is negative for blood by reagent strip method.

pH

The pH is a measure of the degree of acidity or alkalinity of the urine. A pH below 7.0 indicates acid urine; a pH above 7.0 indicates alkaline urine. The pH of urine is affected by diet, medications, kidney disease, and metabolic diseases such as diabetes mellitus. Urine samples from individuals on vegetarian diets usually have alkaline pH. Indicator dyes such as methyl red and bromothymol blue in the pH reagent pad form colors from yellow-orange for acid urine to green-blue for alkaline urine. Normal, recently voided urine has a pH range of 5.0 to 8.0; first morning specimens should have an acid pH (5.0 to 6.0).

Protein

EXERCISE can increase

The condition in which an increased amount of protein is present in the urine is called **proteinuria**. Proteinuria is an important indicator of renal disease. Proteinuria can be caused by urinary tract infection, commonly called UTI, and can also occur following vigorous exercise. Positive tests for protein in urine are due to the presence of **albumin**, the most abundant plasma protein. Because the protein reagent pad is not a good detector of **globulins**, the protein sulfosalicylic acid turbidity test, discussed later in this lesson, should be used to detect proteins other than albumin.

The reagent strip test for protein is based on the principle that proteins can alter the color of some acid–base indicator dyes without changing the pH. This reaction has been called "the protein error of indicators." The protein reagent pad is kept at pH 3.0 by incorporating a buffering dye such as tetrabromophenol blue. At the constant acid pH, the development of any green color on the reagent pad is due to the presence of protein (albumin) and is usually reported using a plus system (neg, trace, 1+, 2+, 3+, 4+). Colors range from yellow for negative to yellow-green or green for positive, depending on the amount of protein present. Rarely, a highly alkaline urine can produce a false positive protein test, because the alkaline urine pH can neutralize the acid pH in the reagent pad. Normal urine is negative or contains just a trace of protein by the reagent strip method.

Urobilinogen

Urobilinogen is a bilirubin degradation product that is formed by the action of intestinal bacteria. Urobilinogen can be increased in hepatic disease or hemolytic disease. The urobilinogen reagent strip test, based on the Ehrlich aldehyde reaction, contains

or liver damage

chemicals that react with urobilinogen to form a pink-red color. Urobilinogen is unstable in acidic urine and when exposed to light; therefore exposure to light or delay in testing can cause a false negative result. The reagent strip method can detect urobilinogen in concentrations as low as 0.1 mg/dL (0.1 Ehrlich unit [EU]). The reference range for urine urobilinogen by the reagent strip method is 0.0 to 1.0 mg/dL (or 0.0 to 1.0 EU/dL).

Nitrite

Gram-negative bacteria produce enzymes that convert urinary nitrate, a normal urine constituent, to nitrite. Nitrite reacts with chemicals in the nitrite reagent pad to form a pink color. A positive nitrite test is an indication of possible bacterial UTI. Examples of bacteria that frequently cause UTI and cause a positive nitrite test are *Escherichia coli, Klebsiella, Proteus,* and *Pseudomonas*. Because certain bacteria are not capable of converting nitrates to nitrite, a negative nitrite result is possible in some UTIs. Normal urine is negative for nitrite by the reagent strip method.

Leukocyte Esterase

Granular leukocytes, primarily neutrophils, contain an enzyme called leukocyte esterase. The presence of this enzyme in urine indicates the presence of leukocytes in urine, usually resulting from infection or inflammation in the urinary tract. The esterase enzyme reacts with esterase substrate in the leukocyte esterase reagent pad to form a purple color. The color intensity is proportional to the number of leukocytes present. Normal urine is negative for leukocyte esterase by the reagent strip method. *Only present in prewritten*

Specific Gravity

The **specific gravity (sp. gr.)** of urine reflects the kidneys' ability to concentrate urine. The specific gravity reagent pad contains an indicator that changes color from blue-green to green to yellow-green depending on the urine ion concentration. Specific gravities between 1.000 and 1.030 can be measured. The reagent strip method is not normally affected by the presence of organic molecules such as glucose, so the reagent strip sp. gr. measurement can be lower than the refractometer measurement in specimens with a positive glucose result. Reagent strip sp. gr. can be affected by pH; neutral or alkaline urines can have falsely decreased sp. gr. by reagent strip and should be checked by another method. The reference range of urine specific gravity in normally hydrated adults is 1.010 to 1.025 by reagent strip method.

Reference Values by Reagent Strip

Normal urine, when tested with a reagent strip, is negative for glucose, ketone, bilirubin, bacteria (nitrite), leukocyte esterase, and blood (see Table 5-11). Normal urine can be negative for protein or contain a trace of protein. Normal, recently voided urine

TABLE 5-11. Reference values for urine chemical tests using reagent strips*

TEST	REFERENCE VALUE	LOWER DETECTABLE LIMIT*
Glucose	Negative	$\geq$ 100 mg/dL
Bilirubin	Negative	$\geq$ 0.4 mg/dL
Ketones	Negative	$\geq$ 10 mg/dL
Blood	Negative	$\geq$ 5–10 RBCs/μL
pH	5.0–8.0	5–9**
Protein	Negative or trace	$\geq$ 15 mg/dL (albumin)
Urobilinogen	0.0–1.0 mg/dL	$\geq$ 0.2 mg/dL
Nitrite	Negative	$\geq$ 0.075 mg/dL
Leukocyte esterase	Negative	$\geq$ 10–15 WBC/μL
Specific gravity	1.010–1.025	1.000–1.030**

*The lower detectable limit can vary slightly among different brands of strips as well as specimen characteristics
**detectable range

has a pH between 5.0 and 8.0 and a specific gravity between 1.010 and 1.025.

Positive or abnormal results should be confirmed according to laboratory policy. Some test results are confirmed by retesting with a single analyte strip or a different brand of strip. Other results must be confirmed using nonreagent strip confirmatory tests. Positive leukocyte esterase or nitrite tests should be confirmed by microscopic examination of urine sediment.

Since urine tests are rarely ordered as STAT tests, most laboratories have few critical urine values. However, a positive reagent strip test for protein, glucose, or ketones in a newborn should be considered a critical value and should be reported immediately, following laboratory protocol.

SINGLE ANALYTE AND SPECIAL REAGENT STRIPS

Reagent strips that detect only one or two constituents of interest, such as glucose or ketones, are useful in certain cases. Examples of these are Diastix and Clinistix, which can be used at home to monitor urine glucose; Ketostix strips, which test for ketones; and Keto-Diastix strips, which test for ketones and glucose on the same strip. Reagent strips are also available for detecting hCG, the hormone of pregnancy.

The Multistix PRO line of strips is particularly useful for detecting or monitoring kidney disease and glomerular complications caused by diabetes mellitus. The strips measure creatinine levels as well as protein, allowing the estimation of the protein-to-creatinine ratio, a value that previously was only possible by testing a 24-hour urine.

Microalbumin test strips are available to detect **microalbuminuria**, urine albumin concentrations between 20 and 200 mg/L urine. This amount of protein is too low to be detected with routine urine chemistry reagent strips. Microalbuminuria is an indicator of early renal disease or damage, such as can occur in nephropathy or as a complication of diabetes. Early detection of microalbuminuria allows kidney damage to be recognized in time to intervene with treatment and slow or prevent further renal damage. Microalbumin values below 20 mg/L are normal.

COPPER REDUCTION TEST AND CONFIRMATORY TESTS

In certain situations, results of reagent strip tests do not provide sufficient information. In these cases, manual confirmatory tests such as a protein precipitation test, ketone tablet test (Acetest), or Ictotest for bilirubin are performed because they are more sensitive than routine reagent strip tests. Another manual test, the copper reduction test, can detect reducing sugars, including glucose, in urine. The principles and procedures of these tests are explained following the reagent strip procedures.

PERFORMING CHEMICAL TESTS BY REAGENT STRIP

Instructions for the use of reagent strips, test interferences, timing of reactions, and a color comparison chart are included with each container of reagent strips. These instructions and the procedure in the standard operating procedure (SOP) manual must be followed precisely. The technician should be familiar with these before performing the test and reporting results.

Safety Precautions

   Standard Precautions must be used when performing all urinalysis procedures. Because urine is a body fluid, all urine specimens must be considered potential biological hazards. Appropriate PPE must be worn. An acrylic safety shield or face shield should be used to protect the eyes and mucus membranes from accidental splashes; the creation of aerosols should be avoided. Urine specimens can be safely discarded in a sink, followed by rinsing the sink with water and cleaning with disinfectant. Contaminated materials should be discarded into appropriate biohazard or sharps containers.

Guidelines for the safe use of a centrifuge must be followed. Tubes for urine centrifugation should be conical and capped, have a 10- to 15-mL capacity, and be able to withstand centrifugation. The Clinitest and protein confirmatory test present special chemical hazards because they use caustic reagents (NaOH) and acids. Chemical-resistant gloves should be worn when performing these tests.

Quality Assessment

   Adherence to a comprehensive quality assessment (QA) program ensures that the results from the chemical analysis of urine are reliable. The QA program must encompass all procedures, from specimen collection to reporting results.

Specimen Collection and Storage

Specimens must be collected, labeled, and stored correctly, and tested within the required time limits to prevent deterioration of urine components. A recently collected midstream specimen is preferred. Testing should be performed within 1 to 2 hours of collection. Specimens can be refrigerated for up to 4 hours but should be allowed to reach room temperature before testing. Specimens should remain tightly covered and in the dark until tested to protect urine components that are volatile, labile, or light-sensitive.

Reagent Strips

Although reagent strip testing appears to be simple, many factors must be kept in mind to ensure that reported results are valid. Manufacturer's instructions include information about the correct storage, use, timing of reactions, and interpretation of results. Technicians should be aware of substances that can possibly interfere with reactions. Interfering substances will be listed in the package inserts accompanying the reagent strips and in the SOP manual.

Reagent strips must be stored at room temperature in their original air-tight container and protected from light, heat, and moisture. Specimens must be mixed well before using the reagent strip to be sure the reagent pads will be exposed to any solid components that have settled out, such as blood cells. Strips are used only once and then discarded; strips must not be used after the expiration date. Because manual tests are interpreted visually using a color comparison chart, technicians must pass a color blindness test before being allowed to report manual urine reagent strip results.

Urine Controls

The reliability of urine reagent strips and confirmatory test reagents is validated by using urine control solutions. Normal and abnormal urine controls must be run and results recorded as specified in the SOP manual. If the control results fall outside the specified ranges, the SOP manual will contain the steps to follow to identify the problem. The control results must be within the manufacturer's stated ranges before patient results can be reported.

Specimen Requirements

A first morning midstream specimen is preferred because the morning specimen is usually the most concentrated and the pH is lower, which protects formed elements.

Reagent Strip by Manual Method

Testing is performed by quickly dipping a reagent strip into recently collected, well-mixed room temperature urine (Figure 5-17A). The excess urine is removed by touching

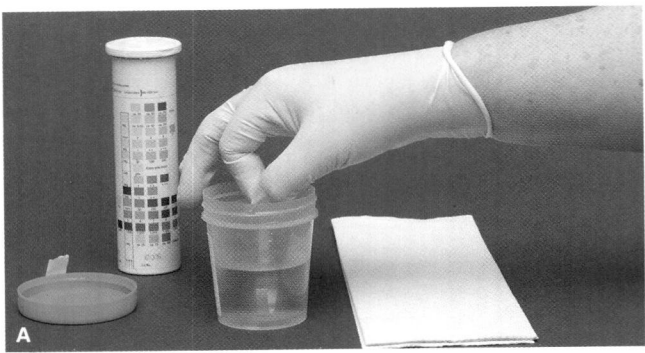
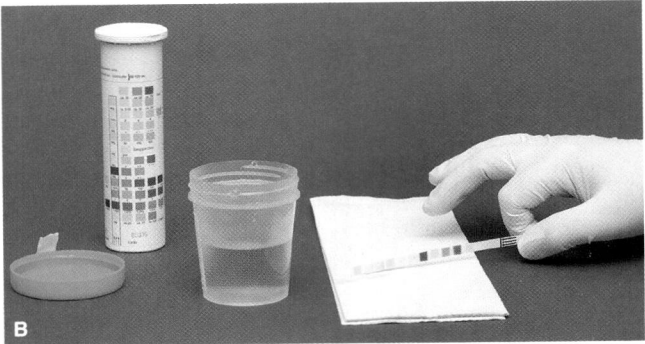
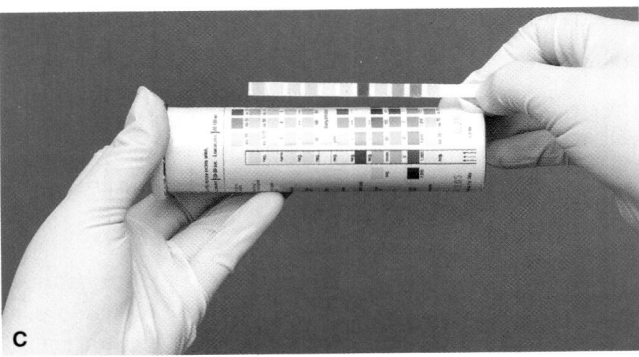

FIGURE 5-17 Manual testing of urine by reagent strip: (A) hold the reagent strip by the top end and dip the strip into the urine specimen; (B) remove the strip from the urine, blot edge of strip to remove excess urine, and begin timer; (C) read reactions at appropriate time intervals by comparing reagent pad colors to color chart

the edge of the strip to the edge of the urine container as the strip is withdrawn from the urine. Timing of reactions should begin as soon as the strip is withdrawn from the urine. The edge of the strip should be quickly blotted on absorbent paper (Figure 5-17B) and the test areas observed at the manufacturer's specified time intervals. The color changes on the reagent pads are visually compared to the color chart provided with the strips (Figure 5-17C) and the results recorded.

Reagent Strip by Instrumentation

Strip readers can be used to read the reactions of urine reagent strip tests (Figures 5-18, 5-19, and 5-20). These readers contain reflectance photometers that detect the colors formed on the reagent pads when urine reacts with the various reagents. Depending on instrument design, results are read directly from the display screen and recorded, printed out, or integrated into the computerized laboratory information system (LIS). Reagent strip readers reduce errors caused by incorrect timing of reactions or incorrect interpretation of colors. However, urine that has an intense color can cause false positive reactions when the reagent strip is read with a strip reader.

To use the simplest reagent strip readers, the technician applies the urine to the reagent strip, inserts the strip into the reader, and reads the results from the instrument display screen or prints the results. This type of reader is ideal for point-of-care and low-volume physician office laboratories (POLs). The

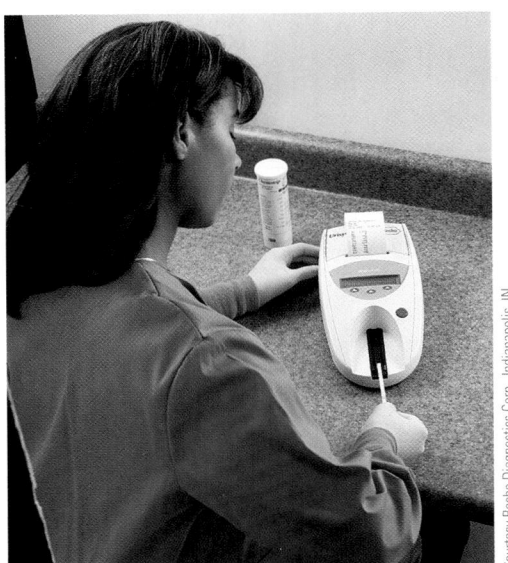

FIGURE 5-18 Urysis 1100 Analyzer

CLIA-waived Urisys 1100 Analyzer from Roche Diagnostics (Diavant) is an example of this type of reader (Figure 5-18). The Clinitek Status (Siemens) can read microalbumin reagent strips and hCG cassettes in addition to urine chemical strips (Figure 5-19). The Clinitek Status is CLIA-waived and can interface with the LIS.

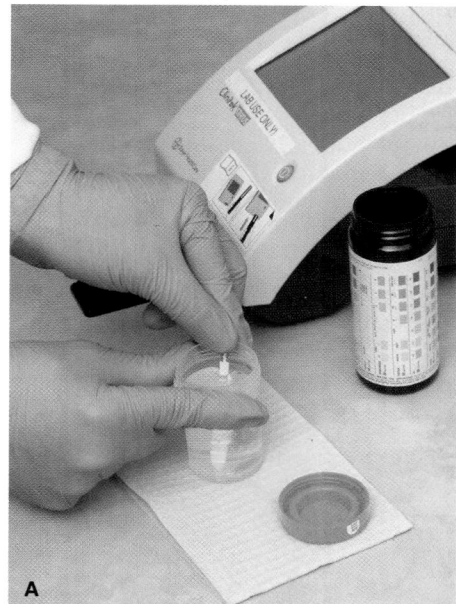
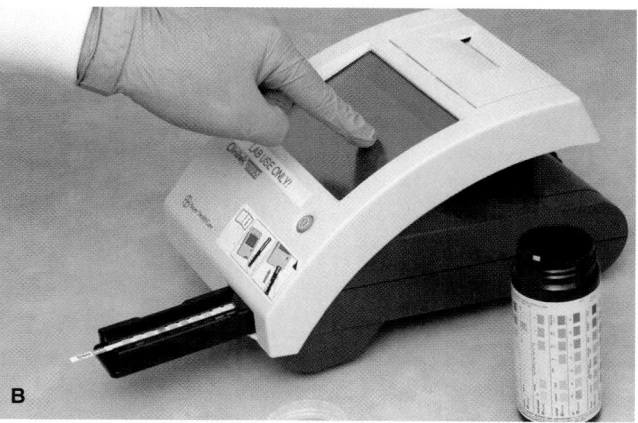
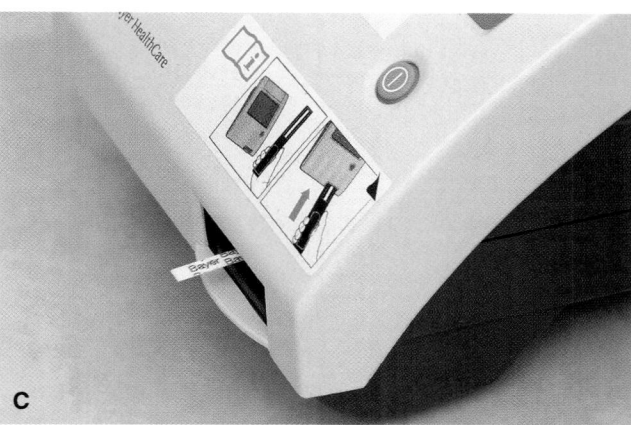
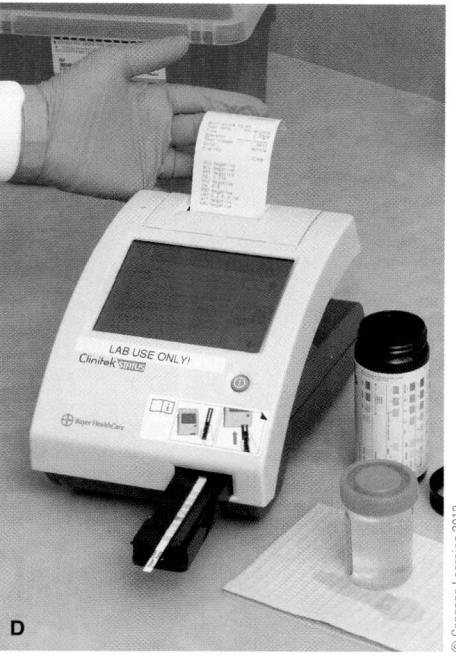

FIGURE 5-19 Reading a urine reagent strip using the Clinitek Status: (A) strip is dipped into urine; (B) strip is placed into carrier and test is selected from the touch-screen; (C) the carrier and strip are taken into the instrument; (D) the carrier ejects and test results are printed when test is complete

Semi-automated and automated strip readers can process several patient samples within a short time. These readers are ideal for higher volume POLs, hospital laboratories, and reference laboratories. For semi-automated readers such as the Criterion II or Urisys 1800 from Roche Diagnostics, the technician enters patient identification and urine color and clarity into the database. The strip is dipped in urine, placed in the carrier, and taken into the reader. The colors of the chemical reactions are measured by reflectance photometry, and the results are printed out or automatically uploaded to the LIS.

The Clinitek Advantus from Siemens (formerly the Clinitek 500) is an automated strip reader that uses a handheld barcode reader to identify the specimen and determine urine color and

clarity (Figure 5-20). Samples can be processed every 7 seconds, and results can be uploaded to the LIS. In the Urisys 2400, a fully automated instrument, tubes of urine are placed in a rack and urine samples are automatically applied to reagent strips.

PERFORMING THE COPPER REDUCTION TEST: CLINITEST

The copper reduction test is a chemical test that detects reducing sugars, including glucose, fructose, lactose, pentose, and galactose. Several other non–sugar reducing substances, such as penicillin, salicylates, ascorbic acid, and cephalosporins,

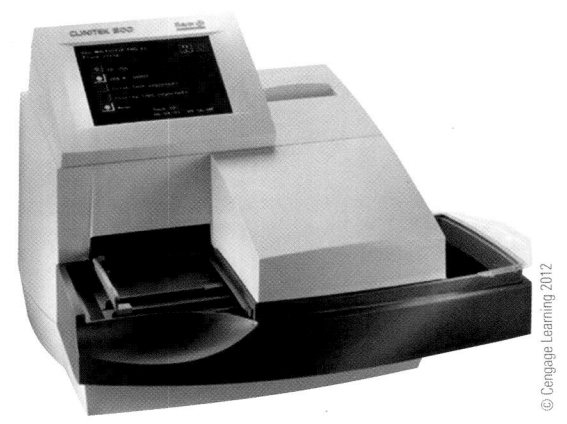

FIGURE 5-20 Clinitek Advantus urine strip reader

© Cengage Learning 2012

can also react in this test when present in high concentrations. The Clinitest tablet contains all of the reagents required for the copper reduction test. The Clintest copper reduction test is CLIA-waived.

Historically, the Clinitest was used to estimate glucose in urine of diabetics. However, with the availability of glucose-specific reagent strips, the Clinitest is no longer used for glucose. It is now used as a simple way to screen urine for other reducing sugars, as when screening newborns or infants for galactosuria. Urine from normal children and adults should be negative by the Clinitest method; urine from normal newborns less than 2 weeks old can contain reducing substances that can cause a positive Clinitest result.

To perform the Clinitest, 5 drops of urine and 10 drops of water are added to a heat-resistant test tube seated in a test tube rack (Figure 5-21). Forceps are used to place the Clinitest tablet into the diluted urine, and the color change is observed while the

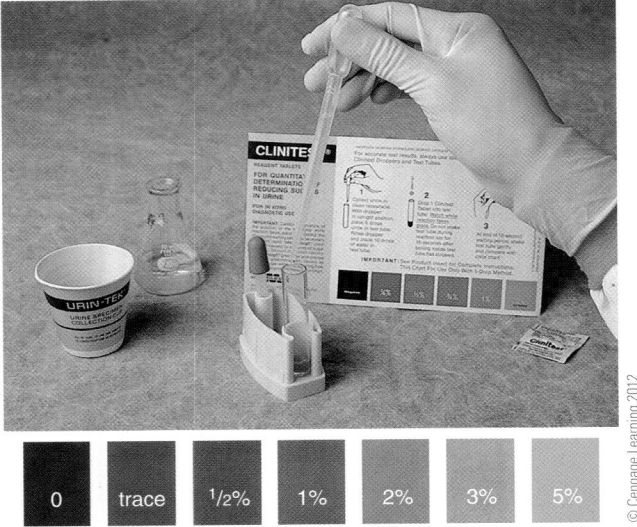

© Cengage Learning 2012

FIGURE 5-21 Clinitest for reducing sugars (top) and example of color chart (bottom). (Note: Do not use chart in this figure to read results—use chart included with package insert)

tablet effervesces. If a reducing sugar is present in the urine, the color changes from blue to green and then to orange, depending on the amount of reducing substance present. When the reaction is complete, the color of the liquid is compared to the color chart included with the Clinitest tablet vial (Figure 5-21), and the results are recorded.

It is important to observe the entire reaction; sugars in high concentration can cause a rapid color change from blue-green to orange and then back to dark green, a reaction called "pass through." Failure to observe pass through might result in a false negative reaction being reported. The 2-drop Clinitest is performed in the same manner as the 5-drop method except that 2 drops of urine are used and the color reaction is compared to the 2-drop color chart.

  Manufacturers' safety recommendations should always be followed when performing the Clinitest method. Care must be taken to avoid burns or injury from the heat and caustic products generated during the reaction. Clinitest tablets (which contain NaOH) should not be handled with bare hands. The test tube opening should be kept pointed away from the face, and face protection should be worn to prevent splashes on the face or into the eyes.

PERFORMING CONFIRMATORY TESTS

The routine use of confirmatory tests has been eliminated in most situations, but occasionally methods other than reagent strips must be used to detect certain urine analytes. These methods are called confirmatory tests because their most common use is to confirm a positive (or negative) result obtained using the reagent strip. Confirmatory tests are simple to perform, but require more technician time and more reagents and equipment than the reagent strip method. Three commonly performed confirmatory tests are the tests for protein, ketones, and bilirubin.

Protein

Most confirmatory tests for urine protein involve treating a portion of supernatant from centrifuged urine with dilute sulfosalicylic acid (SSA) or acetic acid to cause any protein in the urine to precipitate and therefore become visible. Albumins and globulins both react in the protein precipitation test; the amount of precipitate formed is roughly proportional to the concentration of protein present. Precipitate is graded as negative, trace (slightly cloudy), 1+ (turbid), 2+ (turbid with granulation), 3+ (granulation and flocculation), or 4+ (clumps).

Ketones: Acetest

The Acetest is a tablet test for ketones that can be used with urine or serum. The test is based on the same principle as the reagent strip test. If ketones are present in urine, a drop of urine added to the Acetest tablet will produce a purple color (Figure 5-22). Strips such as Ketostix or Ketodiastix are also used to confirm the presence of ketones in urine.

Bilirubin: Ictotest

The Ictotest is a specific test for bilirubin and is four times as sensitive as the reagent strip method. The test uses a tablet and special absorbent mat that causes bilirubin to remain on the mat surface. A few drops of urine are placed on the mat, the tablet is placed on the moist area, and water is dropped on the tablet. If bilirubin is present, a purple color will develop on the mat within 60 seconds (Figure 5-23).

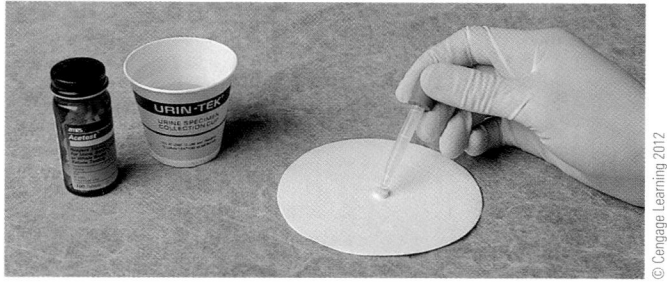

FIGURE 5-22 Acetest for urine ketones

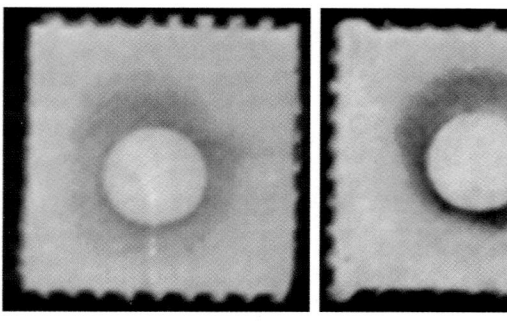

Weak positive   Strong positive

FIGURE 5-23 Ictotest for bilirubin; both tests shown are positive for bilirubin

SAFETY REMINDERS

- Review Safety Precautions section before beginning procedure.
- Observe Standard Precautions.
- Wear appropriate PPE.
- Follow centrifuge safety rules.
- Perform Clinitest procedure with care.

PROCEDURAL REMINDERS

- Review Quality Assessment section before beginning procedure.
- Follow SOP manual.
- Follow manufacturer's directions for reagents and reagent strips.
- Mix urine before performing reagent strip test.
- Observe and record color changes at correct times.

CRITICAL THINKING 1

Megan received two specimens for routine urinalysis. She poured a portion of each specimen into a conical centrifuge tube, recorded the transparency and color, and measured the specific gravity of each. She was then interrupted and had to leave the urinalysis bench. While Megan was away, one of her coworkers centrifuged the urine to prepare it for microscopic examination and left a note stating what she had done. Megan returned and performed chemical testing on the centrifuged specimens. Specimen A had pH 6.0, specimen B had pH 6.5, and both were negative for the remaining tests. Specimen B had a moderate amount of visible sediment at the bottom of the centrifuge tube.

1. Which is the correct action for Megan?
   a. Repeat reagent strip tests on both tubes of centrifuged urine.
   b. Record the reagent strip results and proceed to the microscopic examination.
   c. Retest only specimen B using well-mixed, uncentrifuged urine.
   d. Retest both specimens using well-mixed, uncentrifuged urine.
2. Explain your answer.

CRITICAL THINKING 2

Chemical analysis of a patient's urine using a reagent strip gave negative protein and negative glucose results. However, using a separate microalbumin reagent strip, the result was positive. Earlier in the day, the urine controls gave the expected results with both types of reagent strips.

1. Is there a discrepancy in the patient's test results obtained with the two strips?
2. Should the urine chemistry controls be rerun?
3. What is the most likely explanation for the results?

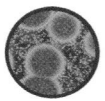

SUMMARY

The chemical examination of urine became greatly simplified with the development of single-use reagent strips that can test for several analytes on one strip. Reagent strip tests that detect up to 10 constituents can be performed and interpreted manually or using semi-automated or fully automated reagent strip readers. Confirmatory tests for protein, ketones, or bilirubin are manual tests used to validate positive or questionable results for these components. Clinitest tablets are used to detect the presence of reducing sugars other than glucose in urine.

Standard Precautions must be observed when performing the chemical examination of urine. For reliable test results, the manufacturers' instructions for using strips, reagents, and instruments must be followed. Urine control solutions must be run as detailed in the SOP manual.

Kidney disease is a silent disease; patients can remain asymptomatic for years before physical symptoms of kidney disease become apparent. If kidney disease is diagnosed early, treatment can begin and irreversible kidney damage can be prevented or postponed. The chemical examination of urine provides valuable information for the diagnosis and treatment of certain kidney diseases as well as other conditions. A recent study conducted throughout several countries compared six urine chemical results in three groups: (1) "normal" patients, (2) outpatients, and (3) hospitalized patients. The importance of urine screening was validated when significant abnormal or pathological findings were present in 16% of normal individuals, 40% of outpatients, and 57% of hospitalized patients. Abnormal chemical test results can be the first indication of a problem in the kidneys or other body systems and can sometimes aid in confirming or ruling out a diagnosis.

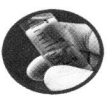

REVIEW QUESTIONS

1. Name 10 chemical tests routinely performed on urine using the reagent strip method.
2. Explain how a reagent strip is used.
3. What type of urine specimen is preferred for chemical testing?

4. What are three confirmatory tests that can be performed on urine?
5. For each of the following, name a condition that can cause the substance to be increased in the urine: protein, ketones, glucose, bilirubin, nitrite, and microalbumin.
6. How can urine protein be estimated other than using a reagent strip?
7. Name a light-sensitive substance that can be present in urine.
8. What is the purpose of the Clinitest? What does it detect?
9. If a reagent strip test yields positive glucose and ketone tests, what condition is suggested?
10. How might interpretation of urine chemical test results be affected if a technician is colorblind?
11. How should a urine specimen be prepared for testing with reagent strip?
12. Explain how controls are used in urine testing and discuss the importance of their use.
13. What are the advantages of using a urine strip reader?
14. How can handling and storage of urine specimens influence the results of chemical tests?
15. What safety precautions should be used when performing urine tests?
16. Define albumin, bilirubin, chromogen, galactosuria, globulins, glycosuria, hematuria, hemoglobinuria, ketones, ketonuria, microalbumin, microalbuminuria, proteinuria, specific gravity, and urobilinogen.

STUDENT ACTIVITIES

1. Complete the written examination on this lesson.
2. Practice performing chemical examinations on several urine specimens as outlined in the Student Performance Guide, using the worksheet.
3. Compare the results of the physical examination of a urine sample with the chemical examination results. Are they as expected? If protein is present in a sample, is specific

gravity also high? If blood is positive on a reagent strip, was it indicated by the urine color in the physical examination?

4. Compare the package inserts of two brands of urine reagent strips. Determine the principles of each reagent pad test and note which tests from the two manufacturers are based on the same chemical principles.

5. Write an explanation of the chemical reactions for the nitrite, hemoglobin, and protein reagent pads, using a reagent strip package insert. Include test sensitivity and substances (if any) that can cause false positive or false negative reactions with the reagent strip.

6. Administer a color blindness test to a fellow student.

WEB ACTIVITIES

1. Find information about two urine strip readers on the Internet. Compare their capabilities: sampling methods, strips used, calibration methods, process times, etc. Can the instruments read reagent strips for microalbumin?

2. Use the Internet to find information on myoglobin. Find out what conditions can cause myoglobinuria (myoglobin in the urine) and what reagent strip reactions indicate presence of myoglobin.

3. Use the Internet to find information on color blindness. How many types of color blindness are there? Find examples of color blindness tests.

4. Use the Internet to search for information on one of the following topics: porphyria, pyuria, glomerulonephritis, or tubular necrosis. Report on the condition listing causes, symptoms, and expected findings in the physical and chemical portions of the urinalysis (urine color, transparency, specific gravity, and reagent strip).

5. Use the Internet to search for information on "inborn errors of metabolism." List three. Select one and report on it, including information on the mechanism, symptoms, treatment, prognosis, and expected findings in the physical and chemical urine examinations.

6. Use the Internet to find information on multiple myeloma and Waldenström's macroglobulinemia. Report on the cause of each disease and state the expected results for the reagent strip protein test and the urine protein precipitation test.

7. Search the internet for self-tests, tutorials, or videos demonstrating chemical testing of urine.

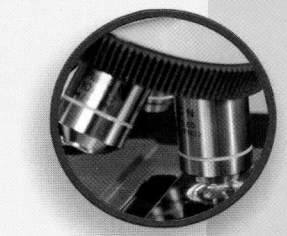

LESSON 5-4
Chemical Examination of Urine

(Individual student results will vary depending on the specimens provided by the instructor.)

Name _____ Date _____

INSTRUCTIONS

1. Practice performing the chemical examination of urine following the step-by-step procedure and using the worksheet.

2. Demonstrate the procedure for the chemical examination of urine satisfactorily for the instructor using the Student Performance Guide. Your instructor will explain the procedures for evaluating and grading your performance. Your performance may be given a number grade, letter grade, or satisfactory (S) or unsatisfactory (U) depending on course or institutional policy.

NOTE: Consult manufacturers' instructions and reagent package inserts before using instruments and reagents or performing tests. Use special precautions when handling acids or caustic reagents; consult MSDS.

MATERIALS AND EQUIPMENT

- gloves (vinyl, for chemical resistance)
- hand antiseptic
- full-face shield (or equivalent PPE)
- acrylic safety shield (optional)
- recently collected urine specimens
- urine controls (normal and abnormal levels)
- reagent grade water (for reconstituting controls)
- micropipetter with disposable tips (if needed to reconstitute controls)
- urine reagent strips with color charts
- paper towels
- laboratory tissue
- timer
- reagent strip reader (optional)
- 15 mL centrifuge tubes (clear, conical, disposable plastic, with caps)
- centrifuge to spin 15 mL conical tubes
- test tube rack
- forceps
- disposable transfer pipets
- Protein precipitation test:
  ○ 20% (or 3%) sulfosalicylic acid (SSA)
  ○ test tubes, 13 × 100 mm (disposable)
  ○ test tube rack
- Clinitest:
  ○ Clinitest tablets with color chart
  ○ distilled water
  ○ borosilicate, heat-resistant test tubes, 16 × 100 mm (disposable)
  ○ test tube rack
- Acetest:
  ○ Acetest tablets
  ○ filter paper
- Ictotest:
  ○ Ictotest tablets
  ○ Ictotest absorbent pads
- worksheet
- urinalysis report form (found at end of Lesson 5-5)
- surface disinfectant (such as 10% chlorine bleach)
- biohazard container
- sharps container

© 2012 Delmar, Cengage Learning. Permission to reproduce for clinical use granted.

PROCEDURE

Record in the comment section any problems encountered while practicing the procedure (or have a fellow student or the instructor evaluate your performance).

S = Satisfactory
U = Unsatisfactory

You must:	S	U	Evaluation/Comments
1. Wash hands with antiseptic and put on gloves and face protection (work behind safety shield if not wearing face protection)			
2. Assemble equipment and materials			
3. Obtain a recently collected urine specimen and urine control solution(s). If specimen has been refrigerated, allow it to reach room temperature before testing			
4. Record specimen I.D. and control I.D. on worksheet			
5. Perform reagent strip test using urine control: a. Obtain reagent strip, accompanying color chart and timer b. Dip reagent strip into urine control, moistening all pads c. Remove strip from control solution immediately, drawing strip across container edge to remove excess urine; quickly blot *edge* of strip on absorbent paper. Start timer as strip is withdrawn from urine d. Observe reagent pads and compare colors to color chart at appropriate time intervals e. Record results on worksheet f. Discard reagent strip and other contaminated materials into biohazard container g. Compare control results to accepted control values h. If values are within acceptable range, repeat 5a-5g with abnormal urine control if available. If not available continue at step 5i i. Repeat 5a–5f using well-mixed patient urine and record patient results on worksheet			
6. Retest the urine specimen and/or urine control(s) if a strip reader is available. Follow manufacturer's instructions for the instrument. Compare the manual test results with those from the strip reader. If no strip reader is available, go to step 7			
7. Perform protein precipitation test: a. Centrifuge 5 to 10 mL of urine b. Place 4 mL of clear supernatant (from 7a) into a 13 × 100 mm test tube c. Add 3 drops of 20% sulfosalicylic acid (SSA). (Alternatively, add 4 mL of 3% sulfosalicylic acid to 4 mL of urine using a large [16 × 100 mm] test tube) d. Mix tube contents thoroughly and estimate the amount of turbidity after 10 minutes			

© 2012 Delmar, Cengage Learning. Permission to reproduce for clinical use granted.

You must:	S	U	Evaluation/Comments
e. Record results as: negative (no turbidity or cloudiness), trace (slight cloudiness), 1+ (turbid), 2+ (turbid with granulation), 3+ (granulation and flocculation), or 4+ (clumps) f. Repeat steps 7a-7e using abnormal control if available			
8. Perform Clinitest for reducing substances: **Caution:** Consult MSDS; Clinitest tablets contain NaOH; avoid direct contact; do not expose tablets to excessive moisture a. Place a heat-resistant 16 × 100 mm test tube into a test-tube rack b. Place 5 drops of urine into the test tube c. Place 10 drops of distilled water into the test tube and gently mix tube contents d. Open the Clinitest tablet package and drop a Clinitest reagent tablet into the urine-water mixture using forceps e. Observe color while tablet effervesces (boils), without touching the test tube and keeping tube opening pointed away from face f. Wait 15 seconds after effervescence (boiling) stops, hold tube with test tube clamp, and mix tube contents gently. Immediately compare color of liquid to color chart NOTE: Tube will be hot and opening should be kept pointed away from your face g. Record results as negative, 1/4%, 1/2%, 3/4%, 1%, or 2% or more as directed on the Clinitest package insert h. Repeat 8a–8g using abnormal urine control solution. Check control instructions for correct number of control drops and water drops to use in the test			
9. Perform Acetest for ketones: a. Use forceps to place an Acetest tablet on a clean piece of filter paper b. Place 1 drop of urine on top of the tablet and start the timer c. Compare color of tablet to Acetest color chart at 30 seconds d. Record results on worksheet as negative or positive e. Repeat 9a–9d using urine control solution(s)			
10. Perform Ictotest for bilirubin: a. Place 10 drops of urine on an Ictotest mat b. Use forceps to place an Ictotest reagent tablet on the moistened area of the mat c. Apply 2 drops of water to the top of the tablet and start timer d. Observe test for 60 seconds and interpret results: a blue to purple color forms on the mat within 60 seconds if bilirubin is present. The rapidity of the color formation and the color intensity are proportional to the amount of bilirubin in the urine. A pink or red color is a negative result e. Record results as negative or positive f. Repeat 10a–10e using urine control solution(s)			

(Continues)

© 2012 Delmar, Cengage Learning. Permission to reproduce for clinical use granted.

You must:	S	U	Evaluation/Comments
11. Dispose of urine specimen(s) as instructed			
12. Discard test tubes and test tube contents as instructed: a. Discard disposable tubes into sharps container b. Discard contents of reusable test tubes as instructed and place tubes into disinfectant			
13. Discard other contaminated materials into appropriate biohazard container			
14. Disinfect and clean equipment/instrument according to manufacturers' instructions and return to proper storage			
15. Clean work area with surface disinfectant			
16. Remove gloves and discard into biohazard container			
17. Wash hands with antiseptic			

Instructor/Evaluator Comments

Instructor/Evaluator _____ Date _____

© 2012 Delmar, Cengage Learning. Permission to reproduce for clinical use granted.

LESSON 5-4
Chemical Examination of Urine

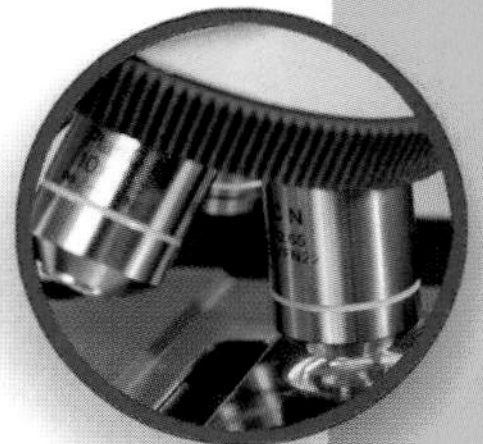

(Individual student results will vary depending on specimens provided by instructor.)

Name _____   Date _____

Specimen I.D. _____

REAGENT STRIP TEST	PATIENT RESULT	CONTROL RESULT	REFERENCE VALUES
Glucose	_____	_____	Negative
Bilirubin	_____	_____	Negative
Ketones	_____	_____	Negative
Blood	_____	_____	Negative
pH	_____	_____	5–8
Protein	_____	_____	Negative, trace
Urobilinogen	_____	_____	0.0 to 1.0 mg/dL (or EU/dL)
Nitrite	_____	_____	Negative
Leukocyte esterase	_____	_____	Negative
Specific gravity	_____	_____	1.010–1.025

REDUCING SUBSTANCES   (Circle Result)

Clinitest	Negative $\frac{1}{4}$% $\frac{1}{2}$% $\frac{3}{4}$% 1% 2% or more	Negative

CONFIRMATORY TEST RESULTS   (Circle Result)

Protein SSA	Negative Trace 1+ 2+ 3+ 4+	Negative
Ketones (Acetest)	Negative Positive	Negative
Bilirubin (Ictotest)	Negative Positive	Negative

Comment: _____

_____

Date _____   Control ID _____

Time _____   Control Lot No. _____

Exp. Date _____

WORKSHEET

© 2012 Delmar, Cengage Learning. Permission to reproduce for clinical use granted.

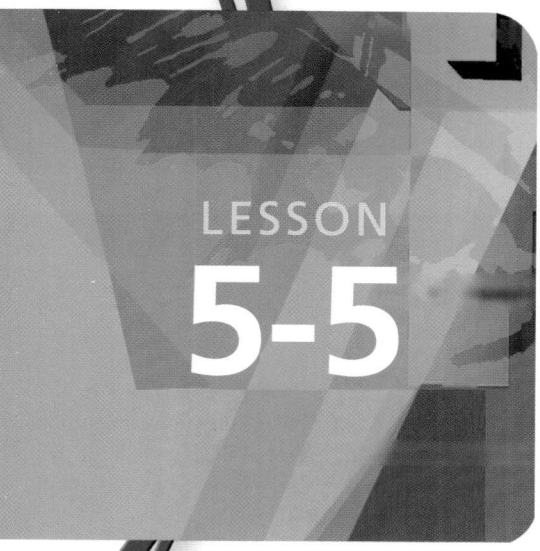

LESSON 5-5

Microscopic Examination of Urine Sediment

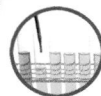

LESSON OBJECTIVES

After studying this lesson, the student will:

◉ Name the preferred urine specimen for the microscopic examination.

◉ Name three categories of cells that can be found in urine sediment and give the significance of each.

◉ Explain how casts are formed.

◉ Name three types of casts that can be present in urine.

◉ List the reference values for red and white blood cells, casts, and bacteria in urine.

◉ Name six crystals that can be present in normal urine and state the pH at which each usually occurs.

◉ List four clinically significant crystals that can occur in urine sediment.

◉ Prepare a urine specimen for microscopic examination.

◉ Perform a microscopic examination of urine sediment and report the results.

◉ Identify cells, casts, crystals, and other sediment components in urine specimens or from visual aids.

◉ Correlate urine microscopic findings with urine physical and chemical test results.

◉ Correlate urine microscopic findings with the presence of certain diseases.

◉ Describe safety precautions that must be observed when performing the microscopic examination of urine sediment.

◉ Discuss the importance of quality assessment procedures in performing the microscopic examination of urine sediment.

◉ Define the glossary terms.

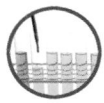

GLOSSARY

cast / in urinalysis, a protein matrix formed in the kidney tubules and washed out into the urine

flagellum (pl., flagella) / slender, lash-like appendage that serves as organ of locomotion for sperm cells and some protozoa

hyaline / transparent, pale

protozoa / unicellular eukaryotic organisms, both free-living and parasitic

sediment / solids that settle to the bottom of a liquid

supernatant / the clear liquid remaining at the top of a solution after centrifugation or the settling out of solid substances in a solution; the liquid lying above a sediment

yeast / a small, single-celled eukaryotic fungus that reproduces by fission or budding

INTRODUCTION

The microscopic examination of urine sediment is the third part of the routine urinalysis. The microscopic examination can provide important information about a patient's health, such as evidence of infection, disease, or trauma in the urinary tract. In addition, certain findings, such as the presence of abnormal crystals, can suggest a metabolic disorder.

Urine **sediment** refers to the solids that settle to the bottom of the urine specimen after centrifugation or when urine is allowed to stand undisturbed. In the laboratory, urine sediment is obtained by centrifuging a standard volume of urine. Most of the **supernatant**, the liquid lying over the sediment, is then removed and the remaining sediment is resuspended and examined microscopically. This lesson explains the procedure for preparing urine sediment and for performing the microscopic examination of the sediment.

COMPONENTS OF URINE SEDIMENT

The components that can be present in urine sediment include blood and epithelial cells, crystals, casts, and microorganisms. These are identified through microscopic examination of the

sediment, and the numbers present are estimated and reported. Urine sediment can be observed unstained or using stains such as Sedi-Stain (Becton, Dickinson and Company) or KOVA Stain (Hycor Biomedical).

Cells

Several types of cells can be present in urine sediment, including blood cells, epithelial cells, and microorganisms (Figure 5-24). Only a few cells are normally seen in urine from healthy individuals. An increase in a particular cell type can indicate the presence of certain pathological conditions. Cells in urine sediment are identified, counted, and reported as part of the microscopic examination of urine.

Blood Cells

Normal urine can contain a few red and/or white blood cells. Blood cells are best identified using the high-power (40×) objective.

- Red blood cells (RBCs) look like pale, light-refractive disks when viewed under high power (Figure 5-24A). RBCs must be differentiated from yeast cells or oil droplets. Hypertonic (high specific gravity [sp. gr.]) urine can cause RBCs to appear crenated. Hypotonic (low sp.gr.) urine can cause

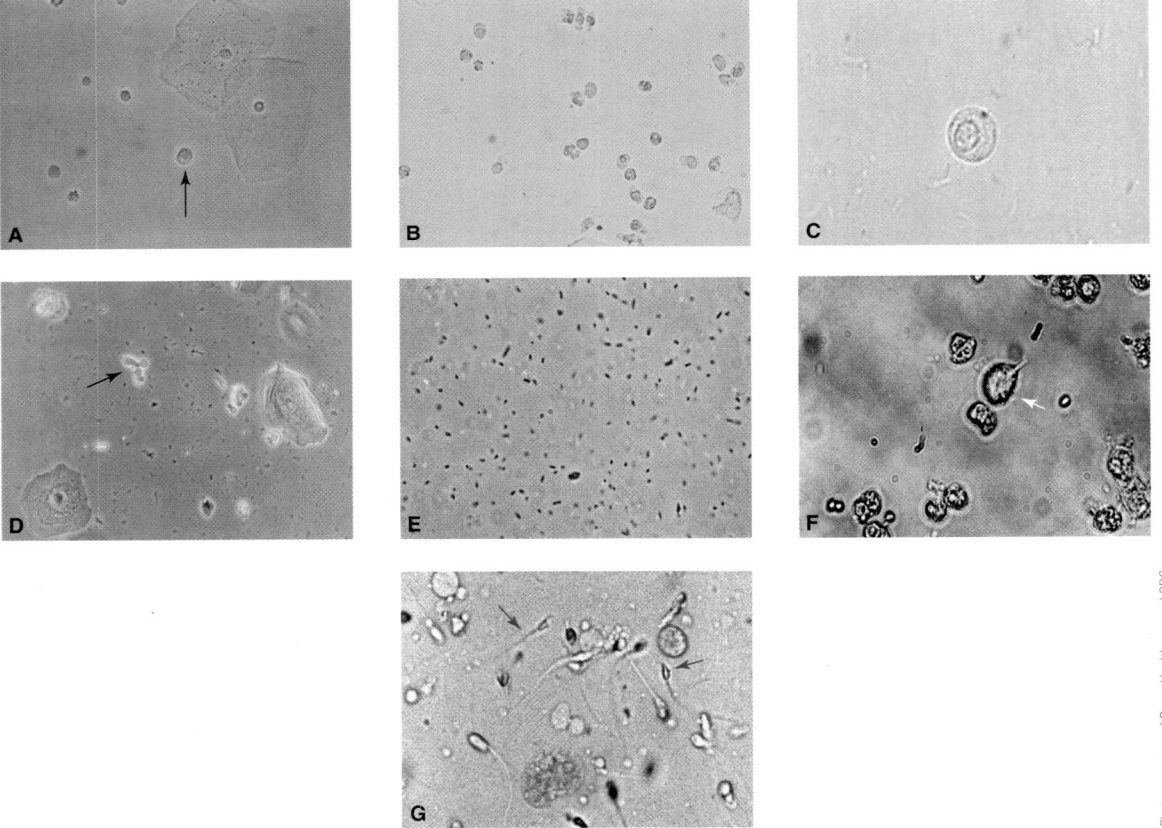

Photos courtesy of Bayer Healthcare and CDC

FIGURE 5-24 Cells in urine sediment: (A) Two squamous epithelial cells (upper right), red blood cells and white blood cell (arrow); (B) white blood cells; (C) renal tubular cell; (D) budding yeasts (arrow) and squamous epithelial cells; (E) bacteria; (F) *Trichomonas* (arrow); (G) spermatozoa (arrows) *Note: images are shown at varying magnifications*

RBCs to lyse. The presence of large numbers of RBCs in urine is called hematuria and is an abnormal condition indicating glomerular damage, other urinary system disease, or urinary system trauma.

- A few white blood cells (WBCs) can be present in normal urine (Figure 5-24A, arrow, and 5-24B). The neutrophil is usually the predominant type. WBCs are slightly larger than RBCs, have a granular appearance, and have a visible nucleus. In dilute urine, WBCs can appear as "glitter cells," cells that shimmer or glitter because of Brownian movement of the cytoplasmic granules. The presence of significant numbers of WBCs in urine is called *pyuria* and is a sign of urinary tract infection (UTI) or inflammation.

Epithelial Cells

Epithelial cells are constantly shed from the lining of the urinary tract and washed into the urine. Epithelial cells are larger than WBCs and appear flattened, each cell having a distinct round to oval nucleus. Epithelial cells are identified and classified using the high-power (40×) objective. The most commonly seen epithelial cell is the squamous epithelial cell (Figure 5-24A and D), which has a large amount of cytoplasm compared to the size of the nucleus; less commonly seen are the smaller bladder and renal tubular cells (Figure 5-24C).

Small renal cells can be differentiated from neutrophilic WBCs by adding a drop of dilute acetic acid to the sediment; this will cause the cell nuclei to be prominent. The nucleus of a renal cell is round; the nucleus of a neutrophil is segmented or lobed.

The presence of large numbers of renal tubular cells (also called renal epithelial cells) indicates possible chronic or acute renal disease, particularly disease affecting renal tubules. In a condition called tubular necrosis, renal tubular cells can contain oval fat bodies. A Maltese cross formation will be visible in the fat bodies when the cells are viewed with a microscope equipped with polarizing light. A fat-specific stain such as Sudan stain can also be used to verify the presence of fat in the renal cells.

Microorganisms

Microorganisms should not be present in normal urine. The presence of large numbers of microorganisms in recently collected urine suggests a UTI. Microorganisms that can be present include bacteria, yeasts or fungi, and protozoa. Microorganisms are observed using the high-power (40×) objective.

- Bacteria appear as tiny round or rod-shaped structures (Figure 5-24E). Rod-shaped bacteria are more easily recognized than are cocci, which can resemble amorphous material.

- **Yeasts** are single-celled, ovoid fungi and are not normally present in urine. When present they are often seen budding or in chains (Figure 5-24D). The yeast most commonly found in urine is *Candida albicans*. Yeast cells are smaller than RBCs, but, in low numbers, can resemble RBCs. A simple method for differentiating between yeasts and RBCs is to add 1 drop of dilute (2%) acetic acid to a drop of urine sediment and then observe the sediment microscopically. The acid will not affect yeast cells; if present, they will still

be visible. The acid will lyse (destroy) the RBCs; if they were initially present, they will no longer be visible.

- **Protozoa** are free-living or parasitic single-celled eukaryotic organisms. *Trichomonas vaginalis*, a parasite of the urogenital tract, can be present in urine (Figure 5-24F). This organism moves through the action of **flagella**, slender, lash-like appendages. *Trichomonas* is usually recognized during the microscopic examination by its characteristic twitching movement.

Spermatozoa

Spermatozoa are occasionally observed in urine and are easily identified by the oval head and single long flagellum (Figure 5-24G). They can be motile or nonmotile.

Casts

Kidney tubules normally secrete small amounts of mucoprotein, also called *Tamm Horsfall* protein. In conditions of slow urine flow, acid pH, and increased solutes, this protein accumulates and begins to gel, forming **casts**. The casts are molds of the tubule in which they form, hence their name. Any substances present in the tubule when the casts form, such as cells or cell remnants, become trapped in the protein. The casts dislodge and wash into the urine, where they are visible in urine sediment.

Casts are cylindrical, with parallel sides and rounded or flat ends, and are classified according to the substances observed in them (Figure 5-25). Casts are counted using low light and the low-power objective (10×) and classified using the high-power (40×) objective.

It is normal to see an occasional hyaline cast in urine. The presence of any other type of cast, such as granular, cellular or waxy casts, indicates possible renal disease or damage. Table 5-12 lists some conditions associated with different types of casts.

- **Hyaline** casts are transparent, colorless cylinders and are best seen by reducing the light on the microscope and/or lowering the condenser (Figure 5-25A).

- A granular cast contains remnants of disintegrated cells that appear as fine or coarse granules embedded in the protein matrix of the cast (Figure 5-25B).

- Cellular casts can contain epithelial cells or red or white blood cells embedded in the protein matrix (Figure 5-25C). WBC casts can be seen in kidney infections.

- Waxy casts usually have flattened ends and irregular or serrated margins (Figure 5-25). They appear more opaque or dense than other casts and are thought to be old casts that formed as a result of prolonged tubular stasis.

Crystals and Amorphous Deposits

A variety of crystals can be present in normal urine (Figure 5-26). Crystal formation is influenced by pH, specific gravity, and temperature. The presence of urine crystals has not been associated with increased incidence of *urolithiasis* (kidney stones). Although most urine crystals have no clinical

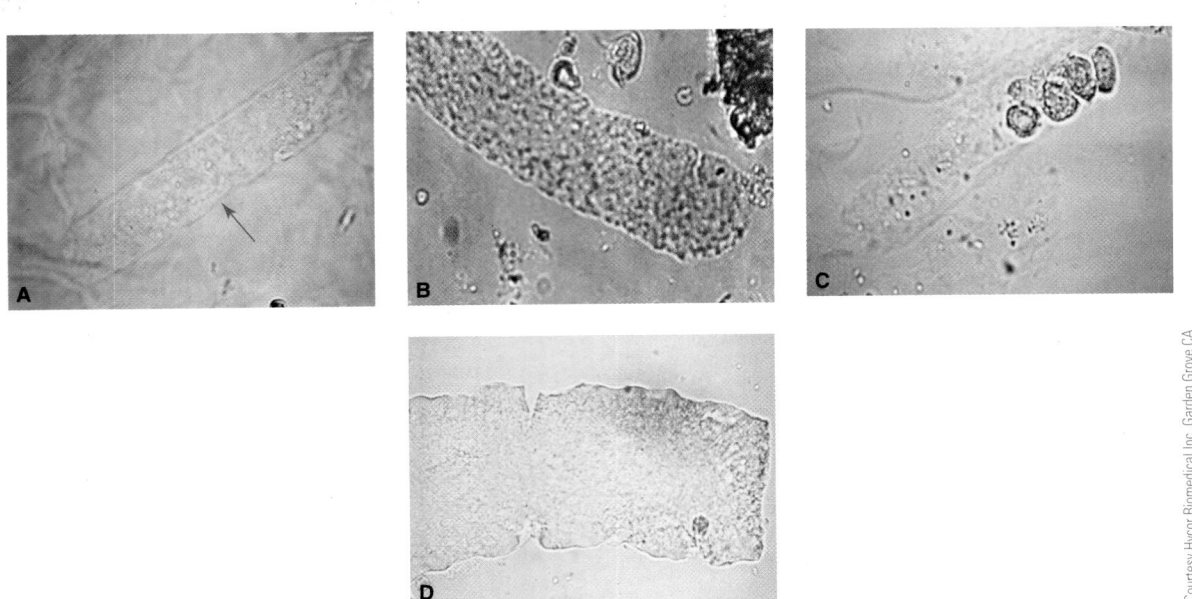

Courtesy Hycor Biomedical Inc, Garden Grove CA

FIGURE 5-25 Casts in urine sediment: (A) hyaline (arrow); (B) granular; (C) cellular; (D) waxy

TABLE 5-12. Examples of conditions associated with the presence of casts in urine sediment

CAST TYPE	ASSOCIATED CONDITIONS
Hyaline	Occasional is normal; increased as a result of stress, strenuous exercise, chronic renal disease, glomerulonephritis, pyelonephritis, congestive heart failure
Granular	Stress, strenuous exercise, pyelonephritis, glomerulonephritis, toxic or viral tubular damage
Cellular:	
Red blood cell	Strenuous exercise, acute glomerulonephritis, pyelonephritis
White blood cell	Pyelonephritis, glomerulonephritis
Epithelial cell	Toxic or viral damage to renal tubules, chronic end stage kidney disease
Waxy	Chronic end stage kidney disease, acute glomerulonephritis

significance, some rare crystals appear in urine because of certain metabolic disorders. Therefore, it is important to be able to recognize both normally occurring and clinically significant crystals. Crystals, when seen, should be identified and reported.

Crystals in Normal Acid Urine

The crystals most commonly seen in normal acid urine are uric acid, amorphous urates, and calcium oxalate (Table 5-13).

- Uric acid can form yellow-brown crystals that have a variety of shapes: irregular, needle-like, rhombic, clusters, or rosettes (Figure 5-26A). Uric acid crystals can be seen in the urine of patients with gout.

- Amorphous urate crystals are called amorphous because they have no specific shape. When amorphous urates are present, the centrifuged sediment often appears pink to the eye, but microscopically the sediment will appear as fine, yellowish granules.

- Calcium oxalate forms colorless, refractile, octahedral crystals. Calcium oxalate crystals can vary in size and have been described as looking like *envelopes*, having an X intersecting the crystal (Figure 5-26C). Calcium oxalate crystals are commonly seen after ingesting large doses of vitamin C or foods high in oxalate, such as tomatoes or spinach. Calcium oxalate crystals can also be seen in neutral pH urine.

Crystals in Normal Neutral or Alkaline Urine

Several types of crystals can occur in neutral to alkaline urine, including amorphous phosphates, calcium phosphate, and triple phosphate. Amorphous phosphates and triple phosphate can also sometimes form in urine that is only slightly acidic, pH 6.5 or higher. Calcium carbonate and ammonium biurate usually occur only in alkaline urine (Table 5-13). Crystals that form in alkaline urine are usually soluble in strong acids.

- Amorphous phosphates appear as white precipitate in the sediment of centrifuged urine having a neutral to alkaline pH. Microscopically they appear as colorless, amorphous, granular particles. Amorphous phosphates are soluble in 10% acetic acid.

- Ammonium magnesium phosphate crystals, commonly called triple phosphate crystals, are six-sided, colorless, highly refractile prisms (Figure 5-26B). They have a very distinctive appearance and are described as coffin-lids. These can be present in neutral to alkaline urine.

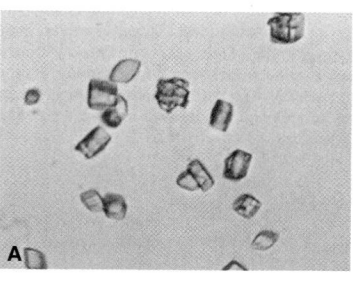 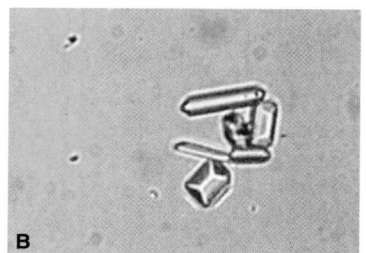 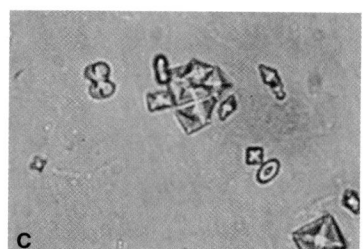

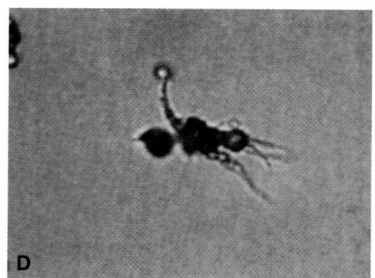

Courtesy Bayer Healthcare

FIGURE 5-26 Crystals in normal urine sediment: (A) uric acid; (B) triple phosphate; (C) calcium oxalate; (D) ammonium biurate

TABLE 5-13. Crystals present in normal urine

CRYSTAL	URINE pH		
	ACID	NEUTRAL	ALKALINE
Uric acid	+		
Amorphous urates	+		
Calcium oxalate	+	+	
Amorphous phosphates		+	+
Calcium phosphate		+	+
Triple phosphate		+	+
Ammonium biurate			+
Calcium carbonate			+

TABLE 5-14. Clinically significant crystals in urine sediment

CRYSTAL	MICROSCOPIC APPEARANCE
Cystine	Colorless, flat, hexagonal crystals
Leucine	Yellow-brown, refractile, oily appearing spheres with concentric circles
Tyrosine	Colorless- to-pale yellow sheaves of needles
Cholesterol	Colorless flat plates with notched or broken corners
Sulfa	Bundles of needles with striations
Hippuric acid	Colorless- to-yellow single needles or prisms
Radiographic media	Flat, colorless plates or slender rectangles

- Calcium phosphate crystals occur in neutral or alkaline urine. They are large, flat, thin plates that can appear granular and can be mistaken for squamous epithelial cells.

- Calcium carbonate forms small, colorless, dumbbell-shaped or leaf-shaped crystals in alkaline urine.

- Ammonium biurate crystals are also called thorn apples because they appear as yellow-brown spheres with thorny projections. These crystals are found in alkaline urine and will revert to uric acid crystals when treated with strong acid (Figure 5-26D).

Clinically Significant Crystals in Urine

Crystals of clinical significance can occur in the urine of patients with certain metabolic diseases or after administration of low solubility drugs such as sulfa drugs. Some abnormally occurring

crystals are cystine, leucine, tyrosine, cholesterol, sulfa, hippuric acid, and crystals of radiographic media (Table 5-14 and Figure 5-27). These crystals are not frequently seen but, when present, are usually in acid urine.

- Cystine forms colorless, refractile, flat, hexagonal crystals, often with unequal sides. Presence of these crystals in urine indicates disease such as *cystinuria*, a condition in which the amino acid cystine is not reabsorbed by the kidney (Figure 5-27A).

- Leucine crystals are refractile, oily-appearing spheres. They can be yellow-brown in color and have concentric striations. Presence of these crystals in urine is an indication of liver disease or damage (Figure 5-27B).

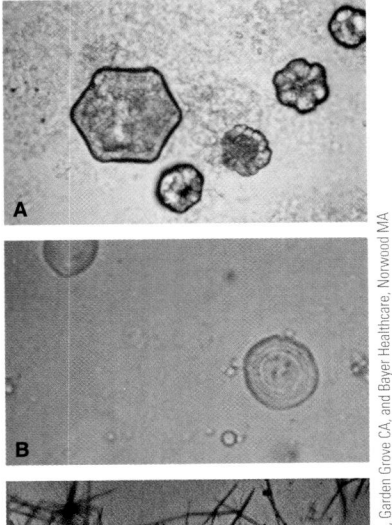
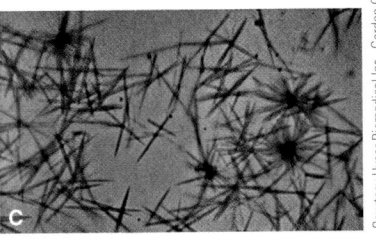
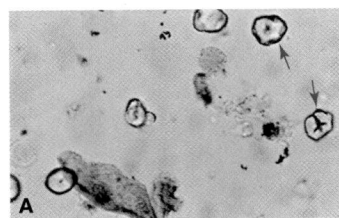
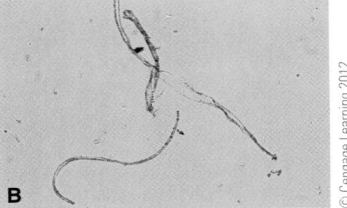

Courtesy Hycor Biomedical Inc., Garden Grove CA, and Bayer Healthcare, Norwood MA

FIGURE 5-27 Clinically significant crystals in urine: (A) cystine; (B) leucine; (C) tyrosine

- Tyrosine forms fine needles arranged in sheaves. Presence of these crystals indicates liver disease or damage (Figure 5-27C).

- Cholesterol crystals are colorless, flat plates with notched or broken corners.

- Sulfa crystals are rarely seen now because of the increased solubility of newer sulfa drugs. When seen, they appear as bundles of needles with striations.

- Hippuric acid is a by-product of the breakdown of benzoic acid and is found in small amounts in normal urine. Hippuric acid is also a metabolic product of organic solvents; levels of hippuric acid can be used to monitor workplace exposure to certain solvents or to monitor substance abuse, such as glue sniffing. When levels of hippuric acid rise, crystals can form in the urine. These appear as colorless, slender needles or prisms.

- Radiographic media crystals can be present in urine for a brief period following intravenous radiographic studies or retrograde cystograms that use diatrizoate dyes. These crystals usually appear as flat, colorless plates or slender rectangles. When present, they can cause urine specific gravity to be especially high (greater than 1.040).

Other Substances in Urine Sediment

Mucus from the urinary tract lining and contaminants such as fibers, hair, starch or talc granules, or oil droplets sometimes are present in urine sediment (Figure 5-28). These substances must be recognized and should not be confused with clinically

© Cengage Learning 2012

FIGURE 5-28 Other substances in urine sediment: (A) starch granules (arrows); (B) cotton fibers

significant substances in the sediment. The presence of mucus is not clinically significant and is reported following the policy in the laboratory's SOP manual. Contaminants or artifacts are not reported.

PERFORMING THE MICROSCOPIC EXAMINATION OF URINE SEDIMENT

The procedure for microscopic examination of urine and the policy for reporting results must be standardized for each laboratory according to equipment and supplies that are available in the particular laboratory.

Safety Precautions

   Because urine is a biological fluid, Standard Precautions must be followed when preparing urine sediment for microscopic examination. Appropriate personal protective equipment (PPE), including gloves and face protection, must be worn during specimen handling, preparation, and evaluation. The creation of splashes or aerosols must be avoided. Safety guidelines for the use of the centrifuge must be followed. The use of microscope slides with beveled corners will decrease the likelihood of injury or tearing gloves when handling slides. Sediment slides must be discarded in a sharps container. Systems such as CenSlide and KOVA eliminate the hazards associated with glass slides and coverglasses.

Quality Assessment

    Each laboratory standard operating procedure (SOP) manual will describe the procedures for microscopic examination of urine, including the volume of urine to be used, the length and force of centrifugation, the sediment volume, quality assessment procedures, and the counting and reporting methods. These guidelines must be followed by all laboratory scientists performing the examinations in order to minimize individual differences in technique.

Because urine sediment components deteriorate rapidly, stable controls for urine microscopy are more difficult to produce than are controls for biochemical tests. However, urine sediment controls such as KOVA-Trol (Hycor Biomedical) contain stabilized RBCs and WBCs.

Specimen Collection and Handling

The preferred specimen is a midstream early morning specimen. The use of a midstream specimen prevents contamination of the specimen with epithelial cells, mucus, and microorganisms. Early morning specimens are usually more concentrated, which increases the chances of finding certain sediment components. In addition, concentrated urines protect some sediment components from deterioration. RBCs, WBCs, and epithelial cells can be damaged or destroyed in dilute urine, causing the numbers of these components to appear falsely decreased during the microscopic examination. All urine specimens should be examined as soon as possible after collection to prevent cellular deterioration and growth of any bacteria present.

Preparing the Sediment

The variables in the procedure for preparing urine sediment must be standardized within each laboratory so that procedures are reproducible. These variables include volume of urine centrifuged, time and speed of centrifugation, and method of resuspending and examining sediment. Typically, procedures call for 10, 12, or 15 mL of well-mixed urine to be poured into a conical centrifuge tube and centrifuged at 400 *g* for 5 minutes. All but 0.5 to 1.0 mL of supernatant is then carefully removed by pouring or pipeting. The sediment is resuspended in the urine remaining in the tube by gently tapping the tip of the tube. One drop of the suspension is pipetted onto a microscope slide and covered with a coverglass.

Several commercial systems are available that standardize the procedure for preparing urine sediment and thus eliminate variations in technique among technicians. The Urisystem (Fisher Scientific), CenSlide 2000 System (IRIS)), and KOVA Urinalysis System (Hycor Biomedical) are examples of such systems (Figures 5-29, 5-30, and 5-31). Depending on the design, the systems can include centrifuge, centrifuge tubes, tube holders, pipets, and standardized slide chambers.

The CenSlide system uses a special centrifuge and a combination test tube/microscope slide. Urine in the capped tube/slide is centrifuged, and sediment is automatically resuspended in the built-in viewing area at the thin, flattened end of the tube (Figure 5-29B). Sediment is viewed microscopically through the thin viewing area by placing the tube/slide directly on the microscope stage (Figure 5-30).

The KOVA Urinalysis System consists of centrifuge tubes and special pipets that are used to standardize the sediment

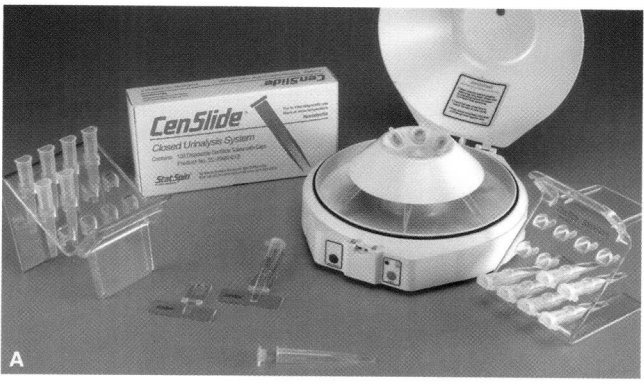

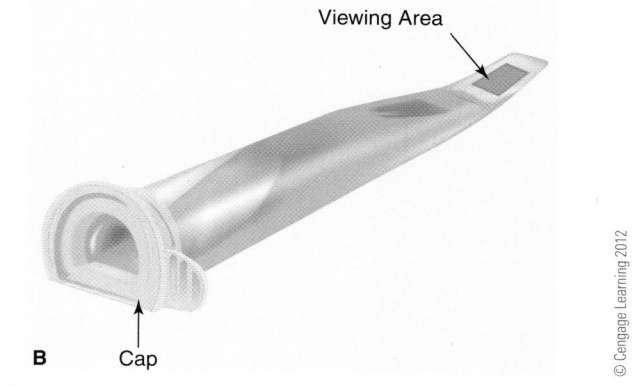

FIGURE 5-29 CenSlide standardized urinalysis system: (A) components of CenSlide system including centrifuge, tubes, tube rack and tube holder; (B) diagram of CenSlide combination test tube-microscope slide

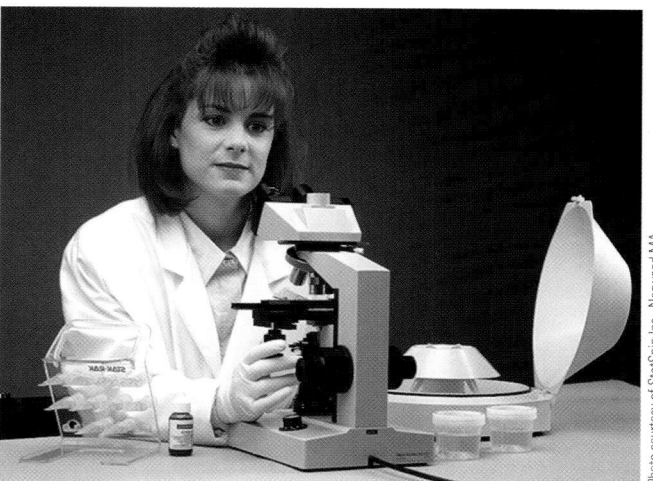

FIGURE 5-30 Using the CenSlide system for microscopic analysis of urine sediment

volume by controlling the volume of urine decanted following centrifugation. The same pipet is used to transfer sediment to slides. Plastic slides with slots for 10 different sediment samples allow multiple specimens to be analyzed from one slide (Figure 5-31).

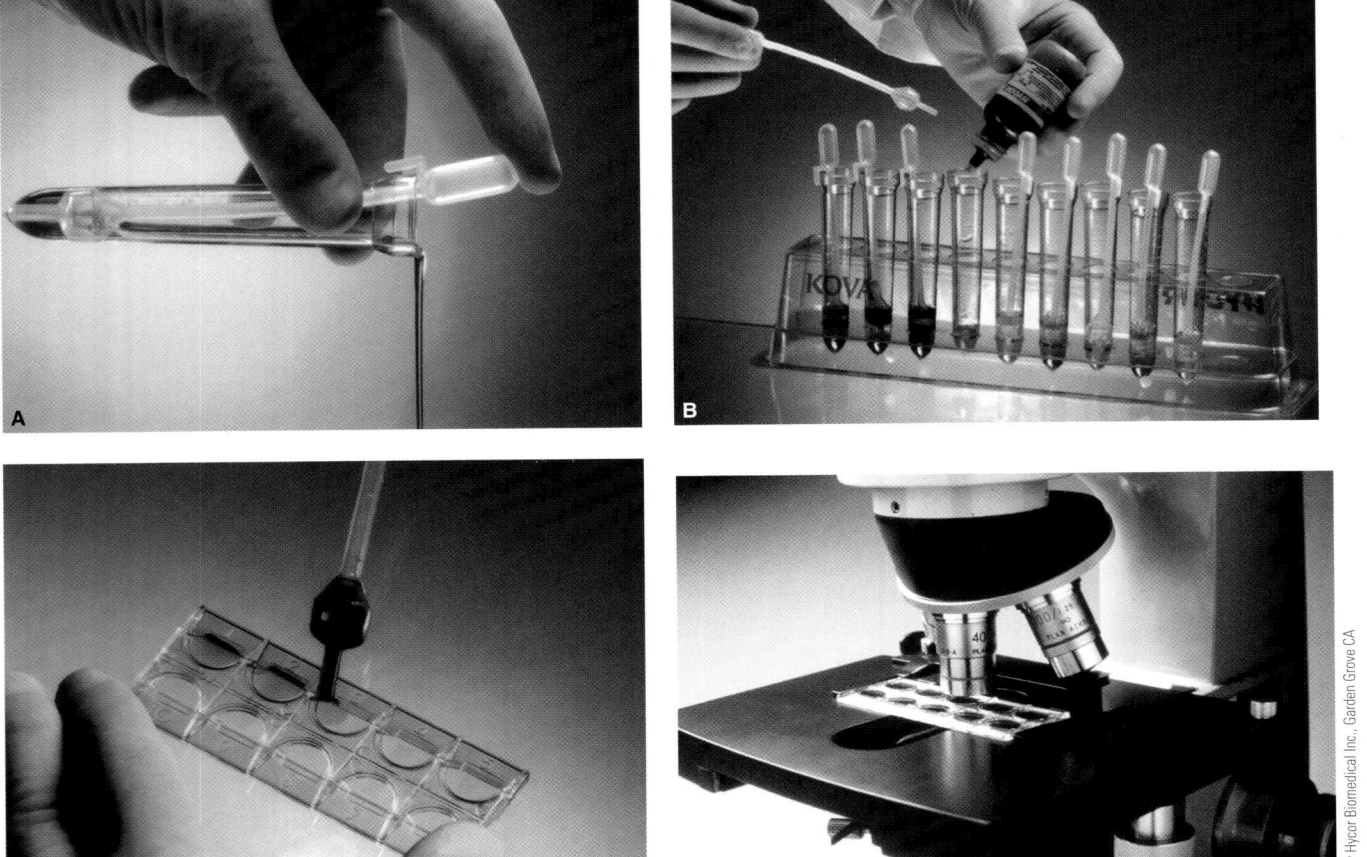

Courtesy Hycor Biomedical Inc., Garden Grove CA

FIGURE 5-31 Using the KOVA® system for standardized urinalysis: (A) pour off supernatant from centrifuged urine using pipet to control remaining volume; (B) stain the sediment (optional); (C) load the slide chamber using the KOVA pipet; (D) observe microscopically

Use of a standardized system ensures that a standard amount of urine is centrifuged and a standard amount of sediment is examined. Some systems include an optional stain to make it easier to identify sediment components.

Counting Sediment Components

Counting and reporting methods can differ slightly among laboratories; therefore, the method used must always be that of the laboratory where the test is being performed. A microscope equipped with phase contrast is preferred for observing urine sediment. If a bright-field microscope is used, the light level and condenser can be adjusted to reduce light and provide more contrast, making it easier to see elements such as casts. During the counting procedure, the fine adjustment should be frequently tweaked to facilitate finding components such as casts.

The sediment slide is examined using the low power objective (10×) to count elements that are few in number, such as casts. The high-power objective (40×) is used to identify and count RBCs, WBCs, epithelial cells, yeasts, bacteria, and crystals and to identify casts. For each component, 10 to 15 consecutive, adjacent microscopic fields are scanned and the numbers of each component present in each field are recorded.

Reporting Results

RBCs, WBCs, and epithelial cells are reported as the number of cells per high power field (HPF) and are usually reported as a range, such as 0–2, 2–4, 4–8, etc. (Tables 5-14 and 5-15). To determine the number to report, the total number of each component recorded from all microscopic fields examined is divided by the number of fields examined. Table 5-16 lists the reference values for urine sediment components.

For example, 10 HPF fields were counted and the numbers of RBCs seen in the 10 fields were 2, 4, 0, 1, 3, 2, 0, 1, 2, and 4. The total number of RBCs seen (19) should be divided by the total number of fields counted (10) to give an average of 1.9 RBCs per HPF. Using the ranges given earlier, this would be reported as *0–2 RBCs/HPF*. When a component is not seen in every field, it can be reported as *occasional* (only 1 seen per 1 to 3 fields) or *rare* (only 1 seen per 5 fields).

Casts are reported as number of casts per low power field (LPF). Casts should also be identified as hyaline, granular, or cellular. Microorganisms such as yeasts and *Trichomonas* should be reported if seen. Bacteria are usually reported only if large numbers are seen in a recently collected urine sample. Bacteria can be reported as negative, $1+, 2+, 3+,$ or $4+$.

Mucus and crystals should be reported if seen, and crystals should be identified. Mucus is usually reported as negative, $1+, 2+, 3+,$ and $4+$. Spermatozoa are reported according to laboratory policy.

Once the microscopic examination is complete, the results of the physical and chemical examination of the specimen should be reviewed to confirm that the microscopic examination results agree or correlate with the physical and chemical tests

TABLE 5-15. Example of a typical method of counting and identifying components of urine sediment

SEDIMENT COMPONENT	IDENTIFY USING	COUNT USING	REPORT
Red blood cells	HP	HP	Average # / HPF
White blood cells	HP	HP	Average # / HPF
Epithelial cells	HP	HP	Average # / HPF
Casts	HP	LP	Average # / LPF
Bacteria/yeasts	HP	HP	0–4+*
Mucus	HP	HP	0–4+
Crystals	HP	—	Type present

HP = high power objective
HPF = high power field
LP = low power objective
LPF = low power field
0 = none seen in 10 fields
Rare = only 1 seen per 5 fields
Occasional = only 1 seen per 1–3 fields
*Usually only reported when large numbers are present

TABLE 5-16. Reference values for components of urine sediment

COMPONENT	REFERENCE VALUE
Red blood cells/HPF	0–4
White blood cells/HPF	0–4
Epithelial cells/HPF	Occasional (can be higher in females)
Casts/LPF	Occasional, hyaline
Bacteria	Negative
Yeasts	Negative
Mucus	Negative to 2+
Crystals	Types present vary with pH (crystals such as cystine, leucine, tyrosine, and cholesterol are considered clinically significant)

HPF = high power field
LPF = low power field

TABLE 5-17. Correlation of results of microscopic findings of urine sediment with physical and chemical examination results

MICROSCOPIC FINDINGS	EXPECTED RESULTS	
	PHYSICAL EXAMINATION	CHEMICAL EXAMINATION
White blood cells*	Turbid	+ Protein
		+ Nitrite*
		+ Leukocytes*
Red blood cells†	Turbid, red color	+ Blood
Large numbers of epithelial cells	Turbid	—
Casts	Clear to turbid	+ Protein
Normal crystals	Turbid	Acid to alkaline pH
Bacteria	Turbid	+ Nitrite

*In cases of bacterial infection, can also see bacteria
†RBCs are not seen if hemolysis has occurred

(Table 5-17). For instance, if the chemical strip test was positive for leukocyte esterase, increased numbers of WBCs should be seen in the microscopic examination. If urine transparency was recorded as hazy, mucus might be present in large amounts. If urine color was reported as red, increased numbers of RBCs would be expected. The results should be examined for unusual findings that warrant making a special note on the report (Table 5-18).

Automated Analysis of Urine Sediment

Several automated and semi-automated urine analyzers are available; most are used to perform only the physical and chemical examinations of urine. These instruments have the advantages of processing large numbers of samples rapidly, improving standardization, and decreasing clerical errors.

A few analyzers are also capable of analyzing urine sediment components. One fully automated analyzer is the IRIS iQ200 Series Urinalysis System manufactured by International Remote Imaging Systems (IRIS), Inc. The iQ200 analyzers perform the physical, chemical, and microscopic parts of routine urinalysis by linking together modules that perform each part of the examination.

The technologist loads a well-mixed, bar-coded aliquot of urine into a sample tray on the analyzer. Physical and chemical examinations are performed first. The instrument mixes the sample again and robotically dispenses urine onto pads of a reagent strip. The reactions are read colorimetrically at the appropriate times. Urine color is determined spectrophotometrically, transparency is determined using a turbidimeter, and specific gravity is read using an internal refractometer.

The specimen is then moved to the microscopy analyzer. There the sample passes through a flow cell, where 500 digital images are taken of each sample. Using particle recognition software, 12 urine sediment components can be identified and categorized into 14 categories based on characteristics such as size, shape, texture, and contrast. The categories are RBC, WBC, WBC clump, hyaline cast, unclassified cast, crystals, squamous epithelial cell, nonsquamous epithelial cell, yeast, bacteria, mucus, sperm, amorphous, and unclassified. Before results are reported, abnormal or unusual results are visually confirmed by a technologist using a video screen. Images are archived and can be viewed at any time; the images also can be used for teaching.

The Clinitek AUWi System combines the Clinitek Atlas analyzer, which performs high-volume physical and chemical urine analyses, with the Sysmex UF-1000i urine particle analyzer to provide a fully automated urinalysis system. The Sysmex UF 1000i uses laser-based fluorescent flow cytometry to differentiate among, and determine numbers of, formed elements in urine sediment (Figure 5-32). This urine sediment analyzer

TABLE 5-18. Correlation of the presence and amount of urine sediment components with examples of physiological and pathological conditions

	CONDITION/DISEASE			
COMPONENT	**STRENUOUS EXERCISE**	**ACUTE CYSTITIS**	**GLOMERULO-NEPHRITIS**	**CHRONIC END STAGE KIDNEY DISEASE**
White blood cells	0–1×	4×	2×	1–2×
Red blood cells	0–1×	2×	4×	1–2×
Bacteria	0	+	0	±
Renal epithelial cells	0	0	1×	1–2×
Hyaline casts	3–4×	1×	1–2×	2×
Granular casts	1×	0	1–2×	1–2×
White blood cell casts	0	0	1–2×	1–2×
Red blood cell casts	0	0	4×	1–2×

0 = count of cells or casts does not exceed reference range
± = small amount present
+ = present
× = a fold increase over reference range. For example, in glomerulonephritis, a two-fold increase (2×) over the normal amount of white blood cells can be seen
1× = one-fold increase over normal
2× = two-fold increase over normal
3× = three-fold increase over normal
4× = four-fold increase over normal

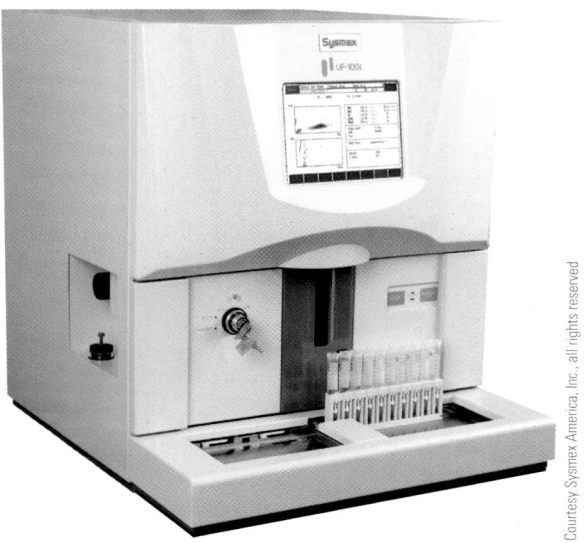

Courtesy Sysmex America, Inc., all rights reserved

FIGURE 5-32 Sysmex UF 100i urine particle analyzer

SAFETY REMINDERS

- Review Safety Precautions section before performing procedure.
- Observe Standard Precautions.
- Wear appropriate PPE.
- Follow centrifuge safety rules.
- Use exposure control methods when discarding specimens.

PROCEDURAL REMINDERS

- Review Quality Assessment section before beginning procedure.
- Follow SOP manual for sediment preparation, counting, and reporting.
- Adjust microscope light, iris diaphragm, and condenser to provide best contrast.
- Use acetic acid to differentiate yeasts from RBCs.

operates similar to hematology flow cytometry analyzers, which are discussed in Lesson 2-10. As stained sediment components flow through the analyzer, a laser excites the fluorescent dye. Measurements are made of fluorescence, scatter, and impedance, providing identification and classification of 10 components. A specimen having unusual results is flagged, and the results are confirmed microscopically by the technician.

CASE STUDY 1

The following results were reported for a microscopic examination of urine from a 31-year-old female patient: 2–4 WBCs, 0–2 RBCs, 0–2 epithelial cells, occasional hyaline cast, occasional uric acid crystal, rare calcium oxalate crystal, and 1+ mucus.

How should these results be interpreted?

CASE STUDY 2

A routine urinalysis was performed on a fresh, random specimen. The results were:

Physical Exam	Patient Results
Clarity	Slightly turbid
Color	Yellow
Sp. gr.	1.015

(Continues)

CASE STUDY 2 (Continued)

Chemical Exam	Patient Results
pH	6.4
Protein	1+
Glucose	Neg
Ketone	Neg
Bilirubin	Neg
Blood	Neg
Urobilinogen	Neg
Nitrite	Neg
Leukocyte esterase	1+

Microscopic Exam	Patient Results
WBCs	6–8/HPF
RBCs	10–15/HPF
Epithelial cells	0–2/HPF
Casts	Rare/HPF
Bacteria	Neg
Yeasts	Neg
Crystals	None seen

1. Which chemical and microscopic results show a discrepancy?

   a. 1+ Leukocyte esterase and 6–8 WBCs/HPF

   b. Negative blood and 10–15 RBCs/HPF

   c. 1+ Protein and 6–8 WBCs/HPF

   d. Neg nitrite and 6–8 WBCs/HPF

2. What follow-up test(s) would be appropriate to resolve the discrepancy?

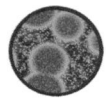

SUMMARY

Microscopic examination of urine sediment is a valuable part of the routine urinalysis and is an important test in the detection of renal disease. Components that can be visible in urine sediment include blood cells, epithelial cells, bacteria, fungal cells, and parasitic organisms. Casts and crystals can also be visible in urine. Laboratory scientists must be able to distinguish clinically significant urine sediment components from artifacts that can also be present in urine sediment.

Experience is required to become proficient in the microscopic identification of urine sediment components. Because there are few controls for urine sediment, it is essential that each laboratory standardize the technique of sediment preparation and counting and reporting procedures. Standardizing these procedures is made easier by the use of commercial systems for preparing sediment or fully automated urine analyzers.

Reproducibility of results is important when tests are performed by different laboratory personnel. For example,

patients with acute or chronic kidney disease can have urinalysis performed frequently to monitor the course of the disease and/ or the effectiveness of treatment. When standardized procedures are used for every patient sample, clinicians can be assured that urinalysis results are reliable indicators of the patient's condition.

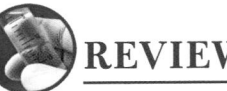

REVIEW QUESTIONS

1. What is the preferred urine specimen for microscopic examination of urine sediment?

2. How is urine sediment prepared for a microscopic examination?

3. Why are microscopic urine tests important?

4. Why is it important to wear gloves and avoid splashes when handling urines?

5. What happens to cells in dilute urine samples?

6. What is the advantage of using a standardized system such as the KOVA System, CenSlide, or UriSystem to prepare urine sediment?

7. Name four types of cells that can be seen in urine sediment.

8. How can yeast cells be differentiated from RBCs?

9. Explain how casts are formed.

10. Name eight crystals that can occur in sediment from normal urine and describe the appearance of each.

11. Name four clinically significant crystals that can be present in urine sediment and describe the appearance of each.

12. What are the reference values for RBCs, WBCs, casts, and bacteria in urine sediment?

13. What is the reference source for the procedure for counting and reporting urine sediment components?

14. The following numbers of WBCs were observed in 15 adjacent HPFs when performing microscopic examination of urine sediment: 6, 5, 6, 2, 7, 1, 3, 4, 8, 6, 9,

7, 6, 5, and 8. How should the WBCs be reported for this specimen?

15. Define cast, flagellum, hyaline, protozoa, sediment, supernatant, and yeast.

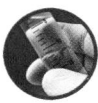

STUDENT ACTIVITIES

1. Complete the written examination for this lesson.

2. Practice identifying components of urine sediment using visuals provided by the instructor.

3. Practice performing a microscopic examination on one or more urine specimens as outlined in the Student Performance Guide, using the worksheet or report form.

4. Compare the microscopic results with the chemical test results on the same specimen. Do they correlate?

5. Draw three components that were found in the urine sediments. Are they normal components of urine?

WEB ACTIVITIES

1. Use the Internet to search for information on glomerulonephritis, nephritis, and cystitis. Discuss the urine sediment components you might expect to see in each condition.

2. Use the Internet to find images of urine sediment components. Make your own reference atlas of sediment components from online images. (Be sure that you do not violate any copyrights; most web sites allow personal use of images.)

3. Search the Internet for tutorials or self-tests on the identification of urine sediment components.

LESSON 5-5
Microscopic Examination of Urine Sediment

(Individual student results will vary depending on specimens provided by instructor and student technique.)

Name _____   Date _____

INSTRUCTIONS

1. Practice preparing and examining urine sediment following the step-by-step procedure and using the worksheet.

2. Demonstrate the procedure for preparing and examining urine sediment satisfactorily for the instructor, using the Student Performance Guide. Your instructor will explain the procedures for evaluating and grading your performance. Your performance may be given a number grade, letter grade, or satisfactory (S) or unsatisfactory depending on course or institutional policy.

NOTE: Follow laboratory SOP manual and manufacturer's instructions for the system or instrument being used

MATERIALS AND EQUIPMENT

- gloves
- hand antiseptic
- full-face shield (or equivalent PPE)
- acrylic splash shield (optional)
- recently collected urine samples
- urine sediment controls (optional)
- centrifuge
- microscope
- worksheet
- timer (if centrifuge lacks timer)
- visuals depicting various components of urine sediment or preprepared slides of urine sediment
- commercial standardized urinalysis system or the following materials:
  - microscope slides and coverglasses
  - disposable transfer pipets
  - 15-mL disposable, conical capped centrifuge tubes and test tube rack
- paper towels
- laboratory tissue
- surface disinfectant (such as 10% chlorine bleach)
- biohazard container
- sharps container
- Optional: materials and equipment for urine physical examination (see Lesson 5-3) and chemical examination (Lesson 5-4) procedures and Urinalysis Report Form

PROCEDURE

Record in the comment section any problems encountered while practicing the procedure (or have a fellow student or the instructor evaluate your performance).

S = Satisfactory
U = Unsatisfactory

You must:	S	U	Evaluation/Comments
1. Wash hands with antiseptic and put on gloves and face protection			
2. Assemble equipment and materials for preparing urine sediment			

(Continues)

© 2012 Delmar, Cengage Learning. Permission to reproduce for clinical use granted.

You must:	S	U	Evaluation/Comments
3. Obtain a urine sample or a urine sediment control			
4. Pour 10 to 15 mL of well-mixed urine into a disposable conical centrifuge tube and cap tube (optional: use tube from standardized system)			
5. Place capped tube in centrifuge, insert balance tube, and close and lock lid			
6. Centrifuge urine for recommended time and at recommended speed (commonly 5 minutes at 1500 rpm or $400 \times g$)			
7. Remove tubes from centrifuge after rotor comes to a complete stop			
8. Pipet or pour off supernatant urine, leaving approximately 0.5 to 1.0 mL of urine in tube (follow system instructions if applicable)			
9. Resuspend urine sediment by lightly tapping the bottom of the tube			
10. Place 1 drop of resuspended urine onto a clean glass slide (or into chamber provided with the system)			
11. Place coverglass over drop of urine if using glass slide			
12. Place slide on microscope stage, focus using low-power ($10 \times$) objective, and adjust light and condenser			
13. Scan 10 to 15 consecutive, adjacent low-power fields (LPF), count the number of casts per field, and record the average number of casts per LPF on the worksheet (divide the total number of casts seen by the number of fields counted)			
14. Rotate the high-power ($40 \times$) objective into position (adjust condenser and/or light if necessary) and record on worksheet			
15. Identify the type(s) of casts present and record			
16. Scan 10 to 15 consecutive, adjacent fields using high power objective: Count the number of RBCs, WBCs, and epithelial cells per high-power field and record; calculate the average for each cell type and record on worksheet			
17. Observe slide for the presence of microorganisms, crystals, or mucus, and record if present. If crystals are present, identify type			
18. Record all results on worksheet			
19. Optional: Perform physical and chemical examinations on the urine used for the microscopic examination, or select another specimen and perform all three examinations: a. Record results on Urinalysis Report Form b. Correlate physical and chemical results with results of microscopic examination			

© 2012 Delmar, Cengage Learning. Permission to reproduce for clinical use granted.

You must:	S	U	Evaluation/Comments
20. Discard specimens as directed, avoiding aerosol formation			
21. Discard used slides and other sharps into sharps container			
22. Discard other contaminated materials into appropriate biohazard container			
23. Clean equipment and return to storage			
24. Wipe work area with surface disinfectant			
25. Remove gloves and discard into biohazard container			
26. Wash hands with antiseptic			
27. Use unlabeled illustrations or preprepared slides of urine sediment provided by the instructor to identify components of sediment not seen on slides			

Instructor/Evaluator Comments:

Instructor/Evaluator _____ Date _____

© 2012 Delmar, Cengage Learning. Permission to reproduce for clinical use granted.

STUDENT PERFORMANCE GUIDE

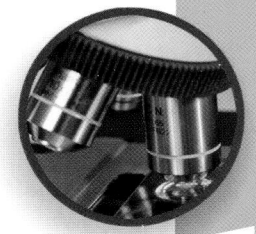

LESSON 5-5
Microscopic Examination of Urine Sediment

(Individual student results will vary depending on specimens provided by instructor and student technique.)

WORKSHEET

Name _____   Date _____

Specimen I.D. _____

MICROSCOPIC EXAM	PATIENT RESULTS	REFERENCE VALUES
White blood cells:	_____ / HPF	0–4
Red blood cells:	_____ / HPF	0–4
Epithelial cells:	_____ / HPF	Occasional (higher in females)
Casts:	_____ / LPF	Occasional, hyaline
Type present	_____	
Yeasts: (circle result)	Negative 1+ 2+ 3+ 4+	Negative
Bacteria: (circle result)	Negative 1+ 2+ 3+ 4+	Negative
Mucus: (circle result)	Negative 1+ 2+ 3+ 4+	Negative to 2+
Amorphous deposits:	_____ None seen _____ Present	
Crystals:	_____ None seen _____ Present	
Type:	_____	

LESSON 5-5
Microscopic Examination of Urine

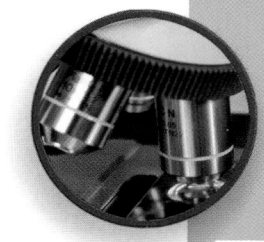

Specimen I.D. _____   Date _____

PHYSICAL EXAM	PATIENT RESULTS	REFERENCE VALUES
Transparency:	_____ Clear	Clear
	_____ Hazy (slightly cloudy)	
	_____ Cloudy (turbid)	
	_____ Milky (opalescent)	
	_____ Other	
Color:	_____	Pale yellow to amber
Specific gravity:	_____	1.010–1.025

REAGENT STRIP

Glucose	_____	Negative
Bilirubin	_____	Negative
Ketones	_____	Negative
Blood	_____	Negative
pH	_____	5.0–8.0
Protein	_____	Negative, trace
Urobilinogen	_____	0.1–1.0 mg/dL
Nitrite	_____	Negative
Leukocyte esterase	_____	Negative
Specific gravity	_____	1.010–1.025

Microscopic Examination

White blood cells:	_____ / HPF	0–4
Red blood cells:	_____ / HPF	0–4
Epithelial cells:	_____ / HPF	Occasional (higher in females)
Casts:	_____ / LPF	Occasional, hyaline
Type present	_____	
Yeasts: (circle result)	Negative 1+ 2+ 3+ 4+	Negative
Bacteria: (circle result)	Negative 1+ 2+ 3+ 4+	Negative
Mucus: (circle result)	Negative 1+ 2+ 3+ 4+	Negative to 2+
Crystals:	_____ None seen _____ Present	
Type:	_____	
Amorphous deposits:	_____ None seen _____ Present	

Comment: _____

© 2012 Delmar, Cengage Learning. Permission to reproduce for clinical use granted.

UNIT 6

Basic Clinical Chemistry

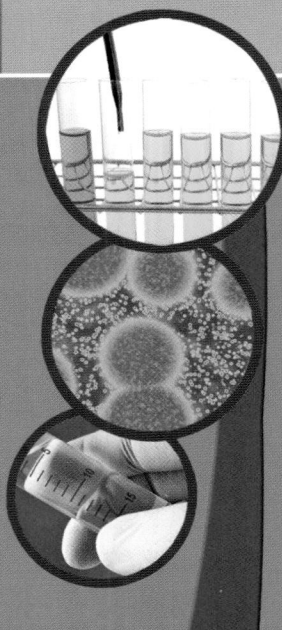

UNIT OBJECTIVES

After studying this unit, the student will:

- Discuss the importance of clinical chemistry.
- Identify 15 frequently performed clinical chemistry tests and explain the significance of each.
- Explain the importance of the proper collection and handling of specimens for clinical chemistry.
- Describe three technologies used in chemistry analyzers.
- Discuss the role of point-of-care testing in health care.
- Discuss the principles and importance of tests for glucose and hemoglobin A1c.
- Explain the significance of tests for cholesterol and triglycerides.
- Explain the principles and importance of electrolyte tests.
- Explain the importance and use of fecal occult blood tests.

UNIT OVERVIEW

Clinical chemistry is the branch of laboratory medicine that uses chemical analysis to study the levels of various body constituents during health and disease. These chemical tests are usually performed on blood samples, but urine and other body fluids are also analyzed. The test results are used by the physician to diagnose disease, institute treatment, and follow the disease's progress. The physician also uses the results to counsel the patient in preventive medicine.

The study of body chemistry has a long history; as far back as Hippocrates, certain physicians emphasized body fluid analysis in patient care. Observations were made on urine and feces because of the ease of collecting these specimens.

Early chemical tests were qualitative in nature in that they could only detect whether or not a constituent was present. As analytical methods were developed, it became possible to measure how much of a substance was present. The results of analyses of some constituents performed by crude manual methods over 100 years ago compare very well with results obtained today using sophisticated methods and technology.

This unit is an introduction to some basic theories and principles of clinical chemistry. To understand the basis of the chemical tests discussed in this unit and the significance of test results, the student must have a fundamental knowledge of human physiology. Before beginning Unit 6, the student may want to review organ systems and functions as well as Lesson 1-9, Quality Assessment.

Lesson 6-1 introduces the topic of clinical chemistry and the relationships between the values of frequently measured blood components and the state of health or disease of the individual. Lesson 6-2 contains general information about collecting and processing blood specimens for laboratory analysis. Lesson 6-3 presents the basic principles of several technologies used in clinical chemistry analyzers.

The increase in testing at sites other than traditional laboratories has resulted largely from the development of small, portable, affordable instruments that can perform a variety of tests. Lesson 6-4 discusses important aspects of point-of-care testing (POCT), also called bedside or near-patient testing.

Because blood glucose is one of the most frequently requested chemistry tests, Lesson 6-5 presents information about glucose metabolism, methods of glucose analysis, and hemoglobin A1c. Lesson 6-6 explains the importance of cholesterol and triglycerides and gives procedures for assaying these at POC. Lesson 6-7 describes the functions of electrolytes and methods and instruments for measuring electrolytes. The fecal occult blood test, explained in Lesson 6-8, is used to screen for intestinal disease and colorectal cancer.

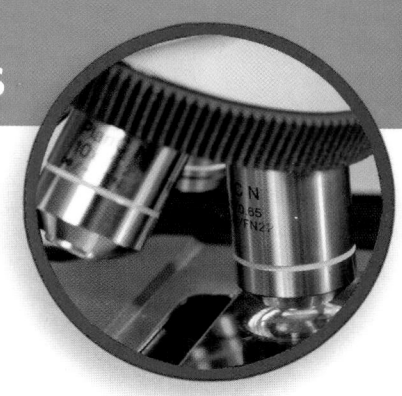

American Diabetes Association. "Executive Summary: Standards of Medical Care in Diabetes—2010." *Diabetes Care.* January 2010; Vol. 33 (Suppl. 1) S4-S10.

American Diabetes Association. "Position Statement: Diagnosis and Classification of Diabetes Mellitus." *Diabetes Care.* January 2010; Vol. 33 (Suppl. 1) S62-S69.

Bishop, M. L. et al. (2009). *Clinical chemistry: Techniques, principles, correlations.* (6th ed.). Baltimore: Lippincott Williams & Wilkins.

Burtis, C. A., et al. (Eds.) (2005). *Tietz textbook of clinical chemistry and molecular diagnosis* (4th ed.). Philadelphia: W. B. Saunders Company.

Burtis, C. A., et al. (Eds.) (2008). *Tietz fundamentals of clinical chemistry* (6th ed.). Philadelphia: W. B. Saunders Company.

Clinical Laboratory Improvement Act of 1988. (Feb. 28, 1992). *Federal Register*, Vol. 7, No. 40.

Daniels, R. (2003). *Delmar's manual of laboratory and diagnostic tests.* Clifton Park, NY: Thomson Delmar Learning.

Helms, J. R. (2009). *Mathematics for medical and clinical laboratory professionals.* Clifton Park, NY: Delmar Cengage Learning.

Hill, B. (2005). Accu-Chek advantage: Electrochemistry for diabetes management. Available at: *currentseparations.com*, Vol. 21, No. 2.

Kaplan, L. A. & Pesce, A. (2009). *Clinical chemistry: Theory, analysis, correlation.* (5th ed.). St. Louis: Mosby.

McPherson, R. A. & Pincus, M. R. (Eds.) (2007). *Henry's clinical diagnosis and management by laboratory methods.* (21st ed.). Philadelphia: Saunders Elsevier.

Nagy, H. et al. (2005). *Case-based pathology and laboratory medicine.* Ames, IA: Blackwell Publishers.

Sacher, R. A. et al. (2000). *Widmann's clinical interpretation of laboratory tests.* (11th ed.). Philadelphia: F. A. Davis Company.

Venes, D., et al. (Eds.) (2009). *Taber's cyclopedic medical dictionary.* (21st ed.). Philadelphia: F. A. Davis Company.

Wadsworth, H. M., et al. (2001). *Modern methods for quality control and improvement.* (2nd ed.). New York: Wiley.

Product Information

A1C NOW Professional Procedure Guide (2008). Tarrytown NY: Bayer Healthcare.

CHOLESTECH. Manufacturer's package insert. Hayward, CA: Cholestech LDX (2004).

ColoScreen package insert. Beaumont, TX: Helena Laboratories.

Hemoccult ICT Product Instructions, 2004. Beckman Coulter Inc., Fullerton CA.

Hemoccult Sensa Product Instructions, 2002. Beckman Coulter Inc., Fullerton CA.

Mayo Clinic (June 2, 2009). "Improved DNA Stool Test Could Detect Digestive Cancers In Multiple Organs." *ScienceDaily.* Available at: http://www.sciencedaily.com /releases/2009/06/090602092251.htm.

Web Sites of Interest

American Association for Clinical Chemistry, www.aacc.org (archives of *Clinical Laboratory News*)

American Cancer Society, www.cancer.org

American Diabetes Association, www.diabetes.org

American Heart Association, www.heart.org

College of American Pathologists, www.cap.org

National Cholesterol Education Program, www.nhlbi.nih.gov/ about/ncep

National Institutes of Health, www.nih.gov

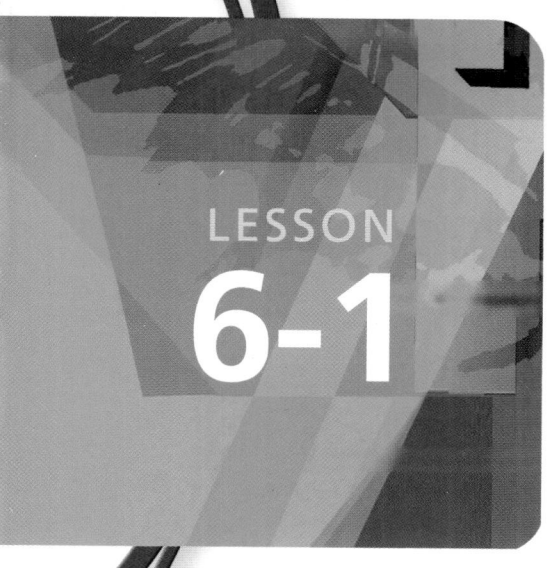

LESSON 6-1

Introduction to Clinical Chemistry

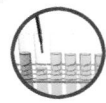

LESSON OBJECTIVES

After studying this lesson, the student will:

⊙ Discuss the history of clinical chemistry.

⊙ List six body fluids tested in clinical chemistry.

⊙ List 15 constituents commonly assayed in a routine chemistry profile.

⊙ Explain the significance or function of each of the constituents commonly included in a routine chemistry profile.

⊙ List the normal or reference values for 15 constituents measured in a routine chemistry profile.

⊙ Give examples of tests performed in kidney, liver, cardiac, thyroid, and lipid profiles.

⊙ Explain how reference ranges are established and how they are used by the laboratory and physician.

⊙ Define the glossary terms.

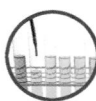

GLOSSARY

alanine aminotransferase (ALT) / an enzyme present in high concentration in the liver and measured to assess liver function; formerly called SGPT

albumins / the most abundant protein in normal plasma; a homogeneous group of plasma proteins that are made in the liver and help maintain osmotic balance

alkaline phosphatase (ALP or AP) / an enzyme widely distributed in the body, especially in the liver and bone

analyte / a chemical substance that is the subject of chemical analysis

anion / a negatively charged ion

aspartate aminotransferase (AST) / an enzyme present in many tissues, including cardiac, muscle, and liver, and measured to assess liver function; formerly called SGOT

bilirubin / a product formed in the liver from the breakdown of hemoglobin

blood urea nitrogen (BUN) / a test measuring urea nitrogen in blood

B-type natriuretic peptide (BNP) / a peptide hormone released primarily from the ventricles of the heart and used as a marker for cardiac function

cardiovascular disease (CVD) / disease of the heart and blood vessels resulting from a variety of causes

cation / a positively charged ion

coronary heart disease (CHD) / a narrowing of the small blood vessels that supply blood and oxygen to the heart; also called coronary artery disease (CAD)

C-reactive protein (CRP) / one of the acute phase proteins found in plasma in inflammation

(continues)

601

creatine kinase (CK) / an enzyme present in large amounts in brain tissue and heart and skeletal muscle and a form of which is measured to aid in diagnosing heart attack

creatinine / a breakdown product of creatine that is normally excreted in the urine

electrolytes / the cations and anions important in maintaining fluid and acid–base balance

gamma-glutamyltransferase (GGT) / an enzyme present in liver, kidney, pancreas, and prostate, and measured to assess liver function

globulins / a heterogeneous group of serum proteins with varied functions

glomerular filtration rate (GFR) / an estimation of how much blood passes through the glomeruli per unit of time (minute); an estimate of the number of functioning nephrons made by using the rate at which molecules such as creatinine and urea are filtered by the kidneys

gout / a painful condition in which blood uric acid is elevated and urates precipitate in joints

HDL cholesterol / high-density lipoprotein fraction of blood cholesterol; *good* cholesterol

homeostasis / the tendency toward steady state or equilibrium of body processes

homocysteine / an amino acid, elevated blood levels of which are associated with increased risk for vascular and cardiovascular disease

hypercalcemia / blood calcium levels above normal

hyperlipidemia / excessive amount of fat in the blood

hyperthyroidism / excessive functional activity of the thyroid gland; excessive secretion of thyroid hormones

hypoalbuminemia / marked decrease in serum albumin concentration

hypocalcemia / blood calcium levels below normal

hypothyroidism / underactive function of the thyroid gland; abnormally low production of thyroid hormones

lactate dehydrogenase (LD or LDH) / an enzyme widely distributed in the body and measured to assess liver function

LDL cholesterol / low-density lipoprotein fraction of blood cholesterol; *bad* cholesterol

lipids / any one of a group of fats or fat-like substances

thyroid-stimulating hormone (TSH) / a hormone that is synthesized by the anterior pituitary gland and regulates the activity of the thyroid gland; thyrotropin

thyroxine / a thyroid hormone, commonly called T_4

triglycerides / the major storage form of lipids; lipid molecules formed from glycerol and fatty acids

triiodothyronine / one of the thyroid hormones, commonly called T_3

troponins / intracellular proteins that are present in skeletal and heart muscle and are released when muscle is injured

uric acid / a breakdown product of nucleic acids

VLDL cholesterol / very low density lipoprotein fraction of blood cholesterol

INTRODUCTION

Chemical constituents in a healthy body are in a delicate balance, or equilibrium, that is influenced by both internal and external factors. This equilibrium, or steady state, is referred to as **homeostasis**. A change in concentration of a chemical constituent will usually trigger a reaction to bring the concentration back to the equilibrium state. For example, when the blood glucose level rises after a meal, the pancreas releases insulin to bring the blood glucose concentration down to a normal level.

In the clinical chemistry laboratory, tests are performed on blood and other body fluids. Formerly chemistry tests were performed primarily on patient serum samples, but instruments that can use plasma are widely available. Specimens are analyzed for the presence or absence of certain substances (qualitative test) or for the level or amount of the substances (quantitative test). The tests can be for **analytes**, substances that have a biological function, or for nonfunctional metabolites or waste products, substances that indicate damage or disease in the body. The test results are compared with values found in health, called normal values or reference values. Therapeutic drugs, drugs of abuse, and other toxic substances can be detected and measured.

Physicians use the results of clinical chemistry tests to aid in the diagnosis, treatment, and prevention of disease. Interpretation of test results is based on understanding the physiological and biochemical processes occurring in health and in disease. Test results must be reliable so the physician can have confidence in using the test results. Reliability of test results is ensured when:

- Specimens are collected, handled, and stored correctly until tests are performed (preanalytical phase)
- Specimens are analyzed using correct procedures and appropriate quality assessment measures (analytical phase)
- Results are calculated and reported accurately (postanalytical phase).

This lesson contains information about several routine clinical chemistry tests often included in chemistry profiles. Included are the expected (reference) ranges for each component and a brief rationale for performing the tests.

TYPES OF CHEMISTRY TESTS

Blood chemistry tests can be organized into the categories of routine and special. The routine tests are those that are frequently ordered, such as a single test for glucose or a chemistry profile. A routine chemistry profile, also called a complete metabolic profile, is a group of tests performed simultaneously on a patient specimen to provide an assessment of the patient's general condition. Tests included in a routine chemistry profile reflect the state of carbohydrate and lipid metabolism, as well as kidney, thyroid, liver, and cardiac function (Figure 6-1).

Profiles or panels that assess one particular biological system, such as renal or liver function, are also performed. Examples of chemistry panels are listed in Table 6-1. Many chemistry analyzers are capable of performing chemistry profiles on hundreds of patient samples per hour.

Tests that are ordered less frequently, such as hormones or certain drug levels, might be performed only on certain days even in the larger laboratories and are sometimes referred to as *special* tests. Many laboratories send these specimens to a regional or reference laboratory. These tests are usually requested when a particular diagnosis is suspected or treatment must be monitored.

Specimens for Chemical Analysis

The most common specimens for chemical analysis are blood and urine. Lesson 6-2 explains the methods of collecting, processing, and handling blood for routine chemical analysis. General techniques for collection of capillary and venous blood are described in detail in Lessons 1-11 and 1-12. Urine collection methods are described in Lesson 5-2. Less frequently tested are cerebrospinal fluid (CSF), synovial fluid, pleural fluid, and pericardial fluid; these specimens are usually collected by the physician. Before specimen collection, it is important to know which tests will be performed so the specimen will be collected and processed appropriately.

Units of Measure

Clinical chemistry test results are usually reported in metric units or SI units (International System of Nomenclature). Commonly used units are milligrams (mg) or micrograms (µg) per deciliter (dL), millimoles per liter (mmol/L), or, in the case of enzymes, enzyme activity units per liter (U/L).

Reference Ranges

The reference (or normal) range of a substance is determined by measuring the level of the substance in a portion of the general population and applying statistical methods to the data. This population should be chosen from the geographical area in which the laboratory is located. For instance, when establishing the reference range for total protein, a laboratory might test 100 random samples from the population and calculate the mean value and the standard deviation (denoted as s, s.d., or SD) of the set of values. The reference range is then determined by adding $2\ s$ to the mean and subtracting $2\ s$ from the mean ($\pm\ 2\ s$). For example, a mean total protein value of 7 g/dL with a standard deviation (s) of 0.5 mg/dL would have a reference range of 6 to 8 g/dL.

Relationship of Patient Values to Reference Ranges

Patient results are compared to the reference range when the results are reported to the physician. Laboratory reports indicate which results fall outside the reference range, but leave it to the physician to determine the significance of these results. The test results for some analytes can differ according to patient gender, time of day, time elapsed after a meal, or drugs or medications a patient is taking. These factors must be considered when comparing patient test results to reference ranges.

Based on the laws of probability, it is expected that, even in the general population, one value of every 20 sampled (5%) will fall outside the reference range, but usually will be only slightly higher or lower. So, a patient's single test result slightly outside the reference range is not necessarily clinically significant.

Factors Affecting Reference Ranges

Reference ranges can differ slightly according to the population sample's geographical area and the age of the population. For example, in an area popular with retirees where a large portion of the population is elderly, the reference values of certain analytes might differ slightly from those in an area having a population of more diverse ages.

Reference ranges for a substance measured in plasma can differ from that measured in serum. Different methods of analysis can also produce slightly different reference ranges. Types of analyzers used and testing methods are not standardized across different laboratories. This means each laboratory must establish its own reference ranges and will supply its reference range when a test result is reported. Examples of reference ranges for common chemical tests, given in Table 6-2, are those for a healthy adult male, using commonly accepted testing methodologies. However, it is important that test results be evaluated using reference ranges supplied by the laboratory that performed the test, rather than a general or theoretical reference range from a book.

LABORATORY ORDER REQUEST

781401 870997

Last Name	First	Middle	Social Security Number	Birthdate
Doe	Jane			

Physician	Date/time drawn	Phlebotomist

ICD-9 code(s)	Bill to: ❏ Insurance ❏ Office ❏ Patient

PROFILES	ICD-9 CODE #		INDIVIDUAL PROCEDURES	ICD-9 CODE #		INDIVIDUAL PROCEDURES	ICD-9 CODE #
☐ BASIC METABOLIC PROFILE		✓	**HEMATOLOGY / COAGULATION**		✓	**CHEMISTRY PROCEDURES**	
			CBC			Potassium (K+)	
Basic Metabolic Profile includes: Calcium Carbon Dioxide Chloride Creatinine Glucose Potassium Sodium Urea Nitrogen			PT (Protime) w/INR			Glucose	
			PTT			BUN (Urea Nitrogen)	
☐ ELECTROLYTE PANEL			Hgb (Hemoglobin)			Calcium	
			HCT (Hematocrit)			Creatinine	
Electrolyte Panel includes: Sodium Potassium Chloride Carbon Dioxide			ESR (sed rate)			PSA (Prostatic Specific Antigen)	
						PSA Screen	
☐ METABOLIC PANEL COMPREHENSIVE			Hemoglobin A1-C			TSH	
		✓	**SEROLOGY**			T-3 Uptake	
						T4, Free (Free Thyroxine)	
Comprehensive Metabolic Panel Includes: Albumin Chloride Potassium Bilirubin,total Creatinine Protein, total BUN Glucose Sodium Calcium Phosphatase, alkaline ALT/SGPT AST/SGOT			RPR			T4, (Total Thyroxine)	
			CRP (C-Reactive Protein)			CK - Total	
			ASO (with titer)			Troponin	
			H. pylori			Iron	
☐ HEPATIC FUNCTION PANEL			RA (Rheumatoid factor)			TIBC (Total Iron Binding Capacity)	
			ANA (anti-nucleic antibody)			Amylase	
Hepatic Function Panel includes: Albumin Phosphatase, alkaline Bilirubin, total Protein, total Bilirubin, direct ALT/SGPT AST/SGOT			SSA/SBB			Vitamin B-12	
		✓	**URINE PROCEDURES**			Folate	
			Urinalysis			Digoxin Level	
☐ LIPID PROFILE			Urinalysis Culture w/sensitivity			Theophylline Level	
			24-hour Urine Protein			**OTHER PROCEDURES**	
Lipid Profile Includes: Cholesterol Triglycerides HDL LDL			24-hour Urine Creatinine with clearance			1.	
MICROBIOLOGY & CULTURES			24-hour Urine, Creatinine			2.	
Culture, Throat			Random Urine, Sodium			3.	
Culture, Sputum			Random Urine, Potassium			4.	
Strep A Screen (swab)			Random Urine, Chloride			5.	
Gram Stain (Note Source)			Random Urine, Myoglobin			6.	
Source:			Random Urine, Osmolality			7.	

Physician's Signature:_____**Date:**_____

Medicare Advanced Beneficiary Notice

Section 1862(a)(1) of the Medicare Law states that Medicare will only pay for services that it determines are "reasonable and necessary."
If the service is determined not to be "reasonable and necessary" by Medicare program standards, payment will be denied.

Medical Record - White Copy   Lab - Yellow Copy   Physician's Office - Pink Copy

Form #1258   Revised 6/02

© Cengage Learning 2012

FIGURE 6-1 An example of a laboratory requisition form with clinical chemistry tests and profiles highlighted

TABLE 6-1. Examples of analytes measured in various chemistry panels

TYPES OF PANELS				
KIDNEY (RENAL)	**LIPID**	**CARDIAC**	**LIVER (HEPATIC)**	**THYROID**
Glucose	Triglycerides	CK-MB	Total protein	T_3
BUN	Total cholesterol	Troponin	Albumin	T_4
Creatinine	Cholesterol fractions	BNP	Bilirubin	TSH (thyroid stimulating
GFR	HDL	hs-CRP	Liver enzymes	hormone)
Electrolytes	LDL	Homocysteine	ALT	
	VLDL		AST	
			ALP	
			GGT	
			LD	

CURRENT TOPICS

HISTORY OF CLINICAL CHEMISTRY

The development of analyzers for use in clinical chemistry has been fairly recent, but physicians have been using crude methods of analysis for centuries. Recorded accounts say that observations were made on urine specimens as early as 400 B.C. Before that time, physicians in Egypt and Mesopotamia made diagnoses by listening to internal body sounds and palpating areas of the body.

In ancient Greece, around 300 B.C., Hippocrates, a physician often called the *Father of Medicine*, began attributing disease to abnormalities in the body fluids. His methods included tasting the patient's urine, listening to the lungs, and observing the patient's appearance. He also made the connection between the appearance of blood and pus in the urine to the presence of disease. In A.D. 50 a physician in Ephesus described hematuria (blood in the urine). Urine testing continued to be important in medicine through the Middle Ages.

In the 1600s, the microscope was invented, allowing scientists to study structures such as plant cells. During this century the circulation of blood throughout the body was described. Also during this time a method of precipitating urine protein by heat and acid was discovered.

In the late 1700s, advances were made in the study of the disease we now know as diabetes when it was proved that sugar was responsible for the

sweetness of urine of some patients. The first tests for sugar in the urine, using yeasts, were also developed. It was not until about 1850 that laboratory medicine became more accepted, and even up to the 1890s, most laboratory tests were performed by physicians using a microscope in their homes or offices.

By 1918, the inspection criteria of the American College of Surgeons required hospitals to have an adequately equipped and staffed laboratory. In the 1920s almost half of US hospitals had laboratories. By this time, several methods for determining urine analytes had been developed, many by Otto Folin. In addition, he did important work on epinephrine, uric acid, ammonia, nonprotein nitrogen (NPN) and protein in blood and established the relationship of uric acid, NPN, and blood urea nitrogen (BUN) to renal function. One reagent he developed, Folin-Ciocalteau, is still used today for protein determination. During this same period, clinical methods for measuring phosphorus and magnesium in serum were introduced.

In the 1930s, methods were developed for the clinical determinations of alkaline phosphatase, acid phosphatase, serum lipase, serum and urine amylase, and blood ammonia. A refractometer also was first used for measuring protein in urine. Beckman Instruments, a company that was to play a large part in laboratory science, was founded and introduced the first pH meter to measure the acidity and alkalinity of fluids.

(Continues)

CURRENT TOPICS (Continued)

The 1940s brought more developments such as photoelectric colorimeters to read color reactions of chemistry analyses and vacuum collection tubes for blood. In addition, the College of American Pathologists (CAP) and the American Association of Clinical Chemistry (AACC), two organizations important to clinical chemistry, were formed.

In 1950, in a move that made tracking quality control easier, Levey and Jennings adapted the Shewhart QC chart for use in the clinical laboratory. Methods to measure several enzymes were developed; these measurements were useful for indicating the site of organ or tissue damage. In the late 1950s, a method was developed to directly measure blood triglycerides. A landmark invention, the *AutoAnalyzer*, was introduced by Technicon Corporation, and flame photometry was applied to automated methods of clinical analysis.

The 1960s were years of rapid development in technology. In one year alone, Perkin-Elmer introduced the atomic absorption spectrophotometer for determination of calcium and magnesium, the laser was developed, and the first mechanical pipetter, the Auto Dilutor, was put into use. Also in this decade, Becton Dickinson introduced the disposable needle and syringe, disk storage for computers was developed by IBM, and the first random-access analyzer for clinical chemistry was introduced by DuPont.

The inventions of the 1960s set the stage for the rapid progression of clinical chemistry instrumentation that continues today. New technologies and methods are constantly being introduced. Analyzers have evolved from being large and complex to smaller counter-top analyzers and handheld instruments, some simple enough to be used at home by the patient.

There are times when the reference range is not the most important consideration, for instance, when cholesterol is tested. Although the high end of the cholesterol reference range is 250 mg/dL, the *recommended* level for good heart health is below 200 mg/dL. There are also some tests for which a reference range is not relevant, such as measuring blood levels of a drug in an unconscious patient. The result will be interpreted in terms of the effect the drug would be expected to have at that level, given the patient's age, size, and physical condition, as well as other factors. (see Lesson 1-9 for a more complete explanation of quality assessment, quality control, statistics and reference ranges.)

ANALYTES COMMONLY TESTED IN CHEMISTRY PROFILES

Routine metabolic or chemistry profiles are used to screen for function of the major organ systems. A selection of 10 to 20 analytes are assayed. Information from the assays can indicate the general status of systems such as heart, kidney, liver, bone, and carbohydrate metabolism. The significance and reference ranges of analytes typically included in a chemistry profile are discussed in this section.

Protein

Proteins are essential components of cells and body fluids. They are formed from chains of amino acids. Some amino acids are made by the body, whereas others must be provided by dietary protein.

Two major groups of serum proteins are the **albumins** and the **globulins**. Albumins comprise approximately 60% of total serum proteins; globulins, about 40%. The albumins are made in the liver and are homogeneous in structure. They serve as transport proteins and help maintain fluid balance in the body.

The globulins are a heterogeneous group of molecules. Antibodies, blood coagulation proteins, enzymes, and proteins that transport iron are all serum globulins.

Total Serum Protein

The reference range for total serum protein is 6.0 to 8.0 g/dL (60 to 80 g/L) and represents the sum of many different blood proteins. Total protein values can provide information about the state of hydration, nutrition, and liver function because most serum proteins are made in the liver. Protein is most commonly measured in serum, but it can also be measured in both urine and CSF, where the concentration is normally low. Total serum protein can be measured chemically or using a refractometer.

Albumin

The reference range for serum albumin is 3.8 to 5.0 g/dL (38–50 g/L). Decreased levels of albumin, or **hypoalbuminemia**, can occur in liver disease, starvation, impaired amino acid absorption, increased protein catabolism, and protein loss through the skin, kidneys, or gastrointestinal tract.

Albumin-to-Globulin Ratio

Total serum protein and albumin are usually measured in a sample simultaneously, and globulin is computed from the difference (total protein − albumin = globulin). A ratio of albumin to globulin (A/G ratio) can be computed and reported.

TABLE 6-2. Table of clinical chemistry reference ranges*

SUBSTANCE MEASURED	REFERENCE RANGES	
	CONVENTIONAL UNITS	SI UNITS
Alanine aminotransferase (ALT)	3–30 U/L	3–30 U/L
Albumin	3.8–5.0 g/dL	38–50 g/L
Alkaline phosphatase (AP)	20–130 U/L	20–130 U/L
Aspartate aminotransferase (AST)	10–37 U/L	10–37 U/L
Bicarbonate (Total CO_2)	22–28 mEq/L	22–28 mmol/L
Bilirubin, total	0.1–1.2 mg/dL	2–21 µmol/L
Bilirubin, direct	0–0.3 mg/dL	0–6 µmol/L
BNP	100 pg/mL	100 ng/L
BUN	8–18 mg/dL	2.9–6.4 mmol/L
Calcium, ionized	4.6–5.3 mg/dL	1.15–1.33 mmol/L
Chloride (Cl–)	98–108 mEq/L	98–108 mmol/L
Cholesterol (Total)	140–250 mg/dL (desirable level <200 mg/dL)	3.6–6.5 mmol/L
High-sensitivity C-reactive protein (hs-CRP)	0.2–12 mg/L	0.2–12 mg/L
Creatine kinase, total	30–170 U/L	30-170 U/L
Creatine kinase (CK-MB fraction)	<5 ng/mL	<5 ug/L
Creatinine	0.7–1.4 mg/dL	62–125 µmol/L
Gamma-glutamyltransferase (GGT)	3–40 U/L	3–40 U/L
Glomerular filtration rate (GFR)	Varies with gender and age	
Glucose	70–110 mg/dL	3.9–6.2 mmol/L
Homocysteine (varies with age)	Less than 8 µmol/L to less than 20 µmol/L	Less than 8 µmol/L to less than 20 µmol/L
Iron	65–165 µg/dL	11.6–29.5 µmol/L
Lactate dehydrogenase (LD)	110–230 U/L	110–230 U/L
Phosphorus (phosphate)	3.0–4.5 mg/dL	0.96–1.44 mmol/L
Potassium (K+)	3.8–5.5 mEq/L	3.8–5.5 mmol/L
Sodium (Na+)	135–148 mEq/L	135–148 mmol/L
Thyroid stimulating hormone (TSH)	0.35–5.0 µIU/mL	0.35–5.0 mIU/L
Total protein	6.0–8.0 g/dL	60–80 g/L
Triglycerides	10–190 mg/dL	0.11–2.15 mmol/L
Uric acid	3.5–7.5 mg/dL	0.21–0.44 mmol/L

*All reference ranges listed are for serum. Laboratories must define their own reference intervals

Electrolytes

In clinical chemistry, the term **electrolytes** refers to the major **cations** *sodium* (Na^+) and *potassium* (K^+), and the major **anions**, *chloride* (Cl^-) and *bicarbonate* (HCO_3^-). These four ions have a great effect on hydration and acid–base (pH) balance, as well as heart and muscle function. Electrolyte measurement is included in most routine chemistry profiles and renal profiles.

Sodium is the cation with the highest serum concentration, having a reference range of 135 to 148 mmol/L (mEq/L). The reference range for serum potassium is 3.8 to 5.5 mmol/L (mEq/L).

Chloride is the anion with the highest serum concentration; the reference range for serum chloride is 98 to 108 mmol/L (mEq/L). The serum bicarbonate reference range (measured as total CO_2) is 22 to 28 mmol/L (mEq/L).

Mineral Metabolism

Minerals are necessary for good health. Calcium, phosphorus (phosphate), and iron are examples of minerals often measured in chemistry profiles. Calcium and phosphorus are necessary for proper bone and tooth formation. Calcium is also required for blood coagulation. Iron is essential for hemoglobin production and is an integral component of some enzymes.

Calcium

The reference range for ionized serum calcium is 4.6 to 5.3 mg/dL (1.15 to 1.33 mmol/L). Of all the minerals in the body, calcium is present in the highest concentration. Approximately 99% of the body's calcium is bound in calcium complexes in the skeleton and is not metabolically active; only unbound calcium ions are metabolically active.

Calcium is required for blood coagulation and for normal neuromuscular excitability. The calcium balance is influenced by vitamin D_3, parathyroid hormone, estrogen, and calcitonin. These control dietary absorption of calcium, calcium excretion by the kidneys, and calcium movement in and out of bone.

Hypercalcemia, an increased level of blood calcium, occurs in parathyroidism, bone malignancies, hormone disorders, excessive vitamin D_3, and acidosis. It can cause calcium to be deposited in soft organs, leading to complications such as kidney stones.

Decreased levels of blood calcium, or **hypocalcemia**, can be life-threatening and should be reported to the physician immediately. Low calcium levels can be due to hypoparathyroidism, vitamin D_3 deficiency, poor calcium absorption due to intestinal disease, and kidney disease.

Phosphorus

The reference range for serum phosphorus (measured as phosphate) is 3.0 to 4.5 mg/dL (0.96 to 1.44 mmol/L). Most phosphorus in the body is in the form of inorganic phosphate. Approximately 80% is in bone, and the rest is mostly in high-energy compounds such as adenosine triphosphate (ATP). Phosphorus levels are influenced by calcium and certain hormones. Children have higher phosphorus levels than adults because they have higher levels of growth hormone.

Iron

Serum iron is normally 65 to 165 μg/dL (11.6 to 29.5 μmol/L). Iron is essential for hemoglobin synthesis. Iron is absorbed from dietary sources and is highly conserved by the body. In blood, iron is transported by *transferrin*, a serum protein. Iron levels differ with age, gender, and time of day, being higher in the AM than in the PM.

Iron deficiency can lead to anemia. The deficiency can be due to insufficient iron in the diet, poor iron absorption, impaired release of stored iron, depletion of storage iron, or increased iron loss as a result of bleeding. Serum iron levels can be elevated with hemolytic anemias, increased iron intake, or blocked synthesis of iron-containing compounds, such as occurs in lead poisoning.

Kidney Function

Good kidney function is necessary for water and electrolyte balance in the body. The kidneys eliminate waste products, help maintain water and pH balance, and produce certain hormones essential to the functions of other organs. Substances are excreted into and reabsorbed from urine to help maintain homeostasis. The serum and plasma concentrations of certain substances such as creatinine, BUN, and uric acid are altered in certain kidney diseases.

Creatinine

The reference range for serum creatinine is 0.7 to 1.4 mg/dL (62 to 125 μmol/L). **Creatinine** is a waste product of creatine phosphate, a substance stored in muscle and used for energy. Creatinine is excreted by the kidney. When renal function is impaired, blood creatinine levels rise, but more than 50% of kidney function must be lost before this happens.

Creatinine levels are not affected by diet or hormone levels. Increases occur when urine formation or excretion is impaired, which occurs in renal disease, water imbalance, or ureter blockage.

Blood Urea Nitrogen

In mammals, surplus amino acids are converted to urea and excreted by the kidneys. This surplus is measured as **blood urea nitrogen (BUN)**. The reference range for serum BUN is 8 to 18 mg/dL (2.9 to 6.4 mmol/L).

The BUN concentration is influenced by diet, hormones, and kidney function. Therefore, the BUN level is not as good an indicator of kidney disease as is the creatinine level. BUN levels can be low during starvation, pregnancy, and a low-protein diet. Increased BUN concentration can occur during a high-protein diet, after administration of corticosteroids, and in kidney disease.

Glomerular Filtration Rate (GFR)

The **glomerular filtration rate (GFR)** is a calculation that estimates nephron function. The GFR is the rate per minute that small molecules such as creatinine and urea are filtered through the glomeruli of the kidneys. The GFR is used to estimate the damage to nephrons in patients with impaired kidney function, such as some diabetic patients.

Uric Acid

The reference range for serum uric acid is 3.5 to 7.5 mg/dL (0.21 to 0.44 mmol/L). **Uric acid** is formed from the breakdown of nucleic acids and is excreted by the kidneys. It has low solubility and tends to precipitate as uric acid crystals, or urates. Uric acid measurement is principally used to diagnose and treat **gout**, a disease in which uric acid precipitates in tissues and joints, causing pain. Uric acid levels can also increase after massive radiation or chemotherapy because of increased cell destruction.

Liver Function

The liver is both a secretory and excretory organ and has numerous metabolic functions. The liver functions in carbohydrate metabolism, synthesizing glycogen from glucose. Most plasma proteins are made in the liver, including albumin, lipoproteins, transport proteins, and several blood coagulation proteins including fibrinogen. The liver is also important in lipid metabolism and is one source of cholesterol.

The liver is a storage site for iron, glycogen, vitamins, and other substances. Other functions include destruction of senescent blood cells by phagocytosis and the detoxification of many substances.

Significant liver function must be lost or impaired before some laboratory tests show abnormality. Numerous tests are used to estimate liver function. Most are not specific for a particular disease but only reflect liver tissue damage or liver dysfunction.

Bilirubin

The reference range for total serum bilirubin is 0.1 to 1.2 mg/dL (2.0 to 21.0 μmol/L); the reference range for direct bilirubin is 0 to 0.3 mg/dL (0 to 6 μmol/L). **Bilirubin**, a waste product from the breakdown of hemoglobin, is formed in the liver and excreted in the bile. In the liver, most bilirubin becomes bound to a glucuronide and is then excreted into the bile—this is called *conjugated bilirubin* or *direct bilirubin*. Bilirubin that is not conjugated is called *indirect bilirubin*. Total serum bilirubin equals direct bilirubin plus indirect bilirubin. Bilirubin assays usually measure both total and direct bilirubin. Indirect bilirubin is then calculated from those two numbers.

Measurement of bilirubin can be used to screen for liver or gall bladder dysfunction. Bilirubin levels are normally low, so only increases in serum bilirubin are significant. Bilirubin can be increased when there is excessive destruction of hemoglobin such as in the hemolytic anemias, impaired excretion by the liver such as in biliary obstruction or gall bladder disease, or impaired bilirubin processing as in hepatitis.

Liver Enzymes

A rise in serum enzymes generally reflects injury to tissue, because most enzymes are intracellular. Some enzymes are widely distributed in many body tissues, whereas others are found in only a few tissues. The measurement of enzyme levels is not always specific for damage to a particular organ but is most helpful when used with other tests, clinical symptoms, and patient history.

Enzymes used to assess liver function include the aminotransferases **alanine aminotransferase (ALT)** and **aspartate aminotransferase (AST)**, **alkaline phosphatase (ALP)**, **gamma-glutamyltransferase (GGT)**, and **lactate dehydrogenase (LD)**.

Aminotransferases. Liver tissue is rich in the aminotransferase enzymes. When liver cells are injured, these enzymes are released. Serum concentrations of these enzymes change with time, rising during acute liver disease and falling as recovery occurs. Generally, only one enzyme need be measured, as levels tend to mirror each other.

ALT was formerly called serum glutamic-pyruvic transaminase (GPT or SGPT). Levels are low in cardiac tissue and high in liver tissue. This enzyme usually rises higher than AST in liver disease, with moderate increases (up to 10 times normal) in cirrhosis, infections, or tumors, and increases up to 100 times normal in viral or toxic hepatitis. The reference range of serum ALT is 3 to 30 U/L.

AST was formerly called serum glutamic-oxaloacetic transaminase (GOT or SGOT). It is present in many tissues, particularly cardiac, muscle, and liver. It is elevated after myocardial infarction, as well as in liver disease. The reference range of serum AST is 10 to 37 U/L.

Alkaline Phosphatase (ALP). ALP, also called AP, is widely distributed in the body, especially in bone and the liver ducts. Serum AP levels can greatly increase with liver tumors and lesions and can show a moderate increase with diseases such as hepatitis. The reference range of serum AP is 20 to 130 U/L.

Gamma-Glutamyltransferase (GGT). GGT is found in the kidney, pancreas, liver, and prostate tissue. GGT can be more helpful than AP in determining liver damage because GGT remains normal in bone disease. It is more useful than AST because it remains normal in muscle disorders. GGT measurement is often used to monitor recovery from hepatitis. The reference range of serum GGT is 3 to 40 U/L.

Lactate Dehydrogenase (LD). LD, also called LDH, is widely distributed in tissue. The LD level increases in blood during liver disease and following myocardial infarction. Hemolysis of a blood sample will cause increased LD levels in the serum because of LD release from red blood cells. The reference range of serum LD is 110 to 230 U/L.

Cardiac Function

Several laboratory tests are used to monitor or assess cardiac function. Some tests detect or measure specific biomarkers that are diagnostic in assessing recent heart damage. Other tests are not specific for heart function but can be used to assess risk for cardiac disease.

Cardiac Markers

Cardiac markers are part of a larger group called biomarkers, substances released in conjunction with events in the body such as muscle injury. Measurement of cardiac markers helps detect acute events such as myocardial infarction or myocardial injury. The measurement of these markers is especially important when the electrocardiogram (ECG) is normal. To be useful a cardiac marker must:

- Be rapidly released from the heart into circulation
- Provide sensitive and specific diagnostic information
- Be detectable by a rapid test method
- Be detectable in low concentrations
- Remain in circulation several days

Three cardiac markers commonly measured are troponin, creatine kinase, and B-type natriuretic peptide (BNP).

Creatine Kinase. **Creatine kinase (CK)** is an enzyme present in large amounts in muscle and the brain but in small amounts in organs such as the liver and kidneys. The reference range for total serum CK is 30 to 170 U/L.

Creatine kinase exists in four forms in heart and skeletal muscle; however, the forms CK-M and CK-B are higher in heart muscle (myocardium). The *CK-MB* test measures blood levels of these two forms. Following heart attack CK-MB enzymes are released from the damaged heart muscle. The serum CK-MB level peaks in about 24 hours, reaching five to eight times the upper limit of normal. It falls rapidly back to normal levels within

3 to 4 days. An elevated CK-MB level is a marker for injury to the heart. CK-MB is present in only trace amounts in healthy individuals, less than 5 ng/mL (or less than 5 ug/L).

Troponins. The action of the heart is generated in bundles of striated muscle fibers. These fibers contain **troponins**, intracellular proteins present in skeletal and heart muscle. Troponins have varying forms called subunits T, I, and C. The C subunits are identical in skeletal and heart muscle so are not useful in cardiac testing. When heart muscle cells die, troponins are released. Therefore, the presence of cardiac troponins in blood is a marker of damage or injury to the heart muscle. Subunits T and I differ structurally according to their muscle source (antibodies can detect the differences), so both cardiac troponin T (cTnT) and cardiac troponin I (cTnI) are useful in cardiac testing. Cardiac troponins remain elevated in blood 7 to 10 days after a myocardial event, which is longer than CK-MB. Cardiac troponins are essentially undetectable in healthy individuals.

B-type Natriuretic Peptide (BNP). The cardiac marker **B-type natriuretic peptide (BNP)** is a hormone released mainly from ventricles of the heart. It is most useful for following the progression of congestive heart failure (CHF). The normal BNP reference value for an adult ranges up to 100 pg/mL. Levels greater than 100 pg/mL can indicate ventricle damage.

C-Reactive Protein (CRP)

C-reactive protein is an acute phase protein and nonspecific indicator of inflammation. CRP can be increased in a variety of diseases, including autoimmune diseases and malignancies. An increase in CRP can also be an indicator of vascular and cardiovascular damage. The *high sensitivity CRP (hs-CRP)* test is used as one of the screening tests for cardiovascular problems; the hs-CRP can detect CRP levels of less than 20 mg/L. (The regular CRP test is ordered for patients at risk for infections or chronic inflammatory diseases; this test detects CRP levels of 10 to 1000 mg/L.)

Total Homocysteine (tHcy)

Homocysteine (tHcy), an amino acid, is associated with increased risk for vascular and cardiovascular disease such as coronary heart disease (CHD), when blood levels are elevated. **Coronary heart disease (CHD)** is a narrowing of the small blood vessels that supply blood and oxygen to the heart. Homocysteine does not normally accumulate in the plasma because it is an unstable molecule. The detectable range can vary with age but in general it ranges from less than 8 μmol/L to less than 20 μmol/L. At this time tHcy is not recommended as a screening test for increased risk for coronary heart disease in the general population; however, it is useful for prognosis of patients that have CHD or are at high risk for CHD.

Lipid Metabolism

Lipids are synthesized in the body from dietary fats. The most commonly measured lipids are cholesterol and triglycerides. These are of interest primarily because of their association with **cardiovascular disease (CVD)**.

Cholesterol and Cholesterol Fractions

Cholesterol is present in all tissues, and serum concentrations tend to increase with age. Elevated cholesterol levels can increase the risk for coronary artery disease. It is widely recommended that total serum cholesterol levels be maintained below 200 mg/dL with some authorities recommending less than 170 mg/dL (reference range is 140 to 250 mg/dL). Cholesterol fractions such as **LDL** (low-density lipoprotein) **cholesterol**, **HDL** (high-density lipoprotein) **cholesterol**, and **VLDL** (very low density lipoprotein) **cholesterol**, are also measured.

Triglycerides

Serum triglyceride reference values range from 10 to 190 mg/dL (0.11 to 2.15 mmol/L). **Triglycerides** are the main form of lipid storage in humans, comprising approximately 95% of fat (adipose) tissue. Triglycerides are transported in the plasma bound to lipoproteins, molecules composed of lipid and protein. The group of lipoproteins called *chylomicrons* transports most of the plasma triglycerides. Increased blood levels of triglycerides cause the plasma to have a milky appearance. Blood to be tested for triglycerides should be collected when the patient has been fasting for 12 to 14 hours, such as in the morning before breakfast. **Hyperlipidemia** is the condition of having high blood levels of triglycerides.

Carbohydrate Metabolism

The reference range for serum glucose is 70 to 110 mg/dL (3.9 to 6.2 mmol/L). Glucose metabolism is largely regulated by insulin, which is produced by the pancreas. It is also influenced by other hormones such as glucagon, growth hormone, and cortisol. Glucose is a commonly tested blood constituent.

Thyroid Function

The thyroid gland synthesizes hormones that stimulate metabolism by increasing protein synthesis and oxygen consumption by the tissues. Thyroid hormones are synthesized from iodide and the amino acid tyrosine. In the blood, more than 99% of thyroid hormones are bound to serum proteins and are metabolically inactive. Graves' disease is an example of a disease caused by **hyperthyroidism**, excessive secretion of thyroid hormones. **Hypothyroidism**, decreased thyroid function, causes a condition called myxedema.

The two major thyroid hormones are **thyroxine**, also called T_4, and **triiodothyronine**, also called T_3. Measurement of thyroid hormones is not usually included as part of a routine chemistry profile. Thyroid profiles or endocrine panels will include measurement of free or total T_4, free or total T_3, and **thyroid-stimulating hormone (TSH)** levels. TSH is an anterior pituitary hormone that regulates thyroid gland activity. The reference range for TSH is 0.35 to 5.0 mIU/mL (mIU/L). Levels of thyroid hormones vary according to age, and the reference ranges can be different depending on the particular assay method. Thyroid hormones are usually measured using immunological techniques.

LESS COMMONLY ORDERED CLINICAL CHEMISTRY TESTS

Many chemistry tests are available that have not been mentioned in this lesson. Several are special tests that measure hormones such as insulin, growth hormone, adrenocorticotropic hormone (ACTH), or follicle-stimulating hormone (FSH). Tests are available to measure vitamins, trace minerals, isoenzymes, and metabolic products. Other tests can monitor therapeutic drug levels or detect drugs of abuse. As advanced testing technologies become more available, special tests such as vitamin assays are being performed more frequently.

CASE STUDY 1

A clinic patient had total protein and albumin assays performed on his serum. When the physician was given the test results, total protein 6.5 g/dL and albumin 3.0 g/dL, she asked the technician to calculate the A/G ratio.

1. What results are used to calculate the A/G ratio?
2. What is this patient's globulin value?
3. Calculate the patient's A/G ratio.
4. The patient's results are:
   a. Both within the reference ranges
   b. Both below the reference ranges
   c. Both above the reference ranges
   d. Normal for total protein and low for albumin

CASE STUDY 2

Dr. Talbot ordered a creatine kinase (CK-MB) and troponin test for a patient he was treating in the emergency room.

Which of the following do you think Dr. Talbot suspects?
   a. Heart disease
   b. Renal disease
   c. Liver disease
   d. Thyroid disease

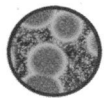

SUMMARY

The majority of clinical chemistry assays are performed using instrumentation. These assays can provide a wealth of information about the status of a patient's health. Tests are available that give information about cardiac, renal, and liver function, as well as the state of mineral, lipid and carbohydrate metabolism. In addition, many specialized tests such as hormone assays and assays of levels of therapeutic drugs are performed in the clinical chemistry department.

Each chemistry laboratory establishes its own reference ranges for the constituents measured in that laboratory. These ranges are based on test results from a sampling of the general population. Patient test results are compared to the reference ranges when the laboratory report is issued; this aids in interpretation of the patient's test results. Comprehensive quality assessment programs must be established and followed to ensure reliable, high-quality chemistry test results. Laboratory personnel must adhere to safety rules and Standard Precautions when performing chemistry assays and operating chemistry analyzers.

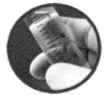

REVIEW QUESTIONS

1. What are the two most commonly tested body fluids in clinical chemistry?
2. What three enzymes are useful in diagnosing liver disease?

3. Give the reference ranges for 15 constituents included in a chemistry profile.

4. What three tests can be useful in diagnosing kidney disease?

5. What enzyme is useful in diagnosing myocardial infarction?

6. What protein is elevated when inflammation is present?

7. Name the four electrolytes commonly measured in serum.

8. What test can be ordered if heart failure is suspected?

9. What problem might be suspected if a physician orders tests for homocysteine and hs-CRP for a patient?

10. What are the two major types of serum proteins and what are their functions?

11. What peptide is released by the ventricles of the heart?

12. Which chemistry profile would include a test for triglycerides?

13. How are reference ranges established? How are they used by the physician?

14. Define alanine aminotransferase, albumins, alkaline phosphatase, analyte, anion, aspartate aminotransferase, bilirubin, B-type natriuretic peptide (BNP), blood urea nitrogen (BUN), cardiovascular disease, cation, coronary heart disease, C-reactive protein (CRP), creatine kinase, creatinine, electrolytes, gamma-glutamyltransferase, globulins, glomerular filtration rate (GFR), gout, HDL cholesterol, homeostasis, homocysteine, hypercalcemia, hyperlipidemia, hyperthyroidism, hypoalbuminemia, hypocalcemia, hypothyroidism, lactate dehydrogenase, LDL cholesterol, lipids, thyroid stimulating hormone, thyroxine, triglycerides, triiodothyronine, troponins, uric acid, and VLDL cholesterol.

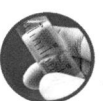

STUDENT ACTIVITIES

1. Complete the written examination for this lesson.

2. Ask what tests are included in chemistry panels in a nearby hospital or laboratory. Find out the laboratory's reference ranges and compare them to those in this lesson.

3. Tour a clinical chemistry laboratory in your area.

WEB ACTIVITIES

1. Use the Internet to find the web site of a university medical center or commercial reference laboratory. Find three types of chemistry panels available and list the analytes included in each panel.

2. Use the Internet to find an example of a high-volume chemistry analyzer for processing chemistry profiles. Write a short report on the analyzer; include the technology used, test menu, and number of samples processed per hour.

3. Use the Internet to look up information on three analytes shown in the form in Figure 6-1. Write a brief report on each analyte, its clinical significance, why it is tested, reference values, etc.

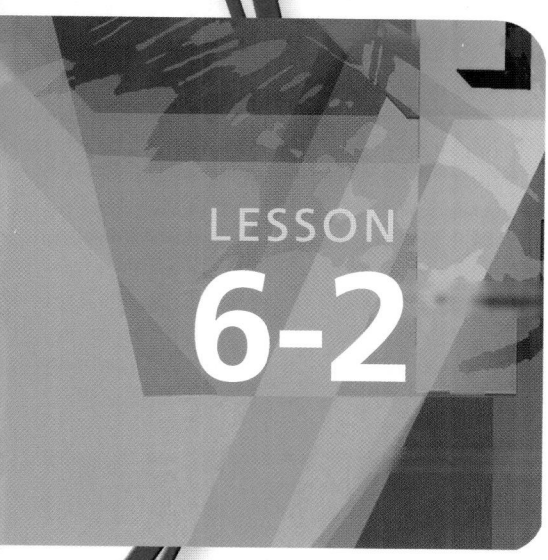

LESSON 6-2

Chemistry Specimen Collection and Processing

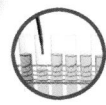

LESSON OBJECTIVES

After studying this lesson, the student will:

⊙ Name six body fluids tested in clinical chemistry.

⊙ Explain the color-coding system used for blood collection tubes.

⊙ List the correct order of draw for commonly used blood collection tubes.

⊙ Discuss the importance of the order of draw when collecting blood samples by venipuncture.

⊙ Explain six problems associated with blood collection and processing that could cause erroneous test results.

⊙ Explain safety precautions that must be followed during specimen collection, handling, and processing.

⊙ Discuss quality assessment procedures involved in specimen collection, processing, and handling.

⊙ Define the glossary terms.

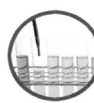

GLOSSARY

anticoagulant / a chemical or substance that prevents blood coagulation

cerebrospinal fluid (CSF) / the fluid surrounding the spinal cord and bathing the ventricles of the brain

diurnal / having a daily cycle

lipemic / having a cloudy appearance because of excess lipid content

order of draw / a standard order of filling blood collection tubes when obtaining blood from a venipuncture in order to avoid cross-contamination between tubes

pericardial fluid / the fluid within the pericardial sac

plasma / the liquid portion of blood in which the blood cells are suspended; the straw-colored liquid remaining after blood cells are removed from anticoagulated blood

pleural fluid / the fluid in the space between the pleural membrane of the lung and the inner chest wall

serum / the liquid obtained from blood that has been allowed to clot

STAT / immediately (from the Latin word *statim*)

synovial fluid / a viscous fluid secreted by membranes lining the joints

INTRODUCTION

The clinical chemistry department performs tests on blood and other body fluids, including urine, **cerebrospinal fluid (CSF)**, **pleural fluid**, **synovial fluid**, and **pericardial fluid**. Depending on the type of specimen, the responsibility for collecting specimens for testing in the central laboratory can be the responsibility of phlebotomists, medical laboratory scientists, nurses, or physicians.

Special attention must be paid to the type of specimen required for each test and to the handling and processing of the specimen. Laboratory analyses can produce useful results only if they are performed on a specimen that has been properly collected and maintained in the appropriate environment until the test is performed.

This lesson describes procedures for collecting and processing blood specimens for clinical chemistry. Lesson 5-2 describes collection procedures for urine specimens. Other body fluids are usually collected by the physician. A review of blood-collection procedures (Lesson 1-11 and 1-12) may be helpful before studying this lesson.

TYPES OF BLOOD SPECIMENS FOR CHEMICAL ANALYSIS

Blood for chemical analysis can be capillary or venous. Blood for testing in clinical laboratories or to be transported is usually drawn in evacuated blood collection tubes. These tubes are available in several sizes and certain tubes contain additives, such as glycolytic inhibitors or **anticoagulants**, chemicals which prevent blood clotting. Tube manufacturers use standard color coding of the tube caps to indicate the type of tube and the tube contents. Examples of some commonly used tubes are shown in Figures 6-2 and 6-3.

Clinical chemistry analyzers can use whole blood, serum, or plasma for testing. Sometimes an analyzer or method requires one particular type of specimen, such as heparinized

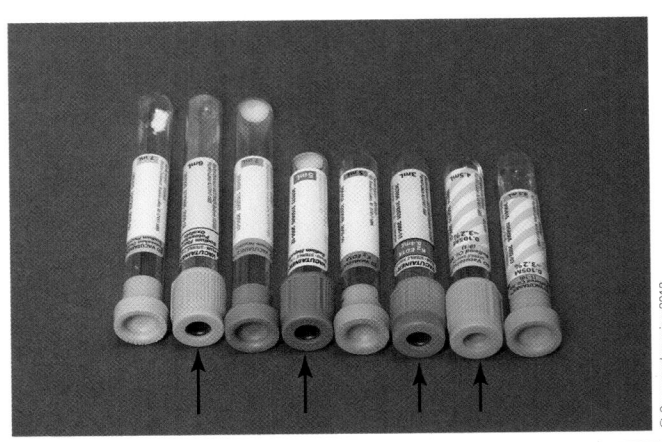

FIGURE 6-2 Assortment of blood collection tubes showing conventional color-coded rubber stoppers and plastic Vacutainer® Hemogard™ color-coded safety caps (arrows)

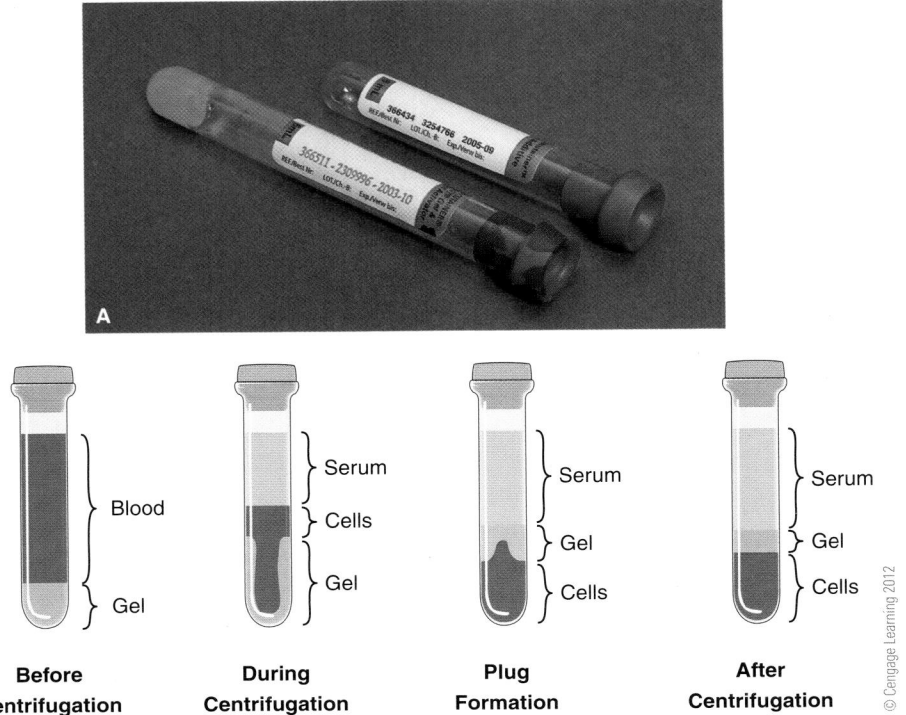

FIGURE 6-3 Serum collection tubes: (A) left, serum separator tube with red/gray mottled stopper, and right, red-top tube; (B) illustration of gel separation of serum from cells during centrifugation of serum separator tube

whole blood. The laboratory standard operating procedure (SOP) manual will specify which type(s) of specimen and collection conditions are required for each test performed in the laboratory.

Serum

Serum is the specimen used for most clinical chemistry tests. **Serum** is the fluid portion that remains after blood has been allowed to clot. It is obtained by collecting blood in a tube without anticoagulant, allowing the blood to clot, centrifuging the clotted sample, and removing the liquid (serum).

Serum is obtained by collecting blood using "red- or orange-top" tubes that can be glass or plastic. The relatively rough interior surface of a glass red-topped tube serves as an activator to initiate blood clotting. Plastic red-topped serum collection tubes have a smoother interior surface and are manufactured with a clotting activator, usually silica particles, coating the interior of the tube to speed up clotting.

Blood can also be collected in serum separator tubes, which have a red-gray cap (Figure 6-3). In these tubes, during centrifugation, the red blood cells displace the gel in the bottom of the tube, and the gel forms a barrier between the serum and the red blood cells. Orange-topped rapid serum tubes (RST) containing thrombin to quickly clot the blood are used for **STAT** tests, those tests that must be done immediately (Figure 6-4).

Plasma

Plasma is obtained by removing the liquid portion of anticoagulated blood following centrifugation. The type of anticoagulant used is determined by the test that is ordered. The color of the cap of the collection tube denotes the anticoagulant present in the tube (Figures 6-2 and 6-4). Plasma separating tubes are available. These contain a gel that becomes displaced by red blood cells during centrifugation, and produces a barrier between red blood cells and plasma.

When either plasma or serum is to be used for testing, the liquid must be removed and placed into another tube to separate it from the blood's cellular portion as soon as possible after collection. This prevents the exchange of substances such as ions and glucose between the cellular and liquid portions, which could alter test results.

Whole Blood

Many of the instruments developed for point-of-care (POC) testing use whole blood for analyses. Whole blood is obtained by capillary puncture (Lesson 1-11) or venipuncture. Whole blood obtained by capillary puncture must be used immediately after collection and is used mostly at POC. When whole blood is to be used in an analysis method, the blood from venipuncture must be collected in an anticoagulant, such as heparin or ethylenediaminetetraacetic acid (EDTA). The tube of anticoagulated whole blood must be mixed well immediately before testing. Detailed procedures for collecting

blood by venipuncture and information on anticoagulants are given in Lesson 1-12.

COLLECTING AND PROCESSING BLOOD SPECIMENS

Collection procedures for capillary or venous blood should be followed as outlined in the laboratory's SOP manual.

Safety Precautions

  Accidental exposure to blood and body fluids is more likely to occur during collection and processing of specimens than during most other laboratory procedures. Standard Precautions must be observed at all times. Appropriate personal protective equipment (PPE), including gloves, face protection, and a buttoned, fluid-resistant laboratory coat, should be worn. Frequent handwashing and changing of gloves are required.

The use of needles and other blood collecting devices with safety features is mandated. Several safety devices that eliminate the need for recapping used needles are available, such as quick-release needles, needles with safety shields, and needles that blunt or retract on exit from the vein. Patient rooms, blood-collection stations, and phlebotomy trays should be equipped with disposal containers so that used sharps can be immediately discarded.

Specimens must occasionally be collected from a patient who is suspected of having, or known to have, a contagious disease. The phlebotomist or technician must stay up-to-date on specific requirements for each transmission-based precaution category. Lesson 7-9 discusses these precautions in more detail.

Safety devices have been developed to reduce the potential for aerosol creation, splatters or tube breakage when uncapping blood collection tubes. Plastic collection tubes should be used whenever possible. Through-the-cap samplers available on many analyzers and sample-processing instruments eliminate the need to uncap tubes and reduce the possibility of aerosol creation. Some collection tubes, such as the Vacutainer Hemogard tubes (BD), have a plastic sleeve that fits over the stopper to contain aerosols or splatters formed when the stopper is removed from the tube (Figure 6-2).

Quality Assessment

   The quality of the specimen is of utmost importance. The SOP manual will have specific instructions for the specimen required, collection procedure, and the processing method for each test. Figure 6-4 lists types of specimen collection tubes and examples of their uses.

Patient Identification

The patient must be identified using two identifiers before a specimen is collected. Patient armbands now have barcodes. Devices incorporating a barcode reader and printer can be carried by the phlebotomist on rounds to scan the patient's

Cap Color	Additive/ Anticoagulant	Examples of use	Inversions required
Various	Various	Blood culture; Discard tube	Per SOP
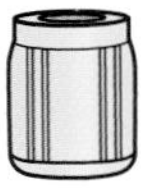 Yellow	Acid-citrate dextrose	DNA, Paternity tests	8
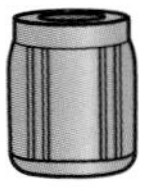 Light blue	Sodium citrate	Most coagulation studies	3-4
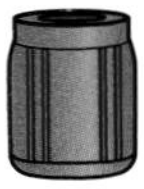 Red	None (glass) Silicon (plastic)	Serum	None (glass) 5 (plastic)
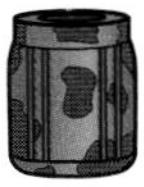 Red/Gray	Gel separator, Clot activator	Serum-separator tube; Tests that require serum	5
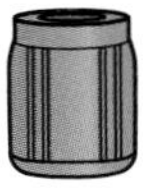 Orange	Thrombin, Gel separator	Rapid clotting	5-6
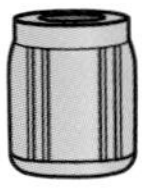 Gold (SST)	Gel separator, Clot activator	Immunology, Endocrine studies	5
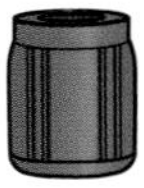 Green	Sodium or lithium heparin	Plasma for routine chemistry	8
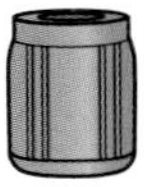 Lavender	K_2EDTA	Most hematological tests	8
Pink	K_2EDTA	Blood banking	8
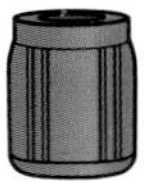 Royal blue	K_2EDTA or silicon	Toxicology, Trace metals	8
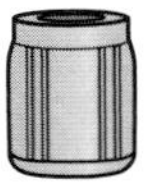 Gray	Potassium oxalate/ sodium fluoride; Sodium fluoride/Na_2EDTA; or Sodium fluoride	Glucose tests; Blood alcohol	8-10
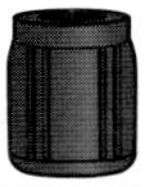 Black	Buffered sodium citrate	Westergren ESR	8

© Cengage Learning 2012

FIGURE 6-4 Standard order of draw for blood collection tubes, tube additives, and examples of uses

armband and print matching bar-coded labels for the tubes of blood. Alternatively, bar-coded labels can be generated at the same time the test is requisitioned (Figure 6-5A).

Specimens must be labeled immediately after collection, while the phlebotomist is still in the patient's presence (Figure 6-5B). The label should include patient name and identification number, the date and time of collection, and the phlebotomist's initials.

Using automated specimen processing systems, blood tubes can be placed in racks on a moving track that transports the tubes to the appropriate analysis area by interpreting the bar codes on the labels. Various machines along the route centrifuge the specimens that need it, transport the tubes to various analyzers, and save samples that are designated to be analyzed out-of-house. Analyzers read the barcode when the tube is inserted into the instrument and code the patient's identification to the test result, reducing transcribing errors.

Criteria for Specimen Acceptability

The laboratory's SOP manual includes a list of specific criteria that must be met in order for a specimen to be accepted for testing. Table 6-3 lists some of these criteria. Tests requiring special collection procedures will have additional criteria for acceptability. Failure to meet these criteria will cause the specimen to be rejected and may require that another specimen be collected. This can be traumatic for the patient, time-consuming for the laboratory, and result in delays in reporting

TABLE 6-3. Examples of some criteria that must be met for a specimen to be acceptable for testing
▶ Label must be complete (name, date, time of collection, person collecting) and attached to the specimen tube correctly
▶ Blood specimens must be free of hemolysis
▶ Anticoagulated blood specimens must be free of clots
▶ Specimens must be delivered to the laboratory within the specified amount of time after collection
▶ Outer surfaces of specimen containers must have no visible contamination
▶ Specimens must be stored properly until the time of testing
▶ Blood specimens cannot be drawn from a site above an IV line
▶ Specimens collected in anticoagulant must have the correct blood- to-anticoagulant ratio.

test findings. Therefore, every effort must be made to ensure that all requirements are met before collecting the specimen.

Order of Draw

The **order of draw** is a set of rules governing the collection order of specimens during venipuncture (Figure 6-4). If blood culture is ordered, those tubes are always drawn first to avoid contamination by bacteria that could be present on tube tops. If blood culture has not been ordered, the first tube collected is the light blue-top citrate tube for coagulation tests. Serum tubes (with or without separator gel or additive) are drawn after the citrate tube. After serum tubes, heparin (green top), EDTA (lavender or pink top), and then gray-top oxalate/fluoride tubes are drawn in that order.

Difficult Collections

Special care must be used in situations in which venipuncture can be difficult, such as collecting blood from children and the elderly. In these cases the specimen must be collected in a manner to ensure that specimen quality is not compromised. The SOP manual will contain specific instructions for specimen collection in these cases. When patients have an intravenous (IV) line, the specimen must be collected from a different arm or from a vein below the IV insertion. Ideally, a blood sample can be drawn by the IV nurse before the IV is started.

Timing of Specimen Collection

Diet, medications, or time of day can influence the levels of certain blood components. Many blood constituents are not changed significantly after eating, so blood used to test for these can be collected at any time. However, concentrations of constituents

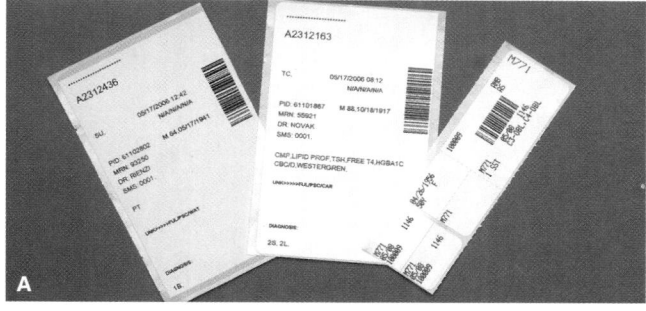

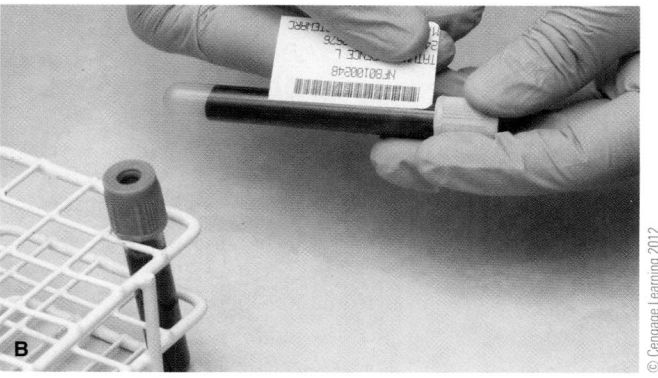

© Cengage Learning 2012

FIGURE 6-5 Specimen labeling: (A) barcoded specimen labels; (B) applying pre-printed barcoded labels to filled tubes immediately after blood collection

such as glucose, triglycerides, and cholesterol increase after eating, and specimens for these tests are collected when the patient has been fasting for a number of hours, generally in the morning before breakfast. Specimens collected from patients with lipid metabolism disorders or shortly after a patient has eaten can appear lipemic. Because **lipemic** serum or plasma is milky or cloudy, it can interfere with certain tests, particularly those that use photometry.

In some conditions, certain blood constituents follow patterns of increase or decrease that make the collection time very important. For example, creatine kinase, an enzyme measured to detect heart attacks (myocardial infarctions), rises rapidly after a heart attack and falls back to normal levels in the days immediately following the attack. If this enzyme is not measured during this critical period, a heart attack can go undiagnosed.

The blood levels of some drugs or medications will fluctuate depending on the dosage time. Some tests for therapeutic drug monitoring must be done at set intervals before or after the medications are administered.

Diurnal variation, changes with the time of day, can occur with certain blood constituents such as iron and corticosteroids. It is important, therefore, to note the collection time of specimens for these tests.

Specimen Transport

The specimen transport method is determined by the distance the specimen must be transported and the type of transport systems available. Specimens for point-of-care testing (POCT) require no transport, one of the benefits of POCT. In hospitals, specimens might require transport to another floor or hospital wing for testing. Many hospitals have pneumatic tube systems for rapid delivery of specimens to the central laboratory in special leak-proof, impact-resistant containers.

Couriers can transport specimens to another laboratory, perhaps in a different city, or specimens can be shipped to a reference laboratory for testing. Regardless of the transport method used, specimens must be packaged in secure containers to prevent contamination (Figure 6-6). Specimen transport methods must meet biosafety regulations and protect the quality of the specimen.

Specimen Processing and Storage

Blood collected to obtain serum should be allowed to clot and then centrifuged according to the SOP manual, to separate serum from blood cells. Serum should be removed from the tube as soon as possible after centrifugation. To obtain plasma, the anticoagulated specimen can be centrifuged immediately after collection.

For most routine tests to be performed within 1 hour, the specimen can remain at room temperature until testing. However, if testing is to be delayed for a few hours, samples should be refrigerated at 4° C. Some enzyme tests require immediate separation of cells from serum or plasma; the serum or plasma must then be frozen as soon as possible to prevent the loss of enzyme activity. Serum and plasma must be removed from cells before freezing, because freezing will cause cell lysis.

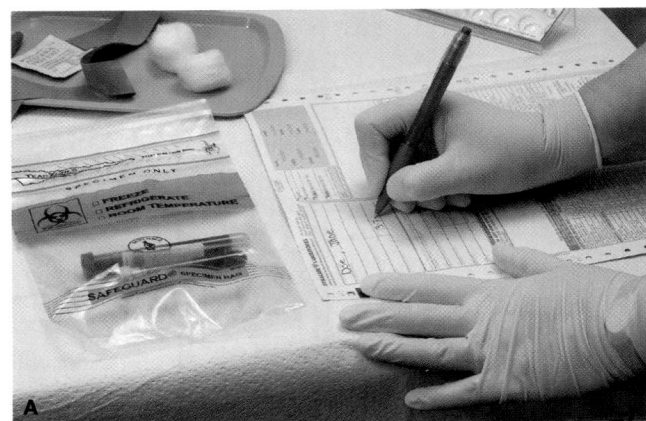

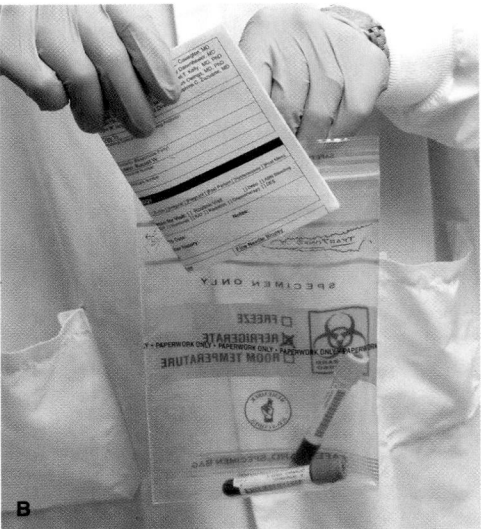

FIGURE 6-6 Specimen transport: (A) seal specimen tubes inside transport bag; complete requisition and (B) place it into a separate sleeve on the transport bag

Most specimens can be stored in capped test or collection tubes until testing. However, certain specimens require special handling. For example, bilirubin is degraded by light, so specimens should be stored in the dark.

Problems Associated with Specimen Collection and Processing

Reliable test results can only be obtained if the laboratory has a suitable specimen (Table 6-3). Erroneous results can be caused by incorrect patient identification or improper collection or handling of specimens; these errors are called *preanalytical errors*. Because a great deal of time is spent on sample preparation it is extremely important that it is done correctly the first time. Specific problems that can be associated with incorrect specimen collection and processing are:

- Hemolysis
- Hemoconcentration

- Overcentrifugation
- Evaporation
- Microbial contamination
- Anticoagulant contamination

Hemolysis

Blood that is hemolyzed during collection or processing cannot be used for most analyses. The destroyed red blood cells will release substances such as hemoglobin, enzymes (LD and AST), potassium (K^+), and other intracellular components, resulting in a blood sample that does not represent the patient's true status. Hemolysis can be caused by overcentrifugation (too long or too fast), excessive turbulence of the sample (shaking, etc.), freezing of cells, or poor venipuncture technique (slow blood flow or needle gauge too small).

Hemoconcentration

Hemoconcentration can occur if the tourniquet is left on too long (more than 1 minute) during venipuncture. This causes blood stasis within the vein, resulting in some blood constituents becoming concentrated (Lesson 1-12).

Overcentrifugation

The SOP manual will specify the correct time and speed of centrifugation required for samples for each type of analysis. Centrifugation at too high a speed or for too long a time can result in red cell hemolysis. In addition, overcentrifugation can cause the gel in plasma or serum separator tubes to be forced back downward into the red cells. In extreme cases, excessive speed and longer times of centrifugation can cause breakage of the specimen tubes or heat up the specimen.

Evaporation

Specimens should remain capped until they are tested. Evaporation will occur in uncapped specimens, resulting in concentration of some constituents or loss of volatile constituents. Gas escape or exchange can also occur and can affect results of tests such as bicarbonate (HCO_3^-) concentration.

Microbial Contamination

Clean pipets or pipet tips must be used to transfer each sample from the collection tube to a tube for analysis. Sample cups must be clean and dry to avoid contaminating or diluting the samples. Bacterial contamination of specimens must be avoided. Single-use disposable products eliminate these problems.

Anticoagulant Contamination

When multiple blood samples are obtained using a vacuum collection system, the order of draw is important. Serum collection tubes must be filled before tubes that contain anticoagulant, with the exception of the sodium citrate (light blue top) tube, which is filled before serum tubes (Figure 6-4).

CASE STUDY

Ms. Tan came to the laboratory for blood tests because her physician suspected renal disease. The tests ordered were serum BUN, creatinine, and electrolytes. The blood specimen was obtained and processed. When the laboratory technician received the serum to perform the tests, he noticed that the serum had a reddish tinge.

1. Was there a problem with this serum sample? If so, what?
2. What conditions could cause this to happen to a serum specimen?
3. Is the sample acceptable for use?

CRITICAL THINKING

What are the advantages of using plasma compared to serum in chemical analyses?

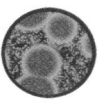

SUMMARY

The tests performed in the chemistry laboratory reveal much about the patient's health status. The physician or other health-care provider uses the results to make decisions about diagnosis, treatment, or prevention of disease. The quality of the specimen can be compromised at any point from collection through analysis. Therefore, the facility must have quality assessment (QA) procedures in place for specimen collection, processing, analysis, and reporting of test results. These QA procedures include positive identification of the patient, correct specimen collection and handling, and utmost attention to the analytical process. Specimens must be collected in the appropriate tube. Separation of serum or plasma from cells should be performed within the time limit specified by the test procedure. Standard Precautions must be observed in all steps of collection and processing for the protection of the patient and laboratory personnel. Advancements in technologies for specimen collection and automated specimen processing promise continued improvements in laboratory safety and in the reduction of specimen identification errors.

 REVIEW QUESTIONS

1. What are the most commonly tested body fluids?
2. How is blood collected for procedures requiring serum?
3. How is blood collected for procedures requiring plasma?
4. Discuss the order of draw and its importance.
5. Place the following collection tubes in the appropriate order of draw: green top, red/gray top, light blue top, dark blue top, gray top, and lavender/pink top.
6. What are the differences between serum and plasma?
7. What safety measures must be observed to avoid accidental needlesticks?
8. What PPE must be worn when collecting and processing specimens?
9. What are three types of tubes (cap colors) that can be used to collect serum?
10. How can the timing of specimen collection affect test results?
11. What can cause hemolysis of a specimen? How will test results be affected if hemolysis occurs?
12. How does freezing of whole blood affect the specimen?
13. Discuss why quality assessment procedures are important in collecting and processing specimens for clinical chemistry.
14. Define anticoagulant, cerebrospinal fluid, diurnal, lipemic, order of draw, pericardial fluid, plasma, pleural fluid, serum, STAT, and synovial fluid.

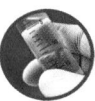 STUDENT ACTIVITIES

1. Complete the written examination for this lesson.
2. Visit a clinical laboratory and obtain information about the specimen collection and processing section. Find out which laboratory personnel are responsible for collecting, transporting, and processing specimens. Request permission to view the specimen collection section of the laboratory's SOP manual.

 WEB ACTIVITIES

1. Select 10 clinical chemistry tests from Table 6-2 in Lesson 6-1. Use the Internet to find specimen collection and handling requirements for each test. Make a table showing the collection requirements for the tests. List the order of draw for the tubes required for the tests.

2. Search the Internet for downloadable wall charts, posters, or other guides to collection tube cap colors and collection tube uses.

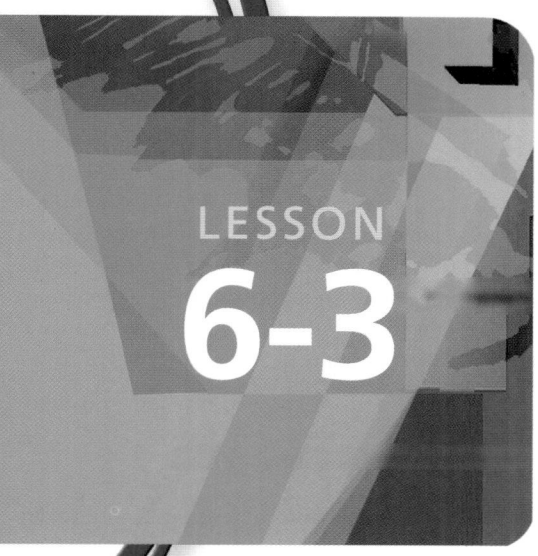

LESSON 6-3

Principles of Chemistry Instrumentation

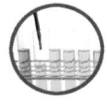

LESSON OBJECTIVES

After studying this lesson, the student will:

⊙ Explain Beer's law.

⊙ Explain how spectrophotometry and photometry are used in clinical chemistry instruments.

⊙ Discuss the major differences between instruments used in small and large laboratories.

⊙ Discuss the reasons for the increase in testing in small laboratories.

⊙ List factors that should be considered when purchasing an instrument.

⊙ Discuss the basic differences among photometers, reflectance photometers, and ion-selective analyzers.

⊙ Discuss how amperometry is used in clinical chemistry analyses.

⊙ Explain what is meant by solid-phase technology.

⊙ Explain the importance of observing all safety precautions when using chemistry instrumentation.

⊙ Discuss the elements that must be included in quality assessment programs for chemistry instrumentation.

⊙ Define the glossary terms.

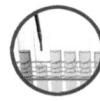

GLOSSARY

absorbance (A) / a logarithmic expression of the amount of light absorbed by a substance containing colored molecules; optical density (O.D.)

amperometry / the technology that uses electrodes and electrode potential to measure electron generation

Beer's law / a mathematical relationship that demonstrates the linear relationship of concentration to absorbance and that forms the basis for spectrophotometric analysis

ion-selective electrode / an electrode manufactured to detect a specific ion and measure its concentration

light spectrum / the portion of the electromagnetic spectrum that is visible to humans; the range of wavelengths of visible radiation

monochromator / a device that isolates a narrow portion of the light spectrum

nephelometry / an analytical technique used to measure light scatter by particles in solution

percent transmittance (%T) / the percentage of light that passes through a solution

reflectance photometer / an instrument that measures the light reflected from a colored reaction product

solid-phase chemistry / an analytical method in which the sample is added to a strip or slide containing all reagents for the procedure in dried form

spectrophotometer / an instrument that measures intensities of light at selected wavelengths

INTRODUCTION

Instrumentation and automation in clinical chemistry make it possible for analyses to be performed much more rapidly and precisely than when they are done manually. Automation is described as a process in which many analytical tests can be performed with little involvement of an analyst. Reduced analysis time and the ability to test each patient specimen for several analytes at the same time are especially important because larger laboratories, such as those in hospitals, process hundreds of specimens daily. When analysis time is reduced, the *turnaround time* (TAT)—time elapsed between ordering a laboratory test and the physician receiving the results—is also usually reduced. Shorter TAT allows for more rapid diagnosis and treatment. Automation also has a place in the smaller clinical laboratory, physician office laboratories (POLs), and point-of-care (POC) testing (Lesson 6-4).

This lesson presents principles of the major technologies used in chemistry instrumentation for measuring various types of analytes. Examples of a few instruments using the technologies presented are also given. Most instruments mentioned are for use in smaller laboratories or at POC and were chosen as examples because they are in use in many laboratories and present different principles of operation.

CURRENT TRENDS IN INSTRUMENTATION

Instrumentation technology is in a continuous state of change. Updated and improved instruments are constantly being developed and introduced. In the past, as the volume of testing increased, the major instrument manufacturers concentrated on developing larger and more diversified instruments designed to meet the needs of larger hospital laboratories and regional reference laboratories. In recent years, however, a revolution has taken place in clinical laboratory instrumentation. Improved electronic, computer, and chemical technology have made it possible for manufacturers to drastically reduce the size of many instruments. In addition, these smaller instruments have other advantages:

- Easy to use
- Produce rapid results
- Require less operator calibration and standardization
- Use prepackaged reagents and test units

CHOOSING AN INSTRUMENT FOR THE LABORATORY

Many factors must be considered before purchasing an instrument for the laboratory. First, the decision must be made concerning which tests will be performed and the expected testing volume. This decision can be based on the patient population being served, which tests would be most helpful to the physicians and patients, and availability of personnel to be trained to operate the instrument.

The most important factor in choosing an instrument is the quality of results. An instrument that produces unreliable results is detrimental to patient care. Other considerations are cost per test, ease of operation, and maintenance costs. The final cost can be more than expected if an inexpensive instrument requires expensive reagents and supplies. The purchase price should be compared to the lease price. Although lease prices sometimes seem more expensive, they often include maintenance, free technical service, and automatic instrument replacement when newer models become available.

Comparison of Methods

When a new instrument is being considered, the methodology of that instrument must be evaluated. If the laboratory has plans to increase the use of automation, the new instrument must have the ability to coordinate with existing or planned instruments in the laboratory as well as the laboratory information system (LIS). Questions that must be considered include: Does the instrument require frequent preventive maintenance? Will the manufacturer provide preventive maintenance for a prescribed period or for the lifetime of the instrument? Will the results produced by the instrument meet the requirements of the laboratory's quality assessment program. The precision, accuracy, detection limits, and sensitivity and specificity of the method performed on the new instrument must be considered.

Safety Precautions

 The operation, maintenance, and repair of laboratory instruments and analyzers expose personnel to biological, physical, and chemical hazards. Standard Precautions must be observed at all times. Care must be taken when handling controls that are made from biological materials. Parts of the instrument that come in contact with specimens and controls must be disinfected regularly. Instruments that incorporate safe technologies, such as through-the-cap sampling, can decrease exposure hazards to personnel.

Instruments must be installed and grounded as recommended by the manufacturer to prevent electrical shocks. The outside case should never be removed except by a person trained in maintenance and repair. Removal of the outer case can expose wiring and other components that carry high voltage electricity and can cause serious harm if touched. Dangling metal jewelry is especially dangerous, because it can inadvertently contact an electrical part. Instructions for operating and maintaining battery-powered instruments, such as those used in POCT, must be followed. The battery used must be the type recommended by the manufacturer; used batteries must be disposed of according to local and state regulations.

Attention must be paid to all MSDS and chemical label warnings to prevent injury from hazardous chemicals. In many cases, chemical hazards can be reduced by using commercially prepared reagents and self-contained reagent packs or cassettes.

Quality Assessment

Quality assessment is an essential part of all laboratory analyses. Analyses using instrumentation are more precise than manual methods of analysis. Use of chemistry instrumentation also increases the laboratory's productivity because many specimens can be analyzed in a short time. Instrumentation results are reliable when an adequate quality assessment (QA) program is in place and is implemented. Details of the QA program must be included in the standard operating procedure (SOP) manual and must encompass all aspects of testing. This includes operator training, maintenance and repair of instruments, patient identification, specimen collection, test procedures, calibration and control methods, and reporting of patient test results.

The operating manual provided with each instrument contains operating procedures, troubleshooting guides, and instructions for simple repairs. Most companies offer a preventive maintenance contract that includes regular scheduled maintenance. A log of all maintenance performed on an instrument must be kept. All personnel who will use the instrument must be trained in its use and the training must be documented.

Instruments must be calibrated and control analyses performed as stated in the manufacturers' instructions and in the SOP manual. Control results must be charted or otherwise entered into the laboratory's QC statistical program; control results must be evaluated at frequent intervals, usually several times daily, as specified in the SOP manual. The manual should also contain the procedures to follow if controls values are out of acceptable range.

CHEMISTRY INSTRUMENTATION PRINCIPLES

Clinical chemistry analyzers utilize different technologies for measuring analytes in patient samples. Some of the technologies used are:

- Photometry
- Spectrophotometry
- Reflectance photometry

- Nephelometry and turbidimetry
- Ion-selective electrodes
- Electrochemical (amperometry)

Photometry and Spectrophotometry

A photometer is an instrument that measures the intensity of light and is used to determine the concentration of colored solutions. This determination is made by passing a beam of light of a specific wavelength through the colored solution contained in a glass or plastic cell called a cuvette.

Different colors of solutions absorb light at different wavelengths, so the wavelength used in the photometer must be matched to the analytical method. Photometers can be used with a variety of "wet" chemistry methods, as long as the test procedure generates a colored product or causes a color change in a solution. The primary difference in photometers and spectrophotometers is in the way the wavelength of light is selected. Instruments that use a diffraction grating or a prism to select the wavelength of light are called **spectrophotometers**; instruments that use a filter to select the wavelength are called *photometers*. For this discussion, the major principles of measurement of colored solutions are the same for photometers and spectrophotometers.

In the simplest design, a light source in the instrument provides a beam of visible light of all wavelengths (Figure 6-7). In spectrophotometers, the visible light passes through a **monochromator** with a diffraction grating or prism that disperses the white light into a **light spectrum** (Figure 6-7). A narrow slit isolates a beam of monochromatic (one wavelength) light; the wavelength is selected by the operator according to the analysis being performed. In the photometer the operator selects the filter to isolate light of the correct wavelength of light.

The monochromatic light is directed through the cuvette containing a colored solution. The portion of light that passes through the colored solution is detected by a photoelectric cell. This light is the **percent transmittance (%T)**. The light that does not pass through is absorbed by the colored solution and is measured

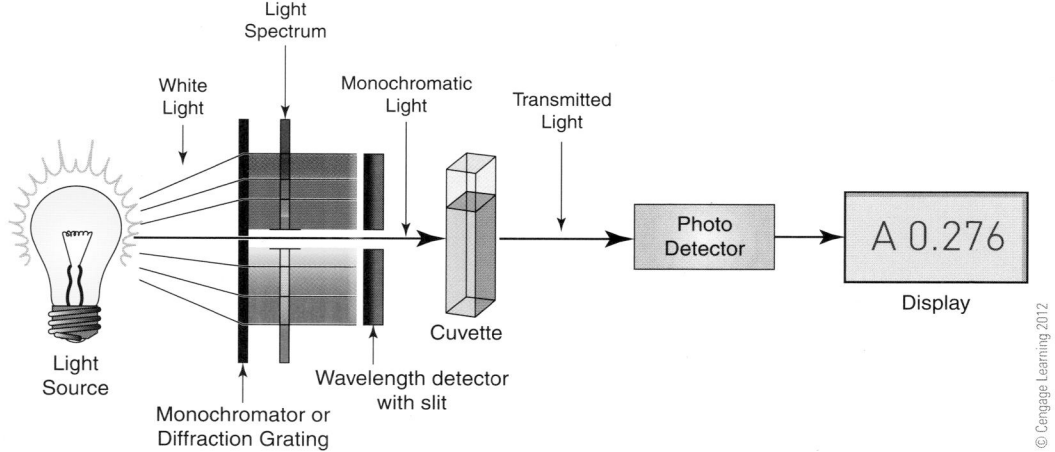

FIGURE 6-7 Diagram of the internal parts of a spectrophotometer

as **absorbance (A)** units. The more concentrated the solution, the greater is its absorbance and the less its transmittance. For most colored solutions, the absorbance increases proportionally with the concentration (Figure 6-8). These solutions are said to follow **Beer's law,** a mathematical relationship that demonstrates the linear relationship of concentration to absorbance and that forms the basis for spectrophotometric analysis.

The light detected by the photoelectric cell is converted to an electrical current that is measured and converted to a digital readout. This information can be displayed as either absorbance (A) or percent transmittance (%T). Spectrophotometers and photometers vary in external design, but the principles are the same whether they are stand-alone instruments or are included as a part of an analyzer.

Photometers and spectrophotometers were the workhorses in laboratories for many years. Designs included spectrophotometers that measured only light in the visible range; others also measured light in the ultraviolet (UV) range. With the increase of automated analyzers, stand-alone photometers are now usually reserved for research laboratories or large reference laboratories. However, most automated chemistry analyzers have incorporated some type of photometric analysis in their design.

Photometry

Several clinical analyzers discussed in this lesson contain simple or modified photometers. These usually operate at only one or a few preset wavelengths. Most clinical laboratory instruments used in small laboratories are *discrete analyzers*, meaning that tests are performed by applying a patient sample a test cartridge, cassette, or reagent strip. After the patient sample is applied to the test unit, the instrument must detect the substance and measure the intensity of the reaction. This is accomplished in different ways, depending on instrument design.

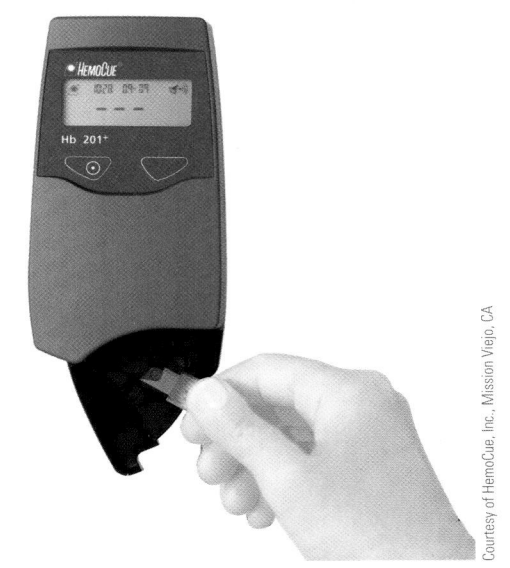

Courtesy of HemoCue, Inc., Mission Viejo, CA

FIGURE 6-9 The HemoCue HB 201+ hemoglobin analyzer uses a photometer to measure blood hemoglobin

The HemoCue glucose and hemoglobin analyzers are small point-of-care testing (POCT) instruments that use principles of photometry (Figure 6-9 and Table 6-4). Special clear disposable cuvettes contain the dried reagents required for a specific analysis. Blood samples are collected directly into the cuvette, and the reagents within the cuvette lyse the blood cells, creating a clear, colored solution. The cuvette is inserted into a chamber in the analyzer. After the sample reacts with the reagent in the cuvette, the photometer measures the intensity of light passing through the solution and converts this to conventional or SI units. Calibration of the analyzer can be performed electronically or by using a control cuvette that is an optical interference filter.

Reflectance Photometry

Reflectance photometers measure light that is *reflected* by a colored product. The reflected light is detected by a photocell, and the information is converted into the appropriate units. Reflectance photometers use **solid phase chemistry** technology, meaning that reagents are present in dried form in the test unit. Solid-phase chemistry analyzers can often use whole blood as the sample. The blood sample is applied directly to the reagent strip, slide, or cartridge that contains all of the reagents needed for the analysis. The reagents are in multiple layers, with each layer having a specific function (Figure 6-10). The area in which the reagents are located is called the *test area* or *reagent pad*. The test cartridges or strips have features that filter out the red blood cells, leaving only plasma to mix with the test reagents. The resulting color of the final product is detected by reflectance photometry. The color intensity is measured and converted to the correct units for the test being performed.

The Cholestech LDX is a small analyzer that uses reflectance photometry to perform lipid profiles, including cholesterol fractions, as well as other blood chemistries (Figure 6-11 and Table 6-4). Some of the tests are packaged individually and some, such as lipid profile tests, are included in one cassette.

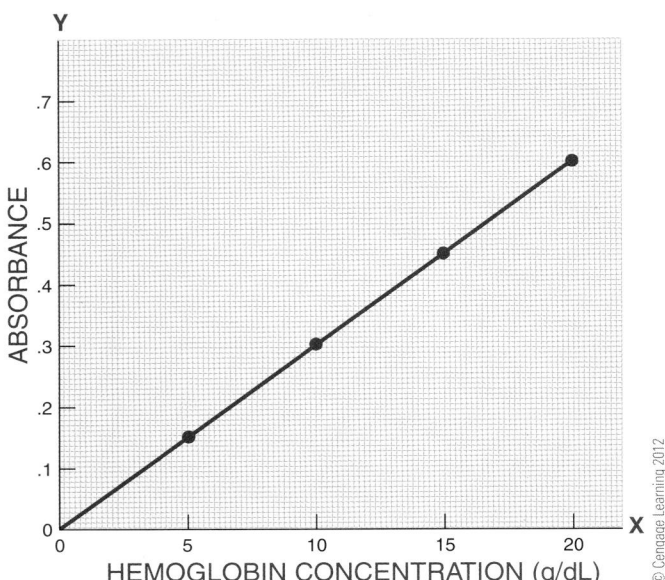

© Cengage Learning 2012

FIGURE 6-8 Illustration of a standard curve showing the relationship of absorbance to concentration

TABLE 6-4. Examples of chemistry analyzers suitable for the small laboratory and point-of-care testing, the technologies used, and their test capabilities

INSTRUMENT	TECHNOLOGIES USED	EXAMPLES OF TESTS
HemoCue Analyzers	Photometry	Hemoglobin, blood glucose
FreeStyle (Abbott)	Electrochemical/amperometry	Blood glucose
ACCU-CHEK (Roche)	Electrochemical/amperometry	Blood glucose
NOVA 16+, NOVA CCX (Nova Biomedical)	Ion-selective electrodes, optical	Electrolytes, blood chemistries
i-STAT (Abbott)	Ion-selective electrodes	Electrolytes, blood chemistries
COBAS Integra 400 Plus (Roche Diagnostics)	Ion-selective electrodes, photometry	Blood chemistries, electrolytes
Cholestech LDX System (Inverness Medical Innovations)	Reflectance photometry	Lipid profiles, blood chemistries
Accutrend (Roche)	Reflectance photometry	Triglycerides, glucose
Urine reagent strip readers	Reflectance photometry	Urine chemistries
IMMAGE (Beckman Coulter)	Nephelometry	Immunology tests, therapeutic drug monitoring
Vitros DT 60 (Johnson & Johnson)	Reflectance photometry	Blood chemistries

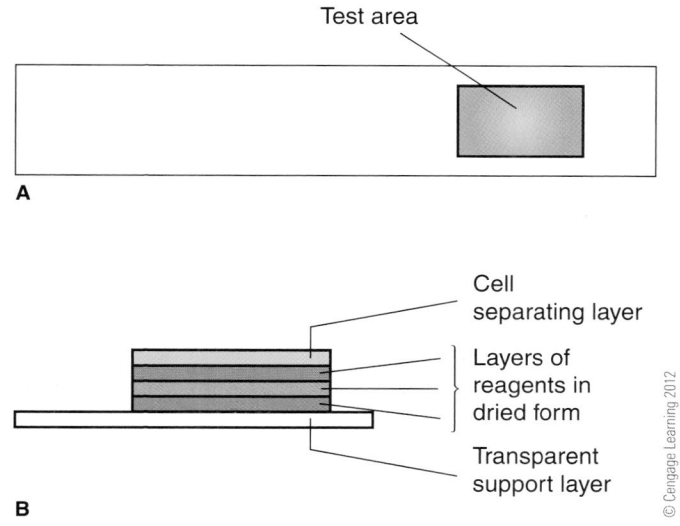

Test area

Cell separating layer

Layers of reagents in dried form

Transparent support layer

© Cengage Learning 2012

A

B

FIGURE 6-10 Illustration of the composition of a solid-phase reagent strip used in reflectance photometry: (A) top view of a strip showing reagent test area; (B) expanded side view of a test area showing the layers

This instrument is CLIA-waived and is especially useful for events such as health fairs that include cholesterol and glucose screening.

Another chemistry analyzer that uses reflectance photometry is the Johnson & Johnson Vitros DT 60 II blood chemistry analyzer, in which each test is contained on a dry reagent slide (Table 6-4). The slide is placed into the sample drawer where the instrument reads the magnetic code on the slide to determine which test is to be performed. The patient sample is dispensed onto the test slide. The colored product produced by the reaction is automatically measured by a reflectance photometer inside the instrument. The DT 60 II can perform more than 30 different test procedures, including blood glucose, total cholesterol and cholesterol fractions, creatinine, bilirubin, amylase, and hemoglobin.

Reflectance photometers can be used in laboratory departments other than chemistry. Urine chemical strip readers such as the Criterion II (Figure 6-11B and Table 6-4) use reflectance photometry. The urine reagent strip pads change colors depending on the composition of the urine. These color changes are detected by reflectance photometry, and the results are displayed or printed.

Nephelometry and Turbidimetry

Nephelometry is a technique used to measure light scatter caused by particles in a solution. Light scatter occurs when the incident light (beam) encounters particulate molecules in suspension. This collision results in the incident light being scattered. The amount of scattering is dependent upon several factors, including particle size, molecular weight of the particle, concentration of particles, wavelength of the incident light, and distance of the light from the cuvette holding the solution. The amount of light scatter measured under standard conditions is proportional to the concentration of the substance being measured. Nephelometry is used for analysis of proteins, antigens, and other immunologic assays. The Beckman Coulter IMMAGE uses nephelometry to perform a broad variety of immunological tests, including tests for several infectious diseases, measurement of immunoglobulin classes and subclasses, and therapeutic drug levels (Table 6-4).

Turbidity in a liquid is caused by the presence of fine, suspended particles. If a beam of light is passed through

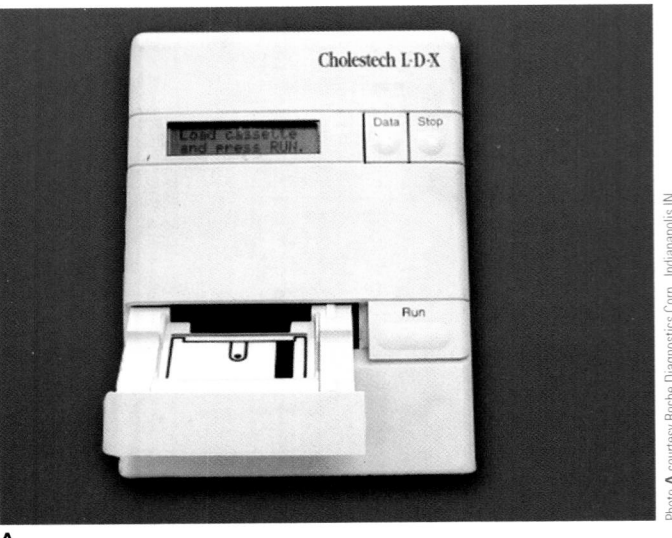

A

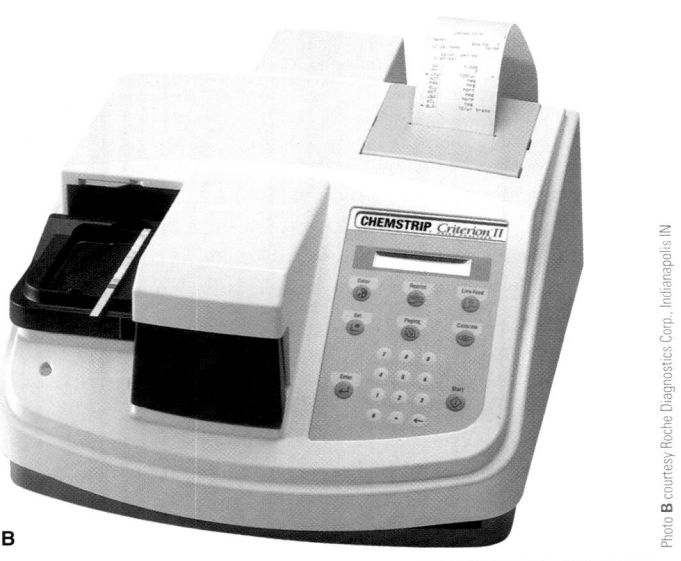

B

FIGURE 6-11 Instruments using reflectance photometry:
(A) Cholestech LDX; (B) Criterion II Urine Analyzer

a turbid sample, the light transmitted through the sample is reduced by scattering of the light, a method of analysis called turbidimetry. The quantity of light scattered is dependent upon the concentration and size distribution of the particles. In nephelometry the intensity of the scattered light is measured; in turbidimetry the intensity of light transmitted is measured. Nephelometry and turbidimety are incorporated into chemistry analyzers that are able to test dozens to hundreds of analytes using multiple test methods in one instrument or linked systems. Nephelometry and turbidimetry are often used in immunological-based tests. Examples of instruments using these technologies are the Advia line of analyzers and the Dimension Vista 500 (Siemens Healthcare Diagnostics).

Ion-Selective Electrodes

Electrodes are probes that measure ions in solution. A common use of electrodes in clinical chemistry is to measure hydrogen ion concentration using a pH meter. **Ion-selective electrodes** selectively detect and measure one particular ion in the presence of other ions; for example, a pH electrode is an ion-selective electrode for hydrogen (H^+).

Two electrodes are required for ion-selective electrode analysis. One electrode contains a known concentration of the ion to be measured and is called the *reference electrode*. The other electrode, which is responsive only to the ion being measured, is exposed to the unknown solution. The difference between the concentration of ions in the reference electrode and the ions in the unknown solution causes an electrical potential to develop. This potential across a membrane in the electrode is proportional to the difference between the two concentrations. A microprocessor converts this voltage into a number representing the concentration of the ion in the unknown solution. Each ion-selective electrode is responsive to a specific ion. For example, the sodium (Na^+) electrode, will measure only Na^+ ions present in a sample. The technology of ion-selective electrodes is used in many clinical instruments and is particularly useful for measuring electrolytes. Analyzers using ion-selective technology include Nova Biomedical's Critical Care Xpress and 16^+ analyzers, Abbott's i-STAT, and Roche Diagnostics' COBAS INTEGRA 400 Plus (Figure 6-12 and Table 6-4).

Nova Analyzers

Nova Biomedical manufactures several analyzers that use ion-selective electrode technology and are suitable for use in smaller laboratories and critical care areas. The Nova 16^+ has a test menu that includes Na^+, potassium (K^+), chloride (Cl^-), glucose, BUN (blood urea nitrogen), and hematocrit. It can analyze more than 50 samples per hour and, depending on the test, requires only 200 μL of whole blood, serum, plasma, or urine. The small size of the instruments is made possible because of the compact size of the electrodes. Nova Biomedical also markets a line of analyzers

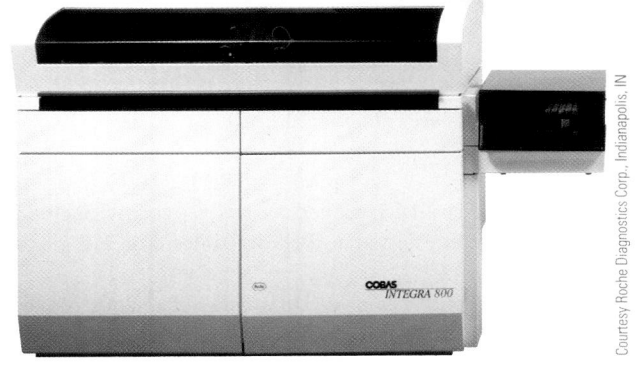

FIGURE 6-12 The COBAS Integra 800 chemistry analyzer which uses photometry and ion-selective electrode technology

called Critical Care Xpress (CCX) for use in POCT areas such as emergency departments. The instruments in the series can perform different combinations of blood gas, electrolyte, and hematocrit analyses.

Control solutions are run in the same manner as patient samples on most of the Nova chemistry analyzers. However, their Stat Profile Critical Care Xpress analyzer has an automated onboard quality control system. Special QC packs containing tri-level controls are loaded into the instrument. The instrument analyzes these packs at preset intervals, and the data are automatically stored. If the controls are not within limits, an audible alarm can alert the technician or an optional feature can put a lockout on the instrument until the problem is corrected. An additional feature is the SmartCheck automated maintenance program that ensures the instrument is operating correctly.

COBAS INTEGRA Analyzers

The COBAS INTEGRA analyzers (Figure 6-12 and Table 6-4) combine a *mix tower* with an ion-selective electrode analyzer. The mix tower is used to ensure that sample and reagents are thoroughly mixed together. With the optional ion-selective electrode module, Na^+, K^+, and Cl^- ions can be measured directly. In addition, the instruments have menus of up to 72 tests, including routine chemistries, hemoglobin A1c, and assays of drugs of abuse. The COBAS 400 can process up to 400 samples per hour, depending on the combination of tests chosen.

Electrochemical Technology

Several handheld analyzers such as glucose meters are based on electrochemical technology (Figure 6-13 and Table 6-4). Other terms used for this technology include **amperometry** and *coulometry*. Analyzers using this technology include ACCU-CHEK meters (Roche Diagnostics), the FreeStyle glucose meters and i-STAT (Abbott Laboratories), and Paradigm Link glucose monitor (Medtronic Minimed).

Analyzers using electrochemical technology incorporate electrodes that measure electrons (current) generated when the sample and reagents react. Patient samples are applied to small disposable biosensor strips that look similar to other types of reagent strips. These biosensors, in addition to containing reagents for the chemical reactions, also contain electrodes called electrochemical sensors. When the sample interacts with the reagents in the biosensor strip, the electrons generated are detected by the meter and converted into glucose units.

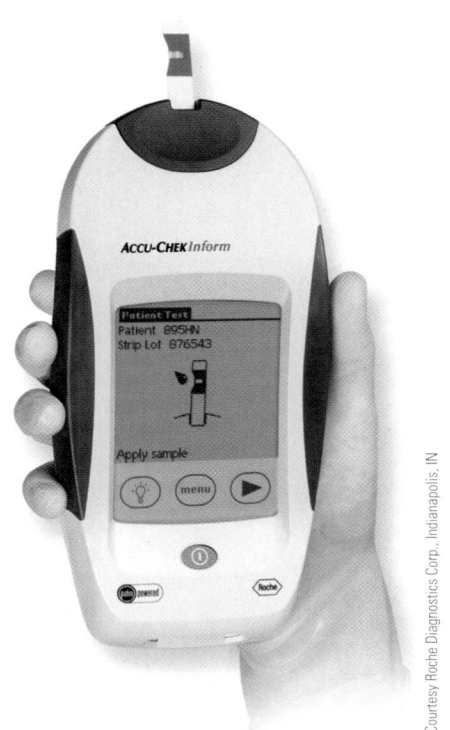

Courtesy Roche Diagnostics Corp., Indianapolis, IN

FIGURE 6-13 Accu-Chek Inform glucose meter which uses electrochemical technology

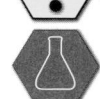

SAFETY REMINDERS

- Review Safety Precautions section before using instruments.
- Wear appropriate PPE.
- Observe Standard Precautions.
- Follow manufacturer's instructions for the instrument being used.
- Consult MSDS and observe chemical and electrical safety rules.
- Allow only trained personnel to perform instrument maintenance

PROCEDURAL REMINDERS

- Review Quality Assessment section before using instrument.
- Follow SOP manual and manufacturer's instructions.
- Perform maintenance and quality control procedures as specified.
- Calibrate instruments according to manufacturer's instructions.

CRITICAL THINKING

Dr. Sharma, a physician in a small group clinic, ordered a triglyceride test on a patient and wanted the results before the patient left the clinic. Latitia, who worked in the clinic laboratory, prepared to perform the test. She calibrated the chemistry analyzer used for triglycerides and found it to be working correctly. However, Latitia found that, although the triglyceride controls had not expired, the reagent packs for the analyzer had expired the previous week.

1. Latitia should:
   a. Run the patient sample because the reagent packs had expired only recently
   b. Use a triglyceride reagent pack from another analyzer to perform the test
   c. Inform Dr. Sharma that the test cannot be run in the clinic laboratory until in-date reagent packs are obtained for the analyzer
   d. Run the controls and, if they are acceptable, perform the patient test
   e. Perform the patient test, but only report the results if they are in the reference range
2. Discuss the choices above and justify your answer.
3. What laboratory policies should have been in place that would have prevented Latitia's dilemma?

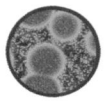

SUMMARY

Instrumentation in the clinical laboratory has changed laboratories' operating procedures. Within the last 40 to 50 years methods have changed from performing all chemistry tests manually to chemistry laboratories becoming almost totally automated. Many different types of chemistry analyzers are available. Factors to consider in choosing an analyzer include reliability of results, the number and kinds of tests to be performed, and the patient population being served. Purchase price, reagent costs, ease of operation, and maintenance requirements also should be considered. In addition, laboratories using the instruments under consideration should be contacted to inquire about analyzer reliability, accuracy and precision, and availability of technical support. Training sessions are offered by manufacturers or distributors or a representative can come to the laboratory to train personnel who will be using the instrument. The operation and maintenance of laboratory analyzers requires the technician to adhere to all biological, chemical, and electrical safety rules. Quality assessment and quality control programs must be maintained for each instrument.

REVIEW QUESTIONS

1. Why might instruments used in small laboratories be different from those used in larger laboratories?
2. What has brought about increased testing in smaller facilities?
3. What are the basic differences between photometers and reflectance photometers?

4. Explain solid-phase technology.
5. Explain how electrochemical analyzers operate.
6. What is the principle of the ion-selective methods?
7. What are the differences between spectrophotometers and photometers?
8. Why is a regular instrument maintenance program important?
9. Discuss the importance of quality assessment programs for chemistry analyzers.
10. What safety hazards are associated with using chemistry analyzers?
11. What is the advantage of an analyzer that can use whole blood specimens instead of only serum or plasma?
12. Explain how instrumentation affects TAT and why this is important.
13. Why is the information in a maintenance logbook important?
14. Define absorbance, amperometry, Beer's law, ion-selective electrode, light spectrum, monochromator, nephelometry, percent transmittance, reflectance photometer, solid-phase chemistry, and spectrophotometer.

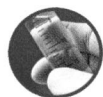

STUDENT ACTIVITIES

1. Complete the written examination for this lesson.
2. Tour a small laboratory to observe the operation of some chemistry analyzers.

3. Visit or contact a local POL and ask what analyzers are used and what quality assessment procedures are performed.

4. Visit a health fair or a cholesterol screening event to observe the analyzers used.

5. Use the information from this lesson and the manufacturer's instructions for an analyzer available in the laboratory to complete the worksheet accompanying this lesson.

WEB ACTIVITY

Using the Internet, find the web site of an instrument manufacturer mentioned in this lesson. List the chemistry analyzers available from the manufacturer. Select an analyzer not discussed in this lesson and report on its principle of operation and test capabilities.

LESSON 6-3

Principles of Chemistry Instrumentation

Select an analyzer available in the laboratory, read the manufacturer's operating manual (or laboratory SOP manual), and answer the following questions about the analyzer:

1. What is the name of the instrument? _____

2. What technology is used? _____

3. What types of test units are used with the instrument? _____

4. List two analytes that can be measured using this instrument. _____
   _____

5. How is the instrument prompted or programmed for the test to be performed? _____
   _____

6. What controls are required for this instrument? Are equivalent or internal controls used _____
   _____
   _____

7. Have Levey-Jennings charts been constructed for each type of analysis performed on this instrument?
   _____

   Are values plotted daily? _____

8. What specimen(s) can be used for the analyses performed on this instrument?
   _____

9. Is a temperature-controlled incubation required for the test(s)? _____ If so, is the temperature
   monitor or chamber integrated into the instrument? _____

10. How are test results obtained (printed out, displayed, uploaded to the LIS, etc.)? _____

11. Are any additional calculations required by the technologist to obtain final test results?
    _____

12. Are maintenance and repair records kept in a logbook? _____

13. List in order the steps for performing a specific analysis using this instrument.

Student/Tech Name _____ Date _____

© 2012 Delmar, Cengage Learning. Permission to reproduce for clinical use granted.

WORKSHEET

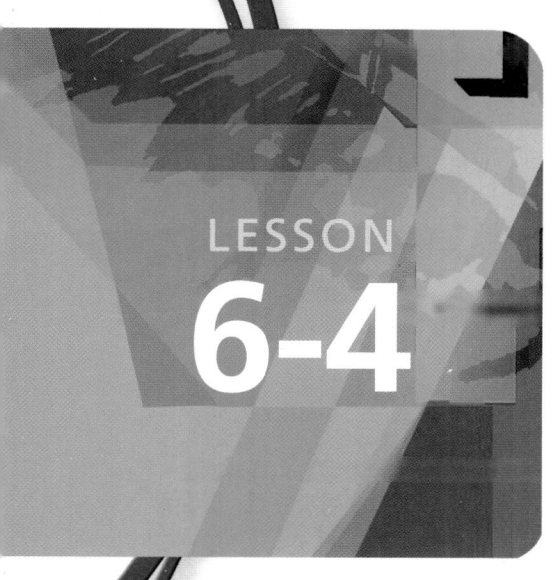

Point-of-Care Testing

LESSON OBJECTIVES

After studying this lesson, the student will:

⊙ Explain what is meant by point-of-care testing (POCT).

⊙ Name three common POCT sites.

⊙ Discuss the advantages and disadvantages of POCT.

⊙ Name the healthcare professionals who are part of the POCT team.

⊙ List five test procedures commonly performed at POC sites.

⊙ Discuss safety procedures that must be followed when performing POCT.

⊙ Explain why compliance with a quality assessment program is important in POCT.

INTRODUCTION

Testing at point of care (POC) is a way of bringing laboratory testing to the patient, rather than sending patients or patient specimens to the laboratory. Point-of-care testing (POCT) is also called near-patient testing (NPT), bedside testing, and alternative testing. POCT has been made possible by the development of small, portable analyzers that give rapid test results. These analyzers are easy to use, give reproducible results, and require little maintenance. The tests performed are regulated by the Centers for Medicare and Medicaid Services (CMS) and the Clinical Laboratory Improvement Amendments of 1988 (CLIA '88).

POCT had its beginning when blood glucose monitors were developed for home use by diabetics. No special expertise was required to operate these first monitors, and the glucose test could be performed using a drop of capillary blood. Patients had daily access to rapid glucose test results and could use these results for adjusting their insulin dosage, diet, or activity levels.

In the 1990s, technological advances in instrument design mushroomed. Today, numerous small, sophisticated, but easy-to-use analyzers are available to perform hematology analyses, urine chemistries, coagulation tests, blood chemistries and immunology procedures. These analyzers are being used in a variety of settings such as hospital bedsides, emergency departments, intensive care units, clinics, physicians' offices, and as back-up instruments in medium-sized laboratories. In addition, rapid immunological test kits that require no instrument have been developed and are used at POC. Some of these, such as urine pregnancy test kits, are available over the counter.

WHO IS INVOLVED IN POINT-OF-CARE TESTING?

Good POCT programs require a multidisciplinary team effort among physicians, laboratory personnel, nursing personnel, and other medical staff (Table 6-5). After thorough training, nurses, medical assistants, emergency medical technicians, licensed practical nurses, physicians and others can perform some of the testing that has traditionally been done by laboratory scientists. The laboratory's usual role in POCT is to provide technical assistance, data management, quality assessment, compliance monitoring, and personnel training.

POINT-OF-CARE TESTING SITES

POCT programs are quite varied. They can be classified as hospital-based or nonhospital-based.

TABLE 6-5. Departments and personnel involved in decision making in point-of-care testing programs

Clinical laboratory	Infection prevention
Nursing	Safety officer
Medical staff	Administration

Hospital Point-of-Care Testing

Hospital POCT programs are usually geared toward providing service to critically ill patients in critical care units, emergency departments, surgical suites, and cardiac units. These patients benefit from quick action by the medical team, which is facilitated by having rapid test results. One example of a hospital POCT program is the use of bedside analyzers that measure glucose, clotting time, and electrolytes in the emergency department, critical care units, and surgery (Figures 6-14 and 6-15). These analyzers are calibrated and maintained by laboratory personnel, who provide procedure manuals, technical assistance, training of testing personnel, and assessment of the training.

A POCT coordinator is responsible for reviewing and analyzing quality control (QC) data, ensuring compliance with accreditation agencies, coordinating staff training, and serving as a liaison among nursing services, testing personnel, and the

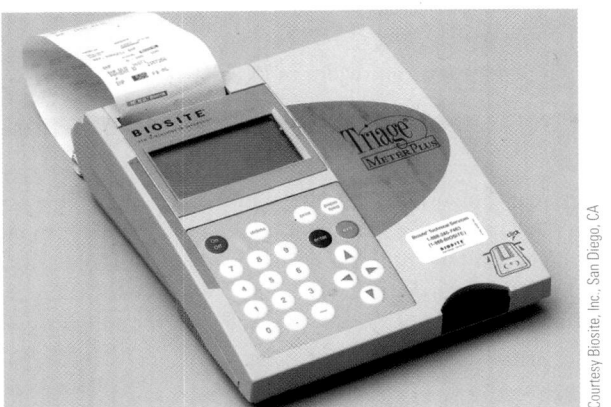

FIGURE 6-14 Triage MeterPlus , an analyzer with a multi-test menu useful in critical care settings

laboratory. One goal in critical care areas of the hospital is to cut down on the TAT (turn-around-time) for laboratory results. Tests usually performed are those for which the results can affect the patient's immediate well-being and treatment. These include blood glucose, blood gases, electrolytes, and coagulation tests.

Nonhospital Point-of-Care Testing Programs

POCT is also used in physician office laboratories (POLs), nursing homes, blood donation centers, health fairs, physical examinations for insurance or employment, and in homes (Figure 6-16). POCT programs outside the hospital have a different purpose from hospital programs. In nonhospital settings, rapid results are usually not critical to patient immediate care, but the on-site testing saves time and costs for the patient as well as the healthcare provider.

Nonhospital POCT programs are designed to provide a small menu of laboratory tests in a convenient, cost-effective, and efficient way. These tests are important in preventive medicine and can be used to screen for anemia, risk for cardiovascular disease (CVD), and kidney disease, as well as to monitor and provide information for managing oral anticoagulant therapy or conditions such as diabetes.

Physician Office Laboratories

Another example of a nonhospital POCT program is a POL that offers tests such as hemoglobin, blood glucose, urine chemistry by reagent strip (dipstick), and prothrombin time. These rapid tests can be performed by medical assistants or nursing staff before the patient sees the physician. The results are available for the physician to use in making decisions concerning further patient treatment or follow-up. This is much more efficient than sending patients to a laboratory for tests, waiting for the results, and calling or having the patient return later to learn their test results. The number of tests performed in POLs has increased in recent years. The availability of testing in the physician's office can be a benefit, especially to the very ill or elderly patient.

Most POLs use CLIA-waived analyzers or test kits that require few routine maintenance and QC procedures. CLIA-waived tests are those laboratory tests and procedures that are simple to perform and have an insignificant risk for an erroneous result. Sites performing only waived tests must keep

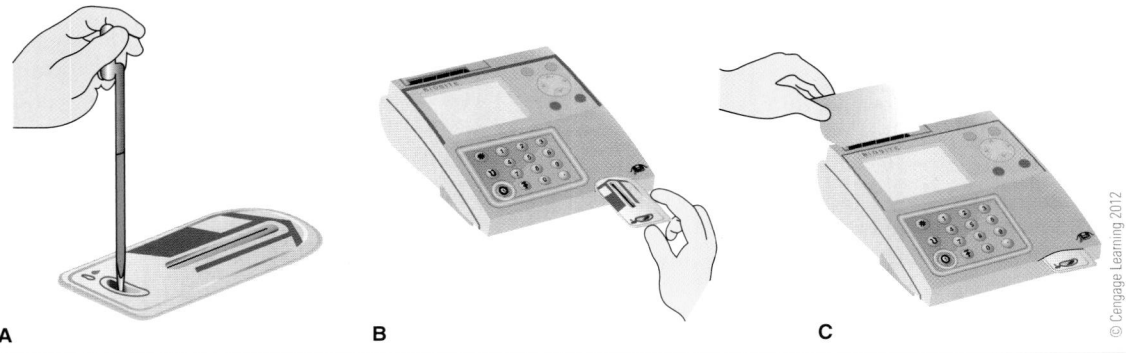

FIGURE 6-15 Using the Triage MeterPlus: (A) Add whole blood to test device; (B) insert device into meter; and (C) read results

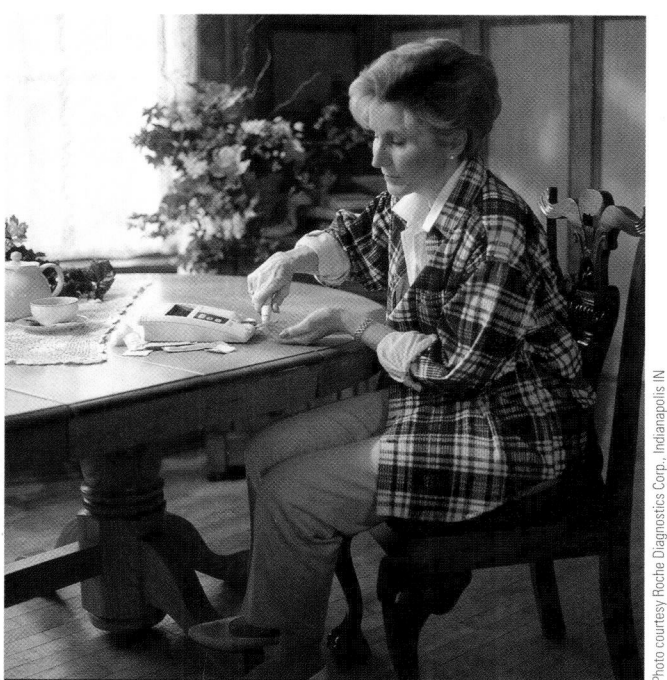

Photo courtesy Roche Diagnostics Corp., Indianapolis IN

FIGURE 6-16 A patient performing at-home coagulation testing

all package inserts on file and keep that file updated with any changes in procedures.

Sites that perform tests of moderate complexity must maintain up-to-date procedure manuals as well as documentation of QC results and instrument maintenance. A laboratory professional can be employed as a consultant to provide periodic review of procedures and technical assistance.

Screening Programs

An example of a POCT screening program is a one-day cholesterol and/or glucose screening program that offers blood cholesterol tests, blood glucose tests, and heart attack risk assessment. Healthcare personnel perform rapid tests on capillary blood using portable glucose and/or cholesterol analyzers. Maintenance, calibration, and QC of these analyzers are performed at the supervising laboratory facility before and after the screening event so that minimal control procedures are required during the screening event. Test results are available immediately so those tested can decide whether or not to consult their physician.

COMPONENTS OF A POINT-OF-CARE TESTING PROGRAM

Whether a POCT program is large-scale or small, there are several components that must be incorporated into the program. These include:

- Compliance with regulatory agencies
- Safety program

- QA program
- Personnel training and assessment
- Technical support
- Data management

Compliance with Regulatory Guidelines

The primary law that regulates POCT is CLIA '88. This law describes the standards that must be met for all testing procedures used in diagnosing and treating human disease. To receive federal Medicare and Medicaid funds, laboratories must obtain a CLIA certificate granting permission to perform certain tests.

Safety Program

   Point-of-care testing programs must adhere to the same Occupational Safety and Health Administration (OSHA) and Centers for Disease Control and Prevention (CDC) safety guidelines and regulations that are required for other medical laboratories. Written safety rules that encompass Standard Precautions must be included in all procedure manuals and must be followed rigorously.

Quality Assessment Program

 A POCT program must be able to provide accurate, reliable test results. This is ensured by having a comprehensive quality assessment (QA) program in place. QA includes procedures that ensure the quality of the test procedure from beginning (test requisition) to end (interpretation and reporting of results). Instrument calibration, up-to-date standard operating procedure (SOP) manuals, testing of control sera or reagents, participation in a proficiency testing program, comprehensive documentation, and employee training and assessment are all part of a QA program. For many POC instruments and kits, the need for performing frequent controls is lessened because internal controls are included in the test systems. Laboratories that operate POCT sites must also ensure that the values obtained at the POCT sites are equivalent to the values obtained in the supervising laboratory.

Personnel Training and Assessment

Depending on the type of POCT program, personnel can be trained by the laboratory or by a technical representative of the instrument manufacturer. Testing personnel must be trained and their competence verified before they can be permitted to report patient test results. Periodic review and documentation of personnel performance is required. Participation in a proficiency testing program is one method of assessing performance.

CURRENT TOPIC

ESTABLISHING A POINT-OF-CARE TESTING PROGRAM

Enhancement of the quality of patient health care should be the primary consideration behind establishment of a POCT program. The Joint Commission (JC) has created National Patient Safety Goals to ensure POC patient safety. POCT programs are not beneficial if test results are not reliable and are not evaluated and acted upon quickly. The healthcare facility must maintain a high-quality program, meet all regulatory requirements, and adequately train and assess testing personnel.

POCT can be performed in the emergency department, operating room, critical care unit, patient hospital room, clinic or POL, or the patient's home (see diagram). Several factors must be incorporated into any successful testing program:

- Testing protocols should be *standardized* across all sites.
- Excellent *communication* is required among testing sites and with the central laboratory.
- All personnel involved should consider themselves to be on a *goal-oriented team*.

- There should be constant *program improvement*, including problem solving and incorporation of new methodologies.
- *Networking* with others in the field and with manufacturers' technical representatives is important.
- Keeping up with *current research* into trends, such as new QA methods, is vital.
- *Connectivity* is essential; this could include automatic documentation of data, electronic posting of POCT data into medical records, and integration of POCT results into overall patient care.
- *Data management* is facilitated using computers incorporated into many analyzers.
- Most of all, a *positive attitude* is required. POCT personnel must be willing to be cross-trained to perform laboratory work in addition to their other duties.

Each POCT site must be self-managed and responsible for its operation. A self-inspection worksheet is helpful for that. The overall responsibility for compliance lies with the individual site and its director.

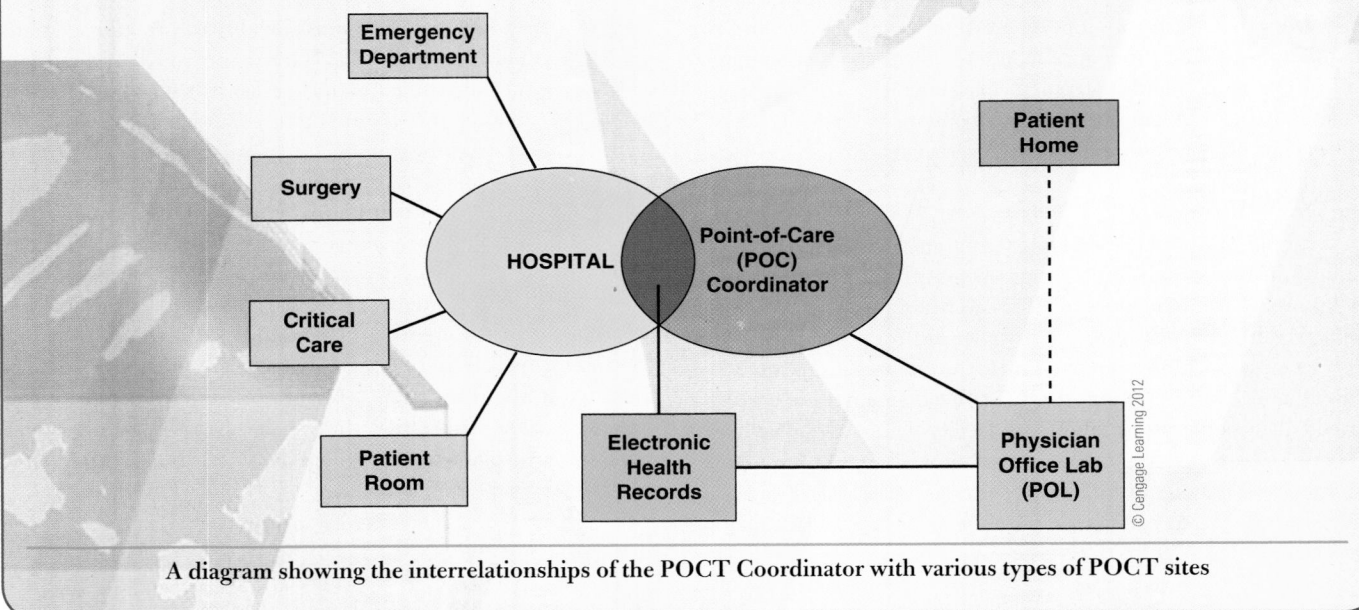

A diagram showing the interrelationships of the POCT Coordinator with various types of POCT sites

Technical Support

Laboratories administering POCT programs must either have a director on site or employ a qualified laboratory consultant. The consultant can provide technical assistance or request technical support from instrument manufacturers, usually through a hotline or local service representative.

Data Management

Data management at POCT sites can be simple or complex. In a POL, test results are usually written directly on the patient's chart, entered electronically into the patient's record, or an instrument printout is inserted into the chart. In a hospital POCT program, the data management system can be more sophisticated.

Testing personnel can use bar-coded identification badges to log in to an analyzer. In this way, only personnel who have proven competency in performing the procedure are permitted to operate the instrument. The analyzers can also be linked directly to the laboratory information system (LIS), with results transferred electronically to the laboratory as soon as they are generated.

ADVANTAGES AND DISADVANTAGES OF POINT-OF-CARE TESTING

Before the advent of widespread computer networks, the results of laboratory tests often were not available until the next day. Now, results of testing can be available within minutes when POCT is used.

POCT has advantages and disadvantages. At first glance the advantages seem to greatly outweigh the disadvantages. However, all factors must be considered; some points to consider are shown in Table 6-6.

Advantages of Point-of-Care Testing

Some benefits of POCT include rapid test results, less trauma to the patient, and reduced errors. These advantages benefit the patient and the physician, and can possibly reduce the need for hospitalization or the length of hospitalization.

Rapid Results

The immediate benefit of POCT is that laboratory test results can be obtained quickly, decreasing TAT. This benefits patients, healthcare workers, and the healthcare system (Table 6-6). Patients can receive required therapy more quickly, which can be especially important for critically ill patients. POCT programs in hospitals can lead to shorter hospital stays, owing to the rapid availability of test results. This has happened at the same time that we have experienced a major change in healthcare delivery, in which more diagnostic procedures are provided at point of care (POC) and test systems available for patient use in the home are on the increase. POC instruments are smaller and portable, making them well suited for the limited space in most POLs and also for use in near-patient testing.

Less Trauma-More Patient Participation

Another benefit of POCT is that these testing methods are less traumatic, requiring only a drop or two of capillary blood. Patients also feel a greater sense of participation in their own care, usually learning of the test results immediately, because the test is performed in their presence.

Multiskilled Personnel

An additional benefit of POCT is that diverse groups of health-care workers can be trained to perform the tests. This is possible because many rapid test kits are simple to use, and POC analyzers are easy to operate and have low maintenance requirements. For

TABLE 6-6. Advantages and disadvantages of point-of-care testing programs

ADVANTAGES OF POC	DISADVANTAGES OF POC
Improved TAT of test results	Increased personnel costs
Increased patient participation in health care	Duplication of costs for standards and controls
Less traumatic specimen collection	Duplication of instruments
Smaller specimen required	Potential for insufficient personnel training
Shorter hospital stays	Repeat tests require repeat capillary collection
Patients receive rapid intervention and/or treatment	Single testing less efficient than automated testing
Improved cooperation and communication among health care team members	Increased cost of single-use test materials
Reduced errors	Inadequate supervision of testing personnel
Reduced need for specimen transport	

instance, in the physician office laboratory (POL), the medical assistant is often trained to perform laboratory tests such as glucose and cholesterol measurements and urine chemical analysis. This is in addition to their regular duties of measuring blood pressure, pulse, temperature and weight and otherwise assisting the physician as needed.

Reduced Errors

The potential for certain errors is decreased in POCT. For example, pre-analytical errors such as sample mis-identification or mishandling, and post-analytical errors such as transcription errors, are reduced.

Improved Communication

Point-of-care testing provides opportunities for increased communication and cooperation among the laboratory staff, nursing staff, and patients, enhancing the overall quality of care.

Disadvantages of POCT

POCT does have some disadvantages. These disadvantages can be attributed to factors such as increased costs, deficiencies in personnel training, failure to adhere to guidelines for quality assessment, and inadequate supervision from the central laboratory (Table 6-6).

Increased Costs

Several POCT components are more costly than tests run in a central laboratory. Duplication of instruments is required because instruments must be placed in several sites. Duplication of control reagents is also required. Because many more individuals will be performing the tests, increased time is required to train personnel. Although POCT instruments are relatively low cost, the single-use test units and cartridges can be expensive.

Deficiencies in Personnel Training

Training of POCT personnel must be consistent; the best scenario is to have one or two coordinators in the central laboratory who are responsible for training all POC testing personnel. This ensures that all testing personnel are trained in the same manner. When a central laboratory is responsible for training personnel at remote sites, or when there is rapid personnel turnover, there is potential for training deficiencies.

Inadequate Quality Assessment Programs

POCT sites are required to have an adequate QA program in place. It is important that careful records are kept of all control and standard results. Absent or incomplete records can indicate that QA is insufficient or not a priority. Problems in this area can be due to laxity of the testing personnel and/or insufficient coordination with the central laboratory.

Inadequate Supervision

The central laboratory POCT coordinator must have good management and communication skills and a strong background in QA. In addition, they must be trained in instrument use by manufacturers' representatives so they are able to troubleshoot problems. All of these characteristics are required to adequately coordinate and supervise the various POCT sites. A breakdown in any of these areas can cause a decline in the quality of results.

CRITICAL THINKING

Community Hospital laboratory has decided to develop several POCT sites both inside and outside the hospital. The plan calls for establishing active POCT programs in the hospital emergency department and intensive care units and in one site in a free clinic. All sites would be supplied with the same instruments and perform the same menu of tests. The laboratory manager has designated an educator in the laboratory to train all employees for the new POCT sites in the operation and maintenance of the instruments. However, the physician at the free clinic also wants to be trained so that he can train personnel who perform the testing at his site.

Explain why it is preferable for the same person to train all employees.

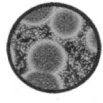

SUMMARY

POCT has become fully integrated into our healthcare system. Although POCT is not the answer for all situations, it is an important component of health care. Careful studies must be done to determine if a POCT program should be implemented and what the scope of the program should be. Improved patient care should be the most important goal. POCT programs must be constantly monitored to ensure they are achieving their goal and that test results are of the highest quality.

Many test procedures have been adapted to POCT use (Table 6-7). Some provide important data useful in acute care facilities, such as electrolyte analysis, activated clotting time assay, and assays for heart attack assessment. Others are more useful in health-screening situations or physician offices. These include hemoglobin, hematocrit, cholesterol, urine dipstick, rapid group A strep tests, pregnancy tests, prothrombin time, and fecal occult blood tests.

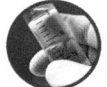

REVIEW QUESTIONS

1. What are four advantages of a POCT program?

2. What are four disadvantages of a POCT program?

3. Name five departments that have decision-making responsibility or otherwise participate in POCT programs.

4. What technological developments have made POCT possible?

5. How do hospital POCT programs differ from nonhospital programs?

6. What are the requirements for a test to be CLIA-waived?

7. What documents must be on file for CLIA-waived tests?

8. Name two hematological tests often performed at point of care.

TABLE 6-7. Tests commonly performed at point-of-care testing sites

Hematology tests
  Hemoglobin
  Hematocrit
Coagulation tests
  Activated clotting time
  Prothrombin time
  Activated partial thromboplastin time
  D-Dimer
Chemistry tests
  Cholesterol
  Electrolytes
  Blood glucose
  Cardiac panel
  Fecal occult blood
  Creatinine
  Hemoglobin A1c
Urine tests
  Urine dipstick
  Pregnancy test (human chorionic
    gonadotropin [hCG])
  Microalbumin
Microbiology/Immunology tests
  Rapid test for group A strep
  Infectious mononucleosis
  Human immunodeficiency virus (HIV)
  Influenza
  Helicobacter pylori

9. Name four chemistry tests often performed at point of care.
10. Discuss the importance of quality assessment in POCT programs.
11. Why is it important for one department to be responsible for training all POCT technicians?
12. What is the primary law that regulates POCT?
13. What safety precautions must be observed when performing POCT?

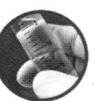 **STUDENT ACTIVITIES**

1. Complete the written examination for this lesson.
2. Inquire about a POCT program in a hospital near you. Find out what tests are performed, who performs them, and how QA is accomplished.
3. Find POCT programs that are in place in your community and comment on the benefits they provide.

 # WEB ACTIVITY

Select two tests from Table 6-7. For each test, use the Internet to find information about a test kit or small analyzer that would be appropriate for use at POC. Report on the test method, its level of complexity (CLIA-waived or not), specimen required, TAT, and reliability of results.

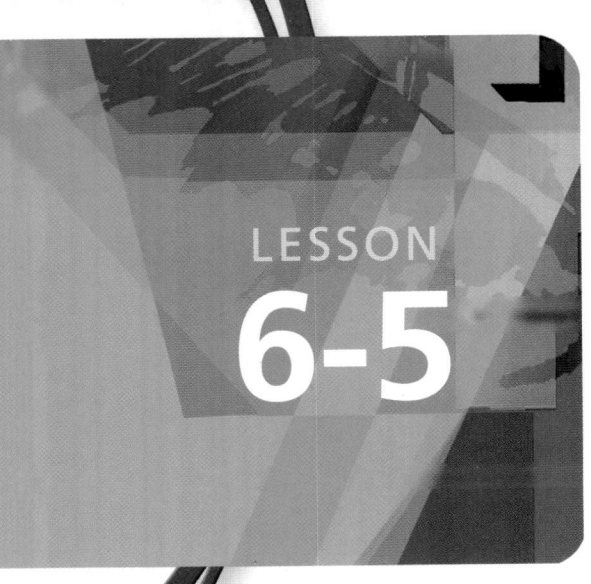

LESSON 6-5

Blood Glucose and Hemoglobin A1c

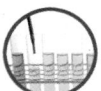

LESSON OBJECTIVES

After studying this lesson, the student will:

- ⊙ Explain the function of glucose in the body.
- ⊙ Explain how blood glucose levels are regulated.
- ⊙ Name two disorders of glucose metabolism.
- ⊙ Name four criteria that can be used for diagnosing diabetes mellitus.
- ⊙ Explain the purpose of a postprandial glucose test.
- ⊙ Describe how a glucose tolerance test is performed.
- ⊙ State the reference values for fasting blood glucose, 2-hour postprandial glucose, and glucose tolerance tests.
- ⊙ Explain the collection requirements for blood glucose specimens.
- ⊙ Explain three principles of glucose test methods.
- ⊙ Perform a blood glucose measurement using a glucose analyzer.
- ⊙ Explain the relationship of hemoglobin A1c (HbA1c) to blood glucose.
- ⊙ Discuss the importance of measuring HbA1c.
- ⊙ Perform a test for HbA1c.
- ⊙ Discuss safety precautions that must be observed when performing tests for glucose and HbA1c.
- ⊙ Discuss the importance of quality assessment programs for glucose and HbA1c testing.
- ⊙ Define the glossary terms.

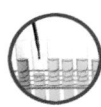

GLOSSARY

alpha cell / a type of cell in the islets of Langerhans that makes and secretes glucagon

beta cell / a type of cell in the islets of Langerhans that makes and secretes proinsulin and insulin

cellular respiration / the series of cellular metabolic processes in which organic substances are oxidized and energy in the form of ATP is released

chromogen / a substance that becomes colored when it undergoes a chemical change

diabetes mellitus / a disorder of carbohydrate metabolism characterized by a state of hyperglycemia resulting from insulin deficiency

glucagon / the pancreatic hormone that increases blood glucose concentration by promoting the conversion of glycogen to glucose

gluconeogenesis / production of glucose from noncarbohydrate sources

(continues)

640

glucose dehydrogenase / an enzyme that converts glucose to gluconolactone and that is used in glucose analytical methods

glucose oxidase / an enzyme that converts glucose to gluconic acid and that is used in glucose analytical methods

glycated hemoglobin (GHb) / see hemoglobin A1c

glycogen / the storage form of glucose found in high concentration in the liver

glycogenesis / conversion of glucose to glycogen

glycogenolysis / the conversion of glycogen to glucose

glycolysis / energy production as a result of the metabolic breakdown of glucose; the breakdown of glucose to pyruvic acid or lactic acid accompanied by the release of energy in the form of ATP

hemoglobin A1c (HbA1c) / hemoglobin modified by the binding of glucose to the beta globin chains of hemoglobin; also called glycated or glycosylated hemoglobin

hexokinase / an enzyme that converts glucose to glucose-6-phosphate and that is used in glucose analytical methods

hyperglycemia / blood glucose concentration above normal

hypoglycemia / blood glucose concentration below normal

insulin / the pancreatic hormone essential for proper metabolism of blood glucose and maintenance of blood glucose levels

islets of Langerhans / irregular-shaped clusters of cells scattered throughout the pancreas that contain alpha cells, beta cells, delta cells, and pancreatic polypeptide (PP) secreting cells

oral glucose tolerance test (OGTT)/ analysis of blood glucose at timed intervals following ingestion of a standard glucose dose

peroxidase / an enzyme that converts hydrogen peroxide to water and oxygen

postprandial / after eating

proinsulin / a precursor of insulin

INTRODUCTION

Glucose, the major carbohydrate in blood, is also the major source of energy for the body's cells. Measurement of blood glucose is one of the most frequently performed clinical chemistry tests.

The most common disorder of glucose metabolism is **diabetes mellitus**, a disease in which the blood glucose is elevated because of lack of insulin regulation. The state of having elevated blood glucose is called **hyperglycemia**. Decreased blood glucose, or **hypoglycemia**, is a less common disorder of glucose metabolism and has several causes, some transient and some pathological.

The glucose test is most often used to aid in diagnosing and managing diabetes, or in managing hypoglycemia. This lesson presents information about glucose metabolism, diagnosis and management of diabetes, and methods of glucose analysis.

GLUCOSE METABOLISM

After a meal, carbohydrates are rapidly converted to sugars that enter the blood stream through the small intestine. The rising blood glucose levels trigger a release of **insulin by beta (ß) cells** in the pancreas. Insulin is a hormone that promotes cellular uptake of glucose through special membrane transport molecules. Most body cells have insulin receptors on their surfaces that bind insulin and allow glucose to enter the cells.

Once inside the cells, the energy-rich glucose is used in the process of **cellular respiration**. During cellular respiration, the energy in glucose is captured and stored in adenosine tri-phosphate (ATP) molecules. **Glycolysis** is the first stage of the three-stage process of cellular respiration. Two molecules of energy-rich ATP are formed from each glucose molecule during glycolysis. Thirty-six more ATP molecules are formed in the second and third stages of cellular respiration.

Certain cells have higher energy needs than others. Muscle cells process glucose at high rates, particularly during periods of exercise. Some tissues can obtain energy from fat or protein in addition to carbohydrates, but brain cells and red blood cells require glucose for energy.

When we take in more food than needed to meet our energy requirements, we convert the extra glucose to **glycogen** which is stored primarily in the liver to be available for later use. This process is called **glycogenesis**. If we did not have energy storage systems, we would have to eat constantly to have enough energy for normal functioning of our body organs. When blood glucose is low, stored glycogen is converted to glucose in a process called **glycogenolysis** and released into the blood. Glucose can also be made from sources other than carbohydrates and glycogen, a process called **gluconeogenesis**.

BLOOD GLUCOSE REGULATION

Although the body has many metabolic pathways that utilize glucose, several hormones work together to keep blood glucose within a fairly narrow range. The maintenance of steady levels of glucose in the body is a necessary and integral part of homeostasis and helps provide a constant environment to the body's cells.

Insulin

The **islets of Langerhans**, part of the pancreas, contain five different cell types, each with its own function. The beta cells of the islets produce **proinsulin** (the inactive form of insulin) and insulin that is secreted by the pancreas. Insulin *lowers* blood glucose by increasing cellular uptake of glucose and increasing the rate of glycolysis. Insulin also increases the rate of conversion of glucose to glycogen.

The blood glucose level, which is due primarily to the amount of carbohydrate in the diet, provides the major signal to cells to produce insulin. In the presence of insulin, cells take up glucose from the circulation, the formation of glycogen from glucose is promoted, and some cells are stimulated to take in and store lipids.

Glucagon and Other Hormones

Hormones such as growth hormone, epinephrine, somatostatin, cortisol, and **glucagon** act in a variety of ways to *increase* blood glucose concentration. These hormones are sometimes called insulin antagonists, because their action is opposite to the action of insulin. Of these insulin antagonists, glucagon has the greatest effect. Glucagon is produced by **alpha cells** in the islets of Langerhans. When blood glucose levels become low, the release of glucagon is stimulated. Glucagon acts by increasing the conversion of glycogen stores to glucose. Together, insulin and glucagon are major hormones that maintain blood glucose concentrations in the normal range.

Hyperglycemia

Diabetes is a chronic, serious disease caused by the body's failure to produce sufficient insulin or to use insulin properly. In the absence of insulin, cells do not take up glucose, and blood glucose levels rise. When insulin is absent or insufficient, as in diabetic patients, the body's cells become starved for fuel even in the presence of a high blood glucose level. These metabolic actions explain one of the symptoms of the onset of diabetes, which is weight loss.

Hypoglycemia

Hypoglycemia, or low blood glucose, occurs most commonly in diabetic patients as a result of overmedication with insulin or other antidiabetic medications. Hypoglycemia in non-diabetic individuals is not common. It can be caused by temporary conditions such as excessive alcohol consumption, missed meals, or fasting. Hypoglycemia can also be due to endocrine disorders or critical illnesses such as cancer or severe liver disease. *Reactive hypoglycemia* is a condition in which the insulin-releasing cells of the pancreas overreact following ingestion of a meal. Too much insulin is released, causing a hypoglycemic event 4 to 6 hours after eating.

DIAGNOSTIC TESTS FOR DIABETES AND HYPOGLYCEMIA

Tests that are used to aid in diagnosis of diabetes or hypoglycemia include the fasting blood glucose, oral glucose tolerance test (OGTT), the 2-hour post-prandial glucose test, and the hemoglobin A1c test.

Fasting Blood Glucose

A fasting blood glucose is performed on a blood sample taken when the patient has not eaten or taken in calories for 8 hours or longer. The fasting specimen is usually obtained before the patient eats breakfast. The fasting glucose can be performed from a fingerstick, and the results can be obtained while the patient is still in the physician's office. The speed of analysis and the relatively low cost of the test make it the diabetes screening test of choice. The American Diabetes Association (ADA) recommends the fasting glucose value as one criterion to be used in the diagnosis of diabetes (Table 6-8).

Oral Glucose Tolerance Test

The 3-hour **oral glucose tolerance test (OGTT)** was used for years to diagnose diabetes mellitus in patients with elevated fasting glucose as well to diagnose hypoglycemia.

For the OGTT, a fasting blood glucose sample was drawn and tested and a urine sample was obtained. Next the patient consumed a beverage containing a standard glucose dose (usually 50 or 75 g). Blood and urine samples were subsequently collected at set intervals, typically 30 minutes and 1, 2, and 3 hours. Glucose was measured in the blood samples, and urine glucose was estimated using a urine glucose reagent strip.

The 3-hour OGTT is no longer recommended for use in diagnosing hypoglycemia because the test can trigger an adverse hypoglycemic event. The 3-hour OGTT is also no longer recommended for use in diagnosing diabetes. However, the OGTT, or a modification of it, can be used to obtain a more complete picture

TABLE 6-8. Criteria for diagnosing diabetes mellitus (From the 2010 American Diabetes Association Position Statement: Diagnosis and Classification of Diabetes Mellitus)

Diagnosis of diabetes/hyperglycemia can be made in any one of the following results:		
HbA1c	≥6.5%	Using standardized and certified method*
Fasting plasma glucose	≥126 mg/dL	Following 8 hour (or longer) fast*
2-hour plasma glucose	≥200 mg/dL	During OGTT using 75 g glucose dose*
Random plasma glucose	≥200 mg/dL	In patient with hyperglycemic symptoms

* In the absence of unequivocal hyperglycemia, results of criteria 1–3 should be confirmed by repeat testing.

of glucose metabolism in pregnant women who have higher than normal fasting glucose levels and are at risk for *gestational diabetes*. The OGTT is expensive and time-consuming, and some patients do not tolerate the glucose beverage. All patients undergoing OGTT should be monitored carefully for adverse reactions.

Two-Hour Postprandial Glucose

ADA guidelines recommend modifying the glucose tolerance test and using just the fasting blood glucose and 2-hour **postprandial** (after eating) blood glucose measurement for diagnosis of diabetes. Postprandial tests are most reliable if the patient is tested following a standard glucose dose (50 or 75 g) rather than a random meal. This is also called the 2-hour OGTT. *When a fasting glucose level is 126 mg/dL or higher, a patient should not be given the glucose dose and the physician should be consulted.*

Hemoglobin A1c

Hemoglobin (Hb) is present in all red blood cells and is the molecule that transports oxygen from the lungs to the tissues. The major hemoglobin in adults is Hb A. Glucose is absorbed from the gastrointestinal tract, enters the circulation, and is taken up by body cells for energy. Within the red blood cells, glucose molecules bind to hemoglobin, forming **hemoglobin A1c (HbA1c)**, which can be easily measured.

The amount of HbA1c is related to the amount of glucose in the blood over time. In hyperglycemic states, the amount of glucose binding to hemoglobin increases. The half-life of red blood cells is approximately 60 days, therefore, the level of HbA1c reflects the average amount of glucose in the blood for that period of time. In reality the HbA1c more closely represents average glucose levels over the 3 to 4 weeks before the HbA1c test is performed. (The HbA1c may not be of use in individuals who have hemolytic disease. The test will not represent glucose levels over time because of the shortened life span of their red blood cells.)

The fasting glucose level indicates the glucose level at the specific time the specimen is collected. The HbA1c value indicates the average blood glucose levels over a period of weeks. The HbA1c test is now recognized as a reliable method for diagnosing diabetes.

GLUCOSE REFERENCE VALUES

The blood glucose reference range is the laboratory's acceptable range of glucose values obtained from statistical analysis of glucose values in the general population (Table 6-9). This reference range is shown on a facility's laboratory report form. Reference ranges can differ slightly from laboratory to laboratory, depending on the type of specimen analyzed and method of analysis. Serum glucose reference values can be as much as 5% higher than plasma glucose reference values, and plasma glucose reference values are higher than whole blood glucose reference values.

CURRENT TOPICS

DIABETES MELLITUS

Diabetes mellitus, commonly called diabetes, is a serious, chronic disease in which the body either produces insufficient insulin or is unable to use insulin properly. The insulin hormone enables the body to convert carbohydrate into energy by unlocking cells to allow glucose to enter and become fuel for the cells. When glucose cannot be used by cells, it accumulates in the blood, causing a condition called hyperglycemia. When allowed to continue over the long-term, hyperglycemia causes damage to blood vessels, tissues, and organs.

Type 1 diabetes results from insufficient insulin or lack of insulin; onset usually occurs during childhood or young adulthood. Type 2 diabetes results when the body fails to properly use insulin and usually has onset later in life, although an increased incidence in adolescents is now being seen. This condition is known as *insulin resistance.* Two additional conditions are *gestational diabetes* and *prediabetes.* Gestational diabetes occurs in about 4% of pregnant women. Prediabetes is the condition in which the blood glucose is above

normal but still below the level of being considered diabetic.

The incidence of diabetes in the United States is increasing at an alarming rate. The 2011 National Diabetes Fact Sheet compiled by the Centers for Disease Control and Prevention (CDC), National Institutes of Health (NIH), ADA, and other organizations estimates that at the end of 2010, 18.8 million people in the United States had been diagnosed with diabetes, approximately 7 million were estimated to have diabetes but not be aware of it, and approximately 79 million were estimated to have prediabetes. These numbers are significantly increased over 2008 estimates. People in the undiagnosed group can have diabetes for up to 10 years without being aware of it until they suffer its complications.

Diabetes causes damage to small blood vessels resulting in problems in the kidneys, the eyes, and extremities such as feet and toes and is a major cause of cardiovascular disease. Early diagnosis is crucial because good management of diabetes can lessen, postpone, prevent, and in some cases even reverse many of these complications.

TABLE 6-9. Glucose reference values*

TEST	GLUCOSE CONCENTRATION	
	mg/dL	mmol/L (SI)
Fasting		
Serum	70–110	3.9–6.1
Whole blood	60–100	3.3–5.6
Plasma	66–105	3.7–5.9
Two-hour postprandial (serum)	≤110	≤6.1
Oral glucose tolerance (serum)		
Fasting	70–110	3.9–6.1
1 hour	20–50 above fasting	1.1–2.8 above fasting
2 hour	5–25 above fasting	0.3–1.4 above fasting
3 hour	Fasting level or below	Fasting level or below

* Values vary slightly among laboratories depending on test method used

TABLE 6-10. Relationship between hemoglobin A1c percentages and average blood glucose values

HEMOGLOBIN A1c (%)	AVERAGE WHOLE BLOOD GLUCOSE (mg/dL)	AVERAGE PLASMA GLUCOSE (mg/dL)	INTERPRETATION
4	61	65	Normal (nondiabetic) range = 4%–5%
5	92	100	
6	124	135	
7	156	170	Target for good diabetes control is 7% or less
8	188	205	Action is required for levels between 8% and 12%
9	219	240	
10	251	275	
11	283	310	
12	314	345	

Venous and capillary glucose levels are about the same in a fasting individual. Reference glucose values are given in Table 6-9.

Fasting Glucose

The reference (normal) fasting blood glucose value for serum in an adult is 70 to 110 mg/dL (Table 6-9). Neonates have lower blood glucose levels because they have less glycogen stored. Plasma and whole blood glucose reference ranges are slightly lower than serum reference ranges. The ADA has recommended that fasting plasma glucose (FPG) values of 126 mg/dL or greater be interpreted as indicating hyperglycemia.

Oral Glucose Tolerance Test

A person with normal glucose metabolism should have a fasting serum glucose level of 70 to 110 mg/dL, a 1-hour level of 90 to 160 mg/dL, a 2-hour level less than 140 mg/dL, and a 3-hour level at or below the fasting level (Table 6-9).

Two-Hour Postprandial

The 2-hour postprandial serum glucose value is normally less than 140 mg/dL. A 2-hour plasma glucose of 200 mg/dL or greater is one criterion for the diagnosis of diabetes.

Hemoglobin A1c

A nondiabetic should have a HbA1c value of 4% to 5%, which represents average plasma glucose values between approximately 65 and 100 mg/dL (Table 6-10). A diagnosis of dia-

betes should be considered when HbA1c values are 6.5% or greater.

Critical Glucose Values

In the clinical laboratory, test results that are extremely high or low are called *critical values, alert values, panic values,* or *action values,* meaning immediate action is required by laboratory staff to alert physicians and/or nursing staff of the test results. Every laboratory must establish its own list of critical values for various tests and a written procedure to follow when a test result falls into this category.

Critical glucose values can differ slightly depending on whether the patient is newborn, less than 1 year old, a child or adult. In general, a patient is considered to be hypoglycemic if the glucose falls below 50 mg/dL and a glucose level of 40 mg/dL or less is considered a critical value. Hypoglycemic patients can experience fainting, weakness, confusion, lack of coordination or seizures, and can lapse into unconsciousness if left untreated (Table 6-11). Hypoglycemia requires treatment to increase the blood glucose value, such as giving the patient a glucose gel or fruit juice (if conscious) or a glucagon injection or intravenous glucose if unconscious.

An extremely high glucose level can lead to diabetic coma and requires immediate treatment to reduce the glucose level. Blood glucose exceeding 400 mg/dL is considered dangerously high. Symptoms of extreme hyperglycemia include confusion, lethargy, extreme thirst, weak pulse, dry skin, and nausea (Table 6-11).

TABLE 6-11. Critical glucose values and symptoms that can accompany them

HYPOGLYCEMIA* ≤40 mg/dL	HYPERGLYCEMIA* ≥40 mg/dL
Faintness	Confusion
Weakness	Coma
Hunger	Nausea
Diaphoresis (sweating)	Intense thirst
Visual disturbances	Ketoacidosis
Palsy	Dry flushed skin
Confusion	Weak pulse
Seizures	
Personality changes	

* Note: Patient may not experience all symptoms.

RECOMMENDED BLOOD GLUCOSE LEVELS

Recommended blood glucose values differ from blood glucose reference ranges. Recommended values are the *ideal* glucose levels recommended by organizations such as the ADA and are used in the differential diagnosis of diabetes (Table 6-8). The recommended glucose value has changed significantly in recent years. The 2010 ADA recommendations for diagnosing diabetes/hyperglycemia are that:

- Patients with a fasting plasma glucose (FPG) less than 100 mg/dL be considered *nondiabetic*
- Patients with FPG between 100 mg/dL and 125 mg/dL be considered *prediabetic* as a result of *impaired fasting glucose* (IFG) and
- Patients with FPG ≥126 mg/dL be considered *hyperglycemic*

DIABETES MANAGEMENT

Good diabetes management is important for preventing complications of diabetes caused by microvascular damage.

Home Glucose Meters

Blood glucose meters for patient use at home were first introduced in the 1970s. Since then, meter accuracy, precision, and ease of use have greatly improved. It is recommended that all diabetic patients use a home glucose monitoring system regularly.

Hemoglobin A1c

The ability of the patient to keep blood glucose levels within acceptable ranges can be assessed by periodic measurement of hemoglobin A1c (HbA1c). It is recommended that the HbA1c in patients with diabetes be measured every 3 or 6 months. HbA1c at or below 7% indicates adequate glucose control.

Recent studies have also shown that HbA1c is the single best test for evaluating the risk for damage to nerves and to the small blood vessels of the eyes and kidneys. This microvascular damage leads to the complications of diabetes, such as blindness and kidney failure. Clinical trials have shown that reducing the HbA1c level in diabetics and maintaining it below 7% will prevent the development of, or further progression of, complications from diabetes (Table 6-10).

PRINCIPLES OF GLUCOSE ANALYSIS

Glucose analysis methods use the enzymes **glucose oxidase**, **hexokinase**, or **glucose dehydrogenase**. These enzyme tests are simple, quick, and specific for glucose and have been adapted for use in many types of glucose analyzers, both large and small. In general, tests that use hexokinase or glucose dehydrogenase are more specific and have fewer interferences than those using glucose oxidase.

Glucose Oxidase Method

The glucose oxidase method of analysis is a two-step reaction. Glucose is converted to gluconic acid and hydrogen peroxide (H_2O_2) in the presence of glucose oxidase and oxygen. The resulting concentrations of gluconic acid and H_2O_2 are proportional to the amount of glucose originally present. In the second part of the reaction, in the presence of the **peroxidase** enzyme and a **chromogen**, the H_2O_2 is converted to water (H_2O) and the chromogen produces a color:

$$(1)\ Glucose + H_2O + O_2 \xrightarrow{\text{Glucose Oxidase}} Gluconic\ acid + H_2O_2$$
$$(2)\ H_2O_2 + Chromogen \xrightarrow{\text{Peroxidase}} 2H_2O + Color\ formation$$

The color intensity is proportional to the amount of H_2O_2 (and thus the amount of glucose) and can be measured using photometry.

Hexokinase Method

The hexokinase method is also a two-step reaction. This method has advantages over the glucose oxidase method, primarily because fewer substances interfere and safer reagents are used. In the first step, hexokinase forms glucose-6-phosphate (G6P) from glucose. In the second step, G6P is converted to 6-phosphogluconate (6PG) by the enzyme glucose-6-phosphate dehydrogenase (G6PD) with the production of NADPH:

$$(1)\ Glucose + ATP \xrightarrow{\text{Hexokinase}} G6P + ADP$$
$$(2)\ G6P + NADP \xrightarrow{\text{G6PD}} 6PG + NADPH$$

NADPH absorbs ultraviolet light at 340 nm. This absorbance can be measured using a spectrophotometer. The increase in absorbance due to NADPH in the solution is proportional to the glucose concentration in the original reaction.

Glucose Dehydrogenase Method

Both the HemoCue and ACCU-CHEK meters use the enzyme glucose dehydrogenase (GDH) to convert glucose to gluconolactone. However, the meters use different detection methods. The glucose dehydrogenase method has few interferences.

PERFORMING BLOOD GLUCOSE AND HBA1c MEASUREMENTS

Tests for blood glucose and HbA1c are frequently performed in the clinical laboratory as well as at POC. The facility's standard operating procedure (SOP) manual, package inserts, and manufacturer's instruction manual will contain detailed information for the test procedures, including specimen collection, test performance, and required quality control checks.

Safety Precautions

  Standard Precautions must be followed when performing blood glucose and HbA1c measurements. Appropriate personal protective equipment (PPE) must be worn when obtaining the blood specimens and performing the tests. All used test materials must be discarded into appropriate biohazard containers.

Quality Assessment

   The manufacturer's instructions must be followed for the particular analyzer used. Test materials such as reagent strips or cuvettes that are made for a particular instrument must be used only with that instrument and must not be used beyond their expiration dates.

Instrument performance is checked using calibrators and controls from the instrument manufacturer. These checks must be performed following the schedule specified in the SOP manual. Control results must be recorded, charted on the QC charts, and compared to the acceptable ranges. Control results must be acceptable before patient samples are tested and results reported.

Specimen Collection

Glucose can be measured in whole blood, plasma, or serum. The laboratory requisition will specify whether the specimen can be random or must be a fasting or other special specimen. Blood cells metabolize glucose and can rapidly lower the specimen's glucose concentration, causing a false low glucose value. Therefore, serum or plasma must be separated from the blood cells as soon as possible after collection. If separation will be delayed, blood can be collected in gray-topped tubes containing a glycolytic inhibitor.

If whole blood glucose is to be measured, the test should be performed immediately following capillary puncture or on blood collected in a suitable anticoagulant, such as ethylenediaminetetraacetic acid (EDTA) or heparin. The anticoagulant must be one that will not interfere with the glucose analysis method being used.

HbA1c methods use whole blood specimens obtained either from a fingerstick or from venous blood collected in appropriate anticoagulant. The patient does not need to be fasting.

Glucose Analyzers

Glucose meters are simple to use, give rapid results, and are appropriate for point-of-care testing (POCT), the physician office laboratory (POL), and home use. Measurement of glucose using a glucose meter is usually a CLIA-waived method. Chemistry analyzers used in larger laboratories measure glucose as well as several other analytes. Most instruments that measure glucose use either photometry or electrochemical principles to measure the end product of the test (Lesson 6-2).

Photometry

The HemoCue Glucose 201 Analyzer is an example of a CLIA-waived analyzer that uses photometry to measure blood glucose (Figure 6-17). The system includes a handheld analyzer and disposable clear microcuvettes that contain the glucose enzyme reagent. The self-filling microcuvette automatically draws up 5 µL of blood from a capillary puncture into the cuvette; the cuvette is then inserted into the analyzer. The plasma equivalent glucose concentration is displayed in milligrams per deciliter (mg/dL) or millimoles per liter (mmol/L) within 45 to 240 seconds. This system is ideal for POLs and POCT because of its calibration stability and the minimal operator training required. Data management programs are available with the HemoCue.

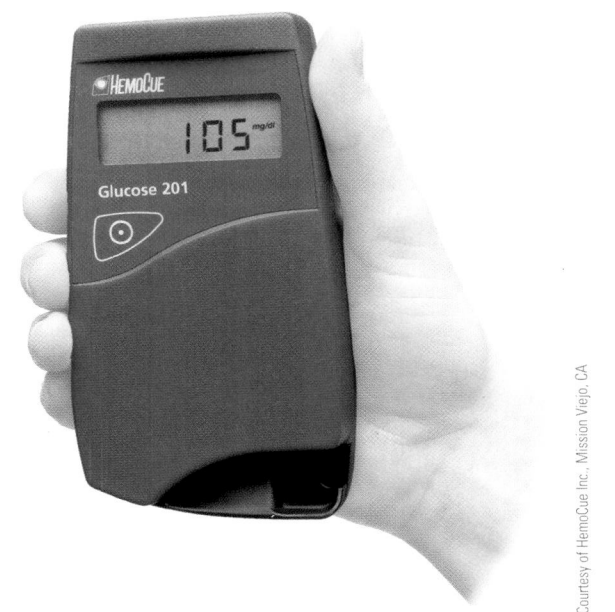

Courtesy of HemoCue Inc., Mission Viejo, CA

FIGURE 6-17 HemoCue Glucose 201 Analyzer

Electrochemical Technology/Amperometry

Electrochemical technology, or amperometry, uses electrodes to detect current (electrons) generated during a chemical reaction. Several glucose meters, including the ACCU-CHEK family of meters (Roche Diagnostics), FreeStyle meters (Abbott Laboratories), and Paradigm Link glucose meter (Medtronic), shown in Figure 6-18A, use this technology. A biosensor strip is inserted into the meter, and a small capillary blood sample is applied to the strip. The glucose dehydrogenase (GDH) enzyme within the strip reacts with glucose in the blood specimen to form gluconolactone, causing a proportional release of electrons. The electrode sensor in the meter detects voltage changes resulting from the electron release, and converts this electrical signal into glucose concentration, which is displayed on the meter screen.

Several glucose meters are designed for home use. Others, such as the ACCU-CHEK Inform, are designed for POCT and can interface with hospital or laboratory information systems, allowing storage and retrieval of patient and quality control (QC) data (Figure 6-18B).

HbA1c Analyzers

Several instruments can quickly measure HbA1c, also called **glycated hemoglobin (GHb)**; many of these methods are CLIA-waived. Most HbA1c analyzers use either immunoassay or chromatography methods. Some home glucose meters calculate HbA1c from the average of the glucose values in memory. Examples of analyzers that can measure HbA1c are the Siemens DCA Vantage Analyzer and the Bayer A1cNow System (Figure 6-19).

The A1cNow measures the HbA1c in less than 5 minutes using just 5 µL of capillary or venous blood. The method is CLIA-waived, certified by the National Glycohemoglobin Standardization Program, and can be performed at home or in POC settings. The DCA Vantage Analyzer uses monoclonal antibody to analyze whole blood samples for HbA1c. Blood is collected from a capillary puncture into a capillary holder supplied with the analyzer. The sample-filled holder is inserted into the reagent cartridge. The analyzer's calibration is verified by sliding the reagent cartridge through the slot and past the integral bar-code reader. The reagent cartridge containing the specimen is then inserted into the instrument. A pull-tab on the cartridge is removed to release buffer into the patient sample, and the analysis is initiated when the instrument door is closed. Results are available within 5 minutes and are displayed on the analyzer. The DCA Vantage can also analyze urine specimens for microalbumin, creatinine, and albumin/creatinine ratio using the appropriate cartridges.

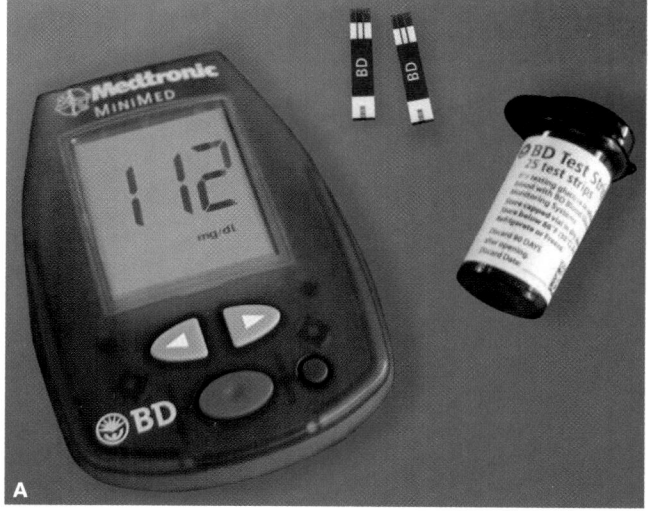

A

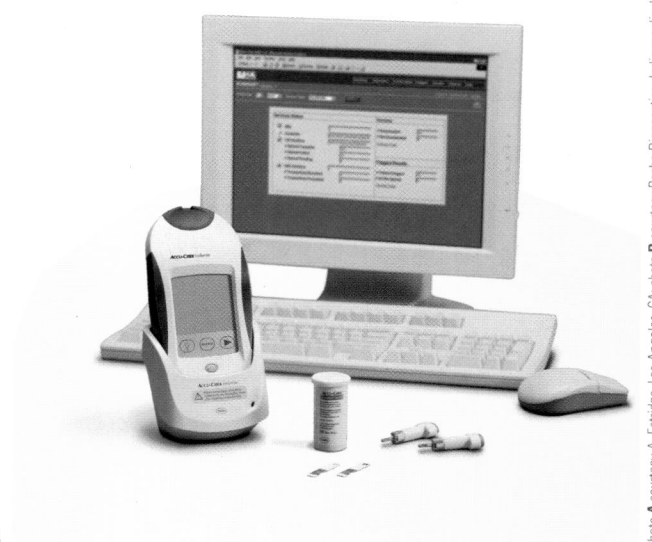

B

*Photo **A** courtesy A. Estridge, Los Angeles, CA; photo **B** courtesy Roche Diagnostics, Indianapolis, IN*

FIGURE 6-18 Glucose monitoring systems: (A) Medtronic Paradigm Link glucose meter; (B) Accu-Chek Inform glucose system can interface with laboratory information systems

---

SAFETY REMINDERS

- Review Safety Precautions section before beginning procedure.
- Observe Standard Precautions.
- Clean and disinfect instruments before returning to storage.
- Discard all used supplies appropriately.

PROCEDURAL REMINDERS

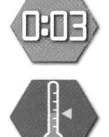

- Review Quality Assessment section before beginning procedure.
- Follow SOP manual and manufacturers' directions.
- Use appropriate controls and calibrators.
- Record control results on QC charts.
- Use specimen appropriate for the test method.
- Do not use reagents and supplies past the expiration dates.

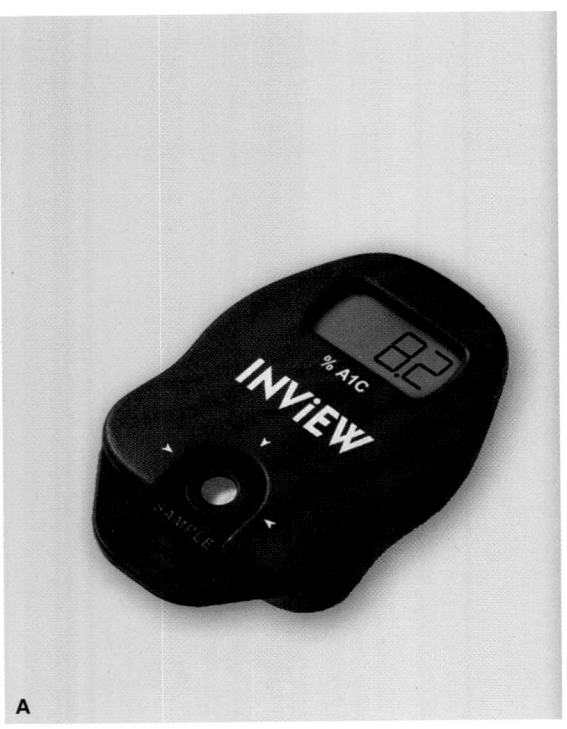
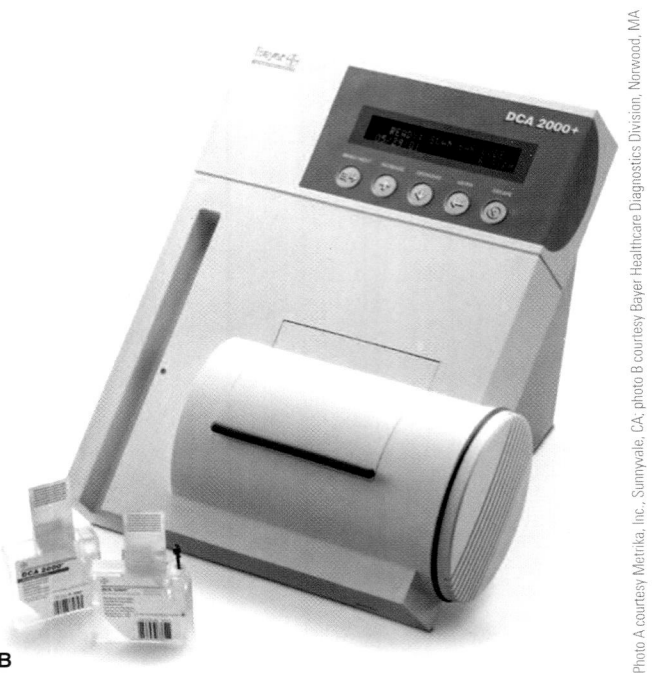

A

B

Photo A courtesy Metrika, Inc., Sunnyvale, CA, photo B courtesy Bayer Healthcare Diagnostics Division, Norwood, MA

FIGURE 6-19 Hemoglobin A1c analyzers: (A) Metrika hemoglobin A1c meter; (B) DCA Analyzer

CASE STUDY 1

José has had insulin-dependent diabetes for 12 years. His physician measures his HbA1c every 3 months. José's latest HbA1c was 6.8.

His physician:

a. Will be concerned because the HbA1c is so high
b. Will compliment José on good management of his diabetes
c. Will advise José to decrease his insulin dosage
d. Will order the test repeated because the results do not make sense

CASE STUDY 2

Mrs. Simpson had the first morning appointment with Dr. Mitchell for her yearly physical. Before seeing the doctor, the nursing assistant drew blood for some routine chemistry tests. Some hours later the laboratory results were received in Dr. Mitchell's office, and showed that Mrs. Simpson's morning whole blood glucose test result was 130 mg/dL.

Dr. Mitchell's nursing assistant should:

a. Call Mrs. Simpson and tell her she has diabetes
b. Interrupt the doctor because the glucose is above the panic value
c. Look on Mrs. Simpson's chart to see if she was fasting when the blood specimen was collected
d. Just chart the glucose results

CASE STUDY 3

Mr. Rodriguez had a fasting glucose specimen drawn in a red-topped serum clot tube at 7 AM in his physician's office. The blood tube was picked up by courier at 10:30 AM and transported to an area reference laboratory for testing. There the specimen was centrifuged, processed and analyzed, and results were reported to Mr. Rodriguez's physician at 1:30 PM on the same day.

Discuss the process of testing Mr. Rodriguez's blood glucose from specimen collection through reporting of results. Is there anything wrong with the process? Will the process affect the glucose value?

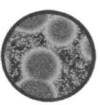
SUMMARY

The measurement of blood glucose is an important test for the diagnosis and management of diabetes mellitus. A fasting glucose level can help to either rule out or confirm a diagnosis of diabetes as well as to indicate how well diabetic patients are controlling their blood glucose levels. Other glucose tests such as the 2-hour postprandial or OGTT can add more detailed information about the state of glucose metabolism in the patient.

The HbA1c test can be used in the diagnosis of diabetes and is also a test of great value in the monitoring the management of diabetes. The HbA1c result estimates the average blood glucose level over a period of several weeks. This information indicates how well patients have been controlling their glucose level and guides the patient and physician in adjusting the diet, amount of exercise, or insulin dosage to achieve better blood glucose control. The HbA1c is also used as a predictor of possible vascular complications of diabetes.

Both the glucose level and the HbA1c can be analyzed rapidly using a small blood sample. Handheld meters measure glucose using a variety of technologies. A number of analyzers can measure the HbA1c. Some glucose meters can calculate estimated HbA1c from the glucose results stored in memory.

Standard Precautions must be observed while performing all glucose and HbA1c tests. The safety recommendations of the instrument manufacturers and of the facility where the test is performed must be followed. Quality assessment procedures must be strictly followed to ensure the reliability of the results obtained.

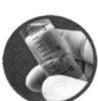
REVIEW QUESTIONS

1. What are two major hormones that influence glucose levels?
2. What is the storage form of glucose?
3. What are two major disorders of glucose metabolism?
4. Why must serum or plasma be separated from cells immediately following collection if the specimen is to be tested for glucose?
5. What is a 2-hour postprandial glucose test?
6. What is the reference range for fasting serum glucose?
7. Explain how the OGTT is performed.

8. Explain the glucose oxidase and hexokinase methods of analyzing glucose. What end product is measured in the glucose oxidase method? In the hexokinase method?
9. What is the purpose of analyzing controls when using glucose analyzers?
10. What is the final product measured in the GDH method?
11. What safety precautions must be observed when using glucose or HbA1c analyzers?
12. Discuss the importance of quality assessment procedures when performing glucose or HbA1c analysis.
13. What are two methodologies used in blood glucose analyzers? Explain how the end product is detected in each methodology.
14. Why is it important for diabetics to maintain blood glucose at or near reference levels?
15. What information is gained from the HbA1c test?
16. What is the difference between reference glucose values and recommended glucose values?
17. What are "critical" glucose values? Why is it important that each laboratory establish these?
18. Give the ADA FPG recommendations for classifying nondiabetic, prediabetic, and hyperglycemic patients.
19. Name four tests that can be used to diagnose diabetes.
20. Define alpha cell, beta cell, cellular respiration, chromogen, diabetes mellitus, glucagon, gluconeogenesis, glucose dehydrogenase, glucose oxidase, glycated hemoglobin, glycogen, glycogenesis, glycogenolysis, glycolysis, hemoglobin A1c, hexokinase, hyperglycemia, hypoglycemia, insulin, islets of Langerhans, oral glucose tolerance test, peroxidase, postprandial, and proinsulin.

STUDENT ACTIVITIES

1. Complete the written examination for this lesson.
2. Practice performing a glucose measurement as outlined in the Student Performance Guide, using the worksheet.
3. Practice performing the test for HbA1c as outlined in the Student Performance Guide and using the worksheet.

WEB ACTIVITIES

1. Explore the ADA web site. Find brochures or resources available to diabetics. Request free information and posters about diabetes and diabetes management.

2. Use the Internet to find three drugs that are used to treat type 2 diabetes. Report on how the drugs work to control blood glucose.

3. Use the Internet to find information on one of the following topics: (1) inhaled insulin, (2) insulin pumps, or (3) continuous glucose monitors. Prepare a report on the chosen topic.

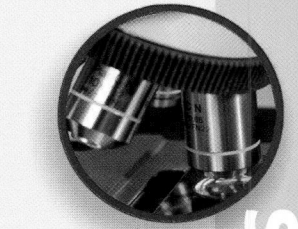

Blood Glucose and Hemoglobin A1c: Blood Glucose Procedure

(Individual student results will vary depending on specimens provided by instructor and available equipment.)

Name _____ Date _____

INSTRUCTIONS

1. Practice measuring glucose following the step-by-step procedure.

2. Demonstrate the procedure for measuring glucose satisfactorily for the instructor, using the Student Performance Guide. Your instructor will explain the procedures for evaluating and grading your performance. Your performance may be given a number grade, letter grade, or satisfactory (S) or unsatisfactory (U) depending on course or institutional policy.

NOTE: The following is a general procedure for using a glucose meter. Consult the laboratory procedure manual, manufacturer's instructions, and package inserts for the instrument and reagents used.

MATERIALS AND EQUIPMENT

- gloves
- hand antiseptic
- full-face shield (or equivalent PPE)
- acrylic safety shield (optional)
- glucose analyzer (such as Accuchek, HemoCue, or other brand) with test strips, cuvettes, or cartridges
- glucose control materials for analyzer(s) used
- capillary puncture materials
- optional: micropipetter (5 to 100 µL capacity) and disposable tips
- paper towels
- laboratory tissue
- surface disinfectant
- biohazard container
- sharps container
- glucose worksheet

PROCEDURE

   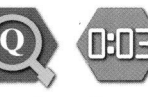

Record in the comment section any problems encountered while practicing the procedure (or have a fellow student or the instructor evaluate your performance).

S = Satisfactory
U = Unsatisfactory

You must:	S	U	Evaluation/Comments
1. Review operating instructions for the glucose analyzer			
2. Assemble materials and supplies			
3. Wash hands with antiseptic and put on gloves			
4. Don face protection or position acrylic safety shield on work surface			
5. Record instrument name, test strip lot number, control lot number, and control ranges on the glucose worksheet			

(Continues)

© 2012 Delmar, Cengage Learning. Permission to reproduce for clinical use granted.

You must:	S	U	Evaluation/Comments
6. Measure blood glucose using a glucose analyzer following steps 6a–6h (to use HemoCue glucose analyzer go to step 8)			
a. Turn the analyzer on and check that the code on the display matches the code on the test strip vial			
b. Run the control tests following the manufacturer's instructions			
(1) Insert a test strip into the analyzer. Be sure the code displayed matches the code on the test strip vial			
(2) Select control level (if applicable)			
(3) Mix contents of the control bottle; dispense 1 drop onto a paper towel and wipe the bottle tip clean			
(4) Apply control to the test strip sample area			
(5) Read the test result from the display, record result on worksheet, and discard the used test strip into biohazard container. Check to see that the control result is within the acceptable range			
(6) Insert a new strip and test the second control in the same manner (steps b1–b5)			
c. Insert a new test strip into the analyzer			
d. Perform a capillary puncture on the patient			
e. Touch the test strip to the drop of patient blood			
f. Read and record the patient's glucose value			
g. Discard the used test strip into biohazard container			
h. Turn off the analyzer, clean or disinfect following manufacturer's instructions, and return it to storage			
7. Perform a blood glucose measurement using the HemoCue following steps 7a–7l and manufacturer's instructions			
a. Turn on the analyzer			
b. Calibrate analyzer according to manufacturer's instructions			
c. Fill a cuvette with a glucose control solution following the manufacturer's directions			
d. Place the cuvette in the carrier and gently push it into the HemoCue. Record the value displayed and verify that control value is within acceptable range			
e. Discard used cuvette into sharps container			
f. Obtain a new cuvette			
g. Perform capillary puncture on patient			
h. Fill the cuvette from the capillary puncture; do not allow air bubbles into the cuvette			
i. Place the cuvette in the carrier and gently push it into the analyzer			
j. Read the patient's glucose value from the display and record			
k. Discard the cuvette into sharps container			
l. Turn off the analyzer, disinfect or clean following manufacturer's instructions, and return it to storage			

© 2012 Delmar, Cengage Learning. Permission to reproduce for clinical use granted.

You must:	S	U	Evaluation/Comments
8. Discard used capillary puncture materials into appropriate sharps or biohazard containers			
9. Wipe work area with disinfectant			
10. Remove gloves and discard into biohazard container			
11. Wash hands with antiseptic			

Instructor/Evaluator Comments:

Instructor/Evaluator _____ Date _____

© 2012 Delmar, Cengage Learning. Permission to reproduce for clinical use granted.

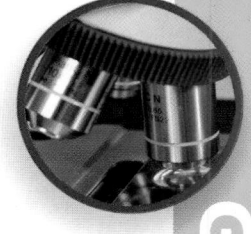

LESSON 6-5
Blood Glucose and Hemoglobin A1c

(Individual student results will vary depending on specimens provided by instructor and available equipment.)

   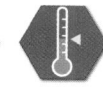

1. Instrument name: _____

2. Record test strip lot No.: _____

3. **Glucose Controls:** Record control lot numbers, acceptable ranges of glucose controls, and results of control test(s). If control results are within acceptable range, mark acceptable (A); if not, mark unacceptable (U).

	Lot No.	Acceptable Range	Control Result	A	U
Normal	_____	_____	_____	_____	_____
Abnormal	_____	_____	_____	_____	_____

Action taken if control test is unacceptable:

_____

_____

4. **Patient test:** Record patient results below and compare with the appropriate reference range.

Patient I.D.	Test Result	**Glucose Reference Ranges**
_____	_____	Serum 70–110 mg/dL
_____	_____	Plasma 66–105 mg/dL
_____	_____	Whole blood 60–100 mg/dL

Comment _____

Student/Tech Name _____ Date _____

© 2012 Delmar, Cengage Learning. Permission to reproduce for clinical use granted.

GLUCOSE WORKSHEET

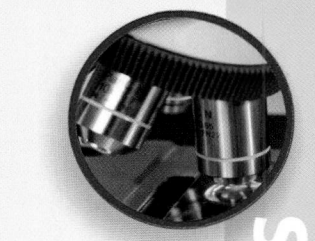

LESSON 6-5

Blood Glucose and Hemoglobin A1c:
HbA1c Procedure

(Individual student results will vary depending on specimens provided by instructor and available equipment.)

Name _____ Date _____

INSTRUCTIONS

1. Practice the procedure for measuring HbA1c following the step-by-step procedure.

2. Demonstrate the procedure for measuring HbA1c satisfactorily for the instructor, using the Student Performance Guide. Your instructor will explain the procedures for evaluating and grading your performance. Your performance may be given a number grade, letter grade, or satisfactory (S) or unsatisfactory (U) depending on course or institutional policy.

NOTE: The following is the general procedure for using a HbA1c analyzer. Consult the manufacturer's instructions, reagent package enclosure, and laboratory procedure manual for exact instructions.

MATERIALS AND EQUIPMENT

- gloves
- hand antiseptic
- full-face shield (or equivalent PPE)
- acrylic safety shield (optional)
- capillary puncture materials
- controls for HbA1c test (normal and high)
- HbA1c analyzer with necessary supplies, including reagent cartridges or test packs and blood sampling devices
- paper towels
- laboratory tissue
- surface disinfectant
- biohazard container
- sharps container
- HbA1c worksheet

PROCEDURE

Record in the comment section any problems encountered while practicing the procedure (or have a fellow student or the instructor evaluate your performance).

S = Satisfactory
U = Unsatisfactory

You must:	S	U	Evaluation/Comments
1. Review the operating instructions for the HbA1c analyzer			
2. Assemble materials and supplies			
3. Wash hands with antiseptic and put on gloves			
4. Don full-face protection (or position acrylic safety shield)			
5. Obtain a HbA1c reagent cartridge			

(Continues)

© 2012 Delmar, Cengage Learning. Permission to reproduce for clinical use granted.

STUDENT PERFORMANCE GUIDE

You must:	S	U	Evaluation/Comments
6. Record the reagent cartridge lot number and patient name on worksheet			
7. Analyze HbA1c controls following manufacturer's instructions. Record control results on worksheet. Confirm that control values are within the acceptable ranges before performing patient test. If acceptable control result is not obtained, consult the trouble-shooting guides in the operating manual			
8. Assemble capillary puncture supplies			
9. Perform the capillary puncture			
10. Collect the required blood sample and apply it to the test cartridge			
11. Insert cartridge into instrument following manufacturer's instructions			
12. Read the result on the display when analysis is complete and record the results on the worksheet			
13. Discard all sharps into sharps containers			
14. Discard other contaminated materials into biohazard containers			
15. Wipe the work area with disinfectant			
16. Return all unused supplies to the storage area			
17. Clean analyzer according to the manufacturer's instructions			
18. Remove gloves and discard into biohazard container			
19. Wash hands with antiseptic			

Instructor/Evaluator Comments:

Instructor/Evaluator _____ Date _____

© 2012 Delmar, Cengage Learning. Permission to reproduce for clinical use granted.

LESSON 6-5

Blood Glucose and Hemoglobin A1c

(Individual student results will vary depending on specimens provided by instructor and available equipment.)

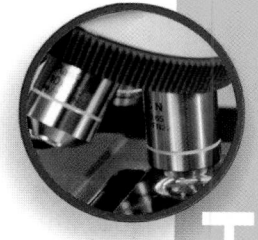

1. Analyzer used _____

2. Reagent pack: Lot No. _____   Expiration Date _____

3. Controls (if applicable):

   Lot No., Normal control _____   Acceptable range _____

   Lot No., High control _____   Acceptable range _____

4. Control values obtained:

   Normal _____   High _____

5. Patient Test:

   Patient ID _____   Result _____

6. Compare the patient results with the reference ranges for HbA1c. Use Table 6-10 to interpret the results.

   _____

   _____

Student/Tech Name _____   Date _____

© 2012 Delmar, Cengage Learning. Permission to reproduce for clinical use granted.

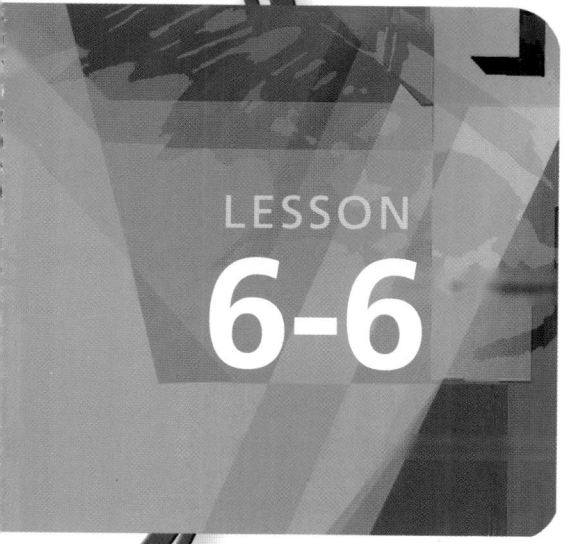

LESSON 6-6

Blood Cholesterol and Triglycerides

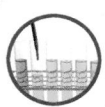

LESSON OBJECTIVES

After studying this lesson, the student will:

- ⊙ Explain the functions of cholesterol in the body.
- ⊙ Explain the differences between exogenous and endogenous cholesterol.
- ⊙ Discuss the risks associated with elevated cholesterol levels.
- ⊙ Explain the importance of high-density lipoprotein (HDL) and low-density lipoprotein (LDL) cholesterol fractions.
- ⊙ Give the reference values for total blood cholesterol levels for males and females in each age group.
- ⊙ Give the mean reference values for HDL cholesterol for males and females in each age-group.
- ⊙ Explain how the risk factor for heart disease can be calculated from the HDL and LDL cholesterol values.
- ⊙ Describe the function and structure of triglycerides.
- ⊙ State the reference range for triglycerides.
- ⊙ Perform a cholesterol determination.
- ⊙ Perform a triglyceride determination.
- ⊙ List the safety precautions that must be followed when performing blood lipid measurements.
- ⊙ Discuss quality assessment policies that must be observed when measuring blood lipids.
- ⊙ Define the glossary terms.

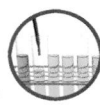

GLOSSARY

atherosclerosis / a form of arteriosclerosis in which lipids, calcium, cholesterol, and other substances deposit on the inner walls of the arteries

chylomicrons / lipoproteins made in the small intestine and released into the blood to transport exogenous (dietary) cholesterol and triglycerides from the small intestines to the liver and other tissues

coronary heart disease (CHD) / a narrowing of the small blood vessels that supply blood to the heart; also called coronary artery disease

endogenous / produced within; growing from within

exogenous / originating from the outside

(continues)

HDL cholesterol / high-density lipoprotein fraction of blood cholesterol; *good* cholesterol

LDL cholesterol / low-density lipoprotein fraction of blood cholesterol; *bad* cholesterol

myocardial infarction (MI) / heart attack caused by obstruction of the blood supply to or within the heart

triglycerides / the major storage form of lipids; lipid molecules formed from glycerol and fatty acids

INTRODUCTION

Measurement of total blood cholesterol and the cholesterol fractions has assumed an important role in assessing risk for and management of coronary artery disease and other atherosclerotic conditions. This lesson presents basic information about the biological sources and functions of cholesterol and triglycerides, as well as their relationship to good health. Total cholesterol, cholesterol fractions, and triglycerides are often included in a routine chemistry profile or are ordered as a lipid profile.

Most people have had cholesterol tests performed, know their cholesterol levels, and are aware of foods especially high in cholesterol. Cholesterol testing is available is settings such as health fairs, pharmacies, or blood donation centers. In addition, over-the-counter (OTC) test kits are available that can estimate the blood cholesterol level and indicate if further testing is needed. The continuing availability of free or inexpensive blood lipid testing is a responsible reaction to the increased awareness of the importance of controlling blood cholesterol and triglyceride levels for cardiac and overall health benefits.

CHOLESTEROL

Structure and Biological Role

Cholesterol, a lipid sterol, is an important component of all body tissues. Cholesterol is a major constituent of all mammalian cell membranes, except those in red blood cells. The chemical structure of cholesterol is shown in Figure 6-20.

Because lipids have limited solubility in water, they help the cell membrane control the flow of water-soluble substances in and out of the cell. A relatively large amount of cholesterol is located in the skin, where it protects against the absorption of water-soluble substances. It also aids in protecting against damaging chemical agents, such as acids, and excessive water evaporation from the skin.

Another major function of cholesterol is to serve as a precursor to bile salts and steroid hormones. The sex hormones, adrenal steroids, and bile salts are synthesized from cholesterol in cells of the ovaries and testes adrenal glands, and liver, respectively.

Sources of Cholesterol

Cholesterol has two main sources. Certain body tissues, especially the liver, synthesize cholesterol. This is called **endogenous** cholesterol and is under genetic control. Everyone consumes at least some cholesterol in their diet. This dietary cholesterol is called **exogenous** cholesterol and is found in fats and fat-rich foods, such as red meat, egg yolks, and some seafood. People who eat a rich, fatty diet can develop dangerously high blood cholesterol levels. However, in some patients pathologically high cholesterol levels are due to genetic factors; dietary restrictions do not signicantly reduce these levels. Cholesterol-lowering medications such as statin drugs are important alternatives for these patients (see Current Topic).

Pathology Associated with Increased Blood Cholesterol

When the blood cholesterol levels remain elevated, it can contribute to **atherosclerosis**, a condition in which lipids and other substances accumulate on the inner walls of blood vessels, narrowing the vessel opening. This is a leading cause of **coronary heart disease (CHD)**. These deposits (plaques) are especially likely to form on any damaged surface of a vessel wall. The major portion of these deposits is made up of cholesterol, although other fats (lipids), calcium, and cells such as macrophages are also found in them.

Once these deposits form, their rough edges can cause blood clots to develop by activating platelets. In addition, parts of the deposit can break off, become emboli and either damage the area in which they originate or travel to small vessels in vital organs such as the brain, heart, kidneys, or liver and cut off the blood supply to these organs. The result can be a cerebrovascular event (stroke), **myocardial infarction (MI)**, and/or damage to other organs.

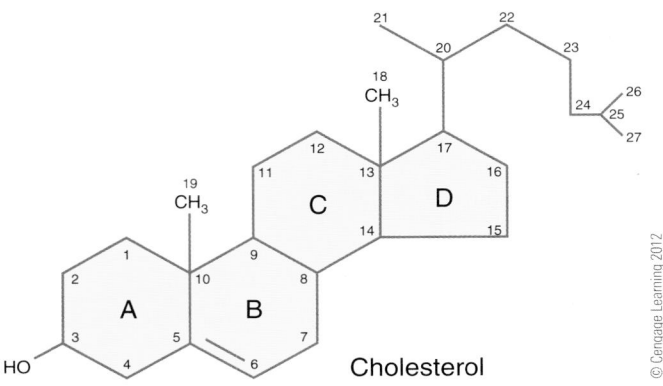

© Cengage Learning 2012

FIGURE 6-20 Structure of the cholesterol molecule

Total Blood Cholesterol and Cholesterol Fractions

It is important to know the levels of total cholesterol and the fractions of cholesterol. The two fractions commonly measured are high-density lipoprotein **(HDL) cholesterol** and low-density lipoprotein **(LDL) cholesterol**. HDL and LDL cholesterol levels are genetically determined to some extent.

HDL transports cholesterol from the tissues to the liver to be broken down, mostly into bile acids. Because of this, HDL cholesterol is called *good* cholesterol. **Chylomicrons**, lipoproteins made in the small intestine, transport cholesterol from the small intestines to the tissues after a meal. The term chylomicron is derived from *chylo*, meaning milky, and *micron*, meaning small. After a meal high in fats, the plasma can appear milky because of the presence of chylomicrons. LDL also transports cholesterol to the tissues to be deposited as fat. LDL cholesterol is sometimes referred to as *bad* cholesterol.

It is recommended that adults have cholesterol screening performed every 5 years. The patient should be fasting for 8 to 12 hours before blood collection for the test. The screening should include total cholesterol, HDL and LDL cholesterol fractions (calculated or measured), and triglycerides. If the patient is not fasting, only total cholesterol and HDL should be measured. If this assay shows the total cholesterol result to be greater than 200 mg/dL or HDL less than 40 mg/dL a fasting lipoprotein profile should be ordered.

Cholesterol Reference Values

At birth, serum cholesterol ranges from about 50 mg/dL to 100 mg/dL. At 1 month, the levels approach 100 to 230 mg/dL and remain at those levels until the age of 20 to 21 years.

Cholesterol levels for adults are affected by age, diet, and gender. In addition, studies have shown that cholesterol values increase 10% to 20% in the nonresting patient compared to the resting patient. Estrogen seems to influence cholesterol levels, because in postmenopausal women the cholesterol level tends to increase.

Cholesterol reference ranges by age-group are shown in Table 6-12. Reference ranges for HDL and LDL cholesterols are shown in Table 6-13. *These are not the recommended levels.* Organizations such as the American Heart Association and the National Cholesterol Education Program (NCEP) recommend that total cholesterol be kept *below* 200 mg/dL (Table 6-14). Total cholesterol of 240 mg/dL or above is considered to present a high risk for heart disease. Cholesterol levels between 200 and 239 mg/dL are considered borderline. There is no known cardiac risk associated with high HDL cholesterol levels.

Using Cholesterol Levels to Determine the Heart Attack Risk Factor

If the total cholesterol concentration is elevated in a patient, the HDL and LDL values can be used to determine the heart attack risk factor. Other factors, such as smoking and

TABLE 6-12. Reference ranges for total blood cholesterol*

AGE (years)	RANGE (mg/dL)	MEAN MALES (mg/dL)	MEAN FEMALES (mg/dL)
0–19	120–230	—	—
20–29	120–240	235	220
30–39	140–270	265	240
40–49	150–310	280	265
50–59	160–330	300	320

* The upper limits of ranges do not represent the desired levels, but represent levels found in the US population.

TABLE 6-13. Reference ranges for HDL cholesterol and LDL cholesterol

AGE (YEARS)	HDL CHOLESTEROL MALE RANGE (mg/dL)	HDL CHOLESTEROL FEMALE RANGE (mg/dL)	LDL CHOLESTEROL* MALE AND FEMALE (mg/dL)
0–19	30–65	30–70	50–170
20–29	30–65	36–78	60–170
30–39	30–59	33–77	70–190
40–49	25–61	40–81	80–190
50–75	29–72	38–91	80–210

* The upper limits of ranges for LDL cholesterol do not represent the desired levels, but represent levels found in the US population.

TABLE 6-14. Recommended cholesterol levels from the National Cholesterol Education Program (NCEP)

TEST	RANGE (mg/dL)	CLASSIFICATION
Total cholesterol	<200	Desirable
	200–239	Borderline
	≥240	High
LDL cholesterol	<100	Optimal
	100–129	Near/above optimal
	130–159	Borderline high
	160–189	High
	≥190	Very high
HDL cholesterol	<40	Low
	>60	High

level of exercise, also influence the risk. When HDL is above the average value, it reduces the risk for MI, a type of heart attack, by as much as one-third. The LDL/HDL ratio is used

CURRENT TOPICS

MANAGING BLOOD CHOLESTEROL

According to the American Heart Association, more than 107 million Americans (over one-third of the U.S. population) have cholesterol levels of 200 mg/dL or higher. Although cholesterol is required for normal cell function, it also contributes to the development of atherosclerosis, a condition in which cholesterol-containing deposits or plaques form within the arteries, reducing blood flow and potentially blocking arteries. This means that a significant portion of the population is potentially at risk for heart disease or stroke.

As part of a good preventive medicine program, individuals should have their cholesterol and triglycerides measured at an early age to establish baseline levels. The levels should then be checked regularly beginning in young adulthood. The goal should be to maintain blood lipid levels at or below the recommended levels (Tables 6-14 and 6-15). If one or more lipids are in the undesirable range, the physician can work with the patient to make changes to diet, medications, and/or lifestyle based on lipid levels and risk factors such as smoking, family history of heart disease, and high blood pressure.

Lifestyle Changes

The first steps to lowering total cholesterol levels are to begin an exercise program, lose weight, and modify the diet. Weight loss is usually accompanied by decreased cholesterol levels. When significantly overweight individuals lose several pounds, the decrease in cholesterol can be dramatic. Frequent participation in a vigorous exercise program can also increase the HDL cholesterol level.

Changing to a diet low in cholesterol-rich foods can also lower cholesterol levels. However, because the body also produces endogenous cholesterol and that level is under genetic control, low-cholesterol diets do not always lead to significantly lower blood cholesterol.

Statin Drugs

Several drugs are available that can lower cholesterol levels. The most widely used drugs belong to the class called statins. Statins interrupt cholesterol production in the liver by blocking the enzyme needed for cholesterol production and by increasing the elimination of cholesterol from the body. Statins primarily lower LDL cholesterol and triglycerides, but statins also cause small increases in HDL cholesterol levels. Use of statins has been shown to reduce the incidence of myocardial infarctions (MIs), strokes, and death and to provide several benefits in addition to lowering cholesterol. These include (1) reduced formation of new plaques; (2) reduction in the size of plaques that already exist; (3) stabilization of plaques, making them less prone to separating or breaking off and forming thrombi or emboli; and (4) reduced inflammation, as early as 2 weeks after starting statin therapy.

In the past, most individuals were only placed on statins because of high levels of cholesterol. Recent research shows, however, that although cholesterol reduction is important, heart disease is complex and other factors such as inflammation can play a role. Over one-third of individuals who have MIs do not have high blood cholesterol levels, yet most of them have atherosclerosis, indicating that high cholesterol levels are not always necessary for plaques to form.

Other Drugs

Other classes of drugs can be used for lowering cholesterol, but are used less frequently than the statins. These include resins and nicotinic acid. Resins act in the intestine to bind and dispose of cholesterol. Nicotinic acid (niacin) is effective in lowering LDL levels and raising HDL levels, but should not be combined with statin therapy. Other drugs aimed at raising HDL levels and/or lowering triglyceride levels include clofibrate and gemfibrozil.

Side Effects of Cholesterol-Lowering Drugs

Cholesterol-lowering drugs can have side effects, so patients taking these drugs should see their physician on a regular basis. Although side effects in most individuals are mild, severe side effects can occur. Liver enzymes can rise to abnormal levels, so they must be monitored at regular intervals in individuals taking cholesterol-lowering drugs. A rare but very serious side effect is damage to muscle, causing breakdown of muscle fibers, a condition called *rhabdomyolysis*. Undesirable interactions can also occur between cholesterol-lowering drugs and other prescription drugs, OTC products, and even certain foods, such as grapefruit. Therefore, it is important that patients inform their physicians of their normal diet and all medications or OTC products taken on a regular basis.

to calculate the heart attack risk factor. As the LDL/HDL ratio increases, the risk for heart attack increases. The calculated risk factor is often included with the laboratory results of cholesterol measurements.

A low risk factor number indicates less risk. As the example in Figure 6-21 shows, the risk factor of a 45-year-old man (patient A) with an LDL cholesterol level of 140 mg/dL and an HDL cholesterol level of 70 mg/dL is compared to the risk factor of a second man (patient B) of the same age and identical LDL level as patient one, but with an HDL of 30 mg/dL. The risk factor is calculated by dividing the LDL by the HDL; in the case of patient B, the risk factor is 4.7 (140/30 = 4.7). As shown in Figure 6-21, patient A has a lower risk factor for heart attack than patient B, even though patient B has a lower total cholesterol level. The example in Figure 6-21 illustrates how an increased HDL level can lower the heart attack risk factor.

TABLE 6-15. Reference values for triglycerides and interpretation of triglyceride levels

TRIGLYCERIDES (mg/dL)	INTERPRETATION
<150	Normal
150–199	Borderline high
200–499	High
≥500	Very high

Patient A: LDL = 140 mg/dL HDL = 70 mg/dL	Patient B: LDL = 140 mg/dL HDL = 30 mg/dL
Patient A : $\dfrac{LDL}{HDL}$ = risk factor $\dfrac{140 \text{ mg/dL}}{70 \text{ mg/dL}} = 2$ *Patient A has risk factor of 2*	Patient B : $\dfrac{LDL}{HDL}$ = risk factor $\dfrac{140 \text{ mg/dL}}{30 \text{ mg/dL}} = 4.7$ *Patient B has risk factor of 4.7*

© Cengage Learning 2012

FIGURE 6-21 Calculating the heart attack risk factor using cholesterol levels

TRIGLYCERIDES

Structure and Function

Triglycerides are the most common form of fat in the body and the major form of stored fat in the body. Triglycerides also comprise the largest portion of fats in the diet. The triglyceride molecule is composed of three chains of fatty acids combined with one molecule of glycerol. Extra calories consumed are converted into triglycerides. Between meals triglycerides are gradually released and metabolized in response to the energy needs of the body.

Triglyceride Reference Values

The reference value for triglycerides is less than 150 mg/dL (Table 6-15). Values from 150 to 199 mg/dL are considered borderline high. Values between 200 and 499 mg/dL are high. Triglyceride values of 500 mg/dL and greater are called very high.

Clinical Considerations

Triglyceride levels have long been thought to be a good predictor for the presence of or development of coronary heart disease (CHD). Levels greater than 200 mg/dL correlate with increased risk for CHD. However, an increased value can also indicate cirrhosis, familial hyperlipoproteinemia, hypothyroidism, or poorly controlled diabetes, especially in type 2 diabetes patients. Many factors other than lipid levels influence development of CHD and must be taken into consideration, such as hypertension, smoking, and family history.

Some researchers now believe that an increased triglyceride value is not so much an indicator for CHD but is often part of a condition called *metabolic syndrome* that is closely related to insulin resistance. Associated with this syndrome are abdominal obesity, increased blood triglycerides, elevated blood pressure, elevated fasting glucose, and a low HDL value. The presence of metabolic syndrome increases the risk for coronary artery disease.

PERFORMING TESTS FOR CHOLESTEROL AND TRIGLYCERIDES

The technology to measure total serum cholesterol has been available for decades, but efficient, easy methods for measuring HDL and LDL cholesterols have been available only since about 1980. Before that time, cholesterol was measured using time-consuming manual chemical methods that required hazardous chemicals. Today's analyzers incorporate enzymatic methods for testing cholesterol, cholesterol fractions, and triglycerides. These methods are simpler, safer, and faster than the chemical methods.

Measurement of triglycerides is a part of a lipid profile but is also offered separately in some screening situations. The analysis can be performed on either venous or capillary blood. Many point-of-care (POC) analyzers include triglyceride measurement in their menu of tests. Examples of analyzers that perform cholesterol and triglyceride measurements include the Accutrend Plus (Roche Diagnostics), the POINTE 180 (POINTE Scientific), and the Cholestech LDX (Inverness Medical Innovations), shown in Figure 6-22.

Safety Precautions

  Standard Precautions must be observed while performing cholesterol and triglyceride tests. Controls manufactured from human blood products should be handled as if potentially infectious. The technician must wear appropriate personal protective equipment (PPE). All contaminated materials must be discarded into appropriate biohazard containers. Manufacturers' instructions must be carefully followed to prevent personal injury or instrument damage. When tests are performed in screening situations such as in a mall, the same safety precautions must be observed that are required in medical facilities.

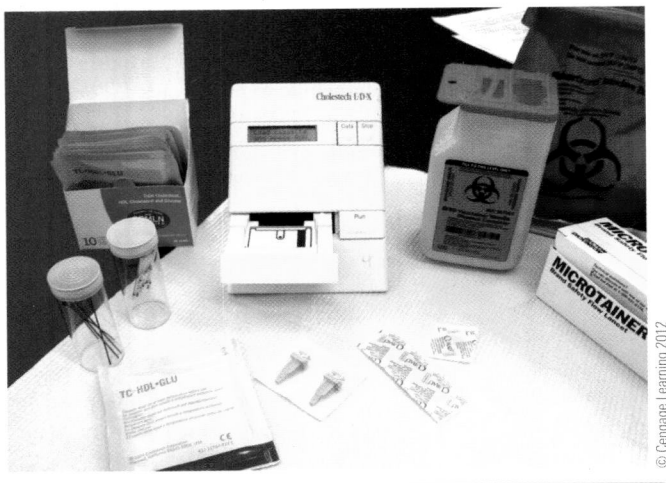

FIGURE 6-22 Cholestech LDX analyzer

Quality Assessment

   The type of specimen required for lipid tests depends on the test to be performed. The laboratory's standard operating procedure (SOP) manual should be followed to determine the appropriate specimen (serum, plasma, whole blood), test method and quality assessment procedures that must be performed.

Manufacturers of chemistry analyzers that perform lipid measurements provide calibrators and/or controls for use with their instruments. The controls are analyzed in the same manner as patient samples. For analyzers that use reagent strips, the liquid control is applied to a separate strip in the same manner as a patient sample and is then analyzed in the instrument. This checks the reliability of the reagent strips, the function of the instrument, and the worker's technique. If control results are not within acceptable limits, the patient specimens should not be analyzed until the problem is found and corrected. Only personnel who have been properly trained on the instrument in use should be allowed to perform lipid testing and report results.

Specimen Collection

Cholesterol, cholesterol fractions and triglycerides should be measured on a fasting specimen. The patient should be fasting for 8 to 12 hours before cholesterol tests; fasting for 12 hours is recommended before testing for triglycerides and lipid profiles.

Cholestech LDX

The Cholestech LDX System can perform a lipid profile, glucose determination, and other blood chemistries (Figure 6-22). The Cholestech LDX System can be used to screen for risk of coronary disease in POLs, POC sites, and corporate wellness programs or community health fairs.

A capillary blood sample is collected and added to the sample well of the test cassette. Each cassette contains the reagents for a specific test or a group of tests, such as total cholesterol; total cholesterol and HDL; or total cholesterol, HDL,

---

SAFETY REMINDERS

- Review Safety Precautions section before beginning procedure.
- Observe Standard Precautions.
- Observe electrical safety.
- Handle controls as if potentially infectious.

© Cengage Learning 2012

and triglycerides. When a single cassette can perform multiple tests, portions of the sample are diverted into different test regions. The test cassette is inserted into the analyzer and the test(s) are complete within minutes. Test results are displayed on the digital screen or can be printed. The instrument can also calculate the cardiac risk factor if the necessary tests have been performed.

PROCEDURAL REMINDERS

- Review Quality Assessment section before beginning procedure.
- Follow manufacturer's instructions and SOP manual.
- Use test kits only with the instruments for which they are intended.
- Do not use test kits past the expiration date.

CASE STUDY

Mr. Chen, 38 years old, attended a health fair at a local mall and had several tests performed. His lipid chemistry results were:

Total cholesterol	220 mg/dL
Total triglycerides	145 mg/dL
HDL cholesterol	50 mg/dL
LDL cholesterol	170 mg/dL

1. Compare Mr. Chen's results to the reference ranges and to desired levels. Are all of his values within the desirable ranges?
2. How can these values be used to calculate the risk factor for heart attack?
3. What is Mr. Chen's risk factor ratio?
4. Which lipid(s) should be targeted for reduction?

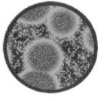

SUMMARY

Lipids play an important role in health. Healthcare advocates recommend that individuals know their blood lipid levels and maintain a healthy lifestyle. With the development of rapid, easy-to-perform, and inexpensive test methods, cholesterol and triglyceride blood tests are available to the general public through venues such as health fairs or pharmacies, precluding the need to go to a laboratory or doctor's office for lipid screening tests.

Cholesterol and triglyceride levels are used for assessing risks for cardiovascular disease and as a basis for recommending treatment regimens. When blood lipids are elevated, the physician can prescribe medication, exercise, change in diet, or some combination of these. Studies indicate that keeping lipid levels at or below recommended levels will provide the possibility of living longer and healthier lives and decrease the incidence of heart disease and stroke.

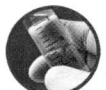

REVIEW QUESTIONS

1. What are the functions of cholesterol in the body?
2. What are the dangers of elevated blood cholesterol?
3. Why are HDL and LDL cholesterol levels important?
4. What are the desirable levels of total cholesterol and LDL cholesterol recommended by the NCEP? Are recommended values the same as reference values?
5. Increased blood levels of what lipid other than blood cholesterol can be a predictor for increased risk of coronary heart disease?
6. How are the HDL and LDL cholesterol values used to calculate the heart disease risk factor?
7. Discuss the function and importance of triglycerides.
8. Explain the value of using an OTC cholesterol test.

9. What classes of drugs can be used to lower LDL cholesterol? What are some side effects of these drugs?

10. Define atherosclerosis, chylomicrons, coronary heart disease (CHD), endogenous, exogenous, HDL cholesterol, LDL cholesterol, myocardial infarction (MI), and triglycerides.

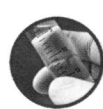

STUDENT ACTIVITIES

1. Complete the written examination for this lesson.

2. If lipid screening is offered in your community, ask about the method of analysis being used.

3. If possible, determine the types of cholesterol analyzers used in local POLs.

4. Have your blood lipids tested at a local health fair.

5. Practice performing cholesterol and triglyceride determinations as outlined in the Student Performance Guide, using available methods.

WEB ACTIVITIES

1. Use the Internet to find online tools for assessing risk for heart disease or coronary artery disease. Use the calculators with these tools to assess your risk or that of a fellow student or family member for whom you have the needed information.

2. Use the Internet to access the National Heart Lung and Blood Institute of the National Institutes of Health. Locate the NCEP Risk Assessment Tool.

    a. Use the risk calculator to determine the risk factor for a nonsmoking 62-year-old woman with total cholesterol of 200 mg/dL, HDL of 80 mg/dL, and systolic blood pressure of 115.

    b. Use the risk calculator to estimate the 10-year risk of having a heart attack for you or a family member.

3. Use the Internet to find information about metabolic syndrome. Write a 1- to 2-page report on the causes, physical symptoms and clinical signs, laboratory findings, and approaches to treatment or management of the condition. Include criteria for diagnosis, risk factors for developing metabolic syndrome, and risks associated with the condition.

LESSON 6-6

Blood Cholesterol and Triglycerides

(Individual student results will vary based on specimens provided by instructor and instruments available.)

Name _____ Date _____

INSTRUCTIONS

1. Practice measuring blood cholesterol and triglycerides following the step-by-step procedure.

2. Demonstrate the procedures for measuring blood cholesterol and triglycerides satisfactorily for the instructor, using the Student Performance Guide. Your instructor will explain the procedure for evaluating and grading your performance. Your performance may be a number grade, a letter grade, or satisfactory (S) or unsatisfactory (U), depending on course or institutional policy.

NOTE: The following procedure is a general procedure for measuring blood lipids using an analyzer. Consult the manufacturer's instructions for the specific analyzer being used.

MATERIALS AND EQUIPMENT

- gloves
- hand antiseptic
- full-face protection (or equivalent PPE)
- acrylic safety shield (optional)
- analyzer for performing cholesterol and triglyceride determinations, including:
  ○ test kits or cassettes for the analyzer
  ○ capillary for collecting specimen (if required)
  ○ controls, standards, or calibrators
  ○ micropipetter with disposable tips (if required by procedure)
  ○ manufacturer's instructions
- blood collection supplies (capillary or venous, depending on analyzer available)
- test tube rack
- pen or pencil
- calculator (optional)
- Levey-Jennings forms (from Lesson 1-9, p. 133)
- laboratory tissue
- paper towels
- surface disinfectant
- biohazard container
- sharps container

PROCEDURE

Record in the comment section any problems encountered while practicing the procedure (or have a fellow student or the instructor evaluate your performance).

S = Satisfactory
U = Unsatisfactory

You must:	S	U	Evaluation/Comments
1. Wash hands with antiseptic and put on gloves and face protection			
2. Assemble equipment and materials			
3. Perform cholesterol/triglyceride measurement using an analyzer following steps 3a–3i: a. Follow manufacturer's instructions for instrument start up and calibration			

(Continues)

STUDENT PERFORMANCE GUIDE

© 2012 Delmar, Cengage Learning. Permission to reproduce for clinical use granted.

You must:	S	U	Evaluation/Comments
b. Obtain appropriate patient specimen for analyzer c. Select test cassette or test unit for cholesterol or tri-glyceride determination d. Add sample to test unit as instructed e. Insert test unit into instrument f. Ensure that correct test name is displayed on analyzer screen g. Wait for results to be displayed or printed out h. Record results i. Repeat steps 3c-3h using control(s) and record results			
4. Discard sharps into sharps container; discard other contaminated materials into appropriate biohazard container			
5. Turn instrument OFF (or leave as manual instructs) and clean or disinfect following manufacturer's instructions			
6. Wipe work area with surface disinfectant			
7. Remove gloves and discard into biohazard container			
8. Wash hands with antiseptic			
9. Construct a Levey-Jennings control chart for each level of control tested, using the acceptable range provided with the control			
10. Plot the control value(s) on the Levey-Jennings chart(s). Determine if the measured control value(s) are within the acceptable range			
11. Optional: if both total cholesterol and HDL were measured on the patient specimen, calculate the patient's cardiac risk factor and report.			

Instructor/Evaluator Comments:

Instructor/Evaluator _____ Date _____

© 2012 Delmar, Cengage Learning. Permission to reproduce for clinical use granted.

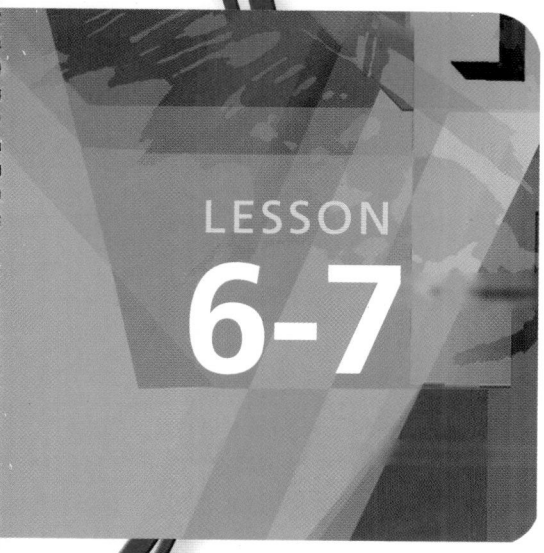

LESSON 6-7

Electrolytes

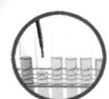

LESSON OBJECTIVES

After studying this lesson, the student will:

- ⊙ Name seven major cations and anions in body fluids.
- ⊙ Name the four electrolytes routinely measured.
- ⊙ Name the major intracellular electrolyte.
- ⊙ List the three major extracellular electrolytes.
- ⊙ State the electrolyte reference ranges.
- ⊙ Measure electrolytes and interpret the results.
- ⊙ Describe safety precautions that must be observed when measuring electrolyte levels.
- ⊙ Discuss how quality assessment policies affect electrolyte analysis.
- ⊙ Define the glossary terms.

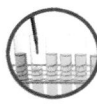

GLOSSARY

acidosis / a condition in which blood pH falls below 7.35

alkalosis / a condition in which blood pH rises above 7.45

anion gap / a mathematical calculation of the difference between the cations and anions measured in the electrolyte assay

hyperkalemia / blood potassium levels above normal

hypernatremia / blood sodium levels above normal

hypokalemia / blood potassium levels below normal

hyponatremia / blood sodium levels below normal

INTRODUCTION

Ions in body fluids are called electrolytes. Major ions include the positively charged cations, sodium, potassium, calcium, and magnesium and the negatively charged anions, chloride, bicarbonate, sulfate, and phosphate. However, a laboratory request for electrolyte measurement usually means the serum levels of four electrolytes are to be measured—sodium (Na^+), potassium (K^+), chloride (Cl^-), and bicarbonate (HCO_3^-).

Electrolyte concentrations in body fluids are maintained within narrow ranges; the correct electrolyte balance within the body's fluid compartments is essential to normal cellular functions. The factors contributing to electrolyte balance are complex. Homeostatic mechanisms regulate the distribution

671

of fluid and ions within various body compartments, as well as their excretion.

Electrolyte imbalances occur when the blood concentration of an electrolyte is either too high or too low. These imbalances can be life-threatening if not brought under control. Therefore, electrolyte measurement is often included in hospital point-of-care testing (POCT) programs and can be ordered as a STAT test, meaning it must be performed immediately.

This lesson provides a brief introduction to the functions of the four major electrolytes and to methods of electrolyte measurement. Other ions such as calcium and phosphorus are discussed in Lesson 6-1.

FUNCTION AND CLINICAL SIGNIFICANCE OF ELECTROLYTES

Changes in electrolyte balance can affect the function of all organ systems. In general, sodium influences body water distribution, blood volume, blood pressure, and fluid retention or loss. Potassium is important in maintaining normal muscular activity in the heart and skeletal muscle through transmission of electrical impulses. Bicarbonate, produced from carbon dioxide (CO_2) which is formed during cellular metabolism, is important in maintaining blood pH.

Electrolyte Reference Ranges

Electrolyte concentrations are expressed either in millimoles per liter (mmol/L), which are SI units, or as milliequivalents per liter (mEq/L). One mEq equals one mmol for monovalent ions such as electrolytes, so the numerical value of an electrolyte test result is the same regardless of which of the two units is used. Reference ranges for serum electrolytes are given in Table 6-16.

The electrolytes are distributed unequally between the intracellular (inside the cell) and extracellular (outside the cell) spaces. As shown in Figure 6-23 and Table 6-16, potassium is higher (↑) inside cells than outside the cells. Sodium, chloride, and bicarbonate are in low concentrations (↓) inside cells and in higher concentrations (↑) outside cells, that is in plasma or other body fluids.

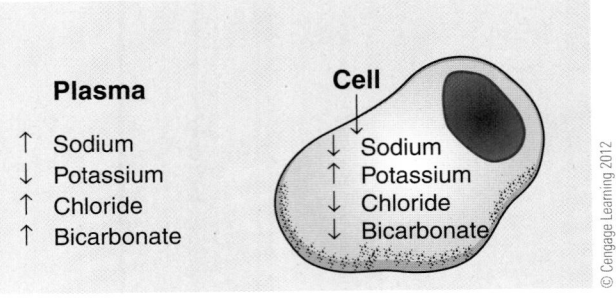

FIGURE 6-23 Relative intracellular and extracellular electrolyte concentrations (↑ indicates an higher concentration; ↓ indicates a lower concentration)

Sodium

The reference range for serum sodium is 135 to 148 mmol/L (mEq/L). Sodium has an important influence on osmotic concentration and determines the extracellular fluid volume. Water moves back and forth across cell membranes to maintain sodium balance; rapid shifts in the water volume in cells can damage or destroy cells. Sodium concentration is influenced by aldosterone levels and kidney function.

Hypernatremia, increased concentration of sodium, occurs in dehydration, hyperadrenalism (Cushing's disease), and diabetes insipidus (a deficiency of antidiuretic hormone). **Hyponatremia**, decreased concentration of sodium, occurs in severe diarrhea, acidosis of diabetes mellitus, decreased aldosterone secretion (Addison's disease), and renal diseases that affect ion excretion or secretion in the kidney tubules.

Potassium

The reference range for serum potassium is 3.8 to 5.5 mmol/L (mEq/L). Potassium is excreted by the kidney. Extremely high or low levels of potassium should be reported immediately to the physician because levels outside normal limits can affect muscle function, particularly in the heart.

Hyperkalemia, increased serum potassium, can occur when potassium leaves cells rapidly; hyperkalemia can occur in anoxia and acidosis. Increased blood potassium levels cause a decrease in muscle function. Aldosterone is an adrenal hormone that stimulates potassium secretion by the renal tubules; increased serum potassium will occur when aldosterone secretion is decreased. Increased potassium can also be associated with circulatory failure (shock) and renal failure. **Hypokalemia**, decreased serum potassium, can be due to decreased intake of potassium, increased levels of aldosterone, or increased loss of potassium caused by excessive vomiting, diarrhea, or use of diuretics.

Chloride

Chloride is the anion with the highest extracellular concentration; the reference range for serum chloride is 98 to 108 mmol/L (mEq/L). Chloride concentration varies inversely with bicarbonate (HCO_3^-) concentration. The concentration of chloride will increase

TABLE 6-16. Reference ranges for serum electrolytes

ELECTROLYTE	REFERENCE RANGE mmol/L (mEq/L)
Sodium (Na⁺)	135–148
Potassium (K⁺)	3.8–5.5
Chloride (Cl⁻)	98–108
Bicarbonate (total CO₂)	22–28

in dehydration or when CO_2 is lost through hyperventilation (respiratory alkalosis). Decreased chloride concentration can occur in acidosis caused by uncontrolled diabetes, renal disease, and excessive vomiting.

Bicarbonate (CO_2 Content)

The bicarbonate anion is part of the blood buffer system that helps maintain a normal blood pH of 7.4; it is usually measured and reported as total CO_2 (carbon dioxide). The reference range for serum total CO_2 (bicarbonate) is 22 to 28 mmol/L (mEq/L). Carbon dioxide is constantly generated by metabolic processes. Combining CO_2 and water (H_2O) creates carbonic acid ($H_2CO_3^-$), which is converted to hydrogen ion (H^+) and bicarbonate (HCO_3^-):

$$H_2O + CO_2 \rightarrow H_2CO_3 \rightarrow H^+ + HCO_3^-$$

The blood pH changes when the ratio of bicarbonate anion to carbonic acid changes. **Acidosis** occurs when the blood pH falls below 7.35 and can be caused by decreased HCO_3^- concentrations. **Alkalosis**, caused by increased HCO_3^- concentrations, occurs when the blood pH is greater than 7.45.

Changes in HCO_3^- concentrations can be caused by several conditions. The bicarbonate concentration is rapidly affected by changes in respiration, the body's way of eliminating CO_2. Lung disease, central nervous system (CNS) depression, or CNS stimulation will also affect HCO_3^- concentrations. Changes in HCO_3^- levels can also occur in diabetic ketosis and renal failure.

Anion Gap

The **anion gap** (AG) is a mathematical calculation of the difference between the cation concentrations (sodium and potassium) and anion concentrations (chloride and bicarbonate) routinely measured in the electrolyte test. The cations *not* measured in the electrolyte test are calcium and magnesium; together these average 7 mmol/L. The anions not measured in the electrolyte test are phosphate, sulfate, and anions of organic acids; together these average 24 mmol/L. The anion gap is calculated using the formula:

$$([NA^+] + [K^+]) - ([Cl^-] + [HCO_3^-]) = AG\,(mmol/L)$$

The normal anion gap is 10 to 17 mmol/L. If the sum of measured anions subtracted from the sum of measured cations is greater than 17 (mmol/L), an abnormal increase in *unmeasured anions* is indicated. Conditions that could cause this are acidosis, diabetic ketosis, starvation, or uremia.

METHODS OF MEASURING ELECTROLYTES

In the past, sodium and potassium were measured by atomic absorption spectrophotometry or flame photometry. Chloride was measured by titration or colorimetry, and CO_2 by manometry or colorimetry. Most analyzers now use ion-selective electrodes and PCO_2 electrodes that can be incorporated into compact instruments suitable for use in POC testing. These analyzers can use serum, plasma, or whole blood for testing, depending on their design. Principles of ion-selective electrodes are discussed in Lesson 6-3, Principles of Chemistry Instrumentation.

Safety Precautions

  Standard Precautions must be observed when performing any laboratory test using blood or other body substances. Gloves and other appropriate PPE must be worn when obtaining the blood specimen and performing the tests. Used test cartridges must be discarded in appropriate biohazard or sharps containers. Chemical and physical safety guidelines must be followed.

Quality Assessment

   Manufacturer's instructions for the instrument used and the required instrument performance checks are detailed in the facility's standard operating procedure (SOP) manual. Test cartridges or cassettes must be stored and tested using abnormal and normal controls or calibrators at the required intervals. Patient specimens should be analyzed only after all quality control procedures have been successfully performed. Training of personnel must be documented, and competency must be verified.

Electrolyte Analyzers

Several small, portable analyzers can be used to measure electrolytes at POC and in physician office laboratories (POLs).

i-STAT Analyzer

The i-STAT analyzer (Abbott Laboratories) is an example of an instrument used in critical care sites (Figure 6-24). It is a handheld analyzer with a test menu that includes sodium, potassium, chloride, and bicarbonate, as well as glucose, BUN, calcium, pH, hemoglobin, and hematocrit. Several parameters can be measured at one time using a sample size of only 2 or 3 drops of blood easily obtained from a capillary puncture and directly applied to a test cartridge. Test results are available within 2 to 3 minutes.

Electrolyte levels are measured by applying the patient's specimen to a single-use cartridge that also contains a calibration solution. The calibrator and the patient specimen are passed over miniaturized ion-specific electrodes within the cartridge that detect and measure the various electrolytes and correlate the whole blood results to values obtained with serum or plasma. Procedural checks within the instrument monitor the cartridge performance and user technique. Quality control cartridges inserted in the instrument monitor the electrical sensors. The i-STAT also contains data management capabilities that simplify reporting patient results and maintaining quality control records.

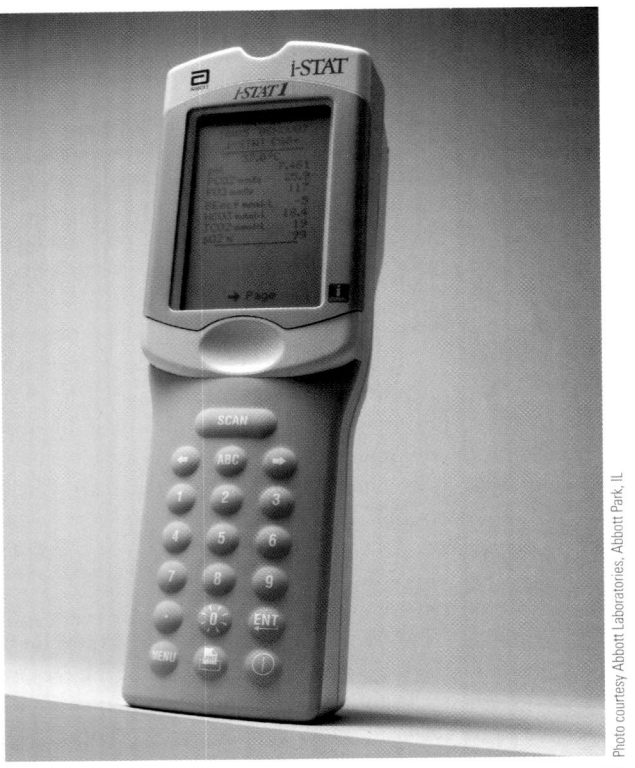

Photo courtesy Abbott Laboratories, Abbott Park, IL

FIGURE 6-24 i-STAT, a small, hand-held POCT analyzer that uses ion-selective electrode technology

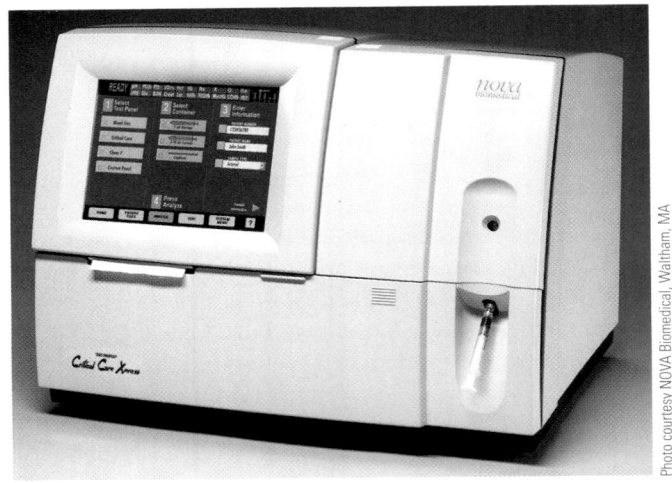

Photo courtesy NOVA Biomedical, Waltham, MA

FIGURE 6-25 Nova CCX analyzer uses ion-selective electrode technology and is small enough to be transported on a cart to patient bedside

GEM Premier

Instrumentation Laboratory's GEM Premier family of instruments analyze blood gases and electrolytes. Tests can be performed on very small volumes of whole blood. The smaller analyzers are useful in sites such as intensive care units, emergency departments, and surgery suites. By adding the GEM PCL Plus coagulation analyzer, the GEM system provides most needs for the critical care setting. A computerized data management system allows central management of information generated by all units.

IRMA System

The IRMA TRUPOINT Blood Analysis System from International Technidyne Corp. (ITC) can be used at the bedside to measure electrolytes, blood gases, glucose, BUN, and hematocrit. The instrument measures Na^+, K^+, and Cl^-, but calculates the HCO_3^- value. The system has single-use cartridges, each with a self-contained calibrator for the specific analyte being tested.

BS-120

The BS-120 automated benchtop chemistry analyzer from MINDRAY performs tests for over 60 analytes. Ion-selective electrodes are used to perform the electrolyte tests. The small instrument footprint makes it useful in smaller laboratories.

Nova Analyzers

The Nova 12^+, 16^+, and CCX analyzers provide chemistry profiles containing frequently ordered STAT chemistry tests. The analyzers are small enough to be portable on a cart and are

useful both in intensive care units in large hospitals and in POLs (Figure 6-25). Most tests are performed using ion-selective electrodes and biosensors within the instruments. These electrodes are self-cleaning and essentially maintenance-free. The instruments aspirate the patient specimens with an automatic sampling probe and complete a profile within minutes.

SAFETY REMINDERS

- Review Safety Precautions section before beginning procedure.
- Observe Standard Precautions.
- Follow instrument safety rules.

PROCEDURAL REMINDERS

- Review Quality Assessment section before beginning procedure.
- Follow manufacturer's instructions and SOP manual.
- Use controls and calibrators as required.
- Store controls and test kits as recommended.

CASE STUDY

Mr. Stein went to an urgent care clinic complaining of lingering "stomach flu," accompanied by severe bouts of diarrhea and vomiting. He said he had almost fainted on the way to the clinic. When Dr. McCloud completed his physical examination, he ordered a laboratory test for serum electrolyte levels.

1. Mr. Stein's sodium levels would be expected to be:
   a. Normal (within reference range)
   b. Below normal (below reference range)
   c. Above normal (above reference range)
2. Mr. Stein's potassium levels would be expected to be:
   a. Normal (within reference range)
   b. Below normal (below reference range)
   c. Above normal (above reference range)
3. Explain why electrolytes are sometimes ordered as a STAT test.

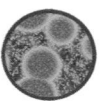

SUMMARY

The measurement of electrolytes is an important analysis. The results can indicate or confirm problems in the body's ability to maintain ion concentrations within the narrow ranges required for good health. Changes in electrolyte balances can affect all organ systems. Electrolyte measurement is often ordered as a STAT test because electrolyte imbalances can be life-threatening. For test results to be of value, all manufacturer's instructions and the SOP manual, including quality assessment procedures, must be strictly followed. Standard Precautions must be observed when collecting the sample, performing the analysis, and disposing of biohazardous materials.

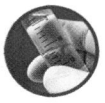

REVIEW QUESTIONS

1. Name the four electrolytes commonly measured and state the reference range for each. Which are anions and which are cations?

2. Which electrolyte is most important in pH balance?

3. Which electrolyte is most important in maintaining fluid balance?

4. Which electrolyte has lower concentration in extracellular fluids than in the intracellular space?

5. What is the importance of potassium in the body?

6. What blood specimens can be used to measure electrolytes?

7. Name four conditions that can cause electrolyte imbalance.

8. What test principle or method is used to measure electrolytes in most analyzers?

9. What is the anion gap and what is the reference range? What ions other than the four major electrolytes influence the anion gap?

10. Discuss the safety precautions that must be observed when performing a test for electrolytes.

11. Why is it important to follow all the quality assessment policies of the institution when performing electrolyte analysis?

12. Define acidosis, alkalosis, anion gap, hyperkalemia, hypernatremia, hypokalemia, and hyponatremia.

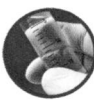

STUDENT ACTIVITIES

1. Complete the written examination for this lesson.

2. Perform measurement of electrolytes as outlined in the Student Performance Guide.

WEB ACTIVITY

Use the Internet to find a web site where electrolyte results are matched to clinical symptoms. Report on the electrolyte results that might be seen in dehydration, dizziness, and confusion.

LESSON 6-7
Electrolytes

(Individual student results will differ based on specimens provided by instructor and instruments available.)

Name _____ Date _____

INSTRUCTIONS

1. Practice measuring electrolytes using an analyzer and following the step-by-step procedure.

2. Demonstrate the procedure for measuring electrolytes satisfactorily for the instructor, using the Student Performance Guide. Your instructor will explain the procedure for evaluating and grading your performance. Your performance may be given a number grade, a letter grade, or satisfactory (S) or unsatisfactory (U) depending on the course or institutional policy.

NOTE: The following is a general procedure for measuring electrolytes. The manufacturers' instructions for the specific method or analyzer being used must be followed.

MATERIALS AND EQUIPMENT

- gloves
- hand antiseptic
- full-face protection (or equivalent PPE)
- capillary blood-collection equipment
- previously collected whole blood, plasma, or serum
- test tube rack
- i-STAT analyzer or other small analyzer capable of measuring electrolytes, including test cartridges, necessary controls, and instructions for instrument use
- paper towels
- laboratory tissue
- surface disinfectant
- biohazard container
- sharps container

PROCEDURE

Record in the comment section any problems encountered while practicing the procedure (or have a fellow student or the instructor evaluate your performance).

S = Satisfactory
U = Unsatisfactory

You must:	S	U	Evaluation/Comments
1. Wash hands with antiseptic and put on gloves			
2. Put on face protection			
3. Assemble equipment and materials			
4. Turn on instrument			
5. Perform calibration or quality control checks according to manufacturer's instructions and record results			
6. Obtain test cartridge or cassette			

(Continues)

© 2012 Delmar, Cengage Learning. Permission to reproduce for clinical use granted.

You must:	S	U	Evaluation/Comments
7. Perform capillary puncture (or use previously obtained blood specimen)			
8. Apply specimen to test cartridge			
9. Insert cartridge into instrument			
10. Read and record test results			
11. Discard test cartridge in biohazard container			
12. Turn off instrument, disinfect or clean following manufacturer's directions, and return instrument to storage			
13. Discard sharps into sharps container			
14. Discard the test cartridge and all other contaminated materials into a biohazard container			
15. Clean work surface with surface disinfectant			
16. Remove gloves and discard into biohazard container			
17. Wash hands with antiseptic			

Instructor/Evaluator Comments:

Instructor/Evaluator _____ Date _____

© 2012 Delmar, Cengage Learning. Permission to reproduce for clinical use granted.

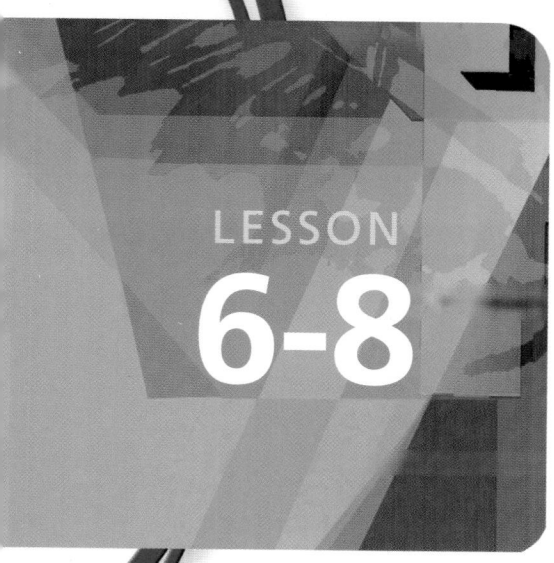

LESSON 6-8

Fecal Occult Blood Test

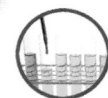

LESSON OBJECTIVES

After studying this lesson, the student will:

- ⊙ Discuss the purpose of the fecal occult blood test.
- ⊙ Explain the principle of the guaiac reaction.
- ⊙ List two causes of false-positive guaiac reactions.
- ⊙ List one cause of a false-negative guaiac reaction.
- ⊙ Explain how the immunochemical test for occult blood differs from guaiac tests.
- ⊙ Instruct a patient on how to collect a specimen for the fecal occult blood test.
- ⊙ Perform a test for fecal occult blood.
- ⊙ Discuss the advantages of the DNA stool test.
- ⊙ List safety precautions to be observed when performing the fecal occult blood test.
- ⊙ Discuss the quality assessment procedures and policies that must be followed when performing the fecal occult blood test.
- ⊙ Define the glossary terms.

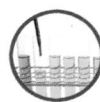

GLOSSARY

guaiac / a chemical derived from the resin of a tree of the genus *Guaiacum*

malignant / cancerous; not benign

occult / concealed or hidden

polyp / growth of tissue projecting from a mucous membrane

INTRODUCTION

The fecal occult blood test is a simple, rapid, and inexpensive screening test that detects bleeding in the gastrointestinal tract. The test is not diagnostic for colorectal cancer or any disease, but it is widely used as a screening test for colorectal cancer, a leading cause of cancer deaths in the United States. The fecal occult blood test is CLIA-waived.

As **malignant** or cancerous cells grow, they can cause microscopic bleeding in the intestine that might not be detected by the naked eye. The fecal occult blood test detects this hidden, or **occult**, bleeding. Fecal occult blood tests use chemical or immunochemical methods to detect blood from a small portion of stool specimen. Early detection of intestinal bleeding aids the physician in discovering diseases of the gastrointestinal tract, including colorectal and other intestinal cancers.

PRINCIPLES OF FECAL OCCULT BLOOD TESTS

The fecal occult blood test is a screening procedure that can detect amounts of blood too small to be visible. Several manufacturers offer test kits for fecal occult blood. Beckman Coulter markets the Hemoccult family of test kits (Figure 6-26). Coloscreen is distributed by Helena Laboratories. Two types of fecal occult blood tests are available—the guaiac test and the immunochemical test.

Guaiac Test

The test for fecal occult blood that has been used for years is also called the guaiac test. It is performed using a slide that contains paper squares coated with **guaiac**, a chemical derived from resin of a tree of the genus *Guaiacum*. A small portion of fecal (stool) specimen is applied to the paper squares in the slide. A developer solution containing hydrogen peroxide (H_2O_2) is added to the paper. If blood is present in the specimen, the iron (Fe) in the hemoglobin catalyzes the reaction between the guaiac in the paper and the H_2O_2, forming a blue color. A simplified reaction equation is:

$$\text{Alpha guaiaconic acid} + H_2O_2 \xrightarrow{\text{hemoglobin (Fe)}} \text{Blue quinone compound}$$

Disadvantages of the guaiac test are that the guaiac reaction is not specific for blood and the test does not detect 100% of colorectal cancers. Another disadvantage is that certain foods and drugs can interfere with the test causing a false result (Table 6-17). Horseradish and turnips contain the peroxidase enzyme and will produce a false-positive result when present in large amounts in the diet. In addition, red meat can cause a (false) positive reaction because of its high iron concentration. Cimetidine, an ulcer medication, contains a blue pigment that can interfere with interpretation of the test result. Excess dietary vitamin C can inhibit the guaiac reaction and cause a false-negative result.

TABLE 6-17. Dietary factors that can cause false guaiac test results

FALSE POSITIVES	FALSE NEGATIVES
Turnips Horseradish	Excess vitamin C (in supplements, citrus)
Excess red meat in diet	
Any food containing peroxidase enzyme	
Nonsteroidal anti-inflammatory drugs	
Excess alcohol consumption	
Cimetidine (blue pigment)	

Immunochemical Test

A method of testing for fecal occult blood has been developed based on the immunochemical detection of hemoglobin in fecal specimens. An example is the Hemoccult ICT (Figure 6-27) by Beckman Coulter, which also manufactures the Hemoccult guaiac-based test kits.

The immunochemical test (ICT) detects fecal occult blood by using an antibody to the globin chain of hemoglobin. The ICT is CLIA-waived and has some advantages over the guaiac test:

- Hemoglobin is stable in a dried fecal specimen, and testing can be delayed for several days without loss of reactivity.

- Dietary restrictions are not necessary because the test is specific for hemoglobin.

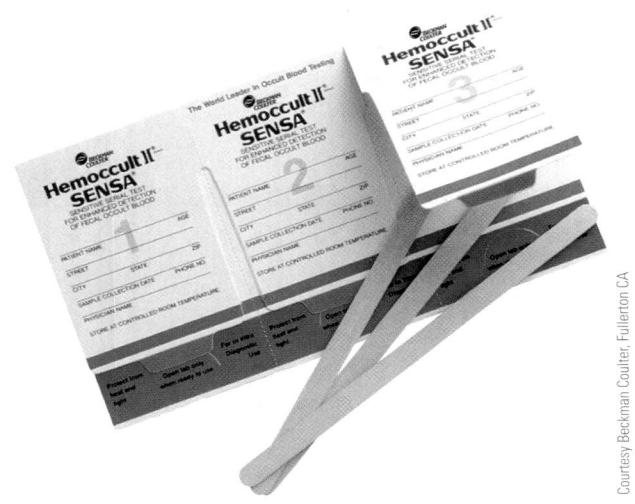

Courtesy Beckman Coulter, Fullerton, CA

FIGURE 6-26 Hemoccult II Sensa slides

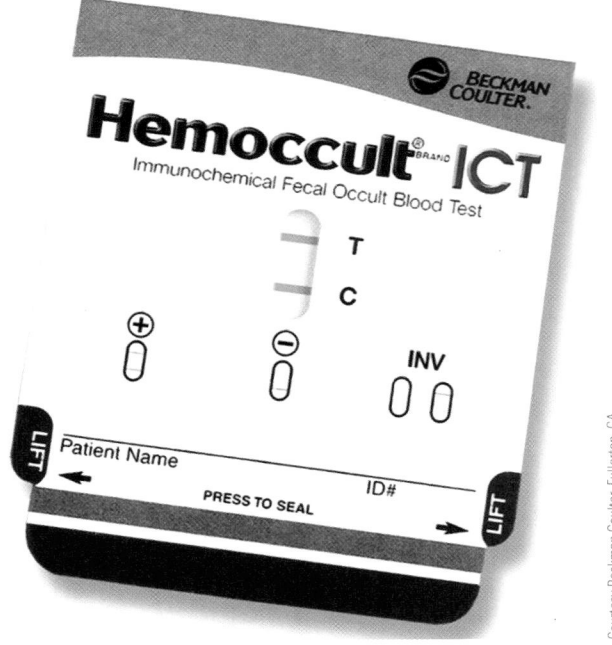

Courtesy Beckman Coulter, Fullerton, CA

FIGURE 6-27 Hemoccult ICT test showing a positive result

- The test has high sensitivity (i.e., it will detect low levels of occult blood).
- The test gives a clear end point, a colored line.

The ICT detects mainly colorectal (lower GI) bleeding, whereas the guaiac test can detect bleeding in the stomach, small intestine, and large intestine as well as in the colorectal area.

PERFORMING THE GUAIAC FECAL OCCULT BLOOD TEST

Fecal occult blood slide tests can differ slightly depending on the test principle and the manufacturer. The manufacturer's instructions must be followed regarding patient preparation, specimen collection, and the procedure for applying specimen to the test slide.

Safety Precautions

  Standard Precautions must be observed when handling fecal specimens or test slides that have had fecal specimens applied

to them. Slides mailed to the laboratory for testing must be shipped in a biosafety container approved by the carrier and labeled as containing a biological specimen. Used slides must be discarded into biohazard containers.

Quality Assessment

   Manufacturer's instructions for the fecal occult blood test being used should be included in the laboratory's standard operating procedure (SOP) manual and must be followed exactly. Dietary substances and certain drugs can interfere with the guaiac reaction, causing false results. Patients must be instructed about diet and drug restrictions that must be followed before and during the fecal specimen collection period. Most procedures require that patients be instructed to eliminate large doses of vitamin C and red meat (beef, lamb, or liver) from their diet for at least 3 days before collecting the fecal specimen(s). Patients are also asked to avoid nonsteroidal anti-inflammatory drugs (naproxen, ibuprofen, and aspirin) for 1 week before the test. Table 6-17 lists factors that can cause false guaiac reactions.

CURRENT TOPICS

DNA STOOL TEST

It is estimated that in 2009 in the United States more than 140,000 new cases of colon and rectal cancer were diagnosed and over 50,000 deaths from colon and rectal cancer occurred. Early detection of these cancers could have prevented many of these deaths. And early detection and treatment of precancerous cells can often prevent development of colorectal cancer. But early detection in the general population is only possible if sensitive screening tests are widely available.

Current colorectal screening methods include:

- Fecal occult blood test
- Rectal examination
- Sigmoidoscopy
- Traditional colonoscopy or virtual colonoscopy
- Barium enema

Of these, the only method that is simple and non-invasive and doesn't require a physical examination is the fecal occult blood test. However, the fecal occult blood test is not sensitive enough to detect all colorectal cancers and there are no reliable noninvasive screening tests for other gastrointestinal cancers.

The cells lining the intestines have rapid turnover, with old epithelial cells being shed daily into

the stool. Researchers have taken advantage of this characteristic and developed a DNA stool test with the potential for use in screening for colorectal cancer and possibly other gastrointestinal cancers. The test can detect genetic changes in the DNA of cells that are shed into the stool; these genetic changes can give early indication of cancer or precancer. No diet restriction or other preparation is required on the part of the patient. And, as with the fecal occult blood test, it is anticipated that patients will be able to collect the stool specimen at home and mail a small sample to a laboratory for testing. In the laboratory, the cells in the stool sample are recovered and subjected to DNA testing.

Preliminary studies have been very promising. It is hoped that the detection level will be high and the test will be as sensitive as a virtual colonoscopy. The DNA test is particularly promising in that it might detect precancerous polyps, growths that often don't bleed in the precancerous stage and thus do not cause positive fecal occult blood tests. It is also believed that the DNA stool test has the potential to detect cancers higher in the intestinal tract, such as in the esophagus, stomach, pancreas, or small intestine. In 2010, several clinical trials of the DNA stool test were begun in many parts of the United States. If the test is approved by the FDA, it can be widely available within a few years.

If the slides are prepared at home by the patient, generally they should be delivered to the laboratory and tested within 1 week, because further delay can cause a false-negative result. This time can vary depending on the test method and brand of slide used. Because the end point of the test is a visible color reaction, technicians must pass a color blindness test before being allowed to report the results.

Slides and developer should be stored at room temperature and protected from light, heat, and volatile chemicals. Slides for the guaiac test contain built-in positive and negative control areas (performance monitors) that should be developed only after the patient specimen is developed and interpreted, to avoid any crossover from the control area to the specimen area. The test must be considered invalid if the performance monitor areas fail to give the expected reactions. Developer from one brand of kit should not be used with slides from a different brand.

Specimen Collection and Slide Preparation

Specimens for the guaiac test can be collected by the physician in the patient examination room or by the patient at home. A very small fecal sample collected by the physician during a rectal examination can be applied directly to the fecal occult blood slides. This slide can be developed while the patient is still in the physician's office, with results available in just a few minutes.

Alternatively, the patient can be given a set of slides to take home. They then collect fecal specimens at home, apply the samples to the test slides, label slides, and bring or send the slides to the laboratory to be developed. The patient's name and date and time of specimen application must be filled out on the slides (Figure 6-28).

If slides are to be prepared at home, the patient should be given a list of preparatory instructions, including dietary and drug restrictions. Detailed instructions can be found in the manufacturers' product inserts and in the SOP manual. Collection containers such as urine cups can be provided to the patient for home use. Patients should be instructed to avoid contaminating the fecal specimen with water, urine, or blood from bleeding hemorrhoids or menstrual periods.

After the specimen has been obtained, the patient should use an applicator stick provided with each kit to apply a thin layer of stool to one of the specimen areas (boxes). The applicator should be reused to obtain a second sample from a different area of the specimen and apply it to the remaining box. To increase the likelihood of detecting occult blood, the patient should prepare three different test slides from fecal specimens collected on 3 successive days.

Developing the Guaiac Test

If the slides were prepared at home, the patient information on the front side of the slides should be confirmed when the slides arrive in the laboratory. The flap on the back of the slide is opened, and two drops of developer are applied to each sample area (Figure 6-29). Any blue color developing around the fecal smears within 60 seconds is a positive test (Figure 6-30). Color photos of positive and negative smears are included with every test kit for comparison.

Using the Performance Monitors

Controls or performance monitors are built into each card. One negative and one positive control monitor are included near the patient test areas. After the patient sample has been tested and interpreted, the control monitors should be developed by applying one drop of developer between the positive and negative spots. If the slide and developer are functioning correctly, a blue color will appear within 10 seconds in the positive control (monitor) area; the negative control (monitor) area will have no blue color (Figure 6-30).

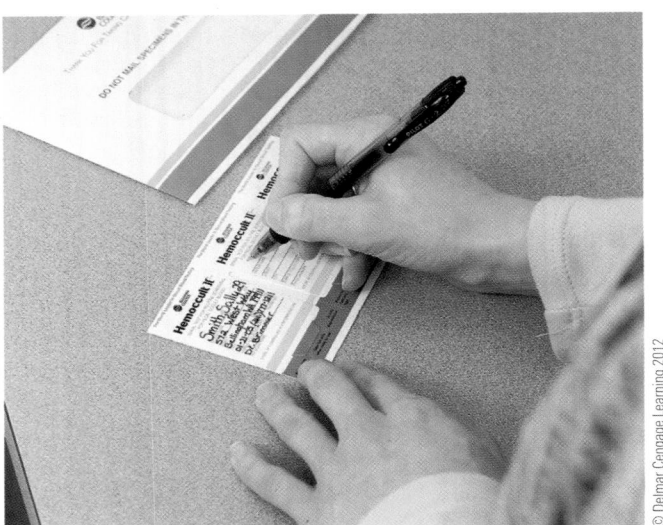

FIGURE 6-28 Write patient name and date and time of specimen application on each fecal occult blood test slide

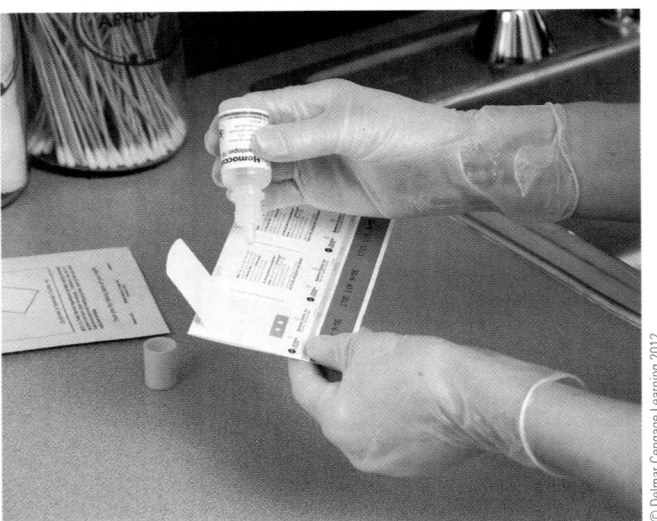

FIGURE 6-29 Hydrogen peroxide developer is added to test area of slide

Test Interpretation

The fecal occult blood test is only a screening test for the presence of blood and is not specific for any one disease. The test has been shown to be very effective in detecting bleeding associated with colon cancer, but detection is not 100%.

Positive tests should be followed with more definitive tests such as colonoscopy or radiographic studies.

Some occult blood tests have a higher sensitivity than others, a factor that should be considered when interpreting the test results. Some minor bowel lesions bleed only intermittently, so a test can be negative even in the presence of disease. For this reason, multiple specimens are usually tested. Patients who continue to have intestinal symptoms and negative occult blood tests should be tested further using more specific methods.

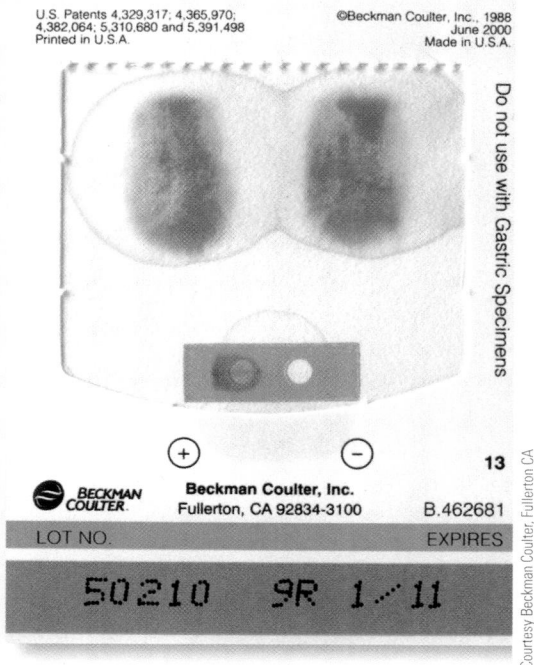

FIGURE 6-30 Positive Hemoccult guaiac test: any trace of blue at the edge of the fecal smear is a positive test; performance monitor area (orange rectangle) shows positive and negative control reactions

SAFETY REMINDERS

- Review Safety Precautions section before beginning procedure.
- Observe Standard Precautions.
- Treat patient specimens as potentially infectious.
- Avoid skin or eye contact with peroxide developer.

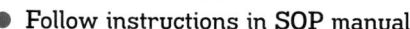

PROCEDURAL REMINDERS

- Review Quality Assessment section before beginning procedure.
- Follow instructions in SOP manual.
- Test slides within the specified time.
- Interpret patient test results before developing the performance monitors.

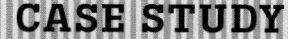

CASE STUDY

At his yearly checkup, Mr. Simpson was given three guaiac test slides. He was instructed to take them home, obtain three different fecal specimens, prepare the slides and return them to the laboratory for developing. He was also given a card listing dietary restrictions. A month later, Mr. Simpson returned to the laboratory with the prepared slides. He apologized for taking so long, but said that the slides had been in his car for a couple of weeks and he had forgotten to drop them off at the laboratory. The technician developed the slides and all three were negative in the patient test areas. On two of the slides both performance monitors were negative; one slide had a positive and a negative performance monitor result.

1. The best explanation for the results is:
   a. The results were correct and should be reported as negative and charted.
   b. The H_2O_2 developer reagent was defective and should be replaced.
   c. The test results are unreliable, likely because of exposure to extreme temperatures and the specimens being more than 1 week old.
   d. The expiration date on the slides had passed.
2. What is the best next step for the technician to take?

CRITICAL THINKING

Ken arrived home from his annual appointment with his primary physician. When his wife asked him how the examination went, Ken told her that all of his blood chemistry tests were normal but that one of his fecal occult blood slides was positive. Then he told her "that means I have colon cancer!"

What do you think of Ken's interpretation of his laboratory results?

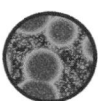

SUMMARY

The fecal occult blood test is a simple, inexpensive screening tool to detect intestinal bleeding, often a symptom of serious intestinal disease, including colorectal cancer. Colon cancer is a leading cause of cancer deaths in the United States. However, it has been shown that a program of regular screening can detect cases early that are treatable and often curable.

Two types of simple tests are currently available to screen for fecal occult blood, one based on the guaiac reaction and the other using immunochemical methods to detect fecal blood. The fecal occult blood test slides can be taken home by patients to apply the fecal specimen and then returned to the laboratory for testing and interpretation of results. Some substances can interfere with guaiac test results, so patient compliance in restricting diet before testing is important. The physician should follow up positive fecal occult blood tests by more definitive diagnostic techniques to determine the exact cause of the bleeding.

REVIEW QUESTIONS

1. What is the purpose of the fecal occult blood test?
2. What is the principle of the guaiac reaction?

3. What are two causes of false-positive guaiac tests and why do they occur?
4. What can cause a false-negative guaiac test result?
5. Explain how to instruct a patient in collecting the fecal specimen and preparing the slides.
6. Why should patient fecal samples be regarded as potentially infectious?
7. Why is colon cancer a leading cause of cancer deaths?
8. Why should the fecal occult blood test be performed in a series of three?
9. How does the Hemoccult ICT test differ from the guaiac test?
10. What is the DNA stool test? Explain its potential usefulness.
11. Define guaiac, malignant, occult and polyp.

STUDENT ACTIVITIES

1. Complete the written examination for this lesson.
2. Practice instructing a patient in collecting the specimen for the fecal occult blood test and in applying the specimen to the slides.
3. Practice performing the fecal occult blood test as outlined in the Student Performance Guide.

WEB ACTIVITIES

1. Use the Internet to search for package inserts for fecal occult blood tests. Find inserts from two different manufacturers. Compare the procedures and sensitivities of the two tests.
2. Use the information from one manufacturer of fecal occult blood tests to prepare a patient instruction card, listing the dietary restrictions and instructions to the patient on how to collect the specimen(s) and prepare the slides.
3. Use the Internet to find information about using the fecal occult blood test as a screening test for colorectal cancer and other gastrointestinal diseases. Visit web sites such as the American Cancer Society site. Report on risk factors for colorectal cancer and compare the advantages and disadvantages of available colorectal screening methods.
4. Search the Internet for information about virtual colonoscopy. Find out the availability and cost. Look for online videos showing images from the procedure.
5. Search the Internet for information on "camera pill endoscopy." Report on how the system works and how effective it is in detecting abnormalities.

LESSON 6-8

Fecal Occult Blood Test

(Results will differ based on specimens provided.)

Name _____ Date _____

INSTRUCTIONS

1. Practice performing the fecal occult blood test following the step-by-step procedure.

2. Demonstrate the fecal occult blood test procedure satisfactorily for the instructor, using the Student Performance Guide. Your instructor will explain the procedures for evaluating and grading your performance. Your performance may be given a number grade, letter grade, or satisfactory (S) or unsatisfactory (U) depending on course or institutional policy.

NOTE: Procedure given is general. Specific instructions in package insert for the test kit in use should be followed.

MATERIALS AND EQUIPMENT

- gloves
- hand antiseptic
- full-face shield (or equivalent PPE)
- timer
- test kits for fecal occult blood
  - test slides, guaiac method with color guide for positive reactions and developer
  - immunochemical test slides (optional) with instructions and developer
- applicator sticks
- cups for collecting fecal specimens
- fecal specimens
- laboratory tissues
- paper towels
- air deodorizer
- fume hood or biological safety cabinet
- surface disinfectant
- biohazard container
- sharps container

PROCEDURE

Record in the comment section any problems encountered while practicing the procedure (or have a fellow student or the instructor evaluate your performance).

S = Satisfactory
U = Unsatisfactory

You must:	S	U	Evaluation/Comments
1. Wash hands with antiseptic and put on gloves and face protection			
2. Assemble materials and equipment			
3. Practice instructing a patient in collecting the specimen and preparing and labeling the slides; show the patient the instructions on the slide cover and ask if there are any questions			
4. If a fecal specimen is available, but not applied to the test slide, follow steps 4a–4g. If the specimen has already been applied to the test slide, skip to step 5			

(Continues)

© 2012 Delmar, Cengage Learning. Permission to reproduce for clinical use granted.

STUDENT PERFORMANCE GUIDE

You must:	S	U	Evaluation/Comments
a. Fill out the patient information on the slide b. Work in a fume hood or biological safety cabinet. Open the slide flap to expose the two paper guaiac squares. c. Obtain a *small* portion of the stool sample on the applicator stick d. Apply a thin fecal smear to box A e. Reuse the applicator stick to obtain a sample from a different part of the fecal specimen and apply a thin smear to box B f. Close the cover and discard applicator into biohazard container g. Wait 3 to 5 minutes for the smears to dry			
5. Turn the slide over and open the perforated flap to expose the backs of boxes A and B, and the performance monitor (control) area			
6. Apply 2 drops of developer onto each test area (boxes A and B) and start the timer			
7. Read the results at the appropriate time			
8. Compare the colors on the slide to the color guide in the package insert (any blue color at the edge of the smear is a positive result in guaiac tests)			
9. Apply 1 drop of developer between the positive (+) and the negative (−) performance monitor areas. Read the results at the appropriate time; the positive performance monitor should have a blue color and the negative monitor should have no blue color. If the performance monitors do not give correct reactions, repeat the test using a new slide or new bottle of developer			
10. Record the results			
11. Optional: If available, perform the ICT test on the fecal specimen following the instructions in the package insert			
12. Discard all specimens and contaminated materials into the appropriate sharps or biohazard container			
13. Return supplies to storage			

© 2012 Delmar, Cengage Learning. Permission to reproduce for clinical use granted.

You must:	S	U	Evaluation/Comments
14. Wipe the work area with surface disinfectant			
15. Remove gloves and discard into biohazard container			
16. Wash hands with antiseptic			

Instructor/Evaluator Comments:

Instructor/Evaluator _____ Date _____

© 2012 Delmar, Cengage Learning. Permission to reproduce for clinical use granted.

UNIT 7

Basic Clinical Microbiology

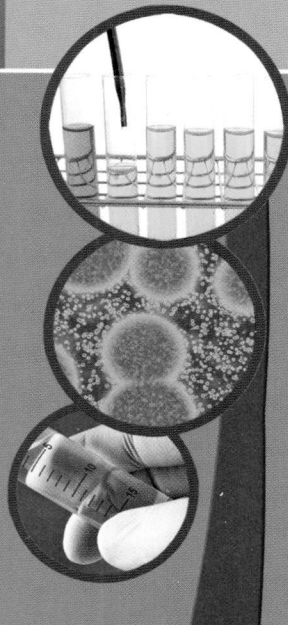

UNIT OBJECTIVES

After studying this unit, the student will:

- Discuss the fields of study included in microbiology.
- Discuss the types of diseases caused by different groups of microorganisms.
- Explain why organisms are classified as normal flora, pathogens, or opportunistic pathogens.
- Explain procedures for collecting and processing specimens for bacteriology.
- Discuss basic culture techniques and culture media used in bacteriology.
- Prepare and Gram stain bacterial smears.
- Describe three basic types of bacterial morphology and identify them microscopically.
- Perform a throat culture and a rapid test for group A *Streptococcus*.
- Perform a urine culture and colony count.
- Explain methods of bacterial identification and antibiotic susceptibility testing.
- Discuss laboratory test methods for the detection of sexually transmitted diseases.
- Discuss the role of transmission-based precautions in preventing infections in healthcare settings.
- List five emerging infectious diseases and explain why they can be a threat to public health.
- List five potential agents of bioterrorism, the diseases they cause, and the role of the clinical laboratory in surveillance and detection.

UNIT OVERVIEW

Unit 7 is an introduction to clinical microbiology, the study of the microorganisms that cause disease and some of the laboratory tests to detect these organisms. The clinical laboratory's microbiology department isolates and identifies medically important bacteria, viruses, fungi, and parasites. The test methods presented in this unit emphasize bacteriological tests suitable for the smaller laboratory or physician's office. Advances in technology are providing an increased number of rapid, easy-to-use tests for bacteriology, virology, and parasitology.

Lesson 7-1 concentrates on history, background information, terminology, and knowledge about the different groups of microorganisms and the diseases they cause. Procedures for collecting specimens for culture in the bacteriology laboratory are discussed in Lesson 7-2 along with explanations of the use of transport media.

Growth requirements of various bacteria and general culture techniques are presented in Lesson 7-3. The differences in primary, selective, and indicator media are described, and explanations and tables are provided to explain the use of each type. Safety in the bacteriology laboratory and use of aseptic technique are emphasized.

The stained bacterial smear is an important tool for identifying bacteria. Lesson 7-4 details how to prepare a smear, perform a Gram stain, and examine the smear microscopically for Gram stain reaction and bacterial morphology.

Rapid tests for group A *Streptococcus,* which causes strep throat, are performed many times a day in most laboratories. The procedures for rapid strep tests and throat culture for group A *Streptococcus,* the cause of strep throat, are given in Lesson 7-5. Lesson 7-6 describes how to perform a urine culture and colony count. Urine culture is another of the most frequently performed laboratory tests. Urine culture can be performed in the small laboratory as long as quality assessment measures are followed and qualified personnel are available. Many smaller facilities send urines to be cultured to a hospital or reference laboratory. Lesson 7-7 describes bacterial identification methods and antibiotic susceptibility testing.

Sexually transmitted diseases (STDs) and the types of STD diagnostic tests available, including those suitable for the small laboratory, are discussed in Lesson 7-8. Methods of preventing healthcare-associated infections (HAIs) and the Centers for Disease Control and Prevention (CDC) categories of transmission-based precautions are discussed in Lesson 7-9.

Lessons 7-10 and 7-11 address two microbiology topics important to public health. Lesson 7-10 reviews several emerging infectious diseases and discusses why these diseases are on the increase and how they pose a threat to public health. Lesson 7-11 addresses the topics of bioterrorism, biological weapons, and the role of clinical laboratories in preparing for and investigating possible threat incidents.

READINGS, REFERENCES, AND RESOURCES

Black, J. G. (2004). *Microbiology principles and explorations.* (6th ed.). New York: John Wiley & Sons.

Centers for Disease Control and Prevention (CDC) and National Institutes of Health (NIH) (2010). *Biosafety in microbiology and biomedical laboratories.* (5th ed.). Washington, D.C.: Government Printing Office. Available free online at www.cdc.gov/biosafety/publications/bmbl5/index.htm

Engelkirk, P. G. & Duben-Engelkirk, J. (2010). *Burton's microbiology for the health sciences, North American edition.* (9th ed.). Philadelphia: Lippincott Williams & Wilkins.

Forbes, B. A., et al. (2007). *Bailey & Scott's diagnostic microbiology.* (12th ed.). St. Louis: Mosby.

Fraise, A. P. & Bradley, C. (2009). *Ayliffe's control of healthcare-associated infections.* (5th ed.). London: Oxford University Press.

Gillespie, S. H. & Pearson, R. D. (Eds.) (2001). *Principles and practice of clinical parasitology.* New York: John Wiley & Sons.

ICON SC Strep package insert. Fullerton, CA: Beckman-Coulter, Inc.

Kiser, K., et al. (2010). *Clinical laboratory microbiology: A practical approach.* Upper Saddle River, NJ: Prentice Hall.

Koneman, E. W. (2005). *Koneman's color atlas and textbook of diagnostic microbiology.* (6th ed.). Philadelphia: Lippincott Williams & Wilkins.

Mahon, C. R., et al. (2010). *Textbook of diagnostic microbiology.* (4th ed.). Philadelphia: W. B. Saunders.

McPherson, R. A. & Pincus, M. R. (Eds.) (2007). *Henry's clinical diagnosis & management by laboratory methods.* (21st ed.). Philadelphia: Saunders Elsevier.

Murray, P. R., et al. (Eds.) (2003). *Manual of clinical microbiology.* (8th ed.). Washington, DC: American Society for Microbiology.

Sachs, J. S. (2007). *Good germs, bad germs.* New York: Hill and Wang.

Web Sites of Interest

Association for Professionals in Infection Control and Epidemiology, www.apic.org

American Society for Microbiology, www.asm.org

Centers for Disease Control and Prevention, www.cdc.gov

Program for Monitoring Emerging Infectious Diseases (ProMed) www.promedmail.org

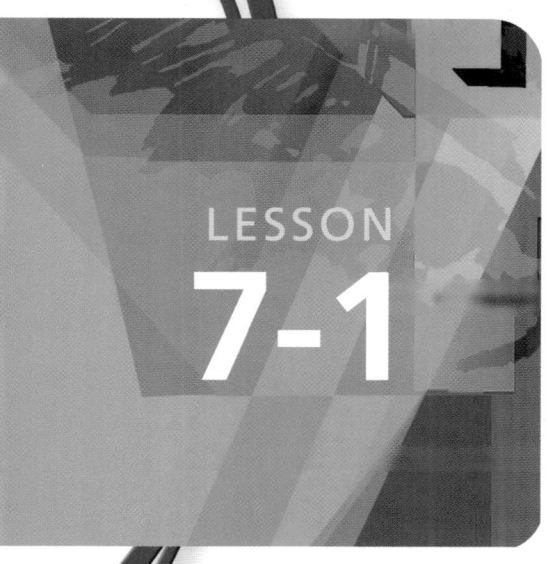

LESSON 7-1

Introduction to Clinical Microbiology

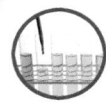

LESSON OBJECTIVES

After studying this lesson, the student will:

- ⊙ List the fields of study included in microbiology.
- ⊙ Discuss the microbiology department's organization and function in small and large laboratories.
- ⊙ Discuss the differences among normal flora, pathogens, and opportunistic pathogens.
- ⊙ Describe the three basic shapes of bacteria.
- ⊙ Explain the importance of microbiology specimen collection and processing techniques.
- ⊙ Discuss methods used to identify bacteria.
- ⊙ Explain the functions of the parasitology laboratory.
- ⊙ Explain how virology diagnostic procedures differ from bacteriology procedures.
- ⊙ Discuss diagnostic methods used in mycology.
- ⊙ Define the glossary terms.

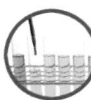

GLOSSARY

aerobic / requiring oxygen for growth

anaerobic / growing in the absence of oxygen

antibiotic susceptibility testing / determining the susceptibility of bacteria to specific antibiotics

bacillus / a rod-shaped bacterium

coccus / a spherical bacterium

colony / a defined mass of bacteria assumed to have grown from a single organism

communicable / able to be transmitted directly or indirectly from one individual to another

culture / growth of microorganisms in a special medium; the process of growing microorganisms in the laboratory

deoxyribonucleic acid (DNA) / the nucleic acid that carries genetic information and is found primarily in the nucleus of all living cells

fastidious bacteria / bacteria that require special nutritional factors to survive

fission / reproductive process in which the parent cell divides into two identical independent cells

gram negative / designation for bacteria that lose the crystal violet (purple) stain and retain the safranin (red) stain in the Gram stain procedure

gram positive / designation for bacteria that retain the crystal violet (purple) stain in the Gram stain procedure

Gram stain / a differential stain used to classify bacteria

(continues)

host / the organism from which a parasite obtains nutrients and in which some or part of the parasite's life cycle is completed

hyphae / filaments of a fungus that make up the mycelium

immunoassay / a diagnostic method using antigen–antibody reactions

infection / a pathological condition caused by growth of microorganisms in the host

medium / a substance used to provide nutrients for growing microorganisms

minimum inhibitory concentration (MIC) / minimum concentration of an antibiotic required to inhibit the growth of a microorganism

mycelium / mass of hyphae that makes up the vegetative body of a fungus

mycosis / infection caused by fungi

normal flora / microorganisms normally present at a specific body site and that do not cause disease in healthy individuals

opportunistic pathogen / a microorganism that causes disease only when the host's normal defense mechanisms are impaired or absent

pathogen / an organism or agent capable of causing disease in a host

progeny / offspring or descendants

ribonucleic acid (RNA) / the nucleic acid that is important in protein synthesis and is found in all living cells

spiral bacteria / motile bacteria having a helical or spiral shape

INTRODUCTION

Microbiology is the study of organisms so small that they can only be seen using a microscope. Louis Pasteur first used the term in the 1860s. However, microorganisms were first observed in 1675 by Antony van Leeuwenhoek, a Dutchman. The term *microbe* was introduced in 1878 to refer to these organisms. The term *microorganism*, as commonly used, includes the bacteria, viruses, some fungi, and some parasites. Viruses are included even though they are not living organisms.

Clinical or medical microbiology encompasses the study of viruses, fungi, bacteria, and parasites that cause disease in humans and other animals. Included are tests to isolate and identify these organisms. In a large hospital laboratory or reference laboratory, each of these specialties might be in a separate department. However, in the small laboratory or physician office laboratory (POL), only the less complicated procedures are performed and most parasitology, virology, and mycology specimens are sent to a reference laboratory. Table 7-1 lists the groups of medically significant microorganisms and the terms used to describe their study.

TABLE 7-1. Groups of medically significant microorganisms and the terms used for their study

MICROORGANISM	FIELD OF STUDY
Bacteria	Medical Bacteriology
Viruses	Medical Virology
Fungi and yeasts	Medical Mycology
Parasites	Medical Parasitology

RULES OF NOMENCLATURE

All living things are classified according to international rules of nomenclature. Species of organisms are given two-part names, according to the rules of the binomial system of nomenclature. The first part is the name of the *genus* to which the organism belongs and is written with the first letter capitalized. The second, uncapitalized name is the *specific epithet*. It is never used without the genus name (or genus abbreviation) preceding it. The scientific names of organisms are underlined when handwritten and italicized in print, for example, *Staphylococcus aureus* (abbreviated *S. aureus*). Nomenclatures for bacteria, fungi, and parasites all follow these rules; because viruses are not living organisms, they are not named using this system of nomenclature.

CLINICAL BACTERIOLOGY

General Characteristics of Bacteria

Bacteria comprise a large, diverse group of single-celled microorganisms. They usually multiply by **fission**, a process in which the parent body divides into two identical independent cells. A bacterium is a single organism. When many bacteria grow from a single organism they form a **colony**.

Bacterial Morphology

Bacteria can be divided into three general groups by their morphology, or shape. The three types are **coccus** (round), **bacillus** (rod), and **spiral bacteria** (Figure 7-1). Certain kinds of cocci occur in pairs and are called diplococci. Some bacilli are filamentous, meaning they form multicelled, branching patterns.

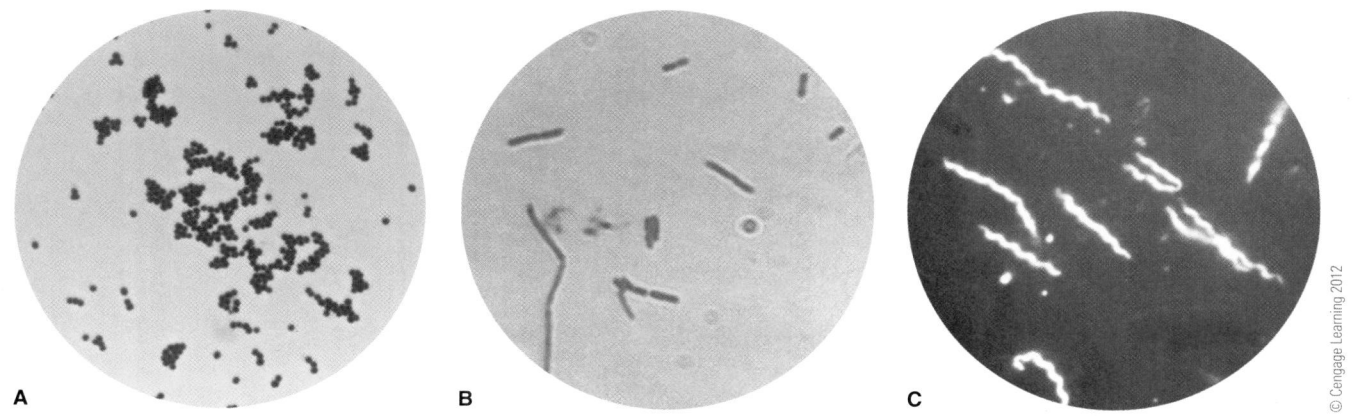

FIGURE 7-1 Three morphological types of bacteria: (A) cocci; (B) bacilli; and (C) spiral. Bacteria shown in A and B are Gram-stained; C is *Borrelia burgdorferi* viewed using dark-field microscopy

Gram Stain Reactions

The **Gram stain** is a procedure that stains bacteria differentially according to the composition of their cell walls. The Gram stain is performed on a bacterial smear by applying crystal violet, Gram's iodine, decolorizer, and the counterstain safranin. The complete procedure is described in Lesson 7-4. Bacteria that retain the crystal violet and appear blue-purple are called **gram positive**. Bacteria that do not retain the crystal violet and stain pink-red with safranin are called **gram negative**.

Growth Requirements

A **medium** is a substance used to provide nutrients for growing microorganisms. Many bacteria can grow on a common medium such as blood agar. However, other bacteria can grow only on a specialized medium and are called **fastidious bacteria**. **Aerobic** bacteria grow in the presence of oxygen, and **anaerobic** bacteria live and multiply in the absence of (or markedly decreased levels of) oxygen. The growth of some types of bacteria is enhanced by growing them in an atmosphere of 5% to 10% carbon dioxide (CO_2). Examples of some

disease-causing bacteria and their growth requirements are shown in Table 7-2.

Pathogenic Bacteria

Clinical bacteriology laboratories isolate and identify bacterial **pathogens**, those bacteria capable of causing disease. Bacterial pathogens cause disease by overcoming the body's normal defenses and invading the tissues causing **infection**. The damage is caused by bacterial growth in tissues or by the toxins bacteria produce. Diseases that can spread from person to person are called infectious or **communicable** diseases.

Pathogens make up only a small portion of the total population of bacteria. Most microorganisms are free-living in soil or water. Some are natural inhabitants of the human body and are thus part of **normal flora**. **Opportunistic pathogens** are microorganisms that invade the body and cause illness only when the body's immune defenses are impaired or absent.

The work of the bacteriology laboratory is to isolate the microorganism that has infected the patient. Once it has been isolated, the microorganism is subjected to various tests to help

TABLE 7-2. Examples of some disease-causing bacteria and their growth requirements

ORGANISM	DISEASE	CULTURE MEDIUM	GROWTH REQUIREMENTS*
Streptococcus	Strep throat	Blood agar	$\downarrow O_2$, 5%–10% CO_2
Neisseria gonorrhoeae	Gonorrhea	Chocolate agar, modified Thayer-Martin (MTM)	$\downarrow O_2$, 5%–10% CO_2
Staphylococcus	Infections, boils	Blood agar	Ambient air
Escherichia coli	Urinary tract infections	Blood agar, eosin methylene blue (EMB), MacConkey's (MAC)	Ambient air
Campylobacter sp.	Gastroenteritis	Campylobacter BAP medium	Anaerobic

* $\downarrow O_2$ = oxygen levels below normal ambient air
* 5%–10% CO_2 = atmosphere in which the carbon dioxide concentration is significantly increased from the normal ambient air CO_2 concentration of < 1%

identify it. **Antibiotic susceptibility testing** is performed to determine the antibiotic that would be most effective in treating the infection.

Bacteriological Procedures in the Smaller Laboratory

Procedures performed in a small laboratory or POL usually include throat cultures or rapid strep tests, urine cultures, and, occasionally, *Neisseria gonorrhoeae* testing. The microorganism(s) in the specimen is cultured, isolated, and either identified on-site or sent to a reference laboratory for identification.

Specimen Collection

Before bacteria suspected of causing an infection can be identified, a specimen must be collected and a culture set up. A **culture** is growth of the bacteria on a medium that provides nutrients to the microorganisms. Each facility's standard operating procedure (SOP) manual will list media that should be used for culturing various types of specimens. The list will categorize media either by the type of bacteria suspected or by the specimen collection site, such as a wound. In addition, the reference or regional laboratory should provide guidelines for the collection and transport of specimens to its laboratory.

The bacterial culture results are only as reliable as the methods used to collect and transport the specimens. Because cotton fibers are toxic to some bacteria, specimens must be collected on rayon or Dacron fibers. Organisms sensitive to drying must be immediately placed in special medium after collection or viability will be lost.

The healthcare provider who collects the specimen must be aware of the oxygen (O_2) requirements for various bacteria. Anaerobic organisms transported in an aerobic atmosphere can die; special anaerobic transport systems should be used. Likewise, if an aerobic organism is subjected to anaerobic conditions, the culture can fail to grow, causing a false negative culture result. For example, *N. gonorrhoeae*, the cause of the sexually transmitted disease gonorrhea, has special growth requirements (Table 7-2). Therefore, immediately after collection, specimens suspected of containing *N. gonorrhoeae* must be inoculated to a special medium, which is then placed in an atmosphere of reduced oxygen and increased carbon dioxide (CO_2).

Identifying Bacteria

Test methods to aid in bacterial identification include microscopic morphology, colony appearance, reactions with Gram stain and other stains, growth on special media, biochemical reactions, gene probes, and antibody reactions (Table 7-3). Four common types of media used to isolate and identify bacteria are shown in Table 7-4.

Antibiotic Susceptibility Testing

Once the bacteria causing the patient's infection has been identified, the bacterial antibiotic susceptibility must be determined. This can be accomplished by finding the **minimum inhibitory concentration (MIC)** of various antibiotics that will inhibit

---

TABLE 7-3. Methods used to identify bacteria

Microscopic appearance
Colonial morphology
Selective or indicating media
Gram and other stains
Biochemical reactions
Gene probes
Antibody reactions

TABLE 7-4. Five types of media used to isolate and identify bacteria

MEDIUM	USE
5% Sheep's blood agar (BA)	Supports growth of most gram-positive and gram-negative organisms, demonstrates hemolysis
Eosin methylene blue (EMB)	Supports growth of gram-negative organisms, inhibits gram-positive organisms, inhibits *Proteus* motility, demonstrates lactose and sucrose use
MacConkey's (MAC)	Supports growth of gram-negative organisms, inhibits gram-positive organisms, demonstrates lactose use
Chocolate agar	Provides heme to fastidious organisms *(Neisseria)*
Thayer-Martin (TM) and modified Thayer-Martin (MTM)	Chocolate agar with antibiotics added to suppress growth of normal flora and contaminants

---

growth of the bacteria or by using the Bauer-Kirby method (Lesson 7-7).

The Bauer-Kirby method is performed on the solid surface of Mueller-Hinton medium. This non-automated procedure is interpreted visually. The MIC can be determined by inoculating a special welled plate with the organism. Dilutions of various antibiotics are added to the wells, the plate is incubated, and the wells are examined for bacterial growth. The minimum amount of antibiotic that inhibits the organism's growth is determined and is used by the physician as a guide to antibiotic choice.

PARASITOLOGY

Clinical parasitology involves studying and identifying parasites and parasitic diseases. Parasites are organisms that live in, on, and at the expense of another organism called the **host** organism.

Parasites can be unicellular (microscopic) or multicellular. They can be present in blood, bone marrow, intestinal tract, liver, spleen, skin, hair, or any organ system. A frequently seen protozoan parasite is *Trichomonas vaginalis* (Figure 7-2A). It can be detected in vaginal or urethral discharge, prostatic secretions, or urine (Table 7-5).

To diagnose parasitic infections, the physician must recognize the symptoms and request the appropriate tests. Smaller laboratories do not perform tests for parasites; instead they process specimens for transport to hospital, state, or reference laboratories for examination and parasite detection and identification. Table 7-5 lists specimens required for detection of some common parasites.

Intestinal Parasites

Roundworms, flukes, and hookworms, all of which are *helminths*, are common intestinal parasites. In addition, certain single-celled protozoa with ameba or cyst forms can be intestinal parasites (Figure 7-2). Intestinal parasites are discovered by examining stool specimens for ova and parasites (O & P). Intestinal worms release ova (eggs) that can be detected in stool specimens. Larvae (immature forms) or adults of some helminths can also be found. When protozoan parasites are suspected, the stool specimen is examined for cysts (nonmotile forms) and trophozoites (motile forms). To increase the likelihood of finding parasites, three stool specimens collected on separate days should be examined for O & P (Table 7-5). One test often performed in small laboratories is the perianal swab or cellophane tape test for pinworm, a common parasite in the United States (see Lesson 8-2).

Stool Examination for Parasites

The O & P test includes microscopic examination of fecal wet mounts and a stained smear. The wet mount is useful for detecting protozoan motility and requires a fresh stool specimen. A wet mount of the specimen is also examined after a concentration technique; this increases the likelihood of finding protozoan cysts and helminth eggs and larvae. The stained smear is for identifying and confirming intestinal protozoa.

TABLE 7-5. Types of specimens examined for parasite detection

ORGANISM	SPECIMEN
Trichomonas vaginalis	Urine, vaginal secretions, urethral discharge, prostatic secretions
Entamoeba histolytica	Stool
Giardia intestinalis	Stool
Cryptosporidium parvum	Stool
Enterobius vermicularis (pinworm)	Perianal swab
Necator americanus (hookworm)	Stool
Plasmodium (malarial parasite)	Blood
Toxoplasma	Tissue, blood

Immunoassays are also available to detect certain parasite antigens in stool specimens.

Preserving and Transporting Specimens

Specimens to be transported to a reference laboratory must be placed in special preservative solutions. The reference laboratory should provide collection vials containing an environmentally safe preservative such as modified polyvinyl-alcohol (PVA).

Blood and Tissue Parasites

Examinations of blood and tissue for parasites are usually performed in large hospital laboratories or in a reference or state laboratory. Although blood and tissue parasitic infections have been seen infrequently in the United States, increases in worldwide travel, military deployments, and immigration are causing them to be seen more frequently.

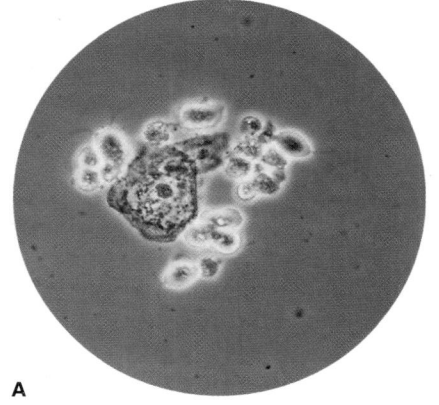 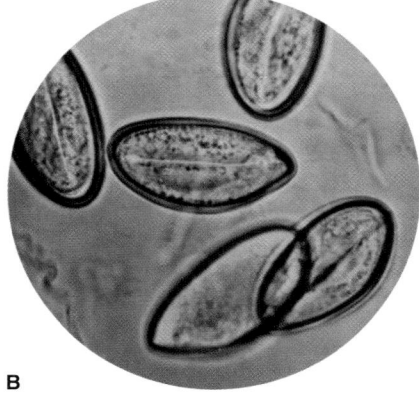 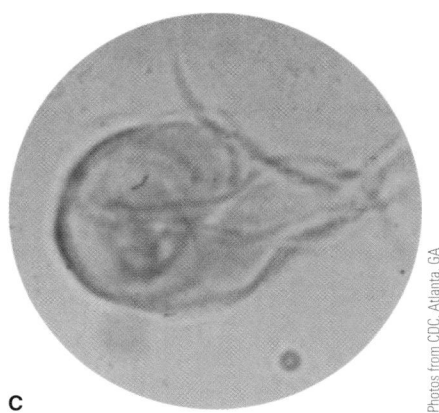

A B C

Photos from CDC, Atlanta, GA

FIGURE 7-2 Examples of three common human parasites (not shown to scale): (A) low magnification view of unstained squamous epithelial cells and the flagellate *Trichomonas vaginalis*, and high magnification views of (B) pinworm ova and (C) unstained *Giardia* trophozoite

Worldwide, the most common blood parasite is the malarial parasite, *Plasmodium* (Lesson 8-4). Blood parasites are discovered and identified by microscopic examination of specially stained blood smears. Although a small laboratory might not perform the actual malaria examinations, personnel must know how to prepare and stain thick and thin blood smears to send to the reference laboratory for examination. Tissue parasites are detected by examination of tissue specimens that are usually processed in the histology/cytology department.

VIROLOGY

Virology is the study of viruses and the diseases they cause. Common viruses that cause disease are influenza viruses, rhinoviruses, rubella virus, mumps virus, measles virus, Epstein-Barr virus, and herpes viruses (Table 7-6). As a group, viruses are the most common cause of human infectious diseases. Some viruses are known to cause cancer.

Characteristics of Viruses

Viruses are not living cells and can only replicate by invading a cell. Once inside the cell, they use the cell's replicative processes to produce multiple virus **progeny**, or offspring.

Each virus consists of a nucleic acid *core* and a protein coat called a *capsid*. Some have an additional component called an *envelope*. Living organisms contain both DNA and RNA, but a virus has only one or the other. **Deoxyribonucleic acid (DNA)** is the nucleic acid that carries genetic information and is found primarily in chromosomes. **Ribonucleic acid (RNA)** is a nucleic acid responsible for protein synthesis. Because viruses are much smaller than bacteria and cannot be seen with a light microscope, electron microscopes are used to study their morphology (Figure 7-3).

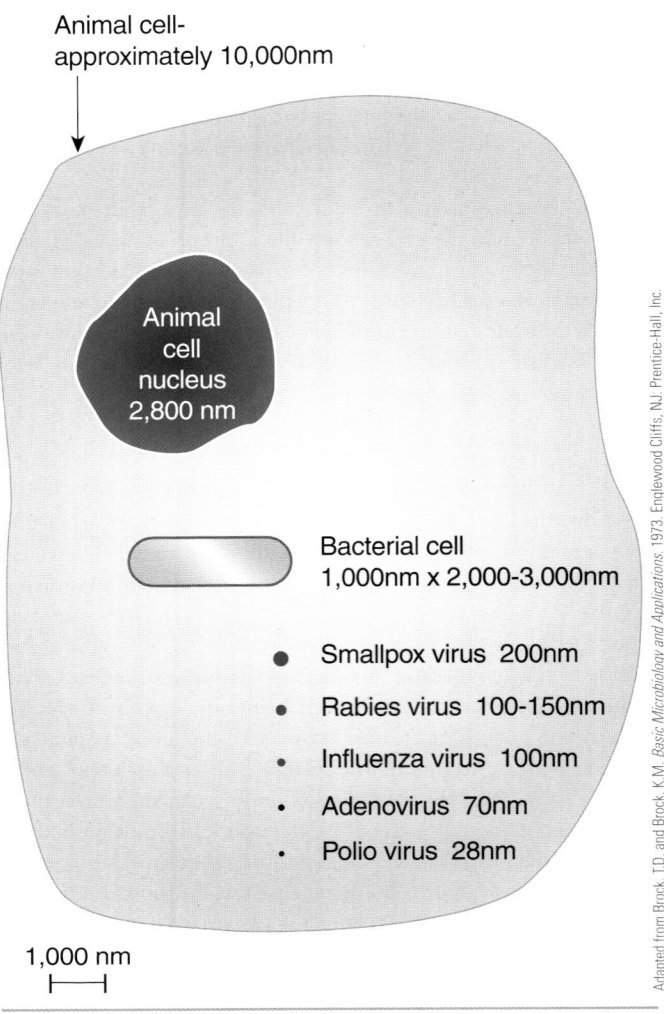

FIGURE 7-3 Relative sizes of viruses compared to the size of a bacterial cell and an animal cell

Adapted from Brock, T.D. and Brock, K.M. *Basic Microbiology and Applications.* 1973. Englewood Cliffs, N.J. Prentice-Hall, Inc.

TABLE 7-6. Common viruses, their abbreviations or acronyms, and the diseases they cause

VIRUS	ABBREVIATION OR ACRONYM	DISEASE
Herpes simplex virus, type 1	HSV-1	Cold sores, fever blisters
Herpes simplex virus, type 2	HSV-2	Genital herpes
Human herpes virus, type 3 (varicella zoster)	HHV-3	Chicken pox, shingles
Epstein-Barr virus	EBV	Infectious mononucleosis
Human papillomavirus	HPV	Warts, tumors, and cancer of genital tract
Hepatitis B virus	HBV	Hepatitis B
Hepatitis C virus	HCV	Hepatitis C
Rhinoviruses	None	Common cold
Influenza A, B, C	None	Influenza (flu)
Rubella virus	None	Rubella (German measles, 3-day measles)
Human immunodeficiency virus	HIV	Acquired immunodeficiency syndrome (AIDS)
Measles virus	None	Rubeola (red measles)

Diagnostic Testing in Virology

Interest in diagnostic clinical virology has increased dramatically because of the demand for more rapid diagnosis of viral diseases caused by influenza viruses, human immunodeficiency virus (HIV), and human papillomavirus (HPV). In addition, increases in cases of hepatitis B and C, which can be chronic or fatal, have helped motivate development of improved laboratory tests for viral infection.

The standard method for isolating and identifying viruses has been cell culture, which is performed in large microbiology departments and reference laboratories. Patient serum can also be tested for anti-viral antibodies using enzyme immunoassays (EIAs). Table 7-7 lists the basic approaches to clinical virology testing. Rapid diagnostic kits are now available for several viral diseases. Many kits are CLIA-waived and are suitable for use in the smaller laboratory.

Most small laboratories do not have the personnel and resources to perform viral cultures. However, they often collect and send specimens to the reference laboratory. The reference laboratory should provide a procedure manual listing available tests, collection methods, and transport media.

MYCOLOGY

Mycology is the study of fungi, a diverse group of organisms that exist in multiple forms, including *molds* and *yeasts*. Most fungi are found in soil and on decaying plant matter. Of more than 100,000 known fungal species, less than 500 are considered capable of causing disease.

Characteristics of Molds

Molds have branching filaments called **hyphae** that make up the vegetative structure, the **mycelium**. They reproduce by forming spores (Figure 7-4A). Most molds are aerobic and grow in the range of 22° to 30° C. They will grow on the usual bacteriological media, but their growth is so slow that bacteria usually overgrow them. Sabouraud's dextrose agar, which contains dextrose, maltose, and peptones, is a medium that selects for growth of pathogenic fungi. Antibiotics can be incorporated into Sabouraud's dextrose agar to inhibit growth of bacteria and nonpathogenic fungi.

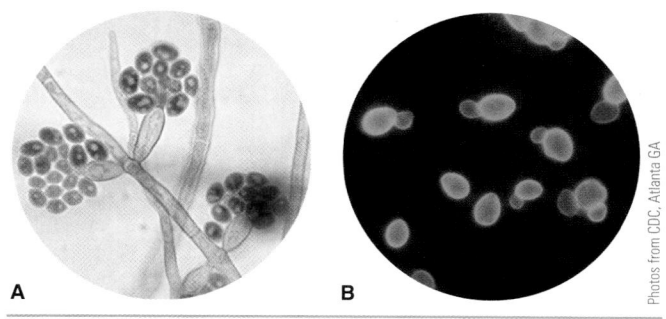

FIGURE 7-4 Reproductive forms of molds and yeasts: (A) spore-producing mold; (B) high-magnification image of budding yeast cells stained with fluorescent stain

Characteristics of Yeasts

Yeast cells are eukaryotic cells that are larger than bacteria. They are easily seen with the light microscope. The most common yeast shape is unicellular (one-celled) and oval. Yeasts usually reproduce by budding instead of forming spores (Figure 7-4B). There are about 350 known species of yeasts. Yeasts are used in fermentation processes such as beer and wine production and leavening of bread. Although yeasts are useful for food and other commercial purposes, some yeasts are pathogenic and some are opportunistic pathogens. Yeasts grow best with an abundant supply of oxygen and grow satisfactorily on common bacteriological media, as well as Saboraud's dextrose agar.

Fungal Diseases: Mycoses

Infection caused by a fungus is called a **mycosis** (pl., mycoses). The mycosis incidence is related to the amount of exposure to fungi in living conditions, occupation, and leisure activities, as well as to immune status. Table 7-8 lists some fungi and the diseases they cause.

TABLE 7-7. Laboratory approaches to detecting viruses

Cell culture: Isolating and identifying the viruses in cell culture

Direct detection: Detecting the viral antigen in a clinical specimen

Immunodiagnosis: Detecting serum antibodies to the virus

TABLE 7-8. Some clinically significant fungi and the diseases they cause

ORGANISM	DISEASE
Tinea species	Ringworm (dermatomycosis)
Candida	Thrush, vaginal infections (candidiasis)
Malassezia furfur	Pityriasis versicolor
Coccidioides immitis	Coccidioidomycosis (valley fever)
Histoplasma capsulatum	Histoplasmosis
Aspergillus, Candida, Cryptococcus, and *Pneumocystis*	Involved in systemic infections, especially in immunocompromised patients

TABLE 7-9. A simplified scheme for culturing and identifying molds and yeasts

GROWTH FORM OF ORGANISM	CULTURE MEDIA	TEMPERATURE OF INCUBATION (°C)	METHOD OF IDENTIFICATION
Molds	Sabouraud's agar	22–27	Macroscopic and microscopic appearance
Yeasts	Blood agar	37	Sugar fermentation, use of carbon or nitrogen, germ tube test

Pathogenic fungi, which can infect any exposed individual, usually fall in the group called *dimorphic* fungi. This means that these fungi can grow in both yeast and mold forms, depending on culture conditions. In the environment, they are found as a mold form; when grown at body temperature, such as when infecting an animal or human, they are found in the yeast form. Three important pathogenic dimorphic fungi are *Blastomyces dermatitidis*, *Histoplasma capsulatum*, and *Coccidioides immitis*, the agent that causes San Joaquin Valley fever.

Other fungi such as *Candida*, *Pneumocystis*, and *Aspergillus* are opportunistic pathogens; they usually cause serious disease only in immunosuppressed (immunocompromised) patients, such as HIV-infected patients. *Candida* can infect the mucous membranes of the mouth and vagina. The *dermatophytes*, the group of fungi that require keratin to grow, can infect hair, nails, and superficial skin. The fungi that cause ringworm and athlete's foot are dermatophytes.

Identifying Molds and Yeasts

Identification techniques for medically important fungi depend on whether the organism grows as a mold or yeast. Molds are largely identified by macroscopic and microscopic study of their morphology and the spores they produce (Figure 7-4). Superficial yeast or dermatophyte infections can be detected by microscopic examination or culturing of skin scrapings or nail clippings. Yeast identification is based on culture and colonial morphology and on the results of biochemical reactions and the organism's ability to ferment certain sugars. *Candida albicans* can be identified by the development of pseudohyphae in a test called the *germ tube test*. Table 7-9 gives a simplified scheme for identifying molds and yeasts.

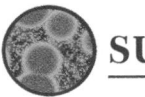

SUMMARY

Microbiology is the study of a wide variety of agents, some helpful to humans and some harmful. The bacteria, fungi, and parasites are named using international rules, so that scientists all over the world use the same nomenclature.

Humans have conquered many infectious diseases, mainly because of the discovery and use of antibiotics. However, new diseases or microbes still are being discovered. Microorganisms and viruses can undergo rapid genetic change. An animal

pathogen can become pathogenic to humans. A bacterium can become resistant to antibiotics. These discoveries lead to more microbiology research in academic institutions and pharmaceutical and research laboratories.

Each discovery causes a trickle-down effect in clinical laboratories. Eventually, if the organism is a pathogen, test methods are developed to detect it or antibodies to it. At the same time, methods to detect more commonplace causes of disease are always being improved and more automated methods are being introduced into the microbiology laboratory.

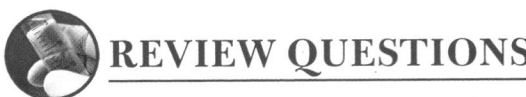

REVIEW QUESTIONS

1. When was the term *microbiology* first used?
2. What four areas of study are encompassed by clinical microbiology?
3. What are the functional differences between a small and large microbiology laboratory?
4. What is the difference between a pathogen and an opportunistic pathogen?
5. How do bacterial pathogens cause host damage?
6. What are the three morphological types of bacteria?
7. What is a Gram stain?
8. What are two morphological forms of fungi?
9. What is the difference between aerobic and anaerobic bacteria?
10. How are viruses different from microorganisms? Name three viral diseases.
11. What type of specimen is required to detect malaria? To detect *Giardia*?
12. List five methods used to help identify bacteria.
13. Define aerobic, anaerobic, antibiotic susceptibility testing, bacillus, coccus, colony, communicable, culture, deoxyribonucleic acid, fastidious bacteria, fission, gram negative, gram positive, gram stain, host, hyphae, immunoassay, infection, medium, minimum inhibitory concentration, mycelium, mycosis, normal flora, opportunistic pathogen, pathogen, progeny, ribonucleic acid, and spiral bacteria.

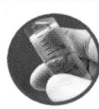

STUDENT ACTIVITIES

1. Complete the written examination for this lesson.

2. Visit a microbiology laboratory in the community. Find out what types of tests are performed in the laboratory and which tests are sent to reference laboratories.

3. Interview an employee of a hospital microbiology laboratory and report on his or her job functions and responsibilities.

WEB ACTIVITIES

Use the Internet to find information on a disease caused by an agent from each microbiology category (bacteria, viruses, fungi, and parasites). For each disease, report on the causative agent, disease symptoms, method of diagnosis, and treatment.

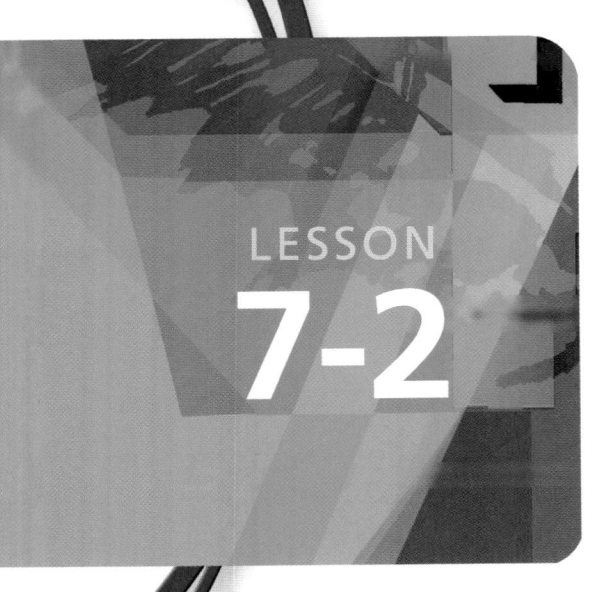

7-2

Bacteriology Specimen Collection and Processing

LESSON OBJECTIVES

After studying this lesson, the student will

- ⊙ List seven specimens that are frequently cultured in the microbiology laboratory.
- ⊙ List five reasons a culture might be ordered.
- ⊙ Discuss the collection and processing of a throat culture.
- ⊙ Explain why a nasal culture would be required.
- ⊙ Explain the procedures for the collection and processing of urine for culture.
- ⊙ List three methods for collecting specimens from wound.
- ⊙ Discuss the collection and processing of a sputum specimen.
- ⊙ Explain how specimens are collected for a stool culture.
- ⊙ Describe the procedure for collecting blood cultures.
- ⊙ Explain the function and importance of transport media.
- ⊙ Explain how the type of specimen must be considered in the choice of transport media.
- ⊙ Discuss safety precautions that must be observed when collecting and processing specimens for bacteriology testing.
- ⊙ Discuss how quality assessment procedures are used in the collection and processing of specimens for bacteriology testing.
- ⊙ Define the glossary words.

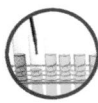 GLOSSARY

carrier / an individual who harbors an organism and is capable of spreading the organism to others, but has no symptoms or signs of disease

culture / growth of microorganisms in a special medium; the process of growing microorganisms in the laboratory

culture medium / a substance used to provide nutrients for growing microorganisms

Escherichia coli (*E. coli*) / a bacterium that is part of the normal flora of the intestines

sepsis / the presence of microorganisms and/or their toxic products in the blood and other tissues

septicemia / the presence and growth of pathogenic microorganisms in the blood

Streptococcus pyogenes / bacterium that causes a common type of streptococcal infection, most notably "strep" throat

(continues)

transport medium / containers specially designed to provide nutrients and an environment that preserves the viability of microorganisms during transport

virulent / highly infectious

wound / a break in the continuity of soft parts of the body structure; trauma to tissues

INTRODUCTION

Specific procedures must be followed when collecting and processing specimens for bacteriology in order for the specimens to yield valid and useful results. Specimens for culture can come from many sources. Any part of the body can become infected. The infection can result from normal flora being depleted and allowing pathogens to multiply; introduction of bacteria by means of a **wound** or surgical incision; direct contact; or through the alimentary tract or respiratory route.

Specimens can be collected during visits to physicians' offices, during outpatient procedures, or in surgery by surgical personnel. Specimens for culture discussed in this lesson include:

- Throat specimens
- Nasal specimens
- Urine specimens
- Wound specimens
- Sputum specimens
- Stool specimens
- Blood cultures

Most specimens collected and cultures performed in smaller laboratories are a combination of throat and urine cultures and collection and processing of stool, blood, and wound samples for **culture**. This lesson describes these specimens and their collection, processing, and preparation for transport. Although this lesson cannot cover the diversity of specimens that are cultured, the general principles and procedures described can be applied to other types of specimens.

REASONS FOR ORDERING CULTURES

Cultures are ordered based on a combination of clinical symptoms and the results of a physical examination.

- Throat cultures are ordered to determine if the patient has strep throat, infection with streptococcal group A (*Streptococcus pyogenes*). Often the healthcare provider first orders a rapid test for *Streptococcus pyogenes*; if the test is negative, a throat swab is collected and cultured to confirm the negative result (Table 7-10).

- Nasal cultures are ordered to screen for carriers of antibiotic-resistant bacteria or to detect infections by the bacteria causing whooping cough or diphtheria.

TABLE 7-10. Reasons for a culture to be ordered

SITE/SPECIMEN CULTURED	REASONS FOR CULTURE
Throat	Sore throat, fever, negative rapid strep test
Nasal	Rule out *B. pertussis*, detect carriers of MRSA
Urine	Repeated urinary tract infections, poor response to antibiotics
Wound	Failure to heal in timely fashion, inflammation, purulent discharge
Sputum	Prolonged cough, fever, suspected lung infection
Stool	Diarrhea with blood and mucous, prolonged bout of diarrhea
Blood	Suspected sepsis or septicemia

- A urine culture and sensitivity (C & S) is ordered when a patient has had recurring urinary tract infections (UTIs) or has completed a regimen of antibiotics but is still symptomatic.

- A wound culture is ordered if symptoms indicate that a wound has become infected and is not healing or responding to treatment.

- Sputum specimens are cultured to detect microorganisms that can cause pneumonia, bronchitis, or tuberculosis.

- A stool culture can be ordered when a patient presents with symptoms of intestinal infection. Stool culture results are particularly important to detect outbreaks with enteric pathogens such as *Salmonella* and to guide treatment of infections by **virulent** (highly infectious) strains of *Escherichia coli* (Table 7-10).

- A blood culture is needed when **sepsis**, the presence of microorganisms or their toxic products in the blood or tissue, is suspected because of the presence of a high fever or other symptoms in the patient. **Septicemia** is a serious situation in which pathogenic microorganisms are growing in the blood.

SPECIMEN COLLECTION MANUAL

The regional reference laboratory or the hospital laboratory should provide a specimen collection manual containing instructions for the collection and processing of bacteriology specimens to be sent to them for culture. Those instructions must be followed; they include information about collection sites, collection procedures, selection of appropriate transport media, and procedures for preparing various specimens for transport (Table 7-11).

COLLECTION AND TRANSPORT SUPPLIES

The laboratory must maintain an assortment of collection supplies and **transport media** to accommodate a variety of specimen types (Figure 7-5). In some cases, the reference laboratory will provide these supplies to the laboratory. The collection supplies must include transport media for aerobic and anaerobic bacteria and sterile swabs contained in kits (Figure 7-6). The collection manual will contain specific instructions regarding the appropriate collection supplies for each specimen collection site or type of culture (Table 7-12).

In general, only sterile rayon or Dacron swabs made for bacterial culture should be used for specimen collection because elements in cotton swabs can be bactericidal or bacteriostatic. Swabs with metal shafts must be used for some specimens because resins in some woods can be eluted into the transport medium and destroy the organisms of interest.

TABLE 7-11. Correlation of site or specimen cultured with the specimen collection method

SITE/SPECIMEN CULTURED	SPECIMEN COLLECTION METHOD
Throat	Swab of pharyngeal surfaces or tonsils
Nasal	Swabs of both nostrils
Urine	Clean-catch urine
Wound	Sterile needle aspirate, biopsy of wound margin, or swab
Sputum	Sputum (not saliva) collected after the mouth is rinsed with water
Stool	One specimen/day for 3 consecutive days; not contaminated by urine or toilet water
Blood	Special cleansing of venipuncture site; drawn first in order of draw

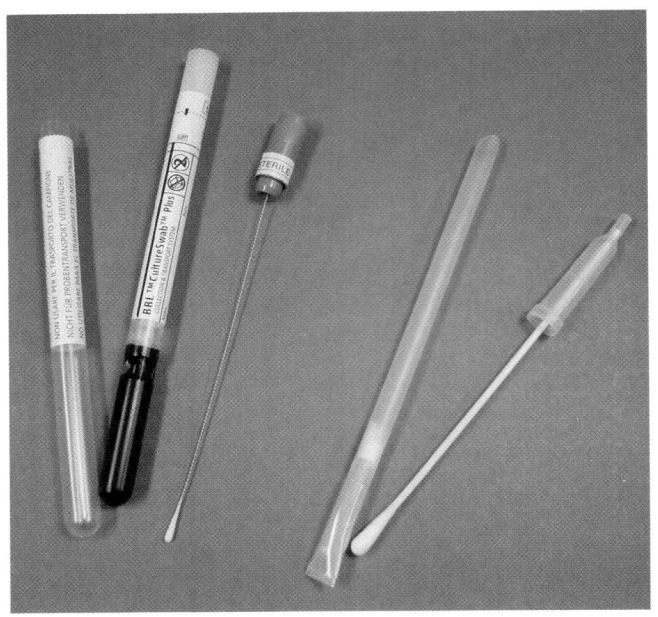

FIGURE 7-6 Culture swabs and transport tubes

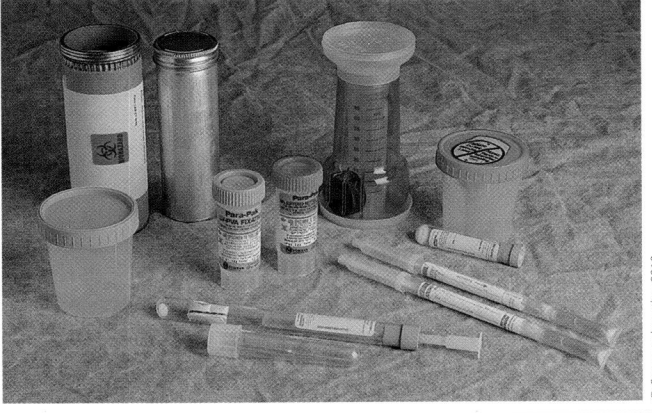

FIGURE 7-5 Specimen containers and transport media

TABLE 7-12. Transport media recommended for various culture sites or types of specimens

SITE/SPECIMEN CULTURED	EXAMPLES OF TRANSPORT MEDIA
Throat	BD CultureSwab Max, Remel BactiSwab; various culturette systems
Nasal	Regan-Lowe, Modified Stuart's
Urine	BD Urine C&S transport kit
Wound	BD BBL Port-A-Cul, A.C.T. II
Sputum	Sterile collection container (culture within 24 hours)
Stool	Para-Pak vial for culture; Cary Blair medium, Amies medium
Blood	Blood culture bottles

The supplies on hand should include sterile containers for urine, stool, or sputum specimens plus blood culture bottles. Additionally, a small supply of nutrient-rich **culture media** should be on hand, such as blood agar, eosin-methylene blue agar (EMB), MacConkey's (MAC) agar, and tubes of thioglycolate broth.

Transport supplies must protect the specimen from contamination as well as protect the transporter and personnel at the receiving laboratory. Depending on the method of transport, the specimen can be placed in a sealed biohazard bag, inside an outer container, or in metal or cardboard tubes (Figure 7-5). All transport containers must be labeled as containing biohazardous material and must meet all governmental transportation regulations.

SAFETY PRECAUTIONS

The procedures for collecting and processing specimens for culture expose the technician to blood and bacteria or other microorganisms. Standard Precautions must be observed. Personal protective equipment (PPE) must be worn, such as gloves; eye protection; and a buttoned, disposable, fluid-resistant laboratory coat. A mask can be worn when a throat or respiratory specimen is being collected. The setup area for specimen collection and processing should be frequently disinfected with surface disinfectant.

QUALITY ASSESSMENT

All procedures of the facility must be followed in the collection and processing of specimens as stated in the SOP manual. It is important that the patient is instructed in any required preparatory procedures. Mislabeling of the specimen can be prevented by applying barcoded labels or using a permanent marker to write patient information, site of specimen collection, and collection time on the specimen containers. Special attention must be given to choosing the correct transport system to ensure survival of the microorganisms until they can be transferred to culture media. Transport and culture media must not be used beyond the expiration dates.

COLLECTING THE SPECIMEN

The physician, technologist, or other healthcare worker collecting the specimen must record the patient identification, source of the specimen and time of collection. Including information about the source of the specimen helps the microbiologist determine the growth medium that should be used for culture and the optimum environment for growth.

Throat Culture

When a patient complains of a sore throat and has a fever the physician considers the possibility of strep throat, an infection by group A *Streptococcus*. Rapid immunological tests that give results within minutes can be performed to test for group A *Streptococcus*. If the rapid test for strep A is negative, many facilities have a policy of performing a throat culture to confirm the negative result. It is important to know if the sore throat is caused by *S. pyogenes* because an untreated infection, especially in children and young adults under the age of 25 years, can cause complications such as scarlet fever, rheumatic fever, rheumatic endocarditis, or glomerulonephritis.

The sterile swab should be touched to the tonsils only; touching the tongue and inside of the mouth will contaminate the swab with the normal flora of the mouth (Figure 7-7A). If the culture is to be performed on-site, the swab can be streaked immediately onto a blood agar plate. The plate must be labeled with a printed barcode label or with permanent marker on the bottom of the plate with the patient's name and date of test.

Preparing a Throat Swab for Transport

When a specimen is to be transported to a reference laboratory, several steps must be taken to ensure that the organism remains viable until being placed on growth medium. The swab must be placed in a container that is capable of providing the correct environment, such as moisture, temperature, and oxygen requirements, until the bacteria present on the swab can be inoculated onto blood agar in the reference laboratory (Figure 7-7B). The test requisition

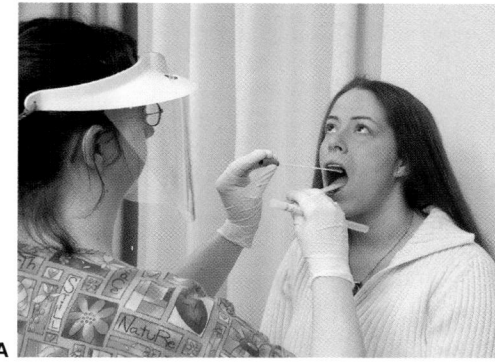

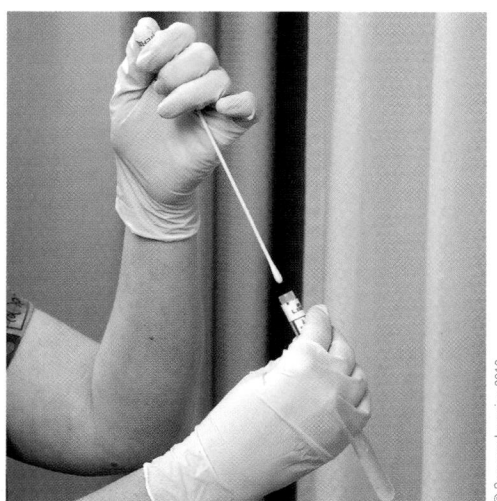

FIGURE 7-7 Throat culture: (A) swabbing the throat; and (B) placing specimen swab into transport media

form and specimen label must be completed and included with the specimen when it is transported to the laboratory (Figure 7-8). Many types of swab/transport systems are available that supply the conditions required to maintain viability of throat organisms until transfer to growth media.

Nasal Cultures

Nasal cultures can be performed for a variety of reasons: to identify **carriers** of drug-resistant bacteria, to aid a physician in ruling out infection by the whooping cough bacterium, *Bordetella pertussis,* and for detection of *Corynebacterium diptheriae,* the bacterium that causes diphtheria. Whooping cough and diphtheria, which occur primarily in children, must be identified so appropriate treatment can begin and prophylactic measures can be taken among close contacts with the infected child. Nasal specimens can also be collected for detection of viruses such as rhinoviruses, influenza viruses, or respiratory syncytial virus (RSV).

Healthcare personnel who are carriers of resistant bacteria, such as the multi-antibiotic resistant *Staphylococcus aureus* known as methicillin-resistant *S. aureus* (MRSA), pose certain risks to patients and coworkers because carriers can unknowingly transmit the bacteria to others. Carriers of MRSA can be identified by culturing nasal swab specimens.

Special nasopharyngeal swabs with flexible shafts are used for collecting nasal specimens. Two swabs are used, one for each nasal cavity. To collect the nasal specimen, a swab moistened with sterile saline is used to gently swab the nasal cavity. The swab is inserted into the anterior nostril about 2 cm and rotated gently against the nasal mucosa to collect material from all surfaces. If any resistance is felt the swab should be withdrawn. Each swab is placed into a separate transport system containing appropriate transport media specified in the SOP manual. If pertussis is suspected, a calcium alginate swab is used; rayon or cotton swabs cannot be used because the fibers are toxic to *B.pertussis.* These swabs must be placed in Regan-Lowe transport medium, a special medium to keep the pertussis organisms viable until they reach the laboratory.

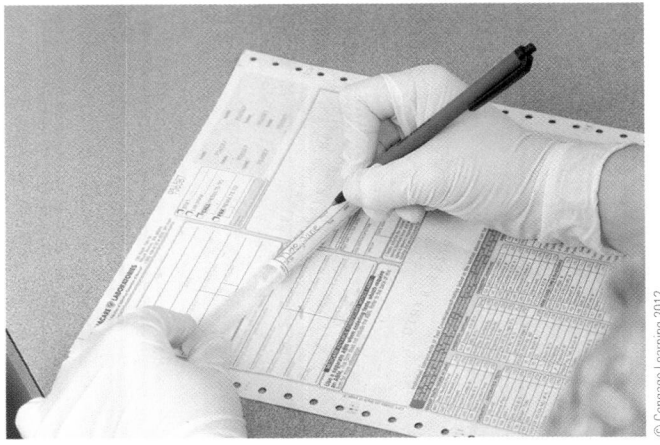

FIGURE 7-8 Labeling the specimen and completing the requisition form

Urine for Culture

The urine specimen for culture must be collected in a sterile container (Figure 7-9A) using the clean-catch method. The patient is instructed to cleanse the area around the urethral opening with antiseptic wipes to avoid contamination of urine by

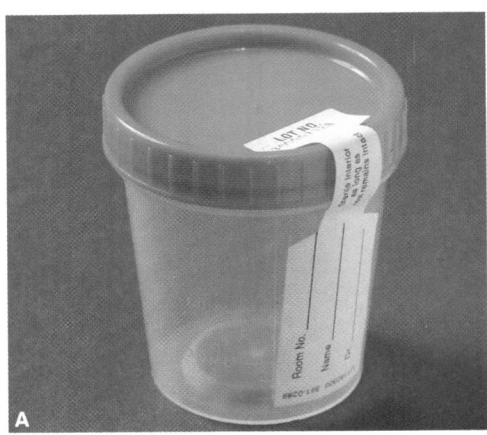

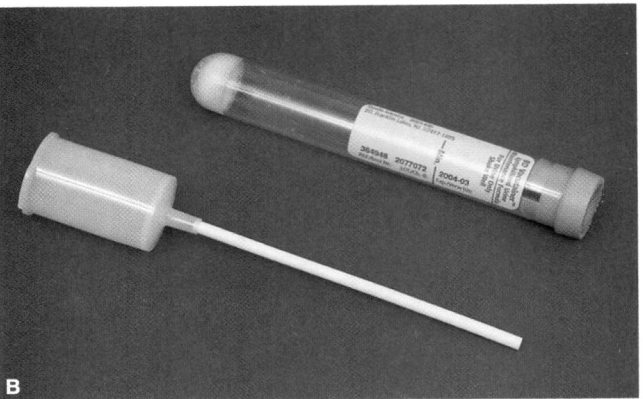

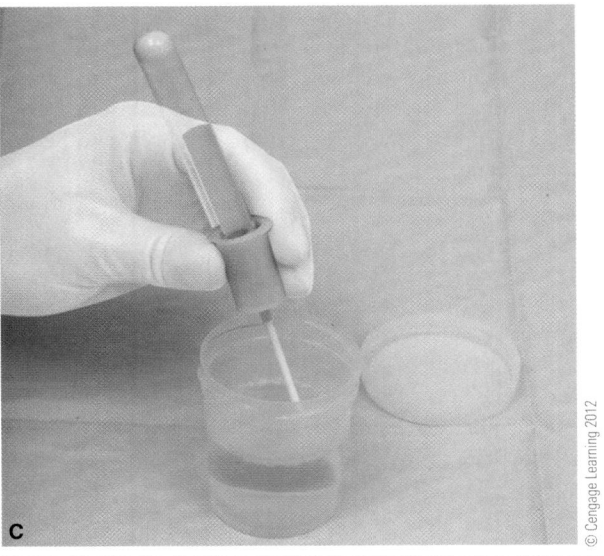

FIGURE 7-9 Collection supplies for urine culture: (A) Sealed, sterile urine cup with lid; (B) sterile urine transport system; and (C) transferring urine into sterile transport tube

skin microorganisms, epithelial cells, and mucus; the urine is then collected midstream. Restrooms used for urine collection should have a poster placed near the toilet with the collection instructions in several languages. The urine container must be labeled on the side of the container, not on the lid, which could be accidentally switched to another container. Collection of urine for culture is detailed in Lesson 5-2 and the urine culture procedure is explained in Lesson 7-6.

Processing the Urine for Transport

The SOP manual should be consulted for urine processing requirements. A general procedure is that if the urine cannot be cultured within 1 hour after collection, a portion of the specimen can be transferred to a sterile tube that contains a special preservative. An example of this kind of container is the B-D Vacutainer Urine C & S Transport kit. The kit includes a sterile vacutainer system that is used to draw an aliquot of well-mixed urine into a tube containing a freeze-dried urine preservative that prevents the overgrowth of bacteria during transport without harming any bacteria present in the specimen (Figure 7-9B, C).

Wound Specimens

A wound is any opening or break in the soft tissue or trauma to the soft tissue. A wound is cultured when it is not healing or when it has the appearance of being infected. Most small laboratories do not culture specimens from wounds because of the many types of microorganism(s) that can cause the infection, the different types of media required, and the varying growth environments that might be required. Facility policy usually allows only the physician or physician's assistant to aspirate material from a wound or to swab a wound. The person collecting the specimen (swab or aspirate) from a wound must have the transport supplies necessary to keep the microorganisms viable until the specimen can be transferred to growth media. The instructions in the SOP manual must be followed; failure to choose the correct system can result in the microorganisms dying before being cultured.

Material aspirated from the wound is preferred to a swab of the wound. The swab is more prone to drying and in addition may not pick up sufficient bacteria for culture. If anaerobic organisms are suspected, a small biopsy sample from the margins of the wound should be collected.

If a swab is used, it should be from a transport system that can support the growth of aerobic and anaerobic microorganisms. Two systems from Remel are the Bacti-Swab, a gel collection and transport system that supports a wide range of bacteria including anaerobes, and the A.C.T. II system, which supports aerobic, anaerobic, and facultative bacteria in a non-nutritive medium that eliminates over-growth of the microorganisms. The BD BBL Port-A-Cul collection and transport system for anaerobic bacteria is designed to keep the miocroorganisms viable for up to 72 hours. Fisherfinest Transport from Thermo Fisher Scientific contains Amies clear, a medium that provides excellent survival for a variety of bacteria. The swab in this system can also be used to make a bacterial smear to be Gram-stained for microscopic examination.

Respiratory Specimens

The causative agents for colds and flu are viruses, and cultures are not normally performed for them. However, if it appears that the patient has developed a secondary bacterial infection of the lower respiratory system (such as pneumonia), a culture of sputum can be performed to identify the organism(s) responsible. *Sputum* is material coughed up from the lungs and is examined to aid in diagnosis of a lower respiratory tract infection, usually in the lungs. Two bacterial species that often cause pneumonia are *Streptococcus pneumoniae* and *Klebsiella pneumoniae.*

The patient can either be given instructions on collecting the specimen or be directed to the respiratory therapy department where a respiratory therapist or technician can assist in collection. The patient first rinses the mouth with plain water to reduce the number of oral bacteria present that can contaminate the sputum sample. For optimum recovery of organisms, it is best to collect two separate specimens in sterile containers with lids. One type of collection container is the BD Sputum Collection System which is a large sterile tube with a funnel-like insert to direct the specimen into the tube (Figure 7-10). The specimen is labeled on the side of the container with the patient's barcode or using a permanent marker.

Sputum specimens are usually sent to the hospital or regional reference laboratory for culture. Liquid specimens such as sputum should be placed in a biohazard transport bag that has a separate compartment for the paperwork. Transport bags are often included with the sputum collection system.

Stool Specimens

Stool cultures can be requested when a patient has had a prolonged period of diarrhea, especially if mucus and blood are present in the stools. Infections can result from ingesting food

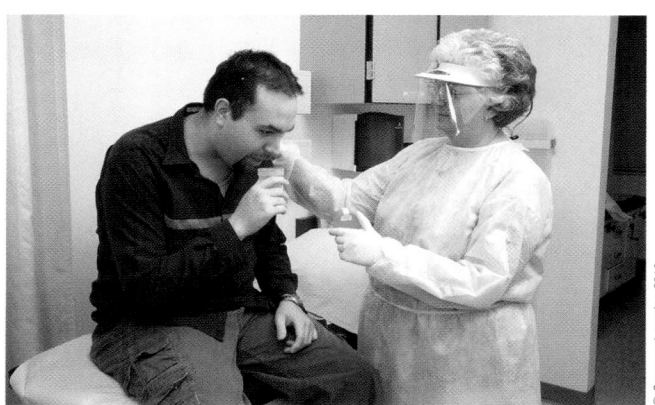

FIGURE 7-10 Assisting a patient in the collection of a sputum specimen

or water contaminated with pathogens such as *Escherichia coli* (*E. coli*), especially *E. coli* 0157:H7, or *Salmonella* species. Other bacteria that can cause intestinal infections are *Clostridium difficile* and species of *Shigella*, *Campylobacter*, and *Vibrio*.

Usually one stool specimen a day is collected on 3 consecutive days. The patient should be given three vials that contain an enteric transport medium such as Cary Blair medium or Amies medium (Figure 7-11). The type of medium used is determined by the organisms that are suspected. The stool specimen is collected so that it is not contaminated with urine or water. One helpful device that can be used fits on the commode seat. A wooden applicator or spork included with some vials can be used to transfer a small portion of the stool into one of the vials. The vial should be placed into a biohazard transport bag to be taken to the laboratory. Stool specimens from babies should not be collected in disposable diapers; these often contain bacterostatic chemicals.

Blood Cultures

Blood cultures are ordered when a patient has symptoms of sepsis or septicemia, conditions that are caused by the presence of microorganisms and their products in the bloodstream. Both conditions are life-threatening; the rapid identification of these causative organisms is essential in order that the patient receive the correct treatment for the infection.

Blood cultures are collected by venipuncture. The venipuncture site must be cleansed much more thoroughly than for a routine venipuncture. If cleansing is not thorough, skin bacteria or fungi can contaminate the culture and produce a false-positive blood culture. This could result in the patient receiving unnecessary treatment or allow a true pathogen to be undetected.

The venipuncture site is cleansed first with alcohol to remove dirt and skin oils. This cleansing is performed in a circular motion, starting at the center of the site and moving outward in a circular motion. The site is next cleansed in a circular motion using a swab containing a 2% solution of tincture of iodine or povidone iodine. The iodine must be allowed to completely dry on the skin to be effective. Kits containing an alcohol scrub pad and iodine swab are available for blood culture collections. If the patient is allergic to iodine products, the venipuncture site can be cleansed with alcohol followed by chlorhexidine.

Sterile gloves should be worn by the phlebotomist collecting blood culture samples. In the order of draw, blood culture bottles are filled first. Two bottles are usually collected for blood cultures, one for culturing aerobic bacteria and one for culturing anaerobes. The facility's collection manual will contain instructions and acceptance criteria for blood culture specimens.

The aerobic bottle is filled first. The protective cap is removed from the top of the bottles, revealing a rubber septum that must be wiped with a sterile alcohol swab before being used. The blood is drawn by venipuncture using a special holder (such as Saf-T holder, Smiths' Medical), to fit the vacuum bottles which have long, narrow necks (Figure 7-12).

BD BBL markets four different types of bottles in their SEPTI-CHEK blood culture systems. BD also makes the Bactec System. In the Bactec system, blood culture bottles are inoculated and placed into the Bactec instrument which contains an incubator with a moving track. Each culture bottle contains a sensor that responds to changes in CO_2, which is released as microorganisms grow. Every few minutes, the bottles pass by a detector that monitors the sensors for increases in CO_2, therefore detecting which bottles contain growing cultures. A smear of the blood from the "positive" bottle can be made and Gram-stained to obtain a preliminary identification on the type of microorganism present.

The Trek Diagnostic ESP EZ Draw is a different type of culture bottle. These bottles draw only 0.1 mL of blood. After thorough mixing these bottles are transported to the laboratory where the blood can be plated directly onto appropriate types of solid media and incubated.

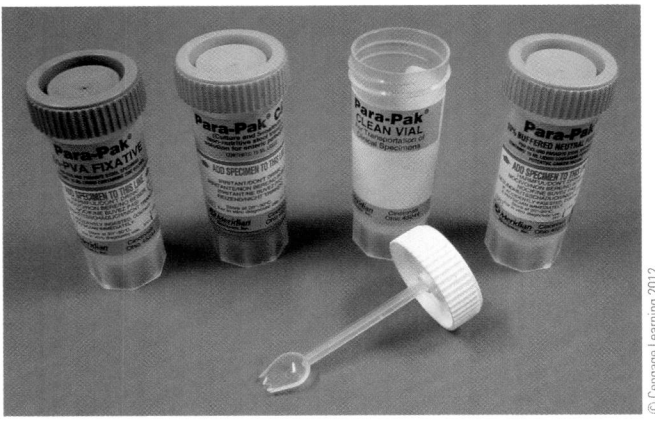

FIGURE 7-11 Examples of containers for collecting stool specimens: the two center containers (orange top and white top) can be used for stool culture; containers such as those on the far left and far right (green top and pink top) cannot be used for culture because they contain preservatives

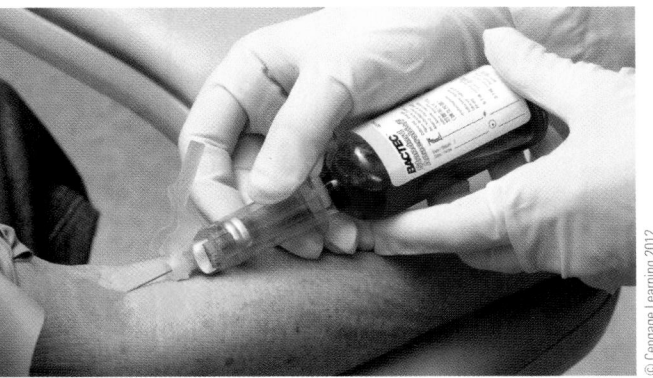

FIGURE 7-12 Collecting a blood culture

TABLE 7-13. Consequences associated with incorrect collection of specimens for culture

SITE/SPECIMEN CULTURED	POTENTIAL COLLECTION PROBLEM(S)	POSSIBLE CONSEQUENCES
Throat	Insufficient specimen; oral/pharyngeal surfaces swabbed	*S. pyogenes* not recovered; contaminating organisms present
Nasal	Swab(s) not premoistened Incorrect type of swab	Insufficient specimen collected Fibers of swab toxic for target organisms
Urine	Insufficient cleansing of urethral opening and surroundings	Contaminating organisms present
Respiratory	Saliva collected instead of sputum	Failure to recover lung pathogen(s)
Stool		
Adult	Collected with urine and/or toilet water	Contamination, failure to recover pathogen(s)
Infants	Collected in disposable, bacteriostatic diapers	No microorganisms survive
Wound	Aspirate or biopsy specimen not collected	Insufficient specimen; specimen dries before culture is set up
Blood	Incomplete cleansing of venipuncture site Failure to sterilize tops of culture bottles	Contamination by skin flora Contamination by environmental bacteria

CASE STUDY 1

Carol was working in a point-of-care testing (POCT) site. A rapid test for group A strep was negative on a 10-year-old boy. The provider ordered a confirmatory throat culture for *S. pyogenes*. Carol collected another throat specimen with a sterile swab. Several patients were waiting for laboratory tests. Carol had to decide whether to set up the culture immediately or wait until after she collected blood samples for the other patients.

1. Carol should:
   a. Place the swab back into the original package until she has time to set up the culture
   b. Place the swab into an open test tube on the counter until she can set up the culture
   c. Let the patients wait while she sets up the culture from the swab
2. How could Carol have avoided her dilemma?

CASE STUDY 2

Rick had performed a rapid test for group A strep on a young child. The result was negative. He knew the laboratory protocol required that a confirmatory culture be performed; however, the child did not seem very ill. His thinking was "Why waste time processing a throat culture when it would probably be negative?"

A. Evaluate the following statements for correctness:
   T F 1. *S. pyogenes* infections have no risk of complications
   T F 2. Rick must follow the laboratory protocol
   T F 3. A throat culture swab should be inoculated to a blood agar plate
B. Have a class discussion about Rick's attitude. Include topics such as professionalism, ethics, best practices for patient care, and job responsibility

CASE STUDY 3

Two different organisms normally found on skin were isolated from a blood culture. No pathogenic organisms were isolated.

Choose from the answers below for the most likely reason(s) for the culture results.

A. The phlebotomist used sterile gloves instead of plain vinyl gloves

B. The phlebotomist cleaned the septum of the culture bottle with alcohol followed by iodine

C. The venipuncture site was cleansed using an alcohol swab

D. All of the above

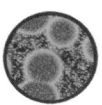

SUMMARY

Collection and processing of specimens for culture is an important component in ensuring that cultures yield useful results. The laboratory's SOP manual contains instructions for collecting the specimen and selecting the transport media. Patient cooperation is essential to culture success for specimens such as urine and stools. Failure to follow the prescribed protocol can result in failure of cultures to grow or contamination of cultures and delay important patient treatment (Table 7-13).

In recent years, incidences of food contamination have received publicity, especially when some infections resulted in fatalities. Infants and the elderly can be especially susceptible to serious illness from foodborne microorganisms. Rapid identification of pathogens in situations such as these can make a difference in patient outcomes. Peanut butter processing plants were contaminated with *Salmonella*, causing shutdown of the plants and recall of peanut butter products. *E. coli* 0157:H7, a virulent strain of *E. coli*, has been found in contaminated ground beef as well as other cases of food contamination. When all protocols are followed, a culture can provide important or critical information to be used in identification and treatment of the microorganism(s) responsible for the patient's illness.

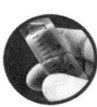

REVIEW QUESTIONS

1. What can cause contamination of a throat swab during collection?

2. What mistakes can occur in the collection of urine for culture?

3. Explain why stool specimens collected in an infant's disposable diaper may not grow microorganisms.

4. Why should the patient rinse the mouth with water before collecting a sputum specimen?

5. Why is an aspirate of a wound preferred over a swab?

6. Why are both alcohol and an iodine preparation used in the collection of blood cultures?

7. Discuss why wound specimens are usually sent to regional reference or hospital laboratories.

8. List three important properties of transport systems for bacteriology specimens.

9. What culture can be performed to determine if a person is a carrier of methicillin-resistant *Staphylococcus aureus* (MRSA)?

10. Define carrier, culture, culture medium, *Escherichia coli*, sepsis, septicemia, *Streptococcus pyogenes*, transport medium, virulent, and wound.

STUDENT ACTIVITIES

1. Complete the written examination for this lesson.

2. Design a patient instruction card explaining how to collect a stool specimen for culture.

WEB ACTIVITIES

1. Search the Internet for infections and complications (other than mentioned in this lesson) caused by *S. pyogenes* infections and prepare a brief report on them.

2. Search the Internet for sputum collection systems for mycobacteria. Choose two and report on their use.

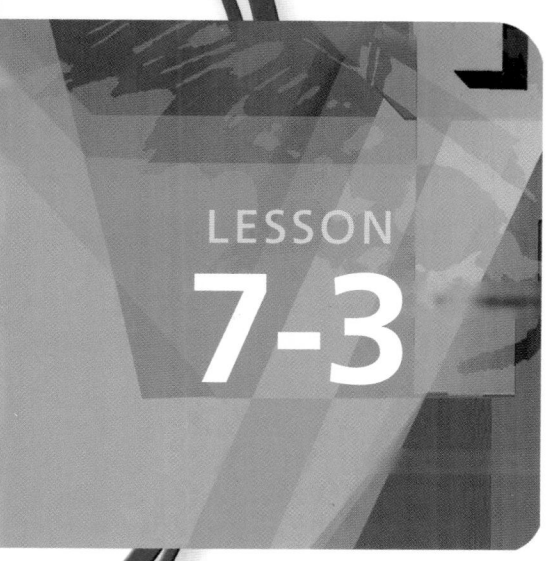

Culture Techniques for Bacteriology

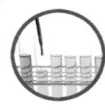

LESSON OBJECTIVES

After studying this lesson, the student will:

- ⊙ Explain the use of aseptic technique in bacteriology.
- ⊙ Explain the differences between antiseptics and disinfectants and discuss how each is used used.
- ⊙ Describe the different types of biological safety cabinets.
- ⊙ Explain the differences in primary, selective, and indicator media.
- ⊙ Describe how to inoculate different forms of media.
- ⊙ Demonstrate the method for inoculating an agar plate and streaking for isolated colonies.
- ⊙ Discuss why different incubation conditions are required for growing cultures of bacterial pathogens.
- ⊙ Discuss safety precautions that must be observed when performing bacterial culture techniques.
- ⊙ Explain the quality assessment procedures involved in culturing bacteria.
- ⊙ Define the glossary terms.

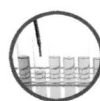

GLOSSARY

agar / a seaweed derivative used to solidify microbiological media

antiseptic / a chemical used on living tissues to control the growth of infectious agents

aseptic technique / work practices used to prevent contamination when working with microorganisms

disinfectant / a chemical used on inanimate objects to kill or inactivate microbes

enriched medium / a medium that contains nutrients to support a wide variety of organisms, including fastidious organisms

hemolysis / the rupture or destruction of red blood cells resulting in the release of hemoglobin

HEPA filter / high-efficiency particulate air filter used in biological safety cabinets

indicator medium / a bacteriological medium that differentiates bacteria on the basis of certain chemical reactions; differential medium

inoculating loop / an instrument used to transfer bacteria

inoculation / the process of transferring microorganisms to a growth medium

inoculum / the microorganisms transferred from one medium to another

isolated colonies / bacterial colonies growing on an agar surface and not touched by other colonies

(continues)

primary medium / a medium that provides nutritional requirements for an microorganism and is used to recover the microorganism from a specimen

quadrant / one-fourth of a circle; one-fourth of an agar plate

selective medium / a bacteriological medium that contains chemicals or substances that allow growth of some organisms while inhibiting growth of others

sterilization / the act of eliminating all living microorganisms from an article or area

INTRODUCTION

Certain basic techniques must be mastered to work in the bacteriology laboratory. Personnel must be trained in the correct selection and use of growth media, equipment, and reagents. Safe work practices must be followed when working with bacterial cultures to prevent contamination of the worker and the environment. Technicians must be proficient in aseptic techniques, use of inoculating loops, and culture techniques. Lesson 1-4 on biological safety should be reviewed before beginning this lesson.

ASEPTIC TECHNIQUE

Aseptic technique is usually thought of as a set of procedures used to prevent spread of infection during surgical procedures. However, in the bacteriology laboratory, aseptic technique includes physical and chemical means of preventing contamination as well as the use of appropriate work practices and bacteriological culture techniques. Aseptic technique incorporates safe work practices to:

- Prevent workers from becoming infected with microorganisms in patient specimens
- Protect workers from exposure to bacteria from cultures
- Prevent contamination of work surfaces with bacteria
- Prevent cross-contamination of cultures
- Prevent contamination of bacterial cultures by environmental contaminants

Physical Barriers

The use of physical barriers is one method of preventing contamination in the bacteriology laboratory. Examples of physical barriers include protective clothing, correct use of equipment and supplies, and the use of biological safety cabinets.

Protective Clothing

There are several ways to incorporate aseptic technique into laboratory procedures. Wearing a fluid-resistant laboratory coat protects the technician from contamination, and the long sleeves protect the culture from contamination. Disposable laboratory coats or gowns should be worn and discarded at the end of the day or anytime they become contaminated. Laboratory coats should not be worn outside the microbiology laboratory.

Safe Use of Equipment

Inoculating loops, used to transfer bacteria, are available as disposable, single-use loops in sterile packages. These come in different styles, so the manufacturer's instructions for their use should be followed. Disposable loops should be discarded into appropriate biohazard containers immediately after used.

If disposable loops are not available, reusable wire inoculating loops can be used. These loops must be heat-sterilized and cooled before and after each use. Loops can be sterilized over an open flame such as a Bunsen burner, but use of an electric incinerator is much safer (Figure 7-13). The loop is sterilized by inserting 2-3 inches of the loop into the incinerator opening. Once the wire loop begins to glow it is carefully withdrawn from the incinerator and allowed to cool without allowing the sterile portion of the loop to touch any surfaces. When the loop has cooled, it is used to transfer an isolated colony from a culture, streak an agar plate, inoculate a tube of media, or make a bacterial smear.

Recent research has shown that the majority of laboratory-acquired infections occur by the respiratory route. Therefore, care must be taken to prevent aerosol formation when the inoculating loop is sterilized. Reusable inoculating loops should never be laid on the countertop but must always be sterilized after use and placed in the loop rack.

Microbiological Safety Cabinets

Microbiological safety cabinets are specially designed laminar flow cabinets that protect the worker from infectious agents. Most laboratories have a class I or class II safety cabinet. Class I cabinets protect the worker and the environment but do not protect the culture. Class II cabinets provide protection to

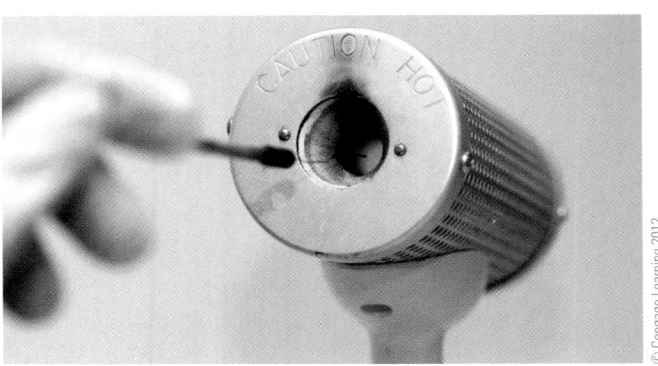

FIGURE 7-13 Sterilizing an inoculating loop using an electric incinerator

© Cengage Learning 2012

the worker, the environment, and the culture (Figure 7-14). Although routine bacteriological work does not require the use of a safety cabinet, all work with pathogenic fungi, *Mycobacterium*, and certain other highly infectious agents must be performed using a class II cabinet.

The class II cabinet operates by drawing air from the room, around the operator, into the front grille of the cabinet, and then into a special *high-efficiency particulate air filter*, called a **HEPA filter**. This filtered air then enters the work chamber from the top and is drawn downward, with the airflow splitting as it nears the work surface. Part of the air is drawn through the front grille and the rest through the back grille, providing a particulate-free environment above the work area inside the cabinet. The air then passes through the exhaust HEPA filter or the supply HEPA filter

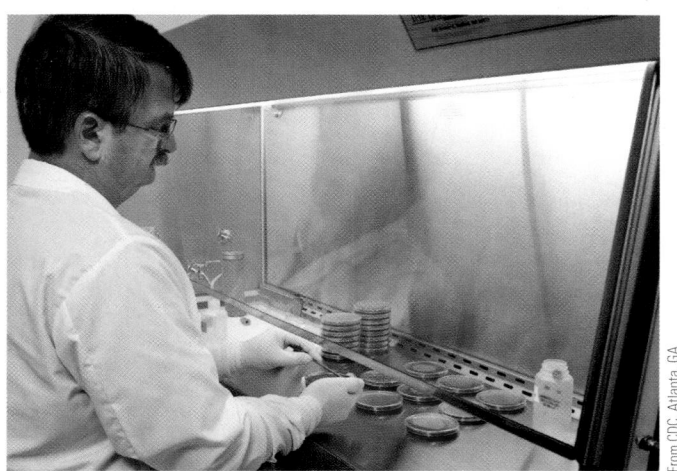

FIGURE 7-14 Working in a biological safety cabinet in the microbiology laboratory

back into the hood. Aseptic technique must still be used when working with cultures, even when using a safety cabinet.

Disinfectants and Antiseptics

Disinfectants, chemicals used to kill or control the growth of microorganisms on inanimate objects, are used liberally and frequently in the bacteriology laboratory. Disinfectants are effective against most bacteria, as well as some viruses and fungi (Table 7-14). Disinfectants labeled *bactericidal* kill bacteria; those labeled *bacteriostatic* only slow or inhibit the growth of bacteria. Disinfectants that kill microorganisms in their active, vegetative states (stages) are not always effective against the more resistant spore (resting) stages.

Disinfectants must be used liberally and *often* on work surfaces. Disinfection does not sterilize a surface; it only reduces the number of microorganisms to a low level, rather than killing all microorganisms present. Disinfectant should be applied to countertops before beginning a procedure and after the work is completed. In addition, work areas should be wiped frequently with disinfectant and any time a spill or splash occurs. The effectiveness of a disinfectant is influenced by its concentration, the numbers and types of microorganisms present, the pH, contact time, and temperature. The presence of protein or other organic material can reduce the effectiveness of disinfectants (Table 7-15).

Antiseptics are chemicals used to control the growth of microorganisms on living tissue. Antiseptic soaps, gels, or foams are used to clean hands before donning gloves, after removing gloves, and any other time hands become contaminated. Labels on disinfectants and antiseptics provide information about the products' effectiveness against various microorganisms. Table 7-14 lists categories of disinfectants and antiseptics and the types of organisms for which they are effective.

TABLE 7-14. Disinfectants and antiseptics commonly used in microbiology

CHEMICAL NAME OR COMMON NAME	EFFECTIVE AGAINST*	USE
Alcohols, 70%–90% (isopropanol, ethanol)	Bacteria, *Mycobacterium*, and some viruses	Antiseptic and disinfectant
Alcohol-based gel or foam hand rubs	Bacteria and viruses, some *Mycobacterium* species	Antiseptic
Iodine, povidone iodine	Bacteria, fungi, viruses, protozoa	Antiseptic
10% chlorine bleach	Especially good for viruses	Disinfectant
Phenolics (Amphyl)	Most bacteria and viruses; *Mycobacterium*	Disinfectant
Quaternary ammonium salts (QUATS)	Bacteria, some fungi	Disinfectant
RelyOn (DuPont)	HAV, HBV, HCV, HIV-1, *E. coli*, MRSA	Disinfectant
Germicidal Surface Wipes (Steris)	*Mycobacterium tuberculosis*, RSV, VRE	Disinfectant

* HAV, HBV, HCV = hepatitis A, B, and C viruses
HIV = human immunodeficiency virus
RSV = respiratory syncytial virus
VRE = vancomycin-resistant enterococci.

TABLE 7-15. Factors influencing the effectiveness of disinfectants and antiseptics

Contact time
Temperature
pH
Concentration of chemical
Number of organisms present
Presence of organic matter, such as protein and blood

Sterilization

Sterilization is a method that frees an article or area from all living organisms. Sterilization is most commonly performed by autoclaving. Bacterial spores, protective forms that certain bacteria can assume, are resistant to many disinfectants and can best be killed by steam sterilization in an autoclave. Although sterilization by autoclave is preferable, items that cannot be heat-sterilized can be sterilized by exposure to chemicals such as aldehydes, peroxides, and chlorine dioxide or ethylene oxide gases.

GROWTH MEDIA FOR CLINICAL BACTERIOLOGY

A bacteriological medium is a nutritive substance used to culture bacteria in the laboratory. The medium can be a liquid broth or a solid medium, such as tubes or plates of media containing agar (Figure 7-15). **Agar** is a derivative of seaweed used to solidify liquid media. In the bacteriology laboratory, the function of media is to help recover, grow, isolate, and identify bacteria.

Primary Media

The **primary medium** is the one first inoculated with the specimen collected from the patient (Figure 7-16A). The choice of primary medium is important and can determine the success of recovering the infection-causing agent. The primary medium is chosen based on the site of the infection; for example, the primary medium selected for a wound culture would be different from that used for a urethral culture (Tables 7-16 and 7-17).

The most common primary medium is sheep's blood agar, commonly called blood agar, which supports the growth of most bacteria. An **enriched medium** is one that supports the growth of a wide variety of organisms, including fastidious organisms—those requiring special nutritional factors. Chocolate agar is an example of an enriched medium; it contains blood that has been heat-treated at 40° to 45° C and is used to support growth of organisms such as *Neisseria*.

Selective Media

A **selective medium** contains ingredients that inhibit the growth of certain microorganisms while allowing the growth of others. Two examples of selective media are eosin methylene blue (EMB) and MacConkey's (MAC), shown in Figures 7-16 and 7-17. Both of these media promote the growth of gram-negative bacteria while inhibiting the growth of gram-positive bacteria. Using a selective medium increases the chances of recovering a particular organism from a mixed bacterial population (Tables 7-16 and

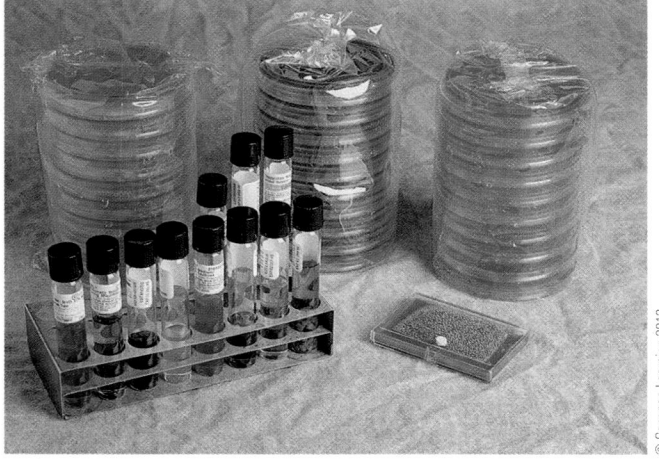

FIGURE 7-15 Various types of media used in bacteriology

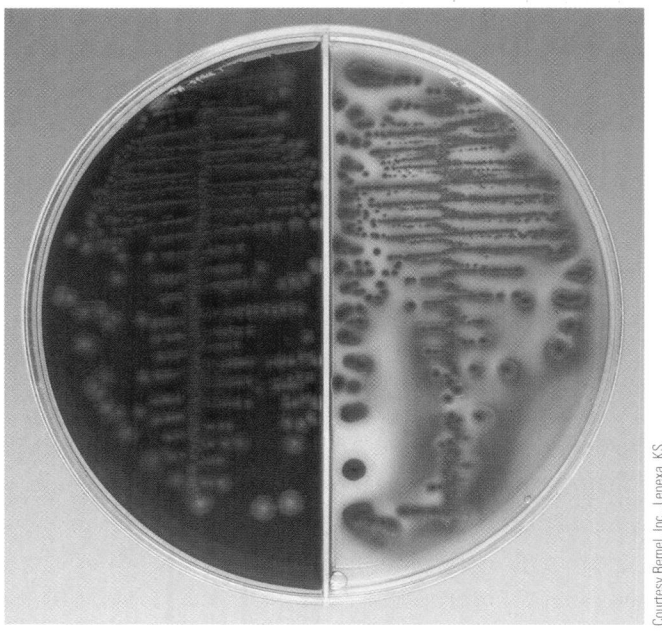

FIGURE 7-16 *Escherichia coli* growth on primary and selective media: gram-negative *E. coli* inoculated to split plate containing blood agar (left side of plate) and MAC (right side of plate)

TABLE 7-16. Common specimens for culture, examples of possible organisms present, media recommendations, and culture conditions, including carbon dioxide requirements

SPECIMEN	POSSIBLE ORGANISMS	RECOMMENDED MEDIA*	CULTURE CONDITIONS†
Urine	*E. coli* *Klebsiella* *Proteus* *Pseudomonas aeruginosa* *Enterococcus*	BA and EMB or MAC	Ambient air‡
Throat	*Streptococcus pyogenes*	BA	$\downarrow O_2$, 5-10% CO_2
Sputum	*Streptococcus pneumoniae*	BA	$\downarrow O_2$, 5-10% CO_2
Wounds	*Staphylococcus* sp. *Streptococcus* sp. *Enterobacter* sp.	BA, CA, and EMB or MAC	$\downarrow O_2$, 5-10% CO_2
Wound	Anaerobic bacteria	Thio, enzyme-reduced agar plates	Anaerobic environment
Vaginal/urethral	*Neisseria gonorrhoeae*	BA, CA, T-M	$\downarrow O_2$, 5-10% CO_2
Stool	*Salmonella* *Shigella* Pathogenic *E. coli*	SS, HE, EMB or MAC, selenite medium	Ambient air
Cerebrospinal fluid	*Neisseria meningitidis* *Haemophilus influenzae* *Streptococcus pneumoniae*	BA, CA, Thio H. isol. Medium BA	$\downarrow O_2$, 5-10% CO_2 $\downarrow O_2$, 5-10% CO_2 Ambient air
Eye, ear	*Neisseria gonorrhoeae* *Haemophilus* species *Pseudomonas aeruginosa* *Staphylococcus aureus* *Streptococcus pyogenes*	BA, CA, T-M H. isol. Medium BA and EMB **or MAC** BA BA	$\downarrow O_2$, 5-10% CO_2 $\downarrow O_2$, 5-10% CO_2 Ambient air Ambient air Ambient air

† All cultures incubated at 35–37° C

‡ Ambient air = normal air, normal atmospheric gas concentrations

* $\downarrow O_2$ = oxygen concentration below normal atmospheric oxygen, BA = blood agar, CA = chocolate agar, MAC = MacConkey, SS = *Salmonella-Shigella,* HE = Hektoen enteric, T-M = Thayer Martin, Thio = thioglycolate, H. isol. medium = *Haemophilus* isolation medium

7-17). Figure 7-18 shows black colonies of *Salmonella* growing on Hektoen agar, a selective medium.

Indicator Media

An **indicator medium,** or differential medium, detects metabolic activity of particular microorganisms. Indicator media show chemical reactions of bacteria (such as fermentation of sugars) demonstrated by a color change in the bacterial colony or in the medium. One example of an indicator medium is MAC, which produces a pink color when inoculated with an organism that ferments lactose (Figure 7-16B). Some media, such as EMB and MAC, contain ingredients that make them function as both indicator and selective media (Table 7-17). The characteristics of growth on primary, selective, and indicator media can be valuable clues to a microorganism's identity. Table 7-17 gives examples of primary, selective, and indicator media, their principal ingredients, and reactions.

Anaerobic Media

Growing and identifying anaerobic cultures requires special expertise. Anaerobic organisms can be cultured using either regular media such as blood agar incubated in an anaerobic environment, or specially manufactured media for anaerobes. Agar plates inoculated with specimens suspected of containing anaerobic bacteria, such as cultures from deep wounds, can be incubated in special sealed bags or containers that include a generator pack to create an anaerobic environment. Anaerobic cultures can also be inoculated to tubed media, such as thioglycolate broth and incubated with the tubes tightly capped to create the anaerobic environment.

TABLE 7-17. Common types of media for bacteriology*

TYPE OF MEDIUM	EXAMPLE	ACTIVE INGREDIENT(S)	PURPOSE
Primary	BA	Sheep or rabbit blood	Supports wide range of organisms; demonstrates hemolysis
Primary	CA, MTM	Heated blood	Provides hemoglobin and growth factors for fastidious organisms
Primary	Thio	Thioglycolate, L-cystine	Anaerobic and microaerophilic organisms
Selective	EMB	Eosin y, methylene blue	Inhibits gram-positive organisms
Indicator	EMB	Eosin-methylene blue complex	Indicates fermentation of lactose, sucrose
Selective	HE	Bile salts, acid fuchsin, bromthymol blue	Isolates and differentiates *Salmonella* and *Shigella*
Selective	SS	Bile salts, phenol red	Isolates and differentiates *Salmonella* and *Shigella*
Selective	MAC	Bile salts, crystal violet	Inhibits gram-positive organisms
Indicator	MAC	Neutral red	Indicates fermentation of lactose

BA = blood agar, CA = chocolate agar, EMB = eosin-methylene blue medium, HE = Hektoen enteric, MAC = MacConkey's medium, MTM = modified Thayer-Martin medium, SS = *Salmonella-Shigella*, Thio = thioglycolate medium.
* These are just a few examples of the common media used in small laboratories or physician office laboratories; there are many other media types with specialized uses.

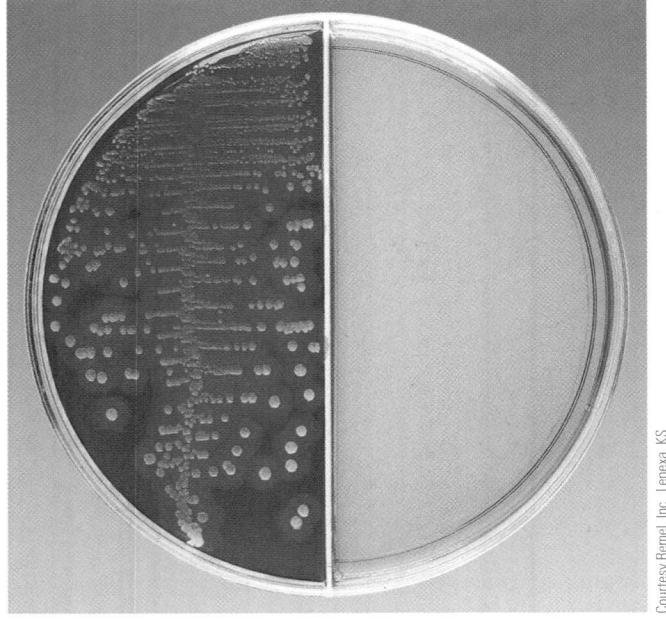

Courtesy Remel, Inc., Lenexa, KS

FIGURE 7-17 *Staphylococcus aureus* inoculated to primary and selective media: gram-positive S. *aureus* grows on blood agar (left side of plate) but growth is inhibited on MAC (right side of plate)

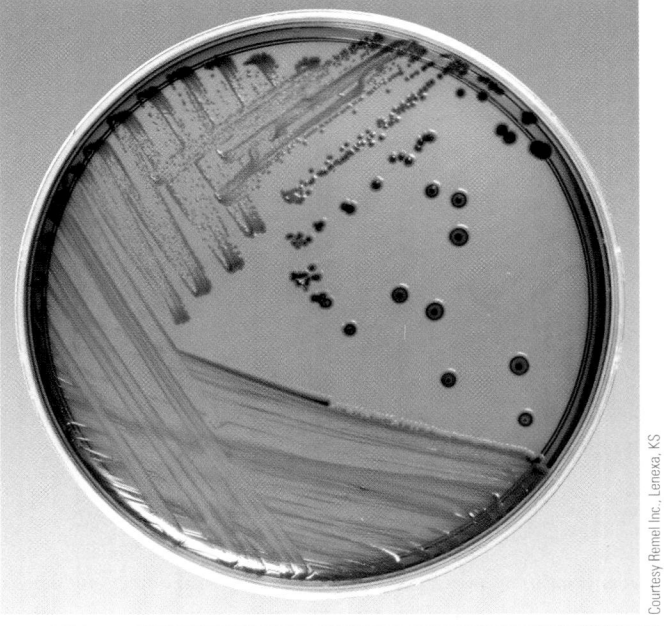

Courtesy Remel Inc., Lenexa, KS

FIGURE 7-18 *Salmonella* growing on Hektoen enteric agar, an indicator medium; note colonies with black centers

Also available are anaerobic media such as OxyPlates and OxyPRAS media (Oxyrase Inc.) OxyPRAS media is pre-reduced-anaerobically sterilized (PRAS) and contains a reducing agent that keeps the agar and the environment inside the plate anaerobic. When the plate is opened, air is introduced. When the lid is replaced, an enzyme reaction chemically reduces the media and the atmosphere above the agar surface. The plates can be incubated in a regular aerobic incubator without the need for special equipment. Tubed media can also have reducing substances such as oxyrase added.

CULTURE TECHNIQUES

In the bacteriology laboratory, culture material must frequently be transferred from one type of medium to another, such as from primary to selective or differential. The process of transferring microorganisms to a growth medium is called **inoculation**. The group of microorganisms being transferred is called the **inoculum**. The first transfer of inoculum is from the site of infection to the primary medium. For example, a throat swab is inoculated to sheep's blood agar. Successful recovery and identification of the disease-causing agent depends on correct collection, processing, and transfer of the inoculum, and use of aseptic technique.

Safety Precautions

  Personnel in the bacteriology laboratory must observe Standard Precautions, remembering that patient specimens can contain bacteria and other potentially infectious material (OPIM). Laboratory personnel should never eat or drink in the laboratory. In addition, makeup, lipstick, lip moisturizers, or lip gloss must not be applied in the laboratory and hands must be washed thoroughly before touching eyes, nose, or mouth.

Personal protective equipment must be worn, including wearing gloves when handling specimens. Hands should be cleansed frequently. Aseptic techniques, physical methods of preventing contamination, and chemical disinfection methods must be combined to ensure that the bacteriology laboratory is a safe working environment. Work surfaces must be wiped with surface disinfectant before and after performing each procedure. Contaminated materials must never be included with general trash. Materials such as used culture media, disposable loops, specimen swabs, and any other supplies that have come in contact with live organisms must be packaged in special biohazard bags and sharps containers, decontaminated, and disposed of according to the facility's protocol. Decontamination is often performed by autoclaving before disposal or by incineration. Medical waste disposal services also are available.

Quality Assessment

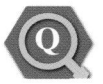   Quality assessment (QA) is an important aspect of bacteriology. A good QA program ensures that media are not contaminated, that they will support growth of organisms, and that indicator and selective media are reacting correctly. A QA program will also help ensure that unknown isolates are correctly identified. The QA program can consist of internal and external components and the requirements of the program are contained in the laboratory's SOP manual.

Internal Quality Assessment Program

The internal QA program includes specimen collection techniques, media checks, reagent quality, equipment performance, and staff proficiency. Commercial sets of control microorganisms can be purchased that meet Clinical Laboratory Standards Institute (CLSI) requirements for testing commercially prepared media, bacterial identification systems, and antibiotic susceptibility testing methods. These commercial controls can also be used to assess personnel performance. A QA program must also include monitoring and recording temperatures of all incubators and refrigerators. Before a new shipment of media is used for patient specimens, one plate or tube from each lot should be incubated in the specified conditions to ensure that no contaminate(s) grow.

External Quality Assessment Program

Laboratories must subscribe to one of several external QA or proficiency testing (PT) programs. Regulatory agencies responsible for laboratory inspections also offer microbiology proficiency programs. These programs ensure that personnel are proficient in isolating and identifying microorganisms.

Collecting and Transporting Specimens

Specimens must be collected correctly to ensure that culture results are valid. Swabs used for most bacteriological procedures are sterile swabs made of polyester (Dacron) or rayon; cotton swabs should not be used because cotton contains ingredients that are toxic to many microorganisms.

Smaller laboratories might only collect the specimens and send them to a reference laboratory for culture. Specimens are sent in a transport medium that provides the necessary nutrients and environment for microorganisms to protect the microorganism from drying and keep them viable during transport. Transport media are available to meet the growth requirements of different types of microorganisms, including aerobic and anaerobic. A variety of transport media and a specimen collection procedure manual are provided by the reference laboratory (see Lesson 7-2). The procedure manual includes recommended uses of the various media and a guide to media selection, based on the site of infection or source of the specimen.

Inoculating the Media

Once the specimen arrives in the laboratory, the specimen should be inoculated to appropriate primary media as soon as possible. Aseptic conditions must be maintained during media inoculation. The risks for aerosol formation can be decreased by careful manipulation of reusable loops or by the use of sterile disposable loops that eliminate the need for heat sterilization. A disposable loop should be discarded into a sharps container immediately after use.

Agar Plate

The agar plate must be labeled with the patient's name and identification number. The plate is always labeled on the *bottom*, not on the lid, because the lid could be accidentally switched from one dish to another.

Inoculating the Plate.
The lid of the agar plate should be lifted just enough to allow inoculation of the agar with the specimen swab or inoculating loop. Otherwise, the lid is always kept on the plate to prevent contaminating the medium and the culture. The agar surface is inoculated by gently rolling the specimen swab onto one **quadrant** of the agar plate (Figure 7-19A). If only one swab is collected, the culture plate should be inoculated first. A bacterial smear can then be prepared by rolling the swab across a sterile glass microscope slide to produce a smear about 0.5 to 1 inch long (Figure 7-19B). The swab is then discarded into a biohazard waste container.

Streaking for Isolated Colonies.
An inoculating loop is used to spread the inoculated material over the agar plate to produce **isolated colonies**, colonies not touching each other. This is accomplished by streaking all four quadrants of a plate, decreasing the amount of culture material as the streaking proceeds into each successive quadrant. Care must be taken to avoid tearing the surface of the agar. The loop is sterilized, cooled, and then is used to spread the material from the first quadrant into the second quadrant (Figure 7-20). The loop is again sterilized and is used to spread material from the second quadrant into the third quadrant, and then from the third into the fourth. In the fourth quadrant, the streaking procedure is done carefully to produce isolated colonies of the bacteria (Figure 7-20).

Agar Slant

Agar slants are prepared by placing tubes of media at an angle while the liquid agar media solidifies. An agar slant tube should be labeled with date and patient information. An agar slant can be inoculated with a specimen directly from a swab, or an inoculating loop can be used to transfer a colony from an agar plate to a slant tube.

To transfer an isolated bacterial colony from an agar plate to a slant tube, a colony growing on an agar plate is touched with a sterile loop (Figure 7-21A). The slant tube is held in the other hand while the fourth and fifth fingers of the hand holding the loop are used to remove the tube's cap (Figure 7-21B). The cap

is not laid down but is held in this way until the tube is recapped after the procedure has been completed. The loop is inserted into the tube and used to make a zigzag pattern on the slant, starting on the slant's far end and ending at the top of the slant, near the mouth of the tube (Figure 7-21C). The loop is withdrawn, the tube is capped, and the loop is sterilized. If the loop or culture material touched the tube's rim, the rim should be sterilized before recapping (Figure 7-21D). If the inoculum is known to be aerobic, the cap should be left slightly loose to allow air to enter the tube; if the tube is being transported, the cap can be screwed tight until it reaches the reference laboratory.

Indicator or Selective Medium

Additional types of media can be required to confirm the identity of bacteria growing on primary media. The isolated colonies growing on the primary plate are transferred to indicator or selective media using a sterile inoculating loop. The lid of the plate of primary medium is raised just enough to insert the sterilized and cooled loop and pick up an isolated colony. The loop is withdrawn, and the indicator/selective medium is inoculated and streaked for isolated colonies. Split plates containing two kinds of media such as BA and EMB or BA and MAC can be used by modifying the streaking method (Figure 7-16).

Incubating the Inoculated Media

Bacteria have different growth requirements depending on the bacterial species. Most human pathogens grow best at 35° to 37° C. Inoculated cultures are usually kept in a 35° to 37° C incubator (Figure 7-22A). Agar plates are incubated inverted (upside down) to prevent the formation of condensate inside the lid. Plates should be stacked in a stabilizing rack. Tubed media such as agar slants are placed in a test tube rack in the incubator.

Bacteria can be aerobic, microaerophilic or anaerobic based on their ability to grow in normal atmospheric oxygen. For aerobic cultures, which are the majority of cultures, the caps of tube cultures should be kept loosened to allow air exchange in the

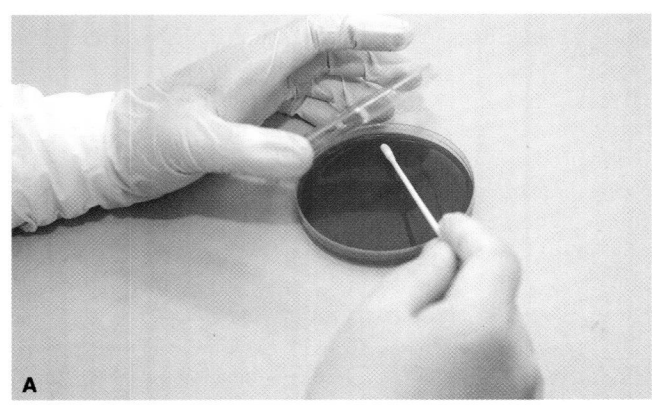
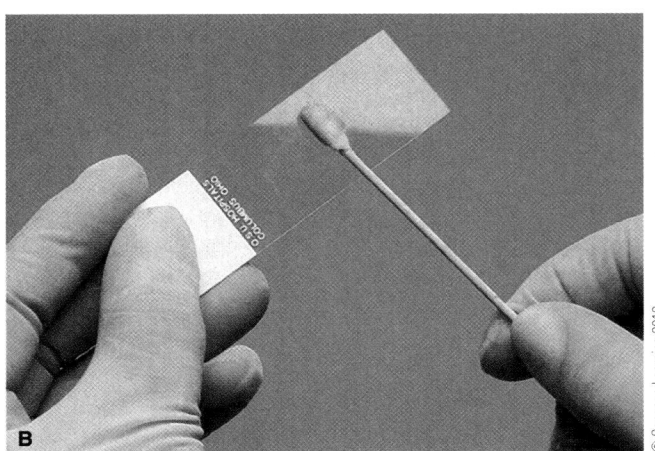

FIGURE 7-19 Inoculating an agar plate and preparing a smear using a specimen swab: (A) one quadrant of an agar plate is inoculated using the swab; (B) a bacterial smear is made by rolling the swab across the slide

© Cengage Learning 2012

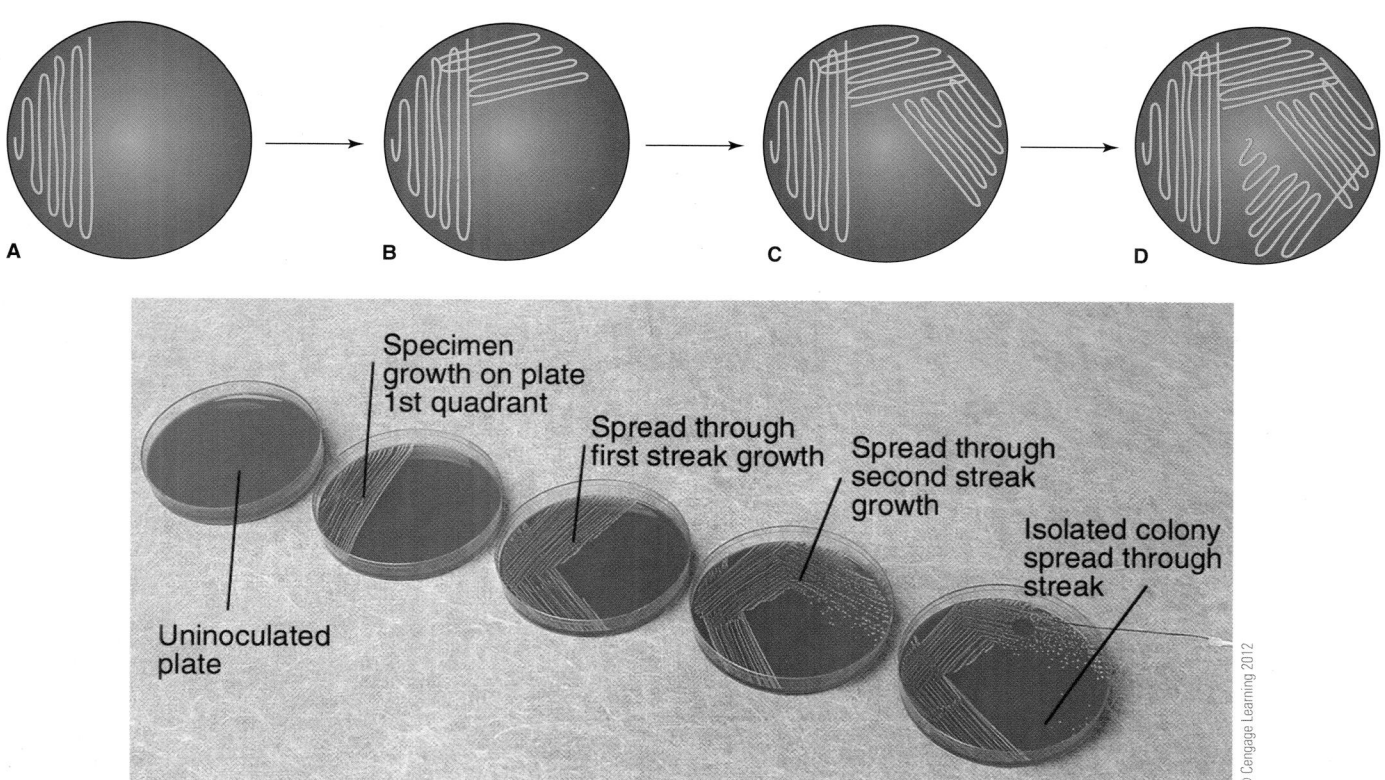

FIGURE 7-20 Streaking an agar plate in four quadrants to produce isolated colonies. Top row: (A) inoculate the first quadrant and streak the first quadrant using a sterile loop; (B) use a sterile loop to streak into the second quadrant; (C) sterilize the loop and streak into the third quadrant; (D) sterilize the loop and make one streak in a "tornado" pattern into the fourth quadrant. Bottom row: bacterial growth in each quadrant when streaked as shown in drawings in top row

tube, and the tubes and plates are incubated in an *aerobic incubator* (ambient air). Certain pathogens grow best in atmospheres with increased carbon dioxide (CO_2); these cultures should be incubated in a *CO_2 incubator* which has an atmosphere of 5% to 10% CO_2 (Table 7-16).

Several methods can be used to create an anaerobic environment for cultures from specimens suspected of containing anaerobes, such as cultures from deep wounds. Agar plates inoculated with such specimens can be incubated in sealed bags or containers that include a generator pack which creates an anaerobic environment (Figure 7-22B). Tubes of media containing possible anaerobes are kept tightly capped. Pre-reduced media that require no special incubator or anaerobic chamber can also be used.

Observing the Culture after 24 Hours

Aerobic cultures and those cultures placed in 5% to 10% CO_2 are incubated 18 to 24 hours (or overnight). If growth is not evident or is insufficient after overnight incubation, the culture is kept and examined after incubating an additional 24 hours. When the plate is removed from the incubator, bacterial growth can be observed through the lid. The plate should be inspected for the presence of isolated colonies (Figure 7-23).

Hemolysis

Growth on blood agar should be observed for **hemolysis**, the lysis of the red blood cells by bacteria growing on the blood agar. Some bacteria can completely lyse red blood cells, making the area around the bacterial growth almost transparent. This is called beta (ß) hemolysis (Figure 7-23B). Other bacteria incompletely lyse the blood cells and produce green discoloration around the colonies. This is called alpha (α) hemolysis. Absence of hemolysis is called gamma (γ) hemolysis. Observation of hemolysis is especially important in diagnosing strep throat, because *S. pyogenes*, which causes strep throat, is beta hemolytic.

Colony Characteristics

Other bacterial colony characteristics that aid in identification are size, color, shape, and even odor. Bacterial colonies can be white, gray, yellow, or even red. Their size can range from almost too tiny to be seen to very large. The colonies can be compact and look dry, or can be spreading and glisten. Colonies are usually round and can be flattened or raised like a dome. Some organisms produce distinctive odors. One *Pseudomonas* species smells like grapes, and *N. gonorrhoeae* smells to some like sweaty tennis shoes. Odors emitted from cultures on agar plates are detectable without opening the plate. *To prevent possible infection with bacteria, never place an open bacterial culture near your face.*

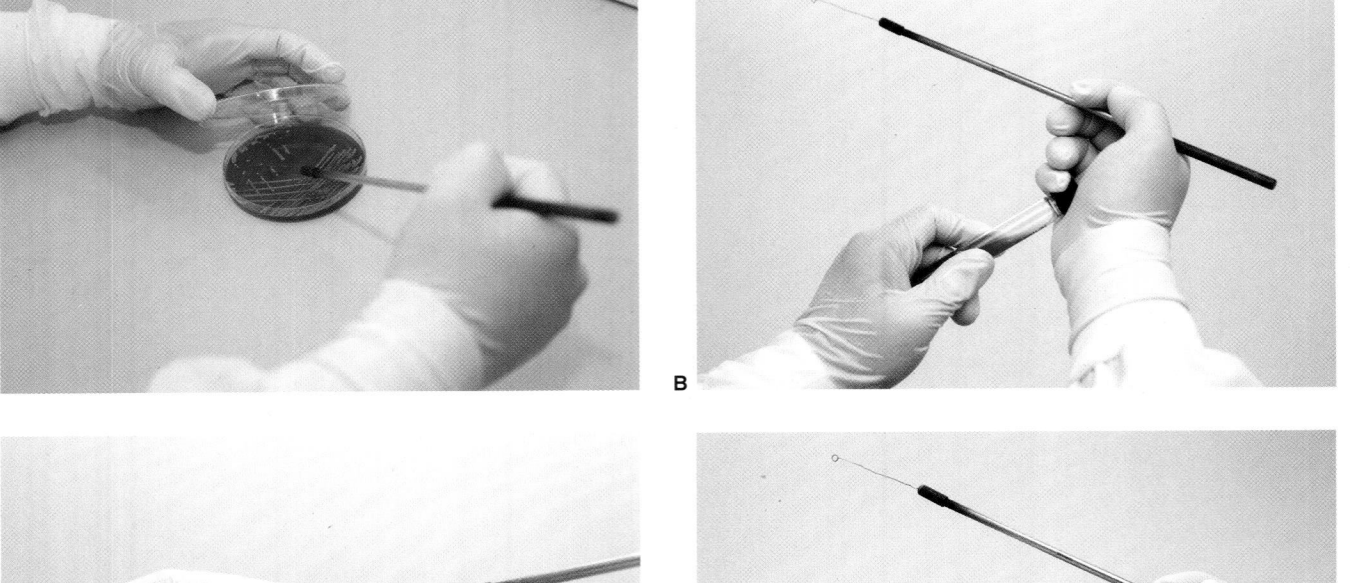

FIGURE 7-21 Transferring bacteria from an agar plate to an agar slant: (A) select a colony from an agar plate; (B) remove cap from tube; (C) inoculate agar slant; and (D) sterilize the mouth of the tube before replacing the cap

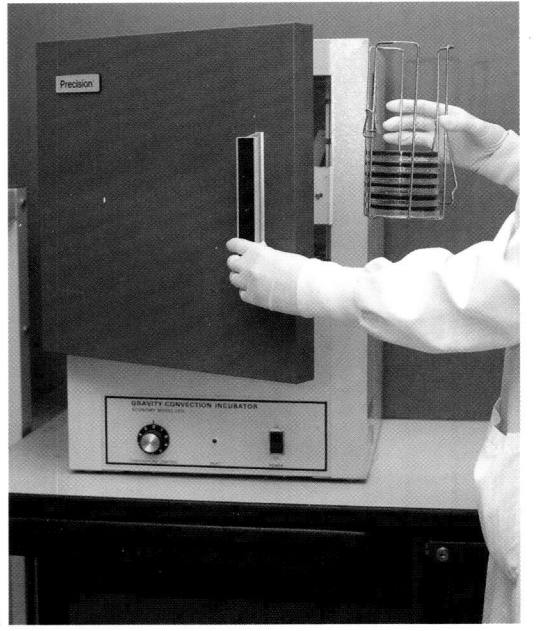

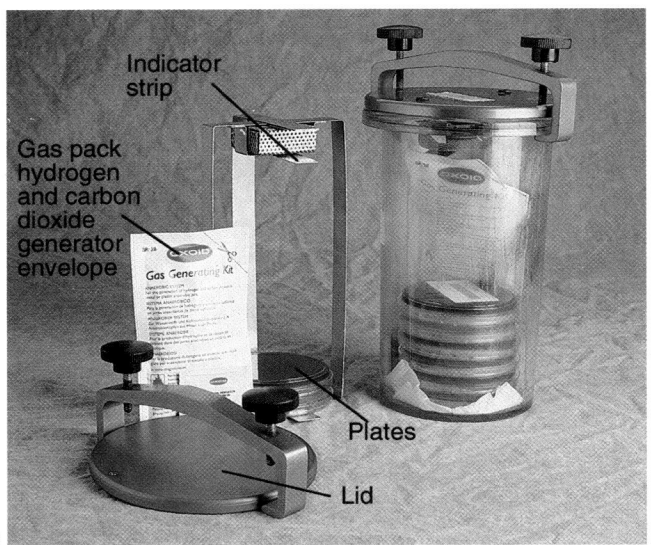

FIGURE 7-22 Incubation chambers for bacterial cultures: (A) A small bacteriological incubator; and (B) a system for incubating anaerobic cultures

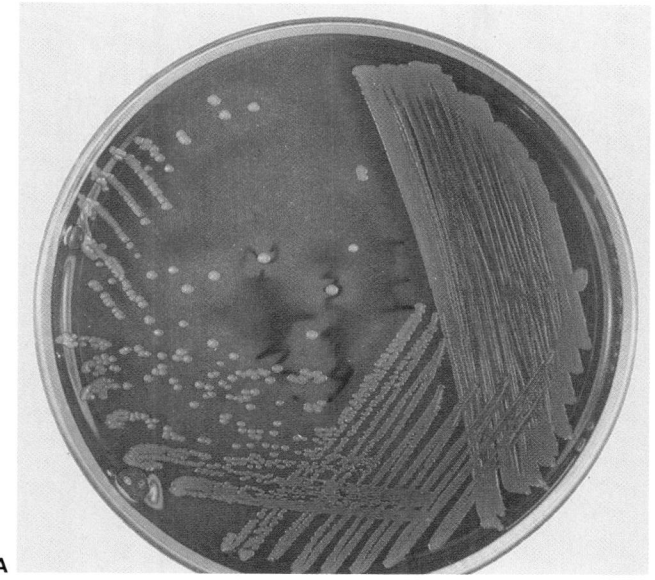
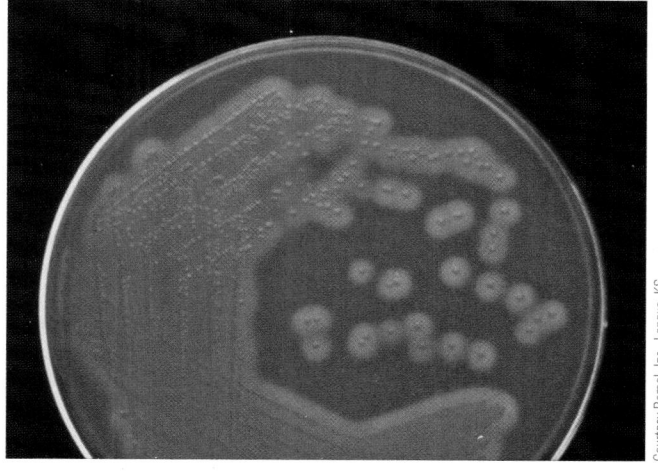

Courtesy Remel, Inc., Lenexa, KS

FIGURE 7-23 Growth of isolated bacterial colonies on blood agar: (A) *Staphylococcus aureus* and (B) beta-hemolytic *Streptococcus*

SAFETY REMINDERS

- Review Safety Precautions section before beginning procedure.
- Observe Standard Precautions.
- Use aseptic technique.
- Use disposable inoculating loops when possible.
- Avoid formation of aerosols.
- Sterilize reusable loops after use and return to holder.
- Disinfect work surfaces frequently.
- Do not wear laboratory coat outside of the laboratory.
- Do not place bacterial cultures near your face.

PROCEDURAL REMINDERS

- Review Quality Assessment section before beginning procedure.
- Follow SOP manual.
- Use aseptic technique.
- Sterilize loop before and after each use.
- Perform quality checks on media and equipment.
- Inoculate specimens to primary media as soon as possible after collection.
- Open agar plates just enough to transfer the culture.

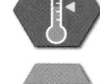

CRITICAL THINKING

Bill's work assignments in bacteriology included wiping down work surfaces and disposing of all contaminated materials and cultures appropriately. He used a surface disinfectant to wipe the counters every hour during the work day. Several times during each shift he gathered all the used culture plates and other contaminated supplies into biohazard bags. After closing the bags securely, he placed them alongside the other trash to be picked up by housekeeping services.

1. Should Bill be commended for ensuring the safety of everyone working in the laboratory?
2. Explain your answer.

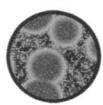

SUMMARY

Good culture techniques are essential for accurate results in the bacteriology laboratory. Safe work practices such as aseptic technique must be used to prevent contamination of personnel, cultures, and the environment. Sterile disposable loops should be used when possible to eliminate the risk for aerosol formation created by sterilizing the loop. Technicians must be able to successfully transfer organisms from the original specimen to primary, selective, and indicator media. The correct medium must be selected based on the source of the specimen and the type(s) of organism normally expected from that type of specimen. The transfer must be accomplished without contamination of the specimen or loss of viability of the organism(s). A comprehensive quality assessment program must be followed. Use of specified culture techniques included in the SOP manual ensures that the organisms causing disease can be cultured and isolated successfully.

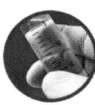

REVIEW QUESTIONS

1. Explain why the use of aseptic technique is important in the bacteriology laboratory.
2. What are the differences between disinfectants and antiseptics?
3. What are two types of safety cabinets used in microbiology?
4. What are the purposes of primary, selective, and indicator media?
5. Describe how to inoculate an agar plate using a swab.
6. Describe how to streak an agar plate for isolated colonies.
7. Describe how to transfer an inoculum from an agar plate to an agar slant.
8. What are important colony characteristics that can be observed?
9. What hemolytic reactions of bacteria can be used to identify the organism?
10. What medium is used to indicate hemolysis?
11. Why are transport media used?
12. Discuss quality assessment programs for the bacteriology laboratory.
13. What safety techniques must be used in the bacteriology laboratory?
14. Define agar, antiseptic, aseptic technique, disinfectant, enriched medium, hemolysis, HEPA filter, indicator medium, inoculating loop, inoculation, inoculum, isolated colonies, primary medium, quadrant, selective medium, and sterilization.

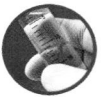

STUDENT ACTIVITIES

1. Complete the written examination for this lesson.
2. Inquire about the types of disinfectants used in local POLs.
3. Practice using aseptic technique to inoculate and streak an agar plate, as outlined in the Student Performance Guide.

WEB ACTIVITIES

1. Search the Internet for disinfectants appropriate for the microbiology laboratory. Select three, and make a table including characteristics, ingredients, and classes of microbes for which they are effective.
2. Search the Internet for information about vancomycin-resistant *Enterococcus* (VRE). Report on the Gram stain reaction and one condition caused by VRE.
3. Examine the labels of two household disinfectants. Use the Internet to compare their active ingredients with those of disinfectants used in healthcare settings. Find out if the household disinfectants are bactericidal or bacteriostatic.

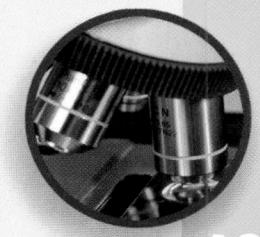

LESSON 7-3
Culture Techniques for Bacteriology

Name _____ Date _____

INSTRUCTIONS

1. Practice using aseptic technique to inoculate and streak an agar plate, following the step-by-step procedure.

2. Demonstrate the procedure satisfactorily for the instructor, using the Student Performance Guide. Your instructor will explain the procedures for evaluating your performance. Your performance may be given a number grade, a letter grade, or satisfactory (S) or unsatisfactory (U) depending on course or institutional policy.

NOTE: If sterile, disposable loops are used, the manufacturer's instructions for use of that specific loop design must be followed.

MATERIALS AND EQUIPMENT

- gloves
- hand antiseptic
- full-face shield (or equivalent PPE)
- Dacron or rayon sterile swabs, or swabs with bacteria already applied, stored in capped culture tubes or transport tubes
- stock cultures of educational or nonpathogenic strains of *Escherichia coli* or *Staphylococcus aureus*
- test tube rack
- blood agar plates
- reusable inoculating loops or sterile disposable loops (preferred)
- loop holder
- electric incinerator such as Bacti-Cinerator
- incubator set at 35° to 37°C
- waterproof marker
- paper towels
- surface disinfectant
- biohazard container
- sharps container

PROCEDURE

Record in the comment section any problems encountered while practicing the procedure (or have a fellow student or the instructor evaluate your performance).

S = Satisfactory
U = Unsatisfactory

You must:	S	U	Evaluation/Comments
1. Wash hands with antiseptic and put on gloves and face protection			
2. Assemble materials and equipment			
3. Turn on the electric incinerator (if using reusable wire loop)			
4. Select an agar plate to be inoculated and label the bottom of the plate			
5. Select an inoculated swab or a sterile swab and the appropriate culture			

(Continues)

© 2012 Delmar, Cengage Learning. Permission to reproduce for clinical use granted.

You must:	S	U	Evaluation/Comments
6. Place package of sterile disposable inoculating loops within reach; if using reusable wire inoculating loop, place it in loop holder within reach			
7. Remove the swab from container; if using a sterile swab, go to step 8; if using a pre-inoculated swab, go to step 11			
8. Pick up tube containing a culture in one hand; use fourth and fifth fingers of the hand holding the swab to remove the cap from the tube (hold cap with fingers for entire procedure; do not lay cap down)			
9. Insert tip of swab into culture and pick up a *small* amount of bacterial culture			
10. Sterilize the mouth of the tube, replace cap, and set tube in test tube rack; do not allow anything to touch the swab tip			
11. Lift the agar plate lid just enough to insert the swab and gently spread the inoculum over the surface of one quadrant of the agar plate			
12. Replace the lid on the agar plate			
13. Discard swab into biohazard container as directed by instructor			
14. Streak the second quadrant of the plate: a. Use the sterile disposable loop following manufacturer's directions; alternatively, sterilize the wire inoculating loop using the electric incinerator and allow the wire to cool b. Lift the lid of the agar plate just enough to be able to insert the inoculating loop c. Touch the sterile loop in the first quadrant and streak all the way across the second quadrant d. Repeat step 14c six to eight times e. Follow manufacturer's instructions if disposable loop is used; or heat-sterilize the reusable loop and allow it to cool			
15. Streak the third quadrant of the plate using the disposable loop or the sterile wire loop: a. Lift the agar plate lid, touch the loop in the second quadrant, and streak all the way across the third quadrant b. Repeat step 15a six to eight times c. Follow manufacturer's instructions if disposable loop is used; or heat-sterilize the reusable loop and allow it to cool			

© 2012 Delmar, Cengage Learning. Permission to reproduce for clinical use granted.

You must:	S	U	Evaluation/Comments

16. Streak the fourth quadrant of the plate to produce isolated colonies:
   a. Use the disposable loop or the sterile wire loop
   b. Lift the agar plate lid, touch the loop to the third quadrant, and spread the inoculum into the fourth quadrant
   c. Use a continuous streak in a *tornado* pattern, decreasing the horizontal width of the streaks and increasing the vertical distance between the streaks			

17. Replace the lid on the plate			
18. Sterilize the loop and replace it in the holder or discard disposable loop into sharps container; dispose of culture as directed by instructor			
19. Turn off the electric incinerator			
20. Place the agar plate upside down in the 35° to 37° C incubator to incubate overnight (18 to 24 hours)			
21. Discard contaminated disposables into appropriate sharps or biohazard containers and clean work area with surface disinfectant			
22. Remove gloves and discard into biohazard container			
23. Wash hands with antiseptic			
24. The next day: Wash hands, put on gloves and wipe work area with surface disinfectant			
25. Remove the inoculated plate from the incubator and examine the growth (do not remove lid)			
26. Observe the colonies. Are they colored? What is the shape? Are they flat or raised? Record observations			
27. Look for hemolysis if blood agar was used. Record as no hemolysis, or alpha (α) or beta (ß) hemolysis			
28. Discard used agar plate into biohazard container			
29. Wipe work area with disinfectant			
30. Remove gloves and discard into biohazard container			
31. Wash hands with antiseptic			

Instructor/Evaluator Comments:

Instructor/Evaluator _____ Date _____

© 2012 Delmar, Cengage Learning. Permission to reproduce for clinical use granted.

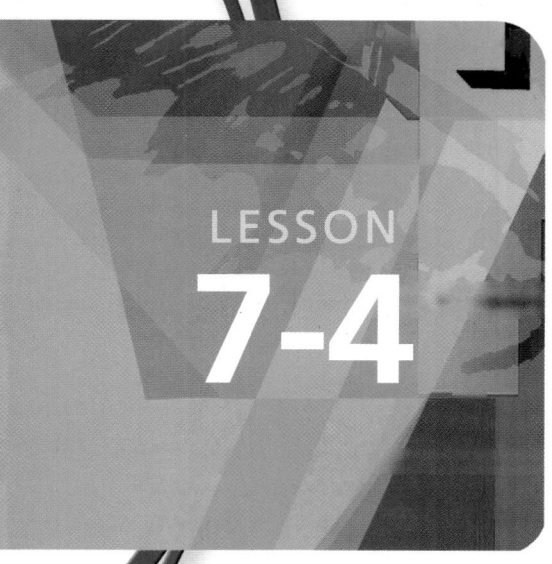

LESSON 7-4

The Gram Stain

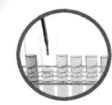

LESSON OBJECTIVES

After studying this lesson, the student will:

- ⊙ Explain the principle of the Gram stain.
- ⊙ Prepare smears of bacteria from a swab and from a bacterial culture.
- ⊙ Perform the Gram stain procedure.
- ⊙ Identify gram-positive organisms on a smear.
- ⊙ Identify gram-negative organisms on a smear.
- ⊙ List the safety precautions to be observed when performing the Gram stain.
- ⊙ Discuss quality assessment procedures that must be a part of preparing smears and performing Gram stains.
- ⊙ Define the glossary terms.

GLOSSARY

bibulous paper / a special absorbent paper used to dry slides; blotting paper

counterstain / a dye that adds a contrasting color

mordant / a substance that fixes a dye or stain to an object

INTRODUCTION

The preparation and staining of a bacteriological smear is an important process. Smears can be prepared from bacteria growing on media or from swabs collected from sites of infection. The smears are then stained to reveal the shape and structure of bacteria present. Bacterial cells are so small and possess so little color, they are difficult to observe microscopically unless they are stained.

The most common bacterial stain is the Gram stain. By gram-staining bacterial smears, bacteria can be separated into two broad groups, Gram positive and Gram negative, based on the structure of the bacterial cell wall. Observation of the

stained bacteria also allows the microbiologist to determine the morphology of the organism—coccus, rod-shaped, spiral, or curved. The Gram stain reaction and bacterial morphology provide clues to bacterial identity and serve as a guide to the selection of culture media and tests that should be used for bacterial identification and determination of antibiotic susceptibility.

PREPARING THE BACTERIAL SMEAR

Bacterial smears can be prepared from specimen swabs or cultures. Correct safety practices and quality assessment procedures must be followed.

Safety Precautions

Standard Precautions must be observed and appropriate personal protective equipment (PPE) worn. In addition, the bacteriology laboratory presents the additional hazards of exposure to bacterial cultures and to patient specimens.

The use of aseptic technique is an essential part of the overall safety plan for the microbiology laboratory. Aseptic technique includes (1) using a sterile loop (disposable or a reusable, heat-sterilizable loop), (2) sterilizing the mouths of culture tubes after opening and before closing them, (3) raising the lids of agar plates only enough to perform a procedure and never placing the lids on the countertop, (4) discarding all contaminated materials into the appropriate sharps or biohazard containers, (5) wiping the work area with surface disinfectant before beginning and after completing a procedure and anytime a spill occurs, and (6) washing hands frequently using antiseptic.

Additional safety guidelines include:

- Wearing gloves when transferring patient specimens to media or slides and when working with other potentially infectious material (OPIM)
- Wearing a disposable buttoned, fluid-resistant laboratory coat to protect clothing and skin from contamination
- Keeping the work area free of clutter
- Decontaminating or sterilizing all specimens and culture materials before disposal, being sure to follow all applicable local, state, and federal disposal regulations

Quality Assessment

The procedures for preparing and Gram-staining smears specified in the facility's standard operating procedure (SOP) manual must be followed. Heat-fixing must be performed carefully to prevent breaking the slide or damaging the organisms. Gram stain reagents should not be used after the expiration date. Control slides should be used to check the reliability of Gram stain reagents and technique of laboratory personnel. Each step in the Gram stain procedure should be timed, with special care taken that the smear is not exposed to decolorizer too long. Oil-immersion microscope lenses must be kept clean and in good condition to allow observation and interpretation of the morphology of the stained organisms.

Preparing a Smear from a Swab

Bacterial smears can be prepared from a specimen swab collected from a patient, such as a swab from a wound or lesion. It is preferable to obtain two swabs from a patient, one for culture and one for smear, but that is not always practical. If only one swab is collected, the culture medium must be inoculated *before* the swab is used to prepare the smear; this prevents contamination of the swab from a nonsterile slide.

Slides can be stored in 95% ethanol and wiped dry with sterile gauze just before use. To prepare a smear of the specimen collected on a swab, a microscope slide is labeled with the patient's identification code. The swab is gently *rolled* across the surface of the slide (Figure 7-24). This should leave just a thin film of material on the slide. When dry, the unstained smear should be barely visible on the slide. The swab should be replaced into its transport container and discarded into a biohazard container.

Preparing a Smear from a Culture

A smear can be prepared from bacteria growing on tube media, such as an agar slant, or on an agar plate.

Using an Agar Slant

To prepare a smear from bacteria growing on a slant, 1 drop of sterile water is placed on a pre-cleaned glass slide. The culture tube is held in one hand and the inoculating loop in the other. The fourth and fifth fingers of the hand holding the loop are used to unscrew the cap of the tube. The loop and the mouth of the tube are sterilized and allowed to cool briefly. Several inches of the loop wire will enter the tube, so the loop and about 2 to 2.5 inches of the wire above the loop should be sterilized.

The loop is used to pick up an isolated bacterial colony from the edge of the streak (Figure 7-25A). These bacteria are mixed with the drop of water on the slide and spread into a circle about the size of a nickel (Figure 7-25B). The mouth of the tube is sterilized again, the lid is replaced, and the tube is set in a test tube rack. The loop is then sterilized and replaced in its holder. The smear is allowed to air-dry.

Using an Agar Plate

A drop of sterile water is placed on a clean glass microscope slide. The agar plate lid should be lifted just enough to insert the sterilized loop and touch it to an isolated colony. The bacteria are then mixed with the drop of water on the slide and spread into a circle about the size of a nickel. The smear is air-dried; the dry unstained smear should be just barely visible.

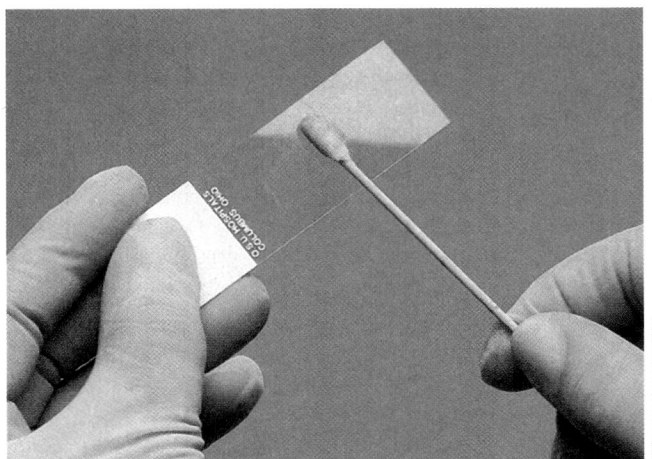

FIGURE 7-24 Preparing a bacterial smear from a specimen swab

© Cengage Learning 2012

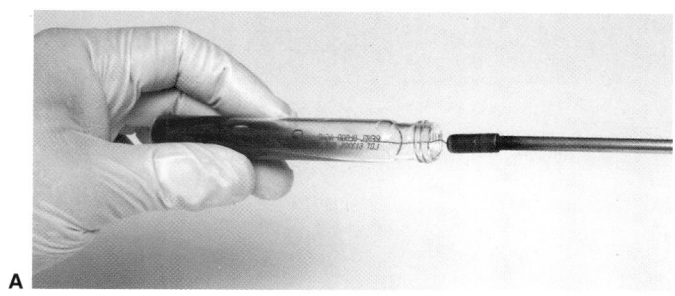

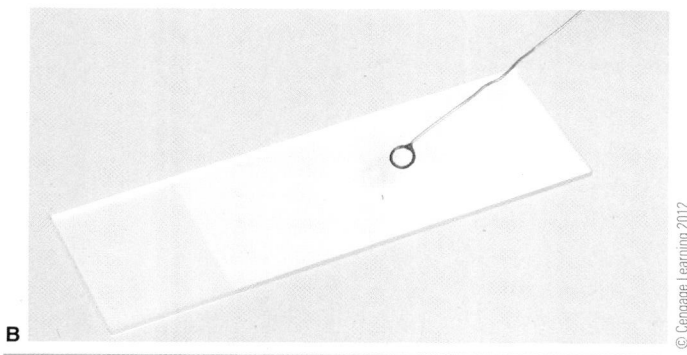

FIGURE 7-25 Preparing a smear from an agar slant: (A) touch sterile loop to bacterial colony; (B) mix bacteria with a drop of sterile water on slide and spread to make a thin smear

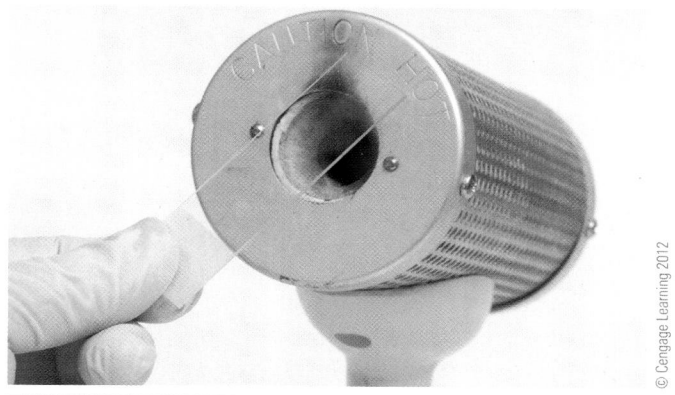

FIGURE 7-26 Heat-fixing a bacterial smear using an electric incinerator

Heat-Fixing the Smear

When the smear is completely dry, it must be heat-fixed. This can be accomplished using an electric incinerator, such as the Bacti-Cinerator (Figure 7-26). The slide is held using forceps or a spring clothespin. The *back* of the slide is placed flat against the opening of the electric incinerator for a few seconds. The slide should not be heated excessively. When a smear has been heat-fixed correctly, the slide should not feel hot if touched to the back of the hand.

Heat-fixing causes the organisms to adhere to the glass slide during the staining. Excessive heating will alter the bacterial morphology or can break the slide. Under-heating will result in the organisms washing off the slide during staining, requiring that the specimen be recollected if the swab has already been discarded.

THE GRAM STAIN

The Gram stain is performed on a thin smear of bacteria that has been air-dried and heat-fixed. The staining procedure consists of applying a sequence of primary stain, Gram's iodine, decolorizer, and **counterstain**, a dye that adds contrasting color to the bacteria.

Gram stain reactions are based on chemical differences in the structures of bacterial cell walls. The walls of gram-negative cells are chemically more complex than the walls of gram-positive cells. Both types of bacteria contain peptidoglycan in their cell walls, but the gram-negative cell wall contains more lipid, polysaccharide, amino acids, and lipoprotein complexes than

gram-positive cell walls. Both types of cell walls take up the primary stain, which is crystal violet. The chemical composition of gram-positive cell walls causes them to retain the crystal violet and resist decolorization. However, the components in the cell walls of gram-negative bacteria allow them to be decolorized (lose the crystal violet stain) and be counterstained by taking up the safranin stain.

Performing the Gram Stain

The air-dried and heat-fixed smear should be placed on a staining rack over a container to catch the staining reagents (Figure 7-27). This can be a beaker, pan, or laboratory sink. Laboratories that have large volumes of work can use automated stainers.

Primary Stain

To begin the Gram stain procedure, the primary stain, crystal violet, is poured on the slide (Figures 7-27 and 7-28). The staining time is usually 1 minute, but the manufacturer's instructions must be followed. After 1 minute, the slide is rinsed by gently pouring tap water on it or by holding the slide with forceps under a gentle stream of tap water. The slide is then returned to the staining rack.

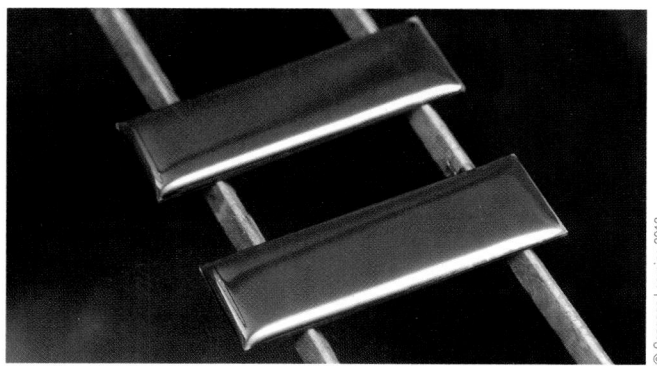

FIGURE 7-27 Slide staining rack

STEP	TIME	PROCEDURE	RESULT
1	one minute	Primary stain: Apply crystal violet stain (purple) ↓ Rinse slide	All bacteria stain purple
2	one minute	Mordant: Apply Gram's iodine ↓ Rinse slide	All bacteria remain purple
3	three to five seconds	Decolorize: Apply alcohol ↓ Rinse slide	Purple stain is removed from Gram-negative cells
4	one minute	Counterstain: Apply safranin stain (red) ↓ Rinse slide	Gram-negative cells appear pink-red; Gram-positive cells appear purple

© Cengage Learning 2012

FIGURE 7-28 Steps in the Gram stain procedure

Gram's Iodine (Mordant)

Gram's iodine, a mordant, is then poured on the slide. A **mordant** is a substance that causes a dye or stain to adhere to the object being stained. After 1 minute, the slide is again rinsed gently with tap water.

Decolorizer

A decolorizer, such as alcohol or an alcohol-acetone mixture, is *briefly* added to the slide. This is best done while the slide is held with forceps and tilted downward at about a 30-degree angle. It is important that this not be done too long—3 to 5 seconds, or until no more purple runs off, is long enough. Immediately after decolorizing, the slide is rinsed with water to remove all decolorizer and stop the decolorization process (Figure 7-28).

The decolorization step is an important one. At this point in the staining process, the gram-positive organisms will be dark purple-blue because their cell wall composition allows penetration and retention of the crystal violet. The gram-negative organisms will be essentially colorless because their cell walls do not retain the crystal violet in the decolorization procedure. However, prolonged decolorization can eventually remove the primary stain from the gram-positive organisms as well, causing incorrect identification of an organism.

Counterstain

In the last step, the slide is flooded with the counterstain safranin. The safranin has no effect on the gram-positive cells, which retained the crystal violet, but the colorless gram-negative cells will be stained pink-red (Figure 7-28).

At the end of the counterstaining time, the slides are rinsed again and the excess water shaken off. The slides are then either placed in a rack to air-dry or dried by blotting between sheets of **bibulous paper** to remove the excess moisture. After the slides are completely dry, they are ready to be viewed microscopically.

OBSERVING THE STAINED BACTERIOLOGICAL SMEAR

The stained smear should be observed using the oil-immersion objective (100×) after the stained area has been located using the low-power (10×) objective. The gram-negative organisms will appear pink-red, and the gram-positive ones will appear

TABLE 7-18. Gram stain reactions of some medically important bacteria

GRAM POSITIVE (+)	GRAM NEGATIVE (−)
Streptococcus pyogenes	*Escherichia coli* (*E. coli*)
Staphylococcus aureus	*Salmonella* species
Lactobacillus species	*Neisseria gonorrhoeae*
Bacillus anthracis	*Pseudomonas* species
Clostridium tetani	*Neisseria meningitidis*

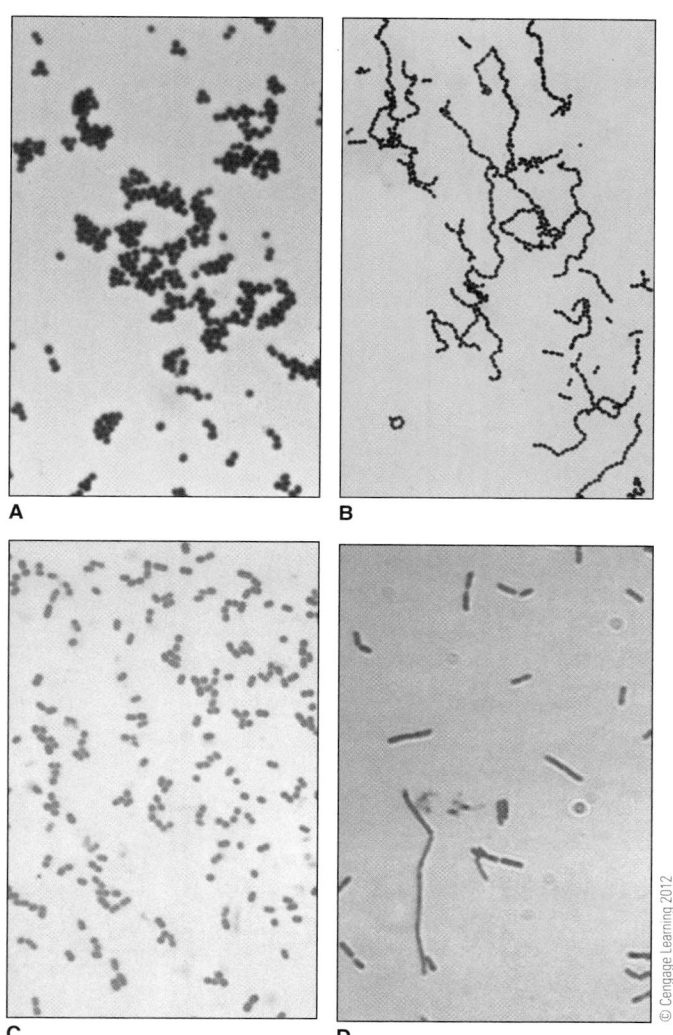

gram-negative rod (Table 7-18). A few other microorganisms, such as the yeast *Candida albicans*, stain dark purple in the gram stain and can be observed microscopically.

If the smear has been prepared correctly, the bacteria should be dispersed evenly on the slide so the morphology is easy to distinguish and the color is crisp and distinct. All bacteria of the same type might not look identical, but the majority will appear similar. Gram-negative rods can be slender and long, fat and long, or fat and short. Some rods are so short that they appear round like the cocci and are called coccobacilli. The round bacteria can appear singly, in pairs, as grape-like clusters (staph), or in chains similar to strings of beads (strep). Figure 7-29 illustrates some of these variations in morphology.

FIGURE 7-29 Variations in bacterial morphology: (A) gram-positive cocci in grape-like clusters; (B) gram-positive cocci in bead-like chains; (C) gram-negative rods, short and fat (coccobacilli); and (D) gram-negative rods, long and slender

dark blue-purple (Figures 7-28 and 7-29). Staphylococci and streptococci are common gram-positive, round (coccus) bacteria (Table 7-18). *E. coli*, an inhabitant of the intestines, is a

© Cengage Learning 2012

SAFETY REMINDERS

- Review Safety Precautions section before beginning procedure.
- Observe Standard Precautions.
- Use aseptic technique.
- Wipe surfaces frequently with disinfectant.
- Use sterile disposable loops when possible.
- Discard used slides in sharps container.
- Autoclave culture materials before disposal.

PROCEDURAL REMINDERS

- Review Quality Assessment section before beginning procedure.
- Follow Gram stain procedure in the SOP manual.
- Use gentle heat to fix the slide.
- Keep microscope objectives and eyepieces clean.

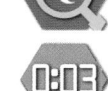
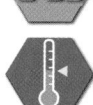

CRITICAL THINKING

Marion made a smear for a Gram stain and left it to dry while she went to lunch. While she was gone Christine had extra time, so she stained it. When she examined it under the microscope bacteria were scarce and large clear areas were present on the slide. Christine prepared another smear, let it dry, heat-fixed it, and stained it. She had no problem observing the morphology of the bacteria present on the second slide.

1. Which of the following is the most likely cause of the problem with the first smear/stain?
   a. Failing to heat-fix the smear

(Continues)

CRITICAL THINKING (Continued)

  b. Rubbing the swab across the slide
  c. Leaving decolorizer on too long
  d. Failing to sterilize the loop
2. Which is most likely the problem—Marion's smear technique or Christine's processing of the slide? Explain.

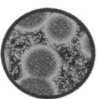

SUMMARY

Preparing a smear and performing the Gram stain are important in the process of identifying bacteria isolated from a specimen. Bacterial morphology and Gram stain reaction are valuable clues to the identity of the organism responsible for an infection. Information learned from the Gram stain is used to determine which bacterial identification tests and antibiotic susceptibility tests need to be performed. The staining process is relatively simple, but each step must be performed carefully. In the preparation of the smear, the facility's SOP manual must be followed. Control slides should be used at prescribed intervals to check personnel technique and the performance of stain reagents. Standard Precautions must be observed because smears are made from patient specimens or from bacterial cultures and are potentially infectious.

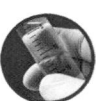

REVIEW QUESTIONS

1. Discuss the use of Standard Precautions and aseptic technique in the bacteriology laboratory.

2. Why is it necessary to wear a laboratory coat when working with bacteria?

3. Why is it important to gently roll the swab across the slide when preparing a smear?

4. Why is the swab used to inoculate the culture medium before it is used to make the smear?

5. Explain the differences in the procedures for preparing smears from tube cultures and from agar plate cultures.

6. Why must the smear for Gram stain be heat-fixed before it is stained?

7. Explain how to perform a Gram stain.

8. Why are some bacteria gram-positive and others gram-negative?

9. What is the appearance of gram-positive cocci? Gram-negative rods?

10. Why is it necessary to wipe countertops often with surface disinfectant?

11. What QA procedures must be followed when making and staining smears?

12. Define bibulous paper, counterstain, and mordant.

STUDENT ACTIVITIES

1. Complete the written examination for this lesson.

2. Obtain Gram-stained bacterial smears and practice identifying bacterial morphology and Gram-stain reactions using the microscope.

3. Practice preparing bacteriological smears, performing the Gram stain, and identifying gram-negative and gram-positive organisms as outlined in the Student Performance Guide.

4. Prepare duplicate smears from a culture of gram-positive organisms. Stain the smears following the Gram stain procedure. Decolorize one smear for the normal time and the other for 30 seconds. Examine the smears microscopically, compare the staining results, and discuss your findings.

WEB ACTIVITIES

1. Use the Internet to find tutorials demonstrating how to perform a Gram stain.

2. Use the Internet to find the morphology and Gram reactions of *Clostridium difficile* and *Haemophilus*.

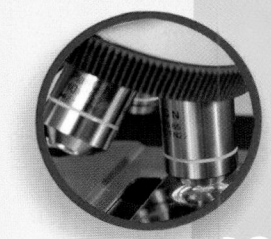
LESSON 7-4
The Gram Stain

Name _____ Date _____

INSTRUCTIONS

1. Practice preparing and staining a bacteriological smear following the step-by-step procedure.

2. Demonstrate the procedure for preparing and staining bacteriological smears satisfactorily for the instructor using the Student Performance Guide. Your instructor will explain the procedures for evaluation of your performance. Your performance may be given a number grade, a letter grade or satisfactory (S) or unsatisfactory (U), depending on the course or institutional policy.

MATERIALS AND EQUIPMENT

- gloves
- hand antiseptic
- full-face shield (or equivalent PPE)
- stock cultures of nonpathogenic or educational strains of *E. coli* and *Staphylococcus aureus* (or other nonpathogenic gram-negative and gram-positive cultures)
- test tube rack
- timer
- microscope with 10×, 40×, and 100× (oil-immersion) objectives
- immersion oil
- electric incinerator
- inoculating loop, disposable preferred
- holder for inoculating loops
- commercially prepared Gram-stained slides of gram-negative and gram-positive organisms
- diamond- or carbide-tip etching pen or other slide-labeling pen
- glass microscope slides stored in 95% ethanol
- sterile H_2O
- sterile gauze
- forceps or spring-type clothespins
- Gram stain kit or individual Gram stain reagents, including tap water for rinse
- staining rack and container or sink
- slide drying rack
- sterile Dacron swabs
- paper towels
- laboratory tissue
- bibulous paper
- pencil (or colored drawing pencils, optional)
- lens paper and lens cleaner
- paper towels
- surface disinfectant
- biohazard containers
- sharps containers

PROCEDURE

    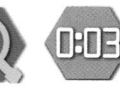

Record in the comment section any problems encountered while practicing the procedure (or have a fellow student or the instructor evaluate your performance).

S = Satisfactory
U = Unsatisfactory

You must:	S	U	Evaluation/Comments
1. Assemble equipment and materials			
2. Obtain commercially prepared and stained slides of gram-positive and gram-negative organisms			

(Continues)

© 2012 Delmar, Cengage Learning. Permission to reproduce for clinical use granted.

You must:	S	U	Evaluation/Comments
3. Observe the prepared slides microscopically and identify the gram-positive and gram-negative bacterial morphologies; sketch representative organisms from each slide examined			
4. Turn on the electric incinerator			
5. Wash hands with antiseptic and put on gloves			

6. Use a swab to prepare one smear of a gram-positive organism (*S. aureus*) and one of a gram-negative organism (*E. coli*) following steps 6a–6i: if not available skip to step 7
  a. Obtain a microscope slide and etch the I.D. (Gm +) onto one end with etching pencil
  b. Obtain a swab that has been inoculated with gram-positive (+) organisms
  c. Roll the swab gently across the surface of the slide to make a smear about the size of a nickel
  d. Return the swab to its container or discard in biohazard container
  e. Allow the smear to air-dry completely
  f. Repeat steps 6a–6e, using a gram-negative organism; label slide Gm (–)
  g. Hold the gram-positive (+) slide by the end using forceps or spring clothespin; place the *back* of the slide flat against the opening of electric incinerator for a few seconds; do not heat slide excessively
  h. Heat-fix the gram-negative slide following step 6g
  i. Allow the slides to cool before staining			

7. Use cultures in tube media to prepare one smear from a gram-positive organism (*S. aureus*) and one from gram-negative organism (*E. coli*) following steps 7a–7l; if tube cultures are not available, go to step 8
  a. Obtain microscope slides and cultures of a gram-positive organism and a gram-negative organism growing on agar slants
  b. Use sterile disposable loop or sterilize and cool a wire loop and transfer 1 drop of sterile water to the center of the microscope slide
  c. Hold the tube of gram-positive culture in one hand and the inoculating loop in the other
  d. Use the fourth and fifth fingers of the hand holding the loop to twist the cap off the tube
  e. Sterilize the loop and 2 to 2.5 inches of the wire above it and cool the loop			

© 2012 Delmar, Cengage Learning. Permission to reproduce for clinical use granted.

You must:	S	U	Evaluation/Comments
f. Sterilize the mouth of the culture tube and use the cooled loop to pick up a small amount of bacteria from the edge of the growth on the slant			
g. Sterilize the mouth of the tube, replace the cap, and set the tube in a test tube rack			
h. Mix the bacteria on the loop with the water on the slide and spread the mixture into a circle about the size of a nickel. Do not make the smear too thick			
i. Repeat steps 7a–7h using the gram-negative culture; label slides Gm (-)			
j. Allow smears to air-dry completely			
k. Heat-fix the smears (as in 6g)			
l. Allow the slides to cool			
8. Use bacteria growing on agar plate to prepare one smear from a gram-positive organism (*S. aureus*) and one from gram-negative organism (*E. coli*) following steps 8a–8k; if agar plate cultures are not available, go to step 9			
a. Obtain microscope slides and a gram-negative and a gram-positive culture growing on agar plates			
b. Label microscope slide; sterilize and cool the inoculating loop and transfer 1 drop of sterile water to the slide			
c. Sterilize and cool the loop again			
d. Lift the lid of the first agar plate just enough so the inoculating loop can fit into it			
e. Touch the sterile loop to a bacterial colony and transfer a small amount to the drop of water on the slide			
f. Replace the lid on the plate			
g. Use the loop to mix the bacteria and water together and spread the mixture into a nickel-sized area			
h. Repeat steps 8a–8g using the second agar plate culture			
i. Allow smears to air-dry completely			
j. Heat-fix the smears (as in 6g)			
k. Allow the slides to cool			
9. Turn off the electric incinerator			
10. Assemble staining rack and stain reagents			
11. Place a set of smears on the staining rack, if space allows			
12. Flood the slides with crystal violet for the manufacturer's recommended time, usually 1 minute			
13. Rinse the stain off the slides with a gentle stream of water from a beaker, faucet, or plastic squeeze bottle and tilt the slides to remove excess water			

(Continues)

© 2012 Delmar, Cengage Learning. Permission to reproduce for clinical use granted.

You must:	S	U	Evaluation/Comments
14. Flood the slides with Gram's iodine for the recommended time			
15. Rinse the slides as in step 13			
16. Decolorize and rinse smears one at a time: a. Hold slide using forceps or clothespin and add the de-colorizer until no more purple color runs off the slide NOTE: Decolorize no longer than a few seconds to prevent over-decolorization b. Rinse the slide with water immediately to remove the decolorizer and stop the reaction; tilt the slide to remove excess water and return slide to staining rack			
17. Counterstain the smears by flooding the slides with safranin for the recommended time			
18. Rinse the slides, tilt to remove excess water; wipe the back of the slide with paper towel to remove stain; stand slides on end or blot between sheets of bibulous paper to dry			
19. Stain remaining heat-fixed smears following steps 11–18			
20. Place a dry stained smear of a gram-positive organism on the microscope stage			
21. Use the low-power (10×) objective to locate the smear area			
22. Observe the smear using the oil-immersion objective			
23. Observe that the *organisms* are gram-positive; describe their morphology (color, shape, arrangement)			
24. Remove the slide and repeat the procedure, using the slide of gram-negative organisms; describe their morphology			
25. Observe the remaining stained slides, record the morphology and Gram stain reactions of the organisms present			
26. Rotate the low-power objective into place and remove the slide			
27. Clean the oil-immersion objective, microscope stage and the top of the microscope condenser with lens paper and lens cleaner			
28. Return equipment to storage; wipe oil off slides gently and store slides, or discard in sharps container			
29. Return cultures to storage or discard into biohazard container as directed by instructor			

© 2012 Delmar, Cengage Learning. Permission to reproduce for clinical use granted.

You must:	S	U	Evaluation/Comments
30. Clean work surfaces with disinfectant			
31. Remove gloves and discard into biohazard container			
32. Wash hands with antiseptic			

Instructor/Evaluator Comments:

Instructor/Evaluator _____ Date _____

© 2012 Delmar, Cengage Learning. Permission to reproduce for clinical use granted.

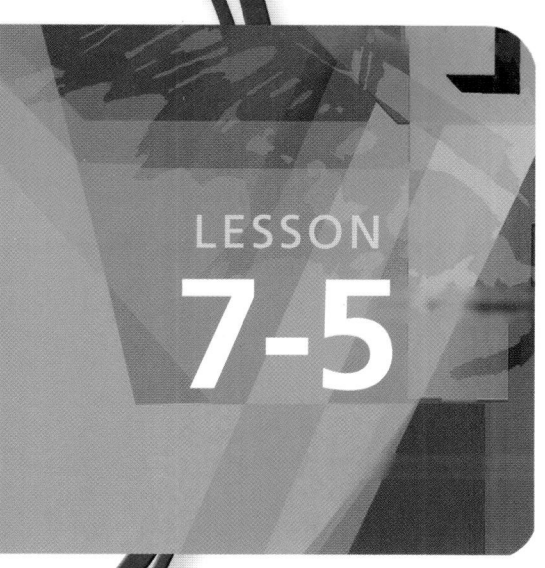

LESSON
7-5

Tests for Group A *Streptococcus*

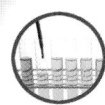

LESSON OBJECTIVES

After studying this lesson, the student will:

- ⊙ Discuss the importance of identifying infections caused by group A *Streptococcus*.
- ⊙ Collect a pharyngeal (throat) swab.
- ⊙ Perform a throat culture and interpret the results.
- ⊙ Use a bacitracin disk to identify group A *Streptococcus*.
- ⊙ List two major types of technology used in rapid tests for group A *Streptococcus*.
- ⊙ Perform a rapid test for group A *Streptococcus*.
- ⊙ Discuss safety precautions that must be observed when performing throat cultures and rapid tests for group A *Streptococcus*.
- ⊙ Discuss quality assessment procedures essential to the performance of throat cultures and rapid tests for group A *Streptococcus*.
- ⊙ Define the glossary terms.

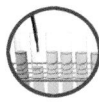

GLOSSARY

fossae / in the throat, shallow depressions where the tonsils were located before surgical removal

hemolysis / the rupture or destruction of red blood cells resulting in the release of hemoglobin

pharyngeal / having to do with the back of the throat or pharynx

INTRODUCTION

The throat culture and rapid strep test are frequently performed microbiology tests, especially in children and young adults. The tests are performed when the patient's clinical symptoms suggest possible strep throat.

Strep tonsillitis is an infection by *Streptococcus pyogenes*, a gram-positive coccus that belongs to Lancefield group A. Therefore, it is often referred to as group A *Streptococcus*. Only 5% to 10% of patients with sore throats test

positive for group A *Streptococcus*. However, because the complications of an untreated streptococcal infection can be serious, all patients who report symptoms should be tested. An untreated group A *Streptococcus* infection can result in scarlet fever, rheumatic fever, rheumatic endocarditis, or glomerulonephritis. These complications are most common in patients under the age of 25 years.

Group A *Streptococcus* (GAS) is just one of several Lancefield groups of streptococci that can cause tonsillitis and other infections in humans. Two other common groups are

Lancefield group C and group G. *Streptococcus* grouping kits can be used to test for the other Lancefield groups if a symptomatic patient tests negative for GAS.

DETECTING GROUP A *STREPTOCOCCUS*

Confirmation of the preliminary diagnosis can be made either by identifying Group A *Streptococcus* in culture or by performing a rapid immunoassay test. The specimen collection is the same for both types of tests.

Safety Precautions

Personnel in smaller laboratories can be responsible for collecting the throat specimen and might also perform the culture or the rapid test for GAS. Appropriate personal protective equipment (PPE) must be worn; a buttoned, fluid-resistant laboratory coat will protect the technician's clothing from contamination. Gloves and protective eyewear should also be worn (Figure 7-30). A mask should be worn while collecting the throat specimen if the patient is coughing excessively. Hands must be washed before gloving, after removing gloves, and any time contamination is a possibility.

The specimen receiving area and other work surfaces should be kept neat and disinfected frequently. Electric incinerators must be used with caution. All culture materials and other contaminated materials must be discarded in the appropriate sharps or biohazard containers and autoclaved before disposal.

Quality Assessment

The facility's standard operating procedure (SOP) manual will specify the procedures for collecting specimens, setting up and incubating cultures, and interpreting and reporting culture results. Quality assessment (QA) programs must be in place to ensure reliability of media and test kits. Each new lot of swabs should be tested to be sure the swabs support viability of GAS and do not interfere with results of rapid strep tests. Each lot of blood agar media should be inoculated with a known culture of GAS to check for support of growth and demonstration of hemolysis. Many commercial check systems are available for use with QA programs.

The manufacturer's instructions must be strictly followed when performing rapid strep tests. Reagents must not be used beyond the expiration dates, and reagents from one kit cannot be used with another. Time limits for setting up the test and observing results must be followed. Most test kits contain built-in (internal) controls. However, if a test system does not have an internal control, an external control must be run at recommended intervals. Patient results cannot be reported unless the controls give the expected reactions.

Performing the Throat Culture

Collecting the Specimen

The **pharyngeal** surfaces are swabbed with a sterile Dacron or rayon swab. The swab should be gently passed across the surfaces of both tonsils or the surfaces of the **fossae** (if tonsils have been removed) and the back of the throat. The swab should not touch the tongue or the inside of the mouth; these surfaces are covered with normal flora of the mouth, which can grow on the medium and contaminate the culture. If transport of specimen to the laboratory will be delayed, the swab must be placed in a transport medium suitable for streptococci.

Inoculating the Media

The throat swab is immediately used to inoculate one quadrant of a blood agar plate (Figure 7-31). A sterile loop is then used to streak for isolated colonies, following the procedure outlined in Lesson 7-3. The loop can also be used to make two or three stabs into the blood agar. This is done by touching the inoculated area in the first quadrant with the sterile loop and then *stabbing* the

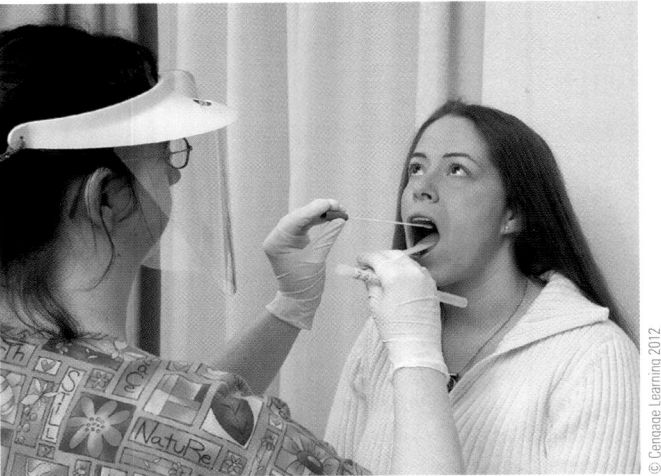

FIGURE 7-30 Wearing a face shield while collecting a throat swab for culture or rapid strep test

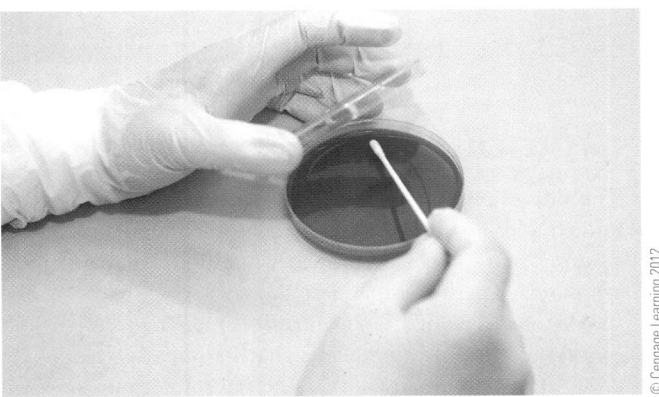

FIGURE 7-31 Inoculating a blood agar plate using a throat culture swab

loop into the agar two or three times in the fourth quadrant. A paper disk (the *A* disk) containing the antibiotic bacitracin can be placed on the concentrated streak in the first quadrant of the newly streaked plate before it is placed in the incubator.

Incubating the Culture

Growth of most streptococci is enhanced by incubation in an increased carbon dioxide (CO_2) environment. A CO_2 concentration of 10% increases the growth of hemolytic streptococci and inhibits the growth of other throat flora (Table 7-19). The culture can be placed in a special CO_2 incubator that has compressed CO_2 pumped into the chamber and the CO_2 level controlled electronically. An enhanced CO_2 environment can also be created using a candle jar (Figure 7-32). To set up a candle jar, culture plates are placed inside a wide-mouth container, a short lighted candle is placed on the top culture plate, and the lid is closed. The candle uses up most of the oxygen before it stops burning, leaving 5% to 10% CO_2 inside the jar. Commercial gas-generating systems are also available that create the increased CO_2 environment by chemical means.

Reading the Throat Culture Plate

After overnight incubation, the blood agar plate is examined for growth, which is noted as scant, moderate, or heavy. The agar is then examined for hemolysis and for growth around the bacitracin disk.

Hemolysis is indicated by clearing of the agar around colonies on the blood agar plate and in the stabs (Figure 7-33A). Complete hemolysis is called beta (ß) hemolysis, and gives a

TABLE 7-19. Characteristics of group A *Streptococcus*

PROCEDURE	CHARACTERISTIC/REACTION
Gram stain	Gram positive
Morphology observations	Coccus, grows in chains
Culture	Enhanced growth in 5% to 10% CO_2
Blood agar	Beta (β) hemolysis
Antibiotic susceptibility	Bacitracin sensitive

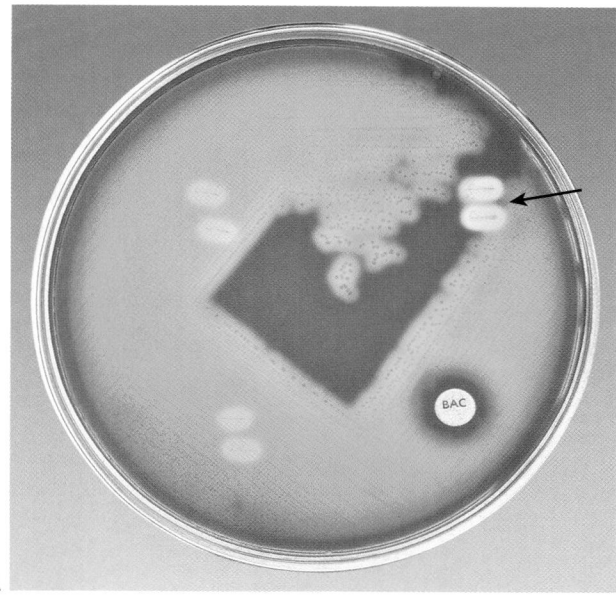

A

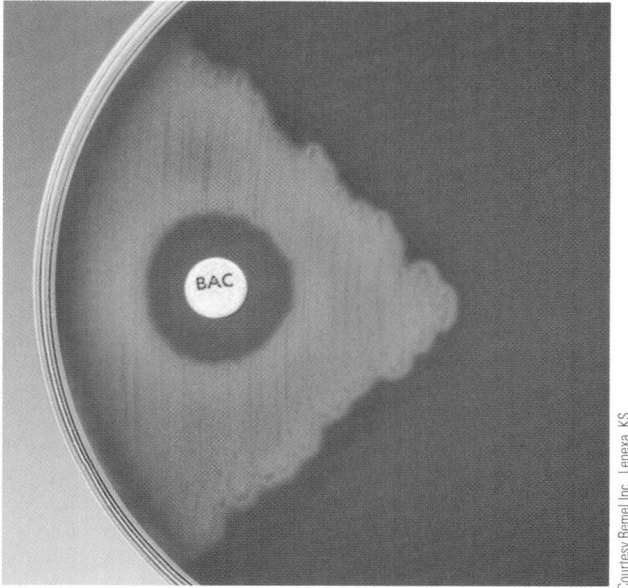

B

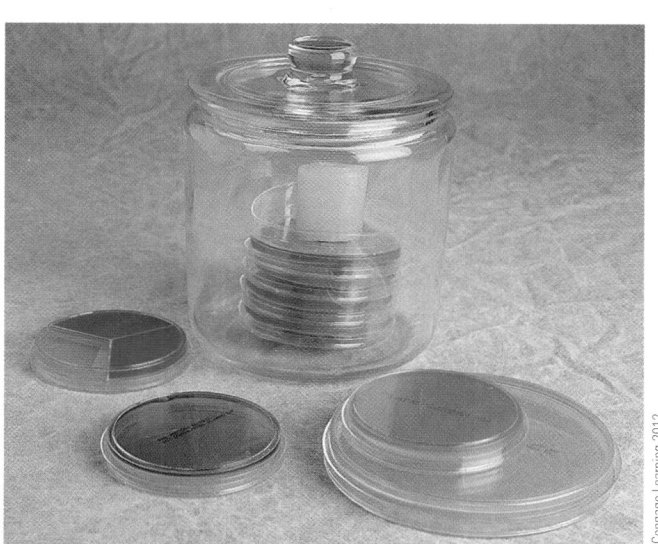

FIGURE 7-32 Candle jar: An atmosphere of 5-10% CO_2 is produced by placing a lighted candle on top of inoculated agar plates and placing lid on the jar

FIGURE 7-33 Beta hemolytic *Streptococcus* growing on blood agar: (A) beta hemolysis around stabs in agar (arrow); (B) inhibition of growth of beta-hemolytic Streptococcus by a bacitracin disk

© Cengage Learning 2012

Courtesy Remel Inc., Lenexa, KS

yellowish appearance to the agar. Incomplete hemolysis produces a green coloration in the agar and is called alpha (α) hemolysis. Absence of hemolysis is referred to as gamma (α) hemolysis (Table 7-20). The stabs in the agar should be closely examined because beta hemolysis will show up in the stabs even if it is difficult to see on the agar surface.

The area around the bacitracin disk is also examined for bacterial growth. Bacitracin inhibits growth of GAS. The presence of a *zone of inhibition* (an area without bacterial growth) around the bacitracin disk, along with the presence of beta-hemolytic colonies, is presumptive identification for Group A *Streptococcus* (Table 7-20 and Figure 7-33B).

Some laboratories do not use a bacitracin disk on the original throat culture plate. If beta-hemolytic colonies are present after incubation of the primary plate, an isolated colony is streaked to another blood agar plate for confluent growth (produced by spreading the inoculum in close or overlapping streaks). A bacitracin disk is placed on the agar to be interpreted after overnight incubation.

If there is a need to confirm GAS or to identify Lancefield groups other than Group A, isolated colonies are tested with a panel of antibodies against the Lancefield groups of *Streptococcus* or with molecular techniques.

Performing a Rapid Test for Group A *Streptococcus*

Although the throat culture continues to be one of the most frequently performed tests, laboratories also use rapid immunological tests to identify GAS. Most of the kits produce test results in about 5 minutes. Two basic technologies used are lateral flow immunoassay and latex agglutination.

Immunoassays for Group A Streptococcus

The majority of rapid strep A tests are immunochromatographic assays that incorporate lateral flow technology. This test method is very sensitive and specific for GAS. All reagents required to perform the test are included in the rapid strep A test kits. The tests use an extract from the throat swab. Some are two-step tests that include an acid extraction and the addition of the extract to the test system. Others have additional steps, such as adding a conjugate or a wash solution.

Results are displayed in different ways, based on the patterns the manufacturers used to apply the antibody to the test membrane. Some test systems produce a plus (+) sign for positive and a minus (-) sign for negative. If no group A antigen is present, the horizontal bar serves as a control to prove that the test is working. Any group A strep antigen present will bind and cause the vertical line to be visible, making a (+) sign. Other test kits use a colored dot or parallel colored lines on the test membrane to indicate results.

ICON Strep A Tests

The Beckman Coulter ICON SC Strep A and ICON DS strep A tests are CLIA-waived rapid immunoassays for detecting GAS antigen from throat swab specimens. In the ICON SC strep A test, strep A specific antibody in the self-contained test device reacts with any strep A antigen extracted from the patient throat swab. The antigen–antibody mixture travels through the membrane and generates a red line visible in the result window. The test device contains an internal control that will always turn red if the test has been performed correctly.

To perform the test, the patient's throat is swabbed using the special swab included in the test kit. Reagents are added to the swab chamber in the cassette. The swab is inserted immediately, agitated 10 times around the chamber, and then is left undisturbed for 1 minute. After 1 minute has elapsed, the swab is rotated around the walls of the chamber while pressed up against the walls to express as much liquid sample from the swab as possible. The swab is then removed and discarded. The valve in the cassette is opened, allowing the mixture to flow into the membrane chamber, and a timer is set for 5 minutes.

TABLE 7-20. Classification of hemolysis on blood agar	
TYPE OF HEMOLYSIS	**APPEARANCE**
Beta (β)	Complete lysis of red blood cells around a colony, making agar almost transparent
Alpha (α)	Green discoloration of agar around a colony
Gamma (γ)	Absence of hemolysis

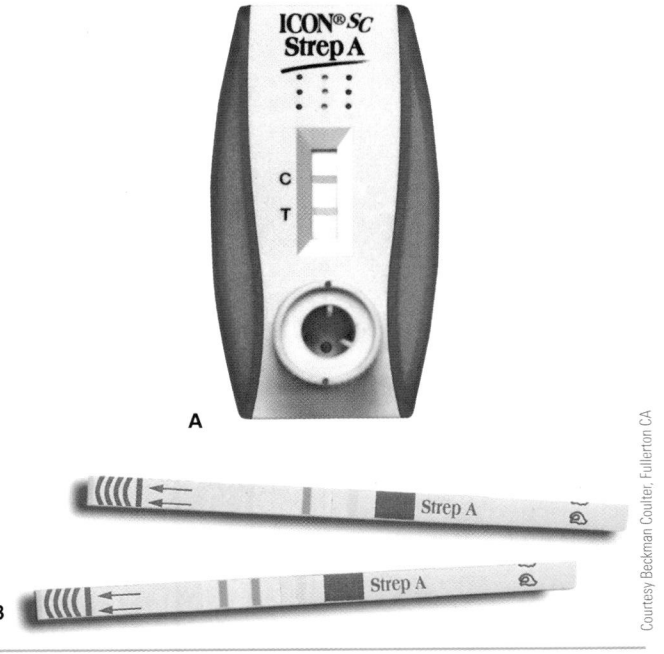

Courtesy Beckman Coulter, Fullerton CA

FIGURE 7-34 Rapid test kits for group A *Streptococcus*: (A) ICON SC Strep A lateral flow immunoassay test device showing positive result; (B) ICON DS Strep A test strips—top strip shows negative result, bottom strip shows positive result

CURRENT TOPICS

INVASIVE GROUP A *STREPTOCOCCUS*

Nothing catches the attention of the public like headlines such as "Victims of flesh-eating bacteria in local hospital" or "Girl loses lower arm to flesh-eating bacteria." News such as this is alarming, especially when readers are led to believe that newly-discovered bacteria are attacking humans and that scientists have no idea how to deal with it. Patients are afraid that their strep throat infection can change into this terrifying new form.

Actually, these invasive bacteria have been around a long time. The condition in which the flesh is damaged is called *necrotizing fasciitis* (NF) and is caused by a subtype of group A *Streptococcus pyogenes*, the same group of bacteria that causes strep throat. Strep infections can be divided into noninvasive and invasive. Infection with noninvasive streptococci can cause strep throat, cellulitis, impetigo, glomerulonephritis, and rheumatic heart disease. Millions of people in the United States have strep throat infections every year and recover. The invasive form of group A *Streptococcus* (GAS) infects only a few thousand people each year.

The two invasive subtypes of GAS differ genetically from the noninvasive types. A method of genotyping bacterial strains of strep is used by researchers to detect these especially virulent types and track the epidemiology of outbreaks. The invasive types can cause NF and streptococcal toxic shock syndrome (STSS), not to be confused with toxic shock syndrome caused by staphylococci. In cases of NF, destruction of muscle and other tissue occurs. Therefore, the news media has called it the *flesh-eating* bacteria.

Invasive strep A infections can begin as a sore or wound that shows redness, pain, drainage, or swelling. The wound rapidly changes to a painful purple or black patch, possibly within an hour. A healthcare provider must be consulted immediately if these symptoms occur. Other symptoms include fever, sweating, chills, nausea, dizziness, profound weakness, and finally shock. Treatment consists of administration of powerful, broad-spectrum intravenous antibiotics as soon as possible. Surgery is required to remove the damaged tissue and open and drain the infected areas. Amputation of an infected limb can be required to prevent spread of the infection. Although fatalities can occur, if infections are treated aggressively and early, patients can have a good prognosis.

Prevention consists of practicing good hygiene such as frequent handwashing, especially after coughing and sneezing. Any skin injuries should immediately be thoroughly cleansed and an appropriate antibiotic applied.

At the end of the 5 minutes, the result, visible on the front of the device, is read and interpreted. Two distinct red lines, one in the test (T) area and one in the control (C) area, indicate a positive result (Figure 7-34). A red line in the control area only indicates a negative result. If no line appears in the control (C) region, the test is invalid and must be repeated after collecting a new specimen.

Latex Agglutination Tests

Latex agglutination kits use the antigen–antibody reaction to identify GAS. Microscopic latex beads coated with *antibodies* to GAS are reacted with an *antigen* preparation made from the throat specimen. Agglutination indicates presence of GAS. Absence of agglutination is a negative result.

SAFETY REMINDERS

- Review Safety Precautions section before beginning procedure.
- Observe Standard Precautions.
- Wear appropriate PPE.
- Treat all used swabs as if infectious.
- Wear mask when collecting a throat swab from a coughing patient.
- Autoclave all specimens and culture materials before disposal.

PROCEDURAL REMINDERS

- Review Quality Assessment section before beginning procedure.
- Follow the manufacturers' directions and the SOP manual.
- Swab only the tonsils and back of the throat.
- Observe expiration dates of reagents and kits.
- Incubate the throat culture in a 5% to 10% CO_2 atmosphere.
- Carefully examine BA plate for hemolysis.

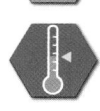

Reliability of Rapid Tests for Group A Streptococcus

Rapid strep kits in general have high sensitivity and specificity. Each brand of kit is different and the package inserts will describe the levels of detection for the kit. Some kits may not be as accurate if numbers of bacteria in the throat are very low or the swabbing is not thorough. The patient should not eat, drink, or gargle in the 30 minutes before the swab is taken. A false-negative result for GAS could cause a strep throat infection to be untreated, which could lead to serious complications in children and young adults. Therefore, negative rapid strep tests should be confirmed by a throat culture.

CRITICAL THINKING 1

Sue was working in the campus health clinic when Tony came in to have a throat swab performed. His healthcare provider had ordered a rapid test for GAS because Tony had a fever and sore throat. The result from the rapid test was negative, so a throat culture for strep was ordered. Sue swabbed Tony's throat, and the healthcare provider gave him a prescription for an antibiotic. Sue inoculated the first quadrant of the plate using the specimen on the swab. She disposed of the swab in the appropriate biohazard container, sterilized the loop, and began to begin to streak the inoculum into the other quadrants. A fellow worker interrupted her, and she laid the loop down momentarily and then continued streaking the plate. After overnight incubation of the plate at 35° to 37° C in a CO_2 incubator, Tom, a coworker, examined the plate and observed atypical colonies that did not look like strep. He performed a Gram stain and saw some gram-positive bacilli, similar in appearance to those commonly found on environmental surfaces.

1. What could be the source of gram-positive bacilli?
2. Were mistakes made in the laboratory procedures? What were they?
3. Which laboratory technician needs a refresher course in culture techniques?
4. Since the rapid strep test was negative, was the throat culture necessary?

CRITICAL THINKING 2

Maria worked the day shift in bacteriology. One of her first responsibilities each day was to examine cultures that had been incubating overnight. She saw that both throat and urine cultures had been set up on specimens from Mrs. Cheng. Maria pulled the plates to read the two cultures and found that the blood agar plate for the throat culture and the blood agar and MAC urine culture plates were all in the 37° C aerobic incubator. The blood agar throat culture plate had scant growth.

Should the results be reported? Explain your answer.

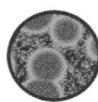

SUMMARY

The rapid test for GAS and the throat culture are frequently performed tests. Both are performed from throat swabs and are important in the detection of group A strep infections. Most rapid strep A kits have a high specificity and high sensitivity. This means that they have the specificity to react only to strep A and are usually sensitive enough to detect light infections. The laboratory's SOP manual and the manufacturer's instructions for performing rapid tests and interpreting results must be strictly followed. Personnel must observe Standard Precautions and wear appropriate PPE while performing the throat swab, the throat culture, and rapid strep tests.

Because the complications from undiagnosed and untreated strep can be serious, a throat culture should be performed if the rapid test for GAS is negative. Throat cultures are performed by inoculating throat swabs to blood agar. This medium supplies the required nutrients for growth of throat isolates and also demonstrates beta-hemolysis, a characteristic of GAS. The culture plates must be incubated in the presence of increased CO_2 for optimum growth of Group A *Streptococcus*.

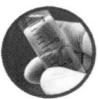

REVIEW QUESTIONS

1. Why is early diagnosis of group A *Streptococcus* (GAS) infection important?

2. Explain why the tongue and mouth should not be touched when collecting a throat swab for strep.

3. Why is a throat culture inoculated to blood agar?

4. What is the purpose of the bacitracin disk?

5. What is the reason for making stabs in the agar?

6. Explain the different types of hemolysis.

7. Explain the principles of agglutination tests and rapid immunoassay tests for GAS.

8. Explain the possible consequence of a false-negative result in a rapid strep A test.

9. List four safety procedures that must be observed when collecting or processing throat culture swabs.

10. What QA procedures are important when testing for GAS?

11. Define fossae, hemolysis, and pharyngeal.

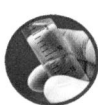

STUDENT ACTIVITIES

1. Complete the written examination for this lesson.

2. Survey local clinics or physician office laboratories to find out which rapid tests for GAS are used and what procedure is followed when a rapid test is negative.

3. Practice performing a throat culture, as outlined in the Student Performance Guide.

4. Practice performing rapid tests for GAS, as outlined in the Student Performance Guide.

WEB ACTIVITIES

1. Use the Internet to find two additional rapid strep tests not mentioned in this lesson. Report on your findings, including information such as test principle, test sensitivity and specificity, and CLIA complexity level.

2. Use the Internet to research a complication that can result from an untreated strep infection.

3. Search the Internet for a video demonstrating the procedures for collecting a throat swab and streaking a throat culture plate.

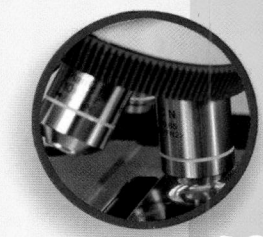

LESSON 7-5

Tests for Group A *Streptococcus*

Name _____   Date _____

INSTRUCTIONS

1. Practice performing a throat culture and rapid test for group A *Streptococcus*, following the step-by-step procedure.

2. Demonstrate the procedures for throat culture and rapid tests for group A *Streptococcus* satisfactorily for the instructor using the Student Performance Guide. Your instructor will explain the procedures for evaluating your performance. Your performance may be given a number grade, a letter grade or satisfactory (S) or unsatisfactory (U) depending on course or institutional policy.

NOTE: The instructions given are for the ICON SC Strep A test (Beckman Coulter). Manufacturer's instructions must be followed for the test kit used. Inclusion of this method does not constitute endorsement by the authors. If disposable loops are used, manufacturer's instructions for use must be followed.

MATERIALS AND EQUIPMENT

- gloves
- hand antiseptic
- full-face shield (or equivalent PPE)
- timer
- sterile Dacron or rayon swabs for performing throat culture
- tongue depressors
- swabs inoculated with Group A *Streptococcus* (from stock culture)–two swabs per student, one for rapid strep test and one for positive culture plate
- rack for culture tubes
- blood agar plate(s)
- inoculating loop, sterile disposable or sterilizable
- loop holder
- electric incinerator
- CO_2 incubator (35° to 37° C) or aerobic incubator (35° to 37° C) with candle jar and candle
- bacitracin disks
- forceps
- rapid test kit for group A *Streptococcus*, with all kit components and manufacturer's instructions
- paper towels
- surface disinfectant
- biohazard container
- sharps container

PROCEDURE

   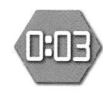

Record in the comment section any problems encountered while practicing the procedure (or have a fellow student or the instructor evaluate your performance).

S = Satisfactory
U = Unsatisfactory

You must:	S	U	Evaluation/Comments
1. Wash hands with antiseptic; put on gloves and face protection			
2. Assemble equipment and materials, including a blood agar plate			

(Continues)

© 2012 Delmar, Cengage Learning. Permission to reproduce for clinical use granted.

STUDENT PERFORMANCE GUIDE

You must:	S	U	Evaluation/Comments
3. Collect throat specimen from a fellow student by swabbing the pharyngeal surfaces			
4. Transfer the throat specimen to the blood agar plate following steps 4a–4e: a. Roll the swab gently on the surface of one quadrant of the blood agar plate. Discard swab into biohazard container b. Sterilize a wire loop or use a sterile disposable plastic loop c. Streak the plate for isolated colonies as described in Lesson 7-3. Make two or three stabs in the fourth quadrant of agar; discard disposable loop as directed or sterilize reusable loop and return to loop holder d. Sterilize forceps; place bacitracin disk on quadrant one; sterilize forceps again e. Label bottom of plate with specimen ID			
5. Obtain a positive control swab (containing GAS) from your instructor, and inoculate a second blood agar plate, following steps 5a–5b a. Label the plate "GAS+"; streak the entire plate for continuous growth b. Sterilize forceps and place a bacitracin disk in the center of the plate; sterilize forceps again			
6. Place both plates upside down (inverted) in the 37° C CO_2 incubator overnight (or use candle jar in aerobic incubator) and proceed to step 7			
7. Perform ICON SC Strep A rapid test for group A *Streptococcus* following steps 7a–7m and instructions in package insert (if another brand of kit is used, follow instructions for that kit) a. Allow test pack to come to room temperature (if not stored at room temperature) b. Remove test device from the foil pouch, check to see that the marks on the chamber are in the position indicated on the package insert, and begin the test immediately c. Invert reagent bottle A, hold vertically and dispense 5 full drops to the swab chamber d. Invert reagent bottle B, hold vertically and dispense 5 full drops to the swab chamber e. Perform the throat swab procedure (or use pre-inoculated swab) and immediately add the swab to the chamber containing the reagents f. Hold the chamber base and vigorously agitate the swab in the chamber about 10 times g. Leave the swab in the chamber 1 minute			

© 2012 Delmar, Cengage Learning. Permission to reproduce for clinical use granted.

You must:	S	U	Evaluation/Comments
h. After 1 minute, hold the base of the chamber firmly with the thumb and index finger of one hand and remove the swab by bringing it halfway up the inside wall of the chamber and pressing it against the ribs on the inside of the wall			
i. Rotate the swab 5 times while continuing to firmly press to expel as much liquid as possible			
j. Discard the swab in the appropriate biohazard container			
k. Open the valve into the device NOTE: If liquid does not appear in the window within 1 minute, discard the device and repeat the test with a new throat swab and new test unit			
l. Set the timer and read the results at 5 minutes. NOTE: Results are not reliable after 10 minutes			
m. Interpret the results: (1) Negative: A negative result will have a single red C line in the top of the window. This indicates that the procedure and reagents were correct but no *Streptococcus* A was detected (2) Positive: A positive result will have a red C line and a red T line (3) Invalid: No red lines are present or only the T line is red			
8. Discard all contaminated materials into appropriate sharps or biohazard container			
9. Return all equipment to storage			
10. Wipe work area with disinfectant			
11. Remove gloves and discard into biohazard container			
11. Wash hands with antiseptic			
12. The next day: Wash hands, put on gloves, and remove plates from incubator a. Observe the GAS+ plate for hemolysis and for a zone of inhibition around the bacitracin disk and record observation: if beta hemolysis and a zone of inhibition (no growth) around the bacitracin disk are present, report as "*beta-hemolytic streptococci present, bacitracin sensitive, presumptive for Group A Streptococcus*") b. Observe "unknown" culture plate: (1) Examine agar surface through the top cover of the plate and estimate the amount of bacterial growth: report as no growth, scant, moderate, or heavy (2) Observe agar for hemolysis and record the type: alpha, beta, or gamma (no hemolysis); be certain to examine the agar stabs			

(Continues)

© 2012 Delmar, Cengage Learning. Permission to reproduce for clinical use granted.

You must:	S	U	Evaluation/Comments
(3) If beta-hemolytic colonies are present and a zone of inhibition (no growth) is present around the bacitracin disk, report as "*beta-hemolytic streptococci present, bacitracin sensitive, presumptive for Group A Streptococcus*" (4) If no beta-hemolytic colonies are observed, report "*no beta-hemolytic colonies present*"			
13. Compare the results from the two plates			
14. Discard cultures into biohazard container as directed by instructor			
15. Wipe work area with disinfectant			
16. Remove gloves and discard into biohazard container			
17. Wash hands with antiseptic			

Instructor/Evaluator Comments:

Instructor/Evaluator _____ Date _____

© 2012 Delmar, Cengage Learning. Permission to reproduce for clinical use granted.

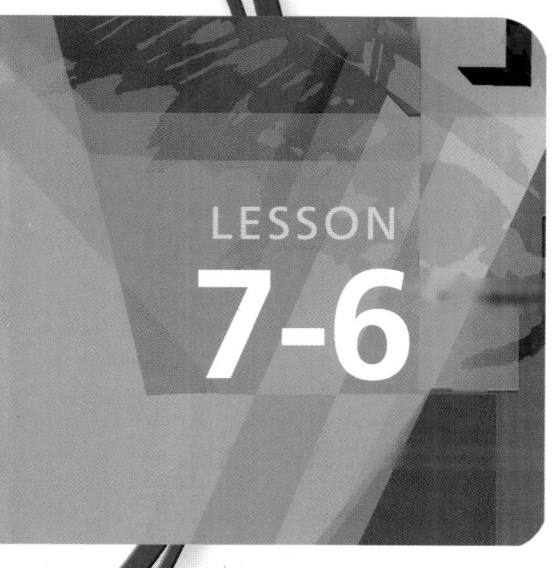

Urine Culture and Colony Count

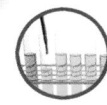

LESSON OBJECTIVES

After studying this lesson, the student will:

⊙ Discuss the reasons why a urine culture and colony count might be requested.

⊙ Select the correct primary medium and indicator medium for a urine culture.

⊙ Demonstrate the streaking technique for urine colony count.

⊙ Perform a colony count on a urine culture.

⊙ Discuss the medical significance of urine culture results.

⊙ Name four bacteria that are common causes of urinary tract infections.

⊙ Discuss aspects of quality assessment that must be considered when performing urine culture and colony count.

⊙ Describe the safety precautions to observe when performing urine culture and colony count.

⊙ Define the glossary term.

GLOSSARY

colony count / an estimation of the number of bacteria in 1 mL of urine made by counting the colonies on a urine culture plate

INTRODUCTION

The urine culture and colony count are frequently performed in the bacteriology laboratory. The physician requests a urine culture and colony count when a patient has urinary tract infection (UTI) symptoms, such as frequent urination, pain and burning during urination, blood in the urine, and sometimes fever and backache (Table 7-21). The **colony count** estimates the number of bacteria in the urine. The colony count is performed by counting the colonies that grow on the urine culture plate.

Urinary tract infections (UTI) are infections occurring in the urinary tract, usually in the urethra. The bacteria can migrate up the urethra into the bladder causing cystitis, or even further into the kidneys. Although females are prone to UTIs because of their anatomy, UTIs also occur in males, particularly in the elderly or when urine flow is partially blocked by a condition such as enlarged prostate.

The most common bacterial species responsible for UTI is *Escherichia coli*, a gram-negative rod that is part of the normal flora of the intestinal tract. Other gram-negative rods, such as *Pseudomonas, Proteus*, and *Klebsiella*, can also cause UTI. *Staphylococcus saprophyticus*, a gram-positive coccus, is also a frequent cause of urinary tract infections (Table 7-22).

TABLE 7-21. Symptoms associated with urinary tract infections

Frequent urination

Pain or burning sensation when urinating

Blood in urine

Fever

Backache

TABLE 7-22. Bacteria that frequently cause urinary tract infections

BACTERIAL SPECIES	MEDIA* SUPPORTING GROWTH
E. coli	BA, EMB, MAC
Klebsiella	BA, EMB, MAC
Proteus	BA, EMB, MAC
Pseudomonas aeruginosa	BA, EMB, MAC
Enterococcus	BA
Staphylococcus saprophyticus	BA

* BA = blood agar
EMB = eosin-methylene blue medium
MAC = MacConkey's medium

PERFORMING THE URINE CULTURE

The urine culture is performed on a clean-catch specimen. The procedure for collecting a clean-catch specimen is described in Lesson 5-2.

Safety Precautions

  The procedures performed in the urine culture and colony count expose the technician to potentially infectious body fluids and to cultures of unidentified bacteria. Standard Precautions must be observed. Gloves and other appropriate PPE must be worn when handling the urine and the bacterial cultures. Calibrated loops that are disposable should be used when possible to eliminate the potential for aerosol formation when sterilizing a wire loop. Work surfaces must be wiped frequently with a surface disinfectant. All contaminated materials and cultures must be discarded into biohazard containers and autoclaved before disposal, following facility guidelines.

Quality Assessment

   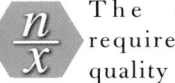 The specimen requirements and quality assessment procedures will be included in the laboratory's standard operating procedure (SOP) manual. The patient must be instructed in the method of collecting a clean-catch urine specimen to prevent contamination of the urine. The specimen for culture must be collected before antibiotic therapy is begun. If a routine urinalysis is also ordered on the specimen, the culture should be set up first to prevent possible contamination of the specimen during the routine urinalysis procedure.

Calibrated inoculating loops must be used for the urine culture; the loop size must be verified to be sure the colony count is calculated correctly. Each new shipment of media should be visually inspected for contamination. One plate or tube from each lot of media should be incubated overnight at 35° to 37° C and then inspected for contamination. In addition, a plate can be inoculated with a known bacterial stock culture to ensure that the media contains all the ingredients required to support bacterial growth. Media must not be used beyond its expiration date.

Collecting the Specimen

The urine must be collected by clean-catch method. In addition, females should be cautioned to avoid contaminating the specimen with vaginal material, which can contain microorganisms. The urine container should be labeled on the side (not on the lid) with the patient's name and identification number and the time of collection. The urine should be inoculated to culture media within 1 hour of collection. If the specimen is to be sent to a reference laboratory for culture, the laboratory's instructions and transport supplies must be used.

Streaking the Plates

Urine specimens are streaked onto two types of media:

- Primary medium, usually blood agar (BA), and
- Indicator/selective medium, such as eosin-methylene blue (EMB) or MacConkey (MAC)

Most urinary tract pathogens will grow on BA. Both EMB and MAC inhibit the growth of gram-positive bacteria and indicate fermentation reactions of gram-negative bacteria (Table 7-22).

A calibrated platinum reusable loop or sterile single-use plastic loop with a capacity of either 0.01 mL or 0.001 mL is used to inoculate the blood agar plate. The loop is sterilized and cooled and then dipped into a well-mixed urine sample. The loop is observed to be sure it is full of urine and then is used to make a vertical streak down the center of the BA plate (Figure 7-35A). Fifteen to twenty horizontal cross streaks are then made across the plate, crossing the vertical streak each time (Figure 7-35B). A second set of horizontal streaks is made at right angles to the first set (Figure 7-35C). The EMB or MAC plate is inoculated in the same manner using another loopful of urine. The loop is sterilized after use and placed in the loop holder. If a sterile, disposable loop is used, it should be discarded into the sharps container. The culture plates are labeled (on the bottom) and placed upside down in the 35° to 37° C aerobic incubator overnight.

Colony Count and Interpretation

After 18 to 24 hours, or overnight incubation, the plates are removed from the incubator and observed for bacterial growth (Figure 7-36). Any distinguishing characteristics of the colonies

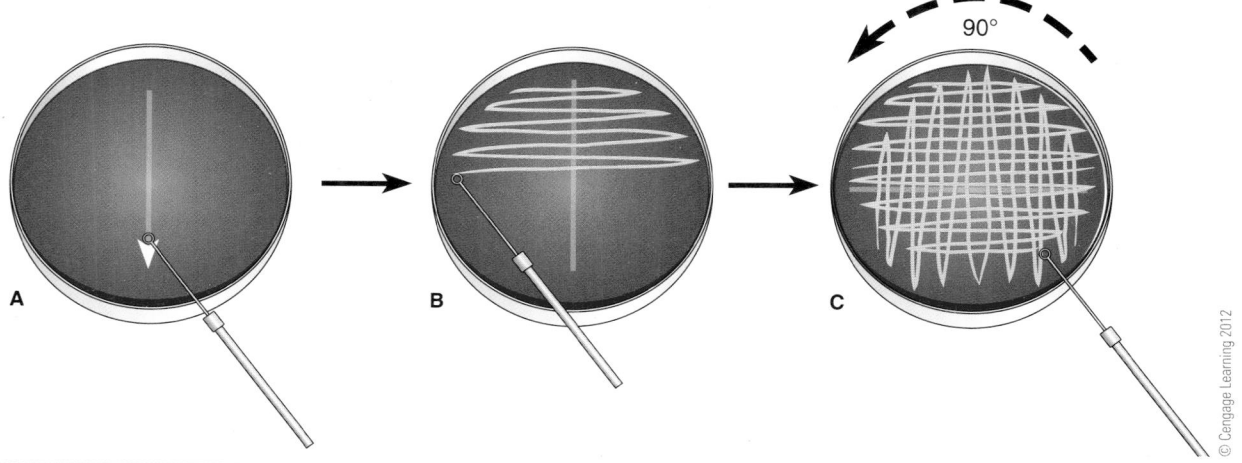

FIGURE 7-35 Streaking a urine culture plate: (A) make one streak down the center of the plate using a calibrated loop; (B) make several streaks at right angles to the initial streak, crossing over the original streak each time; (C) turn plate 90° and make streak at right angles to the previous set of streaks

should be noted, such as colony color, colony morphology, and hemolysis on the BA plate. Both gram-positive and gram-negative bacteria can grow on the blood plate; only gram-negative bacteria should grow on EMB or MAC.

The number of colonies on the BA plate is counted and reported as number of colonies per mL. If a 0.001-mL loop was used to inoculate the plate, the number of colonies counted is multiplied by 1000 to calculate the colony count per mL of urine. If a 0.01-mL loop was used, the number of colonies is multiplied by 100.

Urine cultures that have a significant colony count should be processed for bacterial identification and antibiotic susceptibility. A count of 100,000/mL or greater is evidence of UTI, regardless of whether the patient has symptoms. A colony of 30,000/mL or greater is considered significant in some facilities. In patients who have symptoms or have frequent UTIs, colony counts as low as 1000/mL can be significant.

The presence of three or more different colony types on the primary culture plate suggests that the urine was not clean-catch. The SOP manual of the facility must be followed concerning when to follow up culture results with bacterial identification and antibiotic sensitivity procedures. These procedures can be performed from colonies growing on the urine culture plates.

SAFETY REMINDERS

- Review Safety Precautions section before beginning procedure.
- Observe Standard Precautions.
- Wear appropriate PPE.
- Wipe work area frequently with disinfectant.
- Autoclave all cultures before disposal.

PROCEDURAL REMINDERS

- Review Quality Assessment section before beginning procedure.
- Urine for culture must be clean-catch.
- Use blood agar plate for colony count.
- Consult SOP manual to determine follow-up procedures.
- Report urine culture results following instructions in SOP manual.

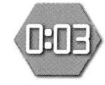

FIGURE 7-36 Examples of isolated colonies from a urine culture

CASE STUDY 1

Shawna was working in a physician office laboratory (POL) when a urine dipstick result indicated presence of blood and WBCs in the urine she was testing. Laboratory protocol specified that a urine culture and sensitivity (C & S) should be set up. Shawna obtained a blood agar plate from stock. On the bottom of the plate she placed the patient's barcode label and streaked the plate for colony count. She then placed the culture plate into the incubator to be read the next morning.

1. Was the urine culture set up correctly?
2. Does blood agar support the growth of both gram-positive and gram-negative organisms?

CASE STUDY 2

Tina is a technician in a small hospital laboratory. She works in the hematology, chemistry, and microbiology sections. On this morning, she was in microbiology examining culture plates that had been set up the previous day. She examined BA and MAC plates set up for a urine culture. Both plates had many colonies growing, and the colonies on each plate appeared to have the same morphology. Tina counted 132 colonies on the MAC plate. From the requisition slip, she saw that the person who set the culture up had used a 0.001-mL loop. Tina reported a colony count of 13,200/mL for the culture.

1. Evaluate Tina's performance in evaluating the urine culture.
2. Does the patient have a urinary tract infection?

CRITICAL THINKING

Mrs. Miller went to her healthcare provider complaining of frequent, painful urination accompanied by a burning sensation, symptoms she had never had before. The provider ordered a routine urinalysis and a urine culture and colony count. In the laboratory, Mrs. Miller gave the laboratory order to John, who handed her a urine collection cup just as the phone rang. Mrs. Miller took the cup to the restroom and brought back a urine specimen, with her ID label on the cup. John set up the urine culture and gave the urine specimen to Timothy, the other technician. Timothy performed a microscopic analysis of the urine sediment and observed 5 to 10 epithelial cells/low power field, mucus threads, and many bacteria. The next morning the BA culture plate had at least four different colony types growing on it.

1. Should the laboratory try to identify all four isolates?
2. What mistake(s) affected the routine urinalysis and culture?

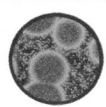

SUMMARY

The urine culture and colony count are frequently ordered tests. If the colony count is significant, the bacteria present will be identified and tested for antibiotic susceptibility as described in Lesson 7-7.

    To ensure the quality of the results, the patient must be given specific instructions for collecting a clean-catch urine. Culturing a contaminated specimen can result in several different microorganisms growing on the culture plates. This complicates the interpretation of the colony count and delays final test results. The facility's SOP manual must be followed in selecting the inoculating loop size, calculating the colony count and reporting the result. Standard Precautions must be observed and aseptic technique must be used. Disposable loops should be used if available. Facility rules for disposal of cultures and other contaminated materials must be followed.

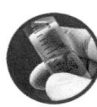

REVIEW QUESTIONS

1. Why must clean-catch urine be used for urine culture?

2. What types of media are used for urine culture?

3. Which culture plate is used to make the colony count?

4. Describe how to streak the BA plate for a colony count.

5. How does the loop used for streaking affect the colony count?

6. What measure(s) should be used in the urine culture procedure to increase safety?

7. Why is it important to perform quality assessment procedures on new shipments of media? How is this done?

8. What are the symptoms of UTIs?

9. What bacterial species is the most common cause of UTIs?

10. Define colony count.

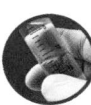

STUDENT ACTIVITIES

1. Complete the written examination for this lesson.

2. Practice performing the urine culture and colony count, as outlined in the Student Performance Guide.

WEB ACTIVITIES

1. Use the Internet to find information on cystitis. Report on the complications that can occur if cystitis is untreated.

2. Search the Internet for tutorials or videos demonstrating how to streak urine culture plates.

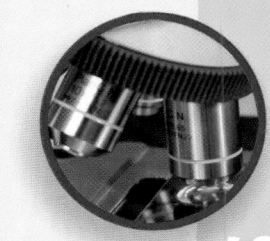

LESSON 7-6
Urine Culture and Colony Count

Name _____   Date _____

INSTRUCTIONS

1. Practice performing the urine culture and colony count following the step-by-step procedure.

2. Demonstrate the urine culture and colony count procedure satisfactorily for the instructor using the Student Performance Guide. Your instructor will explain the procedures for evaluating your performance. Your performance may be given a number grade, a letter grade, satisfactory (S) or unsatisfactory (U) depending on course or institutional policy.

MATERIALS AND EQUIPMENT

- gloves
- hand antiseptic
- full-face shield (or equivalent PPE)
- clean-catch urine specimen(s)
- aerobic incubator set at 35° to 37° C
- blood agar plates
- EMB or MAC agar plates
- Calibrated sterile disposable loop or calibrated platinum loop (0.01 mL or 0.001 mL)
- loop holder (for reusable loop)
- electric incinerator
- wax pencil or marking pen
- paper towels
- surface disinfectant
- sharps container
- biohazard container

PROCEDURE

Record in the comment section any problems encountered while practicing the procedure (or have a fellow student or the instructor evaluate your performance).

S = Satisfactory
U = Unsatisfactory

You must:	S	U	Evaluation/Comments
1. Wash hands with antiseptic and put on gloves			
2. Put on face protection			
3. Assemble equipment and materials			
4. Turn on the electric incinerator			
5. Obtain a clean-catch urine specimen			
6. Mix the urine by swirling, and remove the lid from the urine container carefully, without creating splashes or aerosols			
7. Select a sterile, disposable calibrated loop or sterilize and cool a calibrated platinum loop			

(Continues)

© 2012 Delmar, Cengage Learning. Permission to reproduce for clinical use granted.

You must:	S	U	Evaluation/Comments
8. Insert the loop into the well-mixed urine sample; remove the loop and check to see that the loop is filled with urine			
9. Transfer the loopful of urine to the surface of the blood agar plate by making a streak down the center of the plate			
10. Make 15 to 20 streaks at right angles to the center streak, crossing the center streak each time			
11. Turn the agar plate one-quarter turn (90 degrees) and streak 15 to 20 times at right angles to the first set, crossing all of the streaks each time			
12. Replace the lid on the agar plate			
13 Repeat steps 6–12 using an EMB or MAC plate			
14. Discard disposable loop into sharps container or sterilize the platinum loop and return it to the holder			
15. Label the bottoms of the inoculated plates			
16. Turn off electric incinerator			
17. Return equipment to storage			
18. Place agar plates upside down in 35° to 37° C incubator for 18 to 24 hours (overnight)			
19. Discard contaminated materials into biohazard container to be autoclaved			
20. Wipe work area with disinfectant			
21. Remove gloves and discard into biohazard container			
22. Wash hands with antiseptic			
23. The next day: wash hands and put on gloves			
24. Remove culture plates from the incubator; observe bacterial colonies on the blood agar plate and the EMB or MAC plate through the lids and make a report of the culture results, addressing the questions in steps 24a–27 a. EMB or MAC plate: observe for bacterial growth; if colonies are present, what should be the gram reaction of these colonies? Do all colonies appear of similar morphology?			
b. Blood agar plate: observe for bacterial growth; do all colonies appear of similar morphology?			
25. Count the number of colonies on the blood agar plate			
26. Determine the colony count by multiplying the number of colonies from step 25 by 1,000 if the 0.001-mL loop was used, or by 100 if the 0.01-mL loop was used			

© 2012 Delmar, Cengage Learning. Permission to reproduce for clinical use granted.

You must:	S	U	Evaluation/Comments
27. Record the colony count results and interpret: is the colony count considered to be significant? Does it appear that more than one type of bacteria is present in the urine?			
28. Discard the agar plates as instructed			
29. Wipe the work area with disinfectant			
30. Remove gloves and discard into biohazard container			
31. Wash hands with antiseptic			

Instructor/Evaluator Comments:

Instructor/Evaluator _____ Date _____

© 2012 Delmar, Cengage Learning. Permission to reproduce for clinical use granted.

STUDENT PERFORMANCE GUIDE

759

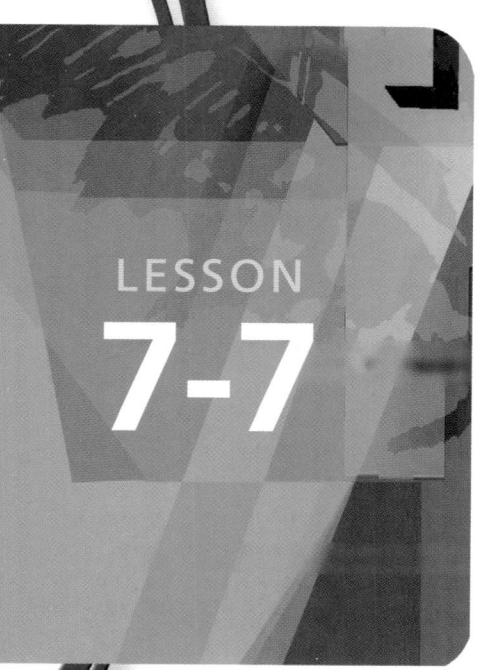

LESSON 7-7

Bacterial Identification and Antibiotic Susceptibility Testing

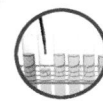

LESSON OBJECTIVES

After studying this lesson, the student will:

⊙ Describe general steps followed to identify gram positive or gram negative bacteria from culture.

⊙ Use the microscope to identify Gram stain reactions of bacteria.

⊙ Explain the purpose of the catalase and coagulase tests.

⊙ Perform the catalase test and interpret the results.

⊙ Perform the coagulase test and interpret the results.

⊙ Explain how to report the presumptive identification of gram-positive and gram-negative bacteria.

⊙ Discuss the use of manual and automated identification systems for bacteria.

⊙ Perform the disk antibiotic susceptibility test and interpret the results.

⊙ Discuss the safety precautions that must be observed when performing bacterial identification and antibiotic susceptibility tests.

⊙ Discuss quality assessment procedures that must be followed when performing bacterial identification and antibiotic susceptibility tests.

⊙ Define the glossary terms.

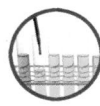

GLOSSARY

catalase test / a test to differentiate between *Streptococcus* and *Staphylococcus* species.

coagulase test / a test to differentiate between *Staphylococcus aureus* and other *Staphylococcus* species

coliform / referring to certain fermentative gram-negative enteric bacteria, including *Escherichia coli*, *Enterobacter*, and *Klebsiella*

minimum inhibitory concentration (MIC) / minimum concentration of an antibiotic required to inhibit the growth of a microorganism

pleomorphic / having varied shapes

zone of inhibition / in the Bauer-Kirby antibiotic susceptibility test, the area around an antibiotic disk in which bacterial growth is inhibited

INTRODUCTION

Identifying bacteria responsible for an infection and determining their antibiotic susceptibility are important steps in the diagnosis and treatment of bacterial infections. For example, when a urine culture yields a colony count considered clinically significant, it is usual to follow up with identification and susceptibility testing of the bacteria present. The identification involves making a Gram stain of an isolated colony to determine if the predominant reaction is gram-positive or gram-negative. Once the Gram reaction and morphology have been determined, biochemical tests are performed to further identify the bacterial species. The identity of the bacteria gives the physician guidance as to which antibiotic would be best, but the antibiotic susceptibility test should be performed to confirm which antibiotic will be most effective.

BACTERIAL IDENTIFICATION

Identification procedures for gram-positive bacteria are different than those for gram-negative bacteria. A combination of criteria including growth and chemical reactions on primary or selective media, type of hemolysis present, colony characteristics, and Gram stain reactions are used in the identification of bacteria.

Common gram-positive cocci, such as staph and strep can often be identified by morphology on Gram stain and results of catalase and coagulase tests or typing tests. Less common gram-positive cocci require additional tests for identification.

Gram-negative rods (bacilli) are identified using tests that demonstrate biochemical reactions such as oxidation or fermentation of sugars. By following organized step-wise identification methods, most common bacteria can be easily identified.

Safety Precautions

   The procedures used in identifying bacteria and determining antibiotic susceptibility expose the technician to reagents and potential pathogens. All safety policies, including Standard Precautions and aseptic techniques, must be followed to prevent contamination of the technician, the environment, and others working in the laboratory. Appropriate personal protective equipment (PPE), such as gloves eye protection, and a disposable, fluid-resistant laboratory coat must be worn. The precautions listed in the material safety data sheet (MSDS) accompanying each reagent must be read and followed.

Quality Assessment

   The facility's standard operating procedure (SOP) manual will contain all quality assessment policies and manufacturer's instructions that must be followed for bacterial identification and antibiotic susceptibility tests. Each new lot of media, identification kits, and reagents must be tested using known microorganisms to ensure that all give the expected reactions.

Gram Stain and Primary Media Results

Observations of growth on the blood agar (BA) plate and the selective or indicator medium plate will give clues as to what type of bacteria are present. Gram-negative bacteria will grow on BA as well as eosin methylene blue (EMB) and MacConkey's (MAC). Gram-positive bacteria will grow only on the BA plate (Figure 7-37). Microscopic examination of a Gram stain performed on a colony will confirm the gram reaction and will reveal

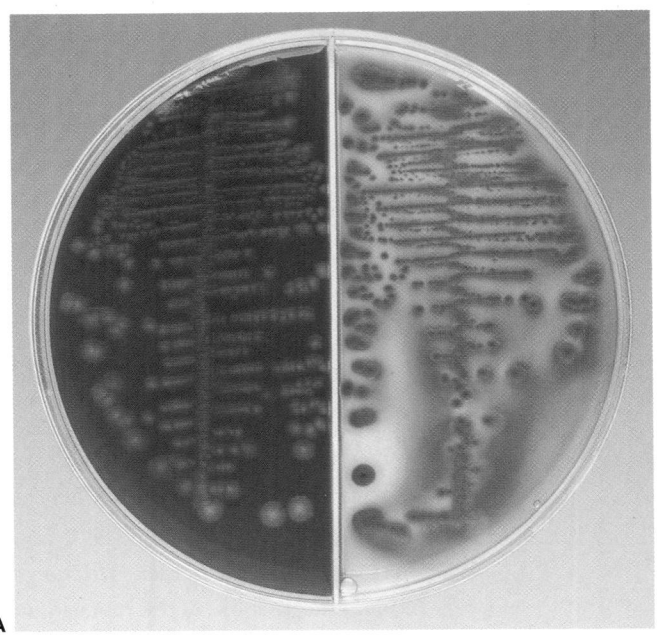

A

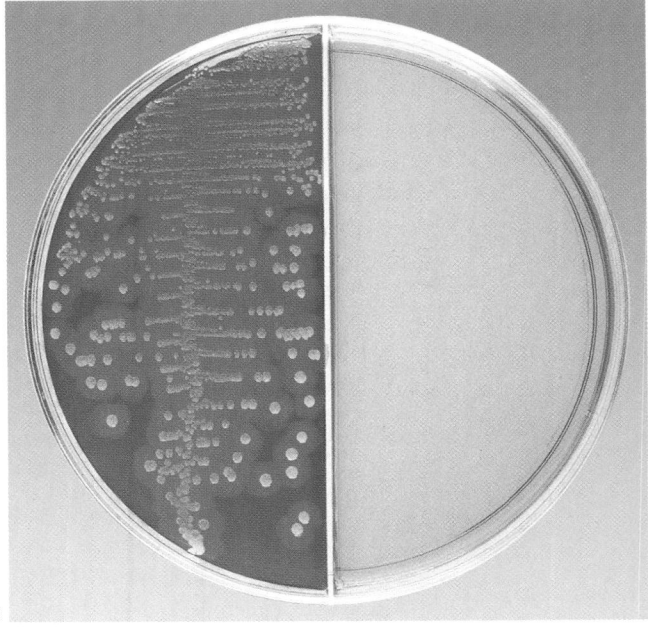

B

FIGURE 7-37 Bacterial growth on selective media: (A) *Escherichia coli* (gram negative) and (B) *Staphylococcus aureus* (gram positive) inoculated to split plates of blood agar (left side of plates and MAC (right side of plates). Blood agar supports growth of both bacteria; MAC selects for gram negatives

or confirm the bacterial morphology—coccus or rod (bacillus). Growth characteristics can also be observed, such as whether the bacteria grows in clusters or chains or is **pleomorphic**, that is, has varied shapes.

Identification of Gram-Positive Bacteria

Two common medically important gram-positive cocci are *Staphylococcus* and *Streptococcus*. Strains of both staph and strep can be beta-hemolytic on blood agar, but the colonies of each have a distinct appearance. In general, colonies of streptococci are small and colorless; colonies of staphylococci are larger and appear white or yellowish (*S. aureus*). On a Gram stain, staphylococci are spherical and appear in grape-like clusters; streptococci are spherical and can appear in chains or in pairs, depending on the species. Although these characteristics are usually reliable, other tests are required for confirming the identification of the bacterial species.

If a colony is found to be a gram-positive coccus, a **catalase test** can be performed to determine if the bacteria are *Staphylococcus* or *Streptococcus* species. Staphylococci are catalase positive, and streptococci are catalase negative. If the catalase test is positive and the bacteria are gram-positive cocci arranged in grapelike clusters, a **coagulase test** can help differentiate between *Staphylococcus aureus* and other *Staphylococcus* species. Latex agglutination tests can also be used to identify *S. aureus*.

Catalase Test

To perform the catalase test, a sterile applicator stick is used to transfer a small portion of a colony to a drop of 3% hydrogen peroxide on a clean microscope slide. Care must be taken that no blood agar is picked up because the hemoglobin in the blood will react with the catalase and cause a false positive reaction.

If bubbles appear within 10 seconds, the colony is catalase positive and can be presumptively identified as *Staphylococcus* species (Figure 7-38). Depending on the facility's microbiology reporting procedure, the preliminary report might read:

"Gram-positive cocci morphologically resembling *Staphylococcus*, catalase positive." A positive catalase test should be followed by a coagulase test.

The absence of bubbles is a negative catalase test and is indicative of *Streptococcus* species. The result might be reported as "Gram-positive cocci, morphologically resembling *Streptococcus* species, catalase negative."

Coagulase Test

The coagulase test is used to differentiate between *S. aureus* and other staphylococci. Pathogenic staphylococci (*S. aureus*) produce the enzyme coagulase that will cause clotting of plasma. The coagulase test can be performed by the slide or tube method, but the tube method is more reliable. Negative coagulase slide tests should be confirmed by a coagulase tube test.

A portion of a bacterial colony is mixed with commercial rabbit *coagulase plasma* on a slide or in a small test tube. The slide is examined for the presence of clumping, which is a positive result. The inoculated tube is incubated at 37° C and checked each hour to see if the plasma has formed a fibrin clot or solidified (Figure 7-39). The tube should be checked every hour because some *S. aureus* can also produce an enzyme that dissolves clots, causing a false-negative result.

A colony that tests positive for coagulase can be reported as "Gram-positive cocci morphologically resembling *Staphylococcus*, coagulase positive." This is a presumptive identification of *S. aureus*.

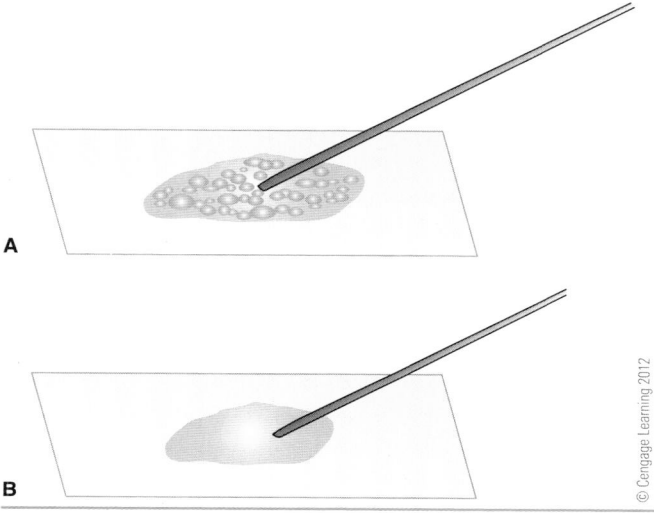

FIGURE 7-38 Catalase test for identifying *Staphylococcus* spp.: (A) bubbles indicate a positive test; (B) absence of bubbles indicates a negative test

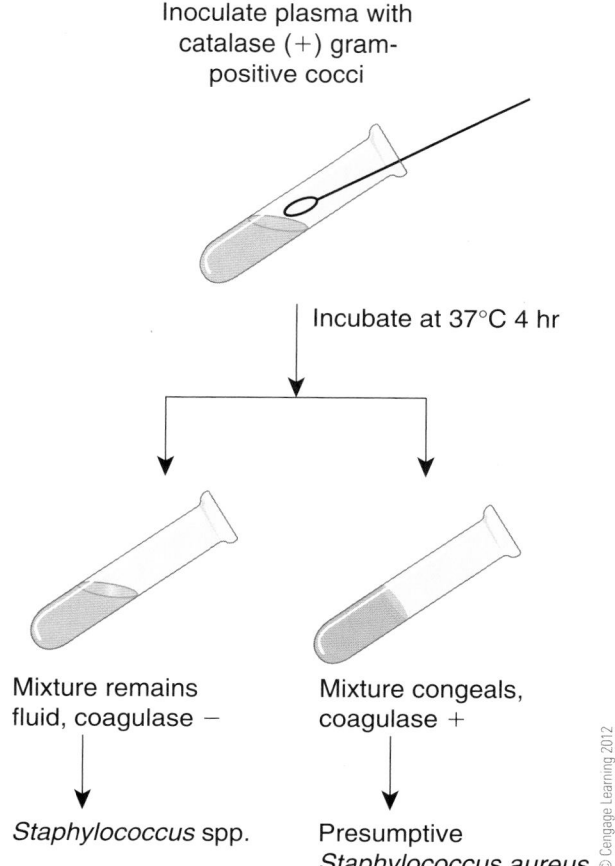

FIGURE 7-39 Schematic of the coagulase test: the formation of a clot is presumptive identification for *Staphylococcus aureus*

CURRENT TOPICS

METHICILLIN-RESISTANT *STAPHYLOCOCCUS AUREUS*

In the nineteenth century, surgeries became more common because of the availability of anesthetics. This increase in surgeries was accompanied by high mortality from hospital-acquired infections. The causative agent was most often *Streptococcus pyogenes*, but *Staphylococcus aureus* also caused these infections. At the end of the century, when the antiseptic methods of Lister were implemented, mortality from infected wounds declined.

In the 1940s penicillin, the miracle antibiotic, was introduced. However, by the 1950s penicillin-resistant strains of *S. aureus* developed and were responsible for additional problems in hospital-acquired infections. The ability of *S. aureus* strains to quickly adapt was demonstrated by their development of resistance to newly introduced antibiotics such as streptomycin, tetracycline, chloramphenicol, erythromycin, and others.

Different forms of penicillin, such as methicillin and cloxicillin, were developed. After the introduction of these, outbreaks of methicillin-resistant *S. aureus* (MRSA) were reported in Europe. The most severe infections were treated with vancomycin, a highly toxic drug. Then, in the 1970s, the number of serious infections caused by MRSA dropped dramatically along with the incidence of MRSA infections in hospitalized populations. In 1970, the incidence of MRSA in the noses of patients was 8.0%, but by 1977 the incidence had dropped to 0.7%.

In the next few years, MRSA returned with a vengeance; in the 1980s a new epidemic strain emerged and spread around the world. The increase has continued into the twenty-first century. Some strains of MRSA have acquired a resistance to vancomycin. Although rare, this resistance is causing serious concern in the world's medical community, because vancomycin is currently the last line of antibiotic defense against MRSA.

Methicillin resistance in *S. aureus* is due to the presence of cell wall proteins called penicillin binding proteins (PBPs) which bind penicillin and prevent it from acting on the bacteria. Rapid tests to identify methicillin-resistant *S. aureus* are based on detection of these proteins (Figure 7-41).

The Centers for Disease Control and Prevention (CDC) has an active role in investigating, tracking, and characterizing strains of MRSA. It has been found that the incidence of MRSA infections is increasing in long-term care facilities. MRSA also occurs in home-bound patients who develop bed sores. This makes it imperative that caretakers change gloves and observe careful handwashing between patients to avoid spreading the infection to other debilitated patients.

An colony that tests coagulase-negative would be reported as "Gram-positive cocci morphologically resembling *Staphylococcus* species, coagulase negative." This result indicates the bacterial species is not *S. aureus* and could be another *Staphylococcus* species such as *S. saprophyticus*, a gram-positive coccus frequently involved in urinary tract infections (UTIs).

Latex Agglutination Tests

Several latex agglutination tests are available to confirm the identification of *S. aureus*. Some examples of these are Staphyloslide (BD BBL), Sure-Vue Color Staph ID Latex Test Kit (Fisher Scientific), and Staphaurex kit (Remel), shown in Figure 7-40. These kits contain a reagent of colored latex particles coated with both human fibrinogen and IgG specific for protein A found in *S. aureus*. A colony suspected of being *S. aureus* is mixed with the latex reagent on the special slide included in the kit. If *S. aureus* is present, the coagulase will react with the fibrinogen and the IgG will react with the protein A to cause or clumping or visible agglutination.

Identification of Gram-Negative Bacteria

Bacterial growth on EMB or MAC and biochemical reactions with the agar after overnight incubation give information about the identify of gram-negative rods that have grown. A Gram stain of colonies growing on EMB or MAC should confirm that bacteria are gram-negative, because both media inhibit growth of gram-positive bacteria.

Many gram-negative bacteria have a characteristic colony appearance on selective and indicator media. *Klebsiella* species form distinctive bubblegum pink, mucoid colonies. *Escherichia coli* colonies form a green metallic sheen on EMB (Figure 7-42) and can be reported as "Gram-negative rods, **coliform** by EMB." Coliform refers to certain gram-negative intestinal (enteric) bacteria. The physician can begin treatment on the basis of these preliminary reports and then check the results of antibiotic susceptibility tests when they become available to be sure that the prescribed antibiotic will be effective. The physician can also request that the laboratory make a definitive identification of the

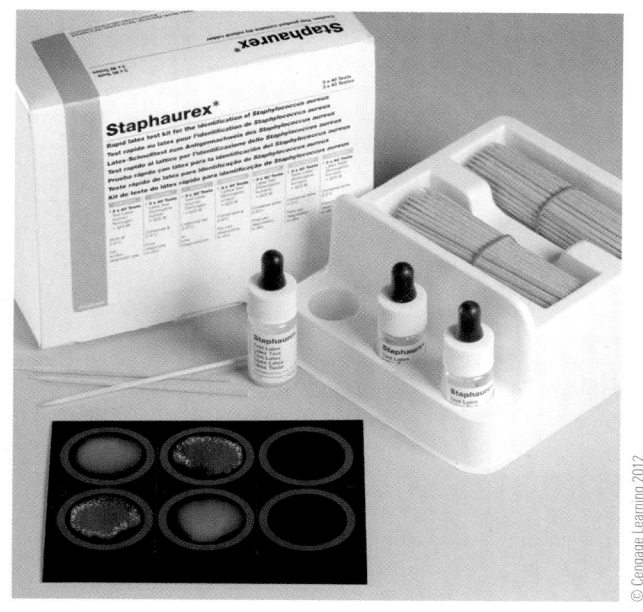

FIGURE 7-40 Staphaurex latex agglutination test kit for identifying *Staphylococcus aureus*

microorganism this is done by subjecting the bacteria to several biochemical tests.

Manual Bacterial Identification Systems

Manual or automated systems can be used to identify bacteria. Manual systems are used in smaller, low-volume laboratories or as a back-up to automated systems in larger laboratories. Manual systems contain several biochemical tests in a strip or tube

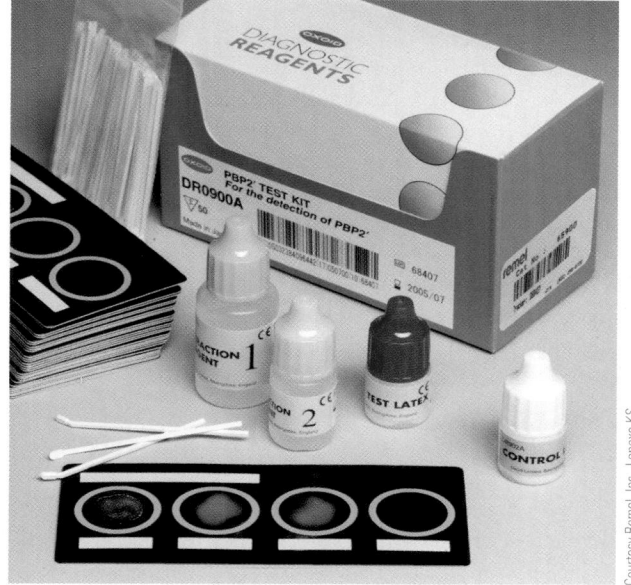

FIGURE 7-41 PBP2' latex agglutination test kit for identifying methicillin-resistant *Staphylococcus aureus* (MRSA)

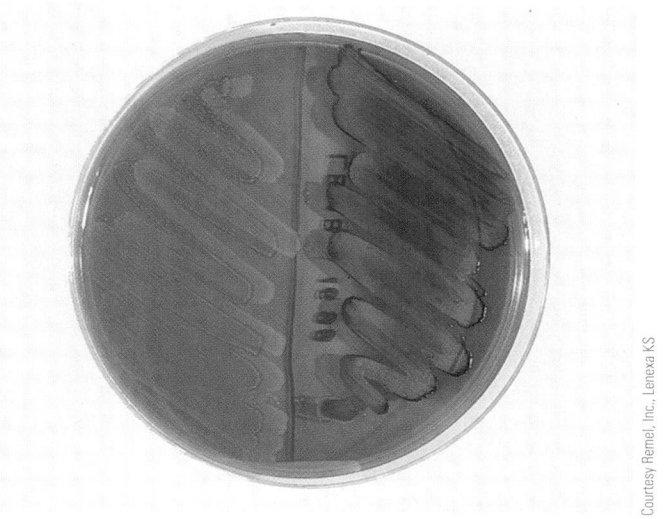

FIGURE 7-42 Metallic sheen produced by coliform bacteria (right half of plate) growing on EMB agar

(Figure 7-43). A bacterial suspension of a specific concentration is made from an isolated bacterial colony; the suspension is used to inoculate the test system.

bioMérieux ChromID Media

ChromID media from bioMérieux is made for manual isolation, enumeration, and identification of several important bacterial pathogens, as well as *Candida* (a yeast). The media formulation

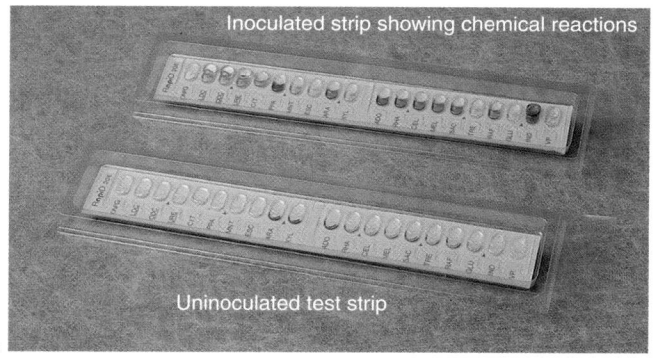

Inoculated strip showing chemical reactions

Uninoculated test strip

A

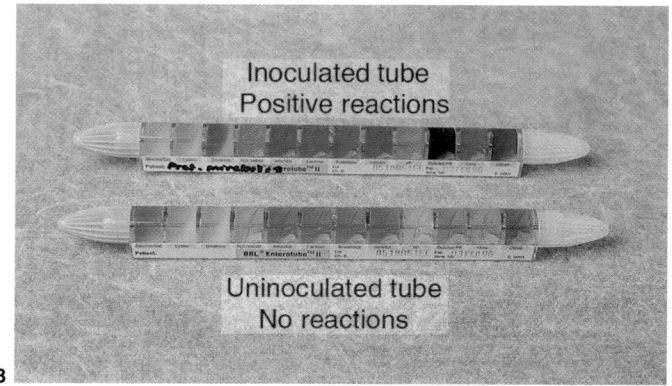

Inoculated tube
Positive reactions

Uninoculated tube
No reactions

B

FIGURE 7-43 Manual bacterial identification systems: (A) the API identification system; (B) Enterotube II

to identify common urinary tract pathogens contains dimethyl-p-phenylene-diamine and certain antibiotics. This medium selects for gram-negatives commonly associated with urinary tract infections. On this medium the following differentiation is made:

- *E. coli* forms pink to burgundy colonies
- *Klebsiella, Enterobacter, Serratia, Citrobacter* (KESC) form green/blue to brownish-green colonies
- *Proteus, Providencia, Morganella* form dark brown to light brown colonies

Other chromID plates are available to identify gram negatives such as Salmonella, and gram positives such as S. aureus (chromID MRSA) and vancomycin-resistant enterococci (chromID VRE).

API Microbial Identification Strips

The API systems from bioMérieux consist of a flat tray with a series of wells containing reagents to test the microorganisms for biochemical reactions such as fermentation of certain sugars. These are actually miniaturized versions of biochemical tube tests used in microbiology for many years. Several types of API strips are available (Figure 7-43A). A few examples are API 20 E (for identifying gram negatives), STAPH (for identifying staphylococci), and API 20 STREP (to identify streptococci).

A standardized suspension of the microorganism to be tested is added into the wells of the strip, and the strip is then incubated at the specified temperature and for the prescribed time, usually 18 to 24 hours. The API 20 STREP can be read at 4 hours and again at 24 hours. The reactions in the wells are recorded. The results are compared to an identification key to identify the microorganism.

Enterotube II

The Enterotube II (BD BBL) is used for rapid differential identification of gram-negative bacteria (Figure 7-43B). It contains 15 tests, such as fermentation of certain sugars and other biochemical reactions. The inoculation is made with a single colony, the system is incubated for 18 to 24 hours at 37° C, and the results are read. The results of the biochemical reactions are recorded and compared to the Enterotube identification guide to make the identification.

Automated Bacterial Identification Systems

Three examples of automated bacterial identification systems are the MicroScan Walk-Away (Siemens Medical Solutions), the Phoenix (Becton Dickinson Diagnostic Systems), and bioMérieux's VITEK-2 (Figure 7-44). These instruments use various methods to detect biochemical reactions as well as antibiotic susceptibility of organisms. Some measure turbidity to detect patterns of susceptibility or resistance to antimicrobials. Others use fluorometry and/or colorimetry to detect gram-positive and gram-negative bacteria.

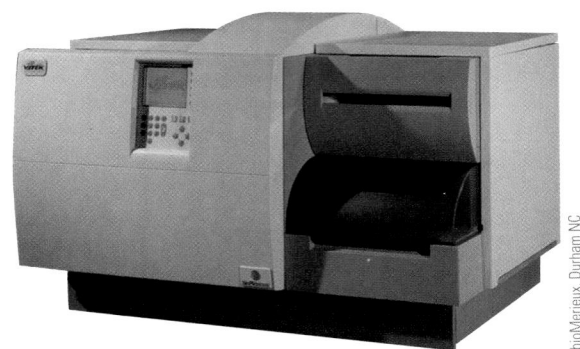

FIGURE 7-44 The VITEK fully automated microbiology identification system

ANTIBIOTIC SUSCEPTIBILITY TESTS

When a culture and antibiotic susceptibility test (C & S) is requested, the susceptibility of the isolate(s) to antibiotics is assessed by exposing the microorganism to varying concentrations of antibiotics. Historically this has been accomplished manually using the method of Bauer and Kirby. Additional methods available are semi-automated **minimum inhibitory concentration (MIC)** and fully automated MIC methods on instruments that also perform bacterial identification. The MIC is the minimum concentration of antibiotic required to inhibit growth of a particular microorganism.

Automated and Semi-Automated Methods

Laboratories with high volumes of cultures that require identification and susceptibility can use automated methods for determining both. Examples are the MicroScan Walk-Away (Siemens), the Phoenix (Becton Dickinson Diagnostic Systems), and the VITEK-2 (bioMérieux). These instruments greatly increase microbiology laboratory efficiency.

Several instruments can perform the MIC test and are suitable for use in smaller laboratories. These instruments require that the technician make a standardized suspension from the culture and add it to wells in a microplate. Predetermined dilutions of selected antibiotics are added to the inoculated wells. The microplate is inserted into the instrument to incubate. At the end of the incubation time, the instrument reads the microplate (Figure 7-45). Wells without bacterial growth will be clear; this indicates the bacteria are inhibited by (susceptible to) that antibiotic concentration. Wells with bacterial growth will be turbid, indicating the bacteria are resistant to that particular antibiotic concentration. The degree of susceptibility for each antibiotic tested is reported as the MIC.

Manual Methods of Antibiotic Susceptibility

Manual methods of performing susceptibility tests involve streaking a Mueller-Hinton agar plate with a dilute suspension of the culture to be tested. Disks or strips containing antibiotics are placed on the surface of the agar. After incubation the plate is

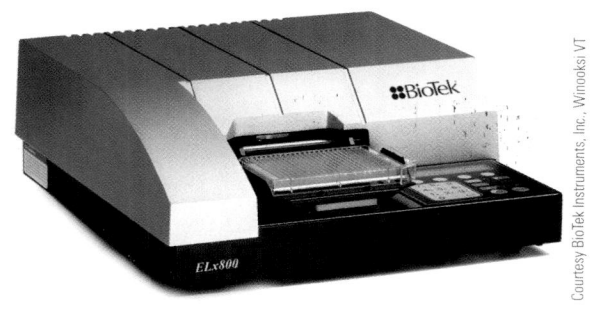

FIGURE 7-45 MIC plate reader system showing the welled microplate in the carrier

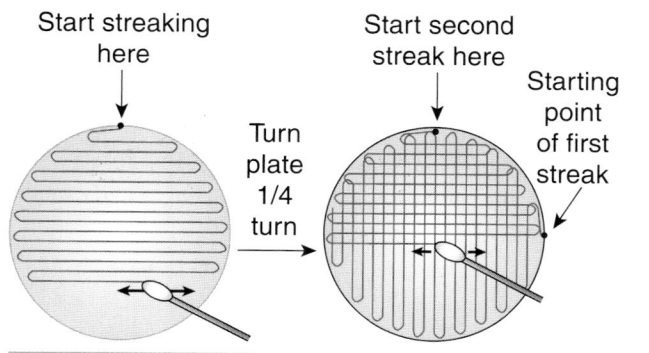

FIGURE 7-46 Streaking the Mueller-Hinton plate

examined to determine which antibiotic inhibits growth of the particular isolate.

Bauer-Kirby Susceptibility Test

The Bauer-Kirby test is a mainstay of smaller laboratories. It does not require the purchase of expensive equipment and the test supplies are readily available.

Performing the Bauer-Kirby Test.
To perform the Bauer-Kirby antibiotic susceptibility test, a standardized bacterial suspension is made by mixing bacteria from isolated colonies with soy broth. The turbidity of the broth suspension is adjusted to be equivalent to a standard, such as a McFarland's standard, available commercially in sets of varying turbidity. Alternatively, commercial kits such as the Prompt by BD-BBL can be used to standardize the procedure.

The bacterial suspension is thoroughly mixed just before use. A sterile swab is wet in the suspension, pressed against the inside of the tube to express excess fluid, and then used to streak

the surface of a Mueller-Hinton plate. The entire plate is streaked by beginning at the top edge and making continuous streaks all the way across the agar to the bottom edge (Figure 7-46). The plate is then turned 90 degrees and streaked from the top edge all the way to the bottom edge, resulting in an almost continuous mat of growth after incubation; this is called a *lawn*.

Antibiotic disks, paper disks impregnated with antibiotics, are placed on the surface of the Mueller-Hinton agar while the surface of the plate is still wet from the inoculum. The disks should be evenly spaced in a circular pattern around the outer edge of the agar using sterile forceps or a disk dispenser that can dispense a set of 12 or more disks at a time (Figure 7-47). The disks are tamped down onto the surface of the agar, so they will not fall off when the plate is turned upside down to incubate overnight.

Interpreting the Bauer-Kirby Test.
After overnight incubation at 35° to 37° C, the plates are examined for bacterial growth around the antibiotic disks (Figure 7-48A). Areas without bacterial growth around the disks are called

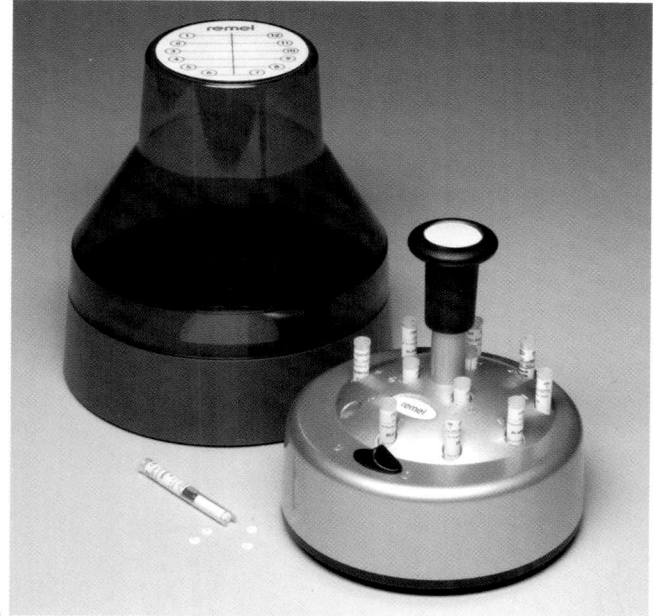

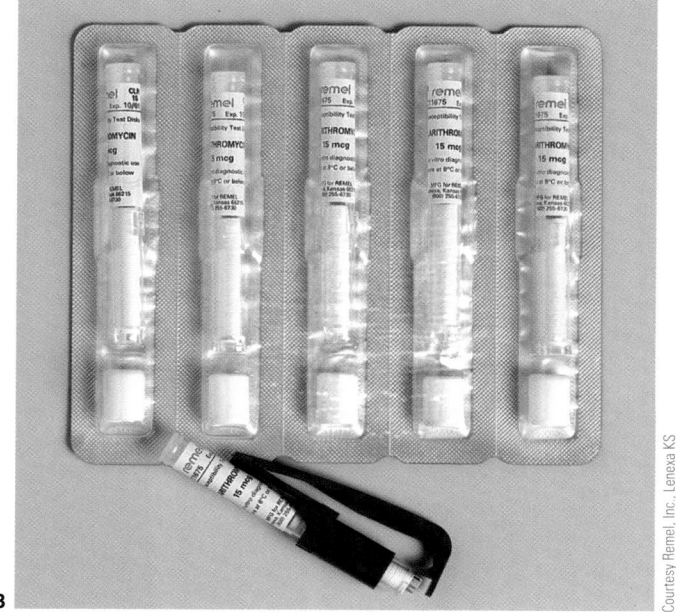

FIGURE 7-47 Antibiotic disk dispensers: (A) multi-disk dispenser and (B) single antibiotic disk cartridge with ejector

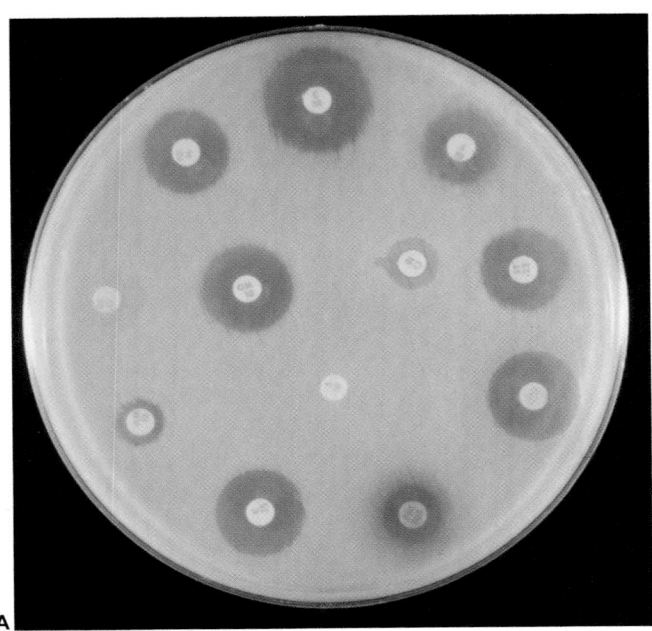

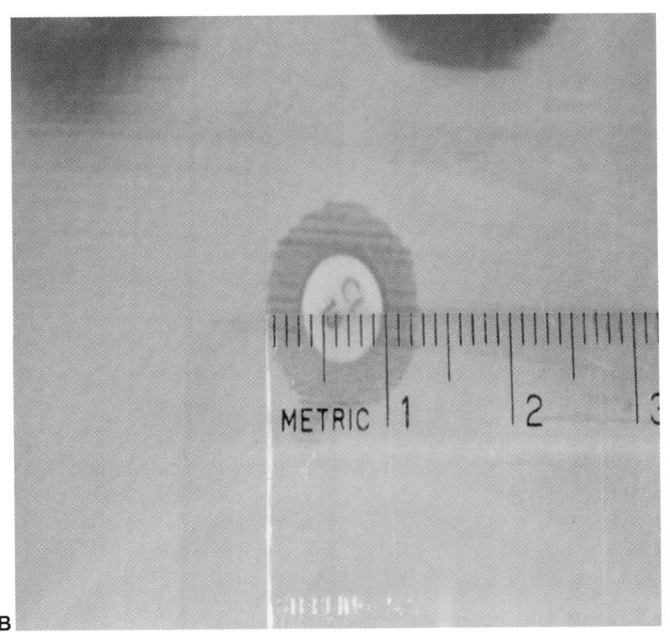

FIGURE 7-48 Antibiotic susceptibility test: (A) Mueller-Hinton plate shows showing zones of inhibition around antibiotic disks after overnight incubation; (B) measuring the zones of inhibition using a ruler

zones of inhibition and are measured using calipers, a ruler (Figure 7-49B), or transparent templates with pre-printed zones for each antibiotic.

Each antibiotic produces a zone size characteristic for each microorganism. The zone size is used to classify the microorganism as *sensitive (S)*, *resistant (R)*, or *intermediate (I)*, based on information in the package insert provided with each cartridge of antibiotic disks. The microorganism is said to be intermediate if the zone size is between sensitive and resistant.

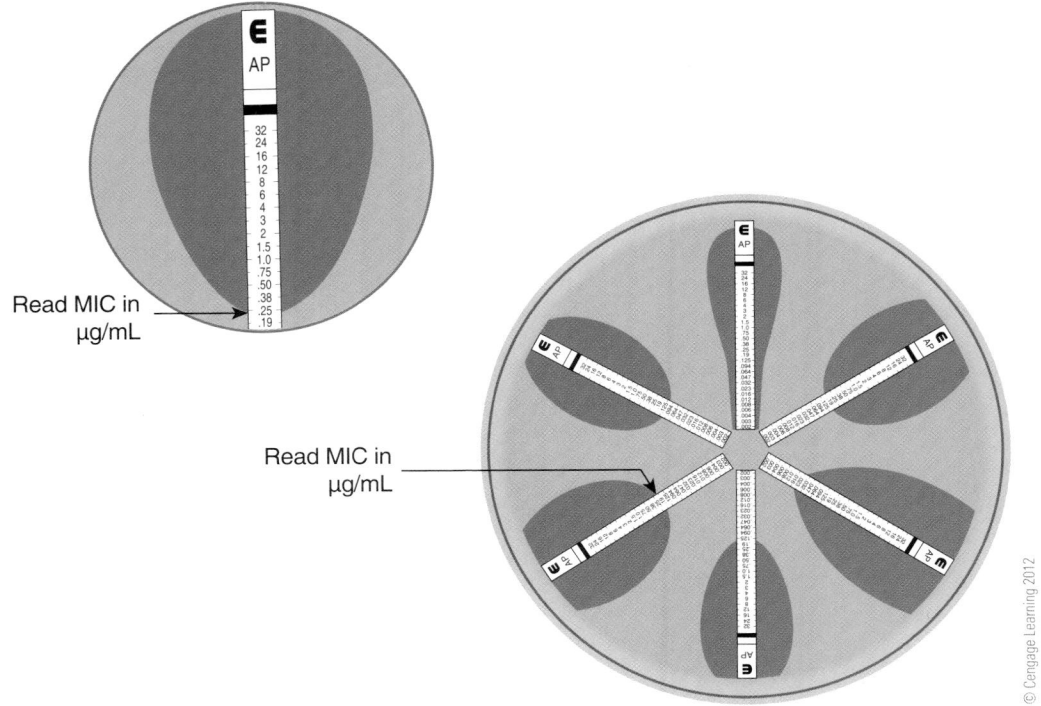

FIGURE 7-49 Diagram of E-test showing elliptical-shaped zones of inhibition (absence of bacterial growth); arrow denotes where MIC value is read (see enlarged view at upper left) with no bacterial growth

AB Biodisk E

The Biodisk E, or E test, is similar to the Bauer-Kirby disk method in that a Mueller-Hinton plate is streaked with a standardized suspension of the microorganism to be tested. The antibiotics are contained on rectangular strips (Epsilometer) that are placed on the inoculated plate, radiating out from the center (Figure 7-49). Each strip contains one antibiotic in a continuous exponential concentration gradient that corresponds to MIC dilutions. Each antibiotic strip is labeled with the antibiotic concentration gradient.

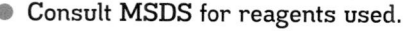

SAFETY REMINDERS

- Review Safety Precautions section before beginning procedure.
- Wear PPE and use aseptic technique.
- Consult MSDS for reagents used.
- Use forceps to place antibiotic disks on inoculated agar.
- Read zones of inhibition through the bottom of the closed plate.

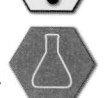

PROCEDURAL REMINDERS

- Review Quality Assessment section before beginning procedure.
- Follow SOP manual and manufacturer's instructions.
- Standardize bacterial suspensions when performing identification and antibiotic susceptibility tests.

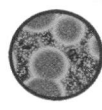

CASE STUDY

It was Natasha's day to read and interpret the urine cultures in the microbiology laboratory. When she examined Ms. Gonzalez's BA and EMB plates, she saw two distinct colony types on the BA plate and only one type on the EMB plate. Natalie counted 74 colonies total on the BA plate, which had been streaked using a 0.001 mL loop.

1. What is the colony count on this patient's urine? Explain your answer.
2. What is the probable Gram-stain reaction of the colony(ies) growing on the EMB plate? Explain your answer.
3. Which colonies should be tested for the catalase reaction? Explain.

SUMMARY

The identification of a microorganism and determination of its antibiotic susceptibility can determine the treatment a patient receives for an infection. Bacterial identification can be as simple as observing a Gram-stained smear and performing catalase and coagulase tests, or as complex as processing the specimen in a semi-automated or automated system that can determine both the identity and the antibiotic susceptibility or MIC.

In some cases, the physician might only need to know the presumptive identity of the microorganism responsible and the antibiotic that is effective. However, in cases of seriously ill patients with infections caused by an unknown microorganism, the most expedient methods should be employed to confirm the bacterial identification and determine the MIC or antibiotic susceptibility.

Aseptic technique and microbiological safety rules must be followed when handling all isolates. The quality assessment procedures in the SOP manual of the microbiology department must be followed to ensure that the identity and antibiotic susceptibility of the microorganism causing infection are correctly determined.

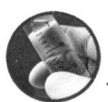

REVIEW QUESTIONS

1. What is known about a culture that grows on both blood agar and EMB?
2. Why is a correctly performed Gram stain important to the process of identifying bacteria?
3. How is the MIC determined?
4. In the Bauer-Kirby susceptibility test, what is indicated by the presence of a large clear area without bacterial growth around an antibiotic disk?
5. Discuss how to presumptively identify bacteria.
6. How is the catalase test performed?

7. How is the coagulase test performed?

8. List two automated methods used to identify bacteria.

9. Give an example of a manual method of identifying bacteria using biochemical reactions.

10. Explain how to set up a disk antibiotic susceptibility test.

11. How are the zones of inhibition around the disks measured in the Bauer-Kirby test?

12. Define catalase test, coagulase test, coliform, minimum inhibitory concentration, pleomorphic, and zone of inhibition.

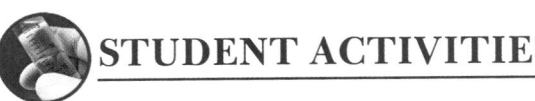

STUDENT ACTIVITIES

1. Complete the written examination for this lesson.

2. Practice performing bacterial identification and antibiotic susceptibility tests as outlined in the Student Performance Guide.

WEB ACTIVITIES

1. Use the Internet to find recent information on microbial resistance to commonly prescribed antibiotics such as the Zithromax Z-Pak, penicillin, or amoxicillin.

2. Search the Internet for information about recent revelations of resistant bacteria, including VRE.

3. Use the Internet to search a web site such as WebMD or Lab Tests Online; find the names of two antibiotics useful for treatment of gram-negative infections with *E. coli* and *Pseudomonas aeruginosa*.

4. Use the Internet to find two antibiotics used in antibiotic susceptibility tests for both gram-negative rods and gram-positive cocci.

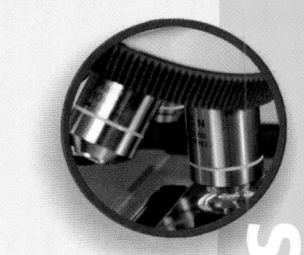

LESSON 7-7

Bacterial Identification and Antibiotic Susceptibility Testing

Name _____   Date _____

INSTRUCTIONS

1. Practice performing bacterial identification and antibiotic susceptibility tests following the step-by-step procedure.

2. Demonstrate the procedures for bacterial identification and antibiotic susceptibility testing satisfactorily for the instructor, using the Student Performance Guide. Your instructor will explain the procedures for evaluating your performance. Your performance may be given a number grade, a letter grade, or satisfactory (S) or unsatisfactory (U) depending on the course or institutional policy.

MATERIALS AND EQUIPMENT

- gloves
- hand antiseptic
- full-face shield (or equivalent PPE)
- Mueller-Hinton (MH) plates
- trypticase soy broth (TSB), 5 mL per tube, and McFarland's standard No. 2; or commercial kit such as Prompt by BBL
- wax pencil or marking pen
- culture tube rack
- electric incinerator
- incubator set at 35° to 37° C

- antibiotic disks (ampicillin, augmentin, norfloxacin, nitrofurantoin, trimethoprim, bactrim, and cephalothin are often used for urines)
- disk dispenser
- forceps
- calipers, ruler, or template to measure zones of inhibition
- sterile swabs
- bacterial cultures growing on blood agar plates:
  - culture of *E. coli*, nonpathogenic strain
  - cultures of gram-positive cocci: catalase positive and negative cultures, and coagulase positive and negative cultures
- materials for catalase and coagulase tests:
  - microscope slides
  - 3% hydrogen peroxide
  - sterile applicators (non-metal)
  - rabbit coagulase plasma (or commercial coagulase kit)
  - 13 x 75 mm test tubes and rack
- paper towels
- surface disinfectant
- biohazard container
- sharps container

(Continues)

STUDENT PERFORMANCE GUIDE

© 2012 Delmar, Cengage Learning. Permission to reproduce for clinical use granted.

PROCEDURE

Record in the comment section any problems encountered while practicing the procedure (or have a fellow student or the instructor evaluate your performance).

S = Satisfactory
U = Unsatisfactory

You must:	S	U	Evaluation/Comments
1. Assemble materials and equipment			
2. Turn on the electric incinerator			
3. Wash hands and put on gloves			

4. Perform presumptive identification of gram-positive colonies growing on a culture plate
   a. Obtain an agar plate containing a culture of a gram positive coccus
   b. Perform the catalase test following steps 4b1–4b3
      (1) Place 1 drop of 3% hydrogen peroxide on a microscope slide
      (2) Touch a sterile applicator to a colony, transfer bacteria to the peroxide drop, and mix the bacteria into the peroxide drop; do not transfer any agar to the slide
      (3) Observe slide for production of gas bubbles: after 10 seconds record as catalase positive (bubbles produced) or catalase negative (no bubbles produced). A positive reaction indicates a presumptive identification of *Staphylococcus* species; a negative reaction indicates a presumptive identification of *Streptococcus*
   c. Repeat the catalase test using the second gram-positive culture, following step 4b1-4b3			

5. Perform the coagulase test on a catalase-positive culture (from step 4) following steps 5a-5e:
   a. Sterilize an inoculating loop; remove cap from a tube of prepared rabbit plasma
   b. Transfer a small amount of catalase-positive colony into the tube of rabbit plasma
   c. Place the inoculated plasma into a test tube rack in a 37° C incubator for 4 hours
   d. Check tube every hour to see if the plasma has clotted (solidified). If clotting occurs, report as "Gram-positive coccus morphologically resembling *Staphylococcus,* coagulase positive." This is a presumptive identification of *Staphylococcus aureus*
   e. Report negative tests as "Gram-positive coccus morphologically resembling *Staphylococcus* species, coagulase negative." This result indicates that the bacteria is a *Staphylococcus* species other than *Staphylococcus aureus*			

© 2012 Delmar, Cengage Learning. Permission to reproduce for clinical use granted.

You must:	S	U	Evaluation/Comments
6. Perform a Bauer Kirby antibiotic susceptibility test following steps 7–13:			
7. Obtain a Mueller-Hinton (MH) plate and label the plate bottom			
8. Prepare a bacterial suspension from a gram-negative bacterial culture following steps 8a–8d or following the manufacturer's instructions if using a commercial system: 　a. Transfer a few colonies from the culture plate using a sterile swab 　b. Remove cap from TSB broth and insert swab into broth, gently swishing the swab around to make a slightly turbid suspension of bacteria 　c. Compare the TSB suspension with a McFarland's No. 2 standard 　d. Press the swab against the side of the tube to express excess liquid as the swab is removed, replace cap on broth tube and set tube in rack			
9. Streak the Mueller-Hinton agar using the swab: Starting at the top edge of the agar, make horizontal streaks the whole width of the plate, from top to bottom (Figure 7-46)			
10. Turn the plate 90 degrees and streak from top to bottom, using the same swab; the agar surface should be almost completely covered with the broth inoculum (Figure 7-46); discard swab into biohazard container			
11. Place antibiotic disks on the surface of the still-wet agar using either a disk dispenser or sterile forceps, tamp disks down if necessary, and replace lid on plate			
12. Sterilize the forceps (if used) and return them to storage			
13. Place the M-H plate upside down in a 35° to 37° C incubator; leave overnight (18 to 24 hours)			
14. Remove gloves and discard into biohazard container			
15. Wash hands with antiseptic			
16. The next day: wash hands and put on gloves			
17. Remove Mueller-Hinton plate from incubator and observe for zones of inhibition through bottom of plate			
18. Measure zones, using a metric ruler, calipers, or a special transparent template			

(Continues)

© 2012 Delmar, Cengage Learning. Permission to reproduce for clinical use granted.

You must:	S	U	Evaluation/Comments
19. Record the susceptibility of the bacteria to each antibiotic disk as sensitive (S), resistant (R), or intermediate (I), following the guidelines included on the package insert for each disk cartridge or the template markings			
20. Discard all contaminated materials into appropriate sharps or biohazard containers			
21. Return equipment to storage			
22. Wipe work area with disinfectant			
23. Remove gloves and discard into biohazard container			
24. Wash hands with antiseptic			

Instructor/Evaluator Comments:

Instructor/Evaluator _____ Date _____

© 2012 Delmar, Cengage Learning. Permission to reproduce for clinical use granted.

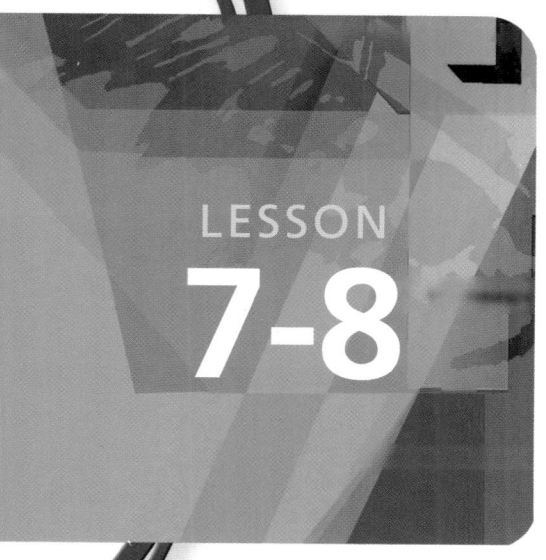

LESSON 7-8

Tests for Sexually Transmitted Diseases

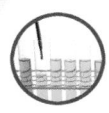

LESSON OBJECTIVES

After studying this lesson, the student will:

⊙ Explain the importance of detecting sexually transmitted diseases (STDs).

⊙ Discuss the incidence of certain STDs in the United States.

⊙ Discuss four basic types of tests used to detect STDs.

⊙ List five STDs common in the United States.

⊙ Name one method of detection for each of the five common STDs.

⊙ Explain the three-slide test for females and list the types of microorganisms that can be detected.

⊙ Explain the special culture conditions for the growth of *Neisseria gonorrhoeae*.

⊙ Explain the safety precautions that must be followed when performing tests for STDs.

⊙ Discuss the quality assessment procedures involved in testing for STDs.

⊙ Define the glossary terms.

GLOSSARY

Candida albicans / yeast that causes vaginitis and other infections, especially following antibiotic therapy

Chlamydia trachomatis / species of gram-negative intracellular bacteria that is a cause of sexually transmitted diseases (STDs)

clue cells / vaginal epithelial cells covered with tiny, gram-variable bacteria and seen in vaginal secretions of patients with bacterial vaginosis

gonorrhea / contagious infection spread by sexual contact and caused by *Neisseria gonorrhoeae*

herpes simplex virus, type 1 (HSV-1) / the virus causing oral herpes

herpes simplex virus, type 2 (HSV-2) / the virus causing genital herpes

human immunodeficiency virus (HIV) / the retrovirus that has been identified as the cause of acquired immunodeficiency syndrome (AIDS)

human papillomavirus (HPV) / a group of DNA viruses, some of which are sexually transmitted

nongonococcal urethritis / gonorrhea-like STD caused by microorganisms other than gonococci

oxidase test / an enzyme test used to identify certain bacteria such as *Neisseria*

sexually transmitted disease (STD) / a disease transmitted by sexual contact; sexually transmitted infection

sexually transmitted infection (STI) / a infection transmitted by sexual contact; sexually transmitted disease

(continues)

spirochetes / motile, helical, or spiral bacteria of the family Spirochaeta

syphilis / an infectious, chronic, sexually transmitted disease caused by a spirochete, *Treponema pallidum*

trichomoniasis / a sexually transmitted genitourinary tract infection caused by the parasitic protozoan, *Trichomonas vaginalis*

urethritis / infection or inflammation of the urethra

vaginitis / infection or inflammation of the vagina

venereal / having to do with, or transmitted by, sexual contact

INTRODUCTION

This lesson introduces basic laboratory methods used to detect STDs in males and females. **Sexually transmitted diseases (STDs)**, also called **sexually transmitted infections (STI)**, are transmitted primarily through sexual intercourse or other intimate sexual contact. STDs can be caused by bacteria, protozoa, fungi, or viruses. Tests for STDs should not be limited to specimens from the genitourinary tract. As sexual practices change, many microorganisms once limited to the genitourinary tract are found in other sites in the body. For example, in suspected cases of gonorrhea, urethral, rectal, and pharyngeal swabs can be collected.

Common STDs detected in the United States are chlamydial infections, gonorrhea, herpes, hepatitis B infection, trichomoniasis, syphilis, human immunodeficiency virus (HIV) infection, human papillomavirus infection, and candidiasis (Table 7-23). In the United States, and in other areas of the world, the incidence of various STDs varies by type of disease and affected age-groups every few years. Statistics show that the numbers of syphilis and gonorrhea cases are on the rise. Chlamydial infections continue to rise. In a recent report, teenage girls in the age-group 15 to 19 years had the largest number of reported cases of chlamydia

and gonorrhea; the next largest group was made up of young women 20 to 24 years of age. The consequences of these infections can be serious, especially for females, which makes testing, detection and treatment important.

Formerly, most STD testing was performed in hospital or state public health laboratories because of the complexity of testing methods. However, several rapid diagnostic kits that produce reliable results have been developed for detecting various STD agents. Many of these diagnostic methods are suitable for use in physician office laboratories (POLs).

Symptoms of Sexually Transmitted Diseases

Venereal disease, or STD, can have long-lasting effects in both males and females. In males, STDs usually produce symptoms such as a penile discharge or burning upon urination. However, evidence indicates that males can be positive for STDs even though asymptomatic. Any male, symptomatic or not, whose sex partner is positive for an STD must be tested or treated. Females can be asymptomatic and go untreated for some STDs, a factor important in disease transmission and in infertility for many women.

DETECTION OF STDS IN FEMALES

Female patients may be tested for STDs because of findings during a routine examination and presence of symptoms or because a partner has tested positive for STDs. Many STDs cause **vaginitis**, an infection or inflammation of the vagina. Vaginitis can be caused by bacteria, fungi, or protozoa. Bacterial and yeast infections may occur because of changes in the vaginal pH or alteration in normal flora. Some of the most common microorganisms causing sexually transmitted infections are *Gardnerella vaginalis* (formerly *Haemophilus vaginalis*), *Mobiluncus* species, *Streptococcus* group B, *Chlamydia trachomatis*, *Neisseria gonorrhoeae*, the protozoan *Trichomonas* and the yeast *Candida albicans*. Detection methods include Gram stain, culture, wet mounts, serum antibody tests, immunoassays, and DNA probes. Table 7-24 gives examples of STD detection methods.

The Three-Slide Test for Vaginitis

The three-slide test is an important tool used to determine the cause of vaginitis. A relatively simple procedure, most results can be

TABLE 7-23. STDs commonly detected in the United States and their causative agents	
DISEASE	**AGENT**
Chlamydial infection	*Chlamydia trachomatis*
Genital warts	Human papillomaviruses (HPV)
Gonorrhea	*Neisseria gonorrhoeae*
Herpes, type 1	Herpes simplex virus, type 1 (HSV-1)
Herpes, type 2	Herpes simplex virus, type 2 (HSV-2)
Hepatitis B	Hepatitis B virus (HBV)
HIV infection	Human immunodeficiency virus (HIV)
Trichomoniasis	*Trichomonas vaginalis*
Candidiasis	*Candida albicans*
Syphilis	*Treponema pallidum*

available in about 30 minutes, while the patient is still in the health-care provider's office. The three-slide test is a CLIA physician-performed microscopy procedure (PPMP). Components of the three-slide test include:

- Saline wet mount preparation of vaginal secretions for *Trichomonas* and clue cells

- KOH (potassium hydroxide) preparation of vaginal secretions for yeasts and fungi

- Gram stain of endocervical secretions for bacteria and yeasts

Specimens for other tests can be collected at the same time, such as a swab for *N. gonorrhoeae* culture, or a swab for *C. trachomatis* or *N. gonorrhoeae* DNA probe tests. If suspected herpes lesions are present, a specimen can be collected from the lesions and sent to the reference laboratory in viral transport medium.

Saline Wet Preparation

The saline wet prep is prepared by mixing a drop of vaginal specimen with a drop of 0.85% saline on a microscope slide and adding a coverslip. A depression slide can also be used. The physician can examine the slide microscopically in the examination room or send it to an on-site laboratory. It must be examined within 30 minutes of collection to detect *Trichomonas vaginalis*, a parasitic protozoan, which causes **trichomoniasis** (Figure 7-50A). If *Gardnerella vaginalis* is present, **clue cells**, which are vaginal epithelial cells covered with the bacteria, may also be seen (Figure 7-50B).

KOH Preparation

A drop of vaginal material is mixed with one to two drops of 10% KOH solution on a microscope slide or in a depression slide to look for fungi that can cause vaginitis, such as *Candida*

TABLE 7-24. STDs and examples of tests available for their detection

DISEASE	TEST METHODS*
Chlamydial infection	EIA, ELISA, DNA probe, cell culture, FA
Gonorrhea	Culture, Gram stain, DNA probe, monoclonal antibody agglutination test
Herpes	Cell culture, EIA, serology for IgG and IgM
Candidiasis	KOH wet prep, culture, Gram stain, rapid chemical confirmation test
Trichomoniasis	Saline wet prep, antibody agglutination
Syphilis	
Screen	VDRL, RPR
Confirmatory	FTA-ABS, MHA-TP, ELISA
HIV infection	
Screen	EIA for anti-HIV-1
Confirmatory	Western blot, culture, p24 antigen
Hepatitis B	Anti-HBcAg (acute), anti-HBsAg (chronic), or hepatitis panel

* EIA = enzyme immunoassay
ELISA = enzyme-linked immunosorbent assay
FA = fluorescent antibody
FTA-ABS = fluorescent treponemal antibody-absorption
HB = hepatitis B
HIV = human immunodeficiency virus
Ig = immunoglobulin
MHA-TP = microhemagglutination assay for *Treponema pallidum*
RPR = rapid plasma reagin
VDRL = Venereal Disease Research Laboratory.

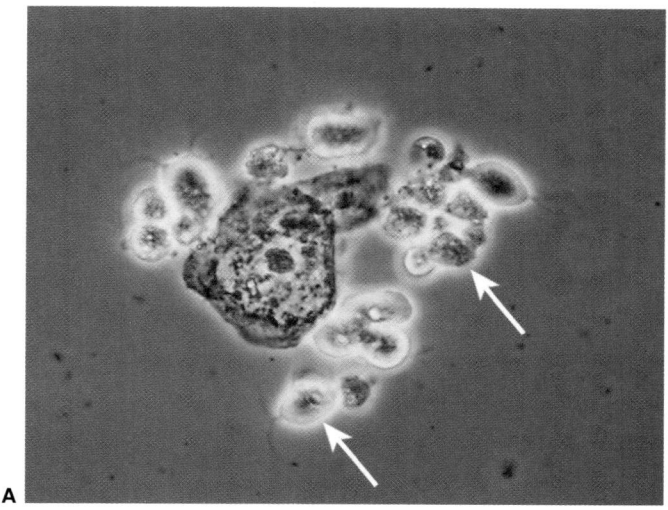

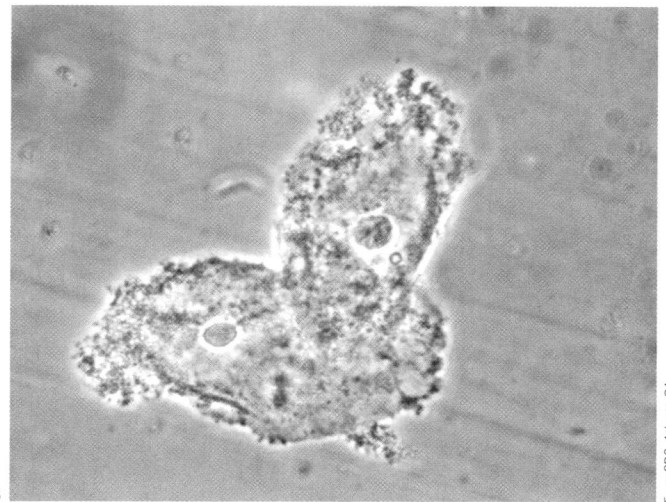

From CDC, Atlanta GA

FIGURE 7-50 Saline wet mounts: (A) wet mount of vaginal discharge viewed with phase-contrast showing *Trichomonas vaginalis* protozoa (arrows); and (B) clue cells, vaginal epithelial cells covered with bacteria indicating bacterial vaginosis

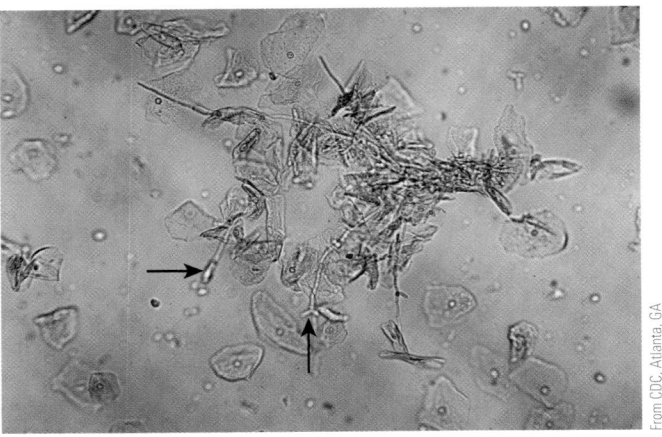

From CDC, Atlanta, GA

FIGURE 7-51 Vaginal smear showing fungal elements (arrows)

albicans. The KOH destroys structures such as epithelial cells and white blood cells; any fungi present will appear as tangled masses resembling hairs or threads. Figure 7-51 shows the microscopic appearance of fungal elements in an unstained smear.

Gram Stain

A smear prepared from an endocervical swab is Gram-stained and examined microscopically for the presence of bacteria and pus cells (white blood cells) using the oil-immersion objective. Smears from uninfected females should have a moderate amount of *Lactobacillus* (gram-positive rods), few or no white blood cells, and few epithelial cells (Figure 7-52A).

    G. vaginalis is a gram-variable bacillus, which can stain either gram-negative or gram-positive. If present the tiny bacteria will be scattered over the other constituents on the smear, especially the vaginal epithelial cells (Figure 7-52B). If yeast cells are present, they will stain dark purple.

    The smear is also examined for the presence of bacteria morphologically resembling *N. gonorrhoeae,* the gram-negative, kidney bean–shaped diplococcus that causes **gonorrhea.** *Neisseria* can be seen inside neutrophilic leukocytes (intracellular) and also extracellular on smears from infected patients (Figure 7-53).

Neisseria gonorrhoeae Culture

A sterile rayon or Dacron swab is used to collect the specimen for culture of *N. gonorrhoeae,* the gram-negative diplococcus that causes gonorrhea. The swab is used to streak a modified Thayer-Martin (MTM) agar plate in the shape of a *Z* or a *W.* The culture must be transported to the laboratory where the plate will be cross-streaked using a sterile loop (Figure 7-54). The culture plate is immediately placed in an increased carbon dioxide environment (5% to 10% CO_2) and incubated at 35° to 37° C to prevent loss of viability of any *N. gonorrhoeae* present. The swab used to inoculate the media for *Neisseria* culture can also be used to prepare the smear for Gram stain.

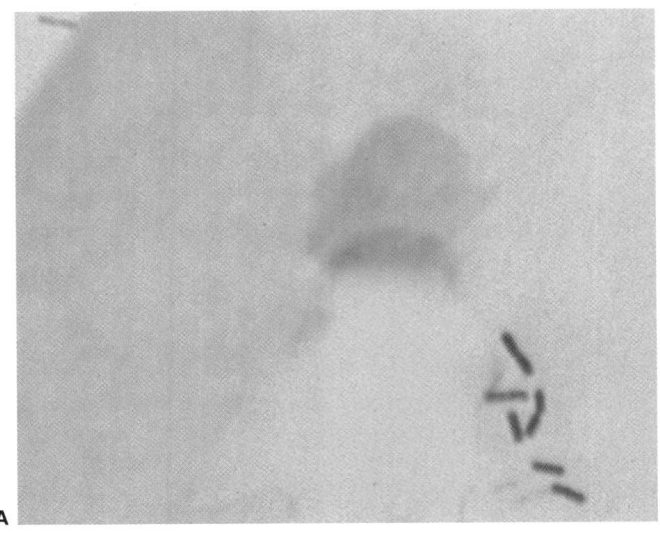

A

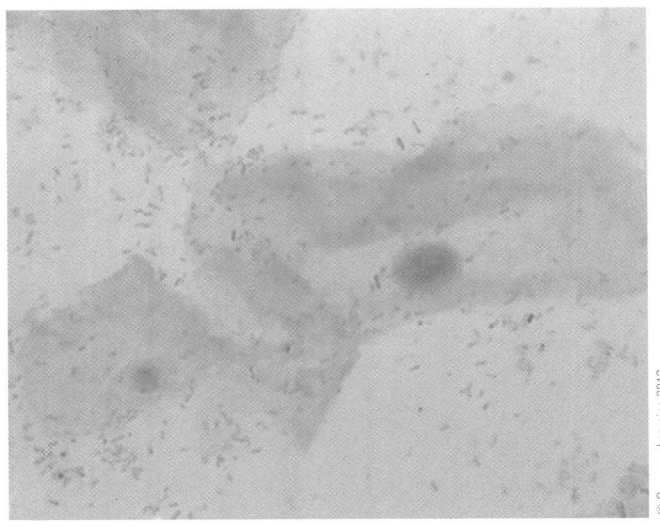

B

© Cengage Learning 2012

FIGURE 7-52 Gram-stained vaginal smears: (A) Gram-positive lactobacilli (normal flora); and (B) vaginal smear from patient with bacterial vaginosis (BV), showing clue cells with large numbers of small gram-variable bacteria, morphologically resembling *Gardnerella vaginalis*

Rapid Tests for Vaginitis and Vaginosis

Many rapid diagnostic tests are available for detection of microorganisms responsible for vaginosis and vaginitis. Several kits are available over the counter without a prescription. The tests are performed directly from the specimen swab. For example, the Genzyme OSOM BV BLUE kit for bacterial vaginosis/vaginitis (BV) can detect *Gardnerella vaginalis, Bacterioides* spp., *Prevotela,* and *Mobiluncus* spp. in less than 10 minutes. The Quidel Quick Vue ADVANCE is specific for *G. vaginalis.* Quidel also has a CLIA-waived kit for vaginal pH and presence of amines, a non-specific test that can indicate the presence of infection. One instrument, the BD Affirm VPIII

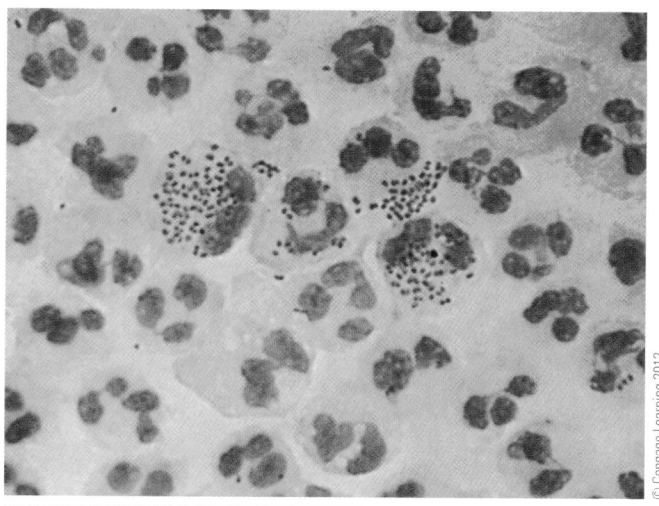

FIGURE 7-53 Gram-negative diplococci: Gram-stained vaginal smear showing white blood cells with intracellular gram-negative diplococci, morphologically resembling *Neisseria gonorrhoeae*

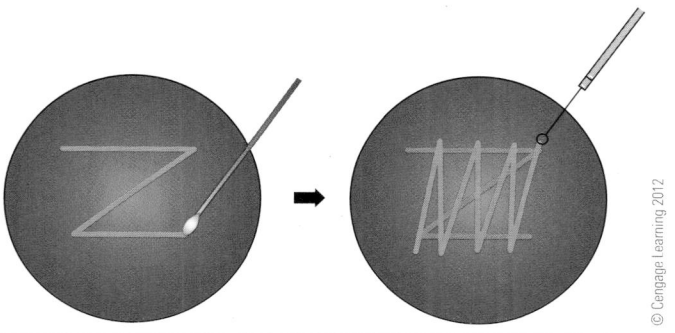

FIGURE 7-54 Inoculating (left) and cross-streaking (right) the modified Thayer-Martin plate for vaginal culture

uses RNA probe technology to detect microorganisms causing BV. This method can detect *Candida, G. vaginalis*, and *T. vaginalis* from the same specimen swab.

DETECTION OF SEXUALLY TRANSMITTED DISEASES IN MALES

Male patients with STDs usually have symptoms of **urethritis**, an inflammation of the urethra. Symptoms of urethritis are a burning sensation on urination or the presence of a penile discharge. Tests can include a urinalysis and culture, a Gram stain, a culture, or DNA probe test for *N. gonorrhoeae*, immunoassay or DNA probe for *C. trachomatis*, and serology tests for herpes simplex virus (HSV), HIV, and syphilis. If symptoms indicate possible STDs in a male patient, the specimens for the STD tests should be collected before the urine specimen is collected.

Males also sometimes develop a *nonspecific* or **nongono-coccal urethritis** in which the microorganisms causing the

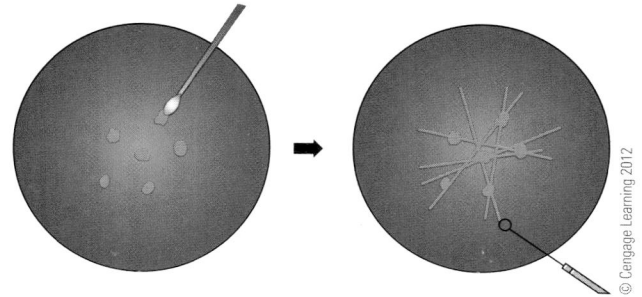

FIGURE 7-55 Inoculating (left) and cross-streaking (right) a modified Thayer-Martin plate for urethral culture

condition cannot be detected. In these cases, the patient is treated for the microorganisms usually implicated in urethritis.

Urinalysis and Urine Culture

A urinalysis can be performed to help determine if symptoms are due to urinary tract infection (UTI) or STD. If the midstream urine specimen contains red blood cells, bacteria, white blood cells, or protein, the patient may have a UTI instead of an STD and a urine culture should be performed. If the urine culture results are negative, the symptoms may be due to an STD.

Urethral Culture

The urethral discharge is collected using a special urogenital swab and cultured for *N. gonorrhoeae*. It is inoculated onto an MTM plate by touching the swab to the plate five or six times. The plate is transported to the laboratory immediately, where it is cross-streaked using a sterile loop and placed into a 35° to 37° C incubator in an increased carbon dioxide (CO_2) environment (Figure 7-55).

Urethral Gram Stain

A smear of the urethral discharge is made from the same swab used to inoculate the culture. The smear is Gram-stained and examined microscopically for evidence of white blood cells and bacteria, especially intracellular and extracellular gram-negative diplococci, with morphology resembling *N. gonorrhoeae*. The presence of many white blood cells on the smear is a strong indicator of infection.

IDENTIFICATION OF *NEISSERIA*
Appearance of Colonies

After overnight incubation, the MTM plate is examined for bacterial growth. *N. gonorrhoeae* appear as tiny, shiny, grayish colonies growing along the streak pattern. If scant or no growth is present, the plate is incubated for an additional 24 hours.

Confirmatory Tests from Culture

The **oxidase test** can be used to aid in identifying colonies of *N. gonorrhoeae*, which is oxidase positive. A purple-black color forms when oxidase-positive colonies are exposed to the oxidase reagent. If a suspected *Neisseria* colony gives a positive oxidase reaction, a smear and Gram stain should be performed on one of the oxidase-positive colonies. The presence of gram-negative diplococci on the smear is *presumptive* for *N. gonorrhoeae* and a confirmatory test must be performed.

Several systems are available to confirm identification of *N. gonorrhoeae*. Examples are Dupont's Gonochek II that identifies *N. gonorrhoeae*, *N. lactima*, and *N. meningitidis*, and GonoGen (BD Microbiology Systems), a 15-minute agglutination test. The Remel BactiCard test can presumptively identify *Neisseria* species. Remel also markets a system of fermentation tubes called Remel mini-ID, which identifies three species of *Neisseria*.

Nucleic Acid Methods for Detection of *Neisseria gonorrhoeae*

Several test methods are available for detecting *N. gonorrhoeae* using RNA or DNA probes or PCR. PCR is more specific and sensitive but technically more difficult to perform than the DNA probe tests. The BD ProbeTec ET System is a DNA amplification assay. It reduces the time required for sample handling and amplification and produces rapid results in the detection of *N. gonorrhoeae*.

TESTS FOR OTHER STDS

Several types of tests are available for detecting other STDs such as herpes, hepatitis, syphilis, HIV, and chlamydial infections. Test methods include negative staining, electron microscopy, fluorescent antibody (FA) techniques, enzyme immunoassays (EIAs),

---

CURRENT TOPICS

HUMAN PAPILLOMAVIRUS

Human papillomavirus (HPV) infects the genital skin and mucus membranes of men and women. More than 30 of approximately 100 types of the virus are sexually transmitted. Most infected individuals have no symptoms, are unaware that they are infected, and unknowingly pass it on to their sexual partners. Most people clear the infection on their own within 2 years. However, some of these viruses are classified as high-risk types and can cause malignant tumors, leading to cancer of the cervix, vulva, vagina, anus, or penis. Data from the Centers for Disease Control and Prevention (CDC) lists HPV as responsible for 85% of cases of anal cancer; 70% of vaginal cancers; 40% of vulvar cancers, and 40% of penile cancers. These high-risk types of the virus can also cause abnormal Papanicolaou (Pap) smears that are indicative of the infection. According to the American Cancer Society, about 10,500 women develop cervical cancer each year and 3,900 die from it. The types of HPV with low cancer risk can cause mild Pap smear abnormalities or genital warts.

Approximately 20 million people in the United States are currently infected with HPV. At least 50% of sexually active men and women will acquire HPV at some point. By age 50 at least 80% of women will have acquired a genital HPV infection. About 6.2 million Americans acquire a new genital HPV infection each year.

According to the CDC, a specific test to detect HPV DNA should be used for women with mild Pap smear abnormalities. Also, it is recommended that women 30 years of age and older be tested for HPV DNA at the time of their annual Pap smear. In 2006, a vaccine to prevent HPV infection was approved for use in pre-adolescent girls. Quadrivalent vaccines have since been developed for both young females and males.

Traditional methods for culturing viruses cannot be used for HPV. Examination of tissue biopsies has been one method of detection, but it is not very specific or sensitive. The Food and Drug Administration (FDA) approved a DNA HPV detection method, the HC 2 from Digene. In this test, the HPV DNA is hybridized to RNA probes. These hybrids are detected by a chemiluminescent system. The sensitivity is similar to polymerase chain reaction (PCR) assays. The NucliSENSEasyQ HPV by the bioMérieux company is an RNA test system for detection of HPV. This system has a high positive predictive value; a positive result indicates with a high level of confidence that the patient has an HPV infection.

serological tests, monoclonal antibody agglutination, and nucleic acid (DNA and RNA) probes (Table 7-24). Tests for one or more of these diseases can be ordered, depending on the patient's symptoms or sexual history.

An increasing number of easy-to-use test systems are becoming available, so that more testing can be performed in the smaller laboratory and the physician office laboratory (POL). However, tests for some STIs are time-consuming, technically advanced, or infrequently requested; specimens for these tests must be sent to a reference laboratory for testing.

Tests for Herpes Infection

Herpes viruses are DNA viruses that cause disease in humans. **Herpes simplex virus, type 1 (HSV-1)** is responsible for cases of oral herpes and **herpes simplex virus, type 2 (HSV-2)** causes genital herpes. However both types can be sexually transmitted. HSV infections have chronic, painful, recurring episodes.

Two methods of testing for herpes infection are cell culture and detection of serum antibody levels of anti-HSV. If herpes lesions are present, a vesicle can be broken with a sterile swab or needle and the vesicle fluid collected using another sterile swab. The swab is then inserted into viral transport medium and sent to a reference laboratory for culture. Cell culture results are available in 24 to 48 hours.

Serum titers of IgG and IgM to HSV-1 or HSV-2 can also be measured. The titers indicate whether the patient has active herpes or has ever had herpes type 1 or type 2 in the past. Several rapid diagnostic tests are available to test for antibodies to HSV-2. One example is the Fisher Sure-Vue, which uses only a few drops of the patient's blood in the test. The result can be read from the test cassette in 7 to 10 minutes.

Tests for *Chlamydia* Infection

Chlamydia trachomatis infection can be detected by EIA, cell culture, fluorescent antibody (FA), and DNA probes. In the female patient, *C. trachomatis* infection may cause the cervix to bleed easily just from the touch of a swab during examination. The cervix is said to be *friable*.

C. trachomatis infection is a common cause of urethritis in males, especially in young adults. Because urination temporarily flushes out any microorganisms inhabiting the urethra, for best chances of detection the patient should not have urinated in the 1 to 2 hours before the specimen collection.

There are several tests for *C. trachomatis*. In DNA probe tests, the same patient swab can be used to test for both *Chlamydia* and *N. gonorrhoeae*. DNA probe tests have high sensitivity and specificity. A piece of DNA with a specific sequence of nucleic acids, called the *probe DNA*, is added to a mixture containing the DNA from microorganisms in the patient specimen. If the patient specimen contains *Chlamydia* or *Neisseria*, the DNA probe will combine with the DNA of the bacteria and produce a color or luminescence. This signal will be measured by the instrumentation and the results printed out or sent to the laboratory computer.

Two immunoassay tests for detection of *C. trachomatis* are are the Premier *Chlamydia* by Meridian and CLEARVIEW *Chlamydia* from Wampole Laboratories. These tests have built-in positive and negative controls. The tests can be used to screen urines for *Chlamydia* in male patients, but has reduced sensitivity when used for testing urine; negative results should be confirmed by another method. The PathoDX *Chlamydia trachomatis* FA direct test is a fluorescent antibody technique from Remel. This test has the advantage of detecting *Chlamydia* directly from urethral and endocervical swab specimens.

Tests for Syphilis

Syphilis is the venereal disease caused by *Treponema pallidum*, a **spirochete**, or spiral bacterium. Early (primary) syphilis is characterized by skin lesions. Organ or tissue damage occurs in the secondary stage. Late-stage (tertiary) syphilis can affect the cardiovascular and central nervous systems.

Because of the difficulty in growing *Treponema* in culture, the screening method of choice has been serum antibody detection. The *Venereal Disease Research Laboratory (VDRL)* test and the *rapid plasma reagin (RPR)* test are screening tests for syphilis. The VDRL test can be performed only by laboratories certified in its use.

Venereal Disease Research Laboratory Test

Patients infected with *T. pallidum* produce non-specific antibodies called reagin. When the VDRL antigen mixture, made of cardiolipin, cholesterol, and lecithin, is reacted with serum containing reagin, a visible reaction—flocculation—occurs. The test is *reactive* in 70% to 99% of primary and secondary syphilis cases, but is usually nonreactive in tertiary cases.

Rapid Plasma Reagin Test

The RPR test has a carbon-containing cardiolipin antigen that reacts with the reagin produced in response to syphilis and some other conditions. The RPR is also a flocculation test, with the carbon causing black clumps on a white background in a *reactive* test. Test results are reported as *reactive* or *nonreactive*. A reactive result is *not* diagnostic for syphilis, but only indicates the presence of reagin.

Confirmation of a Reactive Syphilis Screening Test

A *reactive* result in a serum VDRL or RPR screening test must be confirmed by a more specific test method, because *biological false positives* (BFPs) can occur. Several nonsyphilitic conditions can cause BFPs, including tuberculosis, hepatitis, pneumonia, pregnancy, and rheumatoid arthritis.

The fluorescent treponemal antibody-absorption (FTA-ABS) test is a specific test that uses *Treponema* antigen to detect anti-treponemal antibodies in patient serum. The *T. pallidum* microhemagglutination assay (MHA-TP) also detects serum antibodies to *T. pallidum.* Both the FTA-ABS and the MHA-TP are specific treponemal antigen tests that are used to confirm a reactive RPR or VDRL test. Enzyme-linked immunosorbent assays (ELISA) can be used as screening tests; molecular methods are also available.

Tests for Human Immunodeficiency Virus

Human immunodeficiency virus (HIV) is transmitted sexually and by contact with infectious body fluids. HIV testing methods assay for anti-HIV in the patient's serum. Because this antibody usually does not appear until several weeks or months after exposure, a negative test must be followed by a second test in a few weeks. Tests for HIV are usually performed in reference laboratories and state public health laboratories.

Because saliva and urine from HIV-infected patients contain HIV antibodies, tests have been developed to detect HIV antibodies in saliva, urine, and blood. One rapid blood test for antibodies to HIV-1 is the Trinity Biotech Uni-Gold Recombigen HIV test. The test can be performed on whole blood, plasma, or serum. The sample is added to the sample well in the test cassette, and a wash solution is added. Ten minutes later, the result is shown in the result window. The test is CLIA-waived when whole blood is used. These tests for HIV are *sensitive* to small amounts of antibody. The results of positive antibody tests must be confirmed by a more specific test such as the Western blot test.

As HIV infections progress, the virus multiplies and can be cultured and isolated. Some confirmatory tests detect viral components such as the p24 antigen. The p24 antigen can be detected very early after HIV infection, then disappears and cannot be detected again until the late stages of the disease.

Tests for Hepatitis B Infections

The hepatitis B virus (HBV) can cause serious illness and even be fatal because of its effects on the liver. A patient can remain chronically infected with HBV even when asymptomatic. The chronic infection can lead to liver cancer (hepatocarcinoma).

HBV is highly infectious and can be transmitted through sexual contact, exposure to infectious blood or other body fluids, or exposure to contaminated food. An HBV vaccine is available to provide lifelong immunity for immunocompetent individuals who complete the entire three-shot series. At-risk healthcare workers must be immunized or must sign a refusal statement waiving employer liability.

Many tests are available for detecting HBV antigens and antibodies. Test methods include radioimmunoassays, EIA, and ELISA. A common screening test is the test for HBV surface antigen (HBsAg). A positive result indicates the patient has, or recently has had, an acute HBV infection. The finding of HBsAg several months after infection indicates the person is a chronic HBV carrier. The anti-HBsAg titer is used to check for immunity after receiving the HBV vaccine. Detecting antibody

to the HBV core antigen (anti-HBcAg) is another test for HBV infection.

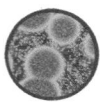 ## SUMMARY

This lesson has introduced basic laboratory methods used to detect STDs. Agents that can cause STDs include bacteria, protozoa, fungi, and viruses. Screening tests for STDs and confirmation of positive results were formerly performed only in large hospitals or state or reference laboratories. However, many STD test kits are now available for use in POLs and other smaller laboratories. Rapid tests are available for detection of BV, HSV-2, and antibodies to HIV-1. Use of these rapid tests makes it possible to screen for some STDs on-site. Most confirmations of STD screening tests are performed by reference or state laboratories.

 ## REVIEW QUESTIONS

1. What is the importance of detecting STDs?
2. When is modified Thayer-Martin (MTM) media used?
3. Why should personnel in POLs and other small laboratories be knowledgeable about STDs and the methods used to detect them?
4. What are five common STDs in the United States?
5. Name one method of detection for each of five STDs.
6. What does the presence of HBsAg indicate about a patient?
7. What is the danger of chronic HBV infection?
8. Why should patients be tested for both HSV-1 and HSV-2?
9. Define *Candida albicans, Chlamydia trachomatis,* clue cells, gonorrhea, herpes simplex virus type 1, herpes simplex virus type 2, human immunodeficiency virus, human papillomavirus, nongonococcal urethritis, oxidase test, spirochetes, sexually transmitted disease, sexually transmitted infection, syphilis, trichomoniasis, urethritis, vaginitis, and venereal.

 ## STUDENT ACTIVITIES

1. Complete the written examination for this lesson.
2. Survey POLs in your community to find out the extent of STD testing performed.
3. Determine how a nearby reference laboratory confirms positive HIV tests and reactive RPR tests.
4. Tour your state's public health laboratory. Ask for copies of their epidemiology reports on STD incidence in your state.

WEB ACTIVITIES

1. Use the Internet to search for the *Morbidity and Mortality Weekly Reports* (MMWR). Find statistics for the incidence of *Chlamydia* cases in the United States for the last 2 years for which reports are available.

2. Use the Internet to find information about PCR or DNA and RNA probe technology. Report on the use of one of these technologies in detecting an STD.

3. Search the Internet for molecular diagnostic tests for a STD.

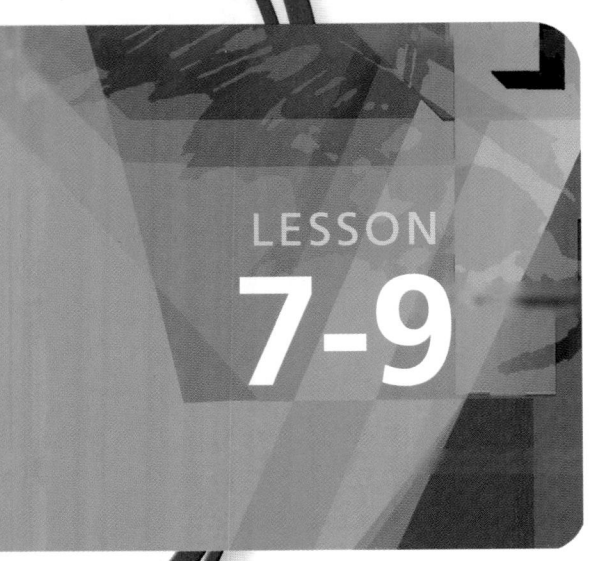

Infection Prevention in Healthcare Settings

LESSON OBJECTIVES

After studying this lesson, the student will:

- ⊙ Discuss the role of the institution's infection prevention department.
- ⊙ List five exposure control methods that are included in Standard Precautions.
- ⊙ Explain why isolation techniques are used.
- ⊙ List the three types of transmission-based precautions and explain the basis for each classification.
- ⊙ Demonstrate handwashing technique.
- ⊙ Demonstrate gowning technique.
- ⊙ Demonstrate the method of putting on a mask.
- ⊙ Demonstrate the technique for donning sterile gloves.
- ⊙ Demonstrate the techniques for removal and disposal of mask, gown, and gloves.
- ⊙ Define the glossary terms.

GLOSSARY

Airborne Precautions / a Centers for Disease Control and Prevention (CDC) isolation category designed to prevent transmission of infectious diseases, such as measles, that are spread by the airborne route

APIC / Association for Professionals in Infection Control and Epidemiology, an organization working across a spectrum of professionals, organizations, and institutions to prevent healthcare-associated infections

carrier / an individual who harbors an organism and is capable of spreading the organism to others, but has no symptoms or signs of disease

Contact Precautions / a CDC isolation category designed to prevent transmission of diseases spread by close or direct contact

Droplet Precautions / a CDC isolation category designed to prevent transmission of diseases spread through the air over short distances

fomites / inanimate objects, such as bed rails, linens, or eating utensils, which can be contaminated with infectious organisms and serve as a means of their transmission

healthcare-associated infection (HAI) / infection acquired while being treated for another condition in a healthcare setting; formerly called nosocomial infection

infection / a pathological condition caused by growth of microorganisms in the host

isolation / the practice of limiting the movement and social contact of a patient who is potentially infectious or who must be protected from exposure to infectious agents; quarantine

nonpathogenic / not normally causing disease in a healthy individual

(continues)

nosocomial infection / an infection acquired in a hospital or healthcare facility; healthcare-associated infection

protective isolation / an isolation category designed to protect highly susceptible patients from exposure to infectious agents; reverse isolation

Standard Precautions / a set of comprehensive safety guidelines designed to protect patients and healthcare workers by requiring that all patients and all body fluids, body substances, organs, and unfixed tissues be regarded as potentially infectious

INTRODUCTION

In today's world, every healthcare institution has an infection prevention program in place, based on regulations and recommendations of agencies such as the Centers for Disease Control and Prevention (CDC), the Joint Commission (JC), the Association for Professionals in Infection Control and Epidemiology (APIC), and state health and regulatory agencies. The goal of the program is to prevent infection transmission in the healthcare setting.

The healthcare facility's infection prevention (infection control) officer or department monitors contagious diseases within the facility. This is accomplished by setting guidelines for managing contagious patients and patients who are highly susceptible to infection (have little resistance or immunity). This department also sets standards to ensure that patients do not acquire **healthcare-associated infections (HAIs)**, those infections acquired while being treated in a healthcare setting, and that infections do not spread to visitors and healthcare personnel.

With new methods of delivering health care, such as increases in POCT, outpatient procedures, home health care, and facilities and services such as hospice, the old way of thinking about "infection control" has changed. The emergence of new infectious diseases and increase in antibiotic resistance among some long-known pathogenic organisms makes it even more important that stringent measures are applied to all healthcare settings to prevent disease transmission.

This lesson provides general information about causes of infection and measures that can be taken to prevent transmission of infection. Guidelines for laboratory personnel such as those who must obtain blood from a potentially contagious patient are emphasized. Exposure control practices are emphasized. The set of guidelines called transmission-based precautions are explained. The laboratory student or employee must follow the particular institution's rules concerning these guidelines.

CAUSES OF INFECTION

Microbes present in the environment and in and on the human body include bacteria, viruses, protozoa, and fungi. Microbes capable of causing disease are called pathogens. Most microorganisms are **nonpathogenic**, meaning they do not normally cause disease in a healthy individual.

Infection occurs when the body is invaded by a pathogenic agent that can, under favorable conditions, multiply and cause disease. Infections usually cause symptoms that can vary greatly depending on the site of infection and characteristics of the infectious agent. Infections in the early stages of incubation, when there are no symptoms, cause particular problems in the healthcare setting, because infections can often be transmitted before the infected person experiences symptoms.

Three components must be present for infection to occur: (1) a source of microorganisms, (2) a susceptible person or host, and (3) a method of transmission from the source to the susceptible host. The source can be an infected person or animal, the environment, or **fomites** (contaminated objects). A source of infection can be contact with a **carrier**, a person who harbors an organism but feels well and displays no symptoms of infection. Infections can be acquired through direct contact; inhaling dust or droplets containing microorganisms; inhaling air droplets produced by coughing or sneezing by an infected person; exposure to infectious body fluids; ingesting contaminated water or food; or through vectors such as insects (Table 7-25).

TRANSMISSION-BASED PRECAUTIONS

In the past, each institution developed **isolation** procedures appropriate for its patient population, taking into consideration newly emerging contagious diseases. In 1992, the CDC issued Universal Precautions, a set of guidelines to assist healthcare providers in reducing the risk for contracting or transmitting infectious agents, particularly HIV and hepatitis B virus.

TABLE 7-25. Methods of acquiring infection

- ▶ Direct contact
- ▶ Inhaling droplets produced by coughing or sneezing
- ▶ Inhaling dust particles containing microorganisms
- ▶ Exposure to infectious body fluids
- ▶ Ingesting contaminated food or water
- ▶ Exposure to disease vectors such as insects or rodents

Standard Precautions

In 1996, **Standard Precautions** were issued by the CDC to augment and synthesize Universal Precautions with the techniques known as body substance isolation (BSI). Standard Precautions represent a comprehensive approach to protecting all healthcare providers, patients, and visitors from acquiring infectious diseases. Standard Precautions apply to:

- All blood
- All body fluids, secretions, and excretions, even if they do not contain visible blood
- Non-intact skin
- Mucous membranes

Standard Precautions must always be observed along with the facility's exposure control plan and CDC safety regulations. Standard Precautions must be used for all patients regardless of diagnosis or presumed health status. The use of Standard Precautions prevents exposure to all blood and body fluids, whether known to be infectious or not. The application of Standard Precautions includes using methods such as safe work practice controls, safety devices, and other engineering controls. These include:

- Using appropriate hand hygiene techniques
- Wearing appropriate personal protective equipment (PPE) whenever exposure to patients' body fluids can occur
- Wearing eye and/or face protection if aerosols or splashes are likely or reasonably anticipated
- Discarding all contaminated sharps into rigid, puncture-proof sharps containers
- Cleaning up spills immediately with an appropriate disinfectant

In addition to issuing Standard Precautions, the CDC also simplified isolation guidelines. The former isolation classification scheme contained five categories: (1) contact isolation, (2) respiratory isolation, (3) acid-fast bacillus (AFB) isolation, (4) strict or complete isolation, and (5) reverse isolation, plus special categories for patients with enteric or drainage secretions. These five categories were reduced to three *transmission-based precautions*, also called *expanded precautions*, classified according to the route of disease transmission. The transmission-based precautions are: (1) **Droplet Precautions**, (2) **Contact Precautions**, and (3) **Airborne Precautions** (Table 7-26).

The first rule is that Standard Precautions are always used! Transmission-based precautions used in addition to Standard Precautions provide additional protection and methods of preventing or interrupting disease transmission in healthcare facilities.

Contact Precautions

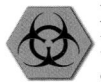

Contact Precautions are used in addition to Standard Precautions when patients have infections that can be spread primarily by close or direct contact (Figure 7-56 and Table 7-27). The patient should be placed in a private room, if possible. Precautions used for this category are

TABLE 7-26. Current CDC transmission-based precautions and former isolation categories

CURRENT TRANSMISSION-BASED PRECAUTIONS*	FORMER ISOLATION CATEGORIES
Droplet precautions*	Contact isolation
Airborne precautions*	Respiratory isolation
Contact precautions*	Acid-fast bacillus (AFB) isolation
	Complete or strict isolation
	Reverse or protective isolation

* Used in addition to Standard Precautions.

intended to protect healthcare workers against infection from contact with infectious material, such as wound or fecal material. Exposure could occur if the patient is incontinent or has diarrhea, an ileostomy, a colostomy, or wound drainage not contained by a dressing. Surfaces and items in the room can become contaminated, so the healthcare worker must wear gloves and gown and remove both before leaving the room to avoid transferring pathogens outside the room. After glove removal, hands must be washed with an antimicrobial agent. Contaminated materials must be discarded in biohazard containers for disposal or disinfection.

Droplet Precautions

Droplet Precautions are used in addition to Standard Precautions when patients are infected with pathogens easily transmitted through the air over short distances (Figure 7-57), a major mode of transmission for certain respiratory infections. Examples include mumps, pertussis (whooping cough), meningococcal pneumonia, and meningitis (Table 7-27). These patients should be in private rooms. Masks are required for those who enter the patient room, because the infectious agents are readily spread by the patient's coughing or sneezing.

Airborne Precautions

Airborne Precautions are used in addition to Standard Precautions when a patient is known to be, or suspected of being, infected with pathogens transmitted by the airborne route (Figure 7-58 and Table 7-27). Persons entering the room of a patient with known or suspected infectious pulmonary tuberculosis must wear an N95 respirator (Figure 7-59). In addition, susceptible personnel should not enter rooms of patients known to have, or suspected of having, measles (rubeola) or chickenpox (varicella) unless an immune caregiver is not available. The patient must be in a private room with negative air

CONTACT PRECAUTIONS
(in addition to Standard Precautions)

 VISITORS: Report to nurse before entering.

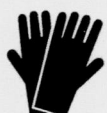

Gloves
Don gloves upon entry into the room or cubicle.
Wear gloves whenever touching the patient's intact skin or surfaces and articles in close proximity to the patient.
Remove gloves before leaving patient room.

Hand Hygiene
Hand Hygiene according to Standard Precautions.

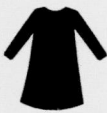

Gowns
Don gown upon entry into the room or cubicle.
Remove gown and observe hand hygiene before leaving the patient-care environment.

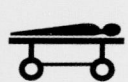

Patient Transport
Limit transport of patients to medically necessary purposes.
Ensure that infected or colonized areas of the patient's body are contained and covered.
Remove and dispose of contaminated PPE and perform hand hygiene prior to transporting patients on Contact Precautions.
Don clean PPE to handle the patient at the transport destination.

Patient–Care Equipment
Use disposable noncritical patient-care equipment or implement patient-dedicated use of such equipment.

Form No. *CPR7*   BREVIS CORP., 225 West 2855 South, SLC, UT 84115   © 2007 Brevis Corp.

Courtesy Brevis Corp.

FIGURE 7-56 Guide to Contact Precautions, a category of transmission-based precautions used in in-patient settings

pressure (Airborne Infection Isolation Room, AIIR). The room must have 6 to 12 air changes per hour and room air must be discharged outside or recirculated through a HEPA filter.

Reverse or Protective Isolation

 Earlier isolation classifications contained a category called reverse or **protective isolation** intended to protect immunosuppressed patients such as transplant recipients or other patients with increased susceptibility. Current standards do not address protective isolation in a direct way. Individual hospitals continue to make it an unofficial category; signs are placed on the room doors of immunosuppressed patients. The signs direct healthcare workers and visitors to wear masks when entering the room if they have a cold or other contagious condition. Laboratory personnel should always clarify any questions about protective isolation by consulting with the floor nurse or the infection prevention officer.

TABLE 7-27. Transmission-based precautions and examples of illnesses and disease agents that require the precautions (adapted from the CDC)

STANDARD PRECAUTIONS

Use for all patients

AIRBORNE PRECAUTIONS

Use in addition to Standard Precautions for illnesses transmitted by airborne droplet nuclei.
Examples:

    Measles (rubeola)

    Infectious pulmonary tuberculosis

    Chicken pox (varicella)

DROPLET PRECAUTIONS

Use in addition to Standard Precautions for illnesses transmitted by large-particle droplets.
Examples:

Mycoplasma pneumonia	Invasive *Neisseria meningitidis*
Pneumonic plague	Rubella
Invasive *Haemophilus influenzae*	Influenza
Diphtheria	Parvovirus B19
Pertussis	Mumps
Adenovirus	Streptococcal pharyngitis

CONTACT PRECAUTIONS

Use in addition to Standard Precautions for illnesses transmitted by direct contact.
Examples:

Wound infections	Enteric infections
Respiratory syncytial virus	Skin infections
Viral hemorrhagic infections	Colonization with multidrug-resistant organisms (MDRO)

COMPLYING WITH THE EXPOSURE CONTROL PLAN

Laboratory personnel must observe their institution's exposure control plan and the CDC's safety regulations, not only in the laboratory but also in patient rooms and all other healthcare situations. These procedures are discussed in depth in Lesson 1-4, Biological Safety. Personnel must always observe Standard Precautions along with transmission-based (expanded) precautions. The types of transmission-based precautions can be combined for diseases that have multiple modes of transmission.

EXPOSURE CONTROL PRACTICES

Healthcare facilities provide specific instructions and necessary supplies outside the room of each patient requiring transmission-based precautions. Exposure control practices that must be used include wearing gloves, masks and gowns and practicing good hand hygiene.

Hand Hygiene

The use of hand hygiene practices is critical to preventing the spread of infection and reducing healthcare-associated infections (HAI). Failure to use appropriate hand hygiene is the leading cause of HAI.

Handwashing or hand antisepsis products include plain soaps and antimicrobial soaps, gel and foam handrubs, and chemical antiseptics. Several factors are considered by institutions when selecting hand hygiene products, including the efficacy against a wide range of microorganisms, the willingness of workers to use the product, and the accessibility or ease of use of the product. Each hand hygiene product has a role in maintaining good hand hygiene. No one product will provide all the necessary protection for all situations.

The effectiveness of hand hygiene techniques depends on frequent hand cleansing and correct use of the product, such as using the correct amount of antiseptic agent and cleansing for the recommended time for the product used. General recommendations for routine hand hygiene are:

- Hands should be decontaminated before and after all procedures
- Alcohol-based hand rubs or antimicrobial soap and water should be used for routine decontamination of hands in most clinical situations
- Visibly soiled hands should be washed with soap and water, followed by use of an antiseptic agent such as an alcohol-based rub
- Hands should be washed with soap and warm water before and after eating and after using a restroom

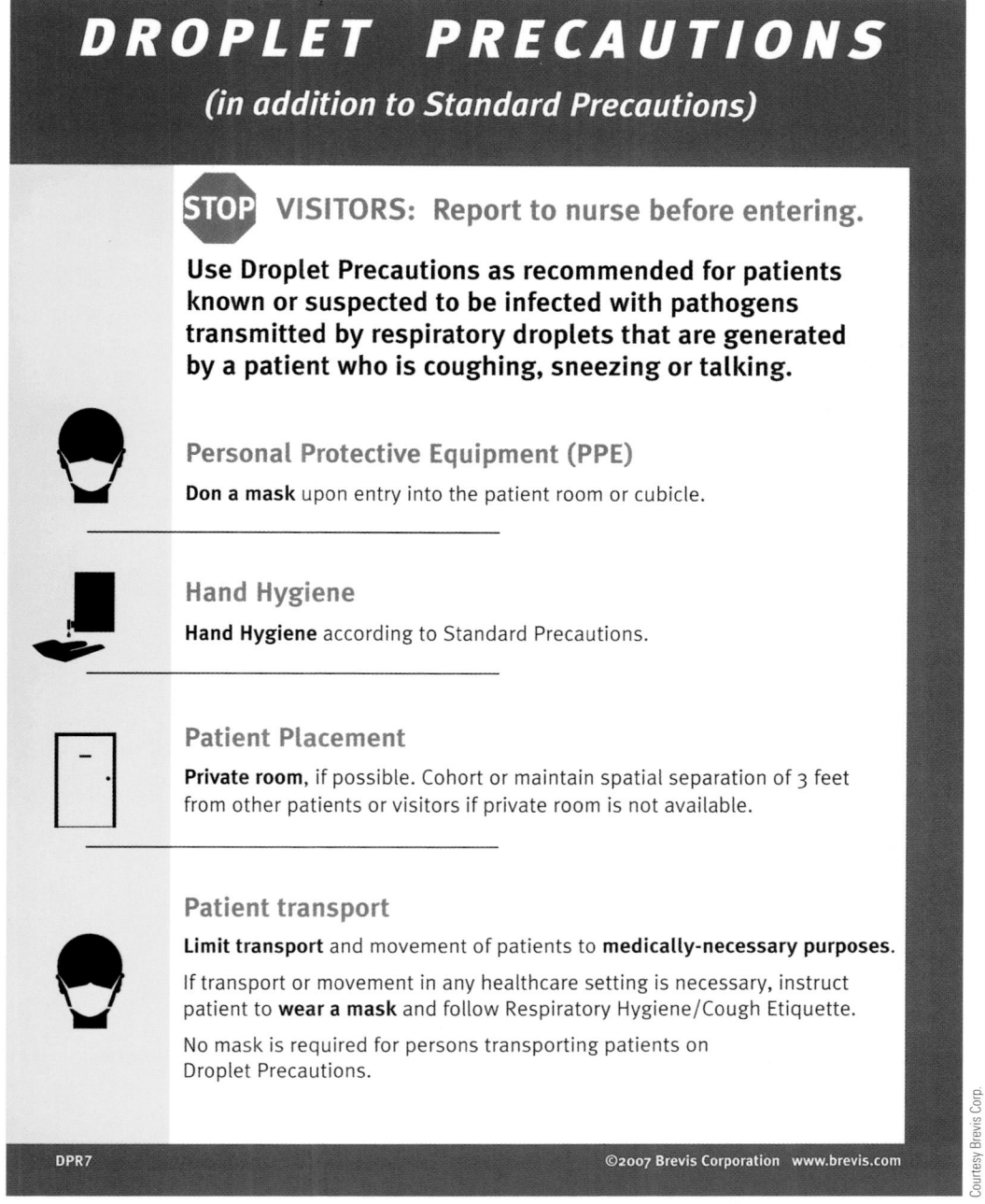

FIGURE 7-57 Guide to Droplet Precautions, a category of transmission-based precautions used in in-patient settings

- Hands should be washed with water and antiseptic or antimicrobial soap after each 5 to 10 hand decontaminations with an alcohol-based waterless handrub
- The institution's hand hygiene policy must be followed

Waterless Handrub Technique

The waterless handrub is applied to the palm of one hand, and the hands are vigorously rubbed together, covering all surfaces of hands, fingers, and between fingers. This procedure is continued until the hands are completely dry. The manufacturer's

recommendations for the volume to use should be followed. One advantage of the waterless handrubs is that a sink is not required for hand decontamination.

Handwashing Technique

To wash hands with soap and water, hands should first be wet with warm or room temperature water, and the amount of soap recommended by the manufacturer applied to the hands. Hot water should not be used because repeated exposure to hot water can increase the risk for dermatitis. The hands and wrists

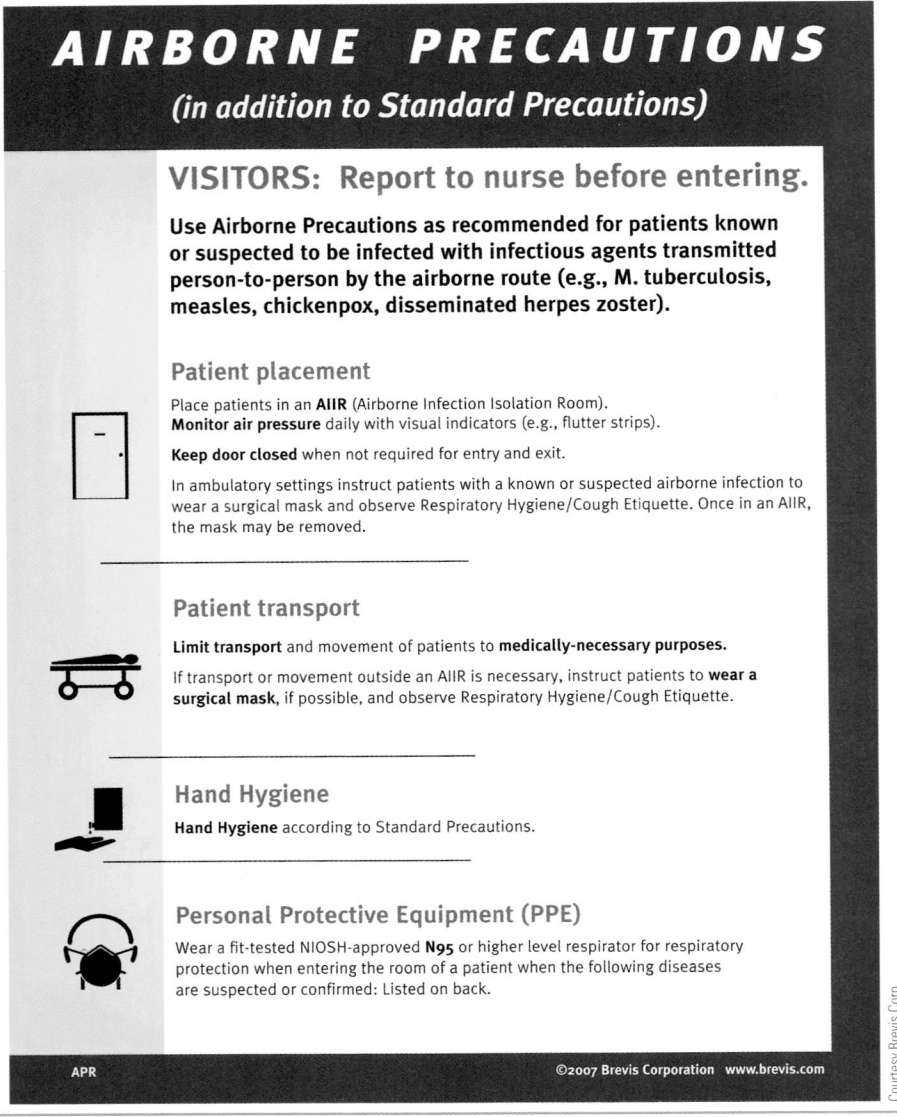

AIRBORNE PRECAUTIONS
(in addition to Standard Precautions)

VISITORS: Report to nurse before entering.

Use Airborne Precautions as recommended for patients known or suspected to be infected with infectious agents transmitted person-to-person by the airborne route (e.g., M. tuberculosis, measles, chickenpox, disseminated herpes zoster).

Patient placement

Place patients in an **AIIR** (Airborne Infection Isolation Room).
Monitor air pressure daily with visual indicators (e.g., flutter strips).

Keep door closed when not required for entry and exit.

In ambulatory settings instruct patients with a known or suspected airborne infection to wear a surgical mask and observe Respiratory Hygiene/Cough Etiquette. Once in an AIIR, the mask may be removed.

Patient transport

Limit transport and movement of patients to **medically-necessary purposes.**

If transport or movement outside an AIIR is necessary, instruct patients to **wear a surgical mask**, if possible, and observe Respiratory Hygiene/Cough Etiquette.

Hand Hygiene

Hand Hygiene according to Standard Precautions.

Personal Protective Equipment (PPE)

Wear a fit-tested NIOSH-approved **N95** or higher level respirator for respiratory protection when entering the room of a patient when the following diseases are suspected or confirmed: Listed on back.

APR   ©2007 Brevis Corporation www.brevis.com

Courtesy Brevis Corp.

FIGURE 7-58 Guide to Airborne Precautions, a category of transmission-based precautions used in in-patient settings

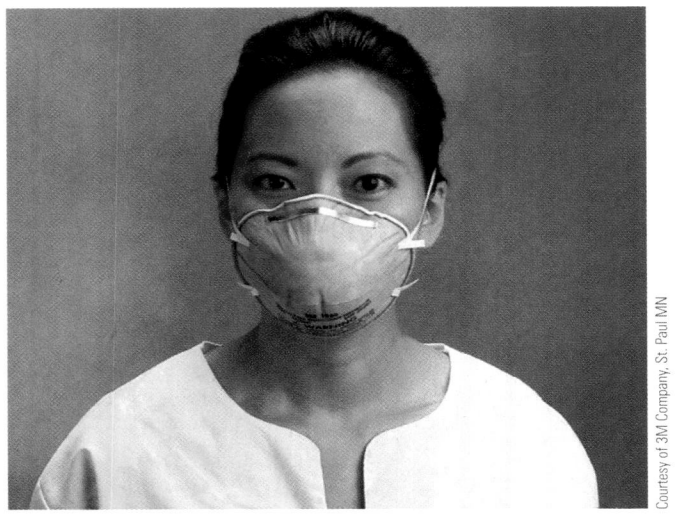

Courtesy of 3M Company, St. Paul MN

FIGURE 7-59 Healthcare worker wearing an N95 respirator

should be lathered, and hands should be rubbed together vigorously for 15 to 30 seconds, covering all surfaces of the hands and fingers (Figure 7-60). Special attention should be given to cleaning fingernails and under rings if a procedure is to be performed that requires sterility. Hands should be held in a downward position and rinsed from the arm or wrist toward the tips of the fingers. The hands should be dried thoroughly with a disposable towel. Hand-operated faucet handles which could have contaminated surfaces should not be touched with the bare hands, but should be turned on and off using a clean disposable towel.

Using Personal Protective Equipment

Standard Precautions require that personnel wear personal protective equipment (PPE) to protect against exposure to potentially infectious material. This PPE includes, but is not limited to, mask, gown, and gloves.

CURRENT TOPICS

CLOSTRIDIUM DIFFICILE

Clostridium difficile (C. difficile) is a gram-positive rod (bacillus) present in the intestines of a small percentage of the population. It is a spore-former, which means it can change into a resistant form called a *spore* when it is in an environment unfavorable for its growth. Spores are more resistant to disinfectants and heat sterilization than the vegetative (non-spore) form.

There are various strains of *C. difficile*; however, the virulent strain that is involved in antibiotic associated diarrhea (AAD) produces an enterotoxin and a cytotoxin that cause disease. This strain has become more prevalent in the last decade. In one study of stool specimens from the decade of 1980–1990 only seven cases of colitis were associated with *C. difficile* out of 6,000 samples. In the years between 2001 and 2007 in an examination of 600 fecal samples *C. difficile* was responsible in eight cases. This is almost a 10-fold increase.

Many theories have been proposed to explain the incidence of *C. difficile* and where it originated. These theories include:

- Environmental sources
- Animal to human transmission
- Human to animal transmission
- Contamination of food animals given antibiotics

The evidence points to transmission from animals; many food animals are given a regimen of antibiotics to keep them healthy. Widespread outbreaks of this strain have occurred in food animals, especially pigs.

At the present time 80% of all *C. difficile* infections are related to healthcare settings, especially long-term care or hospitalization for 2 weeks or more. In 2010, at one hospital 199 patients were diagnosed in 1 year. In Ireland, one hospital had 36 cases, with 4 deaths in a month. In May of 2010 a total of 138 patients were diagnosed among four hospitals all located within a small geographic area.

PATHOLOGY

The greatest rates of infection are in the 45- to 64-year age-group, with the rate decreasing for those 65 years and above. Patients who have been on medications, such as H_2 receptor antagonists and proton pump inhibitors that reduce or suppress gastric acid production seem to be at higher risk. Those who have had antibiotic therapy are also at higher risk. Oral antibiotics reduce the numbers of normal flora in the intestines. The reduced numbers of normal flora allow *C. difficile* to grow and multiply. Although the condition has been found primarily in the adult population new reports indicate the incidence is rising in pediatric patients. It is estimated that 50% of infants are already colonized with *C. difficile* at birth. When these infants and young children are placed on antibiotic therapy for another condition the normal intestinal flora is eradicated and *C. difficile* can easily overgrow. The intestines become over-populated with *C. difficile*, and under stress conditions the organisms produce two toxins, enterotoxin and cytotoxin. The toxins cause production of a pseudo-membrane on the intestinal walls. This thickening of the walls is called pseudomembranous colitis. The membrane is made up of inflammatory cells, fibrin, and necrotic (dead) cells, and serves to protect the bacteria.

TREATMENT

Treatment for pseudomembranous colitis consists of discontinuing antibiotics to allow normal flora to repopulate. If there is no improvement in the patient's condition a regimen of powerful oral antibiotics such as vancomycin and metronidazole (Flagyl) can be prescribed along with some probiotics. Even with treatment the relapse rate is 20%.

PREVENTIVE MEASURES

Studies have shown that *C. difficile* remains on environmental surfaces for a long time. They have been cultured from many surfaces, including door handles, bed frames in patient rooms, and other articles. Evidence indicates that healthcare workers may touch their ungloved hands to commode parts, rectal thermometers, patient sinks and even contaminated hands of the patient. They may then go out, touching the handle on the patient's door and go on to another patient's room. This illustrates the importance of strict adherence to handwashing protocol and changing of gloves between patients. There are some indications that waterless hand antiseptics are not as effective in this scenario because spores may not be removed from the hands. Any contaminated inanimate surfaces can be disinfected using 10% bleach solution. Some common hospital disinfectants are not as effective as bleach because they can cause the bacteria to produce spores which are resistant to sterilization, including autoclaving.

CURRENT TOPICS

HEALTHCARE-ASSOCIATED INFECTIONS

Healthcare-associated infections (HAIs), as the name implies, are infections acquired within healthcare settings. (HAI is the new term replacing nosocomial infections, which was previously used to define infections occurring in hospitalized patients or patients in hospital-like settings, such as long-term care facilities.) An HAI is an infection not present when a patient enters a healthcare facility, but that develops more than 48 hours after admission. If an infection develops within the first 48 hours after admission to a facility, it is considered a community-acquired infection.

It is estimated that more than 2 million HAIs occur annually, with 90,000 deaths. In the United States, the incidence of HAI can be as high as 10% in institutionalized patients. These infections can be acquired through contact with infected personnel, visitors, other patients, or contaminated equipment. HAIs usually present more problems than randomly acquired infections because:

- Hospitalized patients may be more susceptible to infection
- Invasive procedures such as surgery or indwelling catheters provide a portal to infection
- HAIs generally require longer hospital stays, resulting in greater expense
- Bacteria associated with HAIs are often drug-resistant, resulting in some drug treatments being less effective and often requiring more toxic drugs to be prescribed. Multidrug resistant organisms (MDRO) that are becoming more widespread include:
  - Methicillin-resistant *Staphylococcus aureus* (MRSA)
  - *Clostridium difficile*
  - Vancomycin-resistant *Enterococcus* (VRE)

Through the use of effective infection prevention practices, the incidence of HAIs can be kept to a minimum. These practices include:

- Strict adherence to Standard Precautions
- Appropriate use of transmission-based precautions
- Immunization of healthcare workers against vaccine-preventable diseases

A sequence of donning and removing PPE should be used that protects the wearer from becoming contaminated. Generally hands are cleaned with antiseptic and then gown, mask, eyewear or face protection, and gloves are donned in that order. The general order of removal is that gloves are removed first, and then the gown. Hands should then be cleaned with antiseptic before eyewear and mask are removed.

Masks

Masks should be put on after hands are washed, avoiding touching the skin with the hands. Masks can have ties for the upper neck and head or elastic bands to loop over the ears. Masks should be changed after being worn for 15 to 20 minutes.

Gowns

Laboratory coats should be removed before donning gowns. The gown should be touched only on the inside surface and should cover all clothing when tied (Figure 7-61). Gowns are removed by turning the inside of the gown to the outside and folding the contaminated outer side inward.

Gloves

A clean pair of gloves must be used for each patient contact. The gloves are put on by pulling the cuff or wrist area over sleeve ends of gowns or laboratory coats to cover exposed skin. Sharp rings or jewelry that can puncture gloves should not be worn.

Some special instances, such as reverse isolation, require sterile gloves. Sterile gloves are always used to handle sterile equipment or instruments and are used for certain other techniques such as collecting a blood culture. Figure 7-62 shows and describes how to don sterile gloves.

Contaminated gloves can be removed by different methods depending on the preference of the technologist. Whatever method is used, the outside of the glove surface should not be touched with the bare hand. One method of glove removal is to grasp the cuff of one glove with the other gloved hand and pull the glove off over itself, enclosing the removed glove in the palm of the remaining gloved hand. The second glove is removed by inserting bare fingers inside the cuff of the remaining glove and pulling the glove inside out down over the hand, taking care not to touch the outside of glove. The gloves are discarded into a biohazard container. (Figure 7-63). Hands should always be decontaminated with antiseptic after glove removal.

Entering and Exiting a Precaution Room

The procedure used for entering and exiting isolation rooms differs according to the type of precaution. In general, most PPE is located on a cart immediately outside the door of the patient's room and is put on before entering (Figure 7-64).

Only items that will be used for the patient should be taken into the precaution room. Phlebotomists should leave trays and

© Cengage Learning 2012

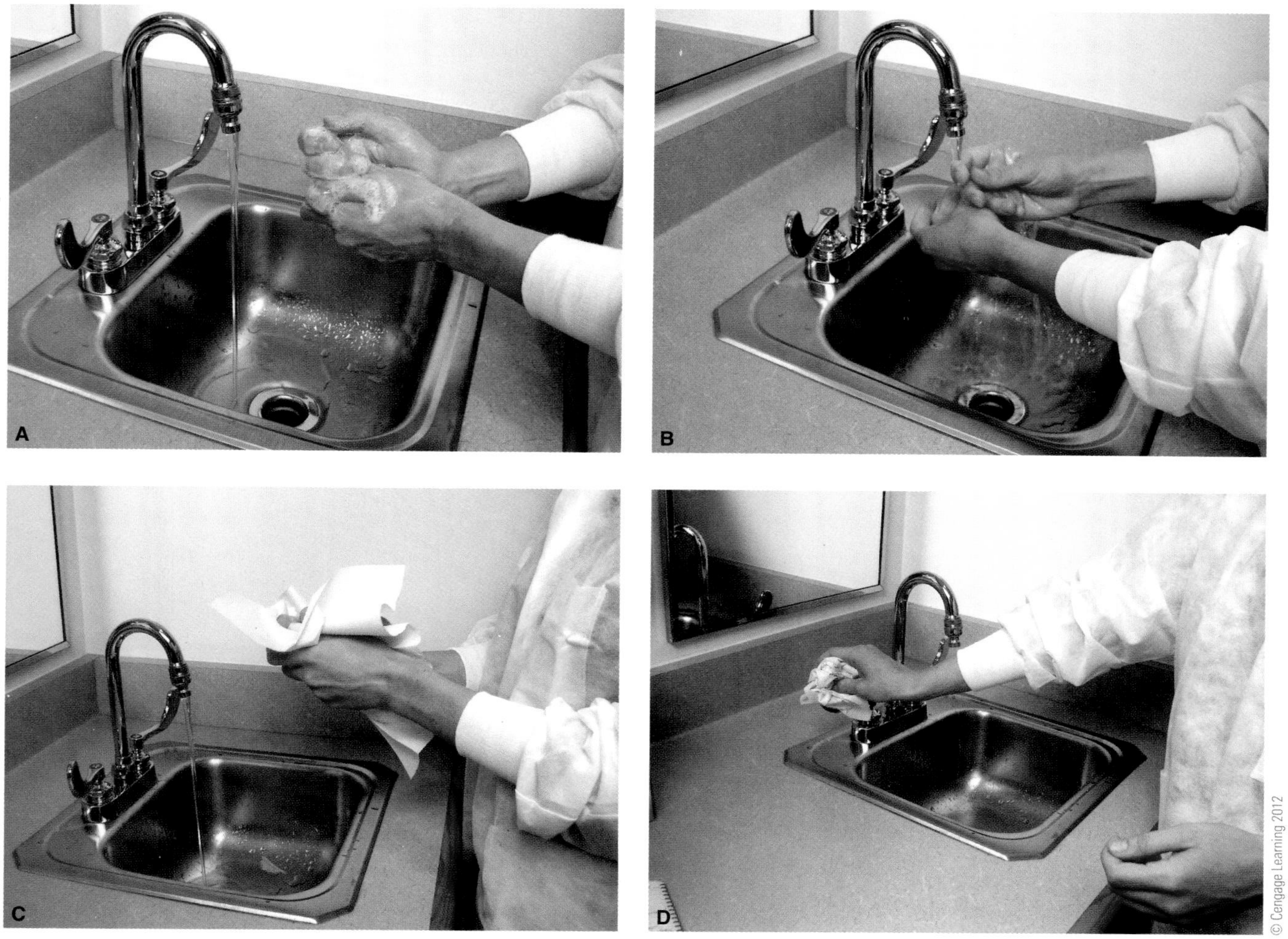

FIGURE 7-60 Handwashing technique: (A) soap hands and interlace the fingers to clean between them; (B) rinse hands and wrists thoroughly; (C) dry hands with disposable towel; and (D) use disposable towel to turn off faucet

© Cengage Learning 2012

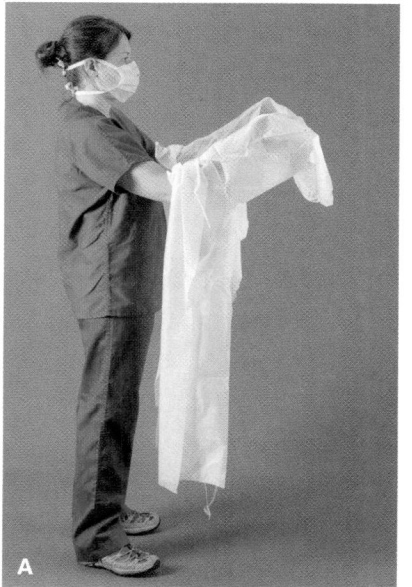

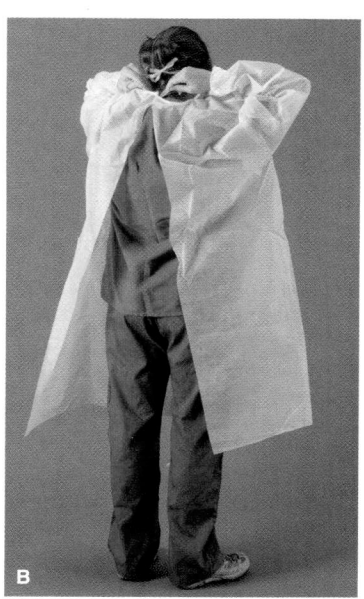

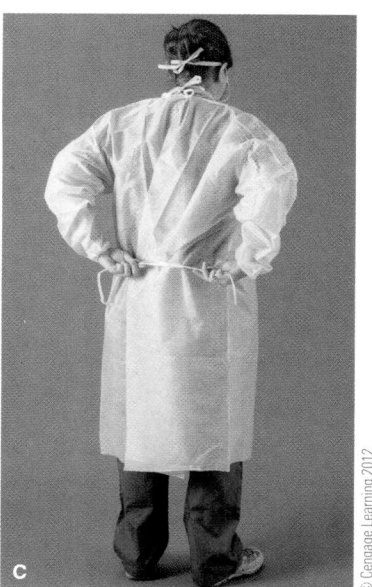

FIGURE 7-61 Putting on cover gown: (A) after mask is on, put on the gown outside the patient's room by placing hands inside the gown shoulders; (B) slip fingers inside the neck-band and tie gown at neck; and (C) overlap the back edges of the gown to cover clothing and secure the waist ties

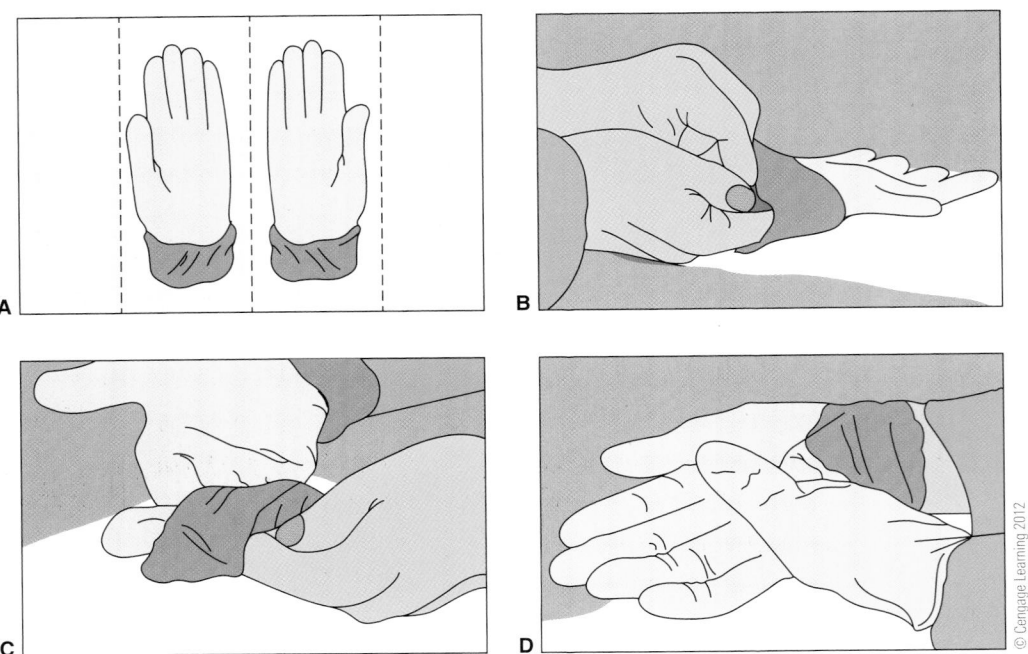

FIGURE 7-62 Donning sterile gloves. (A) Open sterile glove pack, avoiding touching the outer surfaces of gloves; (B) pick up first glove by the cuff to insert hand, taking care not to touch outside of glove; (C) use the sterile gloved hand to don second glove; (D) adjust cuffs of gloves to cover arm and sleeve of gown

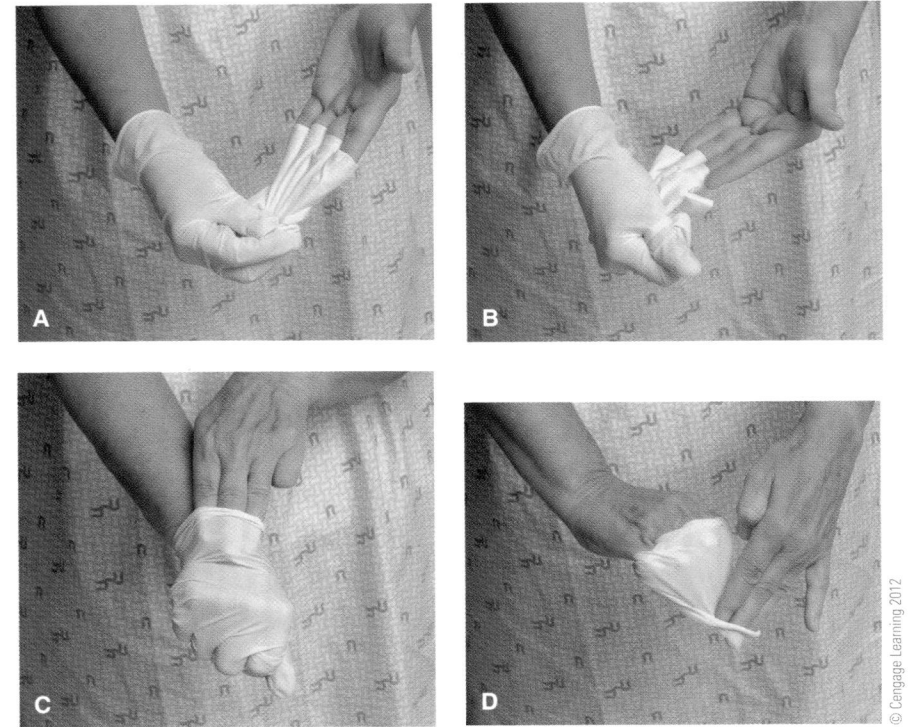

FIGURE 7-63 Removing gloves: (A) hold gloved hands over biohazard container and pull one glove down over the hand (inside out); (B) enclose the removed glove in the palm of the remaining gloved hand; (C) insert bare fingers inside cuff of remaining glove; and (D) pull the glove inside out down over the hand, taking care not to touch the outside of glove; discard gloves

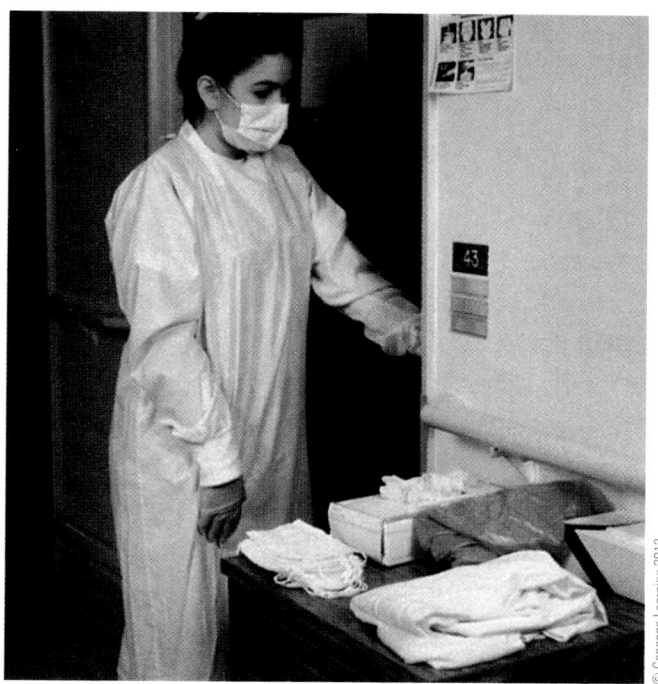

© Cengage Learning 2012

FIGURE 7-64 Healthcare worker wearing gown, gloves, and mask, entering the room of a patient requiring transmission-based precautions

requisition slips outside the room to avoid having them become contaminated. Tourniquets and pens can be left in the room for future use with that patient.

When personnel exit the room, the used supplies should be left in a special disposal container usually located inside the room. Exceptions to this procedure include protective isolation, in which disposables are usually left in a container outside the room for disposal.

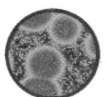 **SUMMARY**

Healthcare-associated infections (HAIs) are a problem nationwide. They cause increased morbidity and mortality in patients, lengthen hospital stays, and increase the costs of medical care. Increased emphasis is being placed on methods of preventing HAIs. Where this formerly was a focus primarily of inpatient facilities such as hospitals, infection prevention methods are being emphasized throughout healthcare, including settings such as outpatient facilities, rehabilitation facilities, hospice, and home health care.

Laboratory personnel must observe their institution's exposure control plan, not only in the laboratory but also in patients' rooms and all other healthcare settings. Standard Precautions

must always be used to prevent exposure to all blood and body fluids, whether known to be infectious or not.

Transmission-based precautions must be used when a patient is suspected of having, or is known to have, a contagious disease or a condition that could expose caregivers or others to infectious agents. Transmission-based precautions protect healthcare workers, visitors, and patients. The disease or type of organism suspected and its mode of transmission determine which exposure control methods must be used, such as gowns, masks, or respirators. The institution's infection prevention department will have a written policy manual to follow when implementing transmission-based precautions.

 REVIEW QUESTIONS

1. What is the function of the institution's infection prevention department?

2. Why are transmission-based precautions used?

3. What are the three categories of transmission-based precautions? Give an example of a condition or disease requiring each type of precaution.

4. Describe correct handwashing technique. When must handwashing be performed?

5. What is the correct technique for putting on and removing a gown?

6. Explain how to put on sterile gloves. How should used gloves be removed to prevent exposure to possible contaminants on glove surfaces?

7. What are five exposure-control methods used to prevent exposure to blood and body fluids?

8. How do Standard Precautions and transmission-based precautions differ? When are Standard Precautions used?

9. What exposure-control methods are used in each of the three categories of transmission-based precautions?

10. Define Airborne Precautions, APIC, carrier, Contact Precautions, Droplet Precautions, fomites, healthcare-associated infection (HAI), infection, isolation, nonpathogenic, nosocomial infection, protective isolation, and Standard Precautions.

 STUDENT ACTIVITIES

1. Complete the written examination for this lesson.

2. Practice the procedures for handwashing and donning and removing mask, gown, and gloves, as outlined in the Student Performance Guide.

WEB ACTIVITIES

1. Explore the web sites of infection prevention organizations to see what publications, alerts, or regulatory information is available. One such site is www.apic.org.

2. Select a disease or condition from the list at the end of this section. Use the Internet to determine which (if any) of the transmission-based precautions should be used for the condition selected. If a disease was selected, use the Internet to research how the disease is transmitted. Outline a scheme, listing the precautions to use for a hospitalized patient with that condition. Include the PPE that must be used, where the PPE should be located, and where and how used materials should be discarded.

Select a topic: Colostomy, chickenpox, tetanus, whooping cough, rubeola, HIV infection, West Nile virus, filovirus.

Infection Prevention in Healthcare Settings

Name _____ Date _____

INSTRUCTIONS

1. Practice the procedures for hand hygiene and donning gown, mask, and gloves following the step-by-step procedure.

2. Demonstrate the procedures for hand hygiene and donning gown, mask, and gloves satisfactorily for the instructor using the Student Performance Guide. Your instructor will explain the procedures for evaluating and grading your performance. Your performance may be given a number grade, a letter grade, or satisfactory (S) or unsatisfactory (U) depending on course or institutional policy.

NOTE: The following procedures are intended as general guidelines for laboratory workers who must have contact with patients in isolation. The appropriate institutional policy manual must be consulted for specific instructions.

MATERIALS AND EQUIPMENT

- sink for handwashing
- antiseptic soap
- waterless antiseptic handrub
- paper towels
- disposable masks and/or face shields
- disposable gowns
- disposable gloves, sterile packs and non-sterile
- biohazard bags or biohazard containers for disposing of used items

PROCEDURE

Record in the comment section any problems encountered while practicing the procedure (or have a fellow student or the instructor evaluate your performance).

S = Satisfactory
U = Unsatisfactory

You must:	S	U	Evaluation/Comments
1. Assemble equipment and materials			

2. Practice hand hygiene:
  a. Using antiseptic soap, perform steps 2a1–2a4:
    (1) Turn on warm water using a paper towel to turn the faucet handle, and discard the towel
    (2) Dispense antiseptic soap onto hands and rub fronts and backs of hands and between fingers vigorously for 15 to 30 seconds
    (3) Rinse hands, holding them with fingertips downward under warm running water
    (4) Use clean towel to dry hands and to turn off faucet. Dispose of towel, touching only the clean side
  b. Cleanse hands using waterless antiseptic handrub, following steps 2b1 and 2b2:			

(Continues)

© 2012 Delmar, Cengage Learning. Permission to reproduce for clinical use granted.

You must:	S	U	Evaluation/Comments
(1) Apply antiseptic to palm of hand and rub hands together vigorously for at least 15 seconds, covering all surfaces of hands, fingers, and between fingers (2) Continue procedure until all of the antiseptic has evaporated and hands are completely dry			

3. Don gown:
  a. Slip arms into the sleeves of a gown, being careful to touch only the inside of gown
  b. Secure gown at neck and back of waist, being careful to completely cover clothing			

4. Don mask:
  a. Pick up a mask and place it over your mouth and nose, being careful not to touch your face with your fingers
  b. Secure the mask by tying or looping over ears			

5. Don sterile gloves:
  a. Open the package of gloves, avoiding touching the outside of the gloves with your hands
  b. Pick up the right glove by the cuff and insert your right hand
  c. Pick up and hold the left glove by inserting the fingertips of your gloved right hand under the cuff of the left glove
  d. Insert your left hand into glove
  e. Position glove cuffs over your wrists by using gloved fingertips to push cuff toward your elbow (consult Figure 7-62)			

6. Remove the gloves by folding them down and turning them inside out, avoiding touching the outside of the gloves (Figure 7-63). Discard gloves in biohazard container			
7. Remove gown by slipping hands back into gown sleeves, touching only the inside of the gown			
8. Fold the gown down over your arms inside-out and discard in biohazard container			
9. Remove mask, touching only the ties			
10. Hold the mask by the ties and discard in biohazard container receptacle			
11. Clean hands with antiseptic			

Instructor/Evaluator Comments:

Instructor/Evaluator _____ Date _____

© 2012 Delmar, Cengage Learning. Permission to reproduce for clinical use granted.

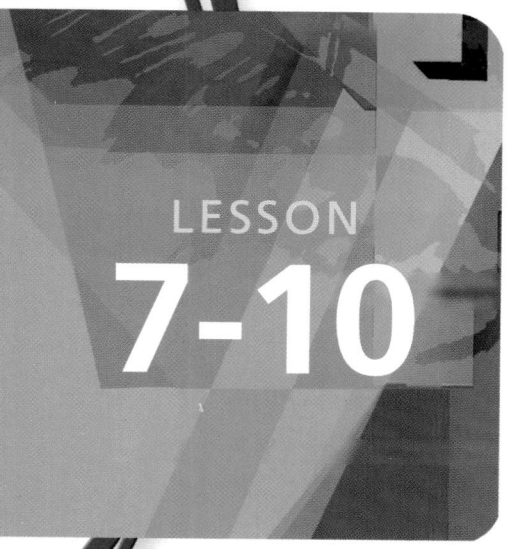

LESSON 7-10

Emerging Infectious Diseases

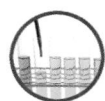

LESSON OBJECTIVES

After studying this lesson, the student will:

- ⊙ Explain what is meant by emerging infectious disease.
- ⊙ List five factors that influence the emergence or re-emergence of disease.
- ⊙ Discuss how emerging infectious diseases present a threat to public health.
- ⊙ Name five emerging diseases and explain transmission, symptoms, precautions for caregivers, and treatment for each disease.
- ⊙ Explain the role of the Laboratory Response Network in responding to emerging diseases.
- ⊙ Explain how natural disasters can create a public health emergency.
- ⊙ Define the glossary terms.

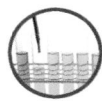

GLOSSARY

avian influenza / an infection of birds with one of the influenza A viruses; bird flu

biosafety level 4 (BSL-4) / a designation requiring the use of a combination of work practices, equipment, and facilities to prevent exposure of individuals or the environment to pathogens that can be transmitted by aerosol and that pose a high risk for life-threatening disease for which treatment or vaccine is not generally available

bovine spongiform encephalopathy (BSE) / a fatal, neurological disease of cattle caused by an unconventional transmissable agent called a prion; commonly called "mad cow disease"

Ebola virus / a highly infectious filovirus that causes a hemorrhagic fever

epidemic / disease affecting many persons at the same time, spread from person to person, and occurring in an area where the disease is not prevalent

epizootic / an outbreak of disease in an animal population

Laboratory Response Network (LRN) / a national network of laboratories coordinated by the Centers for Disease Control and Prevention with the ability for rapid response to threats to public health

Marburg virus / a filovirus that causes a hemorrhagic fever

Mycobacterium tuberculosis / an acid-fast bacillus that causes tuberculosis

pandemic / widespread disease transmitted person to person and occurring over an entire country, continent, or even worldwide

SARS / the acronym for severe acute respiratory syndrome, a condition caused by a coronavirus

zoonotic / infection or disease that can be transmitted from vertebrate animals to humans

INTRODUCTION

Global pandemic, emerging infectious diseases, bioterrorism, weapons of mass destruction, agroterrorism, Ebola, smallpox, anthrax—these are terms that most of us either never worried about or, in some cases, never heard of until recent years. Photographs of citizens wearing surgical masks as they go about their daily life cause apprehension even to those thousands of miles away.

It is estimated that one-third of the 60 million deaths worldwide each year can be attributed to infectious diseases. Because of events happening around the world, the public health systems of every country should have plans for addressing potential threats caused by global disease, natural disasters, or terrorist events. These plans must include outfitting laboratories so that they have the ability to respond rapidly to a potential crisis and training first responders and primary healthcare providers, because these are the people who most often would have the first contact with affected individuals.

Recognizing the existence of several types of global threats, agencies such as the World Health Organization (WHO) are partnering with health agencies of governments around the world to plan for, train for, coordinate responses to, and share information about disease outbreaks. It is imperative that governments provide the leadership, expertise, and funding to address these threats that could have significant clinical and public health consequences.

The agents recognized in recent years as presenting a danger to public health can be divided into two broad groups: *emerging infectious disease agents* and *bioweapon/bioterrorism agents*. In many cases the groups overlap. Emerging infectious diseases are diseases that have increased in humans or threaten to increase in the near future. Re-emerging diseases are those that were on the decrease for a time but have again become major health threats. This lesson introduces the topic of emerging infectious diseases, giving a brief summary of several agents of concern and outlining public health preparedness. Lesson 7-11 discusses potential biological threat agents, as well as preparedness.

EMERGING INFECTIOUS DISEASES

In recent years the number of diseases classified as an emerging infectious disease has been on the increase. These diseases have gained our attention because they are usually associated with high morbidity and mortality, and no reliable preventive measure such as a vaccine exists. A variety of factors contribute to the emergence of these diseases. A combination of factors such as global climate changes, natural disasters, movement of populations to more crowded living conditions, increase in international travel and trade, failures of public health policies or disease surveillance, and mutations or adaptations of pathogens can all contribute to increases in a disease (Table 7-28).

In some cases, the focus on a disease such as **SARS** (severe acute respiratory syndrome), occurred because it was newly recognized. In other cases, an animal disease gained attention because of its potential to spread to humans, such as **avian influenza** and **bovine spongiform encephalopathy (BSE)**, commonly

TABLE 7-28. Factors that contribute to emergence or re-emergence of infectious disease

CAUSATIVE FACTOR	DISEASE EXAMPLE
Environmental change	Lyme disease, cholera
Population concentrations	Dengue fever, polio
International travel/commerce	Cholera, hepatitis A, cyclosporiasis, antibiotic-resistant gonorrhea
Public health/policy failures	Bovine spongiform encephalopathy (BSE), hepatitis B and C
Pathogen adaptation/mutation	SARS, avian influenza, H1N1, tuberculosis, infections with strains of antibiotic-resistant *Staphylococcus* and *Streptococcus*
Natural disaster/flooding	Cholera, hepatitis A, malaria

called mad cow disease. In still other cases, re-emergence of a previously known pathogen gained attention because of mutations or changes in virulence or drug resistance, as has been the case with the tuberculosis bacterium.

Whatever the reason, we are seeing an emergence of infectious diseases that pose a threat to public health and, in some cases, have the potential to develop into a **pandemic**. Pandemics occur when a disease spreads to a wide area, sometimes even worldwide. The threat of pandemic H1N1 influenza in 2009 mobilized governments and laboratories to produce vaccines for worldwide distribution in a very short time. Fortunately, the outbreak of H1N1influenza did not prove much more severe than influenza seen during regular flu season. However, it was a great opportunity for agencies responsible for preparedness to discover deficiencies in planning and execution of their strategies to deal with a pandemic.

Natural disasters such as the 2004 south Asia tsunami, the 2005 hurricanes in the United States, the 2010 earthquake in Haiti, and the 2011 earthquake in Japan also can create the potential for public health crises. Increases in foodborne illnesses such as cholera can occur due to contamination of water and food supplies. Failures of wastewater treatment plants can also occur, resulting in contamination of waters by sewage. Natural disasters such as floods also create environments favoring the growth and spread of insects and pathogens. An increase in malaria was seen in aid workers in Haiti following the earthquake. A virulent cholera epidemic began in Haiti several months after the earthquake, and by the beginning of 2011 had killed over four thousand and hospitalized over 100,000. This outbreak was unexpected because cholera outbreaks had not been seen in Haiti in several decades. In some instances, the infection was spread to other countries when infected aid workers returned home.

Because we live in a global society, measures to control or prevent epidemics require new techniques and more attention. Several pathogens cause diseases that can be categorized as emerging infectious diseases. A sampling discussed in this lesson includes SARS-associated corona virus, avian influenza virus, *Mycobacterium tuberculosis,* West Nile virus (WNV) and the hemorrhagic fever viruses (Ebola, Marburg, and Rift Valley viruses). In some cases, such as the Ebola, Marburg, and Rift Valley fever viruses, these disease agents are also considered potential bioterrorism agents.

West Nile Virus

WNV, a member of the flavivirus family, was first isolated in 1937 in the West Nile district of Uganda (Figure 7-65). Until it surfaced in New York City in 1999, causing mortality in several types of birds, it had only been found in Asia, Africa, the Middle East, and Europe. WNV quickly became a cause of illness and mortality in humans, causing subclinical infection in the majority (80%) of infected individuals, mild febrile illness or flu-like symptoms in about 20%, and severe encephalitis or meningitis in less than 1%. Elderly patients are at greatest risk for severe illness, which can cause permanent neurological damage or death.

West Nile infection is spread geographically by virus-infected migratory birds. Since 1999, the virus has spread over most of the United States and has also been documented in Canada, the Caribbean, and Mexico. In 2002 it caused the largest WNV **epidemic** and animal **epizootic** ever reported before that time, resulting in over 4,000 human cases with 284 deaths (all in the United States). In 2003, U.S. cases more than doubled over 2002, with almost 10,000 human cases reported.

The virus is normally transmitted by mosquitoes, but blood transfusion, transplacental transmission, organ transplantation, and breastfeeding-associated cases have all been documented. In the United States, donated blood is now tested for evidence of West Nile Virus infection. There is currently no specific treatment for WNV infection, and prevention is based on limiting mosquito exposure in enzootic and epidemic areas. Although an equine vaccine is available, as of this writing no human vaccine is available, although several are in research trials.

Viral Hemorrhagic Fevers

The viral hemorrhagic fevers (VHFs) make up a group of febrile illnesses that have similar symptoms, ranging from mild to severe. Onset is often abrupt. Symptoms include fever, fatigue, and bleeding or hemorrhaging under the skin, internally, or from body orifices. These symptoms are caused by multiple organ damage, especially vascular system damage. Some of the hemorrhages are life-threatening. Fatality rates vary according to which virus is involved, but range from less than 5% for some VHFs, to a 70% to 90% death rate from Ebola (Zaire) virus.

The VHFs are caused by RNA viruses in four families—arenaviruses, filoviruses, bunyaviruses, and flaviviruses (Table 7-29). These viruses are **zoonotic**, meaning they are found in vertebrate animals or arthropods. Of the known hosts/vectors, most are rodents or arthropods. The reservoirs for some, such as Ebola virus and Marburg virus, remain unproven (Figure 7-66), but animals native to the African continent, particularly the rain forest, are believed to be a possible source. The African fruit bat has been shown to harbor Marburg virus. Although hemorrhagic fever viruses are found all over the globe, most are associated with a particular geographical area and host/reservoir. Therefore, only residents of or visitors to a particular area would have the potential for exposure. Potential for infection can also occur when exotic animals harboring the viruses are imported into a new area.

Once human disease occurs, some VHFs can be transmitted person to person. It is important to control disease spread by avoiding close physical contact with infected individuals and

TABLE 7-29. Viral hemorrhagic fevers (VHFs) grouped by virus family

ARENA VIRUSES
Lassa fever (Lassa virus)
Bolivian hemorrhagic fever (Machupo virus)
Argentine hemorrhagic fever (Junin virus)
Venezuelan hemorrhagic fever (Guanarito virus)
Brazilian hemorrhagic fever (Sabia virus)

FLAVIVIRUSES
Dengue
Yellow fever
Omsk hemorrhagic fever

FILOVIRUSES
Ebola hemorrhagic fever
Marburg hemorrhagic fever

BUNYAVIRUSES
Crimean-Congo hemorrhagic fever
Rift Valley fever
Hantavirus pulmonary syndrome

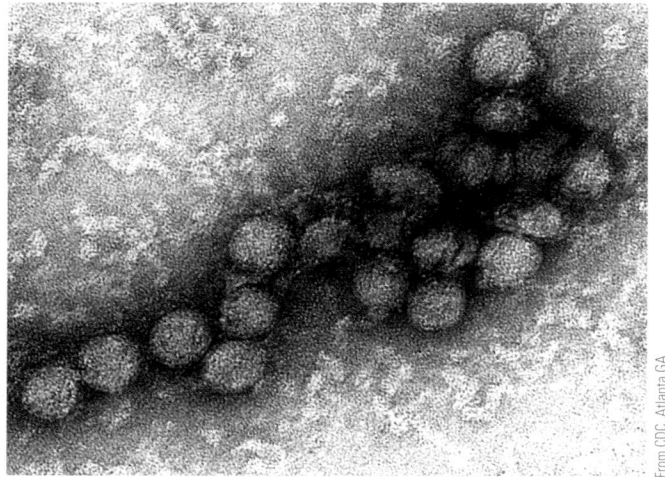

From CDC, Atlanta GA

FIGURE 7-65 Electron micrograph of West Nile virus

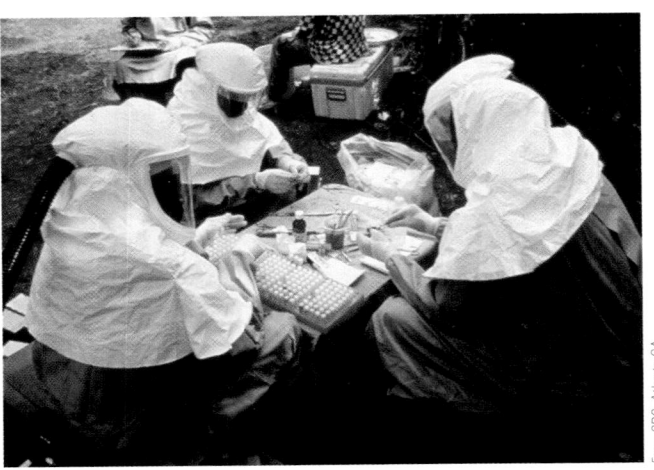

FIGURE 7-66 Centers for Disease Control and Prevention (CDC) and Zairian scientists collect animal samples during a 1995 Ebola outbreak near Kitwit, Zaire.

their body fluids. Infection control precautions for healthcare personnel include using personal protective equipment (PPE), disinfecting or disposing of all materials and equipment that contact the patient, and instituting airborne precautions when possible (Figure 7-66).

For the most part, there is no vaccine, cure, or treatment for VHFs, with the exception of yellow fever and Argentine fever. Prevention efforts focus on rodent and arthropod control measures, as well as discouraging cultural practices that bring populations in close contact with potential reservoirs. The viruses that cause the most severe hemorrhagic fevers are classified as **biosafety level 4 (BSL-4)** pathogens. Only a few laboratories worldwide have the BSL-4 facilities required to work with these pathogens (Figure 7-67). (Some hemorrhagic fever viruses, such as the dengue and yellow fever viruses are not considered BSL-4 pathogens.)

Sporadic outbreaks of VHFs are expected to continue. To decrease morbidity and mortality from these diseases, improvements are needed in:

- Containment methods and facilities, especially in developing countries
- Antiviral drugs and supportive therapies
- Vaccine development
- Tools for rapid diagnosis
- Understanding the pathology of disease
- Understanding the ecology of the viruses and the natural reservoirs

Rift Valley Fever

Rift Valley Fever occurs in livestock and humans in Africa and Arabia. It is caused by a virus of the Bunyaviridae family and is normally transmitted by mosquitoes. Human outbreaks are usually associated with animal disease outbreaks and can occur in rural and urban areas (Figure 7-68). Infected individuals who develop an acute, febrile form of the disease can transmit the virus to other humans through aerosols.

The virus has also been shown to be transmitted to humans by aerosols created in animal husbandry practices or through livestock slaughtering. Infection rates can reach as high as one-third of a population. Rift Valley fever is a much more severe disease than West Nile disease. Unlike West Nile disease, 90% of

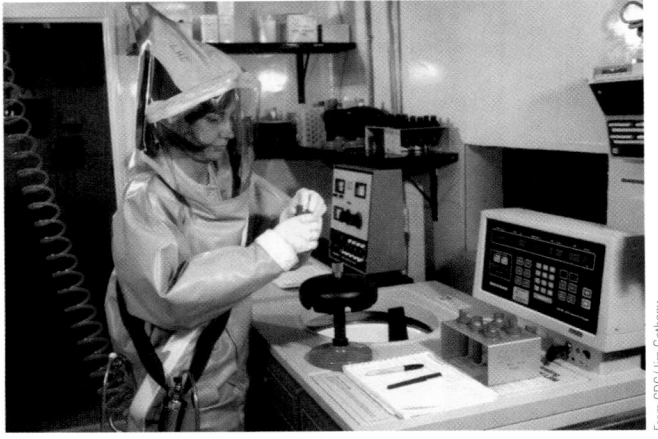

FIGURE 7-67 A Centers for Disease Control and Prevention (CDC) scientist wears a protective suit with helmet and face mask as she studies pathogens in the CDC BSL-4 laboratory

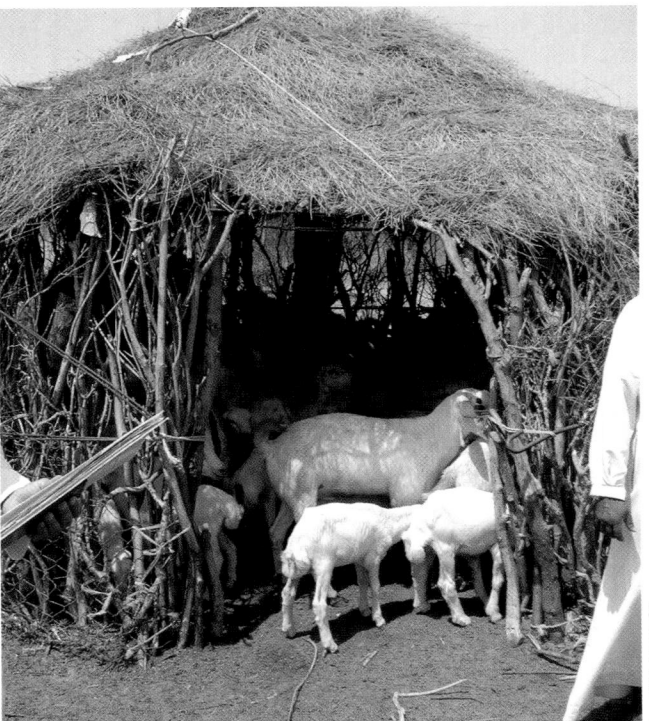

FIGURE 7-68 Rift Valley Fever can affect domesticated animals such as these goats in Saudi Arabia; the disease can be spread to humans after exposure to blood or body fluids of infected animals

patients with Rift Valley fever are very ill, and the fatality rate is 10 times that of West Nile disease. The RVF outbreak in Kenya in the winter of 2006–2007 affected animals and humans, with a 25% to 30% human fatality rate. In 2010, an outbreak occurred in South Africa, which had not seen a major outbreak in over 30 years; transmission to humans was through contact with infected animal parts.

Rift Valley fever is considered a threat both as a natural emerging disease and as a potential biological weapon because it can be spread by aerosols as well as by the mosquito vector. Rift Valley fever vaccines for livestock are available; military-developed human Rift Valley fever vaccines are not licensed for the public. Antiviral drugs have not been effective, and some have caused severe side effects.

Ebola and Marburg Viruses

Two deadly viruses that always seem to gain attention in the news are the **Ebola** and **Marburg viruses** (Figure 7-69). Marburg and Ebola viruses are the only known filoviruses and are considered to have potential as biological weapons. These have caused several deadly outbreaks in Central Africa, and small sporadic outbreaks continue. The filoviruses cause high mortality and morbidity, can be spread person to person, and are highly infectious in aerosol form. Several subtypes of Ebola have been identified, and most have caused disease in humans. Through 2004, the WHO had documented 17 Ebola outbreaks in humans, totaling 1,848 cases and 1,287 fatalities, a fatality rate averaging 70%. A 2006 Ebola outbreak is believed to have killed more than 5,000 gorillas in West Africa. Outbreaks continue to occur sporadically in Congo, but are not as severe as early outbreaks now that methods to prevent person-to-person transmission are known.

Ebola was first recognized in 1976 in the Democratic Republic of the Congo (formerly Zaire) (Figure 7-70). The natural reservoir of Ebola and initial route of infection remain unconfirmed, despite extensive investigation. Once an individual becomes infected, secondary transmission of the virus can occur through direct exposure to blood or body secretions from that

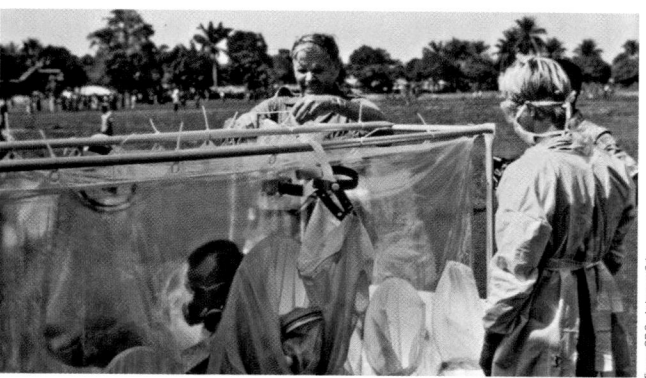

From CDC, Atlanta GA

FIGURE 7-70 Evacuating a patient from an Ebola "hot zone" in 1976: this archival photo illustrates the primitive isolation techniques used during early outbreaks of Ebola, which occurred before guidelines such as BSI, BBP, or Universal and Standard Precautions were developed

infected individual. Airborne transmission between humans has not been documented, although it has been documented between research animals in a primate quarantine facility in Reston, Virginia. Infection control measures, such as using Standard Precautions; wearing PPE, including gloves, gown, mask, and eye protection; and decontamination of all materials and equipment that come in contact with the patient is vitally important.

Although most outbreaks of Ebola and Marburg have been limited to their geographic region in Africa, the viruses have unintentionally been transported to other countries. In 1996, a health care professional who had been treating Ebola patients in Gabon traveled to South Africa and became ill. In the hospital the virus was transmitted to a nurse, who subsequently died. This secondary transmission can occur through close contact, exposure to infected body fluids or contaminated instruments, or inhalation of aerosolized virus particles.

Marburg virus has also been transported from its natural habitat. In fact, the virus was unknown until it was discovered in 1967 during simultaneous outbreaks among laboratory personnel in Marburg and Frankfurt, Germany, and Belgrade, Yugoslavia. These workers became infected by handling infected research monkeys that had been imported from Uganda. Since then, small outbreaks have occurred periodically in Africa. The African fruit bat has been found to be a host for the Marburg virus, but is unconfirmed as a sole source of virus transmission. Whatever the method of initial infection, secondary transmission of the virus others can occur. The fatality rate is approximately 25%.

Severe Acute Respiratory Syndrome

In 2002, news of fatalities associated with acute respiratory diseases surfaced in Asia. This disease came to be known as **SARS** (**s**evere **a**cute **r**espiratory **s**yndrome) and was found to be caused by a previously unknown variant of the coronavirus family (Figure 7-71). Members of the coronavirus family are responsible for the common cold. The SARS-associated coronavirus

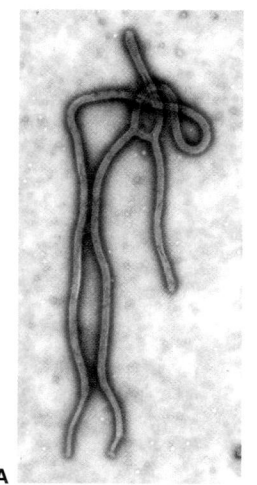
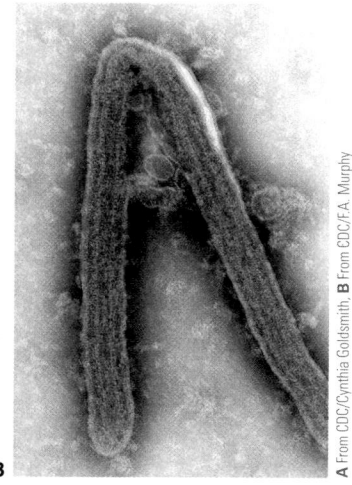

A From CDC/Cynthia Goldsmith, B From CDC/F.A. Murphy

A **B**

FIGURE 7-69 Electron micrographs: (A) Ebola virus and (B) Marburg virus; both are filoviruses

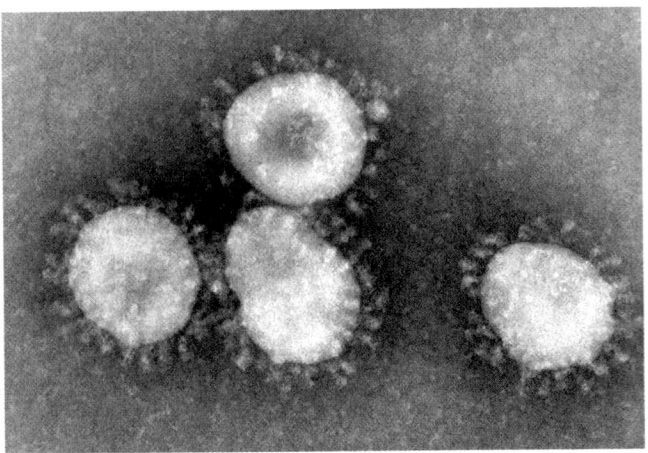

FIGURE 7-71 Electron micrograph of coronavirus, showing its characteristic crown-like (corona) appearance

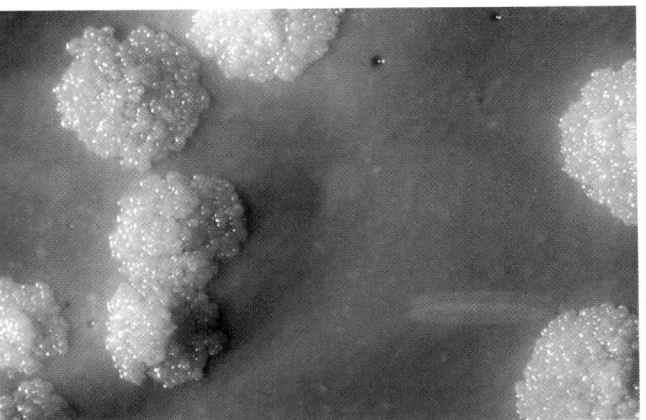

FIGURE 7-72 Colonies of *Mycobacterium tuberculosis* growing on special medium; colonial morphology is one component of identification

(SARS-CoV) is thought to have originated in the Guangdong Province of China. It spread regionally and then was spread to Hong Kong by a physician who treated patients for flu and then subsequently traveled to Hong Kong. International travelers staying at the same hotel as this physician also became ill with SARS.

In the following weeks, SARS spread to parts of Asia, the Americas, and Europe, presumably through close contacts with air travelers, hospital workers, and relatives of infected individuals. In the first 9 months of the outbreak, over 8,000 cases of SARS were reported, with 774 deaths. Most cases occurred in China and Southeast Asia; only eight confirmed cases were identified in the United States. In early 2004, several new cases of SARS were confirmed in China, causing public health officials to launch intense surveillance measures to detect spread of this virus. Symptoms of SARS included fever, headache and other body aches, respiratory symptoms such as cough, and pneumonia.

SARS was quickly recognized to be a highly contagious disease that spread rapidly by person-to-person contact unless recognized early and strict infection prevention precautions put in place. These included Standard Precautions, especially hand hygiene, droplet precautions, contact precautions, airborne precautions in a room with negative pressure, and use of an N-95 filtering respirator for all persons who entered the room. SARS disappeared almost as quickly as it appeared. As of 2011, it has been several years since any SARS cases have been documented, although health agencies continue surveillance and reporting.

Mycobacterium tuberculosis

Estimates are that, worldwide, 3 billion people are infected with *Mycobacterium tuberculosis*, the bacterium that causes tuberculosis, a disease of the lungs (Figure 7-72). In the last half of the twentieth century, cases of tuberculosis were cured by the use of new drugs developed against the bacterium. However, to obtain a cure, patients were required to take the drugs over a period of several months. It is believed that this prolonged exposure to antibiotics contributed to the emergence of multidrug-resistant

M. tuberculosis (MDR TB) strains in the 1980s. As the incidence of immunosuppressive diseases such as human immunodeficiency virus (HIV) infections has increased worldwide, the incidence of tuberculosis has also increased and has reached crisis levels in some parts of the world. Currently, in some places, 20% of the strains tested are antibiotic resistant. In sub-Saharan Africa, where infection with HIV is very high, 60% of the children and 70% of the adults who have tuberculosis also are infected with HIV. In 2006, an extensively drug-resistant form of tuberculosis (XDR-TB) emerged that has a very high mortality rate. The outlook for controlling this disease is sobering. Although *M. tuberculosis* was identified more than 100 years ago, it is still a major cause of death, causing 1 to 2 million deaths per year.

Avian Influenza

Influenza A viruses of several different types, strains, genetic differences, and pathogenicity levels can infect humans, swine, birds, horses, and other animals. The natural reservoir for these viruses is wild birds, so it is called avian influenza or *bird flu*. Although wild birds do not necessarily become ill when infected, domestic poultry can become sick and die, especially when infected with a highly pathogenic form. Avian influenza viruses have been identified in human influenza cases that have high morbidity and mortality rates. In recent years public health professionals worldwide have been concerned that one of these avian influenza strains could cause an influenza pandemic against which humans would have little or no immunity.

Bird Flu Outbreaks

In early 2004, a widespread outbreak of a highly pathogenic H5N1 strain of avian influenza occurred in poultry across many Asian countries; 35 human cases were reported (Thailand and Vietnam), with 24 deaths. These cases occurred in persons with close association with poultry, and transmission was suspected to be bird-to-human. New bird outbreaks of H5N1 influenza began in late June 2004 across China and other parts of Asia, with sporadic human cases and more human deaths. By February 2007, outbreaks of H5N1 avian influenza in wild birds and domestic poultry had been reported in most Southeast Asian countries, several Middle Eastern countries, as well as Russia, Ukraine, Turkey, Romania, and England. Human cases with fatalities were reported in several countries. In May 2006, the World Health Organization (WHO) confirmed that a cluster of cases of human H5N1 infections in Indonesia was caused by human-to-human transmission. Concern began to mount about a possible **pandemic.** Pandemic influenza refers to a global influenza outbreak due to emergence of an influenza virus that can be transmitted from person to person and can rapidly spread worldwide.

Prevention

Prevention focused on eliminating infected poultry flocks and limiting human contact with infected birds. Importation of potentially infectious birds was banned by most countries. Infection control precautions recommended by the Centers for Disease Control and Prevention (CDC) included Standard Precautions, Contact Precautions, eye protection, and Airborne Precautions. In 2007, the first vaccines against the H5N1 strain were approved for human use. The drug oseltamivir (Tamiflu) was shown to be effective in some H5N1 infections. However, some H5N1 viral isolates exhibited genetic changes and oseltamivir-resistant strains emerged. H5N1 strains resistant to other antivirals (rimantidine, zanamivir, and amantadine) that are active against influenza A viruses were also seen.

PANDEMIC INFLUENZA

Scientists, worried about the potential for spread of H5N1 influenza virus to a susceptible population, had been developing preparedness plans to deal with H5N1 virus for sometime. Meanwhile, a stealth virus called H1N1 suddenly emerged and began a rapid worldwide spread.

In the United States, the H1N1 virus was first found in California in April 2009. The virus had not been seen before, but was related to viruses found in swine (as well as being similar to a virus that had caused an outbreak almost half a century previous). So at the beginning of the outbreak the infection was called "swine flu," even though the virus was not a problem in swine herds and humans were not infected by contact with swine. Within 2 weeks, in the United States efforts toward vaccine production had begun. By the end of April 2009, the WHO, along with other major public health agencies agreed that an H1N1 pandemic was imminent.

In June 2009, a worldwide H1N1 pandemic was declared and all preparedness plans were operational. A public health emergency was declared worldwide. Vaccine producers hurriedly worked to grow the virus, develop a vaccine, conduct trials for effectiveness and safety, and get the vaccine out to the public. Public health infomercials were broadcast; schools and businesses were urged to close if several employees became ill, and simple procedures such as frequent handwashing and shielding a cough were emphasized. As vaccines became available in the summer of 2009, free clinics were held nationwide to attempt to vaccinate the majority of the most susceptible population. As increasingly more vaccine became available

and many became vaccinated, the peak infection began to fall off in 2010.

On August 10, 2010, WHO announced an end to the H1N1 pandemic. Along the way, as theory of how to plan for pandemic was put to practice, public health agencies and governments were able to adapt to unforeseen developments, especially in vaccine production. Although much of the general public expressed that in the end it was "much ado about nothing," the worldwide mobilization to deal with the pandemic was a valuable experience with a good outcome. We will never know what the outcome would have been had world health agencies not worked together to quickly respond to the pandemic.

Pandemics may be a greater possibility today than ever before because of global travel. Whether H1N1 or another agent as yet unknown can cause another pandemic is uncertain. Public health agencies worldwide have the responsibility to be vigilant as infectious agents emerge or re-emerge with genetic changes and as infections in animal reservoirs spread. Immunity to influenza is short-lived. Influenza viruses undergo frequent genetic change so vaccinations must be given annually, and the vaccine mixture must be changed based on predictions of which virus outbreak might occur in the near future.

Although a viral pandemic might have a mortality of only 1% to 20%, that would represent a huge number of fatalities worldwide. During the twentieth century, pandemics have included:

- 1918–1919: Spanish flu. This was caused by H1N1 influenza A virus and was the worst recorded in modern history, with more than 500,000 deaths in the United States and an estimated 50 million deaths worldwide.

- 1957–1958: Asian flu. This outbreak originating in China was caused by H2N2 influenza A virus. In the United States, 70,000 deaths were recorded.

- 1968–1969: Hong Kong flu. Caused by H3N2 influenza A virus, this outbreak resulted in 34,000 deaths in the United States.

- 2009–2010: H1N1 virus. The first global pandemic in 40 years resulted in much lower mortality than was feared at its onset.

Because human influenza viruses can be spread efficiently from person to person, it can be almost impossible to prevent all influenza pandemics. Measures the general public and public health agencies can take to prevent disease spread include frequent handwashing; staying home when ill; closing schools and businesses when necessary; instituting travel restrictions; promoting vaccinations; increasing vaccine production; including new strains in vaccines; and stockpiling vaccines and antiviral drugs.

ROLE OF THE CLINICAL LABORATORY IN EMERGING DISEASES

Clinical laboratories must have a comprehensive plan in place for rapidly responding to the appearance of an emerging infectious disease. In the United States, the CDC and state public health departments are the leaders in organizing and

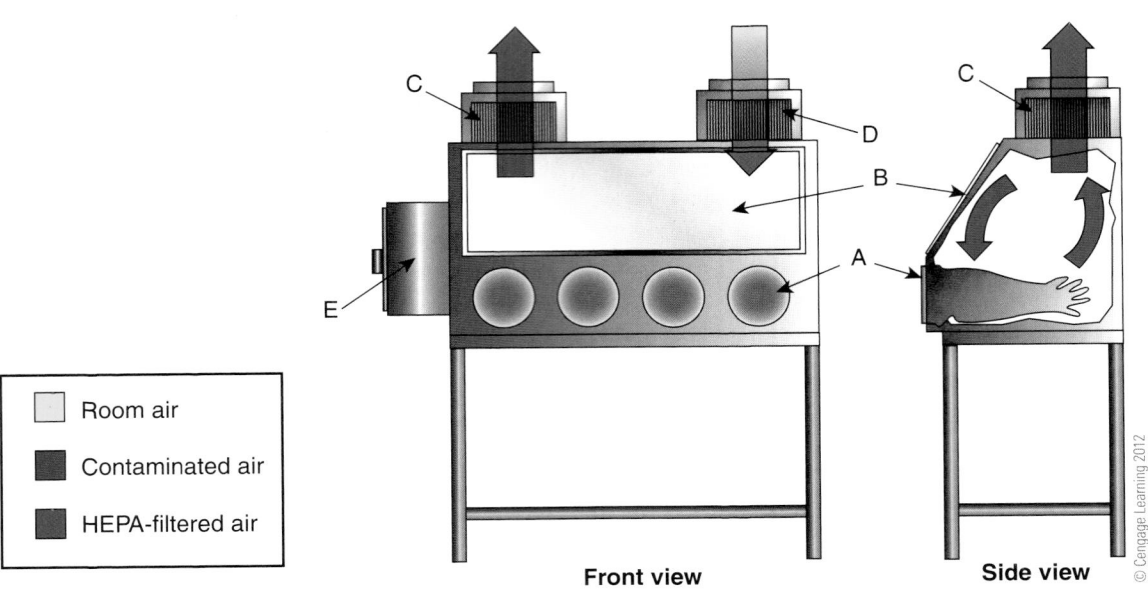

FIGURE 7-73 Diagram of air flow in a Class III biological safety cabinet (BSC): the cabinet exhaust must be connected to the building exhaust system; (A) glove ports for attaching arm-length gloves to cabinet; (B) sash; (C) HEPA exhaust filter; (D) HEPA supply filter; and (E) pass-through box to autoclave

training laboratory personnel for this possibility. The **Laboratory Response Network (LRN)** is a national network of laboratories organized by the CDC, Federal Bureau of Investigation (FBI), and Association of Public Health Laboratories. The LRN has the ability to respond rapidly to public health threats such as emerging diseases and acts of bioterrorism. Included in this network are federal laboratories such as the CDC, U.S. Department of Agriculture (USDA), and Food and Drug Administration (FDA) laboratories; state and local public health laboratories; and veterinary, military, and environmental/water/food testing laboratories. The LRN also partners with international laboratories.

Three levels of laboratories have been designated as part of the LRN:

- National laboratories
- Reference laboratories
- Sentinel laboratories

The national laboratories include federal laboratories such as the CDC and USDA laboratories. These agencies are responsible for bioforensics and handling and characterizing highly infectious biological agents. The more than 140 reference laboratories have installed BSL-3 facilities. These laboratories have the capability to perform confirmatory testing of BSL-3 agents, those agents transmitted by the respiratory route, such as *Mycobacterium tuberculosis* (Figure 7-73). Sentinel laboratories provide routine diagnostic services and preliminary testing to determine if specimens need to be sent to a reference laboratory for further testing. The LRN provides these laboratories with:

- Standardized reagents and controls
- Agent-specific protocols
- Laboratory referral directory
- Secure communications

- Electronic laboratory reporting
- Training and technology transfer
- Proficiency testing
- Appropriate vaccinations for laboratory workers

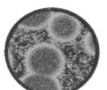 ## SUMMARY

Awareness of the threat of emerging infectious diseases is becoming a part of everyday life. Global changes in the environment, population movements, and travel have created environments favoring the emergence or re-emergence of diseases. Vaccines for certain of these diseases have become available or are in the research stage. It is the task of public health agencies to develop plans to contain and treat diseases when they surface, as well as to find ways to prevent disease occurrence.

 ## REVIEW QUESTIONS

1. What is the difference between an emerging infectious disease and a re-emerging infectious disease?

2. What five factors can influence the emergence of a disease?

3. The most serious emerging infectious disease pathogens are currently not a problem in the United States. What conditions could cause the spread of these pathogens to the United States?

4. What characteristics do most emerging infectious diseases have in common?

5. Why is avian influenza, or bird flu, a problem for humans?

6. What must happen to an animal virus in order for it to cause a pandemic?

7. What are three viral hemorrhagic fevers? Why are they given this designation?

8. Why are insect control programs important in developing nations?

9. Why has tuberculosis resurfaced as a disease on the increase?

10. Explain the role of the LRN in responding to emerging diseases.

11. Explain how natural disasters can create a public health emergency.

12. Name five emerging diseases and explain transmission, symptoms, precautions for caregivers, and treatment.

13. Define avian influenza, biosafety level 4, bovine spongiform encephalopathy, Ebola virus, epidemic, epizootic, Laboratory Response Network, Marburg virus, *Mycobacterium tuberculosis*, pandemic, SARS, and zoonotic.

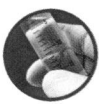

STUDENT ACTIVITIES

1. Complete the written examination for this lesson.

2. Find articles about emerging diseases in news magazines, newspapers, and other periodicals. Report on your findings.

WEB ACTIVITIES

1. Use the Internet to look up information on emerging infectious diseases on web sites of the CDC, WHO, FDA, or USDA. Note how many diseases the CDC categorizes as emerging infectious diseases. Report on a an emerging infectious disease that is not discussed in this lesson. Include information about where it is endemic, how it is transmitted, and describe the symptoms, treatment, and prevention.

2. Search the CDC web sites to find current information on tuberculosis in the United States. Get information on which states report the highest numbers of infections.

3. Polio has not been a problem in the United States since the development of effective vaccines and institution of childhood vaccinations. Use the Internet to search for information on recent outbreaks of polio around the world. Report on the cause(s) of these outbreaks.

4. Search the Internet for information on recent contagious disease outbreaks associated with natural disasters, such as the 2010 Haiti earthquake or Pakistan floods. Report on what diseases created problems, or what diseases health agencies were most concerned about.

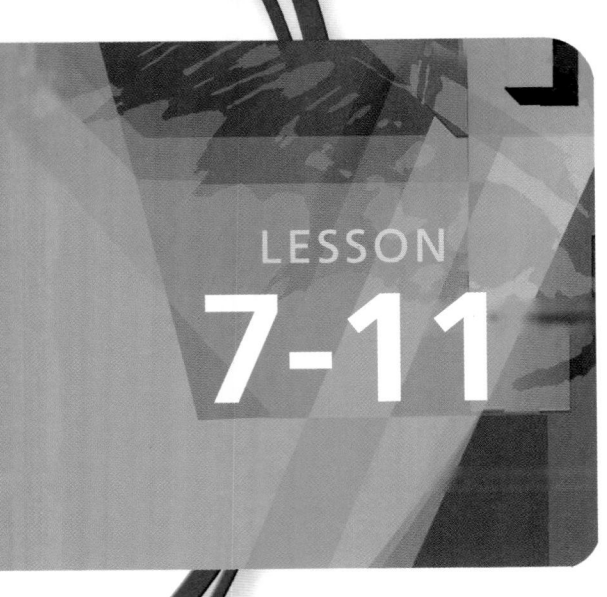

Biological Threat Agents

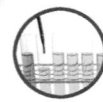

LESSON OBJECTIVES

After studying this lesson, the student will:

- ▶ List five pathogens that have potential use in bioterrorism or as biological weapons and explain how they are transmitted.
- ▶ Name six characteristics that make an agent useful as a biological weapon.
- ▶ Explain how the threat of bioterrorism affects the agricultural industry.
- ▶ Explain the role of laboratories and primary healthcare providers in recognizing and responding to potential bioterrorism agents.
- ▶ Define the glossary terms.

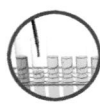

GLOSSARY

agroterrorism / acts of terrorism involving threats to agricultural products, including food animals and crops

botulinum intoxication / a condition in which body tissues are affected by the botulinum toxin

botulinum toxin / a neurotoxin produced by *Clostridium botulinum*

Department of Homeland Security / a federal agency whose primary mission is to prevent, protect against, and respond to acts of terrorism on U.S. soil

intoxication / poisoning

virion / the infectious form of a virus

virulent / highly infectious or highly pathogenic

INTRODUCTION

For the past several decades, discussions about threats of biological weapons and bioterrorism have occasionally surfaced. However, since the September 11, 2001, attacks on the World Trade Center and the rise of terrorist activities around the world, serious attention is being given to these subjects. Investigations into the response to the 9/11 attacks showed that the United States was unprepared to handle a large-scale emergency.

In response to these concerns, the U.S. government created the **Department of Homeland Security** and charged it with the responsibility of planning for natural and man-made disasters as well as working to eliminate potential terror threats. Billions of dollars were distributed to state, city, and local governments and emergency preparedness agencies to help them plan, equip, and train for preparedness. However, hurricanes Katrina and Rita, which ravaged the Texas, Louisiana, Mississippi, and Alabama coasts in 2005, demonstrated an alarming lack of disaster preparedness at all levels of government. Workable plans for evacuating, relocating, housing, feeding, and providing health care to large numbers of displaced persons were practically nonexistent. Backup communication systems failed. Systems to provide medical care were compromised. Although these disasters directly affected one geographic region, they brought the realization that disaster preparedness plans nationwide would likely have been deficient if faced with the same circumstances.

Federal, state, and local governments and public and private healthcare systems must be prepared to deal with the possibility that agents of terrorism might appear in civilian society. These terrorism threats could come in many forms, including chemical agents, radioactive agents, and biological agents. This lesson presents information about some biological agents that have the potential for use as weapons or bioterrorism agents and outlines the role of clinical laboratories in preparedness and reaction to a possible threat event.

BIOLOGICAL WEAPON AGENTS

The Centers for Disease Control and Prevention (CDC) have identified pathogens that they consider to have high potential for use as biological weapons. These have been placed on a high-priority list (class A list) that includes some pathogens rarely seen in the United States and some that have been considered eradicated (Table 7-30). Characteristics that cause these pathogens to be considered useful as biological weapons or terror agents include:

- Easily transmitted person-to-person transmission
- Easily disseminated or dispersed
- Cause high mortality
- Outbreak would have potential for major public health impact
- Require special measures to reach a state of preparedness
- Might cause panic or disrupt society

Pathogens in the high-priority category that are discussed in this lesson include the bacteria and viruses that cause anthrax, smallpox, plague, tularemia, botulism, and viral hemorrhagic fevers.

TABLE 7-30. Class A agents recognized by the Centers for Disease Control and Prevention (CDC) as having potential for use as biological weapons

AGENT	DISEASE
Bacillus anthracis	Anthrax
Variola virus	Smallpox
Francisella tularensis	Tularemia
Clostridium botulinum	Botulism
Yersinia pestis	Plague
Hemorrhagic viruses	Hemorrhagic fevers

Anthrax

Anthrax is caused by infection with the spore-forming bacterium *Bacillus anthracis* (Figure 7-74). The disease occurs in domestic, wild, and exotic animals, including goats, sheep, cattle, hippos, elephants, lions, zebras, and camels. Humans become infected by contact with infected animals or contaminated articles and animal products, such as animal skins. Depending on the route of exposure, the victim can develop inhalation anthrax, gastrointestinal anthrax, or cutaneous anthrax. Because anthrax spores persist in the environment, infection can occur when the spores deposited in the past become disturbed and aerosolized. Anthrax cases occur sporadically around the world in humans and livestock.

Anthrax has a long history. It is thought that the plagues described in Exodus were caused by anthrax in domestic animals and humans. In Europe, during the 1500s and the 1700s, anthrax was an important agricultural disease. Wool sorters in fifteenth-century England were described as having inhalation anthrax, caused by inhaling aerosols containing anthrax spores generated during the processing of goat wool. Louis Pasteur, in 1881, reported success in developing a vaccine for anthrax using live attenuated bacteria.

For decades, attention has been focused on the potential for anthrax to be used as a biological weapon. During World War I, attempts were made to use anthrax spores as a weapon against horses. Before and during World War II, the Japanese military developed the first relatively sophisticated anthrax biological weapons. Since World War II, many countries, including Russia, Great Britain, Canada, the United States, and Iraq, have shown an interest in the possible use of anthrax as a weapon.

Anthrax is uniquely suited for use as a weapon because:

- It is easy to produce large quantities. Using simple equipment, even an individual can produce gram quantities, as discovered when anthrax-contaminated letters were sent to the Hart Senate building in 2001.
- It has a long shelf life; dried spores remain viable for years.
- It is dispersed easily and effectively.
- It is environmentally stable. Areas can remain contaminated for months or years.

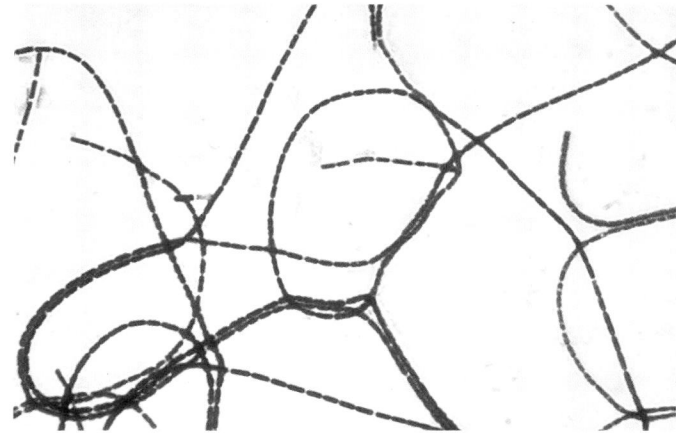

FIGURE 7-74 Gram stain of *Bacillus anthracis*, the agent that causes anthrax

- It has a high mortality rate, with systemic infection approaching 100% mortality within a few days after onset of symptoms.

- Effective treatment for inhalation anthrax is lacking, especially once symptoms appear.

In 1979, the accidental release of anthrax spores from a production facility in Sverdlosk, Russia, demonstrated on a small scale what the effects might be if anthrax were to be used as a weapon. Winds carried the spores 50 km from the facility, and at least 66 deaths resulting from inhalation anthrax were acknowledged, although some believe the number to be much higher.

Smallpox

Smallpox is a highly contagious, **virulent**, and often fatal disease caused by variola virus, a member of the family of pox viruses (Poxviridae). It is considered one of the most dangerous of the potential biological weapons. Smallpox also has a long history. It was endemic in India for over 2,000 years and spread to other parts of Asia, including China and Japan, and also to Africa. In the twentieth century, the less virulent form of smallpox spread from Africa to the Americas and Europe.

A worldwide smallpox eradication program began in 1956 using vaccination with vaccinia virus, a related pox virus. Unvaccinated patients contracting the virulent form of the disease had a greater than 30% fatality rate. Smallpox was shown to have considerable potential as a biological weapon when outbreaks occurred in Europe in the 1970s and spread rapidly, despite a vaccinated population. In Yugoslavia in 1972, the last major outbreak of smallpox, more than 170 individuals contracted the disease. The outbreak began when a traveler infected with the deadly virus returned home from the Middle East to the Kosovo region of Yugoslavia.

In 1972, smallpox was considered eradicated in the United States and routine smallpox vaccinations were discontinued. From 1972 until 2001, the vaccine was provided to only a few hundred research scientists and medical professionals working with smallpox and similar viruses. After 9/11 and the anthrax scare of October 2001, the U.S. government developed a smallpox response plan. As part of this plan, enough vaccine has been stockpiled to vaccinate every person in the United States in the event of a smallpox emergency. In addition, a vaccination program that includes certain healthcare personnel and the military was initiated (Figure 7-75).

At one time, only two high-security laboratories in the world were believed to have stores of the smallpox virus, the CDC in the United States and the Vector laboratory in the U.S.S.R (now Russia). Although these stocks were supposed to be destroyed in 1999 (by resolution of the 1996 World Health Assembly), destruction was postponed and still has not occurred. However, with the dissolution of the Soviet Union, it is believed that stocks of the virus may have been taken out of the country illegally. The U.S. government maintains a list of nations and groups suspected of having clandestine stocks of smallpox or of trying to obtain the virus. In 1999, this list was said to include Russia, China, India,

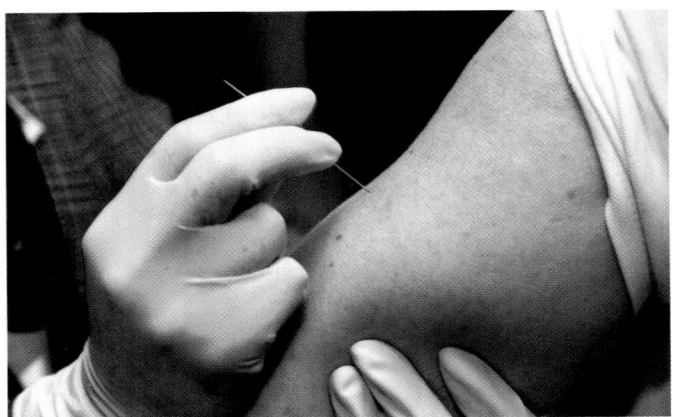

FIGURE 7-75 Demonstration of smallpox vaccination technique

Pakistan, Israel, North Korea, Iraq, Iran, Cuba, and Serbia, as well as terrorist organizations such as al Qaeda.

Characteristics that make the smallpox virus of potential use as a terror agent include:

- The infective dose is small, only 10 to 100 **virions**.

- Virions are stable in aerosols, which is a good way to deploy biological weapons.

- The disease has a short incubation period and progresses rapidly.

- The duration of the disease is long.

- Treatment requires complex transmission-based precautions and extensive medical support.

- A large portion of the civilian population is susceptible because vaccinations of the general public ended in 1972 in the United States.

However, smallpox virus is not as readily available and not as easily handled as some potential bacterial agents of bioterrorism such as anthrax (*Bacillus anthracis*) or plague (*Yersinia pestis*) organisms.

Plague

Plague is a zoonotic infection of rodents caused by the gram-negative bacillus *Yersinia pestis*. Rodents are the reservoir host; infection is spread by fleas that feed on rodents and then transmit the bacteria when they bite other animals or humans. Plague was the cause of the Black Death in mid–fourteenth-century Europe, killing one-third of the European population (Figure 7-76). Worldwide, cases of plague still occur. From 1970 to the present, in the United States, between 5 and 15 human cases occur each year, mostly in the southwestern states.

The disease normally occurs in three forms:

1. Bubonic plague, characterized by swollen lymph nodes (buboes), usually in the groin

2. Septicemic plague, blood infection

3. Pneumonic plague, development of secondary lung infection in patients with bubonic plague; the pneumonic form can be spread from person to person

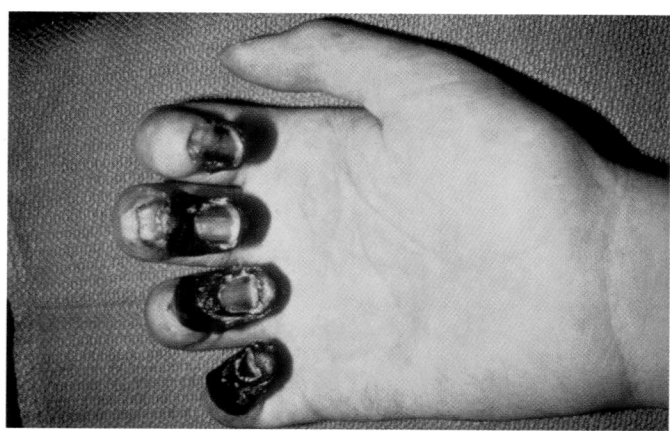

FIGURE 7-76 Gangrenous fingertips of a plague patient, showing why this disease was called the "Black Death"

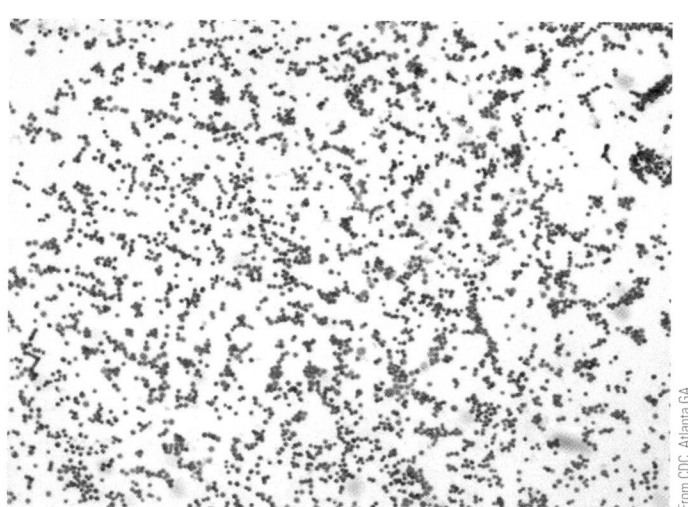

FIGURE 7-77 Gram stain of *Francisella tularensis*, a tiny Gram-negative coccobacillus that causes tularemia

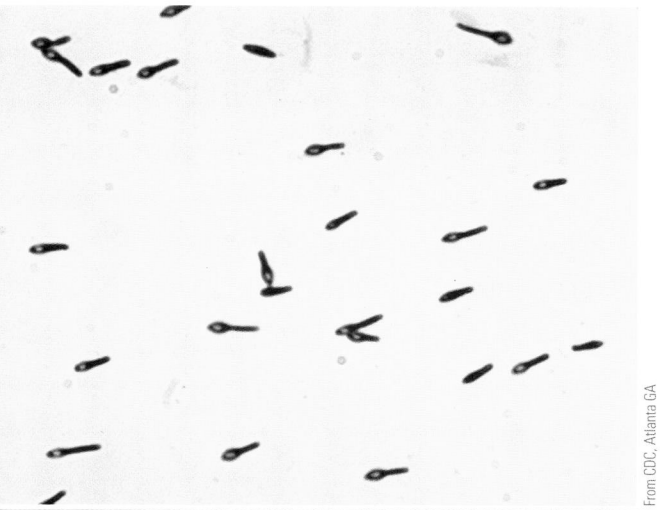

FIGURE 7-78 A photomicrograph of Gram-positive, spore-forming *Clostridium botulinum*

Several times in human history there have been attempts to use the plague organism as a biological weapon. During the years of the Black Death, Tartars, whose population was stricken with plague, catapulted corpses of their infected soldiers at the Genoese enemy. When plague broke out, the Genoese troops fled back to Italy. During World War II, the Japanese army secretly studied the plague organism for purposes of biological warfare, developing a way to use fleas to disseminate plague in a bomb or spray. Reports show that the Japanese used plague as a weapon in China at least three times during World War II. In the 1970s and 1980s, the Soviet Union also developed weapon forms of *Y. pestis*, using a dry, genetically engineered, antibiotic-resistant form of the bacterium. Other countries, including North Korea, Canada, and the United States, have had active plague research programs. Although plague has never been used as a weapon against U.S. forces, troops have been deployed in areas where plague is endemic, such as Hawaii and Vietnam. It was official policy during World War II to vaccinate U.S. troops with a killed plague vaccine.

Tularemia

Tularemia, also called rabbit fever, is caused by *Francisella tularensis*, a small, gram-negative coccobacillus (Figure 7-77). The organism occurs in wild and domestic animals in America, Europe, and Asia. Humans, such as rabbit hunters, become infected by contacting infected animals or animal products. Depending on the route of exposure, the organism can cause cutaneous infection, gastrointestinal symptoms (if ingested), or pneumonic disease (if inhaled). Tularemia has a short incubation period and causes symptoms that can be difficult to distinguish from anthrax or plague. Person-to-person transmission has not been documented.

F. tularensis has been considered a potential biological weapon for decades. It can be cultured easily, is stable in liquid and dry form, and causes infection at a low dose, less than 100 organisms. After World War II, weapons were developed by the United States with the capability of disseminating the organism. The Soviet Union was also developing weapons using tularemia

from that period to the early 1990s. In both countries the work included modifying the organism's genetic makeup to create antibiotic-resistant strains or to enhance virulence.

A World Health Organization (WHO) committee estimated that dispersal of 50 kg of virulent *F. tularensis* in a city of 5 million inhabitants would result in approximately 19,000 deaths and cause long-lasting and/or relapsing illness in as many as a quarter million people. A study by the CDC estimated that the economic cost of an aerosol attack of *F. tularensis*, including treating the disease and decontaminating the area, would be $5.4 billion for every 100,000 persons exposed.

Botulism

Botulism is a life-threatening condition caused by **botulinum toxin**, a neurotoxin produced by the gram-positive, spore-forming bacterium *Clostridium botulinum* (Figure 7-78).

It is said that these neurotoxins are the most potent toxins known. They produce a muscular paralysis that can lead to respiratory failure. The botulinum toxin can be inactivated by heat. Botulism is not contagious and is not spread person to person. **Botulinum intoxication** is a public health emergency and must be immediately treated without waiting for laboratory confirmation. This includes notification of public health officials, administration of antitoxin, and hospitalization in a critical care unit with close monitoring for respiratory failure.

Natural cases of botulism occur as a result of ingestion of the toxin (foodborne cases), wound contamination with the bacteria, or intestinal proliferation of *Clostridium*. The toxin cannot penetrate intact skin. Nearly three-fourths of the more than 100 yearly botulism cases in the United States are infant botulism, caused by ingestion of *Clostridium* from sources such as contaminated honey. Infant botulism differs from foodborne botulism in that the bacteria survive and grow in the infant gut, producing toxins that are absorbed and cause gradual symptoms.

The remaining natural cases of botulism are acquired either through ingestion of food contaminated with the toxin or by contamination of a wound by the *Clostridium* organism. Food botulism is usually associated with low-acid canned foods (beans, carrots, corn, etc.) that have not been heated properly. Botulinum toxin (Botox) is also approved for some medical and cosmetic uses. Cases of botulinum intoxication have occurred as a result of injections of incorrectly prepared botulinum toxin.

Another potential method of acquiring botulism is by inhalation of aerosolized toxin. Biological weapons programs that include the production of botulinum toxin have been carried out by several nations. Before the 1991 Gulf War, Iraq is said to have produced thousands of liters of botulinum toxin, with more than half of its stock being incorporated into weapons designed to deliver aerosols of the toxin. This method of toxin dissemination has also been attempted by bioterrorists. Botulinum toxin can be produced using crude technology, so it is of potential use to bioterrorist groups.

In a bioterrorism attack, the routes of exposure to botulinum toxin would most likely be oral or by inhalation. The toxins are rather unstable, so the range of an aerosol attack would be limited. It is estimated that toxin in concentrations as low as 0.01 mg/kg of body weight is lethal to humans by inhalation, and 1.0 mg/kg is lethal by the oral route.

Hemorrhagic Fever Viruses

The viral hemorrhagic fevers (VHFs) are a group of viral diseases associated with significant hemorrhaging. Many of these diseases are considered emerging infectious diseases. Viruses included in the VHF group include Ebola virus, Marburg virus, and the viruses causing Lassa Fever, Rift Valley fever, dengue, and yellow fever. (See the information on emerging infectious diseases in Lesson 7-10.) Naturally occurring outbreaks of these viral diseases, and subsequent person-to-person transmission in some cases, have shown that they could potentially be used as weapons (Table 7-31). In natural outbreaks of Ebola and Marburg, person-to-person spread has been prevented by use of contact and airborne precautions. Case fatality rates vary according to the

TABLE 7-31. Four families of hemorrhagic viruses that have potential as biological weapons

VIRUS FAMILY	DISEASES
Arenaviruses	Lassa fever New World hemorrhagic fevers
Filoviruses	Marburg VHF Ebola VHF
Bunyaviruses	Crimean-Congo hemorrhagic fever Rift Valley fever
Flaviviruses	Dengue, yellow fever

virus, ranging from approximately 25% for Marburg to 70% to 90% for the Ebola Zaire subtype.

Ebola and Marburg viruses, both members of the filovirus family, are considered to be the most dangerous and are categorized as *category A* bioweapon agents. Characteristics of these viruses include:

- High mortality and morbidity
- Person-to-person transmission
- Highly infectious at a low dose by the aerosol route
- Environmentally stable
- Large-scale production possible

Several governments have shown interest in hemorrhagic fever viruses as weapons. The Soviet Union produced large quantities of Marburg, Ebola, and Lassa viruses, as well as others. During the Kikwit Ebola outbreak in Zaire in the 1990s, the Aum Shinrikyo cult in Japan attempted to gain access to Ebola virus.

THREATS TO AGRICULTURE

Although it is imperative to prepare for events that directly and immediately affect the health of citizens, it is also important to put measures in place to protect food sources from plant and animal diseases and from acts of terrorism on agriculture, or **agroterrorism**. Routine monitoring and surveillance programs of crops and livestock must be in place so that the presence of an exotic pathogen is detected rapidly and its source discovered. Enhanced security measures should also be adopted. In the United States, surveillance is primarily a function of the U.S. Department of Agriculture's (USDA) Animal and Plant Health Information Service (APHIS). This department has the tools to control the entry of foreign pests and to manage infestations, should they occur.

Plant and Animal Diseases

Several diseases affecting plants and animals can result in diminished food productivity. Animal diseases of concern include diseases such as bovine spongiform encephalopathy (BSE or mad cow disease), foot-and-mouth disease, and avian influenza. Insects present a bioterrorism/agroterrorism risk because most of the economically important insect pests in North America are not native but are introduced. Insects that can infect either livestock or crops are both of concern. If a new insect pest were discovered, it would be difficult to determine the source and whether it was deliberately introduced.

Whether a disease is brought in as an act of agroterrorism, or whether it is brought in accidentally, agricultural authorities must be prepared to respond promptly. Livestock illness and death can sometimes be noticed before authorities become aware of human health problems resulting from the same exposure. Farmers must be vigilant about security and report any abnormalities to veterinarians, law enforcement, or appropriate USDA authorities immediately to prevent problems from spreading. Introduction of harmful agents that would compromise farm products could be accomplished using low technology, but the impact and cost could be high. Losses from infectious agents would include animal suffering, injury, or death, as well as economic damage and public health danger from an unsafe food supply.

Foot-and-Mouth Disease

Foot-and-mouth disease (FMD) is a highly contagious viral disease of livestock and other hoofed animals. Concern has been expressed over the ease with which a disease such as FMD might be brought to America from countries where it is endemic, such as Afghanistan. About one-third of the al Qaeda September 11, 2001 hijackers had agricultural training; some had demonstrated an interest in aerial spraying of crops.

Threats to agriculture have also been used to try to influence or change government policies. For example, the agent causing foot-and-mouth disease has been used in extortion threats. In 2005, in New Zealand, a group demanding money and changes in governmental policy threatened to release the agent causing foot-and-mouth disease in a farming area, and claimed to have already released it on an island.

FOOD AND WATER SAFETY

Several pathogenic organisms have the potential to contaminate food or water supplies. These include the bacteria *Escherichia coli, Salmonella typhi, Shigella,* and *Vibrio cholerae.* The botulinum toxin is not stable in treated (chlorinated) water but is relatively stable in beverages. Heightened security measures and increased surveillance methods are needed to detect these organisms when they first occur. Municipal water supplies should have security measures installed.

LABORATORY ROLE IN BIOTERRORISM RESPONSE

The Laboratory Response Network (LRN), described in Lesson 7-10, is a nationwide network of laboratories trained for rapid response to both biological and biochemical threats. Partners in the LRN include several governmental agencies and organizations, such as the CDC, Federal Bureau of Investigation (FBI), Defense Department, Agriculture Department, Environmental

Protection Agency (EPA), Energy Department, Food and Drug Administration (FDA), Homeland Security, American Society of Microbiology (ASM), Association of Public Health Laboratories (APHL), and American Association of Veterinary Laboratory Diagnosticians (AAVDL). The LRN has played and will continue to play an important role in responding to biological threats.

Laboratory Response Network in Action

2001 Anthrax Attack

In October 2001, shortly after the World Trade Center attacks in New York City and the Pentagon attack in Washington, D.C., letters containing anthrax spores were delivered to Florida, New York, and Washington D.C. Twenty-two people subsequently became infected—11 with inhalation anthrax—and five died.

In Florida, a clinical specimen from one of the first victims revealed the anthrax bacillus. The identification was quickly confirmed by the Florida public health laboratory (an LRN member) and the CDC, setting in motion a large-scale investigation. Environmental and clinical samples were collected from the hospital, the victim's place of work, and places in North Carolina that he visited shortly before becoming ill. LRN laboratories performed tests on the samples and helped to determine that he had been exposed at work by a letter containing anthrax. As part of the investigation, testing was performed on samples from postal facilities, the U.S. Senate office buildings, and offices of news organizations.

By the time the investigation was completed in December 2001, 125,000 samples had been tested, which translates into more than 1 million separate tests. Before the recent cases of anthrax terrorism in 2001, only 15% of patients with inhalation anthrax would have been expected to survive. Because of rapid response and awareness, however, 6 of the 11 patients with inhalation anthrax survived that event.

Severe Acute Respiratory Syndrome (SARS)

The CDC and the LRN also played an important role in the investigation of the SARS outbreak (Lesson 7-10). CDC laboratories sequenced the viral DNA of the coronavirus that caused SARS and laboratories of the LRN-developed tests and test materials that could be used by member laboratories to identify the virus.

BioWatch

The Department of Homeland Security has initiated an around-the-clock environmental surveillance program to sample air in certain densely populated cities. The samplers are maintained by the EPA, and filters are removed daily and analyzed by LRN BioWatch laboratories. Using polymerase chain reaction (PCR) technology, biological agents can be rapidly identified. If a harmful agent were found, it would trigger a set of emergency response procedures.

Laboratory Preparedness

Members of the LRN have also developed materials to help smaller laboratories and sentinel laboratories reach a state of preparedness. Documents such as the Clinical Laboratory

Bioterrorism (BT) Readiness plan, prepared by the ASM, provide a template for laboratories to follow to ensure that their readiness plan is comprehensive. Included in this material are detailed instructions for the handling and transport of the identified threat agents, as well as communication protocols, containment levels, detailed identification procedures, and training checklists.

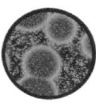 **SUMMARY**

Several agents are currently recognized as having the potential to be used in biological weapons or as bioterrorism agents. Some of these are well-known pathogens that have been around a long time. Others cause diseases that have only been recognized in recent years. All have the potential to cause high mortality as well as to disrupt society. Many government agencies and scientific organizations have joined together to coordinate comprehensive readiness plans to respond rapidly to the emergence of a threat agent.

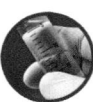 **REVIEW QUESTIONS**

1. What is meant by agroterrorism? What is one example of an agent that might be used in this way?

2. What is the causative agent and reservoir for each of the following disease threats: plague, tularemia, and smallpox?

3. What are six characteristics that make an agent useful as a threat agent?

4. Why is bioterrorism a hot topic?

5. What was the role of the LRN in the 2001 anthrax outbreak in the United States?

6. What is BioWatch?

7. What two threat agents have an ancient history of causing disease?

8. Define agroterrorism, botulinum intoxication, botulinum toxin, Department of Homeland Security, virion, and virulent.

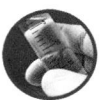 **STUDENT ACTIVITIES**

1. Complete the written examination for this lesson.

2. Visit a regional hospital, reference laboratory, or state public health laboratory. Find out what procedures they would follow if they suspected the presence of a threat agent. Ask if the laboratory is a sentinel or reference laboratory.

3. Look in newspapers, news magazines, or periodicals for information on recent natural outbreaks of agents such as the anthrax or plague bacterium. Find out what kind of disease was caused and what the mortality was.

 WEB ACTIVITIES

1. Use the Internet to explore the Homeland Security web site or another web site with information about bioterrorism response. List six biological threat agents. Report which, if any, of these agents have caused animal or human illness in the last 5 years.

2. Use the Internet to search for outbreak information. Use reliable web sources such as the CDC's *Morbidity and Mortality Weekly Reports* or Pro Med (Program for Monitoring Emerging Diseases) at www.promedmail.org.

UNIT 8

Basic Parasitology

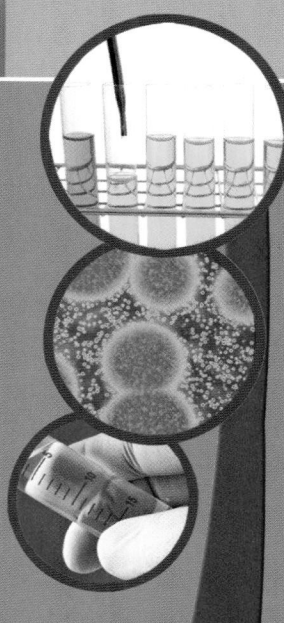

UNIT OBJECTIVES

After studying this unit, the student will:

- Discuss the functions of the parasitology section of the clinical laboratory.
- Discuss mechanisms of parasitic infection.
- Describe parasite control methods.
- Explain why knowledge of parasite life cycles is necessary to detect parasitic infections.
- Describe diagnostic techniques for blood, tissue, and intestinal parasites.
- Explain procedures for collection and processing of specimens for parasite examination.
- Perform a test for pinworms.
- Prepare fecal specimens for microscopic parasite examination.
- Prepare blood smears for parasite examination.

In a hospital laboratory, the parasitology section can be part of the microbiology department or a stand-alone department. Because of the variety of parasites and the relative infrequency of tests for parasites, most laboratory personnel do not gain much experience in parasite identification. Therefore, many laboratories routinely prepare specimens for parasite examination and then send the specimens to a reference laboratory or a state health laboratory for examination and identification.

The stool, or fecal, specimen is the specimen most frequently examined for parasites. However, parasites can be present in and on all parts of the body, so the correct specimen required for testing is determined by the patient's symptoms and medical history. Because the malarial parasite infects red blood cells, the parasite is often first detected during examination of a stained blood smear. *Trichomonas*, a flagellated protozoan parasite, can inhabit the genitourinary tract and can be detected during the microscopic part of a routine urinalysis. Parasites such as lice can infest body hair. Tapeworms, roundworms, intestinal amebae, *Giardia*, and *Cryptosporidium* infect the intestinal tract and can be detected in fecal specimens. Parasites such as *Toxoplasma* are found in tissue and can be detected by immunological methods.

Many types of Parasites cause human disease. Most parasitic diseases in the United States have been brought under control with education, improved sanitation techniques, and insect control measures. However, worldwide millions of people are infected with parasites and parasites remain a major cause of disease and death in many parts of the world.

As worldwide travel has become commonplace, parasitic infections are detected more frequently in U.S. laboratories. Additionally, microorganisms such as *Toxoplasma* and *Cryptosporidium* are becoming an increasing problem because they can cause severe disease in immunocompromised individuals, such as HIV-infected patients, or those who have had transplants or are undergoing chemotherapy treatments.

Unit 8 provides information about basic parasitology concepts and laboratory procedures. Lesson 8-1 is a brief introduction to the field of parasitology. Groups of the more common human parasites, modes of transmission, life cycles, and diagnostic methods are outlined. Lesson 8-2 describes specimen collection and processing for parasite examination and explains the procedure for the pinworm test. Methods of preparing fecal specimens for microscopic examination for parasites are presented in Lesson 8-3. Lesson 8-4 describes the procedure for preparing, staining, and examining blood smears for parasites.

This unit represents only an introduction to the field of clinical parasitology. Much practice and study are required to become expert in parasite identification. Specimens must be collected and processed correctly to increase the likelihood of detecting any parasite(s) present. Personnel should also have a solid knowledge of parasites and be able to recognize parasitic forms. Technicians in laboratories that do not perform frequent parasitology procedures might not be able to identify all parasites but must be alert enough and sufficiently trained to recognize something unusual in the specimen that requires expert evaluation.

READINGS, REFERENCES, AND RESOURCES

Ash, L. R. & Orihel, T. C. (2007). *Atlas of human parasitology.* (5th ed.). Chicago: ASCP Press.

Bogitsh, B., et al. (2005). *Human parasitology.* (3rd ed.). San Diego: Academic Press.

CDC. "Cryptosporidiosis Surveillance—United States, 2003-2005." *Morbidity and mortality meekly report.* September 7, 2007. 56(SS07):1–10.

CDC. "Giardiasis Surveillance—United States, 2003–2005." *Morbidity and mortality weekly report.* September 7, 2007. 56(SS07):11–18.

Forbes, B. A., et al. (2007). *Bailey & Scott's diagnostic microbiology.* (12th ed.). St. Louis: C. V. Mosby.

Garcia, L. S. (2001). *Diagnostic medical parasitology.* (5th ed.). Washington, DC: American Society for Microbiology.

Heelan, J. S. & Ingersoll, F. W. (2001). *Essentials of human parasitology* . Clifton Park, NY: Delmar Cengage Learning.

Leventhal, R. & Cheadle, R. F. (2002). *Medical parasitology: A self-instructional text.* (5th ed.). Philadelphia: F. A. Davis Company.

McPherson, R. A. & Pincus, M. R. (Eds.) (2007). *Henry's clinical diagnosis and management by laboratory methods.* (21st ed.). Philadelphia: Saunders Elsevier.

Mahon, C. R. et al. (2011). *Textbook of diagnostic microbiology* . (4th ed.). Maryland Heights, MO: Saunders Elsevier.

Ridley, J. (2010). *Parasitology for medical laboratory technicians.* Clifton Park, NY: Delmar Cengage Learning.

Roberts, L. S. & Janovy, Jr., J. (2008). *Foundations of parasitology.* (8th ed.). St. Louis: McGraw-Hill.

Zeibig, E. A. (2010). *Clinical parasitology: A practical approach.* (2nd ed.). Philadelphia: W. B. Saunders.

Web Sites of Interest

Centers for Disease Control and Prevention, www.cdc.gov
National Institutes of Health, www.nih.gov
World Health Organization, www.who.int

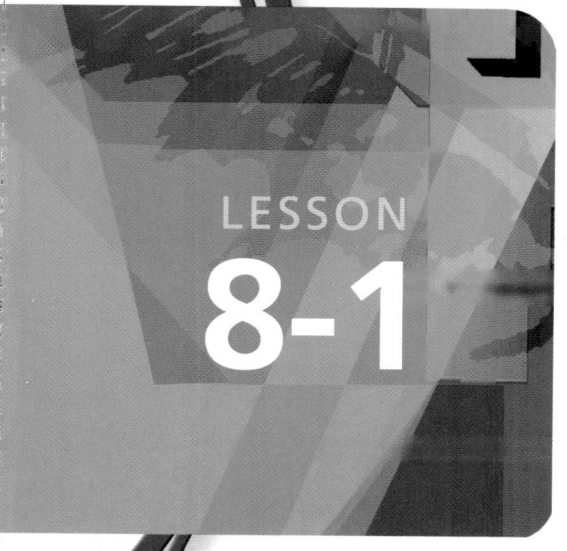

Introduction to Parasitology

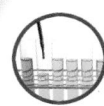

LESSON OBJECTIVES

After studying this lesson, the student will:

- ⊙ Name the three major morphological groups of parasites.
- ⊙ Explain three ways in which parasite infections are transmitted.
- ⊙ Describe four ways to control or prevent parasitic infections.
- ⊙ Discuss types of waterborne and foodborne outbreaks caused by parasites.
- ⊙ List three methods used to diagnose parasitic infections.
- ⊙ Name four types of specimens that can be examined for parasites.
- ⊙ Name three blood parasites.
- ⊙ Name three intestinal protozoan parasites.
- ⊙ Name three types of parasitic helminths.
- ⊙ Explain how immunological tests are useful in the parasitology laboratory.
- ⊙ Explain how eradication of guinea worm is a successful model for eradication of parasitic disease.
- ⊙ Define the glossary terms.

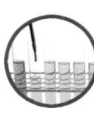

GLOSSARY

ameba (pl. amebae) / a single-celled eukaryotic organism lacking a definite shape and moving by means of pseudopodia; also spelled amoeba (pl. amoebae)

arthropod / a member of the phylum Arthropoda, which includes crustaceans, insects, and arachnids

atrial / of or relating to a body cavity

cestode / tapeworm; member of the class Cestoda

commensal / an organism that lives with, on, or in another organism, without injury to either

congenital / acquired during fetal development, and present at the time of birth, but not inherited

cyst / the dormant stage of an organism surrounded by a resistant covering; the nonmotile, nonfeeding stage of a protozoan parasite; a closed sac-like structure within a tissue

definitive host / the host in which the sexual or adult form of the parasite is found

ectoparasite / a parasite that lives on the outer surface of a host

endemic / recurring in a specific location or population

endoparasite / a parasite that lives within the host

helminth / a worm, especially a parasitic worm; in parasitology, the group comprising the roundworms and flatworms

(continues)

host / the organism from which a parasite obtains nutrients and in which some or part of the parasite's life cycle is completed

immunocompromised / having reduced ability or inability to produce a normal immune response

intermediate host / the host in which the asexual, immature, or larval form of the parasite is found

larva / immature stage of an invertebrate

mechanical vector / a vector (usually an arthropod) that is not essential to a parasite's life cycle but that can transfer an infective parasite to a noninfected host

nematode / roundworm; any unsegmented worm of the class Nematoda

opportunistic parasite / an organism that causes disease only in immunocompromised hosts

ova / eggs

parasite / an organism that lives in or on another species and at the expense of that species

pathogenic / capable of causing damage or injury to the host

primary amebic encephalitis (PAM) / rare and usually fatal central nervous system infection caused by *Naegleria fowleri* ameba

proglottid (pl. proglottids) / the tapeworm body segment that contains the male and female reproductive organs

protozoa / unicellular eukaryotic organisms, both free-living and parasitic

reservoir host / a host, other than the usual host, in which the parasite lives and is infectious

sporozoite / the banana-shaped motile infective stage of certain apicomplexan protozoa such as *Toxoplasma*, *Cryptosporidium*, and *Plasmodium*; in *Plasmodium*, the stage present in mosquito salivary glands that is introduced into blood by mosquito bite

trematode / fluke; any parasitic flatworm of the class Trematoda

trophozoite / the motile feeding stage of protozoan parasites

trypomastigote / the characteristic developmental stage of trypanosomes, which has a leaf-like form, an undulating membrane, and usually a free flagellum

vector / an agent that transports a pathogen from an infected host to a noninfected host

INTRODUCTION

Parasites are organisms that live in or on another organism, the **host**, and live at the expense of the host organism. The parasite depends on the host for nutrients, which causes injury to the host. Clinical parasitology is the study of parasites and parasitic diseases, including methods of diagnosing, treating, and controlling parasitic diseases.

Some parasites cause little obvious harm to the host, for example, head lice. Others, such as the malarial parasite, can cause severe disease and even death if untreated. Parasites that cause disease in healthy individuals are called **pathogenic** parasites. **Opportunistic parasites** are those parasites that cause few or no symptoms in healthy hosts but can cause severe disease in **immunocompromised** hosts.

Parasites can be classified in several ways. They can be grouped according to the site in which they normally are found; for example, intestinal parasites, blood parasites, or **ectoparasites** (parasites on the exterior of the host). Or they can be grouped according to morphological characteristics; for example, worms (tapeworms, roundworms, and flukes), protozoa, and arthropods (insects and arachnids).

Parasitic infections are usually diagnosed by finding and identifying the parasite, either macroscopically or microscopically, or by immunological tests. This lesson presents an overview of the field of clinical parasitology as it relates to clinical laboratory procedures. Clinical parasitology textbooks and atlases should be consulted for more comprehensive information.

CHARACTERISTICS OF PARASITES

Several characteristics are considered when identifying parasites. These include morphology, host specificity, geographical distribution, life cycle, and vectors.

Morphological Classification

Parasites, like other living organisms, can be grouped according to international rules of zoological classification based on morphology and other characteristics. Although organisms are often called by various common names, such as hookworm or beef tapeworm, they have two-part latinized scientific names that are recognized internationally. The scientific name of an organism is always italicized, with the genus name also capitalized. For example, the scientific name for one species of malarial parasite is *Plasmodium ovale*.

Types of Hosts

Most parasites require specific conditions to complete their life cycles. Although essentially all animal species have parasites, these parasites are often very host-specific. However, if conditions are right, parasites normally found in one host can survive or even thrive in an unnatural host. An example of this is the dog heartworm, *Dirofilaria immitis*. This parasite is considered to be host-specific, with dogs being the natural host. However, the dog heartworm can infect other animals, such as cats. These infections are not usually as serious as infections in dogs.

The **definitive host**, or main host, is the organism in which the sexually mature (adult) form of a parasite is found. Some parasites require two or more different host species to complete their life cycle.

The **intermediate host** is an organism required to complete a parasite's life cycle in addition to the definitive host. The intermediate host usually harbors an asexual or **larval** (immature) form of the parasite. For example, malarial parasites (*Plasmodium*) live in both humans and mosquitoes. In humans, *Plasmodium*'s intermediate host, the parasite reproduces asexually. Sexual reproduction of *Plasmodium* occurs in the mosquito, the definitive host.

A **reservoir host** is an organism other than the main host that can harbor a parasite and serve as a source of infection. A **vector** is a living carrier that transfers the infective parasite to an uninfected host. A *biological vector* is a vector that is also essential to the parasite's life cycle. For example the mosquito is both the definitive host and the biological vector for *Plasmodium*. **Mechanical vectors** transfer parasites mechanically without being infected themselves. For example, flies that land on infected feces and then land on food can carry infective parasite stages from one site to another.

Geographical Distribution

Parasites are only found where the appropriate hosts, vectors, or animal reservoirs are available to allow the parasite's life cycle to develop and be perpetuated. Environmental factors such as humidity and temperature are important to the survival of most parasites, especially those that require arthropod vectors. Temperature extremes and dry conditions are often detrimental to parasitic forms. Therefore, the majority of parasites are found in temperate to tropical climates.

Parasite Life Cycles

A parasitic life cycle is the complete developmental process of a parasite infecting (or infesting) a host, growing, reproducing, and being transmitted to a new host (Figure 8-1). Parasite life cycles can be simple or complex. Some parasites spend their entire life in one type of host. Others require different types of hosts during various parts of their life cycles. Still others are only parasitic for a portion of their life and are free-living at other times. Knowledge of the specific life-cycle requirements of each parasite is valuable in preventing parasitic infections and determining the appropriate specimen to examine when parasitic infection is suspected.

Infective Stage versus Diagnostic Stage

The *infective stage* of the parasite is the stage of the life cycle during which the parasite is capable of infecting a host. The *diagnostic stage* is the life cycle stage that can be detected in a specimen

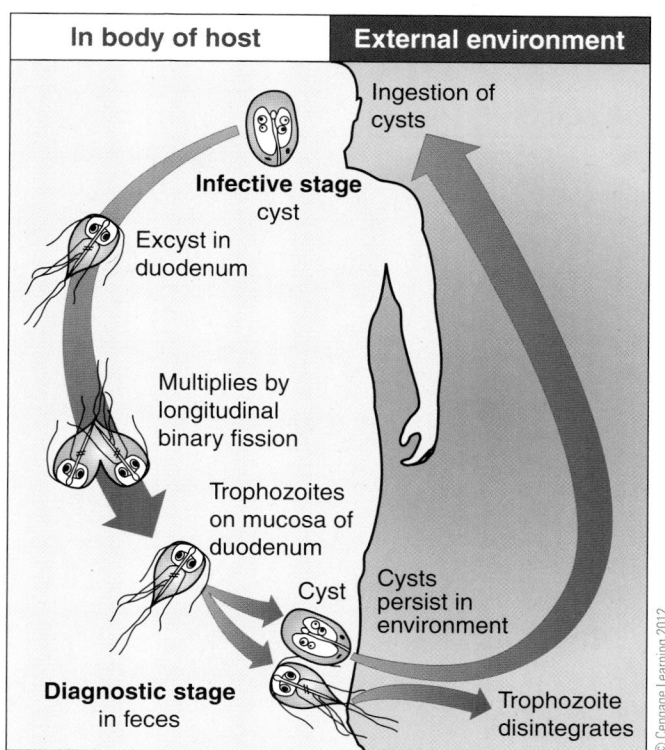

FIGURE 8-1 Example of parasite life cycle diagram: shown is life cycle of *Giardia intestinalis*

and aids in diagnosis. Knowledge of the infective stage is required to understand how to prevent transmission. Knowledge of the diagnostic stage is required to select the correct specimen and diagnostic test method. Sometimes the diagnostic stage and infective stage are the same, particularly for the intestinal parasites. For example, in the life cycle diagram of *Giardia* shown in Figure 8-1, the **cyst** is the infective stage as well as a diagnostic stage.

Infection versus Infestation

Parasites such as lice that live on external body surfaces cause *infestations*. Parasites that live within the host cause *infections*. Parasites can infect (or infest) external body surfaces, external body cavities, the intestinal tract, and tissues and organs such as the blood, bone marrow, brain, lung, or liver. Many parasites have specific tissue requirements and will migrate through the body to locate in a specific organ. The site infected by a parasite is determined by characteristics of the particular type of parasite, how the parasite enters the body, the parasite's tissue specificity, and the host's immunity.

Transmission of Parasitic Infections

Most parasitic infections are acquired through contact with an infected person, ingestion of an infective form in food or water, or arthropod (primarily insect) bites. A few parasites can be acquired through **congenital** infection, and some parasites such as hookworm can penetrate intact skin. Table 8-1 lists some parasitic diseases, their usual routes of transmission, and their infective stages.

TABLE 8-1. Examples of parasitic diseases, causative organisms, transmission routes, and infective stages

DISEASE	CAUSATIVE ORGANISM	TRANSMISSION ROUTE	INFECTIVE STAGE
Amebiasis	Entamoeba histolytica	Ingestion	Cyst
Giardiasis	Giardia intestinalis	Ingestion	Cyst
Malaria	Plasmodium	Mosquito bite	Sporozoite
Toxoplasmosis	Toxoplasma gondii	Ingestion, congenital	Oocysts, tissue cyst, tachyzoite
Trichomoniasis	Trichomonas vaginalis	Sexual contact	Trophozoite
Babesiosis	Babesia	Tick bite	Sporozoite
Cryptosporidiosis	Cryptosporidium	Ingestion	Oocyst
Cyclosporiasis	Cyclospora	Ingestion	Oocyst
Trichinosis	Trichinella spiralis	Ingestion	Larva
Enterobiasis	Enterobius vermicularis	Ingestion	Ova
Primary amebic meningoencephalitis (PAM)	Naegleria fowleri	Penetration of cells lining nasal cavities	Trophozoite
Hookworm	Necator, Ancylostoma	Skin penetration	Larva
Ascariasis	Ascaris lumbricoides	Ingestion	Ova
Chagas disease	Trypanosoma cruzi	Ingestion, mucous membrane, blood	Trypomastigote
Dracunculiasis	Dracunculus medinensis	Ingestion	Larva

ORGANISMS PARASITIC FOR HUMANS

The parasites that infect humans can be grouped into three large groups: **protozoa**, **helminths**, and **arthropods** (Figure 8-2).

Protozoa

Protozoa are single-celled eukaryotic organisms that are larger than most bacteria. Parasitic protozoa include **amebae**, flagellates, ciliates, and apicomplexans (formerly sporozoa; see Table 8-2). All four of these protozoan groups contain parasites of humans and other animals. Protozoa can infect most body sites, including blood and other tissues, the intestinal and genitourinary tracts, and the oral cavity.

Helminths

Helminth is the common name used for parasitic worms. These include **trematodes** (flukes), **cestodes** (tapeworms), and **nematodes** (roundworms; Table 8-3). Most helminth infections occur in the intestinal tract. However, other tissues are sometimes infected by certain helminths.

Arthropods

Arthropods include arachnids such as spiders, ticks, and mites, and insects such as lice, bugs, fleas, flies, and mosquitoes (Table 8-4). Some arthropods, such as lice, fleas, and mosquitos, are parasitic to humans; others, such as flies, are important as vectors in transmitting the infective stages of parasites to humans.

HOW PARASITES CAUSE DISEASE

Parasitic disease occurs when the damage caused to the host by the parasite becomes severe enough to cause pathologic changes in the host. Parasitic infections can be asymptomatic (without symptoms), cause to mild to moderate symptoms, or even cause death.

Many factors determine the effect a parasitic infection will have on the host, including the parasite numbers (dose), size, location, and toxicity. The host's condition is also a factor. Damage can be mechanical, such as obstruction of an organ or vessel; irritative or toxic, caused by substances produced or released by the parasite; or damage can be caused by an allergic reaction. Some infections are self-limiting. Common problems seen with parasitic infections include anemia, jaundice, secondary bacterial infections, organ dysfunction, and interference with normal physiological processes.

Immunity to Parasites

Absolute immunity to parasites is rare unless the individual (species) is an unsuitable host. In general, resistance to parasitic infection increases with age. Hosts with good nutrition and health are less likely to develop severe symptoms than hosts from impoverished socioeconomic conditions.

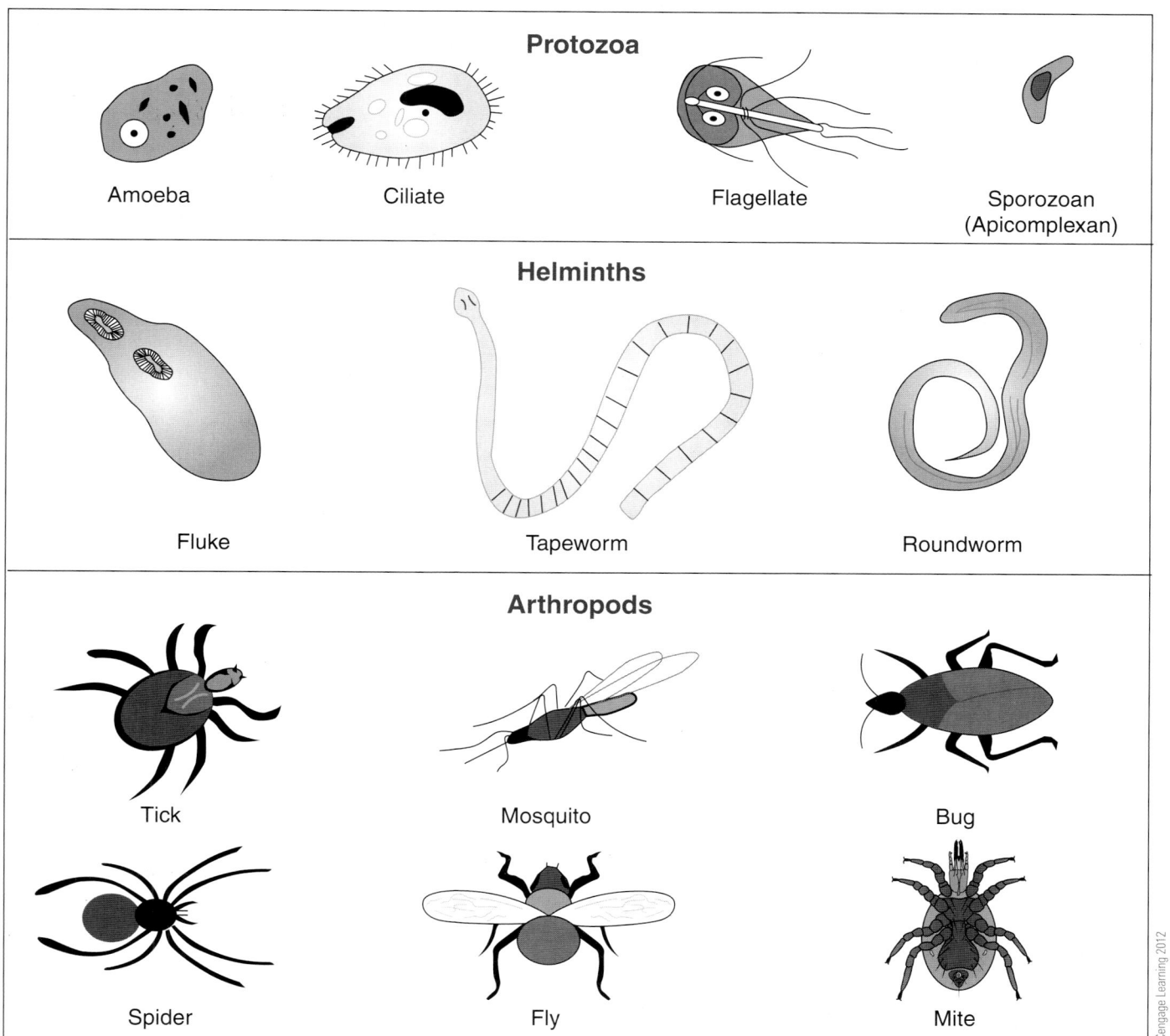

FIGURE 8-2 Three major groups of parasites: protozoa, helminths, and arthropods (not drawn to scale)

TABLE 8-2. Examples of medically important protozoa

PROTOZOAN GROUP	EXAMPLES
Amebae	*Entamoeba, Naegleria, Acanthamoeba*
Flagellates	*Trichomonas, Giardia*
Ciliates	*Balantidium*
Apicomplexa	*Plasmodium, Toxoplasma*

TABLE 8-3. Examples of medically important helminths

HELMINTH GROUP	EXAMPLES
Trematodes (flukes)	Liver fluke, lung fluke
Cestodes (tapeworms)	Beef tapeworm, pork tapeworm
Nematodes (roundworms)	Pinworm, hookworm, whipworm

TABLE 8-4. Medically important arthropods

ARTHROPOD GROUP	EXAMPLES
Arachnids	Spiders, ticks, mites
Insects	Lice, bugs, fleas, flies, mosquitoes

Parasites stimulate immune responses much like those stimulated by viruses or bacteria. This means antibodies can develop against the infecting parasite and the cell-mediated immune response can be stimulated. Immunological tests can be used to aid in diagnosing some parasitic infections. These are especially useful when it is difficult to obtain a specimen for examination, such as in tissue or organ infections. For example, toxoplasmosis is a parasitic disease that can be diagnosed by measuring serum antibody to *Toxoplasma*.

Treating Parasitic Infections

Several drugs are effective against parasites but most have some level of toxicity. The success of treatment depends on the infecting parasite, the magnitude of the infection, the host's health, and the infection site. In some cases, surgery is required to remove the parasite.

Parasitic Infections in Immunocompromised Patients

Immunocompromised patients, such as HIV-positive, organ transplant, chemotherapy, or radiation patients, are especially vulnerable to parasitic infection. Infections with parasites such as *Toxoplasma* and *Cryptosporidium* can be life-threatening to these patients and must be treated with vigorous drug therapy. Immunodiagnosis of parasitic infections can be unsuccessful in immunocompromised patients because blood antibody levels can be below detection limits.

CURRENT TOPICS 1

OUTBREAKS OF PARASITIC INFECTIONS

Although the incidence of parasitic infections in the United States is not as high as bacterial and viral infections, a small lapse in sanitation or other preventive measures can allow parasite infections to emerge and cause disease and sometimes death. Most U.S. parasite outbreaks can be traced to failures in infrastructure, such as water or sewage treatment, or to unsafe food processing and preparation procedures, such as use of reclaimed wastewater for irrigation of food crops. Another potential source of outbreaks is natural disasters, such as major flooding and hurricanes. These increase the risk for contamination of drinking water with untreated sewage or animal wastes, creating potential for parasitic infections. Examples of recent foodborne and waterborne parasitic outbreaks in the United States include:

- In the 1990s, a water treatment plant failure in Milwaukee, Wisconsin, caused more than 400,000 people to become infected with *Cryptosporidium*, an intestinal protozoan parasite. *Cryptosporidium* causes severe diarrhea of 1- to 2-week duration in healthy, immunocompetent individuals and can cause life-threatening illness in immunocompromised individuals. Several fatalities occurred as a result of the Milwaukee cryptosporidiosis outbreak.
- Between 1999 and 2003, all 50 states reported cryptosporidiosis cases, averaging more than 3,000 cases annually. *Cryptosporidium* is one of the most frequent causes of gastroenteritis associated with treated (disinfected) recreational waters such as swimming pools, because of its resistance to chlorine disinfection. In 2007-2008, 60 outbreaks resulted in over 12,000 reported cases of cryptosporidiosis; 99% of these outbreaks occurred after exposure to treated recreational waters.

- In recent years, several outbreaks of cyclosporiasis have been reported in the United States and Canada. Cyclosporiasis is caused by infection with *Cyclospora*, a coccidian parasite causing symptoms similar to those caused by *Cryptosporidium*. Most of these outbreaks were traced to ingestion of contaminated raw produce, primarily raspberries. Improved sanitation techniques in food harvesting and processing could have prevented most of these outbreaks.
- In California, in 2006, lung infections with *Paragonimus*, the lung fluke, were diagnosed in patients who had eaten raw or undercooked imported freshwater crabs.
- Outbreaks of giardiasis, caused by the intestinal flagellate *Giardia intestinalis*, are reported fairly frequently in the United States. Examples include:
  - Waterborne outbreaks in New York State (1975, 1995, 1997); New Hampshire and Montana (1980), Colorado, (1981), Nevada (1982), Oregon (1997), Florida (1998), and Ohio (2004)
  - Foodborne outbreaks (1990s) caused by contaminated salad bars and taco ingredients
  - Outbreaks after playing in recreational waters such as swimming pools, lakes, or public spraying fountains (Florida, 2006)
  - Outbreaks in institutions such as nursing homes and day care centers
  - Between 2006 and 2008 over 19,000 *Giardia* cases were reported annually in the United States. Several were classified as outbreaks.

DIAGNOSIS OF PARASITIC INFECTIONS

Most parasitic diseases have generalized symptoms such as fever, pain, chills, diarrhea, or fatigue and loss of vitality, symptoms that could be caused by a variety of conditions or diseases. A definitive diagnosis of parasitic infections usually depends upon finding and identifying the parasite's diagnostic stage.

Specimens that are examined for evidence of parasites include stool, urine, sputum, aspirations, and blood and other tissues. For some parasites, immunological tests are available. Patient history is also very important in the diagnosis of parasitic infections, particularly if the patient has any history of travel to **endemic** areas, areas where the parasite occurs naturally.

PREVENTING PARASITIC INFECTIONS

The key to prevention of parasitic infections is to understand transmission methods and know the location of the parasite's infective stages. Parasite-control methods include:

- Blocking transmission of the infective form
- Providing health education
- Improving sanitation
- Identifying and treating infected individuals to prevent the spread of infection
- Developing vaccines

Blocking Transmission

One of the most effective ways of preventing parasite infections is to block transmission of the parasite's infective stage by breaking a link in its life cycle. For this reason, it is important to understand the life history of the parasite, where it is found, the host required for its reproduction, and how transmission occurs.

When the infective stage of the parasite is known, it is possible to plan effective control and prevention methods. For example, in the 1800s in North America, malaria was found as far north as southern Canada. When it was discovered that the malarial parasite was transmitted to humans through the bite of infected mosquitoes, mosquito control measures were implemented in the United States. The use of DDT and other pesticides rapidly and drastically reduced the malaria infection rate, so that by the 1950s, the United States was not considered endemic for malaria. However, because of the banning of effective, but toxic, pesticides such as DDT and increases in worldwide travel, occasional new cases of malaria have been seen in the United States since 2000. Some of these have occurred in individuals who have no history of travel to endemic areas.

Health Education and Improved Sanitation

Emphasis on education about personal hygiene, handwashing, and safe food handling has contributed to a drop in foodborne parasitic diseases. Improved sanitation techniques and strict standards in water quality, sewage treatment, and waste disposal have reduced the incidence of infection with waterborne parasites. Table 8-5 lists parasites associated with foodborne and waterborne infections.

TABLE 8-5. Parasites associated with foodborne and waterborne infections

PARASITE	PARASITE GROUP	INFECTION CAUSED	USUAL INFECTION ROUTE*
Giardia intestinalis	Protozoa	Giardiasis	Ingestion of contaminated water
Cryptosporidium parvum	Protozoa	Cryptosporidiosis, "Crypto"	Ingestion of contaminated water
Cyclospora cayetanensis	Protozoa	Cyclosporiasis	Ingestion of contaminated food or water
Toxoplasma gondii	Protozoa	Toxoplasmosis	Ingestion of infected raw/undercooked meat or infective oocysts from cat feces
Trichinella spiralis	Nematode (roundworm)	Trichinosis, trichinellosis	Ingestion of infected raw/undercooked meat such as pork or game
Taenia saginata	Cestode (tapeworm)	Beef tapeworm infection, taeniasis	Ingestion of infected raw/undercooked beef
Taenia solium	Cestode (tapeworm)	Pork tapeworm infection, taeniasis, cysticercosis	Ingestion of infected raw/undercooked pork

* Other infection routes or sources are possible with most parasites, but are not as common as those listed

CURRENT TOPICS 2

ERADICATING PARASITIC DISEASES: GUINEA WORM DISEASE—A SUCCESS STORY

Parasitic diseases such as malaria cause millions of deaths worldwide each year. Parasites also cause painful, debilitating disease and loss of productivity for millions worldwide. However, efforts by various organizations such as the Centers for Disease Control and Prevention (CDC), World Health Organization (WHO), UNICEF, Bill and Melinda Gates Foundation, and The Carter Center, to name a few, are succeeding in controlling, reducing, and in some cases eradicating some parasitic diseases. Partnering with these organizations are industry, drug companies, and governments of many countries around the world. Three parasitic diseases that are currently targeted for eradication by worldwide cooperation are *dracunculiasis* caused by the guinea worm, lymphatic *filariasis*, and *onchocerciasis*, also called river blindness.

Guinea Worm Disease

Guinea worm disease is an ancient disease, known to have been around for thousands of years. The worm has been found in ancient Egyptian mummies. Before eradication efforts began, Guinea worm was found in Africa, Asia (including India and Pakistan), and some parts of South America. Rather than being a rapid killer disease, Guinea worm disease causes painful crippling, resulting in children who cannot attend school and adults who cannot work. This spells economic disaster for agricultural communities.

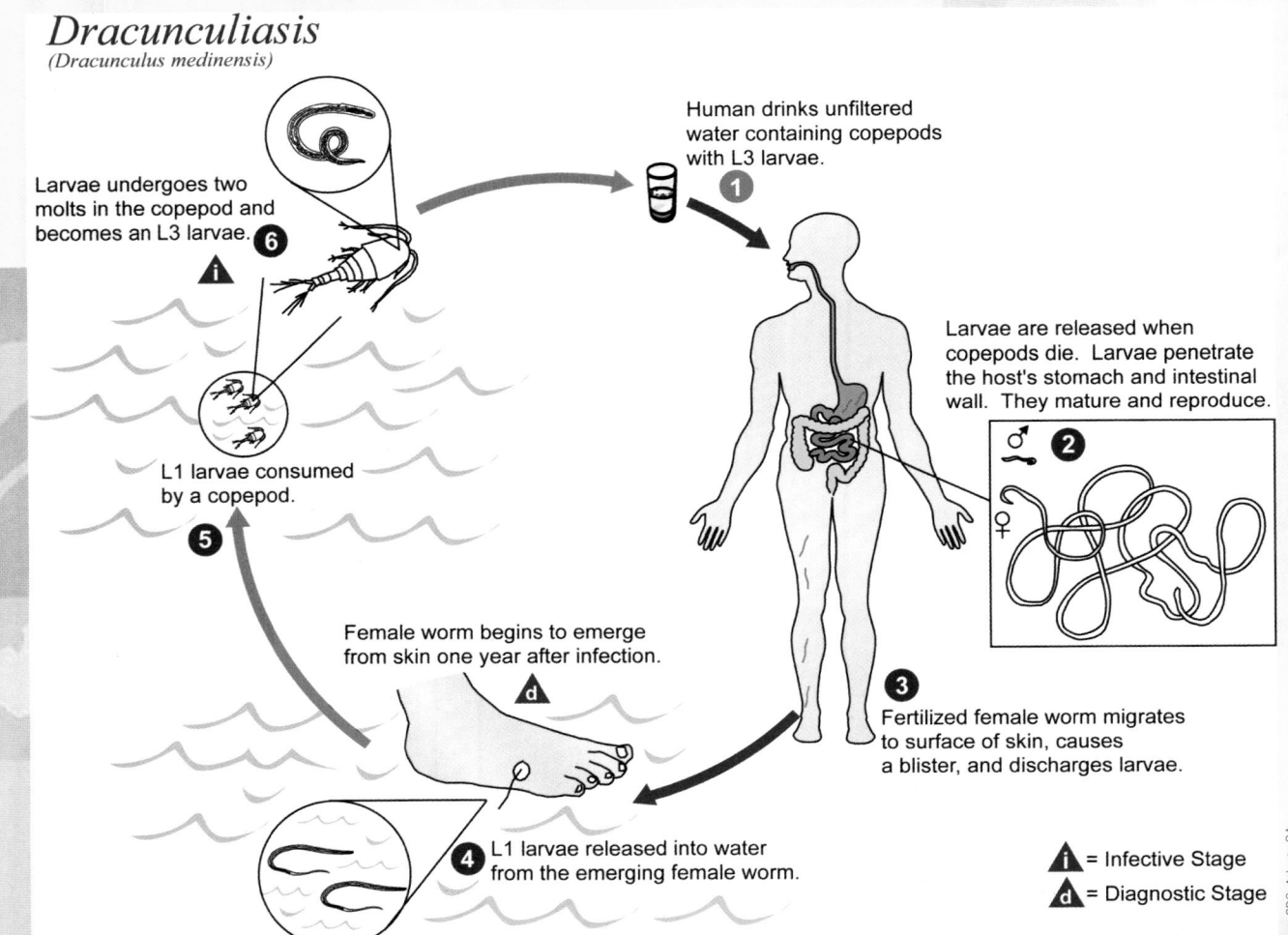

Guinea worm life cycle

From CDC, Atlanta GA

(Continues)

CURRENT TOPICS 2 (Continued)

Life Cycle

Guinea worm disease (dracunculiasis) is caused by the roundworm *Dracunculus medinensis*. It is contracted by ingesting water contaminated with microscopic water fleas (copepods) carrying infective larvae, as shown in the life cycle diagram. Once ingested, the larvae migrate to the small intestine, penetrate the wall of the intestine, and pass into the body cavity. There, over a period of about a year, the female Guinea worm matures to an adult approximately 2 to 3 feet long and the diameter of a cooked spaghetti noodle. She then migrates to a subcutaneous site, usually on the lower leg, where she emerges through a painful, burning skin blister, creating a lesion in which a secondary infection can occur.

The Guinea worm life cycle is perpetuated when victims immerse their affected limbs in water to relieve pain caused by the emerging worm, or when they wade into water to collect drinking water. When an emerging Guinea worm senses water, the worm releases millions of immature larvae into the water, thus contaminating the water supply. The worm is capable of doing this for several days when it comes in contact with water after emerging from the ulcer. The larvae are ingested by microscopic copepods, where they develop into the infective stage in about 2 weeks. The transmission cycle continues when people drink water containing copepods harboring the infective Guinea worm larvae.

Once an individual is infected with Guinea worm, there is no effective drug treatment. Instead, once the adult worm begins emerging from the blister, it is removed by wrapping the end of the worm around a small stick and extracting it gradually over a period of weeks, a slow and painful process.

Disease Control and Eradication

Guinea worm disease is expected to be the first infectious disease eradicated from the world without a vaccine or treatment. Efforts to control Guinea worm disease have focused on education about disease transmission and use of low technology methods. Because infection only occurs by drinking contaminated water, education of communities about measures to create safe drinking water can eliminate disease. These include:

- Preventing people with open Guinea worm ulcers from entering waters used for drinking
- Obtaining drinking water from deep, uncontaminated wells
- Filtering drinking water to remove copepods
- Treating unsafe drinking waters with larvicides

Because of eradication efforts beginning in 1986, Guinea worm disease has been reduced worldwide by more than 99.5%. In 1986, there were an estimated 3.5 million cases annually; in 2005, reported cases numbered less than 11,000; in 2010, only 1,700 cases were reported. By 2010 according to WHO, more than 170 countries had been declared free of Guinea worm disease, and only a handful of African countries—including Sudan, Ghana, Ethiopia, and Mali—accounted for the remaining pockets of disease. Through continued cooperative efforts, this debilitating disease can be completely eradicated.

LABORATORY IDENTIFICATION OF PARASITIC INFECTIONS

One useful parasite classification used in the laboratory diagnosis of parasites is based on the organ system in which the parasites are found. The ectoparasites are usually easily seen and identified. However, **endoparasites** living within the host present more of a problem and require special specimen preparation. Two broad categories of endoparasites are:

- Intestinal and atrial parasites
- Blood and tissue parasites

Intestinal and Atrial Parasites

Of the several types of organisms that can infect the intestinal tract (Table 8-6), some are pathogenic and others are **commensal**, that is, they are not harmful.

Atrial Protozoa

Atrial parasites infect body cavities. *Entamoeba gingivalis* is an ameba that can be present in the mouth but is usually considered commensal. *Trichomonas vaginalis* is a flagellate that can infect the urogenital tract.

Intestinal Protozoa

Pathogenic intestinal protozoa include *Entamoeba histolytica, Giardia intestinalis, Cyclospora, Isospora belli*, and *Cryptosporidium. Giardia* is the most common intestinal protozoan pathogen in the United States and is a frequent cause of diarrhea in children in day care centers.

Nonpathogenic protozoa common to the intestinal tract include other *Entamoeba* sp., *Endolimax, Chilomastix*, and *Iodamoeba*.

TABLE 8-6. Examples of pathogenic intestinal parasites

PROTOZOAN GROUP	EXAMPLES
Amebae	*Entamoeba histolytica*
Ciliates	*Balantidium*
Flagellates	*Giardia, Trichomonas*
Apicomplexans	*Cryptosporidium, Isospora, Cyclospora*
HELMINTH GROUP	**EXAMPLES**
Trematodes	*Fasciolopsis*
Cestodes	*Taenia, Dipylidium, Hymenolepis*
Nematodes	*Enterobius, Ascaris*

Intestinal Helminths

The most common helminths are nematodes. These include *Enterobius vermicularis* (pinworm), *Trichuris trichiura* (whipworm), *Ascaris lumbricoides* (large roundworm), and hookworms (*Necator* and *Ancylostoma*). Trematodes found in the intestinal tract include *Fasciolopsis, Fasciola, Heterophyes, Metagonimus*, and *Clonorchis*.

The most common tapeworm infection in the United States is caused by the dwarf tapeworm, *Hymenolepis nana*. Other tapeworms that can infect humans include the beef tapeworm (*Taenia saginata*), the pork tapeworm (*Taenia solium*), the fish tapeworm (*Diphyllobothrium latum*), and the dog tapeworm (*Dipylidium caninum)*. Examples of pathogenic intestinal helminths are listed in Table 8-6.

Detection of Intestinal and Atrial Parasites

Two methods of detecting and identifying intestinal and atrial parasites are morphology and immunological tests.

Parasite Morphology. Microscopic examination of fecal or oral specimens is a valuable tool for identifying intestinal and atrial parasites and is the only method of identification in some cases. Atlases of parasite morphology are indispensable references in the parasitology laboratory.

Intestinal protozoa are identified by the morphology of cysts, **trophozoites**, or oocysts in fecal specimens. Because protozoa are so small, identification of genus and species can be difficult. However, it is very important to distinguish pathogenic protozoa from commensals.

Roundworm infections are diagnosed by identifying **ova** (eggs), larvae, or adults in fecal or perianal specimens. Trematode infections can also be diagnosed by identifying ova in fecal specimens. *Paragonimus* and *Schistosoma* worms inhabit the lungs and blood vessels, respectively, but their eggs are often found in stool or urine (*Schistosoma*). Tapeworms are identified by finding ova or **proglottids** (tapeworm segments) in fecal specimens.

Immunological Tests. Immunological tests have been developed to detect a few intestinal protozoa. These tests are coming into wider use because they have some advantages over traditional microscopic methods. The technician does not need to have morphological expertise to be able to interpret the results of immunoassays. The assays often have high sensitivity. That is, they can detect low levels of antigen, levels that might require microscopic examination of several specimens before the parasite could be visually detected.

Antigen capture immunoassays (modified enzyme immunoassays) are available for detecting some parasite antigens in fecal specimens. An example is the Triage Parasite Panel by Biosite Diagnostics (Figure 8-3). *Entamoeba histolytica, Giardia*, and *Cryptosporidium* antigens can be detected in less than 20 minutes using a single self-contained test cassette that also includes antigen controls for each of the three parasites.

Other immunological tests available include kits that detect serum antibody to *E. histolytica* and fluorescent antibody kits to detect *Giardia* and *Cryptosporidium* in fecal specimens as well as in water supplies.

Blood and Tissue Parasites

Worldwide, parasites of blood and other tissues are a diverse group (Table 8-7). However, only a few blood and tissue parasites are endemic in the United States. The most common blood parasite worldwide is the malarial parasite (*Plasmodium* sp.). Other blood parasites include the trypanosomes, *Babesia*, and the filarial worms.

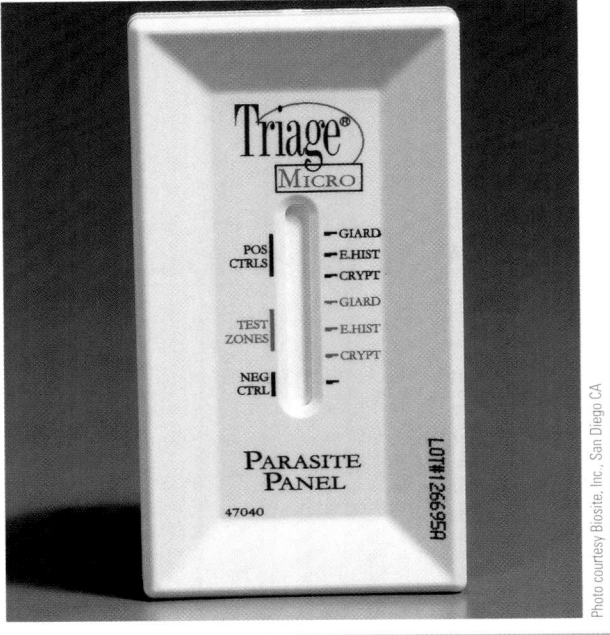

FIGURE 8-3 Biosite Triage® Parasite Panel, a chromatographic immunoassay for detection of *Giardia, Entamoeba* and *Cryptosporidium* antigens in fecal specimens

BLOOD PARASITES	PARASITES OF TISSUES OTHER THAN BLOOD
Plasmodium	Toxoplasma
Babesia	Trichinella
Trypanosoma	Leishmania
Filarial worms	Trypanosoma
	Amebae
	Schistosoma
	Filarial worms

TABLE 8-7. Examples of blood and tissue parasites

Tissue parasites include *Toxoplasma*; free-living and parasitic amebae such as *Naegleria*, *Acanthamoeba*, and *Balamuthia*; *Leishmania*; *Schistosoma*; some filarial worms; microsporidia; trypanosomes; and *Trichinella*.

Pneumocystis jiroveci, an opportunistic pathogen found in the lungs, causes pneumonia in immunocompromised individuals and has been responsible for many deaths of patients with acquired immunodeficiency syndrome (AIDS). *Pneumocystis jiroveci* was formerly called *Pneumocystis carinii* and was considered to be a type of protozoa because it can be identified with stains typically used for protozoan parasites. Although it is now accepted that *Pneumocystis* is a yeast-like fungus some parasitology laboratories continue to provide diagnostic testing for *Pneumocystis*.

Laboratory Detection of Blood Parasites

The specimen required to detect blood and tissue parasites is determined by the location or site of infection and the parasite suspected. Blood parasites are identified by microscopic examination of stained blood smears, described in Lesson 8-4.

Laboratory Detection of Tissue Parasites

Tissue parasites can be identified by microscopic examination of stained biopsy material, aspirates, sputum, skin snips, or immunological tests, such as tests for serum antibody to *Toxoplasma*.

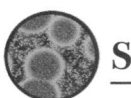 ## SUMMARY

Parasites capable of infecting humans are quite diverse and belong to three major groups—protozoa, helminths, and arthropods. Knowledge of parasite life cycles, geographical distribution, infective stages, and diagnostic stages are all key to understanding, diagnosing, treating, and preventing parasitic infections. In the laboratory, most parasitic infections are diagnosed by finding a parasitic form in a clinical specimen. However, in recent years, immunochemical tests have been developed for some intestinal and tissue parasites.

In the United States, parasites are not frequently observed in clinical specimens. Because of this, many laboratory personnel do not have much experience in parasite identification and specimens for parasite examination are often sent to reference or state public health laboratories.

Clinical laboratory personnel should be familiar with characteristics of common parasitic infections so the appropriate specimens are collected and correctly processed for examination. This greatly increases the chances of discovering parasites in the laboratory examination.

 ## REVIEW QUESTIONS

1. How are parasitic infections usually diagnosed?
2. What are the three major groups of organisms that contain human parasites?
3. How does geography or climate affect the incidence of parasites?
4. What body sites can be infected by parasites?
5. Name three factors that affect the severity of parasitic infections.
6. What are three ways parasitic diseases can be transmitted?
7. Name four methods used to prevent or control parasite infections.
8. Name four groups of protozoan parasites.
9. Name three groups of parasitic helminths.
10. How are intestinal parasitic infections usually diagnosed?
11. Name four parasites that cause foodborne or waterborne infections.
12. How are infections with blood or other tissue parasites usually diagnosed?
13. What is Guinea worm disease? What measures have been used to eradicate the disease?
14. To what group of organisms does *Pneumocystis* belong?
15. Define ameba, arthropod, atrial, cestode, commensal, congenital, cyst, definitive host, ectoparasite, endemic, endoparasite, helminth, host, immunocompromised, intermediate host, larva, mechanical vector, nematode, opportunistic parasite, ova, parasite, pathogenic, primary amebic meningoencephalitis (PAM), proglottid, protozoa, reservoir host, sporozoite, trematode, trophozoite, trypomastigote, and vector.

 ## STUDENT ACTIVITIES

1. Complete the written examination for this lesson.
2. Research a parasitic disease caused by a helminth other than Guinea worm. Report on the parasite's life cycle, transmission, symptoms, diagnostic methods, and recommended course of treatment.

WEB ACTIVITIES

1. Use the Internet to search the CDC or National Institutes of Health (NIH) web sites and find the sections on parasitic diseases. Report on a protozoan intestinal parasite. Include life cycle, diagnostic stage, and infective stage information. Find photographs of the parasite to include in your report.

2. Use the Internet to find the section on the CDC web site that archives the *Morbidity and Mortality Weekly Report.* Find out which parasitic diseases are considered reportable.

3. Use the Internet to find information about the incidence of leishmaniasis in the United States. Discuss the reason(s) for increased findings of parasites in U.S. clinical laboratories in recent years.

4. Use the Internet to find reports of outbreaks of waterborne parasites in the last 15 years. Report on why the outbreaks occurred, which parasites were involved, and how the outbreaks could have been prevented.

5. Use the Internet to find information on human infections with free-living amebae. Report on disease caused, geographical distribution, method of transmission, organ(s) infected, diagnosis, treatment, and prognosis.

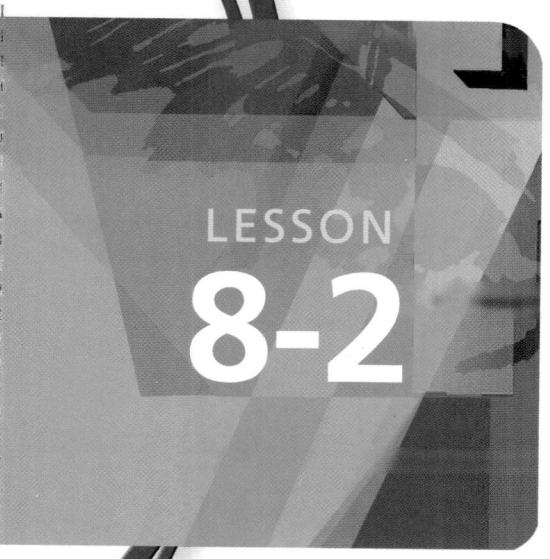

LESSON 8-2

Collecting and Processing Specimens for Parasite Detection

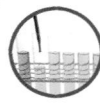

LESSON OBJECTIVES

After studying this lesson, the student will:

- ⊙ Explain the procedure for collecting fecal specimens for parasite examination.
- ⊙ Name two preservatives commonly used for fecal specimens.
- ⊙ Describe transport procedures for fecal specimens.
- ⊙ Demonstrate the preparation of a cellophane tape swab.
- ⊙ Name two nonfecal specimens that can be examined for parasites.
- ⊙ Discuss transmission and detection of enterobiasis.
- ⊙ Discuss how immunological tests are used to detect parasite infections.
- ⊙ Explain how toxoplasmosis is transmitted and how it can be prevented.
- ⊙ Discuss how free-living amebae cause disease in humans.
- ⊙ Explain safety precautions to observe when handling fecal specimens.
- ⊙ Discuss why adhering to quality assessment policies is important to specimen collection and processing procedures.
- ⊙ Define the glossary terms.

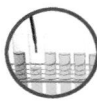

GLOSSARY

ameba (pl. amebae) / a single-celled eukaryotic organism lacking a definite shape and moving by means of pseudopodia; also spelled amoeba (pl. amoebae)

bradyzoite / a slowly multiplying form of coccidian parasite found within tissue cysts and typical of chronic infection with *Toxoplasma gondii*

formalin / a 37% solution of formaldehyde used for fixing and preserving biologic specimens

granulomatous amebic encephalitis (GAE) / rare and usually fatal brain infection caused by *Acanthamoeba* species and usually occurring only in immunocompromised individuals

micrometer / a ruled device for measuring small objects

ocular micrometer / a clear glass disk that fits in the microscope eyepiece, is etched with an arbitrary scale, and is used to measure objects viewed with the microscope; also called ocular reticle

oocyst / the infectious, thick-walled, resistant stage of coccidian parasites, such as *Toxoplasma* and *Cryptosporidium*, which is found in the definitive host of the parasite

pinworm / *Enterobius vermicularis*, a small parasitic nematode; seatworm

primary amebic encephalitis (PAM) / rare and usually fatal central nervous system infection caused by *Naegleria fowleri* amebae

(continues)

proglottid / the tapeworm body segment that contains the male and female reproductive organs

pseudopod/pseudopodium (pl. pseudopods/pseudopodia) / a temporary extension of cytoplasm of certain single-celled organisms such as ameba, that is used for movement and feeding

PVA / polyvinyl alcohol, a preservative used for fecal specimens

tachyzoite / a rapidly multiplying stage in the development of the tissue phase of certain coccidians, as in acute *Toxoplasma gondii* infections

tissue cyst / intracellular cysts located within host tissues and containing organisms in a state of reduced metabolism that can survive and remain infectious for years

trophozoite / the motile feeding stage of protozoan parasites

INTRODUCTION

Tests for parasites are not the most frequently performed laboratory tests. However, large laboratories should have the capability of preparing specimens for examination and detecting and identifying at least the most commonly encountered parasites. For cases in which parasite identification is more complex, the specimen might be sent to a reference laboratory or public health laboratory.

Small laboratories do not usually have the capability of performing the tests for parasites, but the laboratory personnel must be able to instruct patients in the correct procedures for specimen collection. They must also process specimens for parasite examination before the specimens are sent to a reference laboratory. A basic understanding of parasite life cycles is required to be sure the most appropriate specimen is obtained, and thus increase the chances that any parasites present will be discovered.

Two of the most common parasitology laboratory test requests are:

- Tests for fecal examination for ova and parasites (O & P) and
- Blood examination for malarial parasites

The O & P test requires a fecal specimen, and the malarial test requires a fresh blood specimen and freshly made blood smears. Less frequently performed tests include examination of tissues or other body fluids for evidence of parasites.

This lesson describes routine specimen collection and processing to detect intestinal parasites and the procedure for detecting pinworms. Lesson 8-3 describes the procedures for preparing fecal wet mounts and fecal smears for staining, as well as fecal-concentration techniques. The procedure for preparing and staining blood smears for detection of blood parasites is described in Lesson 8-4.

TYPES OF SPECIMENS FOR PARASITE EXAMINATION

Fecal (Stool) Specimens

The fecal specimen is examined when infection with intestinal parasites is suspected. Helminths, amebae, and other intestinal protozoa can be identified during microscopic examination of unstained, stained, and concentrated fecal specimens. Fecal specimens are also used for immunological tests that detect *Giardia*, *Cryptosporidium*, and *Entamoeba histolytica* antigens.

Blood Specimens

Blood is examined when infection with blood parasites such as the malarial parasite, filarial worms, or certain trypanosomes is suspected. Specially prepared and stained blood smears or wet mounts of blood are prepared. Blood to be tested for malaria must be collected at timed intervals. The collection of blood and preparation of blood smears for examination for parasites is described fully in Lesson 8-4.

Specimens for Immunological Tests

Although immunological tests are being developed for many parasites, only a few have widespread use. Kits to detect and differentiate parasitic diarrheal diseases caused by *Cryptosporidium*, *Giardia*, or *Entamoeba histolytica* are used by many laboratories. Fresh fecal specimens are centrifuged and filtered for use in the kits. Parasite antigens in the filtered specimen, if present, are detected using a rapid colorimetric enzyme immunoassay that contains antibodies against specific parasite antigens.

Immunological tests can also be used to detect the presence of anti-parasite antibody in patient serum, as in the test for *Toxoplasma*. In the case of suspected acute infection, paired serum samples (samples collected 2 to 3 weeks apart) are tested for the presence of IgM and IgG, or for a rising antibody titer. Toxoplasmosis is discussed further in Current Topics 2 in this lesson. Immunological tests are also becoming available for other parasites, such as the test for antibody to *Trypanosoma cruzi* used to screen donor blood. Many of the immunological tests to detect antibodies to parasites are still in the research phase or are only available through CDC, public health laboratories, or large reference laboratories.

Other Specimens

Specimens other than blood or stool can be tested or examined for parasites. The type of specimen required depends on which organism(s) are suspected based on the patient's symptoms and medical history. For example:

- Sputum specimens are examined for *Paragonimus*.
- Vaginal secretions are examined for *Trichomonas*.

- Tissue or biopsy specimens, usually processed and stained by the histology laboratory, are examined when *Trichinella* or other tissue parasites are suspected.

- Cerebrospinal fluid (CSF) is examined when certain parasitic protozoa or free-living amebae such as *Naegleria* or *Acanthamoeba* are suspected.

Examples of organisms that can be found in nonfecal specimens are listed in Table 8-8. Specific requirements for collecting, processing, and submitting these specimens for parasite examination should be in each laboratory's standard operating procedure (SOP) manual.

COLLECTING AND PROCESSING FECAL SPECIMENS

Safety Precautions

   Several potential hazards are present when collecting and processing specimens for parasite examination. These include possible exposure to infective parasite cysts, oocysts, eggs, or larvae in stool specimens as well as to pathogens such as intestinal bacteria that can be present in stool and biological fluids. Standard Precautions as well as standard microbiology safety practices must be observed when handling specimens. Standard Precautions must be used even with preserved (fixed) specimens, because some parasite forms can remain viable for weeks after placed in preservative.

Good safety practices include, but are not limited to, wearing fluid-resistant protective clothing and gloves; using biological safety cabinets; decontaminating work surfaces frequently with disinfectant; washing hands before donning gloves, after removing gloves, and any other time hands become soiled; and discarding all sharp objects into a sharps container.

Specimens should be processed in a fume hood to avoid inhaling preservative fumes and to minimize unpleasant odors. All specimens and processing materials should be decontaminated

TABLE 8-8. Examples of organisms found in nonfecal specimens	
TYPE OF SPECIMEN	**POSSIBLE ORGANISMS**
Sputum	*Paragonimus, Ascaris*
Blood	*Plasmodium, Babesia, Trypanosoma*
Cerebrospinal fluid	Amebae, *Toxoplasma, Trypanosoma*
Liver	Amebae, *Leishmania, Schistosoma*
Urine	*Trichomonas, Schistosoma*
Muscle	*Trichinella*
Duodenal aspirates	*Giardia, Isospora*
Vaginal secretions	*Trichomonas*

or sterilized before disposal, in the same manner as bacterial or other biohazardous specimens.

Quality Assessment

  Specimens must be collected and processed according to established laboratory procedures outlined in the laboratory's SOP manual.

- The timing of specimen collection is critical for some tests, such as the pinworm test.

- Specimens must be collected from patients before antiparasite drugs are administered.

- Fecal specimens should not be collected within 7 days after administration of antacids, mineral oil, barium, bismuth, or antidiarrheal medications or within 3 weeks after certain antimicrobial agents.

- Fecal specimens should not be contaminated with soap, water, or urine.

- Specimens must be processed as quickly as possible after collection to ensure that parasite morphology is maintained.

- Microscopic examination of unfixed specimens must be performed within 30 minutes to 1 hour of collection to increase the chance of finding motile forms.

Fecal Specimen Collection

Fecal samples should be collected in a clean, dry, wide-mouth, leakproof container that has a tight-fitting lid. Specimens can be collected in a bedpan and transferred to the container, but the sample *must not* be contaminated with urine, water, soap or disinfectant.

The specimen container must be labeled with the patient's name and the date and time of collection. It is recommended that at least three separate specimens be collected over a period of 3 to 5 days. If amebiasis is suspected, as many as 6 specimens can be required because the organism is often difficult to find.

Specimens should be delivered to the laboratory as soon as possible and should arrive at the laboratory within 2 hours of collection. If specimen transport must be delayed, kits containing vials with preservatives (Figure 8-4) and containers for mailing (Figure 8-5) are available.

Fecal Specimen Processing

Specimens should be processed and examined as soon as possible after arrival at the laboratory. Specimen consistency should be observed and recorded as watery, loose, soft, or formed. In helminth infections, adult worms or tapeworm **proglottids** can sometimes be seen and should be reported. If blood or mucus is present in the fecal sample, portions of these areas should be selected for examination.

It is especially important to process watery or liquid specimens within 30 minutes, because forms such as protozoan **trophozoites** deteriorate rapidly. Specimens of soft

CURRENT TOPICS 1

DISEASES CAUSED BY FREE-LIVING AMEBAE

Amebae are microscopic, single-celled protozoa that have no definite form and move by pseudopodia. Free-living amebae that can cause parasitic infection are most frequently found in soil, freshwater lakes and ponds, tap water, or standing waters such as found in air-conditioning units. Free-living amebae do not frequently cause disease in humans. However,

when humans do acquire an infection with a free-living ameba, it is very serious, is often untreatable, and can be fatal. *Naegleria fowleri,* several species of *Acanthamoeba,* and *Balamuthia mandrillaris* are the most commonly identified free-living amebae that cause disease in humans.

Naegleria infections are rare amebic infections that occur when individuals are swimming and diving in stagnant or warm ponds, a good environment for

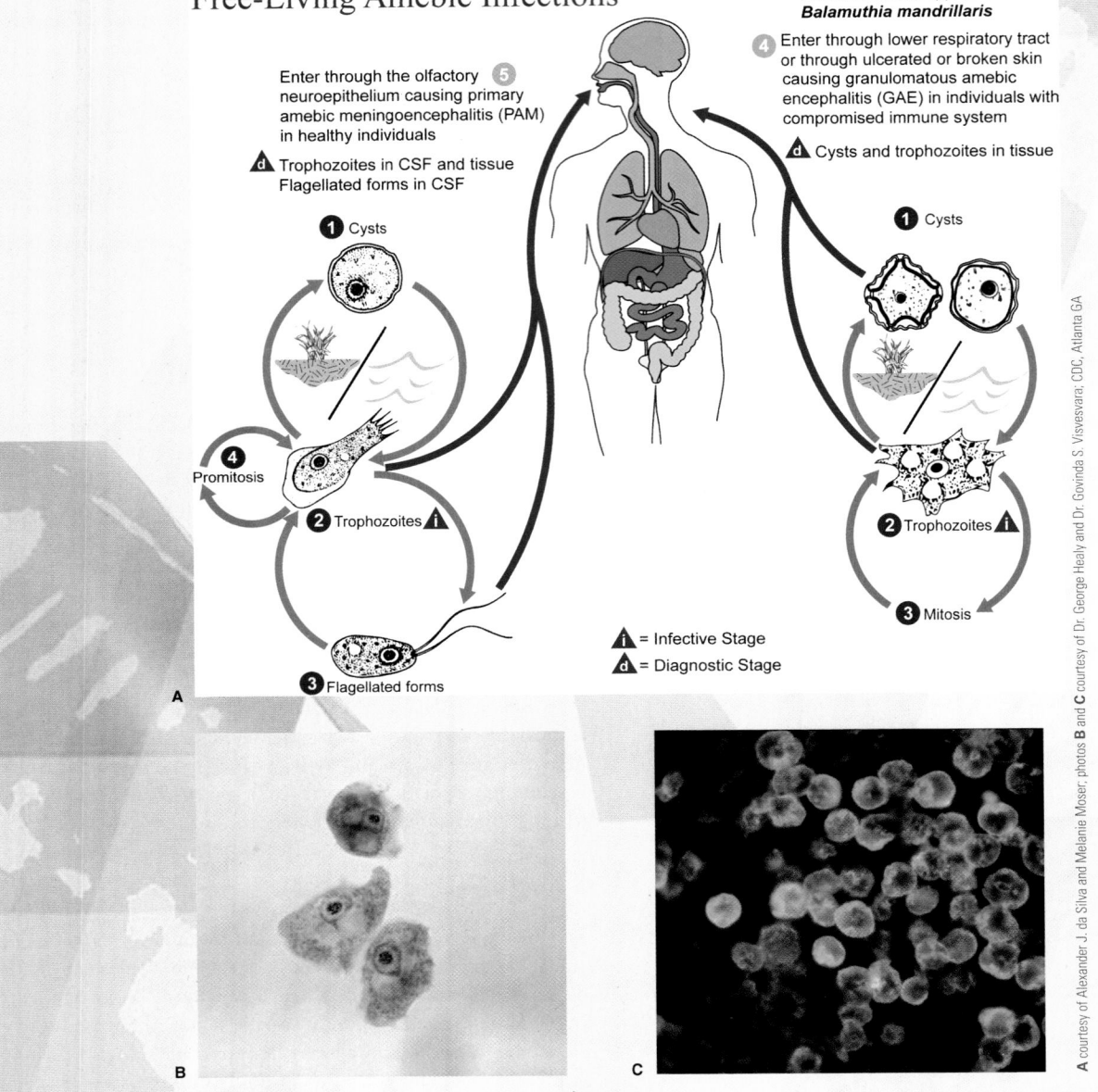

Free-Living Amebic Infections

Enter through the olfactory ⑤ neuroepithelium causing primary amebic meningoencephalitis (PAM) in healthy individuals

🔺d Trophozoites in CSF and tissue
Flagellated forms in CSF

❶ Cysts

❹ Promitosis

❷ Trophozoites 🔺i

❸ Flagellated forms

Acanthamoeba spp. and
Balamuthia mandrillaris

❹ Enter through lower respiratory tract or through ulcerated or broken skin causing granulomatous amebic encephalitis (GAE) in individuals with compromised immune system

🔺d Cysts and trophozoites in tissue

❶ Cysts

❷ Trophozoites 🔺i

❸ Mitosis

🔺i = Infective Stage
🔺d = Diagnostic Stage

A

B

C

A courtesy of Alexander J. da Silva and Melanie Moser; photos **B** and **C** courtesy of Dr. George Healy and Dr. Govinda S. Visvesvara; CDC, Atlanta GA

Free-living amebic infections: (A) life cycle diagram of parasites causing "free-living" amebic infections; (B) typical microscopic appearance of three *Naegleria* trophozoites showing pseudopodia and single nucleus in each cell; (C) lower magnification photomicrograph showing immunofluorescently stained *Naegleria* from a case of primary amebic meningoencephalitis

(Continues)

CURRENT TOPICS 1 (Continued)

the amebae. The organisms penetrate cells lining the nasal cavities, migrate to the brain and cause primary amebic meningoencephalitis (PAM) in otherwise healthy individuals. The disease usually follows an acute course. Amebae rapidly destroy brain tissue, and death can occur in as few as 3 days.

Acanthamoeba and *Balamuthia* are opportunistic amebae, causing infection primarily in immunocompromised individuals. Both can cause granulomatous amebic encephalitis (GAE), which follows a more chronic neurological course than PAM and can progress to death after several weeks. The amebae can enter the host through broken skin or by inhalation or ingestion of the organism.

Acanthamoeba species can also cause skin lesions and has in particular been implicated in corneal infections caused by using amebae-contaminated contact lens solutions. Corneal lesions can occur in healthy individuals because the cornea receives little blood supply and thus can have a low immune response to foreign agents.

Diagnosis of *Naegleria* infections can be made by finding amebae in cerebrospinal fluid (CSF), either by observing a wet mount to detect motile amebae or by examination of a Giemsa-stained or immunofluorescently-stained smear. Typical appearance of the amebic (trophozoite) phase of free-living amebae can be seen in micrograph B. Visible are pseudopodia and one nucleus in each cell.

Diagnosis of *Acanthamoeba* infections can be made by microscopic examination of stained smears from biopsy of skin or cornea. Both trophozoites and cysts can be seen. Immunofluorescent antibody techniques are also used to identify some species. A micrograph showing immunofluorescent staining of *Naegleria* in a case of PAM is shown in micrograph C. In addition, molecular diagnostic techniques have been developed and are being improved.

Most cases of PAM and GAE result in death, although a few have been treated successfully using antifungal drugs or special drug formularies. Rapid diagnosis of the cause of the encephalitis is crucial to a positive outcome. Skin and eye *Acanthamoeba* infections are usually treatable. Eye infections should be diagnosed and treated early to prevent permanent corneal damage.

CURRENT TOPICS 2

TOXOPLASMOSIS

One of the most common human infections worldwide is toxoplasmosis, caused by the protozoa *Toxoplasma gondii*. In the United States, over 20% of the population (more than 60 million people) test positive for *Toxoplasma* antibodies. The two infective forms of *Toxoplasma* are oocysts and tissue cysts.

Life Cycle and Epidemiology

The definitive hosts of *Toxoplasma gondii* are domestic and wild cats. Humans and many other animal species are intermediate hosts. Cats become infected by ingesting *T. gondii* tissue cysts present in meat/animals or by ingesting oocysts. After ingestion, parasites released from the tissue cysts or oocysts invade the epithelial cells of the cat's small intestine, replicate, and form oocysts, which are excreted in the cat feces. One to 5 days after excretion, the oocysts develop to the infective stage (sporulate). *Toxoplasma* oocysts are resistant to disinfectants, freezing, and drying. They can remain viable for months in the environment, but are destroyed by heating to 70° C for 10 minutes.

Humans and other animals become infected by ingesting viable oocysts or tissue cysts. This can occur by:

- Accidentally ingesting viable oocysts from hands or food contaminated with cat feces (such as by touching hand to mouth after cleaning a litter box, gardening, or touching anything that has contacted cat feces)
- Eating contaminated raw or undercooked meat or touching hands to mouth after handling raw meat, especially pork, lamb, or venison. This foodborne transmission accounts for a large portion of U.S. cases and is estimated to be the third leading cause of death resulting from a foodborne organism
- Ingesting water contaminated with *Toxoplasma*
- Transplacental transmission
- Organ transplant or blood transfusion from infected donor (rare occurrence)

(Continues)

CURRENT TOPICS 2 (Continued)

Once the infective form is ingested by an intermediate host, the parasites released, called tachyzoites, invade tissue and form tissue cysts—usually in skeletal muscle, heart muscle, or brain—that can remain for the host's lifetime. In the dormant tissue cysts, the parasites are called bradyzoites. In the healthy individual, tissue cysts are usually few in number and are kept dormant by the host's immune system.

Clinical Symptoms and Complications

Symptoms of toxoplasmosis vary depending on the health and immune competency of the individual. For the healthy population, toxoplasmosis is rather benign. Most people have very few symptoms, and some are not even aware they have an infection. Others experience mild flulike symptoms, with muscle aches and swollen lymph nodes.

For immunocompromised individuals and pregnant women, *Toxoplasma* infection can cause serious complications. *Toxoplasma* can cause brain, eye, and organ damage in patients with human immunodeficiency virus (HIV) infections, transplant patients, or patients undergoing chemotherapy treatments. Inactive infections can be reactivated if the immune system becomes unable to keep the infection dormant and allows tissue cysts to rupture, releasing parasites. Complications develop, such as disseminated disease or toxoplasmic encephalitis, the most frequent severe neurological infection among persons with AIDS in the United States.

Congenital toxoplasmosis can occur in infants born to women who become infected during (or just before) pregnancy. Many infants with congenital toxoplasmosis are born with serious eye or brain damage, including hydrocephaly. The severity of the complications can be reduced by prompt diagnosis and treatment of the mother. Infants can also be born with

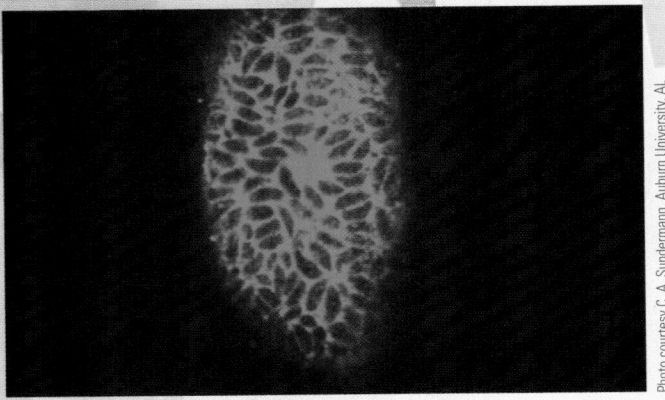

Photo courtesy C. A. Sundermann, Auburn University, AL

Toxoplasma cyst stained with immunofluorescent stain and showing numerous banana-shaped bradyzoites in the cyst

subclinical infection and remain asymptomatic until their teens or twenties, when ocular toxoplasmosis develops causing a condition called *retinochoroiditis*.

Laboratory Diagnosis of Toxoplasmosis

Toxoplasma gondii antibodies appear early in infection and remain detectable for life; the primary method of detecting *T. gondii* infection in immunocompetent individuals is serological testing. Patient serum is tested for IgG and/or IgM *T. gondii*-specific antibodies using immunofluorescent assay (IFA) methods available in various commercial kits. In adults, a rising IgG titer, or presence of IgM in acute serum and IgG in convalescent serum indicates recent or active infection.

In immunocompromised patients, serology results are not always reliable because antibody levels are often low even when infection is present. In these patients, the parasites can be observed in blood, body fluids, bronchoalveolar lavage fluids, and lymph node or other biopsy tissue. If congenital toxoplasmosis is suspected, the newborn should be tested for IgA as well as IgM, because the test for IgA is more sensitive in infants. Molecular methods such as polymerase chain reaction (PCR) can be used for detecting congenital infections *in utero*.

Prevention

Females, before becoming pregnant, and individuals with weakened immune systems should be tested for *Toxoplasma*-specific IgG antibodies. For immunocompetent females, a positive IgG test means that they have been infected sometime previously, have immunity, and generally do not need to worry about passing the infection to the fetus, should they become pregnant. For immunocompromised individuals who test positive, drug therapy might be prescribed to prevent reactivation of infection. A negative test for either of these patient populations indicates that they have not been infected, are most likely susceptible to infection, and should take precautions to avoid exposure to the parasite. These precautions include:

- Wearing gloves when gardening or handling soil
- Washing hands with soap and water after outdoor activities
- Having someone else change the cat's litter box daily, before oocysts have time to become infectious
- Washing hands thoroughly after handling raw meat and before eating or preparing other foods
- Thoroughly washing cutting boards, knives, and all utensils used to prepare raw meat
- Cooking all meat to an internal temperature of 160° F until it is no longer pink or the juices become colorless.

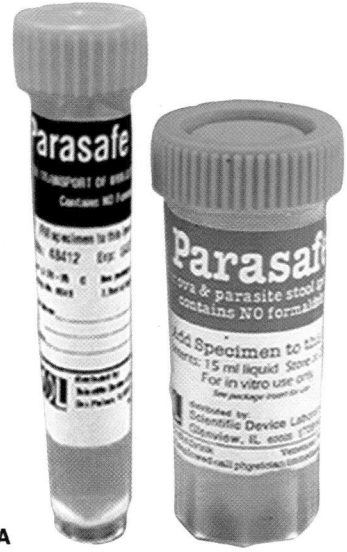

A

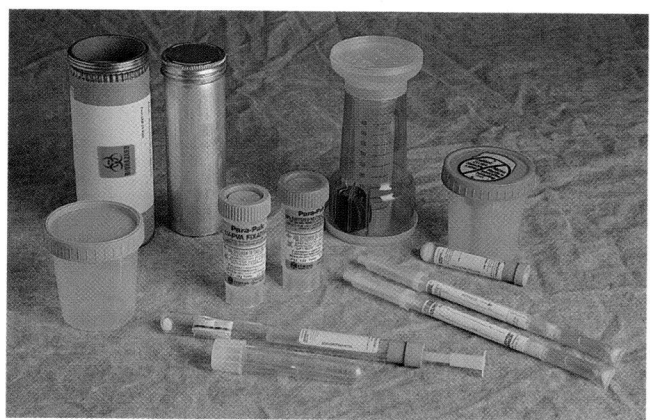

© Cengage Learning 2012

FIGURE 8-5 Containers for transporting or mailing biological specimens

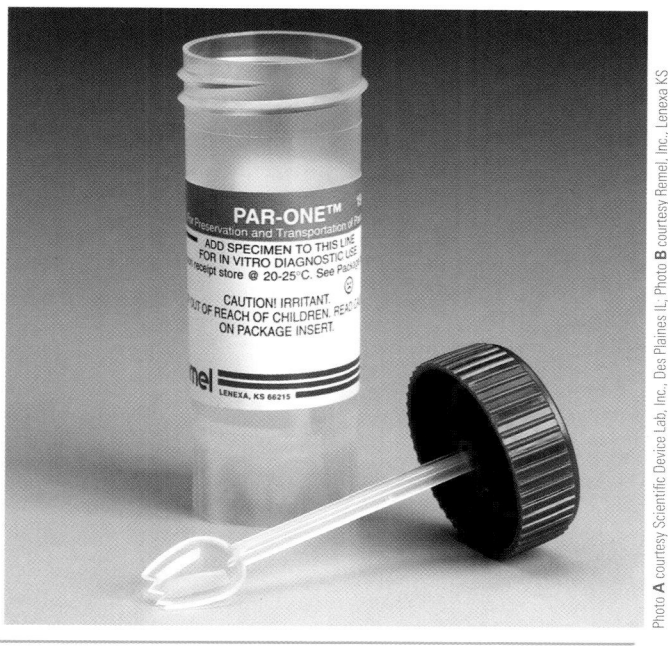

B

Photo **A** courtesy Scientific Device Lab, Inc., Des Plaines IL, Photo **B** courtesy Remel, Inc., Lenexa KS

FIGURE 8-4 Fixative vials for preserving fecal specimens: several types of vials come with spork (shown in B) for measuring correct specimen size

trichrome parasite stain and immunochemical tests. Because formalin and PVA have the disadvantages of producing toxic fumes (formalin) and containing mercury (PVA), much effort has gone into research to find suitable replacements for these preservatives. To meet Occupational Safety and Health Administration (OSHA) requirements for safety and disposal, formalin- and mercury-free, environmentally-safe zinc and copper-based PVA preservatives are now available (Figure 8-4). For most parasites, preservatives such as ParaPak EcoFix (Meridian Diagnostics), Proto-*fix*™ (Alpha-Tec Systems, Inc., Vancouver, WA), and Parasafe® (Scientific Device Laboratory) provide satisfactory morphology, staining, and immunochemical results using just one preservative.

Specimen Transport

Fecal specimens to be mailed or otherwise transported should be placed in fixative and appropriately labeled. The sealed vial should be enclosed in a leakproof container or bag and placed in a labeled mailing/transport carton (Figure 8-5). Transport containers must be approved for biological materials by the United States Postal Service or other carrier.

PROCEDURE: DETECTION OF PINWORM (*ENTEROBIUS*) INFECTION

Enterobiasis

The most common roundworm infection in the United States is enterobiasis, which is caused by infection with *Enterobius vermicularis*, the human **pinworm** or seatworm. This parasite is frequently found in young children in day care centers and elementary schools. It is estimated that, in the United States, approximately 40 million people are infected at any one time. The parasite can be found worldwide in temperate regions.

consistency should be processed within 1 hour. In protozoan infections, trophozoite forms are more likely to be found in the more fluid specimens and cyst forms in the more formed specimens.

Preservation of Fecal Specimens

Portions of the specimen should be preserved for future examination and for staining. Traditionally, two separate preservatives, **formalin** and **PVA** (polyvinyl alcohol) have been used because a single preservative was not available that could preserve parasite morphology and also provide satisfactory results with the

Life Cycle, Transmission, and Clinical Symptoms

Pinworm infections are acquired by ingesting pinworm ova. The ova hatch in the host's small intestine, releasing larvae that mature into tiny adult worms within about 30 days. The adult female pinworm lives in the colon and migrates out of the anus during the night to deposit microscopic-size ova in the perianal folds. The ova are not immediately infective when they are deposited, but become infective within a few hours. The migration of the female worm leads to the characteristic symptom, anal itching, and contributes to re-infection when children scratch and their hands become contaminated. Pinworm infections are also easily spread when ova from contaminated clothing and bedding become airborne and are inhaled and then ingested.

Humans are the only host for *Enterobius* so infections are passed from person to person. Infections are usually self-limiting, lasting about two months, but re-infection is possible. Because the symptoms are mild or nonexistent, there is no effort to eradicate this disease.

Specimen Collection

Pinworm infections are rarely detected by examining fecal specimens. Rather, the specimen for pinworm is a perianal specimen. A simple collection technique is to provide a perianal *paddle* swab for the patient or parent to take home. A typical commercial pinworm collection device consists of a flat plastic paddle or spatula with one sticky surface in a sterile sealed container (Figure 8-6). The perianal specimen is obtained by gently spreading the buttocks apart and pressing the paddle swab several times around the anal opening between 9 PM and midnight or in the early morning before bathing. It can be necessary to collect several specimens over a period of days because the female worm does not migrate every night.

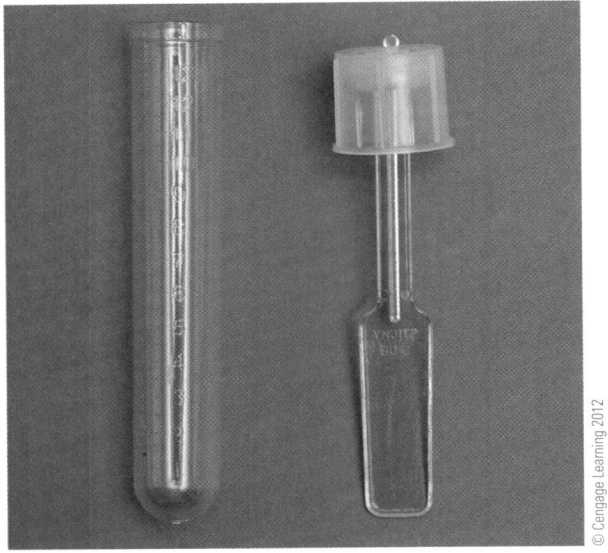

FIGURE 8-6 Commercial perianal "paddle" kit: pinworm ova adhere to surface of paddle

The specimen should be delivered to the laboratory the morning of collection.

If a commercial collection device is not available, a perianal swab can be prepared from clear cellophane tape, a microscope slide, and a wooden tongue depressor. A piece of cellophane tape 4 to 5 inches long is attached to the back of a microscope slide, wrapped around the end of the slide, and smoothed into place on the top of the slide. A paper tab is attached to the free end of the tape for labeling (Figure 8-7). These prepared slides can be stored at 20 to 25° C in a dust-free place for several weeks.

To collect the perianal specimen using the cellophane tape slide, the slide is placed against a tongue depressor, and the tape is lifted and looped over the end of the depressor, sticky side out (Figure 8-7). The sticky surface of the tape is gently pressed against the perianal region several times. The tape is then smoothed back onto the slide, sticky side down, and the slide is delivered to the laboratory for examination.

Microscopic Identification

Because the location and appearance of *Enterobius* ova are so characteristic, identification of pinworm ova is a parasitology procedure that can be performed in most laboratories and usually does not require the services of a reference laboratory. Diagnosis is confirmed by finding *Enterobius* ova in the perianal swab specimen. The paddle (or slide) is microscopically examined for ova using the 10× objective. When examining a cellophane tape preparation, a nontoxic clearing agent (xylene substitute) can be placed under the tape to dissolve the adhesive and make ova identification easier.

Enterobius ova have a characteristic microscopic appearance (Figure 8-8). They are 20 to 32 µm × 50 to 60 µm in size, colorless, flattened on one side, have a thick-walled shell, and contain a developing larva.

 An **ocular micrometer** can be used to measure the size of any ova seen. An ocular micrometer is a clear glass disk that can be fitted into a microscope eyepiece. The disk is etched with an arbitrary scale (Figure 8-9). Before using the ocular micrometer, the scale must be calibrated for each objective by focusing on a stage micrometer, a glass slide placed on the microscope stage that has a scale divided into divisions as small as 10 µm. Use of ocular micrometers is very helpful in parasitology because parasitic forms have definite size characteristics which aid in identification.

Special Precautions

  Pinworm ova remain viable for weeks as do other helminth ova. Infection is easily transmitted when airborne ova are accidentally ingested or when the mouth is touched with contaminated fingers. Therefore, special care must be taken when collecting the specimen, handling the swab, and examining the swab for ova. The microscope must be decontaminated after examining the preparation. The used collection device or slide should be discarded into a biohazard sharps container.

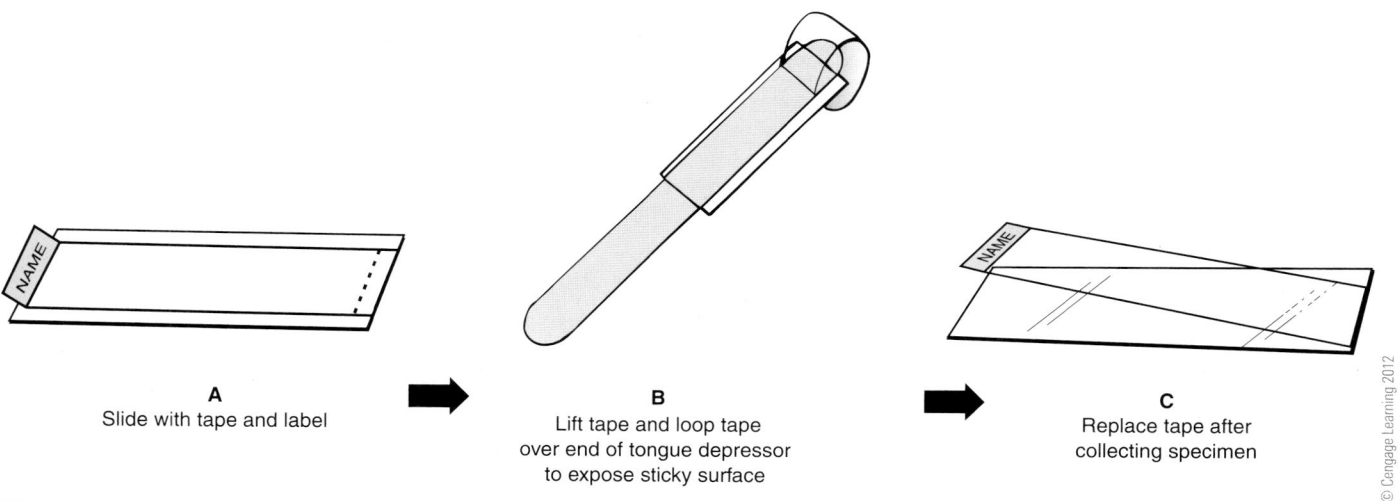

FIGURE 8-7 Technique for preparing a cellophane tape swab

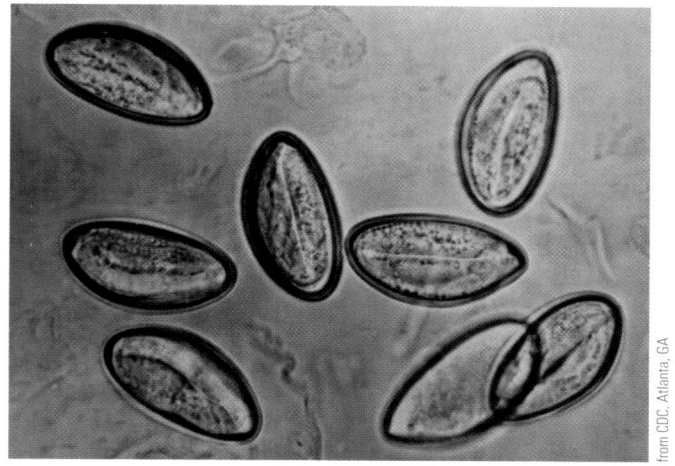

FIGURE 8-8 Microscopic appearance of *Enterobius vermicularis* ova from cellophane tape prep

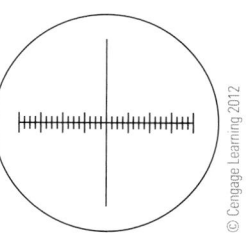

FIGURE 8-9 Ocular micrometer scale

CRITICAL THINKING

Jan visited her nurse practitioner and told her she had just found out she was pregnant by using an over-the-counter pregnancy test. Jan said she had an indoor cat for about five years, but had heard that cats were a risk to pregnant women. She asked her nurse practitioner for advice.

1. Advise Janet to immediately get rid of her cat.
2. Advise Janet to put her cat outside and not allow it in the house until the pregnancy is over.
3. Perform a serological test for *Toxoplasma* antibodies on Janet.
4. Perform a serological test for *Toxoplasma* antibodies on the cat.
5. Examine the cat feces for parasites.

Of the following choices, which is the most appropriate action to recommend? Explain your answer and explain why you did not select the remaining choices.

SAFETY REMINDERS

- Review Safety Precautions section before performing procedure.
- Observe Standard Precautions.
- Wear appropriate PPE.
- Avoid skin contact with preservatives and inhalation of fumes.
- Treat preserved specimens as if infectious.
- Dispose of specimens appropriately.

PROCEDURAL REMINDERS

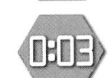
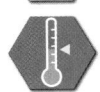

- Review Quality Assessment section before performing procedure.
- Follow procedures in SOP manual.
- Collect specimens at correct time intervals.
- Process specimens promptly.
- Measure ova using ocular micrometer.

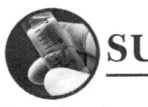

SUMMARY

Examinations of stool, blood, tissues, and other biological specimens are essential to the diagnosis of parasitic infections. Successful detection of parasites depends on having properly collected and prepared specimens. Although parasite examination is often performed in a reference laboratory, the local laboratory must provide instructions for specimen collection, process the specimens, and prepare them for transport. Established procedures for specimen collection and processing will be included in the SOP manual and must be carefully followed to ensure that specimens meet criteria for acceptability. Standard Precautions must be used when handling all specimens in case infective parasite forms or other infectious agents are present.

Some tests for parasites can be easily performed in local laboratories. The pinworm test is one such test because the distinguishing characteristics of pinworm ova and the symptoms of pinworm infection make it easily identified and diagnosed. Tests to detect antigens of intestinal protozoa that cause diarrheal disease such as *Cryptosporidium, Giardia,* and *Entamoeba histolytica,* are available as rapid enzyme immunoassay kits. Tests for *Toxoplasma* based on the detection of anti-toxoplasma antibodies in patient serum are, in general, more complex to interpret and should be performed by personnel experienced in testing for toxoplasmosis. Tissue specimens (other than blood) for parasite examination are usually processed by a histology laboratory.

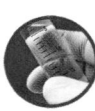

REVIEW QUESTIONS

1. Explain the factors that must be considered for correct collection of fecal specimens.
2. Which type of fecal specimen must be processed quickly? Why?
3. What terms are used to describe the consistency of fecal specimens?
4. What safety precautions must be observed when handling and processing fecal specimens? Why?
5. What characteristics are required of a preservative that is to be used with fecal specimens?
6. What parasite is best detected from a perianal swab?
7. How are commercially available sticky paddles used to collect perianal specimens?
8. Explain how to prepare and use a cellophane tape swab.
9. What specimens other than fecal specimens are examined for parasites?
10. Name three parasites found in nonfecal specimens.
11. Explain why the timing of specimen collection and rapid processing of the specimen can be important to recovery of the parasite.
12. What free-living amebae can cause disease in humans? How do individuals become infected with free-living amebae?
13. How are pinworm infections transmitted? How are they diagnosed?
14. What is the scientific name of the pinworm? To what parasite category does it belong?
15. How is *Toxoplasma* transmitted to humans? How is transmission prevented?
16. Define ameba, bradyzoite, formalin, granulomatous amebic encephalitis (GAE), micrometer, ocular micrometer, pinworm, primary amebic meningoencephalitis (PAM), proglottid, pseudopod, PVA, tachyzoite, tissue cyst, and trophozoite.

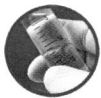

STUDENT ACTIVITIES

1. Complete the written examination for this lesson.
2. Practice instructing a patient to collect a fecal specimen for parasite examination as outlined in the Student Performance Guide.
3. Practice preparing a perianal swab (cellophane tape swab) as outlined in the Student Performance Guide.

4. Practice instructing a patient to collect a perianal specimen using a paddle or slide preparation as outlined in the Student Performance Guide.

5. Practice processing fecal specimens for parasite examination as outlined in the Student Performance guide.

6. Prepare a card instructing patients how to collect a fecal specimen.

7. Prepare a card instructing patients how to collect a perianal specimen for pinworm.

8. Optional: If ocular micrometer and stage micrometer are available, practice calibrating the ocular micrometer for each objective. Measure several objects using different objectives and compare the measurements.

WEB ACTIVITIES

1. Use the Internet to find distributors of parasitology supplies. Report on preservatives that are used in the collection vials.

2. Use the Internet to find information about the preferred treatment for enterobiasis.

3. Use the Internet to find information about the treatment for toxoplasmosis.

4. Use the Internet to research and report on one of the following parasites: *Paragonimus*, *Trichinella*, *Trichomonas*, or *Entamoeba histolytica*. Include life cycle, method of infection, diagnostic procedure, and treatment in your report. Find a photograph of the diagnostic stage of the organism to include in your report. Report on recently documented cases.

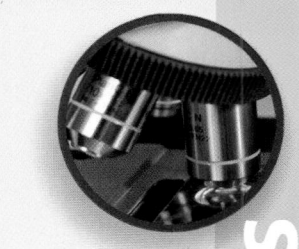

LESSON 8-2
Collecting and Processing Specimens for Parasite Detection

Name _____ Date _____

INSTRUCTIONS

1. Practice giving instructions or practice the procedures for collecting and preserving fecal specimens for parasite examination, following the step-by-step procedure.

2. Practice preparing a cellophane tape slide and instructing a patient to collect a perianal specimen using a pinworm paddle or cellophane tape slide following the step-by-step procedure.

3. Demonstrate these procedures satisfactorily for the instructor, using the Student Performance Guide. Your instructor will explain the procedures for evaluating and grading your performance. Your performance may be given a number grade, letter grade, or satisfactory (S) or unsatisfactory (U) depending on course or institutional policy.

NOTE: Consult product package inserts, manufacturer's instructions, and procedure manual for specific instructions for the procedure being performed.

MATERIALS AND EQUIPMENT

- gloves
- hand antiseptic
- full face shield (or equivalent PPE)
- fume hood (recommended) or biological safety cabinet (optional)
- microscope
- ocular micrometer (optional)
- disposable applicator sticks
- fecal collection containers with lids
- fecal preservative vials (environmentally safe brand)
- leakproof transport containers
- waterproof marker
- fecal specimens (students can bring pet specimens for practice)
- commercial perianal paddle swabs
- materials for preparing cellophane tape swabs
  - microscope slides with beveled edges
  - clear (not frosted) cellophane tape
  - wooden or plastic tongue depressors
- digital images, other visuals, and prepared microscope slides of *Enterobius* ova
- atlas of parasite morphology containing illustrations of *Enterobius* ova
- paper towels
- surface disinfectant (such as 10% chlorine bleach)
- biohazard container
- sharps container

PROCEDURE

Record in the comment section any problems encountered while practicing the procedure (or have a fellow student or the instructor evaluate your performance).

S = Satisfactory
U = Unsatisfactory

You must:	S	U	Evaluation/Comments
1. Instruct a patient in the procedure for collecting a fecal specimen (steps 1a and 1b):			

(Continues)

© 2012 Delmar, Cengage Learning. Permission to reproduce for clinical use granted.

843

You must:	S	U	Evaluation/Comments

a. Give patient a lidded fecal specimen container, label, and transport container
b. Explain the fecal collection procedure to the patient, emphasizing the following precautions:
   1. Specimen must not be contaminated with urine or water
   2. Outer surface of specimen container must not be contaminated
   3. Container must be labeled with the patient's name, date, and the time of collection
   4. Labeled specimen container must be placed in outer transport container
   5. Unpreserved specimens must be transported to a laboratory immediately following collection (within 2 hours)
   6. Specimens should not be collected until at least 7 days after ingesting interfering substances such as mineral oil laxatives, barium or radiopaque contrast media, antimicrobial or antidiarrheal medications			

2. Preserve a fecal specimen (steps 2a through 2n)
  a. Wash hands with disinfectant and put on gloves and face protection. Work in a fume hood or biological safety cabinet
  b. Obtain a fecal specimen, preservative vial, and transport container. Check specimen label to be sure required patient information is present (name, date, time of collection)
  c. Open container and observe consistency of specimen. Record as watery, loose, soft, or formed
  d. Use applicator in cap of preservative vial or disposable applicator to obtain a small portion of specimen
  e. Add specimen to the *fill* line on the preservative vial, or add amount of specimen equal to approximately one-third the volume of the preservative in vial
  f. Mix specimen with preservative thoroughly using applicator
  g. Replace cap on vial and tighten
  h. Discard used applicator (if applicable) into biohazard container
  i. Label vial with patient information
  j. Insert labeled vial into transport container, seal container, and label
  k. Discard remaining specimen into biohazard container
  l. Disinfect work area with disinfectant
  m. Remove gloves and discard into biohazard container
  n. Wash hands with antiseptic			

© 2012 Delmar, Cengage Learning. Permission to reproduce for clinical use granted.

You must:	S	U	Evaluation/Comments

3. Prepare a cellophane tape slide following steps 3a through 3e. (If materials are not available, skip to step 4.)
   a. Obtain clear cellophane tape, clean microscope slide, and paper tab
   b. Attach a 4- to 5-inch section of tape to one end of the back of the slide
   c. Bring the tape over the end of the slide and smooth the tape down over top surface of the slide, leaving a small portion of tape free at the end (see Figure 8-7)
   d. Attach a small paper tab to the free end of the tape for use as a label and lifting tab
   e. Store the slide in a cool, dust-free location			

4. Explain how to collect a pinworm specimen using a commercial pinworm paddle following steps 4a through 4e. (If commercial paddle is not available, skip to step 5.)
Instruct patient (or parent) to:
   a. Wash hands and put on gloves
   b. Remove paddle from sterile container
   c. Obtain specimen by gently touching the sticky surface of the swab/paddle to the perianal region several times upon first arising in the morning and before bathing
   d. Return the swab to its container being careful to avoid touching the sticky swab, and seal the container
   e. Label container with name, date, and time and transport to the laboratory			

5. Practice instructing and demonstrating to a patient (or parent) how to collect a pinworm specimen using a cellophane tape slide following steps 5a through 5j. (If cellophane tape slide is not available, skip to step 6.)
Instruct patient (or parent) to:
   a. Wash hands and put on gloves
   b. Obtain cellophane tape slide, tongue depressor, and transport container
   c. Label tab on slide with patient information
   d. Place slide against tongue depressor near the end, tape side up
   e. Lift the cellophane tape and form a loop around the end of the tongue depressor, sticky side of tape to the outside (see Figure 8-7)
   f. Obtain specimen by gently touching the sticky surface of the tape to the perianal region several times upon first arising in the morning and before bathing
   g. Lift the tape from the tongue depressor carefully and smooth the sticky side back down onto the microscope slide, being careful not to touch the sticky surface			

(Continues)

© 2012 Delmar, Cengage Learning. Permission to reproduce for clinical use granted.

You must:	S	U	Evaluation/Comments
h. Place slide in transport container and seal i. Remove and discard gloves and wash hands j. Label transport container with name, date, and time and arrange for transport to the laboratory			
6. If available, practice identifying *Enterobius* ova by examining prepared microscope slides using the 10× objective (Figure 8-8). Make several drawings of the ova seen; if an ocular micrometer is available, measure length and width of five ova			
7. Practice the procedure for microscopic examination of the pinworm swab/slide following steps 7a–7e a. Wash hands with antiseptic and put on gloves b. Place the pinworm paddle on the microscope stage, sticky side up and scan the paddle area using the 10× objective; discard paddle into biohazard container after observations c. Place the cellophane tape slide on the microscope stage and demonstrate how to observe for ova using the low-power (10×) objective d. Discard used slide into sharps container e. Disinfect microscope stage with surface disinfectant			
8. Return supplies and equipment to storage			
9. Wipe work area with disinfectant			
10. Remove gloves and discard into biohazard container			
11. Wash hands with antiseptic			

Instructor/Evaluator Comments:

Instructor/Evaluator _____ Date _____

© 2012 Delmar, Cengage Learning. Permission to reproduce for clinical use granted.

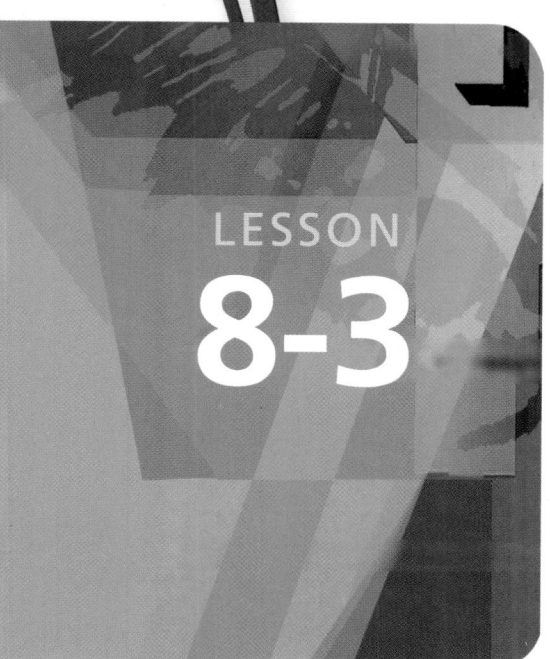

Microscopic Methods of Detecting Intestinal Parasites

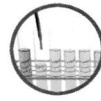

LESSON OBJECTIVES

After studying this lesson, the student will:

⊙ Name three types of preparations used for the microscopic examination of fecal specimens.

⊙ Explain how to prepare saline and iodine wet mounts for microscopic examination.

⊙ Explain the use of flotation and sedimentation procedures to concentrate fecal specimens.

⊙ Prepare fecal smears from fresh or fixed fecal specimens.

⊙ Discuss giardiasis, including modes of transmission and methods of diagnosis.

⊙ List safety precautions to be observed when preparing fecal specimens for microscopic examinations.

⊙ Discuss why adherence to quality assessment policies is important when preparing fecal specimens for microscopic examination.

⊙ Define the glossary terms.

GLOSSARY

trichrome stain / a stain commonly used to identify parasites in fecal smears

INTRODUCTION

The majority of parasitic infections are diagnosed by the microscopic identification of the parasite in blood, tissue, or fecal specimens. Much experience is required to become expert in parasite identification.

This lesson describes methods of preparing fecal specimens for microscopic parasite examination. The procedures for examining blood for parasites are described in Lesson 8-4. The preparation of tissues for parasite examination is usually performed in the histology laboratory, where tissues are fixed, sectioned, and stained with special stains for parasite detection.

MICROSCOPIC EXAMINATION OF FECAL SPECIMENS

The routine fecal specimen examination for parasites includes three types of preparations for microscopic examination:

● Direct wet mounts from fresh or fixed specimens

● Wet mounts of concentrated specimens

● Stained fecal smears

A schematic illustrating how to prepare fecal specimens for microscopic examination is shown in Figure 8-10.

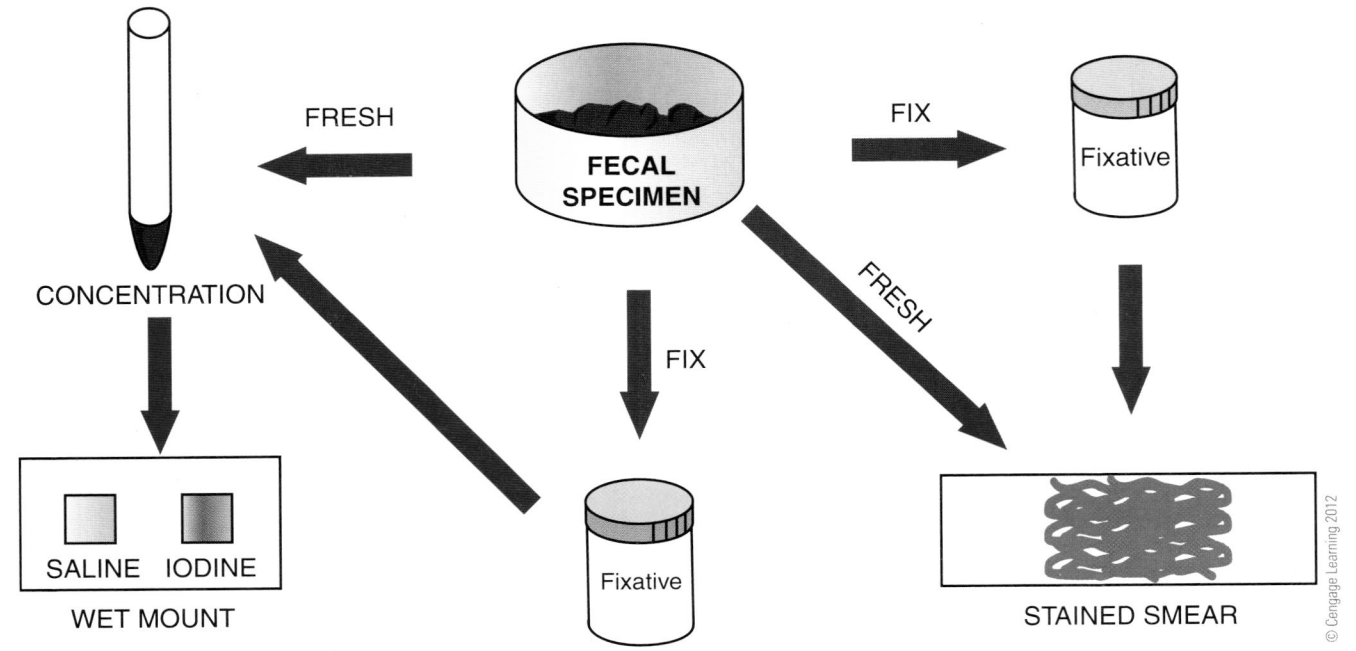

FIGURE 8-10 Schematic for processing fecal specimens for microscopic examination of wet mounts, fecal concentrates, and stained fecal smears

Safety Precautions

   Preparing fecal specimens for microscopy exposes the technician to biological and chemical hazards. Standard Precautions must be followed when handling fecal specimens. Even after fixative is added, specimens are still potentially infectious, because some parasites (particularly helminth eggs and protozoan cysts) are not immediately killed by fixatives. Procedures that use fixatives and volatile chemicals should be performed in a fume hood to eliminate the possibility of inhaling fumes. Appropriate personal protective equipment (PPE), including chemical-resistant gloves, must be worn to prevent exposing skin to the fixatives. Specimens and chemicals must be discarded following each laboratory's written procedure. Centrifuge safety rules must be followed when performing fecal concentration techniques. The rotor load must be balanced. The centrifuge lid must remain closed until the rotor has completely stopped.

Quality Assessment

   The laboratory standard operating procedure (SOP) manual and manufacturer's instructions must be carefully followed when preparing fecal specimens for examination. Specimens must be processed promptly to prevent deterioration of any viable organisms in the specimen. Reagents should not be interchanged between fecal concentration kits or diagnostic kits. Reagent containers must remain tightly capped when not in use to prevent evaporation or changes in specific gravity. Centrifuge speed should be checked and recorded at designated intervals using a tachometer. Timing requirements of concentration techniques must be followed.

Wet Mounts

Wet mounts (direct mounts) can be prepared from fresh or preserved fecal specimens, but fresh specimens are preferred. The two solutions used to prepare wet mounts are physiological saline and iodine. A weak iodine solution such as Lugol's, D'Antoni's, or Dobell and O'Connor's solutions must be used. These are specifically formulated for parasite identification; Gram's iodine is too concentrated for parasite identification.

Preparing Wet Mounts

Wet mounts are prepared by mixing a small amount of fresh or fixed stool specimen with a drop of saline on one end of a 2- × 3-inch microscope slide (Figure 8-11). A similar-sized portion of specimen is mixed with a drop of iodine solution on the other end of the slide and a coverglass is placed over each mixture. If desired, the coverglass edges can be sealed with petroleum jelly to retard drying. The preparations should be thin enough to read newsprint through the specimen when the slide is placed on newspaper (Figure 8-11).

Examining Wet Mounts

Both saline and iodine wet mount preparations should be examined for ova and larvae using the 10× or 20× objective and for protozoan forms using the 40× (high-power) objective. Saline wet mounts are particularly useful to aid in finding motile protozoan trophozoites (trophs) in *fresh* specimens. Observing motility is helpful, because preserved trophozoites are very small and lack many distinguishing characteristics. Protozoan trophozoites can be easily overlooked by the microscopist in the iodine wet mount because the iodine kills the trophozoite.

Protozoan cysts and helminth ova and larva can be detected in wet mounts from fixed specimens. Iodine stains cysts and nuclei, as well as most helminth ova. Helminth ova retain better morphology in the saline mount; protozoan cysts have better morphology in iodine. An ocular micrometer can be used to measure the size of any organisms or structures seen.

Concentration Techniques for Fecal Specimens

Concentration techniques are used to increase the likelihood of detecting parasites by concentrating the parasite forms and separating parasites from some of the fecal debris, making the parasites easier to see. Fresh or preserved specimens can be concentrated by *sedimentation* or *flotation* techniques. However, trophozoites are not recovered using concentration techniques because they cannot withstand the specific gravity of the concentration solutions.

Sedimentation Techniques

Sedimentation techniques use solutions of lower specific gravity (sp. gr.) than the sp. gr. of the parasites, causing the parasites to collect in the sediment when the specimen is centrifuged. Parasites such as helminth ova and larvae and protozoan oocysts can be detected. In the sedimentation technique, the fecal specimen is filtered, washed by centrifugation, and then mixed with ethyl acetate. The mixture is centrifuged, the top layers of supernatant are removed, and the sediment in the bottom of the tube is used to prepare saline and iodine wet mounts for microscopic examination (Figures 8-11 and 8-12).

The formalin-ethyl acetate sedimentation method has been modified for use in several commercially available fecal concentrator kits. Some commercial kits are Para-Pak CON-trate by Meridian Bioscience, Fecal Concentrator II by Remel, CONSED by Alpha-Tec Systems, Inc. (Vancouver, WA), and Parasep by Diasys Corporation. These disposable kits filter and concentrate fecal specimens, using modified sedimentation techniques. Some kits are designed as completely closed systems, in which the concentrator tube fits onto the preservative vial and all steps take place within the closed system. This minimizes exposure of the technician to the specimen.

Flotation Techniques

Flotation techniques use solutions of high sp. gr. to cause the less dense parasitic forms to float to the solution's top while heavier fecal debris settles to the bottom (Figure 8-12). Flotation methods give cleaner concentrates than sedimentation methods, but some helminth eggs become distorted and difficult to recognize. Flotation methods are useful for isolating protozoan cysts and oocysts.

Two solutions used for flotation are zinc sulfate ($ZnSO_4$) and Sheather's sucrose solution, which is particularly useful for *Cryptosporidium* oocysts and *Giardia* cysts. In flotation techniques, the fecal specimen is filtered, washed by centrifugation, and mixed with a solution such as zinc sulfate (sp. gr. 1.18) or Sheather's solution (sp. gr. greater than 1.2). It is then either allowed to sit, giving parasite forms time to rise to the top of the solution, or centrifuged to accelerate flotation. The fluid surface is collected using a loop or coverglass, and wet mounts are prepared for microscopic examination.

Fecal Smears

Smears should be prepared from all fecal specimens. The smears can be made from fresh or fixed specimens.

Preparing Fecal Smears

Smears from modified polyvinyl alcohol (PVA)-fixed specimens are prepared by removing a small portion of well-mixed specimen and spreading thinly on a microscope slide. A wooden applicator stick can be used to roll or dab the specimen on the slide, keeping the specimen layer very thin (Figure 8-13). The smear should extend from the top edge to the bottom edge of the slide (Figure 8-14). Smears should dry for at least 4 hours (or overnight) at 35° C before staining. Smears from fresh specimens are prepared similarly. A portion of the specimen is spread over a large area of the slide. Smears of fresh specimens must be placed in modified-PVA fixative *before* they are allowed to dry. Smears can remain in fixative several days. After fixation and drying, the smears can be stained.

Staining Fecal Smears

Stained smears are particularly important for positive identification of protozoan parasites. Most laboratories use a modification of the **trichrome stain**, which is both relatively easy to perform and gives consistent results. Trichrome-stained protozoa are blue-green to purple with red nuclei; helminths are purple.

© Cengage Learning 2012

FIGURE 8-11 Wet mounts of fecal material for microscopic examination: density of saline and iodine wet mounts is checked by placing slide over newsprint

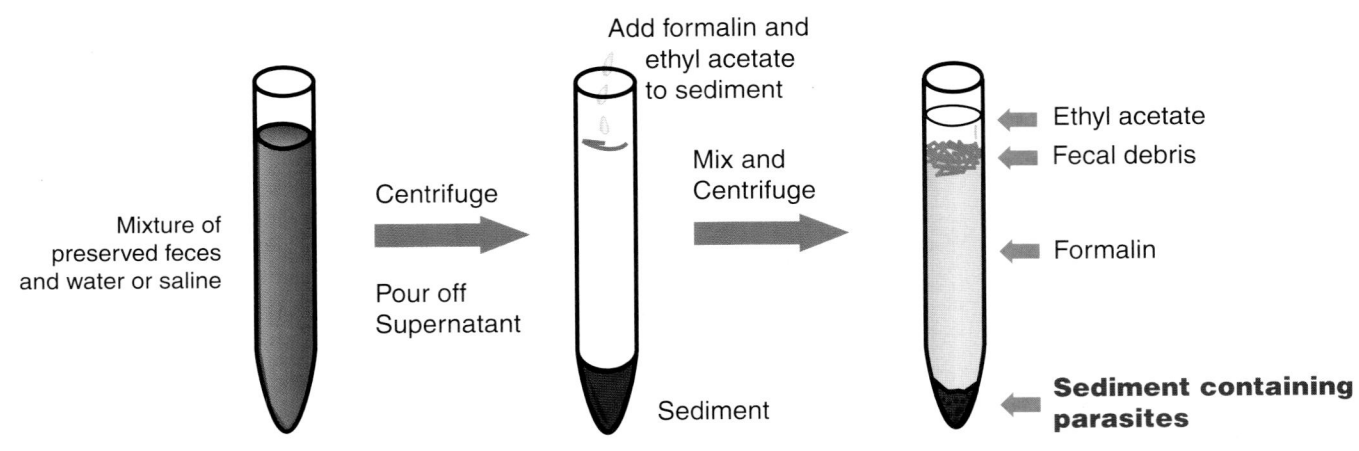

SEDIMENTATION

Mixture of preserved feces and water or saline

Centrifuge

Pour off Supernatant

Add formalin and ethyl acetate to sediment

Mix and Centrifuge

Sediment

Ethyl acetate
Fecal debris
Formalin
Sediment containing parasites

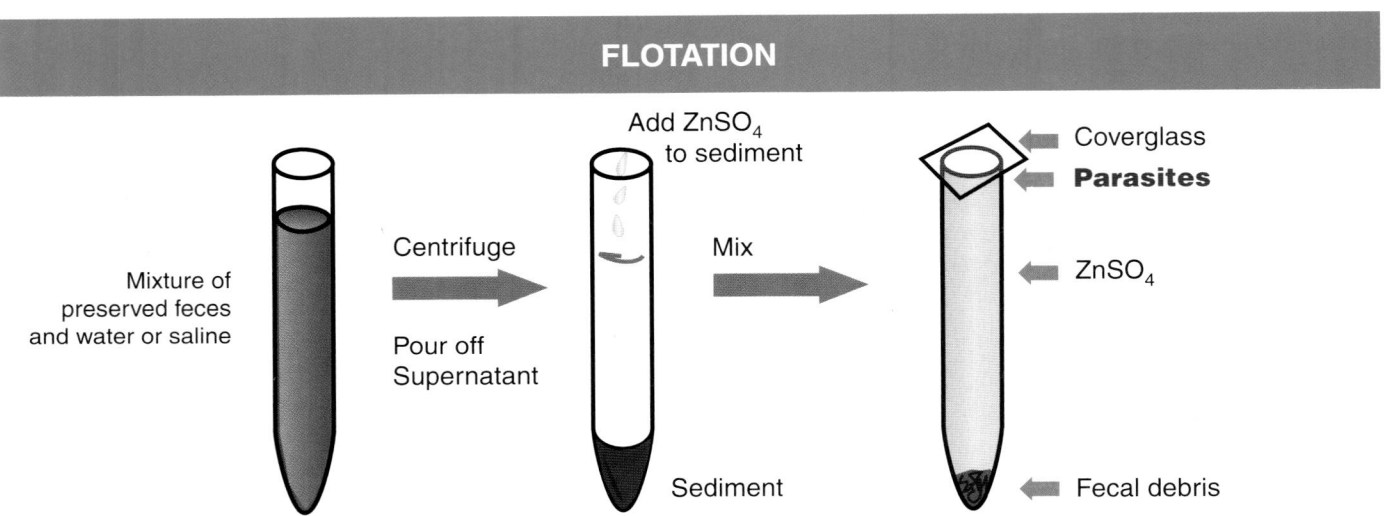

FLOTATION

Mixture of preserved feces and water or saline

Centrifuge

Pour off Supernatant

Add ZnSO$_4$ to sediment

Mix

Sediment

Coverglass
Parasites
ZnSO$_4$
Fecal debris

FIGURE 8-12 Fecal concentration methods: sedimentation (top) and flotation (bottom)

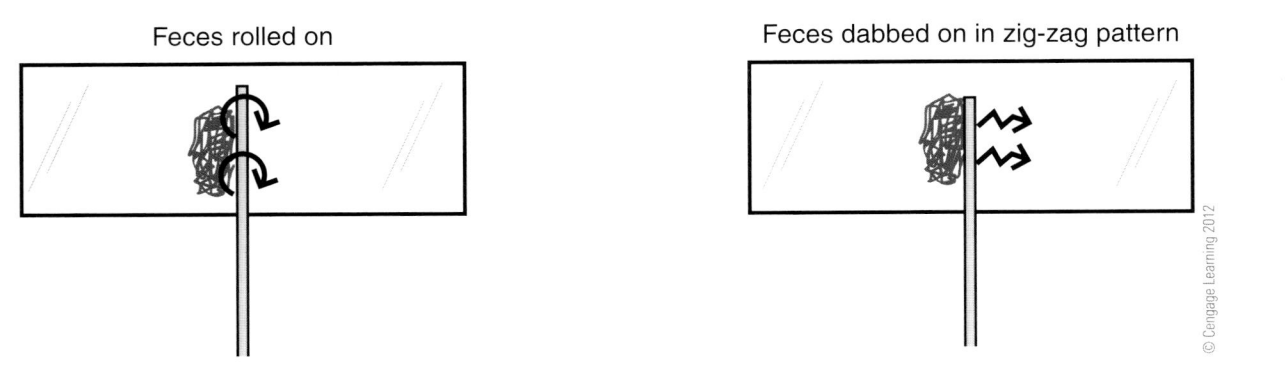

Feces rolled on

Feces dabbed on in zig-zag pattern

FIGURE 8-13 Two methods of preparing fecal smears

© Cengage Learning 2012

Immunofluorescent stains or modified acid-fast stains are used to identify *Cryptosporidium*, which do not stain reliably with trichrome.

Staining techniques for fecal specimens are time-consuming. Most laboratories prepare the smears when processing the specimens and save the smears to stain in a batch. For this reason, final laboratory ova and parasites (O & P) reports are often not available until several days after the specimen is received.

Organisms Seen in Fecal Specimens

Intestinal protozoa are identified by the morphology of trophozoites, cysts or oocysts in fecal specimens. Pathogenic

intestinal protozoa include *Entamoeba histolytica, Dientamoeba fragilis, Giardia intestinalis, Balantidium coli, Isospora belli, Cryptosporidium, Cyclospora*, and possibly *Blastocystis hominis*. Nonpathogenic intestinal protozoa include other *Entamoeba* sp., *Endolimax, Chilomastix*, and *Iodamoeba*.

Helminths are identified by finding ova, larvae, or adults in fecal specimens. Any helminth found in a fecal specimen is considered of clinical importance.

Figures 8-15, 8-16, and 8-17 contain diagrams of amebic, flagellate, ciliate, apicomplexan, and helminth forms of the more common human parasites. More information on these parasites can be found in Lesson 8-1 and textbooks of clinical parasitology.

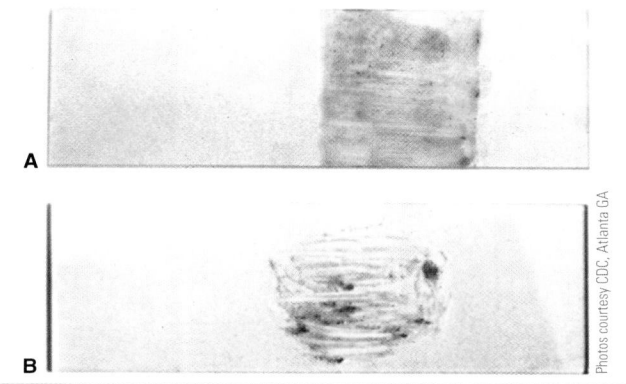

Photos courtesy CDC, Atlanta GA

FIGURE 8-14 Fecal smears of correct thickness ready to be stained: (A) smear from PVA-fixed specimen and (B) smear from unfixed specimen

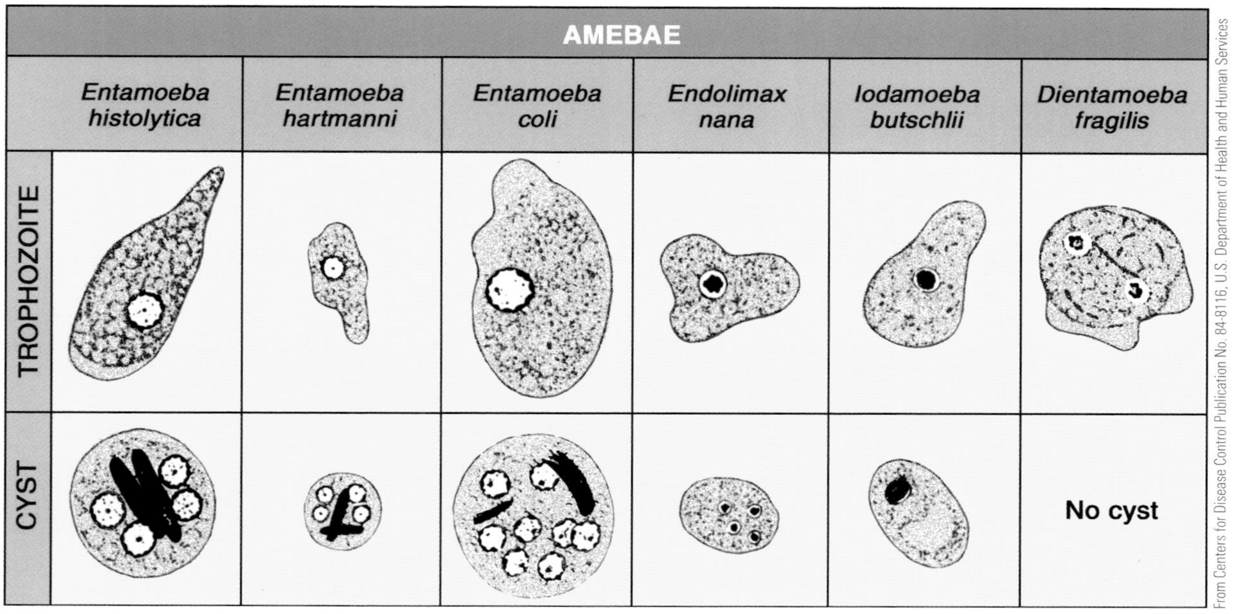

AMEBAE					
Entamoeba histolytica	*Entamoeba hartmanni*	*Entamoeba coli*	*Endolimax nana*	*Iodamoeba butschlii*	*Dientamoeba fragilis*
TROPHOZOITE					
CYST					No cyst

From Centers for Disease Control Publication No. 84-8116, U.S. Department of Health and Human Services

FIGURE 8-15 Intestinal amebae (except for *Dientamoeba,* which is a flagellate)

From Centers for Disease Control Publication No. 84-8116, U.S. Department of Health and Human Services

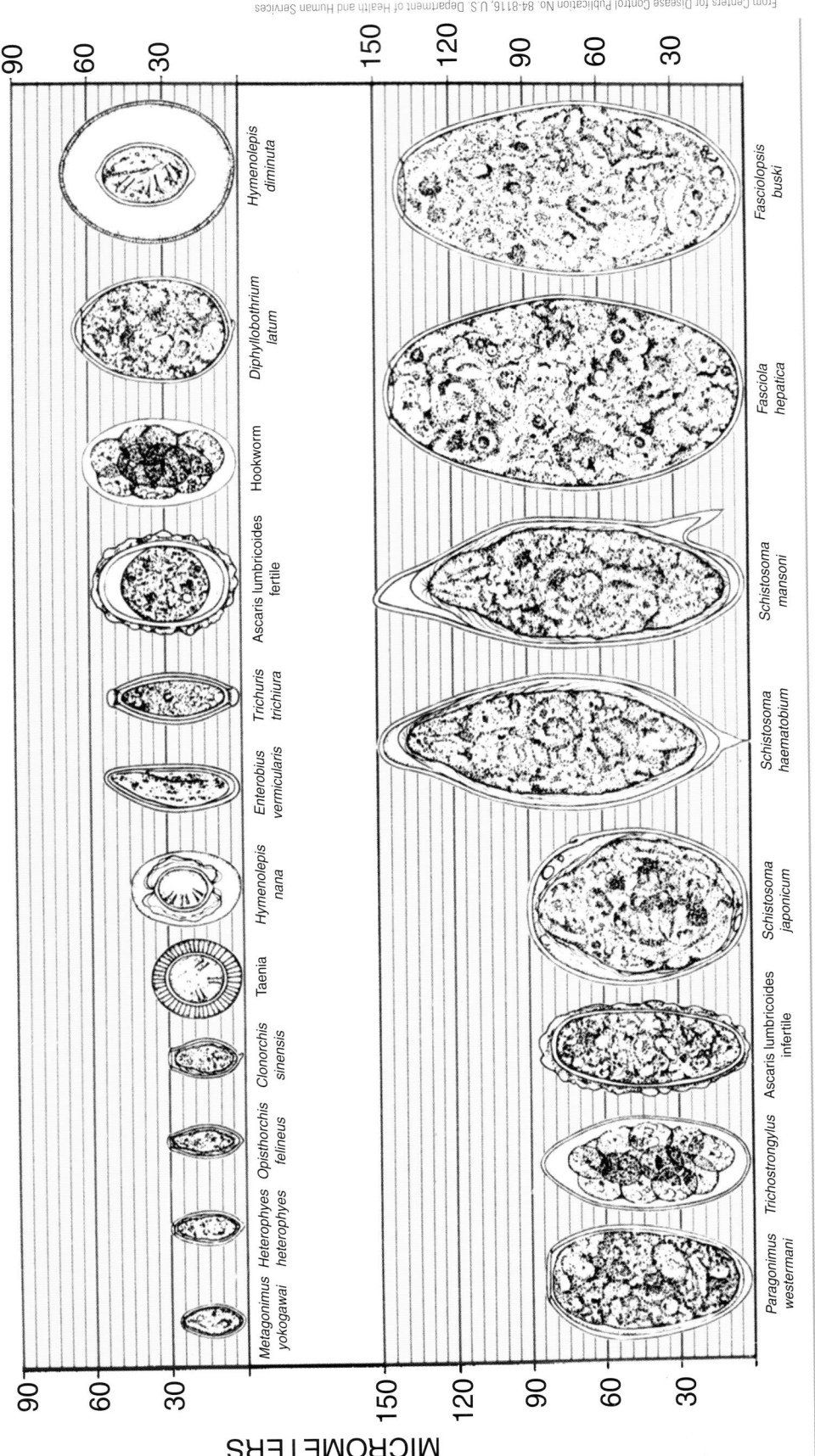

FIGURE 8-16 Helminth ova

MICROMETERS

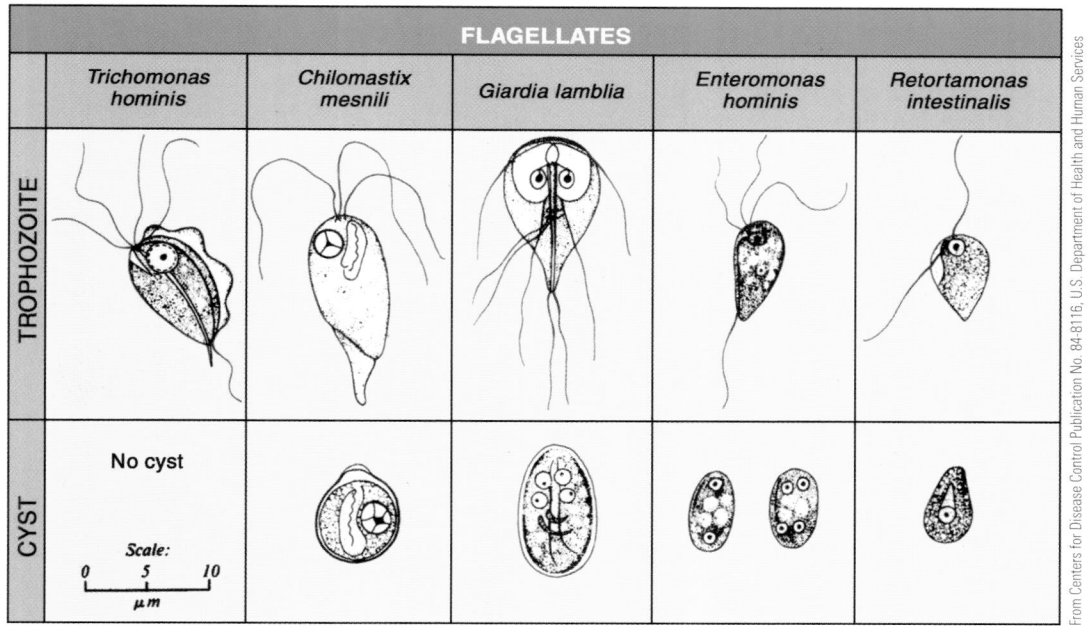

FIGURE 8-17 Intestinal ciliates, coccidia and flagellates

From Centers for Disease Control Publication No. 84-8116, U.S. Department of Health and Human Services

CURRENT TOPICS

GIARDIASIS

Giardiasis is caused by infection with the single-celled flagellated protozoan *Giardia intestinalis* (also called *Giardia lamblia* or *Giardia duodenalis*). *Giardia,* a cause of diarrheal disease worldwide and a common cause of diarrhea in travelers, is found in every region in the United States. It is one of the most common causes of waterborne enteric disease in the United States and is the most common intestinal protozoan identified in U.S. public health laboratories. Giardiasis is a nationally notifiable disease. The incidence of *Giardia* in the U.S. population is estimated to be 2% by the Food and Drug Administration (from FDA *Bad Bug Book,* May 2009).

Transmission

Giardia infections are transmitted by the fecal–oral route, most commonly by eating or drinking contaminated food or water. *Giardia* parasites live in the small intestine of infected humans and animals in a motile form called a *trophozoite*. As trophozoites move through the intestine, they form protective, resistant cysts (shown in micrographs A and B) that are eliminated in the feces into the environment. Infection occurs when the cysts are ingested by:

- Swallowing recreational water (swimming pools, hot tubs, fountains, lakes, springs, etc.) contaminated with animal or human feces or sewage containing *Giardia*
- Eating uncooked food contaminated with *Giardia*
- Accidentally swallowing *Giardia* picked up from surfaces (such as bathroom fixtures, changing tables, diaper pails, or toys) contaminated with feces from an infected person

Clinical Symptoms and Laboratory Diagnosis

Symptoms of giardiasis begin a week or two after infection and include diarrhea, nausea, flatulence, abdominal cramps, and fatty stools that tend to float. In healthy individuals the symptoms can last from a couple of weeks to several weeks, and the infection can become chronic. In immunocompromised individuals, the disease can be long-lasting and debilitating, requiring supportive therapy as well as drug treatment.

Giardiasis is diagnosed by microscopic examination of fecal specimens for the presence of Giardia cysts. Examination of wet mounts (iodine-stained or unstained) using the high-power objective is sometimes all that is required to find Giardia cysts. If wet mounts are negative, the specimen can be concentrated and re-examined, providing a higher probability of finding the organism in light infections. The figure below shows an iodine-stained *Giardia* cyst (A) and a trichrome-stained cyst (B).

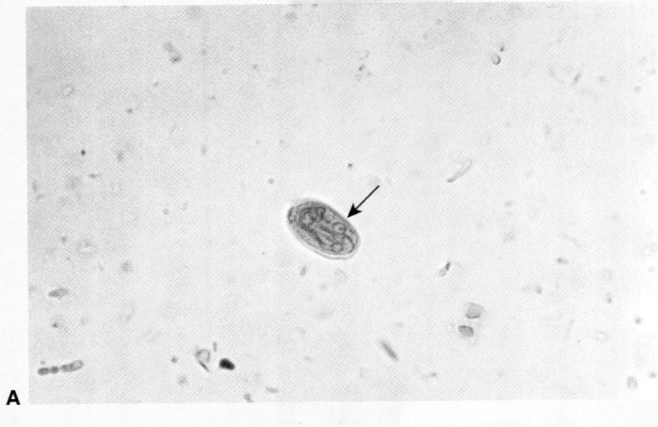

A

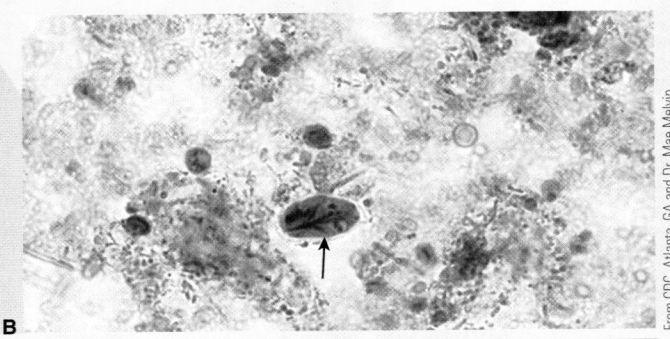

B

From CDC, Atlanta, GA and Dr. Mae Melvin

Giardia intestinalis: (A) iodine-stained cyst in fecal wet mount; (B) cyst (arrow) in a fecal smear stained with trichrome stain

SAFETY REMINDERS

- Review Safety Precautions section before beginning procedure.
- Observe Standard Precautions when handling all fecal specimens.
- Balance rotor load before turning on centrifuge.
- Do not open centrifuge lid until rotor has completely stopped.
- Wear appropriate PPE.
- Work in a fume hood.
- Discard specimens into biohazard containers.

PROCEDURAL REMINDERS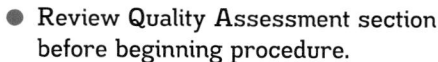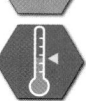

- Review Quality Assessment section before beginning procedure.
- Follow SOP manual.
- Check specific gravity of concentrating solutions.
- Do not use reagents after expiration dates.

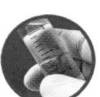 # SUMMARY

Intestinal parasites are discovered and identified by microscopic examination of direct wet mounts of fresh or fixed fecal specimens, wet mounts prepared from concentrated fecal specimens, and trichrome-stained fecal smears. Large laboratories generally perform these procedures in house, but many smaller laboratories process specimens and send them to a reference laboratory for analysis.

One intestinal parasite that is common worldwide, including in the United States, is *Giardia intestinalis*. Infection with *Giardia* occurs through ingestion of infectious cysts present in contaminated food or water. *Giardia* cysts have a characteristic appearance and are easily identified in fecal specimens.

Standard Precautions must always be observed when handling all fecal specimens, even preserved ones, because some parasite forms remain infective even in preservative. Use of a concentration method increases the likelihood of finding parasites in light infections. Kits for fecal concentration that use closed systems provide technicians protection from exposure to the specimen.

 # REVIEW QUESTIONS

1. What three types of preparations are used for microscopic examination for intestinal parasites?

2. What specimens are used for wet mounts?

3. What diluents are used for wet mounts?

4. Name two methods of concentrating fecal specimens. Where are the concentrated parasites found in each method?

5. What type(s) of iodine are used for staining wet mounts?

6. How are fecal smears prepared for staining?

7. What stain is used for fecal specimens?

8. What are symptoms of giardiasis? How is it acquired?

9. Why must Standard Precautions be used when handling preserved fecal specimens?

10. What is the best method for identifying intestinal protozoa?

11. Define trichrome stain.

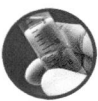 # STUDENT ACTIVITIES

1. Complete the written examination for this lesson.

2. Practice preparing fecal specimens for microscopic examination as outlined in the Student Performance Guide.

WEB ACTIVITIES

1. Use the Internet to search the CDC web site. Find out how many *Giardia* cases have been reported in the United States in the last 10 years.

2. Use the Internet to find the drug of choice (trade name and generic name) for treating *Giardia* infections. For what other conditions is the drug used?

3. Use the Internet to find information about intestinal amebiasis. Report on the causative organism and how it is diagnosed. What organism has a similar appearance and must be differentiated from the parasite causing amebiasis?

4. Search for information on the Entero-Test, also called the "string test." Describe the test procedure and explain when it would be used and the organism(s) is it used to detect.

LESSON 8-3

Microscopic Methods of Detecting Intestinal Parasites

Name _____   Date _____

INSTRUCTIONS

1. Practice preparing fecal specimens for microscopic examination for parasites, following the step-by-step procedure.

2. Demonstrate the procedure for preparing fecal specimens for microscopic examination satisfactorily for the instructor, using the Student Performance Guide. Your instructor will explain the procedures for evaluating and grading your performance. Your performance may be given a number grade, letter grade, or satisfactory (S) or unsatisfactory (U) depending on course or institutional policy.

NOTE: Consult package inserts, manufacturer's instructions, and procedure manual for specific instructions for the methods being used.

MATERIALS AND EQUIPMENT

- gloves
- hand antiseptic
- full-face shield (or equivalent PPE)
- plastic-backed absorbent bench paper
- applicator sticks
- preserved fecal specimens
- fume hood or biological safety cabinet
- microscope
- paper towels
- surface disinfectant (such as 10% chlorine bleach)
- biohazard container
- sharps container

Materials for Wet Mounts:

- coverglasses, 22 mm^2
- glass microscope slides, 2 × 3 inch preferable
- saline (0.85% NaCl)
- iodine solution for fecal wet mounts (Lugol's, Dobell and O'Connors, or D'Antoni's)
  Recipe for D'Antoni's iodine:
  - add 1.0 g potassium iodide (KI) and 1.5 g iodine crystals to 100 mL distilled water in a dark bottle. Shake well and filter daily before use
- disposable transfer pipets

Materials for Preparing Fecal Smears for Staining:

- 35° C incubator or laboratory oven
- microscope slides, 1 × 3 inch
- applicator sticks

Materials for Fecal Concentration:

- fecal concentrator kit(s) and package insert
- clinical centrifuge capable of spinning conical tubes at 500 × g
- applicator sticks

OPTIONAL: Preserved fecal specimens containing parasites; commercially prepared stained microscope slides containing parasites; atlases, diagrams, photographs, digital images, or videos of intestinal parasites.

(Continues)

© 2012 Delmar, Cengage Learning. Permission to reproduce for clinical use granted.

PROCEDURE

Record in the comment section any problems encountered while practicing the procedure (or have a fellow student or the instructor evaluate your performance).

S = Satisfactory
U = Unsatisfactory

You must:	S	U	Evaluation/Comments
1. Wash hands with antiseptic			
2. Put on gloves and face protection			
3. Assemble equipment and materials			
4. Prepare a work area by placing absorbent laboratory paper on counter or in fume hood			
5. Demonstrate the procedure for preparing a fecal smear for staining, following steps 5a–5d: a. Obtain preserved fecal specimen and two 1- × 3-inch microscope slides b. Use applicator stick to mix specimen and remove a small portion c. Spread specimen evenly on slide by rolling applicator stick across slide or smearing in a zigzag fashion (as in Figure 8-13). Smear should cover one-third to half the length of the slide and should extend from the slide's top edge to bottom edge. Prepare a second slide from the same specimen d. Label slides and place them in 35° C incubator to dry for at least 4 hours, preferably overnight			
6. Demonstrate the procedure for preparing saline and iodine wet mounts from a preserved fecal specimen, following steps 6a–6i: a. Obtain a preserved specimen b. Place a 2 × 3 inch glass slide on work area c. Place 1 drop of saline on left half of slide and 1 drop of iodine solution on right half of slide d. Use applicator stick to mix specimen e. Remove a small portion of specimen with applicator stick and mix with saline drop. Place a coverglass over the drop f. Remove another small portion of fecal specimen and mix with iodine drop. Place a coverglass over the drop. Discard applicator in biohazard container g. Place slide over newsprint and check thickness of wet mounts (letters should be readable through the specimen) h. *Optional:* Place slide on microscope stage and scan specimens with the low-power and high-power objectives. Use visual aids to help recognize parasitic forms i. Discard slide in biohazard sharps container			

© 2012 Delmar, Cengage Learning. Permission to reproduce for clinical use granted.

You must:	S	U	Evaluation/Comments

7. Perform a fecal concentration procedure, following steps 7a–7k. (If not available, skip to step 8)
  a. Obtain a preserved fecal specimen and a fecal concentrator kit
  b. Follow the manufacturer's specific directions (general directions are given below)
  c. Add surfactant to the preservative vial that contains the specimen
  d. Attach the filtration unit with conical tube to the vial securely
  e. Invert unit and tap to force specimen into the tube
  f. Remove filtration unit and vial and discard appropriately
  g. Add appropriate volumes of ethyl acetate, or other solutions indicated, to the tube
  h. Cap tube tightly and shake the tube
  i. Centrifuge the tube at the speed and for the time specified in the package insert
  j. Decant supernatant as directed
  k. Resuspend pellet, prepare wet mounts (as in step 6), and examine microscopically			

8. Discard all contaminated materials into appropriate bio-hazard containers and used slides into sharps containers			
9. Discard or store preserved specimens, as directed by instructor			
10. Optional: Use the microscope to examine commercially prepared slides containing fecal parasites; use parasitology atlases and figures in this lesson to identify parasite forms			
11. Wipe work area with disinfectant			
12. Remove gloves and discard into biohazard container			
13. Wash hands with antiseptic			

Instructor/Evaluator Comments:

Instructor/Evaluator _____ Date _____

© 2012 Delmar, Cengage Learning. Permission to reproduce for clinical use granted.

STUDENT PERFORMANCE GUIDE

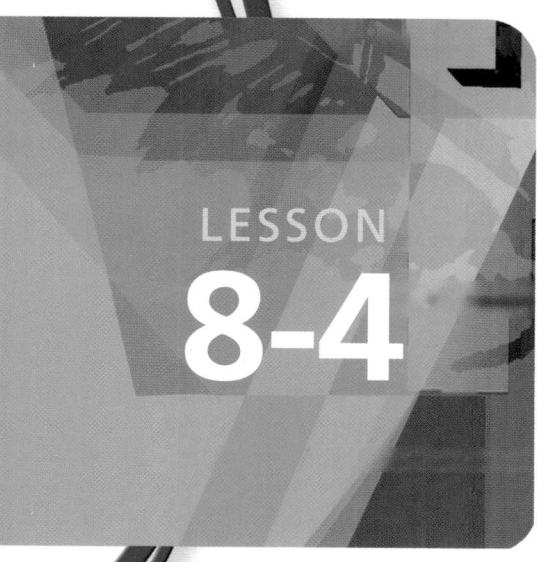

LESSON 8-4

Blood Smears for Parasite Detection

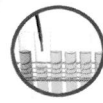

LESSON OBJECTIVES

After studying this lesson, the student will:

- ⊙ Describe how to collect a blood specimen for parasite examination.
- ⊙ Diagram the *Plasmodium* life cycle.
- ⊙ Describe the symptoms of malaria.
- ⊙ Name three types of tests for malaria.
- ⊙ Discuss the epidemiology and symptoms of Chagas disease.
- ⊙ Explain the purpose of preparing thin and thick blood smears for detecting blood parasites.
- ⊙ Prepare and stain thin and thick blood smears.
- ⊙ List safety precautions to be observed when preparing and staining blood smears for parasites.
- ⊙ Discuss quality assessment procedures to follow when preparing blood smears for parasite examination.
- ⊙ Define the glossary terms.

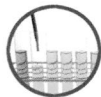

GLOSSARY

Anopheles / the genus of mosquito that is the definitive host for the human malaria parasites (genus *Plasmodium*) and that is capable of transmitting the organism to humans

babesiosis / an infection spread by tick bite and caused by protozoan parasites of the genus *Babesia*

Giemsa stain / a polychromatic stain used for staining blood cells and blood parasites

malaria / in humans, a disease caused by infection with protozoan parasites of the genus *Plasmodium*

microfilaria (pl. microfilariae) / immature form of a filarial worm

parasitemia / parasites in the blood

paroxysm(s) / the cycle(s) of chills and fever associated with malaria that occur 36 to 72 hours apart, depending on the *Plasmodium* species

Plasmodium / the protozoan genus that includes the organisms causing human malaria

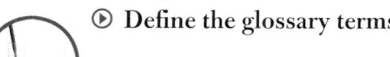

INTRODUCTION

Several parasites have forms or stages that are present in the blood of infected individuals during part of the parasite's life cycle. Examples of these are the parasites that cause malaria, sleeping sickness (African trypanosomiasis), Chagas disease (American trypanosomiasis), and babesiosis.

The best method for detecting blood parasites is microscopic examination of the blood. This lesson explains the techniques of preparing and staining blood smears for detecting and identifying blood parasites. Much experience is required to recognize and identify the various species of blood parasites.

BLOOD PARASITES

Parasites found in blood during some part of their life cycle include *Plasmodium, Babesia, Trypanosoma,* and *Leishmania.* Table 8-9 gives information about blood parasites, including modes of transmission.

Malaria

Human **malaria** is caused by any one of four species of parasitic protozoa of the genus *Plasmodium* (Table 8-10). The parasites are transmitted to humans through the bite of *Anopheles* mosquitoes (the definitive host) or, rarely, through transfusion of infected blood. Mosquitoes become infected when they ingest blood from an infected person. Figure 8-18 shows a malarial parasite's life cycle.

Malaria is the most widely known parasitic disease of the blood and has high morbidity and mortality rates. Forty-one percent of the world's population live in malaria endemic areas, which include parts of Africa, Asia, the Middle East, Central and South America, Hispaniola, and Oceania. The World Health Organization (WHO) estimates that about 300 million cases of malaria occur each year, with over 1 million deaths annually, the majority of them children. The recent increase in insecticide-resistant mosquitoes and drug-resistant *Plasmodium* strains has made malaria prevention and treatment more difficult. Despite over 60 years of research, an effective malarial vaccine for widespread human use has yet to be approved, although some have shown promise in trials.

Malaria has been considered eradicated in the United States since the early 1950s, but an average of more than 1,000 cases are still reported annually. A few of these cases are due to locally transmitted outbreaks of mosquito-borne malaria that still occur. These are caused when local mosquitoes become infected after taking a blood meal from an infected individual who acquired the parasite in an endemic area. If these mosquitoes bite other individuals, the organisms can be transmitted to local residents. Because the two species of *Anopheles* mosquito that can transmit malaria are still widely found in the United States, there is a risk that malaria could be reestablished.

Most of the approximate 1,000 annual cases of malaria in the United States are imported, acquired by travelers to malaria-endemic countries. After the magnitude 7.0 earthquake that struck Haiti in 2010, several cases of malaria were confirmed in both military and civilian emergency responders. These infections occurred even though the individuals had been given doxycycline as a prophylaxis. *Plasmodium falciparum* is the predominant malaria-causing species endemic in Haiti and infection risk among Haitians and emergency workers increased as people were required to live and work in temporary shelters.

Since the early 1960s, only rarely have cases of confirmed malaria in the United States been traced to transmission by blood transfusion. If donor and testing guidelines are followed, transfusion-transmitted malaria should not be a risk for blood transfusion.

Other Blood Parasites

Among the other blood parasites infecting humans are the filarial worms and the protozoa *Babesia* and *Trypanosoma* (Table 8-9). Infection with any of the *Babesia* species causes **babesiosis**, which occurs following the bite of an infected tick. In infected humans,

TABLE 8-9. Examples of parasites found in blood, their modes of transmission, and the diseases they cause

ORGANISM	TRANSMISSION	DISEASE CAUSED
Plasmodium spp.	Mosquito bite	Malaria
Babesia	Tick bite	Babesiosis
Trypanosoma brucei	Tsetse fly bite	African sleeping sickness, trypanosomiasis
Trypanosoma cruzi	Reduviid bug bite contaminated with bug's infected feces	Chagas disease (American trypanosomiasis)
Wuchereria bancrofti	Mosquito bite	Filariasis, elephantiasis
Brugia	Mosquito bite	Filariasis, elephantiasis
Leishmania donovani	Sand fly bite	Visceral leishmaniasis, kala azar, dumdum fever
Toxoplasma gondii	Ingestion of oocysts, congenital, eating under-cooked infected meat	Toxoplasmosis

TABLE 8-10. *Plasmodium* species that cause human malaria

SPECIES	DISEASE CAUSED	PAROXYSMS
P. vivax	Benign tertian malaria	Every 48 hours
P. ovale	Ovale malaria	Every 48 hours
P. malariae	Quartan malaria	Every 72 hours
P. falciparum	Malignant malaria	Every 36 to 38 hours

Babesia parasites can be seen inside red blood cells on blood smears and must be distinguished from malarial parasites (Figure 8-19).

Trypanosoma brucei causes African sleeping sickness (also called trypanosomiasis) and is transmitted through the bite of the tsetse fly. It is found in areas where the tsetse fly is endemic. *Trypanosoma cruzi* causes American trypanosomiasis, also called Chagas disease. This disease had been confined mostly to Latin America. However, its incidence in the United States and other countries is increasing primarily because of population mobility. More information about Chagas disease is in Current Topics 2, p. 866.

The filarial worms that infect humans are not endemic in the United States. However, the dog heartworm, *Dirofilaria immitis*, is a filarial animal parasite transmitted by mosquitoes and is common in the United States. Heartworm infection is diagnosed by examination of dog blood for **microfilariae**, immature forms of the heartworm (Figure 8-20).

LABORATORY DETECTION OF BLOOD PARASITES

Safety Precautions

Standard Precautions must be observed to protect health-care workers and patients. Appropriate personal protective equipment (PPE) must be worn when collecting blood specimens and handling any biological

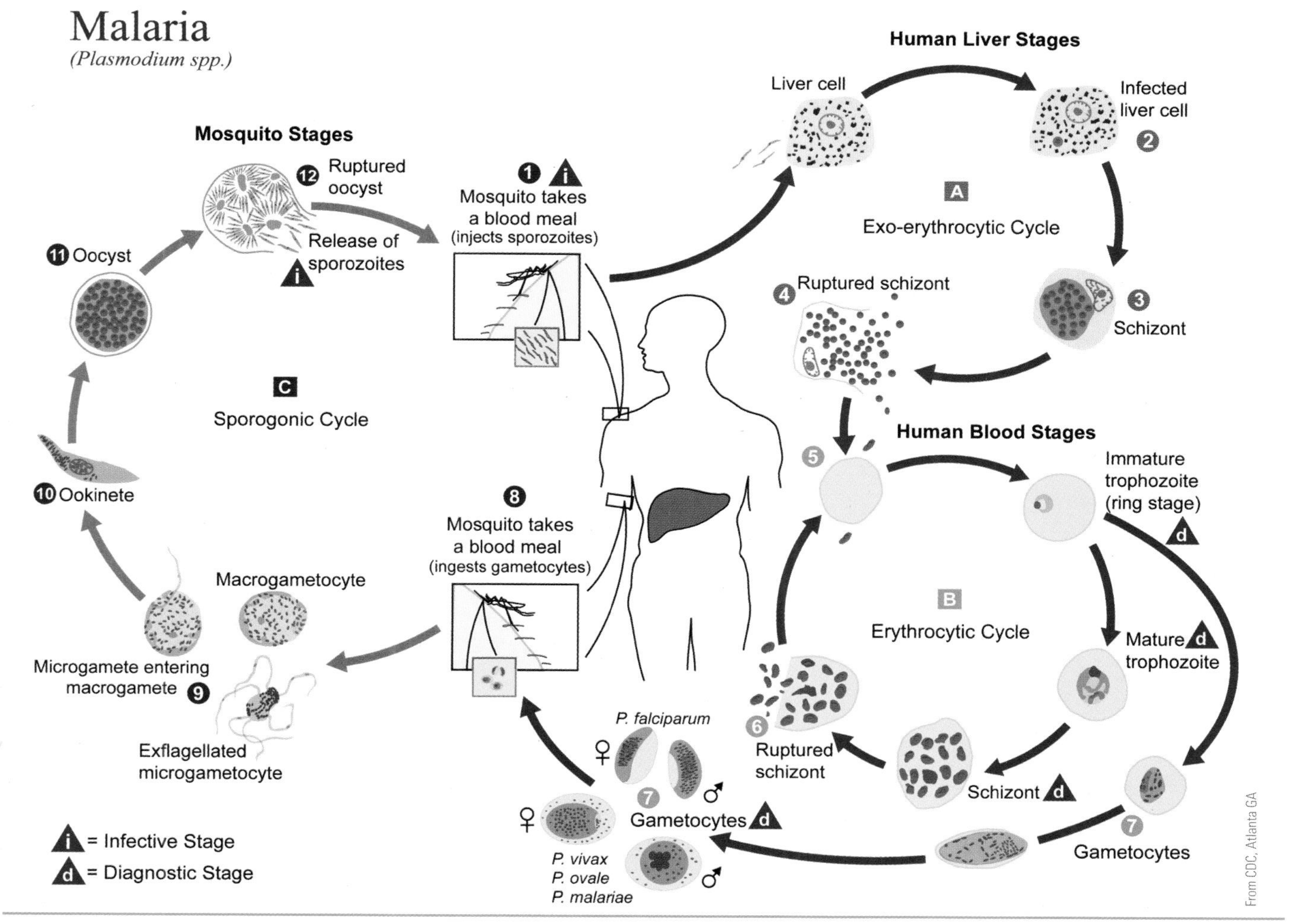

FIGURE 8-18 Life cycle of *Plasmodium*, the organism causing malaria

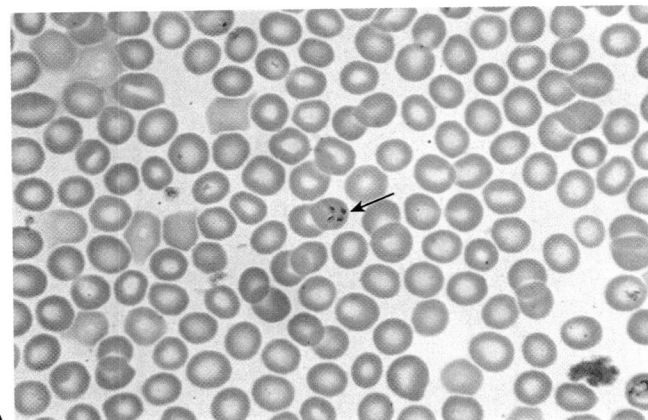

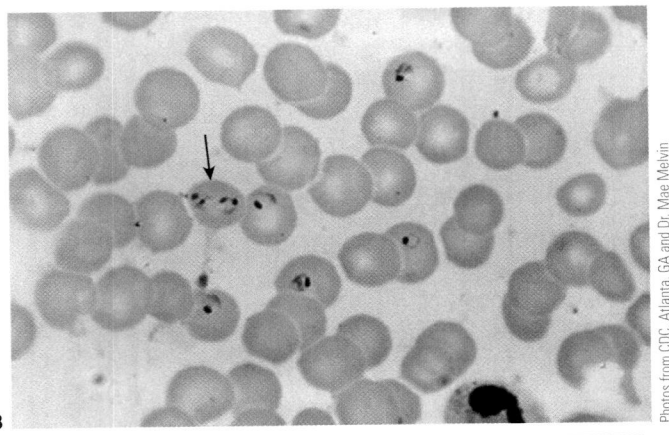

FIGURE 8-19 Intraerythrocytic parasites: (A) tetrad configuration of intraerythrocytic *Babesia* trophozoites (arrow) resembles (B) multiple intraerythrocytic *Plasmodium falciparum* ring stage trophozoites (arrow). One identifying characteristic of *Plasmodium falciparum* infections is that erythrocytes often contain multiple ring forms

Photos from CDC, Atlanta, GA and Dr. Mae Melvin

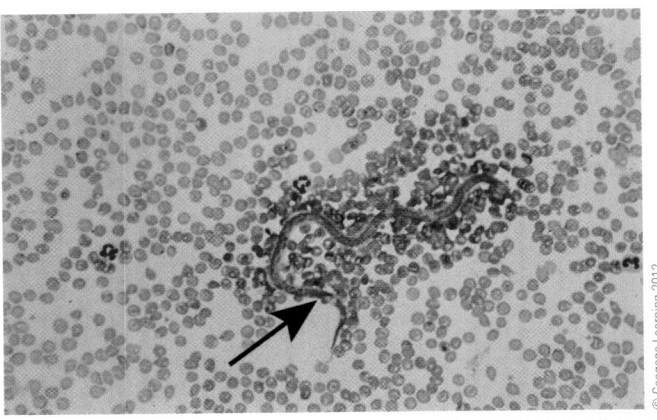

© Cengage Learning 2012

FIGURE 8-20 Canine heartworm microfilaria in stained blood smear

specimens. Hands should be washed before donning and after removing gloves. Safety needles and lancets must be used and should be discarded into a sharps container immediately

after use. Skin contact with chemicals and inhalation of chemical fumes should be avoided.

Quality Assessment

The procedures for preparing and staining blood smears for parasite examination will be explained in each laboratory's standard operating procedure (SOP) manual and must be followed. Only qualified personnel shown to be competent in parasite identification should interpret and report results from blood smears for parasites. Considerations unique to preparing and staining these smears include:

- Timing of blood collection: Some **parasitemias**, such as malaria, exhibit periodicity (the number of parasites in the blood fluctuates with time), making the timing of blood collection critical. Blood should be collected between paroxysms. Collection at several intervals over a period of 2 to 3 days can be required to ensure obtaining a specimen containing the parasites.

- Blood specimens should be collected before any drug treatment is initiated.

- Capillary blood is the preferred specimen, especially for malaria, because anticoagulants can alter parasite morphology and staining characteristics.

- Smears should be prepared at least in duplicate, with only one set being stained initially.

- Blood smears should be stained and examined as soon as possible after collection because parasite morphology deteriorates with time.

- Positive control smears should be stained with each fresh dilution of Giemsa stain.

Specimen Collection

Blood for parasite examination should be obtained by capillary puncture. If it must be obtained by venipuncture, the blood should *not* be anticoagulated. Anticoagulants distort parasite morphology and interfere with staining of parasitic stages.

The timing of blood collection in suspected malaria cases is important. Blood should be collected between paroxysms, which can occur from 36 to 72 hours apart depending on the infecting species (Table 8-10).

Preparing the Blood Smears

Thick and thin blood smears are prepared (Figures 8-21, 8-22, and 8-23). The thick smear is used for screening; it contains 10 to 30 times as much blood per microscopic field as a thin smear. Therefore, examining thick smears increases the chance of detecting parasites in a light infection because of the greater volume of blood screened. The thin film or smear is used to identify the parasite because the morphology is better in thin than in thick smears.

CURRENT TOPICS 1

LABORATORY DIAGNOSIS OF HUMAN MALARIA

Human malaria is usually associated with distinct, recognizable symptoms. Malarias can range from mild to fatal, depending on the species of *Plasmodium* causing the infection. *Plasmodium falciparum* is the most deadly species. Diagnosis of the type of malaria can be confirmed by identification of the malarial parasite in a blood smear.

Symptoms

Plasmodium infection causes anemia, enlarged spleen, and cycles of chills, fever, and sweats called paroxysms. The parasites infect liver cells and red blood cells. As the parasites develop in red blood cells, they eventually cause the infected cells to rupture, releasing toxins and parasites and initiating the cycle of paroxysms. Malaria should be considered a possible cause of unexplained fever even for patients in malaria-free countries, and these patients should be questioned about their recent travel history.

Laboratory Identification

Rapid species identification is important because treatment can vary according to the species of malarial parasite. Thin and thick blood smears prepared from blood obtained at carefully timed intervals are stained with Giemsa stain. In general, blood is collected shortly after a paroxysm and every 6 to 8 hours after the paroxysm so that different stages of the parasite will be present to aid in species identification.

Plasmodium species can be identified by careful microscopic examination of both types of smears by experienced personnel. The smears are examined extensively using the oil-immersion objective and the back-and-forth serpentine motion to scan adjacent fields as for the differential count. A minimum of 100 to 200 microscopic fields are examined in the thick smear, looking for the presence of parasitic forms (see micrographs right). Thin smears are examined for at least 30 minutes, looking for parasitic red blood cell inclusions. Malarial species identification is beyond the scope of this lesson. However, the photos shown here depict blood stages of *P. falciparum* and *P. vivax* as they appear in thin and thick smears.

Malarial species determination can also be made by detecting parasite DNA in a peripheral blood sample using molecular methods such as polymerase chain reaction (PCR). Several days can be required before these tests results are available, but the tests can provide definitive results.

Rapid diagnostic tests have been developed that detect malarial parasite antigens in blood using immunochemical methods. These tests do not require that a technician have microscopic expertise, but the tests are not as sensitive for detecting low-level infections as are blood smear examinations or nucleic acid tests. The immunodiagnostic tests do not distinguish among all the malarial species and, in the United States, they are currently used primarily as research tools or preliminary screening tests that must be confirmed by blood smear or DNA test.

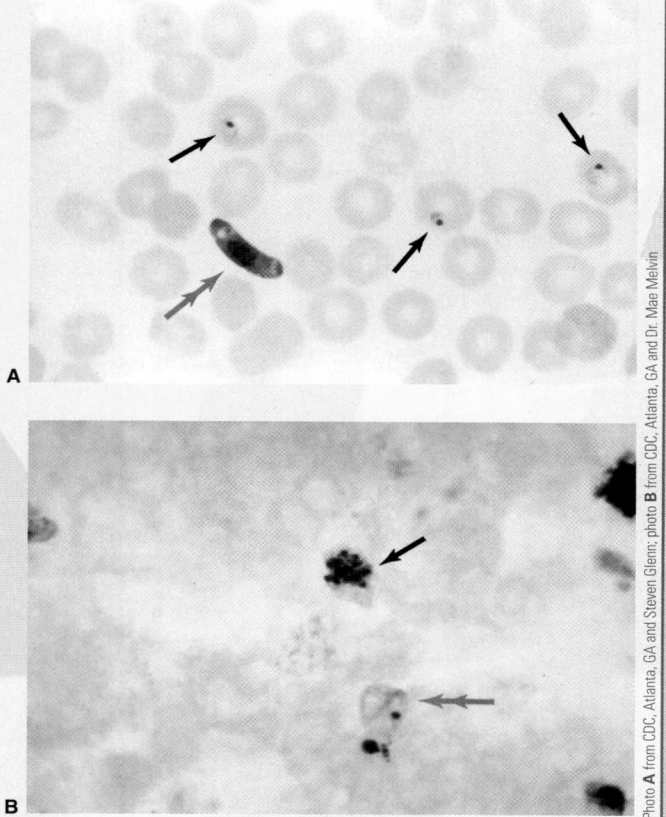

Photo **A** from CDC, Atlanta, GA and Steven Glenn; photo **B** from CDC, Atlanta, GA and Dr. Mae Melvin

Malarial parasites in blood smears: (A) micrograph of Giemsa-stained thin smear showing a *Plasmodium falciparum* gametocyte (double arrow) and erythrocytes containing malarial ring forms (single arrows); (B) thick film micrograph showing a mature *Plasmodium vivax* schizont (single arrow), a growing trophozoite (double arrow), and "ghost" red blood cells

CURRENT TOPICS 2

AMERICAN TRYPANOSOMIASIS: CHAGAS DISEASE

American trypanosomiasis, also called Chagas disease, is caused by the protozoan parasite *Trypanosoma cruzi*. The disease is found in the Americas from the southern United States through Central and South America to southern Argentina. Chagas disease is a major health problem in many Latin American countries, affecting an estimated 8 to 11 million people and causing approximately 50,000 deaths per year. In the United States, in 2009, over 300,000 people were estimated by the Centers for Disease Control and Prevention (CDC) to have Chagas disease.

As immigration from Latin and South America has increased, the potential of transmission of Chagas disease by blood transfusion has become more substantial in the United States, with some transfusion-related cases being reported in North America. In addition, the infection has been shown to be transmitted to organ transplant recipients through infected donated organs.

In the United States, national screening of donated blood for *T. cruzi* antibodies was begun in 2007. In the first 3 years of screening, more than 1,000 positives were identified and eliminated as potential blood donors. More than half of the states have reported *T. cruzi*–positive blood donor applicants. In addition, this screening identified previously unknown cases of *T. cruzi*, allowing the patients to receive counseling and treatment. By 2010, two companies were producing Food and Drug Administration (FDA)-approved tests for use in screening blood, tissue, and organ donors for *T. cruzi* antibodies. These tests have been shown to be both specific and sensitive and, if used for screening donated blood, should prevent transfusion- or transplant-transmitted Chagas disease.

Epidemiology

T. cruzi can be transmitted to both humans and animals by a bug called the reduviid, triatomine, or kissing bug (shown in image A, below), which lives primarily in cracks and holes of substandard housing in the tropics and subtropics of the Americas. The bug becomes infected by taking a blood meal from an infected individual. The infective stage then develops in the bug and is passed in its feces. People can become infected by:

- Touching eyes, mouth, or open cuts after hands have come in contact with infective bug feces
- Bugs directly depositing infected feces in eyes
- Congenital infection acquired from mother during pregnancy or at birth
- Receiving transfused blood or transplanted tissue or organ containing the parasite

Clinical Symptoms and Laboratory Diagnosis

Chagas disease is a serious disease that develops over many years. Infection often begins in childhood, and victims often do not experience severe symptoms in the early stages. If symptoms are

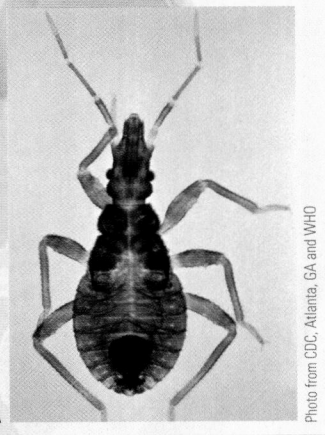

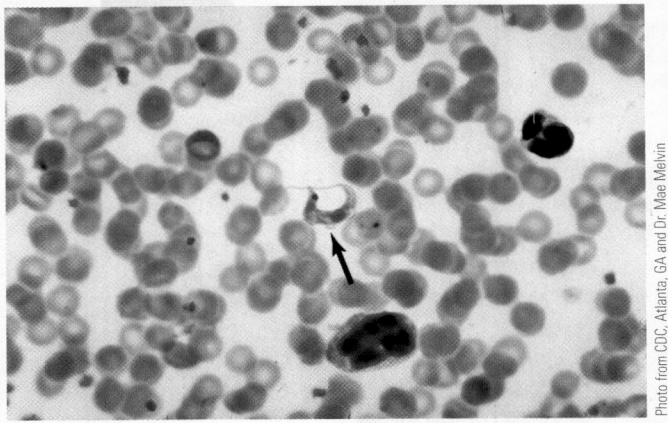

Photo from CDC, Atlanta, GA and WHO

Photo from CDC, Atlanta, GA and Dr. Mae Melvin

A   **B**

Chagas disease: (A) the kissing bug, *Triatoma infestans,* **a vector for Chagas disease; (B) micrograph of Giemsa-stained** *Trypanosoma cruzi* **trypomastigote in a blood smear**

(Continues)

CURRENT TOPICS 2 (continued)

present during the acute phase, they can include fever, enlarged spleen and lymph nodes, and fatigue. Diagnosis is made by microscopic examination of a fresh blood specimen to look for motile forms, examination of a stained blood smear (shown in B), or by blood culture. Drug treatment is usually successful in the early acute phase.

About one-third of infected persons develop chronic disease 10 to 30 years after initial infection. Enlarged

heart, heart failure, and cardiac arrest can occur, all caused by growth of the parasite in the heart tissue. In chronic disease, parasite numbers in the blood are usually too low to be detectable in smears, so culture, immunological, or molecular testing methods are used for diagnosis. Drug treatment is usually not successful in the chronic phase.

Preparing a Thin Smear

A thin smear is prepared from freshly collected *anticoagulant-free* blood in the manner described in Lesson 2-7.

- A small drop of blood is spread on a clean glass slide in the same way as for a differential count (Figure 8-21).
- The smear is allowed to air-dry in a slide rack.
- The dry smear is immersed in absolute methanol for 30 to 60 seconds to fix the smear and is again allowed to air-dry.
- A minimum of two thin smears should be prepared from each blood collection.

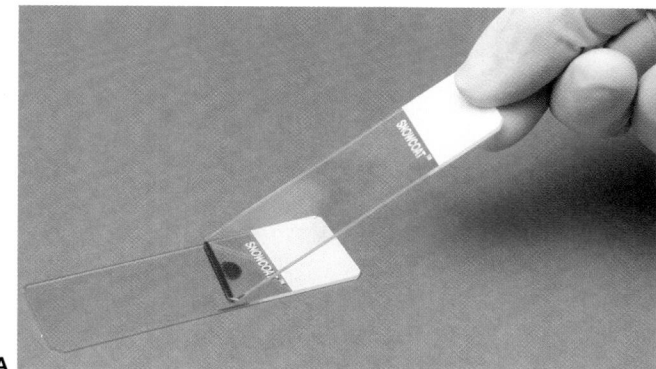

A

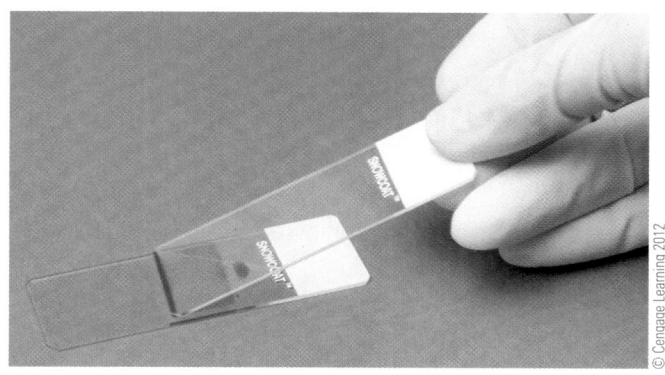

B

© Cengage Learning 2012

FIGURE 8-21 Preparing a thin blood smear: (A) gently bring the back side of a spreader slide into contact with a drop of blood; (B) quickly and gently push the spreader slide forward to make the smear

Preparing a Thick Smear

Two methods of preparing thick blood smears are shown in Figure 8-22. A few small drops of blood can be placed on a slide and spread into a nickel-sized (approximately 2 cm) circle with the corner of another glass slide; or a large drop of capillary blood can be touched from a fingerstick to a slide and spread in a circular motion using slight pressure against the finger.

- A *minimum* of two thick smears should be prepared from each blood collection.
- Thick smears should be allowed to dry flat at room temperature several hours or overnight before staining.
- A thick film should be thin enough to read through when the slide is laid on a newspaper; smears that are too thick can peel off the slide during staining.
- Thick smears are *not* fixed before staining.
- Thick smears should be stained within 24 hours of preparation.
- Thick and thin smears can be prepared on the same slide (Figure 8-23), but only the thin smear should be fixed with methanol.

Staining the Blood Smears

The preferred stain for identifying parasites in blood is **Giemsa stain**. This polychromatic stain is similar to Wright's stain but does not have fixative incorporated into it. Wright's stain, which is routinely used for hematological studies, can be used for thin smears if rapid results are needed. However, parasites do not stain as well with Wright's stain as with Giemsa stain and results from Wright's-stained smears should be confirmed by examination of a Giemsa-stained smear.

Giemsa stain can be purchased as a stock solution to be diluted before use. Optimal dilutions and staining times should be determined for the brand and stain lot used. Staining times range from 20 minutes to 2 hours, depending on the stain dilution (Table 8-11). Quick Giemsa stains are available that do not require the long staining times, but staining results are usually not as good as with traditional Giemsa stain.

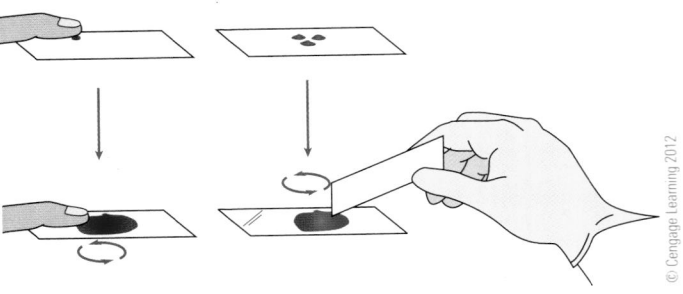

FIGURE 8-22 Two methods of preparing thick blood smears: (left) make smear directly from finger puncture; (right) use corner of slide to spread a few drops of blood to form a thick smear

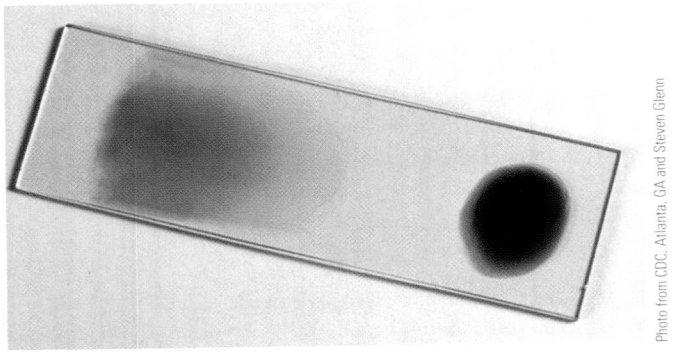

FIGURE 8-23 Thin (left) and thick (right) smears prepared on the same slide and ready for staining with Giemsa stain

TABLE 8-11. Dilutions and staining times for blood smears using commercial Giemsa stain

GIEMSA DILUTION	STAINING TIME	DIRECTIONS FOR MAKING DILUTION
1:20	20 minutes	2 mL Giemsa* + 38 mL bH₂O**
1:40	45–50 minutes	1 mL Giemsa* + 39 mL bH₂O**
1:50	50–60 minutes	1 mL Giemsa* + 49 mL bH₂O**
1:100	2 hours	1 mL Giemsa* + 99 mL bH₂O**

*stock Giemsa stain, available commercially
**0.0067 M phosphate-buffered water, pH 7.2

Since thick films are not fixed, the red blood cells will be lysed (destroyed) during the staining procedure and only white blood cells, platelets, and parasites (if present) will remain intact. The lysed red blood cells will appear as "ghosts" (see micrograph B in Current Topics 1). This makes it possible to microscopically scan the thick areas without the red blood cells obscuring the field of view.

Preparing the Stain

A fresh dilution of Giemsa stain should be made daily. The stock Giemsa solution should be diluted with 0.0067 M phosphate-buffered water, pH 7.2. Commonly used dilutions are 1:20, 1:40, 1:50, or 1:100, with 1:40 and 1:50 being the most common (Table 8-11).

Staining the Smears

Only one set of smears should be stained initially. This leaves a backup set in case a problem occurs during staining or unstained smears must be sent to a reference laboratory.

Thin Smears. A thin smear previously fixed in absolute methanol should be immersed in freshly diluted Giemsa stain for the appropriate time (see Table 8-11). After staining, the slide should be rinsed briefly by dipping 3-4 times in phosphate-buffered water and then air-dried in a slide rack. Stained slides should be stored in covered slide boxes protected from light.

Thick Smears. The dry smear should be immersed in diluted Giemsa stain (for staining options see Table 8-11). The stained smear is then rinsed for 5 minutes in buffered water and allowed to air-dry in a slide rack. Dry, stained smears should be stored in slide boxes.

SAFETY REMINDERS

- Review Safety Precautions section before beginning procedure.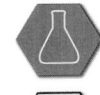
- Observe Standard Precautions.
- Do not inhale methanol fumes or allow skin contact.

PROCEDURAL REMINDERS

- Review Quality Assessment section before beginning procedure.
- Follow directions in SOP manual.
- Make smears from fresh anticoagulant-free blood.
- Make fresh dilutions of Giemsa stain daily.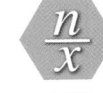
- Stain positive control slides with new batches of stain.
- Allow only qualified personnel to screen and interpret stained smears.

CRITICAL THINKING

Tommy Rogers, a regular patient at a small internal medicine clinic, came in complaining of episodes of chills, fever, and sweats. Upon questioning, he revealed that he had returned from India 3 weeks previously. Tommy's physician ordered blood smears to be prepared and stained so that she could examine them for malarial parasites. Adrian, the laboratory assistant, prepared thin and thick smears. Not finding Giemsa stain in the laboratory, he stained both smears using Wright's stain. Before the physician even looked at the smears microscopically, after a glance at the stained smears, she immediately said that new smears needed to be made and stained.

1. Was anything wrong with the types of smears prepared? If so, what?
2. Was anything wrong with the staining procedure? If so, what?
3. What did the physician see by glancing at the stained smears that caused her to request that the new smears be prepared?

SUMMARY

Several parasites are identified by microscopic examination of specially prepared and stained blood smears. Human blood parasites include *Plasmodium*, the organisms causing malaria; the trypanosomes, which cause African sleeping sickness and American trypanosomiasis or Chagas disease; and *Babesia*, which causes babesiosis. Animal blood parasites, such as the dog heartworm, are also diagnosed by microscopic examination of blood.

In diseases such as malaria, patients' clinical symptoms, such as the interval between paroxysms, must be considered when scheduling blood collection times. The procedures for collecting the blood specimen and preparing and staining smears must be carefully followed to ensure the best chance of finding and identifying parasites. Examination of both thin and thick smears increases the chances of finding parasites in light infections. All safety precautions must be observed and quality assessment policies must be followed for reliable results. Smear results must be reviewed, interpreted, and reported only by qualified personnel trained in parasite identification.

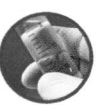

REVIEW QUESTIONS

1. What blood specimen is preferred for preparing smears for parasite examination?
2. Why are both thin and thick smears prepared?
3. Explain the procedure for making the thin blood smear.
4. Explain the procedure for making the thick blood smear.
5. What is the preferred stain for blood smears for parasite examination?
6. What safety precautions must be observed when preparing malarial smears?
7. Why is the blood collection time important when malaria is suspected?

8. Diagram the life cycle of malaria. Indicate points where the life cycle could be interrupted to stop transmission of the parasite.
9. Name two test methods other than blood smear examination that can be used to detect malarial infections.
10. What intraerythrocytic parasite can appear similar to the malaria parasite in a stained blood smear?
11. What organism causes Chagas disease and how is it transmitted? Where is Chagas disease endemic?
12. Explain why cases of malaria and Chagas disease might increase in the United States.
13. What type of screening test can be used to detect *T. cruzi* infections? When is the test used?
14. How is babesiosis acquired?
15. Define *Anopheles*, babesiosis, Giemsa stain, malaria, microfilaria, parasitemia, paroxysm, and *Plasmodium*.

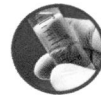

STUDENT ACTIVITIES

1. Complete the written examination for this lesson.
2. Practice the procedure for preparing and staining smears for blood parasites as outlined in the Student Performance Guide.
3. Optional: Heartworm infection is diagnosed by examining dog blood for microfilariae, which are immature forms (larvae) of the heartworm. To examine blood for heartworm, obtain freshly collected canine blood (less than 1 day old) from a local veterinary practice. Prepare and stain thin and thick smears from the blood. If the dog is infected with heartworm (*Dirofilaria*), the stained microfilariae can be seen with the low-power objective. Microfilariae will stain even in anticoagulated blood and will appear as long, purple worm-like organisms. Wet preparations can also be performed: Place a small drop of blood on a glass slide and place a coverglass over it. Observe the specimen using the low-power objective. If the blood specimen is fresh and contains microfilariae, they will be seen moving under the coverglass.

WEB ACTIVITIES

1. Search the Internet to find recommendations for malaria prevention for U.S. citizens traveling to foreign countries. Find out where malaria is endemic. Report on prophylactic drugs that are prescribed for travelers and list countries that have a risk for malaria transmission.

2. Report on a blood parasite other than *Plasmodium* or *Trypanosoma cruzi* (Table 8-9 lists some examples). Search the Internet for information about the parasite, including geographical distribution, life cycle, symptoms of infection, diagnosis, and treatment.

3. Find a life cycle diagram of *T. cruzi* on the Internet. Identify the infective stage and the diagnostic stage and tell where each is found.

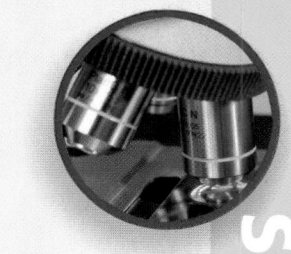
LESSON 8-4

Blood Smears for Parasite Detection

Name _____   Date _____

INSTRUCTIONS

1. Practice preparing and staining smears for blood parasites, following the step-by-step procedure.

2. Demonstrate the procedure for preparing and staining smears for blood parasites satisfactorily for the instructor, using the Student Performance Guide. Your instructor will explain the procedures for evaluating and grading your performance. Your performance may be given a number grade, letter grade, or satisfactory (S) or unsatisfactory (U) depending on course or institutional policy.

MATERIALS AND EQUIPMENT

- gloves
- full-face shield (or equivalent PPE)
- hand antiseptic
- timer
- slide drying rack
- materials for capillary puncture
- microscope slides
- staining jars (Coplin jars) for methanol, stain, and buffer
- absolute methanol
- stock Giemsa stain

- 0.0067 M phosphate-buffered water, pH 7.2

  Recipe for Giemsa buffer (phosphate-buffered water):
  - 39 mL 0.067 M NaH_2PO_4
  - 61 mL 0.067 M Na_2HPO_4
  - 900 mL distilled water
  - check pH; should be 7.2
- microscope with high power and oil immersion objectives
- immersion oil
- lens paper and lens cleaner
- slide box
- paper towels
- surface disinfectant (such as 10% chlorine bleach)
- biohazard container
- sharps container

OPTIONAL VISUAL AIDS: commercially prepared stained slides of *Plasmodium, Trypanosoma,* and *Babesia*; commercially prepared stained slides of filarial worms, such as dog heartworm (*Dirofilaria*); charts, digital images, slides, and figures showing morphology of blood parasites.

NOTE: Consult manufacturer's instructions accompanying Giemsa stain for recommended optimal dilution and staining time.

PROCEDURE

Record in the comment section any problems encountered while practicing the procedure (or have a fellow student or the instructor evaluate your performance).

S = Satisfactory
U = Unsatisfactory

You must:	S	U	Evaluation/Comments
1. Assemble equipment and materials for capillary puncture			
2. Wash hands with antiseptic and put on gloves and face protection			

(Continues)

© 2012 Delmar, Cengage Learning. Permission to reproduce for clinical use granted.

You must:	S	U	Evaluation/Comments
3. Perform a capillary puncture			
4. Wipe away the first drop of blood			

5. Prepare thick smears:
  a. Allow 1 or 2 large drops of blood from the capillary puncture to fall onto the center of a microscope slide
  b. Spread the blood evenly into a nickel-sized circle using *slight* pressure against the slide with the finger-tip (or use the corner of a clean glass slide to spread the blood)
  c. Make a second thick smear
  d. Check the thickness of the smears by placing slides on printed material. The print should be readable through the blood film
  e. Place the slides on a flat surface in a dust-free place and allow them to completely air-dry at room temperature for several hours, or overnight. DO NOT FIX			

6. Prepare thin smears:
  a. Apply a small drop of blood to a glass slide and use a clean spreader slide to form a thin blood film
  b. Make a second thin smear and set both smears aside to air-dry
  c. Immerse dried thin smears in absolute methanol for 30 to 60 seconds and air-dry			

7. Apply pressure to puncture site with sterile gauze when satisfactory smears have been obtained. (If staining is to be done another day, disinfect work area, remove gloves, and wash hands. Reglove before handling smears for staining slides)			
8. Discard capillary puncture materials into appropriate bio-hazard and sharps containers			

9. Stain smears (instructor will provide stain dilution and exact staining and rinsing times):
  a. Immerse slides in a freshly prepared 1:50 dilution of Giemsa stain for 50 to 60 minutes. (Be sure thin smear has been fixed and thick smear has dried for several hours)
  b. Rinse stained smears in buffered water: rinse thin smear by dipping several times in buffer; rinse thick smear 5 minutes in buffer
  c. Place rinsed slides in slide rack and allow to air-dry			

10. Place thin smear on microscope stage and observe cells using oil-immersion objective. Observe quality of stain: red blood cells should be pinkish; white blood cell nuclei should be blue-purple			
11. Examine red blood cells for stained intracellular parasitic inclusions (Refer to charts, figures, or commercially prepared slides, if available)			

© 2012 Delmar, Cengage Learning. Permission to reproduce for clinical use granted.

You must:	S	U	Evaluation/Comments
12. Remove thin smear from microscope stage and place thick smear in position			
13. Examine thick smear using oil-immersion objective: white blood cells and platelets should be visible, but red blood cells should have been destroyed in the staining process and appear as red cell ghosts. If parasites were present in the blood specimen, they will be stained (Refer to charts, figures, or commercially prepared slides, if available)			
14. Examine commercially prepared malaria smears, if available. Use an atlas to aid in identification of parasite forms			
15. Remove slide from microscope stage and clean oil from microscope objective with lens cleaner			
16. Store slides in covered slide box			
17. Clean microscope and return to storage			
18. Wipe work area with disinfectant			
19. Remove gloves and discard into biohazard container			
20. Wash hands with antiseptic			

Instructor/Evaluator Comments:

Instructor/Evaluator _____ Date _____

© 2012 Delmar, Cengage Learning. Permission to reproduce for clinical use granted.

STUDENT PERFORMANCE GUIDE

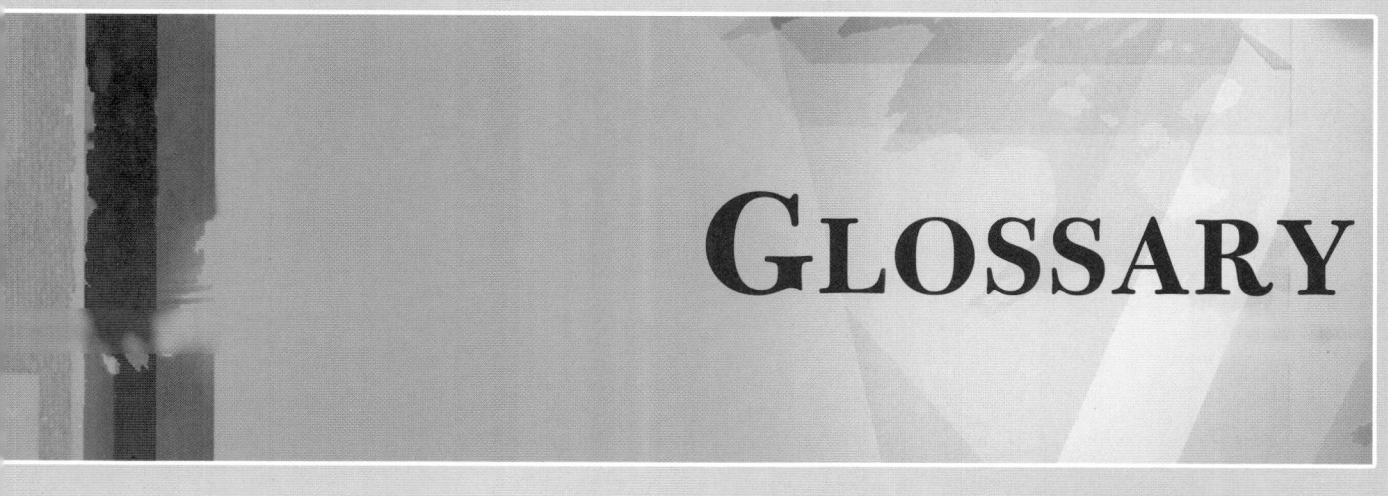

GLOSSARY

A

abbreviation / the shortening of a word, often by removing letters from the end of the word

absorbance (A) / a logarithmic expression of the amount of light absorbed by a substance containing colored molecules; optical density (O.D.)

accessioning / the process by which specimens are logged in, labeled, and assigned a specimen identification code

accreditation / a voluntary process in which an independent agency grants recognition to institutions or programs that meet or exceed established standards of quality

accuracy / the closeness of agreement of a measured value with the true value

acidosis / a condition in which blood pH falls below 7.35

acquired immunodeficiency syndrome (AIDS) / a form of severe immunodeficiency caused by infection with the human immunodeficiency virus (HIV)

acronym / combination of the first letters or syllables of a group of words to form a new group of letters that can be pronounced as a word

activated clotting time (ACT) / a test that assesses the effect of heparin on the ability of blood to clot

activated partial thromboplastin time (APTT) / the time required for a fibrin clot to form when $CaCl_2$ is added to citrated plasma that has been activated with partial thromboplastin reagent

acute phase proteins / proteins that increase rapidly in plasma during acute infection, during inflammation, or following tissue injury

adhesion / the act of two parts or surfaces sticking together

aerobic / requiring oxygen for growth

aerosol / liquid in the form of a very fine mist

agar / a seaweed derivative used to solidify microbiological media

agglutination / the clumping or aggregation of particulate antigens result from reaction with specific antibody

agglutination inhibition / interference with, or prevention of, agglutination

aggregate / the total substances making up a mass; a cluster or clump of particles

aggregation / the collecting of separate objects into one mass

agroterrorism / acts of terrorism involving threats to agricultural products, including food animals and crops

Airborne Precautions / a Centers for Disease Control and Prevention (CDC) isolation category designed to prevent transmission of infectious diseases, such as measles, that are spread by the airborne route

alanine aminotransferase (ALT) / an enzyme present in high concentration in the liver and measured to assess liver function; formerly called SGPT

albumin / the most abundant protein in normal plasma; a homogeneous group of plasma proteins that are made in the liver and help maintain osmotic balance

albumins / the most abundant protein in normal plasma; a homogeneous group of plasma proteins that are made in the liver and help maintain osmotic balance

alimentary tract / the digestive tube from the mouth to the anus

alkaline phosphatase (ALP or AP) / an enzyme widely distributed in the body, especially in the liver and bone

alkalosis / a condition in which blood pH rises above 7.45

allele / one of two (or more) forms of a gene responsible for genetic variation

allergy / a condition resulting from an exaggerated immune response; hypersensitivity

alpha cell / a type of cell in the islets of Langerhans that makes and secretes glucagon

ameba (pl. amebae) / a single-celled eukaryotic organism lacking a definite shape and moving by means of pseudopodia; also spelled amoeba (pl. amoebae)

American Association of Blood Banks (AABB) / international association that sets blood bank standards, accredits blood banks, and promotes high standards of performance in the practice of transfusion medicine

American Association of Medical Assistants (AAMA) / professional society and credentialing agency for medical assistants

American Medical Technologists (AMT) / professional society and credentialing agency for several categories of medical laboratory personnel

American Society for Clinical Laboratory Science (ASCLS) / professional society for clinical/medical laboratory personnel

American Society for Clinical Pathology (ASCP) / professional society for clinical/medical laboratory personnel and allied health personnel

American Society of Phlebotomy Technicians (ASPT) / professional society and credentialing agency for phlebotomists, as well as credentialing agency for specialty areas such as point-of-care technician

amorphous / without definite shape

amorphous phosphates / granular crystals without uniform shape that can form in alkaline urine, give urine sediment a whitish appearance after contrifugation, and appear clear microscopically

amorphous urates / granular crystals without uniform shape that can form in acid urine, can give urine sediment a pink appearance after centrifugation and appear yellowish microscopically

amperometry / the technology that uses electrodes and electrode potential to measure electron generation

anaerobic / growing in the absence of oxygen

analyte / a chemical substance that is the subject of chemical analysis

anamnestic response / rapid increase in blood immunoglobulins following a second exposure to an antigen; also called booster response or secondary response

anemia / a condition in which the red blood cell count or hemoglobin level is below normal; a condition resulting in decreased oxygen-carrying capacity of the blood

anion / a negatively charged ion

anion gap / a mathematical calculation of the difference between the cations and anions measured in the electrolyte assay

anisocytosis / marked variation in the sizes of erythrocytes

Anopheles / the genus of mosquito that is the definitive host for the human malaria parasites (genus *Plasmodium*) and that is capable of transmitting the organism to humans

antibiotic susceptibility testing / determining the susceptibility of bacteria to specific antibiotics

antibody (Ab) / protein that is induced by, and reacts specifically with, a foreign substance (antigen); immunoglobulin

anticoagulant / a chemical or substance that prevents blood coagulation

antigen (Ag) / foreign substance that induces an immune response by causing production of antibodies and/or sensitized lymphocytes that react specifically with that substance; immunogen

anti-human globulin test / a sensitive test that uses a commercial anti-human globulin reagent to detect human globulin coated on red blood cells; antiglobulin test; Coombs' test

antiseptic / a chemical used on living tissues to control the growth of infectious agents

antiserum / serum that contains antibodies

anuria / absence of urine production; failure of kidney function and suppression of urine production

aperture / an opening

apheresis / the process of removing a specific component, such as platelets, from donor blood, and returning the remaining blood components to donor circulation

APIC / Association for Professionals in Infection Control and Epidemiology, an organization working across a spectrum of professionals, organizations, and institutions to prevent healthcare-associated infections

arteriole / a small branch of an artery leading to a capillary

arteriosclerosis / abnormal thickening and hardening of the arterial walls, causing loss of elasticity and impaired blood circulation

artery / a blood vessel that carries oxygenated blood from the heart to the tissues

arthritis / inflammation of the joints, due to several causes

arthropod / a member of the phylum Arthropoda, which includes crustaceans, insects, and arachnids

ASCP Board of Certification (ASCP BOC) / a separate body within the ASCP organizational structure, formed in 2009 by merging NCA with the ASCP BOR and providing certification for medical laboratory personnel

aseptic technique / work practices used to prevent contamination when working with microorganisms

aspartate aminotransferase (AST) / an enzyme present in many tissues, including cardiac, muscle, and liver, that is measured to assess liver function; formerly called SGOT

atherosclerosis / a form of arteriosclerosis in which lipids, calcium, cholesterol, and other substances deposit on the inner walls of the arteries

atrial / of or relating to a body cavity

atypical lymphocyte / lymphocyte, usually large, that occurs in response to viral infections and is common in infectious mononucleosis; reactive lymphocyte

autoantibody / an antibody directed against self (one's own tissues)

autoclave / an instrument that uses pressurized steam for sterilization

autoimmune disease / disease caused when the immune response is directed at one's own tissues (self-antigens)

average / the sum of a set of values divided by the number of values in the set; the mean

avian influenza / an infection of birds with one of the influenza A viruses; bird flu

azidemethemoglobin / a stable compound formed when azide combines with methemoglobin

azurophilic / a term used to describe the reddish-purple staining characteristics of certain blood cells; the quality of staining with azure dyes

B

B lymphocyte (B cell) / the type of lymphocyte primarily responsible for the humoral immune response

babesiosis / an infection spread by tick bite and caused by protozoan parasites of the genus *Babesia*

bacillus / a rod-shaped bacterium

bacteriology / the study of bacteria

band cell / an immature granulocyte with a nonsegmented nucleus; a "stab cell"

basilic vein / large vein on inner side ("pinky" side) of arm

basophil / a leukocyte containing basophilic-staining granules in the cytoplasm

basophilia / abnormal increase in the number of basophils in the blood; basophilic leukocytosis; also, the affinity of cellular structures for basophilic dyes

basophilic / blue in color; having affinity for the basic stain

basophilic stippling / remnants of RNA and other basophilic nuclear material remaining inside the red blood cell after the nucleus is lost from the cell; small purple granules in red blood cells stained with Wright's stain

beaker / a wide-mouthed, straight-sided container with a pouring spout formed from the rim and used to make estimated measurements

Beer's law / a mathematical relationship that demonstrates the linear relationship of concentration to absorbance and that forms the basis for spectrophotometric analysis

Beral pipet / a disposable plastic pipet with a built-in bulb on one end that usually can deliver up to 2 mL and can have a graduated stem; also called a transfer pipet

beta cell / a type of cell in the islets of Langerhans that makes and secretes proinsulin and insulin

bibulous paper / a special absorbent paper used to dry slides; blotting paper

bilirubin / a product formed in the liver from the breakdown of hemoglobin

binocular / having two oculars or eyepieces

biohazard / risk or hazard to health or the environment from biological agents

biological safety cabinet / a special work cabinet that provides protection to the worker while working with infectious microorganisms

biosafety level 4 (BSL-4) / a designation requiring the use of a combination of work practices, equipment, and facilities to prevent exposure of individuals or the environment to pathogens that can be transmitted by aerosol and that pose a high risk for life-threatening disease for which treatment or vaccine is not generally available

birefringence / the characteristic of double refraction; the characteristic of being able to split a beam of polarized light into two light beams

blast cell / an immature blood cell normally found only in the bone marrow

blind sample / an assayed sample that is provided as an unknown to laboratories participating in proficiency testing programs

blood bank / clinical laboratory department where blood components are tested and stored until needed for transfusion; immunohematology department; transfusion services; also the refrigerated unit used for storing blood components

blood group antibody / a protein (immunoglobulin) that reacts specifically with a blood group antigen

blood group antigen / a substance or structure on the red blood cell membrane that stimulates antibody formation and reacts with that antibody

blood urea nitrogen (BUN) / a test measuring urea nitrogen in blood

bloodborne pathogens (BBP) / pathogens that can be present in human blood (and blood-contaminated body fluids)

Bloodborne Pathogens (BBP) Standard / OSHA guidelines for preventing occupational exposure to pathogens present in human blood and body fluids, including, but not limited to, HIV and hepatitis B virus (HBV); final OSHA standard of December 6, 1991, effective March 6, 1992

borosilicate glass / nonreactive glass with high thermal resistance commonly used to make high-quality labware

botulinum intoxication / a condition in which body tissues are affected by the botulinum toxin

botulinum toxin / a neurotoxin produced by *Clostridium botulinum*

bovine spongiform encephalopathy (BSE) / a fatal, neurological disease of cattle caused by an unconventional transmissible agent called a prion; commonly called "mad cow disease"

Bowman's capsule / the portion of the nephron that receives the glomerular filtrate

bradyzoite / a slowly multiplying form of coccidian parasite found within tissue cysts and typical of chronic infection with *Toxoplasma gondii*

B-type natriuretic peptide (BNP) / a peptide hormone released primarily from the ventricles of the heart and used as a marker for cardiac function

buffer / a substance that lessens change in the pH of a solution when acid or base (alkali) is added

buffy coat / a light-colored layer of white blood cells and platelets that forms on top of the red blood cell layer when a sample of blood is centrifuged or allowed to stand undisturbed

C

calibration / the process of checking, standardizing, or adjusting a method or instrument so that it yields accurate results

Candida albicans / yeast that causes vaginitis and other infections, especially following antibiotic therapy

capillary / a minute blood vessel that connects the smallest arteries to the smallest veins and serves as an oxygen exchange vessel

capillary action / the action by which a fluid enters a tube because of the attraction between the fluid and the tube

capillary tube / a slender glass or plastic tube used for laboratory procedures

carcinogen / a substance with the potential to produce cancer in humans or animals

cardiopulmonary circulation / the system of blood vessels that circulates blood from the heart to the lungs and back to the heart

cardiovascular disease (CVD) / disease of the heart and blood vessels resulting from a variety of causes

carrier / an individual who harbors an organism and is capable of spreading the organism to others, but has no symptoms or signs of disease

cast / in urinalysis, a protein matrix formed in the kidney tubules and washed out into the urine

cation / a positively charged ion

catalase test / a test to differentiate between *Streptococcus* and *Staphylococcus* species

caustic / a chemical substance having the ability to burn or destroy tissue

cell diluting fluid / a solution used to dilute blood for cell counts

cell-mediated immunity / immunity provided by T lymphocytes and cytokines

cellular respiration / the series of cellular metabolic processes in which organic substances are oxidized and energy in the form of ATP is released

Celsius (C) scale / temperature scale having the freezing point of water at 0° C and the boiling point at 100° C

Centers for Disease Control and Prevention (CDC) / central laboratory for the national public health system

Centers for Medicare and Medicaid Services (CMS) / the agency within the Department of Health and Human Services (DHHS) responsible for implementing CLIA '88

centi / prefix used to indicate one-hundredth (10^{-2}) of a unit

centrifuge / an instrument with a rotor that rotates at high speeds in a closed chamber

cephalic vein / a superficial vein of the arm (thumb side) commonly used for venipuncture

cerebrospinal fluid (CSF) / the fluid surrounding the spinal cord and bathing the ventricles of the brain

cestode / tapeworm; member of the class Cestoda

chemical hygiene plan / comprehensive written safety plan detailing the proper use and storage of hazardous chemicals in the workplace

Chlamydia trachomatis / species of gram-negative intracellular bacteria that is a cause of sexually transmitted diseases (STDs)

chromogen / a substance that becomes colored when it undergoes a chemical change

chronic fatigue syndrome (CFS) / a syndrome characterized by prolonged fatigue and other nonspecific symptoms, and for which the cause remains unknown

chylomicrons / lipoproteins made in the small intestine and released into the blood to transport exogenous (dietary) cholesterol and triglycerides from the small intestines to the liver and other tissues

clean-catch urine / a midstream urine sample collected after the urethral opening and surrounding tissues have been cleansed

Clinical and Laboratory Standards Institute (CLSI) / an international, nonprofit organization that establishes guidelines and standards of best current practice for clinical laboratories; formerly National Committee for Clinical Laboratory Standards (NCCLS)

clinical chemistry / the laboratory section that uses chemical principles to analyze blood and other body fluids

Clinical Laboratory Improvement Amendments of 1988 (CLIA '88) / a federal act that specifies minimum performance standards for clinical laboratories

clinical laboratory science / the health profession concerned with performing laboratory analyses used in diagnosing and treating disease, as well as in maintaining good health; synonymous with medical laboratory science and medical (laboratory) technology

clinical laboratory scientist (CLS) / the NCA term for a professional who has a baccalaureate degree from an accredited college or university, has completed clinical training in an accredited clinical/medical laboratory science program, and has passed a national certifying examination; also called medical laboratory scientist (MLS) or medical technologist (MT)

clinical laboratory technician (CLT) / the NCA term for a professional who has completed a minimum of 2 years of specific training in an accredited clinical/medical laboratory technician program and has passed a national certifying examination; also called medical laboratory technician (MLT)

clue cells / vaginal epithelial cells covered with tiny, gram-variable bacteria and seen in vaginal secretions of patients with bacterial vaginosis

coagulase test / a test to differentiate between *Staphylococcus aureus* and other *Staphylococcus* species

coagulation / the process of forming a fibrin clot

coagulation factors / a group of plasma proteins (and the mineral calcium) involved in blood clotting

coarse adjustment / control that adjusts position of microscope objectives and is used to initially bring objects into focus

coccus / a spherical bacterium

codocyte / target cell

codominant / in genetics, a gene that is expressed in the heterozygous state, that is, in the presence of a different allelic gene

coefficient of variation (CV) / a calculated value that compares the relative variability between different sets of data

COLA / agency that offers accreditation to physician office laboratories, hospitals, clinics, and other healthcare facilities; formerly the Commission on Office Laboratory Accreditation

coliform / referring to certain fermentative gram-negative enteric bacteria, including *Escherichia coli, Enterobacter,* and *Klebsiella*

collagen / a protein connective tissue found in skin, bone, ligaments, and cartilage

College of American Pathologists (CAP) / organization that offers accreditation to clinical laboratories

colony / a defined mass of bacteria assumed to have grown from a single organism

colony count / an estimation of the number of organisms in 1 mL of urine made by counting the colonies on a urine culture plate

commensal / an organism that lives with, on, or in another organism, without injury to either

Commission on Accreditation of Allied Health Education Programs (CAAHEP) / agency that accredits educational programs for allied health personnel; formerly CAHEA

communicable / able to be transmitted directly or indirectly from one individual to another

community-acquired infection (CAI) / infection acquired through contact with friends, family, and the public or by contact with contaminated environmental surfaces

complement / a group of plasma proteins that can be activated in immune reactions, can cause cell lysis, and can help initiate the inflammatory response

complete blood count (CBC) / a commonly performed grouping of hematological tests

condenser / apparatus located below the microscope stage that directs light into the objective

confocal laser scanning microscope / a microscope using a laser as the light source and producing images of very high resolution

congenital / acquired during fetal development, and present at the time of birth, but not inherited

Contact Precautions / a CDC isolation category designed to prevent transmission of diseases spread by close or direct contact

controls / commercially available assayed solutions that are chemically and physically similar to the unknown and are tested in the same manner as the unknown to monitor the precision of a test method

coronary heart disease (CHD) / a narrowing of the small blood vessels that supply blood and oxygen to the heart; also called coronary artery disease (CAD)

cortex / the outer layer or portion of an organ

Coumadin / an anticoagulant derived from coumarin that is administered orally to prevent blood clotting; or to reduce the risk of clots a trade name for warfarin

Coumadin / an anticoagulant drug derived from coumarin that is administered orally to prevent blood clotting or to reduce the risk of clots; a trade name for warfarin

counterstain / a dye that adds a contrasting color

C-reactive protein (CRP) / one of the acute phase proteins found in plasma in inflammation

creatine kinase (CK) / an enzyme present in large amounts in brain tissue and heart and skeletal muscle and a form of which is measured to aid in diagnosing heart attack

creatinine / a breakdown product of creatine that is normally excreted in the urine

crenated cell / a shrunken red blood cell with scalloped or toothed margins

critical measurements / measurements made when the accuracy of the concentration of a solution is important; measurements made using glassware manufactured to strict standards

culture / growth of microorganisms in a special medium; the process of growing microorganisms in the laboratory

culture medium / a substance used to provide nutrients for growing microorganisms

cyanmethemoglobin / a stable colored compound formed when hemoglobin is reacted with Drabkin's reagent; hemiglobincyanide (HiCN)

cyst / the dormant stage of an organism surrounded by a resistant covering; the nonmotile, nonfeeding stage of a protozoan; a closed sec-like structure within a tissue

cystitis / inflammation of the urinary bladder, usually caused by an infection

cytokines / any of various nonantibody proteins secreted by cells of the immune system and that help regulate the immune response; lymphokine

cytoplasm / the fluid portion of the cell surrounding the nucleus

D

D-dimer / one of the products formed from the breakdown of cross-linked fibrin by plasmin

deci / prefix used to indicate one-tenth (10^{-1}) of a unit

deep vein thrombosis (DVT) / occurrence of a thrombus within a deep vein, usually of the leg or pelvis

definitive host / the host in which the sexual or adult form of the parasite is found

deionized water / water that has had most of the mineral ions removed

dendritic cells / cells in lymphoid tissues that form a network to trap foreign antigens

deoxyhemoglobin / the hemoglobin formed when oxyhemoglobin releases oxygen to tissues

deoxyribonucleic acid (DNA) / the nucleic acid that carries genetic information and is found primarily in the nucleus of all living cells

Department of Health and Human Services (DHHS) / the governmental agency that oversees public healthcare matters; also called HHS

Department of Homeland Security / a federal agency whose primary mission is to prevent, protect against, and respond to acts of terrorism on U.S. soil

diabetes mellitus / a disorder of carbohydrate metabolism characterized by a state of hyperglycemia resulting from insulin deficiency

dialysate / in kidney dialysis, a solution used to draw waste products and excess fluid from the body

differential count / a determination of the relative numbers of each type of white blood cell when a specified number (usually 100) is counted; leukocyte differential count; white blood cell differential count

differential interference contrast (DIC) microscope / a microscope equipped with special Normarski optics that enhance contrast in unstained, transparent specimens, producing a three-dimensional image

diluent / a liquid added to a solution to make it less concentrated

dilution / a solution made less concentrated by adding a diluent; the act of making a dilute solution; the degree to which a solution is made less concentrated

dilution factor / reciprocal of the dilution

disinfectant / a chemical used on inanimate objects to kill or inactivate microbes

disseminated intravascular coagulation (DIC) / a hemostasis emergency characterized by widespread circulatory thrombotic events coexisting with fibrinolytic events

distal convoluted tubule / the portion of a renal tubule that empties into the collecting tubule

distilled water / the condensate collected from steam after water has been boiled

diurnal / having a daily cycle

Drabkin's reagent / a hemoglobin diluting reagent that contains iron, potassium, cyanide, and sodium bicarbonate

drepanocyte / sickle cell

Droplet Precautions / a CDC isolation category designed to prevent transmission of diseases spread through the air over short distances

E

Ebola virus / a highly infectious filovirus that causes a hemorrhagic fever

ectoparasite / a parasite that lives on the outer surface of a host

ectopic pregnancy / development of fetus outside the uterus; extra-uterine pregnancy

EDTA / ethylenediaminetetraacetic acid; an anticoagulant commonly used in hematology

electrolyte solution / a solution that contains ions and conducts an electrical current

electrolytes / the cations and anions important in maintaining fluid and acid-base balance

electron microscope / a microscope using an electron beam to create images from a specimen and that is capable of much greater magnification and resolving power than a light microscope

electronic health record (EHR) / comprehensive, portable electronic patient health record

electronic medical record (EMR) / a digital form of a patient chart created in a physician's office or a hospital where a patient received treatment

elliptocyte / elongated, cigar-shaped red blood cell

embolus (pl. emboli) / a mass (clot) of blood or foreign matter carried in the circulation

endemic / recurring in a specific location or population

endogenous / produced within; growing from within

endoparasite / a parasite that lives within the host

endothelium / the layer of epithelial cells that lines blood vessels and the serous cavities of the body

engineering control / use of available technology and equipment to protect the worker from hazards

English system of measurement / system of measurement in common use in the United States for nonscientific measurements; sometimes called U.S. customary system

enriched medium / a medium that contains nutrients to support a wide variety of organisms, including fastidious organisms

enzyme / a protein that causes or accelerates changes in other substances without being changed itself

enzyme immunoassay (EIA) / an assay that uses an enzyme-labeled antibody as a reactant

eosin / a red-orange stain or dye

eosinophil / a leukocyte containing eosinophilic granules in the cytoplasm

eosinophilia / abnormal increase in the number of eosinophils in the blood

epidemic / disease affecting many persons at the same time, spread from person to person, and occurring in an area where the disease is not prevalent

epidemiology / the study of the factors that cause disease and determine disease frequency and distribution

epistaxis / nosebleed

epitope / the portion of an antigen that reacts specifically with an antibody; antigenic determinant

epizootic / an outbreak of disease in an animal population

Epstein-Barr virus (EBV) / a virus that infects lymphocytes and is the cause of infectious mononucleosis

erythrocyte / red blood cell; RBC

erythrocytosis / an excess of red blood cells in the peripheral blood; sometimes called polycythemia

erythropoiesis / the production of red blood cells

***Escherichia coli* (*E. coli*)** / a bacterium that is part of the normal flora of the intestines

ethics / a system of conduct or behavior; rules of professional conduct

ethylenediaminetetraacetic acid (EDTA) / an anticoagulant commonly used in hematology

exogenous / originating from the outside

exposure control plan / a plan identifying employees at risk for exposure to bloodborne pathogens and providing training in methods to prevent exposure

exposure incident / an accident, such as a needlestick, in which an individual is exposed to possible infection through contact with body substances from another individual

eyepiece / ocular

F

Fahrenheit (F) scale / temperature scale having a freezing point of water at 32° F and boiling point at 212° F

fastidious bacteria / bacteria that require special nutritional factors to survive

FDPs / fibrinogen or fibrin monomer degradation products formed when plasmin cleaves fibrinogen or fibrin monomers into protein fragments; formerly called fibrin split products

femto / prefix used to indicate 10^{-15}

femtoliters (fL) / 10^{-15} liter

feto-maternal hemorrhage (FMH) / the occurrence of fetal blood cells entering into the maternal circulation before or during delivery

fibrin / a protein formed from fibrinogen by the action of thrombin

fibrinogen / a plasma protein produced in the liver and converted to fibrin through the action of thrombin

fibrinolysis / enzymatic breakdown of a blood clot

field diaphragm / adjustable aperture attached to microscope base

fine adjustment / control that adjusts position of microscope objectives and is used to sharpen focus

fission / reproductive process in which the parent cell divides into two identical independent cells

fixative / preservative; a chemical that prevents deterioration of cells or tissues

flagellum (pl., flagella) / slender, lash-like appendage that serves as organ of locomotion for sperm cells and some protozoa

flask / a container with an enlarged body and a narrow neck

flint glass / inexpensive glass with low resistance to heat and chemicals

fluor / a substance that absorbs short-wavelength (exciting) light and emits longer wavelength (emitting) light

fluorescent / having the property of emitting light of one wavelength when exposed to light of another wavelength

folic acid / a member of the B vitamin complex

fomites / inanimate objects, such as bed rails, linens, or eating utensils, which can be contaminated with infectious organisms and serve as a means of their transmission

Food and Drug Administration (FDA) / the division of the Department of Health and Human Services (DHHS) responsible for protecting the public health by ensuring the safety and efficacy of foods, drugs, biological products, medical devices, and cosmetics

formalin / a 37% solution of formaldehyde used for fixing and preserving biological specimens

formula weight (F.W.) / weight of the entity represented by a chemical formula; molecular weight

forward grouping / the use of known antisera (antibodies) to detect unknown antigens on a patient's cells; forward typing; direct grouping

fossae / in the throat, shallow depressions where the tonsils were located before surgical removal

fume hood / a device that draws contaminated air out of an area and either cleanses and recirculates it or discharges it to the outside

G

galactosuria / the presence of galactose in the urine; the condition in which galactose is excreted into the urine

gamma-glutamyltransferase (GGT) / an enzyme present in liver, kidney, pancreas, and prostate, and measured to assess liver function

gauge / a measure of the internal diameter (or bore) of a needle

Gaussian curve / a graph plotting the distribution of values around the mean; normal frequency curve

genes / segments of DNA that code for specific proteins and that are the structural units of heredity

genotype / the genetic makeup of a cell or organism

Giemsa stain / a polychromatic stain used for staining blood cells and blood parasites

globin / the protein portion of the hemoglobin molecule

globulins / a heterogeneous group of serum proteins with varied functions

glomerular filtrate / the fluid that passes from the blood into the nephron and from which urine is formed

glomerular filtration rate (GFR) / an estimation of how much blood passes through the glomeruli per unit of time (minute); an estimate of the number of functioning nephrons made by using the rate at which molecules such as creatinine and urea are filtered by the kidneys

glomerulonephritis / inflammation of the glomeruli

glomerulus (pl. glomeruli) / a small bundle of capillaries that is the filtering portion of the nephron

glucagon / the pancreatic hormone that increases blood glucose concentration by promoting the conversion of glycogen to glucose

gluconeogenesis / production of glucose from noncarbohydrate sources

glucose dehydrogenase / an enzyme that converts glucose to gluconolactone and that is used in glucose analytical methods

glucose oxidase / an enzyme that converts glucose to gluconic acid and that is used in glucose analytical methods

glycated hemoglobin (GHb) / see hemoglobin A1c

glycogen / the storage form of glucose found in high concentration in the liver

glycogenesis / conversion of glucose to glycogen

glycogenolysis / the conversion of glycogen to glucose

glycolysis / energy production as a result of the metabolic breakdown of glucose; the breakdown of glucose to pyruvic acid or lactic acid accompanied by the release of energy in the form of ATP

glycoprotein / a protein molecule having a carbohydrate component

glycosuria / glucose in the urine; glucosuria

gonorrhea / contagious infection spread by sexual contact and caused by *Neisseria gonorrhoeae*

gout / a painful condition in which blood uric acid is elevated and urates precipitate in joints

graduated cylinder / an upright, straight-sided container with a flared base and a volume scale

gram (g) / basic metric unit of weight or mass

gram equivalent weight / the number obtained by dividing the formula weight by the valence

gram negative / designation for bacteria that lose the crystal violet (purple) stain and retain the safranin (red) stain in the Gram stain procedure

gram positive / designation for bacteria that retain the crystal violet (purple) stain in the Gram stain procedure

Gram stain / a differential stain used to classify bacteria

granulocyte / a white blood cell containing granules in the cytoplasm; any of the neutrophilic, eosinophilic, or basophilic leukocytes

granulomatous amebic encephalitis (GAE) / rare and usually fatal brain infection caused by *Acanthamoeba* species and usually occurring only in immunocompromised individuals

guaiac / a chemical derived from the resin of a tree of the genus *Guaiacum*

H

hand antisepsis / decontamination of hands using antiseptic soap or waterless antiseptic handrub

hand hygiene / a set of techniques that includes handwashing with soap and water, washing with antiseptic soap, or cleansing with a waterless antiseptic product

HDL cholesterol / high-density lipoprotein fraction of blood cholesterol; *good* cholesterol

Health Care Financing Administration (HCFA) / see Centers for Medicare and Medicaid Services (CMS)

Health Insurance Portability and Accountability Act (HIPAA) / 1996 act of Congress, a part of which guarantees protection of privacy of an individual's health information

healthcare-associated infection (HAI) / infection acquired while being treated for another condition in a healthcare setting; synonym for healthcare-acquired infection; formerly called nosocomial infection

helminth / a worm, especially a parasitic worm; in parasitology, the group comprising the roundworms and flatworms

hemacytometer / a heavy glass slide made to precise specifications and used to count cells microscopically; a counting chamber

hemacytometer coverglass / a special coverglass of uniform thickness used with a hemacytometer

hemagglutination / the agglutination of red blood cells

hematocrit / the volume of red blood cells packed by centrifugation in a given volume of blood and expressed as a percentage; packed cell volume (PCV)

hematology / the study of blood and the blood-forming tissues

hematoma / the swelling of tissue around a vessel resulting from leakage of blood into the tissue

hematopoietic stem cell / see hemopoietic stem cell

hematuria / the presence of blood in the urine

heme / the iron-containing portion of the hemoglobin molecule

hemiglobincyanide (HiCN) / cyanmethemoglobin

hemoconcentration / increase in the concentration of cellular elements in the blood

hemoglobin (Hb, Hgb) / the major functional component of red blood cells that is the oxygen-carrying molecule

hemoglobin A1c (HbA1c) / hemoglobin modified by the binding of glucose to the beta globin chains of hemoglobin; also called glycated or glycosylated hemoglobin

hemoglobinuria / the presence of hemoglobin in the urine

hemolysis / the rupture or destruction of red blood cells resulting in the release of hemoglobin

hemolysis / the rupture or destruction of red blood cells resulting in the release of hemoglobin

hemolytic disease of the newborn (HDN) / a condition in which maternal antibody targets fetal red blood cells for destruction

hemophilia / a bleeding disorder resulting from a hereditary coagulation factor deficiency or dysfunction

hemopoiesis / the process of blood cell formation and development; hematopoiesis

hemopoietic stem cell / an undifferentiated bone marrow cell that gives rise to blood cells

hemorrhage / uncontrolled bleeding

hemostasis / the process of stopping bleeding, which includes clot formation and clot dissolution

HEPA filter / high-efficiency particulate air filter used in biological safety cabinets

heparin / an anticoagulant used therapeutically to prevent thrombosis; also used as an anticoagulant in certain laboratory procedures

hepatitis B virus (HBV) / the virus that causes hepatitis B infection and is transmitted by contact with infected blood or other body fluids

hepatitis C virus (HCV) / the virus that causes hepatitis C infection and is transmitted by contact with infected blood or other body fluids

hepatosplenomegaly / enlargement of the liver and spleen

herpes simplex virus, type 1 (HSV-1) / the virus causing oral herpes

herpes simplex virus, type 2 (HSV-2) / the virus causing genital herpes

heterophile antibodies / a group of multispecific antibodies that are increased in infectious mononucleosis and that react with heterogeneous antigens *not* responsible for their production

hexokinase / an enzyme that converts glucose to glucose-6-phosphate and that is used in glucose analytical methods

HIPAA / Health Insurance Portability and Accountability Act of 1996

histocompatibility testing / assays to determine if donor and recipient tissue are compatible

histogram / a graph that illustrates the size and frequency of occurrence of articles being studied

homeostasis / the tendency toward steady state or equilibrium of body processes

homocysteine / an amino acid, elevated blood levels of which are associated with increased risk for vascular and cardiovascular disease

host / the organism from which a parasite obtains nutrients and in which some or part of the parasite's life cycle is completed

Howell-Jolly body / nuclear remnant remaining in red blood cells after the nucleus is lost and commonly seen in pernicious anemia and hemolytic anemias

human chorionic gonadotropin (hCG) / the hormone of pregnancy, produced by the placenta; also called uterine chorionic gonadotropin (uCG)

human immunodeficiency virus (HIV) / the retrovirus that has been identified as the cause of acquired immunodeficiency syndrome (AIDS)

human leukocyte antigen (HLA) / one of several antigens present on leukocytes and other body cells that are important in transplant rejection

human papillomavirus (HPV) / a group of DNA viruses, some of which are sexually transmitted

humoral immunity / immunity provided by B lymphocytes and antibodies

hyaline / transparent, pale

hypercalcemia / blood calcium levels above normal

hypercoagulation / a greater tendency than normal for blood to coagulate

hyperglycemia / blood glucose concentration above normal

hyperkalemia / blood potassium levels above normal

hyperlipidemia / excessive amount of fat in the blood

hypernatremia / blood sodium levels above normal

hyperthyroidism / excessive functional activity of the thyroid gland; excessive secretion of thyroid hormones

hyphae / filaments of a fungus that make up the mycelium

hypoalbuminemia / marked decrease in serum albumin concentration

hypocalcemia / blood calcium levels below normal

hypochromic / having reduced color or hemoglobin content

hypodermic needle / a hollow needle used for obtaining fluid specimens or for injections

hypoglycemia / blood glucose concentration below normal

hypokalemia / blood potassium levels below normal

hyponatremia / blood sodium levels below normal

hypothyroidism / underactive function of the thyroid gland; abnormally low production of thyroid hormones

I

immune thrombocytopenic purpura (ITP) / a blood disorder characterized by purpura in skin and mucous membranes and low platelet count caused by the destruction of blood platelets by antiplatelet autoantibodies; also called idiopathic thrombocytopenic purpura

immunity / resistance to disease or infection

immunoassay / a diagnostic method using antigen–antibody reactions

immunocompetent / capable of producing a normal immune response

immunocompromised / having reduced ability or inability to produce a normal immune response

immunoglobulins (Ig) / antibodies; proteins that are induced by and react specifically with antigens (immunogens)

immunohematology / the study of the human blood groups; in the clinical laboratory, often called blood banking or transfusion services

immunology / the branch of medicine encompassing the study of immune processes and immunity

immunosuppression / suppression of the immune response by physical, chemical, or biological means

impedance / resistance in an electrical circuit

implantation / attachment of the early embryo to the uterus

incubation period / the time elapsed between exposure to an infectious agent and the appearance of symptoms

index of refraction / the ratio of the velocity of light in one medium, such as air, to its velocity in another medium

indicator medium / a bacteriological medium that differentiates bacteria on the basis of certain chemical reactions; differential medium

infection / a pathological condition caused by growth of microorganisms in the host

infectious mononucleosis (IM) / a contagious viral disease occurring in primarily the 15- to 25-year-old age-group and caused by infection with Epstein-Barr virus

inflammation / a nonspecific protective response to tissue injury that is initiated primarily by the release of chemicals such as histamine and serotonin and the actions of phagocytic cells

inhibitor / a substance that retards or stops a process or chemical reaction

inoculating loop / an instrument used to transfer bacteria

inoculation / the process of transferring microorganisms to a growth medium

inoculum / the microorganisms transferred from one medium to another

insulin / the pancreatic hormone essential for proper metabolism of blood glucose and maintenance of blood glucose levels

intermediate host / the host in which the asexual, immature, or larval form of the parasite is found

international normalized ratio (INR) / a way of reporting a prothrombin time that takes into consideration the sensitivity of the prothrombin thromboplastin reagent used and the mean prothrombin time of a normal population

international sensitivity index (ISI) / a value assigned to each lot of prothrombin thromboplastin reagent to compensate for variations in sensitivities of thromboplastin from different sources

intoxication / poisoning

intravascular / within the blood vessels

ionized calcium / in the body, a mineral that plays an important role in hemostasis

ion-selective electrode / an electrode manufactured to detect a specific ion and measure its concentration

iris diaphragm / device that regulates the amount of light striking the specimen being viewed through the microscope

islets of Langerhans / irregularly shaped clusters of cells scattered throughout the pancreas that contain alpha cells, beta cells, delta cells, and pancreatic polypeptide (PP) secreting cells

isolated colonies / bacterial colonies growing on an agar surface and not touched by other colonies

isolation / the practice of limiting the movement and social contact of a patient who is potentially infectious or who must be protected from exposure to infectious agents; quarantine

isotonic solution / a solution with the same concentration of dissolved particles as the solution or cell with which it is compared

J

Joint Commission (JC) / an independent agency that accredits hospitals and large healthcare facilities; formerly known as the Joint Commission on Accreditation of Healthcare Organizations (JCAHO)

K

keratocyte / a red blood cell deformed by mechanical trauma

ketones / a group of chemical substances produced during increased fat metabolism; ketone bodies

ketonuria / ketones in the urine

kidney / the organ in which urine is formed

kilo / prefix used to indicate 1000 (10^3) units

Köhler illumination / alignment of illuminating light for microscopy; double diaphragm illumination

L

Laboratory Response Network (LRN) / a national network of public and private laboratories coordinated by the Centers for Disease Control and Prevention (CDC) with the ability for rapid response to threats to public health

labware / article(s) or container(s) intended for laboratory use

lactate dehydrogenase (LD or LDH) / an enzyme widely distributed in the body and measured to assess liver function

lancet / a sterile, sharp-pointed blade used to perform a capillary puncture

larva / immature stage of an invertebrate

laser / a narrow, intense beam of light of only one wavelength going in only one direction

latent / dormant; in an inactive or hidden phase

lateral / toward the side

LDL cholesterol / low-density lipoprotein fraction of blood cholesterol; *bad* cholesterol

lens / a curved transparent material that spreads or focuses light

lens paper / a special nonabrasive material used to clean optical lenses

leukemia / a cancer of white blood cells characterized by an abnormal increase of white blood cells and their precursors in bone marrow, tissue, and peripheral blood

leukocyte / white blood cell; WBC

leukocytosis / increase above normal in the number of leukocytes (white blood cells) in the blood

leukopenia / decrease below normal in the number of leukocytes (white blood cells) in the blood; leukocytopenia

Levey-Jennings chart / a quality control chart used to record daily quality control values

light spectrum / the portion of the electromagnetic spectrum that is visible to humans; the range of wavelengths of visible radiation

lipemic / having a cloudy appearance because of excess lipid content

lipids / any one of a group of fats or fat-like substances

liter (L) / basic metric unit of volume

loop of Henle / the U-shaped portion of a renal tubule between its proximal and distal portions

lumen / the open space within a tubular organ or tissue

lymphadenopathy / a condition in which the lymph glands are enlarged or swollen

lymphocyte / a small basophilic-staining leukocyte having a round or oval nucleus and playing a vital role in the immune process

lymphocytosis / an increase above the normal number of lymphocytes in the blood

lymphokines / nonantibody proteins produced by lymphocytes in response to antigen stimulation and that play a role in regulating the immune response; cytokines

lyophilize(d) / remove water from a frozen solution under vacuum; freeze-dry

M

macrocytic / having a larger-than-normal cell size

macrophages / long-lived phagocytic tissue cells that are derived from blood monocytes, function in destruction of foreign antigens, and serve as antigen-presenting cells

magnification / in microscopy, the size of the image produced compared to the actual size of the object being viewed

major histocompatibility complex (MHC) / the group of genes responsible for producing antigens such as HLA that are important in organ and tissue transplants

malaria / in humans, a disease caused by infection with protozoan parasites of the genus *Plasmodium*

malignant / cancerous; not benign

maple syrup urine disease (MSUD) / a rare metabolic condition in which the amino acids leucine, isoleucine, and valine are not metabolized, causing the urine to have the odor of maple syrup

Marburg virus / a filovirus that causes a hemorrhagic fever

material safety data sheet (MSDS) / written safety information that must be supplied by manufacturers of chemicals and hazardous materials

mean / the sum of a set of values divided by the number of values in the set; the average

mean cell hemoglobin (MCH) / average red blood cell hemoglobin expressed in picograms (pg); mean corpuscular hemoglobin

mean cell hemoglobin concentration (MCHC) / comparison of the weight of hemoglobin in a red blood cell to the size of the red blood cell, expressed in percentage or grams per deciliter (g/dL); mean corpuscular hemoglobin concentration

mean cell volume (MCV) / average red blood cell volume in a blood sample, expressed in femtoliters (fL) or cubic microns (μ^3); mean corpuscular volume

mechanical vector / a vector (usually an arthropod) that is not essential to a parasite's life cycle but that can transfer an infective parasite to a noninfected host

median cubital vein / a superficial vein located in the bend of the elbow (cubital fossa) that connects the cephalic vein to the basilic vein

medical laboratory science / the health profession concerned with performing laboratory analyses used in diagnosing and treating disease, as well as in maintaining good health; synonymous with clinical laboratory science and medical (laboratory) technology

medical laboratory scientist (MLS) / a professional who has a baccalaureate degree from an accredited college or university, has completed clinical training in an accredited medical laboratory science program, and has passed a national certifying examination; synonymous with medical technologist (MT) or NCA certified clinical laboratory scientist (CLS)

medical laboratory technician (MLT) / a professional who has completed a minimum of 2 years of specific training in an accredited medical laboratory technician program and has passed a national certifying examination; synonymous with NCA certified clinical laboratory technician (CLT)

medical technologist (MT) / a term gradually being replaced but referring to the professions of medical laboratory scientist (MLS) or clinical laboratory scientist (CLS)

medical technology / synonymous for clinical laboratory science and medical laboratory science

medium / a substance used to provide nutrients for growing microorganisms

medulla / the inner or central portion of an organ

megakaryocyte / a large bone marrow cell from which platelets are derived

melanin / a dark pigment of skin, hair, and certain tumors

meniscus / the curved upper surface of a liquid in a container

meter (m) / basic metric unit of length or distance

methylene blue / a blue stain or dye

metric system / the decimal system of measurement used internationally for scientific work

micro / prefix used to indicate one-millionth (10^{-6}) of a unit

microalbumin / a small amount of albumin in urine that is not detectable by routine reagent strip

microalbuminuria / condition in which small amounts of albumin are present in the urine but are not detectable by routine reagent strip

microbiology / the branch of biology dealing with microbes

microcytic / having a smaller-than-normal cell size

microfilaria (pl. microfilariae) / immature form of a filarial worm

microfuge / a centrifuge that spins microcentrifuge tubes at high rates of speed; microcentrifuge

micrometer / a ruled device for measuring small objects

microhematocrit / a hematocrit performed in capillary tubes using a small quantity of blood; packed cell volume (PCV)

microhematocrit centrifuge / an instrument that spins capillary tubes at a high speed to rapidly separate cellular components of the blood from the liquid portion of blood

micrometer / a ruled device for measuring small objects

micropipet / a pipet that measures or holds 1 mL or less

micropipetter / a mechanical pipetter that can measure or deliver very small volumes, usually 1 mL or less

microscope arm / the portion of the microscope that connects the lenses to the base

microscope base / the portion of the microscope that rests on the table and supports the microscope

midstream urine / a urine sample collected from the mid-portion of a urine stream

Miller reticle / a reticle that imposes two squares over the field of view and that is used for reticulocyte counts

milli / prefix used to indicate one-thousandth (10^{-3}) of a unit

minimum inhibitory concentration (MIC) / minimum concentration of an antibiotic required to inhibit the growth of a microorganism

molar solution (M) / solution containing 1 mole of solute per liter of solution

mole / formula weight of a substance expressed in grams

molecular weight (M.W.) / the sum of the atomic weights of the atoms in a molecule or compound formula; formula weight

monochromator / a device that isolates a narrow portion of the light spectrum

monoclonal antibody / antibody derived from a single cell line or clone

monocular / having one ocular or eyepiece

monocyte / a large leukocyte usually having a convoluted or horseshoe-shaped nucleus

mordant / a substance that fixes a dye or stain to an object

morphology / the form and structure of cells, tissues, and organs

mucus / a substance secreted by cells lining the urethra and vagina and that can be present in urine

mutagen / a substance or agent, such as radiation, certain chemicals, or some viruses, that causes a stable change in a gene that can then be passed on to offspring

mycelium / mass of hyphae that makes up the vegetative body of a fungus

Mycobacterium tuberculosis / an acid-fast bacillus that causes tuberculosis

mycology / the study of fungi

mycoplasma / the smallest free-living group of bacteria (class Mollicutes) that lack a cell wall and grow in the absence of oxygen; mollicutes

mycosis / infection caused by fungi

myocardial infarction (MI) / heart attack caused by obstruction of the blood supply to or within the heart

myoglobin / a pigmented, oxygen-carrying protein found in muscle tissue

N

nano / prefix used to indicate one-billionth (10^{-9}) of a unit

National Accrediting Agency for Clinical Laboratory Sciences (NAACLS) / agency that accredits educational programs for clinical laboratory personnel

National Committee for Clinical Laboratory Standards (NCCLS) / see Clinical and Laboratory Standards Institute (CLSI)

National Credentialing Agency for Laboratory Personnel (NCA) / a credentialing agency for clinical laboratory personnel that merged with the ASCP Board of Registry (BOR) in 2009 to form the ASCP Board of Certification (BOC)

National Institute for Occupational Safety and Health (NIOSH) / federal agency responsible for workplace safety research and that makes recommendations for preventing work-related illness and injury

National Institute of Standards and Technology (NIST) / a federal agency that promotes international standardization of measurements; formerly the National Bureau of Standards

National Phlebotomy Association (NPA) / professional society and credentialing agency for phlebotomists

nematode / roundworm; any unsegmented worm of the class Nematoda

nephelometry / an analytical technique used to measure light scatter by particles in solution

nephron / the structural and functional unit of the kidney composed of a glomerulus, Bowman's capsule, and its associated renal tubule

nephropathy / general term for kidney disease

nephrotoxic / toxic or destructive to kidney cells

neutrophil / a leukocyte containing neutral-staining cytoplasmic granules and a segmented nucleus; also called polymorphonuclear cell (PMN), poly, or seg

neutrophilia / abnormal increase in the number of neutrophils in the blood

nocturia / excessive urination at night

noncritical measurements / estimated measurements; measurements made in containers that estimate volume (such as beakers)

nongonococcal urethritis / gonorrhea-like STD caused by micro organisms other than gonococci

nonpathogenic / not normally causing disease in a healthy individual

normal flora / microorganisms normally present at a specific body site and that do not cause disease in healthy individuals

normality (N) / the number of gram equivalents of a compound per liter of solution

normochromic / having normal color

normocytic / having a normal cell size

nosepiece / revolving unit to which microscope objectives are attached

nosocomial infection / an infection acquired in a hospital or health-care facility; healthcare-associated infection

NSAIDs / acronym for nonsteroidal anti-inflammatory drugs

nucleated red blood cell (NRBC) / an immature red blood cell that has not yet lost its nucleus

nucleus (pl. nuclei) / the central structure of a cell that contains DNA and controls cell growth and function

numerical aperture (N.A.) / a mathematical expression of the resolving power of a lens

O

objective / magnifying lens closest to the object being viewed with a microscope

occult / concealed or hidden

Occupational Safety and Health Act (OSH Act) / congressional act of 1970 created to help reduce on-the-job illnesses, injuries, and deaths and requiring employers to provide safe working conditions

Occupational Safety and Health Administration (OSHA) / the federal agency that creates workplace safety regulations and enforces the Occupational Safety and Health Act of 1970

ocular / eyepiece of the microscope that contains a magnifying lens

ocular micrometer / a clear glass disk that fits in the microscope eyepiece, is etched with a precise scale, and is used to measure objects viewed with the microscope; also called ocular reticle

oliguria / decreased production of urine

oocyst / the infectious, thick-walled, resistant stage of coccidian parasites, such as *Toxoplasma* and *Cryptosporidium*, which is found in the definitive host of the parasite

opalescent / having a milky iridescence

opportunistic parasite / an organism that causes disease only in immunocompromised hosts

opportunistic pathogen / a microorganism that causes disease only when the host's normal defense mechanisms are impaired or absent

oral glucose tolerance test (OGTT) / analysis of blood glucose at timed intervals following ingestion of a standard glucose dose

order of draw / a prescribed order for filling vacuum tubes during blood collection to prevent contaminating one tube with the additive of another

other potentially infectious materials (OPIM) / any and all body fluids, tissues, organs, or other specimens from a human source

ova / eggs

oxidase test / an enzyme test used to identify certain bacteria such as *Neisseria*

oxyhemoglobin / the form of hemoglobin that binds and transports oxygen

P

packed cell column / the layers of blood cells that form when a tube of whole blood is centrifuged

palpate / to examine by touch

pandemic / widespread disease transmitted person to person and occurring over an entire country, continent, or even worldwide

parasite / an organism that lives in or on another species and at the expense of that species

parasitemia / parasites in the blood

parasitology / the study of parasites

parenteral / any route other than by the alimentary canal; intravenous, subcutaneous, intramuscular, or mucosal

parfocal / having objectives that can be interchanged without varying the instrument's focus

paroxysm(s) / the cycle(s) of chills and fever associated with malaria that occur 36 to 72 hours apart, depending on the *Plasmodium* species

partial thromboplastin / the lipid portion of thromboplastin, available as a commercial preparation; formerly called cephaloplastin

pathogen / an organism or agent capable of causing disease in a host

pathogenic / capable of causing damage or injury to the host

pathologist / a physician specially trained in the nature and cause of disease

percent solution / a solution made by adding units of solute per 100 units of total solution

percent transmittance (%T) / the percentage of light that passes through a solution

pericardial fluid / the fluid within the pericardial sac

peritoneum / a membrane lining the abdominal cavity and containing a fluid that keeps abdominal organs from adhering to the abdominal wall; parietal peritoneum

peroxidase / an enzyme that converts hydrogen peroxide to water and oxygen

personal protective equipment (PPE) / specialized clothing or equipment used by workers to protect from direct exposure to blood or other potentially infectious or hazardous materials; includes, but is not limited to, gloves, laboratory apparel, eye protection, and breathing apparatus

petechiae / small, purplish hemorrhagic spots on the skin; very small purpura

petri dish / a shallow, round covered dish made of plastic or glass primarily used to culture microorganisms

pH / a measurement of the hydrogen ion concentration expressing the degree of acidity or alkalinity of a solution

phagocytosis / the engulfing of a foreign particle or cell by another cell

pharyngeal / having to do with the back of the throat or pharynx

phenotype / the observable characteristics in a cell or organism as determined both by genetic makeup and environmental factors

phenylketonuria (PKU) / an inherited condition in which the amino acid phenylalanine is not metabolized, but is excreted into the urine and causes urine to have a mousy or musty odor

phlebotomist / a healthcare worker trained in blood collection

phlebotomy / venipuncture; entry of a vein with a needle

physician office laboratory (POL) / small medical laboratory located within a physician office, group practice, or clinic

physiological saline / 0.85% (0.15 M) sodium chloride solution

pico / prefix used to indicate 10^{-12} of a unit

picogram / 10^{-12} gram

pinworm / *Enterobius vermicularis*, a small parasitic nematode; seatworm

pipet / a slender calibrated tube for measuring and transferring liquids

plasma / the liquid portion of blood in which the blood cells are suspended; the straw-colored liquid remaining after blood cells are removed from anticoagulated blood

plasma / the liquid portion of blood in which the blood cells are suspended; the straw-colored liquid remaining after blood cells are removed from anticoagulated blood

plasma cell / a differentiated B lymphocyte that produces antibodies

plasmin / an enzyme that binds to fibrin and initiates breakdown of the fibrin clot (fibrinolysis)

plasminogen / the inactive precursor of plasmin

Plasmodium / the protozoan genus that includes the organisms causing human malaria

platelet / a formed element in circulating blood that plays an important role in blood coagulation; a small disk-shaped fragment of cytoplasm derived from a megakaryocyte; a thrombocyte

pleomorphic / having varied shapes

pleural fluid / the fluid in the space between the pleural membrane of the lung and the inner chest wall

poikilocytosis / significant variation in the shape of red blood cells

point-of-care testing (POCT) / testing outside the traditional laboratory setting; also called bedside testing, off-site testing, near-patient testing or alternative-site testing

polychromatic / having many colors

polyclonal antibodies / antibodies derived from more than one cell line

polycythemia / an excess of red blood cells in the peripheral blood

polyethylene / plastic polymer of ethylene used for containers

polyp / growth of tissue projecting from a mucous membrane

polypropylene / lightweight plastic polymer of propylene that resists moisture and solvents and withstands heat sterilization

polystyrene / clear, colorless polymer of styrene used for labware

polyuria / excessive production of urine

population / the entire group of items or individuals from which the samples under consideration are presumed to have come

porphyrins / a group of light-sensitive, pigmented, ringed chemical structures that are required for the synthesis of hemoglobin

postprandial / after eating

precipitation / formation of an insoluble antigen–antibody complex

precision / reproducibility of results; the closeness of obtained values to each other

prefix / modifying word or syllable(s) placed at the beginning of a word

primary amebic encephalitis (PAM) / rare and usually fatal central nervous system infection caused by *Naegleria fowleri* amebae

primary lymphoid organs / organs in which B and T lymphocytes acquire their special characteristics; in humans, the bone marrow and thymus

primary medium / a medium that provides nutritional requirements for an microorganism and is used to recover the microorganism from a specimen

proficiency testing (PT) / a program in which a laboratory's accuracy in performing analyses is evaluated at regular intervals and compared to the performance of similar laboratories

progeny / offspring or descendants

proglottid (pl. proglottids) / the tapeworm body segment that contains the male and female reproductive organs

proinsulin / a precursor of insulin

proportion / relationship in number or amount of one portion compared to another portion or to the whole; ratio

protective isolation / an isolation category designed to protect highly susceptible patients from exposure to infectious agents; reverse isolation

proteinuria / protein in the urine, usually albumin

prothrombin / the precursor of thrombin; factor II

prothrombin ratio / a comparison of a patient's prothrombin time result with the mean of the prothrombin time of a normal population

prothrombin time test / a coagulation screening test used to monitor oral anticoagulant therapy

protozoa / unicellular eukaryotic organisms, both free-living and parasitic

Provider-Performed Microscopy Procedure (PPMP) / a certificate category under CLIA '88 that permits a laboratory to perform waived tests and also permits specified practitioners to perform on-site microscopy procedures

proximal convoluted tubule / the portion of a renal tubule that collects the filtrate from Bowman's capsule

pseudopod/pseudopodium (pl. pseudopods/pseudopodia) / a temporary extension of cytoplasm of certain single-celled organisms such as ameba, that is used for movement and feeding

pulmonary embolism (PE) / occlusion of a pulmonary artery or one of its branches, usually caused by an embolus that originated in a deep vein of the leg or pelvis

purpura / purple-colored areas that can occur in the skin, mucous membranes, or organs and that are caused when small blood vessels leak

PVA / polyvinyl alcohol, a preservative used for fecal specimens

pyelitis / inflammation of the renal pelvis, usually caused by an infection

pyelonephritis / inflammation of the kidney and the renal pelvis, usually caused by an infection

Q

quadrant / one-fourth of a circle; one-fourth of an agar plate

quality assessment (QA) / in the laboratory, a program that monitors the total testing process with the aim of providing the highest quality patient care

quality control (QC) / a system that verifies the reliability of analytical test results through the use of standards, controls, and statistical analysis

quality systems (QS) / in an institution, a comprehensive program in which all areas of operation are monitored to ensure quality with the aim of providing the highest quality patient care

quartz glass / expensive glass with excellent light transmission; glass used for cuvettes; silica glass

R

radioisotope / an unstable form of an element that emits radiation and can be incorporated into diagnostic tests, medical therapies, and biomedical research; radioactive isotope

random error / error that is inconsistent and whose source cannot be definitely identified

random urine specimen / a urine specimen collected at any time, without regard to diet or time of day

ratio / relationship in number or degree between two things

reagent / substance or solution used in laboratory analyses; substance involved in a chemical reaction

reactive lymphocyte / see atypical lymphocyte

reagent / substance or solution used in laboratory analyses; substance involved in a chemical reaction

reciprocal / inverse; one of a pair of numbers (as 2/3 and 3/2) that has a product of one

recombinant / referring to molecules or cells created as a result of genetic engineering

red blood cell (RBC) / blood cell that transports oxygen (O_2) to tissues and carbon dioxide (CO_2) to the lungs; erythrocyte

red blood cell indices / calculated values that compare the size and hemoglobin content of red blood cells in a blood sample to reference values; erythrocyte indices

reference laboratory / an independent regional laboratory that offers routine and specialized testing services to hospitals and physicians

reflectance photometer / an instrument that measures the light reflected from a colored reaction product

refractive index / the ratio of the speed of light in air to the speed of light in a solution

refractometer / an instrument for measuring the refractive index of a substance; also called a total solids meter

renal hilus / the concavity in the kidney where nerves and vessels enter or exit

renal pelvis / the funnel-shaped expansion of the upper portion of the ureter that receives urine from the renal tubules

renal threshold / the blood concentration above which a substance not normally excreted by the kidneys appears in urine

renal tubule / a small tube of the nephron that collects and concentrates urine

reservoir host / a host, other than the usual host, in which the parasite lives and is infectious

resolving power / the ability of a microscope to produce separate images of two closely spaced objects

reticle / a glass circle etched with a pattern of calibrated grids, lines, or circles and inserted into a microscope eyepiece to allow the etched pattern to be imposed on the field of view

reticulocyte / an immature erythrocyte that still contains RNA remnants in the cytoplasm

reticulocytopenia / a decrease below the normal number of reticulocytes in the circulating blood

reticulocytosis / an increase above the normal number of reticulocytes in the circulating blood

reticulum / a filamentous network

reverse grouping / the use of known cells (antigens) to identify unknown antibodies in the patient's serum or plasma

reverse osmosis / purification of water by forcing water through a semi-permeable membrane

Rh D immune globulin (RhIG) / a concentrated, purified solution of human anti-D antibody used for injection

rheumatoid arthritis (RA) / an autoimmune disease characterized by pain, inflammation, and deformity of the joints

rheumatoid factors (RF) / autoantibodies directed against the Fc fragment of human immunoglobulin G (IgG) and often present in the serum of patients with rheumatoid arthritis

ribonucleic acid (RNA) / the nucleic acid that is important in protein synthesis and is found in all living cells

rotor / the part of a centrifuge that holds the tubes and rotates during the operation of the centrifuge

rouleau(x) / group(s) of red blood cells arranged like a roll of coins

S

sample / in statistics, a subgroup of a population

SARS / the acronym for severe acute respiratory syndrome, a condition caused by a coronavirus

schizocyte / a fragmented red blood cell; formerly called schistocyte

scleroderma / a systemic or localized autoimmune connective tissue disease characterized by a chronic hardening (*sclero*) of skin (*derma*) and connective tissue

secondary lymphoid tissue / tissues in which lymphocytes are concentrated, such as the spleen, lymph nodes, and tonsils

sediment / solids that settle to the bottom of a liquid

sedimentation / the process of solid particles settling to the bottom of a liquid

selective medium / a bacteriological medium that contains chemicals or substances that allow growth of some organisms while inhibiting growth of others

sepsis / the presence of microorganisms and/or their toxic products in the blood or other tissues

septicemia / the presence and growth of pathogenic microorganisms in the blood

sequestered / isolated or set apart from the whole

seroconversion / the appearance of antibody in the serum to plasma of an individual following exposure to an antigen

serological centrifuge / a centrifuge that spins small tubes such as those used in blood banking; serofuge

serology / the study of antigens and antibodies in serum using immunological methods; laboratory testing based on the immunological properties of serum

serum / the liquid obtained from blood that has been allowed to clot

sexually transmitted disease (STD) / a disease transmitted by sexual contact; also sexually transmitted infection

sexually transmitted infection (STI) / a infection transmitted by sexual contact; also sexually transmitted disease

shift / an abrupt change from the established mean indicated by the occurrence of all control values on one side of the mean

shift to the left / the appearance of an increased number of immature neutrophil forms in the peripheral blood

SI units / standardized units of measure; international units

sickle cell / crescent- or sickle-shaped red cell; drepanocyte

sickle cell disease / inherited blood disorder in which red blood cells can form a sickle shape because of the presence of hemoglobin S

Sjögren's syndrome / a systemic autoimmune disease affecting moisture-producing glands such as tear, sweat, and saliva glands but also affecting organs

solid-phase chemistry / an analytical method in which the sample is added to a strip or slide containing all the reagents for the procedure in dried form

solute / the substance dissolved in a given solution

solution / a homogeneous mixture of two or more substances

solvent / a dissolving agent, usually a liquid

specific gravity (sp. gr.) / the ratio of the weight of a solution to the weight of an equal volume of distilled water; a measurement of density

spectrophotometer / an instrument that measures intensities of light at selected wave lengths

spiral bacteria / motile bacteria having a helical or spiral shape

spirochetes / motile, helical, or spiral bacteria of the family Spirochaeta

sporozoite / the banana-shaped motile infective stage of certain apicomplexan protozoa such as *Toxoplasma*, *Cryptosporidium*, and *Plasmodium*; in *Plasmodium*, the stage present in mosquito salivary glands that is introduced into blood by mosquito bite

stage / platform that holds the object to be viewed microscopically

stage micrometer / a transparent glass slide marked with a precise scale in micrometers and used to calibrate ocular micrometers by aligning the ocular scale with the stage scale

standard / a chemical solution of a known concentration that can be used as a reference or calibration substance

standard deviation (*s*) / a measure of the spread of a population of values around the mean

standard operating procedure (SOP) / established procedure to be followed for a given operation or in a given situation with the purpose of ensuring that a procedure is always carried out correctly and in the same manner

Standard Precautions / a set of comprehensive safety guidelines designed to protect patients and healthcare workers by requiring that all patients and all body fluids, body substances, organs, and unfixed tissues be regarded as potentially infectious

STAT / immediately (from the Latin word *statim*)

statistics / the branch of mathematics that deals with the collection, classification, analysis, and interpretation of numerical data; a collection of quantitative data

stem / main part of a word; root word; the part of a word remaining after removing the prefix or suffix

stem cell / an undifferentiated cell

sterilization / the act of eliminating all living microorganisms from an article or area

stomatocyte / red blood cell with an elongated, mouth-shaped central area of pallor

Streptococcus pyogenes / bacterium that causes a common type of streptococcal infection, most notably "strep" throat

suffix / modifying word or syllable(s) placed at the end of a word

supernatant / the clear liquid remaining at the top of a solution after centrifugation or the settling out of solid substances in a solution; the liquid lying above sediment

supravital stain / a nontoxic dye used to stain living cells or tissues

synovial / of, or relating to, the lubricating fluid of the joints

synovial fluid / a viscous fluid secreted by membranes lining the joints

syphilis / an infectious, chronic, sexually transmitted disease caused by a spirochete, *Treponema pallidum*

syringe / a hollow, tube-like container with a plunger, used for withdrawing fluids or for injections

systematic error / error that is introduced into a test system and is not a random occurrence

systemic circulation / the system of blood vessels that carries blood from the heart to the tissues and back to the heart

T

T lymphocyte (T cell) / the type of lymphocyte responsible for the cell-mediated immune response

tachyzoite / a rapidly multiplying stage in the development of the tissue phase of certain coccidianas, as in acute *Toxoplasma gondii* infections

tare / in chemical analysis, a determination of the net weight of a chemical by subtracting the weight of the container from the overall weight of the container and the chemical being weighed

target cell / abnormal red blood cell with target appearance; codocyte

TC / on pipets, a mark indicating *to contain*

TD / on pipets, a mark indicating *to deliver*

teratogen / a substance or agent capable of causing birth defects by direct harm to a fetus or embryo, or by interfering with normal fetal development

teratogenic / relating to a substance or agent capable of leading to birth defects by causing change or harm to a fetus or embryo, or interfering with normal fetal development

terminology / terms used in any specialized field

thalassemia / a genetic disorder involving underproduction of the globin chains of hemoglobin and resulting in anemia

thrombin / a protein formed from prothrombin by the action of thromboplastin and other factors in the presence of calcium ions; factor II_a

thrombocyte / a blood platelet

thrombocytopathy / abnormal platelet function

thrombocytopenia / abnormally low number of platelets in the blood

thrombocytosis / abnormally high number of platelets in the blood; thrombocythemia

thromboembolism / blockage of a blood vessel by a clot (thrombus) that formed in another vessal

thromboplastin / a lipoprotein found in endothelium and other tissue; coagulation factor III; also called tissue factor

thrombotic thrombocytopenic purpura (TTP) / a blood disorder with varied causes and characterized by formation of clots in the small vessels, consumption of platelets, and skin purpura

thrombus (pl. thrombi) / a blood clot that obstructs a blood vessel

thymus / a gland located in the upper chest that is the primary lymphoid tissue in which T lymphocytes mature and acquire T cell characteristics

thyroid-stimulating hormone (TSH) / a hormone that is synthesized by the anterior pituitary gland and that regulates the activity of the thyroid gland; thyrotropin

thyroxine / a thyroid hormone, commonly called T_4

tissue cyst / intracellular cysts located within host tissues and containing organisms in a state of reduced metabolism that can survive and remain infectious for years

titer / in serology, the reciprocal of the highest dilution that gives the desired reaction; the concentration of a substance determined by titration

tourniquet / a band used to constrict blood flow

Transmission-Based Precautions / specific safety practices used in addition to Standard Precautions when treating patients known to be or suspected of being infected with pathogens that can be spread by air, droplet, or contact

transplant / living tissue placed into the body; the placing of living tissue into the body

transport medium / containers specially designed to provide nutrients and an environment that preserves the viability of microorganisms during transport

trematode / fluke; any parasitic flatworm of the class Trematoda

trend / an indication of error in the analysis, detected by increasing or decreasing values in the control sample

trichomoniasis / a sexually transmitted genitourinary tract infection caused by the parasitic protozoan *Trichomonas vaginalis*

trichrome stain / a stain commonly used to identify parasites in fecal smears

triglycerides / the major storage form of lipids; lipid molecules formed from glycerol and fatty acids

triiodothyronine / one of the thyroid hormones, commonly called T_3

trophoblastic / relating to embryonic nutritive tissue

trophozoite / the motile feeding stage of protozoan parasites

troponins / intracellular proteins present in skeletal and heart muscle and that are released when muscle is injured

trypomastigote / the characteristic developmental stage of trypanosomes, which has a leaf-like form, an undulating membrane, and usually a free flagellum

tubular necrosis / death of the tissue comprising the renal tubules

turbid / having a cloudy appearance

U

Universal Precautions (UP) / a method of infection control in which all human blood and other body fluids containing visible blood are treated as if infectious

ureter / the tube carrying urine from the kidney to the urinary bladder

urethra / the canal through which urine is discharged from the urinary bladder

urethritis / infection or inflammation of the urethra

uric acid / a breakdown product of nucleic acids

urinary bladder / an organ for the temporary storage of urine

urinary tract infection (UTI) / an infection of the urinary tract, usually of the urethra

urine / excretory fluid produced by the kidneys

urinometer / a float with a calibrated stem used for measuring specific gravity of urine; hydrometer

urobilinogen / breakdown product of bilirubin formed by the action of intestinal bacteria

urochrome / the yellow pigment that gives urine its color

V

vacuole / a membrane-bound compartment in cell cytoplasm

vaginitis / infection or inflammation of the vagina

valence / the positive or negative charge of a molecule; a number representing the combining power of an atom

variance (s^2) / the square of the standard deviation; mean square deviation

vasoconstriction / narrowing of the diameter of a blood vessel

vector / an agent that transports a pathogen from an infected host to a noninfected host

vein / a blood vessel that carries deoxygenated blood from the tissues to the heart

venereal / having to do with, or transmitted by, sexual contact

venipuncture / entry of a vein with a needle; a phlebotomy

venule / a small vein connecting a capillary to a vein vessel

virion / the infectious form of a virus

virology / the study of viruses

virulent / highly infectious or highly pathogenic

vitamin B$_{12}$ / a vitamin essential to the proper maturation of blood cells and other cells in the body

vitamin K / a vitamin essential for production of coagulation factors II, VII, IX, and X

VLDL cholesterol / very low density lipoprotein fraction of blood cholesterol

von Willebrand's disease (vWD) / an inherited platelet disorder associated with decreased platelet adhesion and a bleeding tendency

W

waived test / a category of test defined under CLIA '88 as being simple to perform and having an insignificant risk for error

warfarin / an anticoagulant drug taken to prevent blood clotting or to reduce the risk of clots

Westergren pipet / a slender pipet marked from 0 to 200 mm, used in the Westergren erythrocyte sedimentation rate method

Westgard's rules / a set of rules used to determine when a method is out of control

white blood cell (WBC) / blood cell that functions in immunity; leukocyte

winged collection set / a short, small-gauge needle with attached plastic tabs (wings), 6 or more inches of tubing, and a Luer-Lok or vacuum tube holder connector; sometimes called a "butterfly" set

Wintrobe tube / a slender, thick-walled tube used in the Wintrobe erythrocyte sedimentation rate

work practice controls / methods of performing tasks that reduce the worker's exposure to blood and other potentially hazardous materials

working distance / distance between the microscope objective and the microscope slide when the object is in sharp focus

wound / a break in the continuity of soft parts of the body structure; trauma to tissues

Wright's stain / a combination of eosin and methylene blue in methanol; a polychromatic stain

X

XDPs / degradation products formed by plasmin action on cross-linked fibrin and containing the D-dimer cross-linked region

Y

yeast / a small, single-celled eukaryotic fungus that reproduces by fission or budding

Z

zone of inhibition / in the Bauer-Kirby antibiotic susceptibility test, the area around an antibiotic disk in which bacterial growth is inhibited

zoonotic / infection or disease that can be transmitted from vertebrate animals to humans

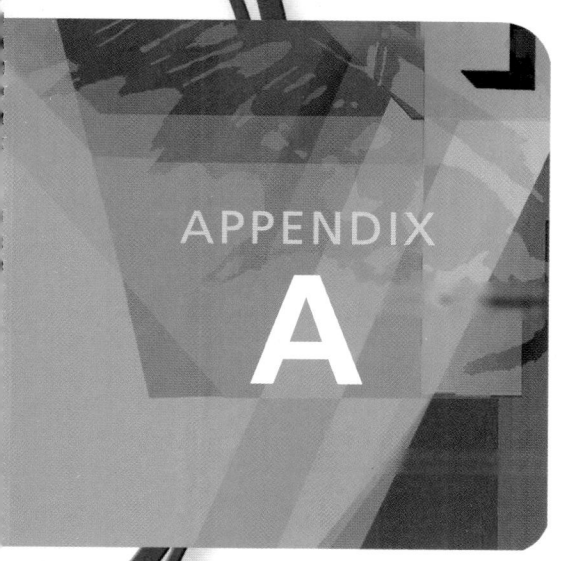

APPENDIX A

Guide to Standard Precautions

STANDARD PRECAUTIONS

A set of preventive measures used as the primary method of preventing transmission of infection in healthcare settings.

Standard Precautions:

- Apply to all persons, both patients and staff, in healthcare facilities
- Assume that every person is potentially infectious and susceptible to infection
- Assume that all body fluids, tissues, secretions, and excretions are potentially infectious
- Use physical, mechanical, and chemical barriers to prevent the spread of infection

KEY COMPONENTS OF IMPLEMENTING STANDARD PRECAUTIONS

Hand Hygiene—the most important procedure for preventing cross-contamination

Wash hands with soap and water when visibly soiled or contaminated, and after every 10-12 uses of antiseptic handrubs or foams.

Wash hands or use antiseptic handrub:

- immediately before gloving and after removing gloves
- between patient contacts

- after touching blood, body fluids, secretions, excretions and contaminated items with gloved hands
- immediately after removing damaged gloves

Use Physical Barriers if Splashes or Spills of Any Body Fluids are Likely

Physical barriers include personal protective equipment (PPE) such as gloves, gown, mask, goggles, and face shield.

- Wear PPE when contact with any body fluid is reasonably anticipated
- Wear gloves before touching broken skin, mucous membranes, any body fluids, soiled instruments, contaminated waste materials, and before performing invasive procedures
- Wear gown to protect skin and prevent contamination of clothing
- Wear mask and goggles or face shield to protect mucous membranes of eyes, nose and mouth during procedures that can generate aerosols or sprays of blood or other body fluids
- Educate patients and healthcare personnel in cough etiquette
- Remove gown, discard PPE, and perform hand hygiene before leaving the patient's environment

Needlestick Prevention and Sharps Disposal

Discard used needles, scalpels and other sharps into rigid, puncture-proof containers immediately after use. Locate sharps containers near the point of use.

889

- Use safety needles and needle safety devices
- Do not attempt to recap used needles
- Do not remove used needles from disposable syringes
- Do not attempt to manipulate used needles by hand

Patient Placement

Place patients who can contaminate the environment or cannot maintain appropriate hygiene in private rooms.

Patient Environment and Equipment

Routinely clean and decontaminate furniture in patient care areas and surfaces (fomites) of mobile equipment, reusable equipment, and items that are used by patients or are used in delivery of patient care. Wear PPE when handling and disinfecting patient-care equipment and instruments.

Decontamination and Sterilization of Instruments

Process instruments, and other sterilizable items after use by first decontaminating and thoroughly cleaning them; the items must then be either sterilized or disinfected using high-level disinfection, following the recommended procedures.

Laundry

Handle used linens and fabrics with minimum agitation to prevent contamination of air, surfaces and persons. Do not allow soiled linens to contact skin or mucous membranes.

Infectious Waste Disposal

Dispose of infectious waste materials in a manner that protects and prevents injury or possible infection to personnel and to the community.

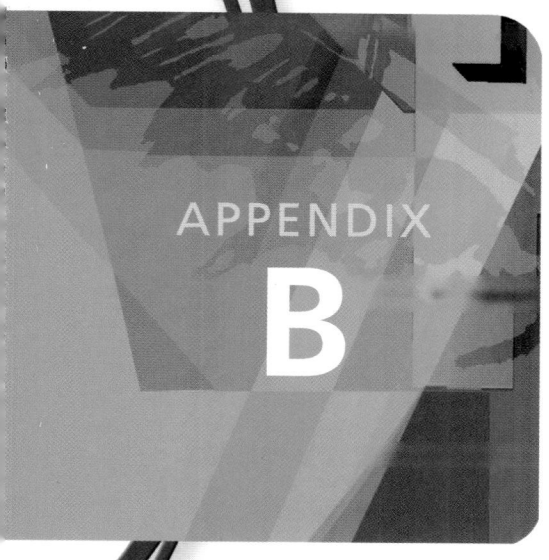

Laboratory Reference Values

HEMATOLOGY AND COAGULATION

TEST	REFERENCE RANGE	
Hemoglobin:	**CONVENTIONAL UNITS**	**SI UNITS**
Newborn	16–23 g/dL	160–230 g/L
Children	10–14 g/dL	100–140 g/L
Adult males	13–17 g/dL	130–170 g/L
Adult females	12–15 g/dL	120–150 g/L
Microhematocrit:		
Newborn	51–61%	0.51–0.61
One year	32–38%	0.32–0.38
Six years	34–42%	0.34–0.42
Adult males	42–52%	0.42–0.52
Adult females	36–48%	0.36–0.48
Red Blood Cell Counts:		
Adult males	$4.5\text{–}6.0 \times 10^6/\mu L$	$4.5\text{–}6.0 \times 10^{12}/L$
Adult females	$4.0\text{–}5.5 \times 10^6/\mu L$	$4.0\text{–}5.5 \times 10^{12}/L$
Newborn	$5.0\text{–}6.3 \times 10^6/\mu L$	$5.0\text{–}6.3 \times 10^{12}/L$
White Blood Cell Counts:		
Newborn	$9.0\text{–}30.0 \times 10^3/\mu L$	$9.0\text{–}30.0 \times 10^9/L$
One year	$6.0\text{–}14.0 \times 10^3/\mu L$	$6.0\text{–}14.0 \times 10^9/L$
Six years	$4.5\text{–}12.0 \times 10^3/\mu L$	$4.5\text{–}12.0 \times 10^9/L$
Adult	$4.5\text{–}11.0 \times 10^3/\mu L$	$4.5\text{–}11.0 \times 10^9/L$
Platelet Count	$1.5\text{–}4.0 \times 10^5/\mu L$	$1.5\text{–}4.0 \times 10^{11}/L$

White Cell Differential Count:					Absolute Cell Counts (cells/µL)
White Blood Cell	*1 month*	*6-year-old*	*12-year-old*	*Adult*	*Adult*
Neutrophil (seg)	15%–35%	45%–50%	45%–50%	50%–65%	2250–7150
Neutrophil (band)	7%–13%	0–7%	6%–8%	0–7%	0–770
Eosinophil	1%–3%	1%–3%	1%–3%	1%–3%	45–330
Basophil	0–1%	0–1%	0–1%	0–1%	0–110
Monocyte	5%–8%	4%–8%	3%–8%	3%–9%	135–990
Lymphocyte	40%–70%	40%–45%	35%–40%	25%–40%	1125–4400
Platelets	An average of 7–20 platelets per oil-immersion field is considered normal				

(continues)

TEST	REFERENCE RANGE
Red Blood Cell Indices:	
Mean Cell Volume (MCV)	80–98 fL
Mean Cell Hemoglobin (MCH)	27–32 pg
Mean Cell Hemoglobin Concentration (MCHC)	32–37%
Reticulocyte Percentages:	
Newborn	2.5–6.5%
Adult	0.5–1.5%
Erythrocyte Sedimentation Rate (ESR)	
Wintrobe method (one-hour)	
Adult males	0–9 mm/hr
Adult females	0–20 mm/hr
One-hour Sediplast ESR	
Males < 50 years	0–15 mm/hr
> 50 years	0–20 mm/hr
Females < 50 years	0–20 mm/hr
> 50 years	0–30 mm/hr
ZSR (all ages)	
Normal	40–51%
Borderline	51–54%
Elevated	≥55%

COAGULATION TEST	REFERENCE RANGE
Bleeding Time:	
Ivy method	2–9 min
ACT (Hemochron Jr.)	81–125 sec
Prothrombin Time – Citrated plasma	
Plasma	10–13 sec
INR	1.0–1.4
Prothrombin Time – Hemochron Jr.	
Whole blood	20–26 sec
Plasma equivalent*	8–15 sec
INR*	0.8–1.5
Activated Partial Thromboplastin Time – Plasma	
Citrated plasma	24–34 sec
Activated Partial Thromboplastin Time – Hemochron Jr.	
Whole blood	93.2–116.8 sec
Plasma equivalent*	20.6–38.6 sec

mathematically derived

URINE REFERENCE VALUES

URINE VOLUME (AGE)	REFERENCE RANGE (mL/24 HOURS)
Newborn	20–350
One year	300–600
Ten years	750–1500
Adult	750–2000

URINALYSIS	REFERENCE VALUES
Color	pale yellow to amber
Transparency	clear
Specific gravity	1.010–1.025
pH	5.0–8.0
Protein	Negative to trace
Glucose	Negative

(continues)

URINALYSIS	REFERENCE VALUES
Ketone	Negative
Bilirubin	Negative
Blood	Negative
Urobilinogen	0.0–1.0 mg/dL
Bacteria (nitrite)	Negative
Leukocyte esterase	Negative
RBC/HPF*	0–4
WBC/HPF	0–4
Epith/HPF	Occasional (may be higher in females)
Casts/LPF**	Occasional hyaline
Bacteria	Negative
Yeasts	Negative
Mucus	Negative to 2+
Crystals	Only crystals such as cystine, leucine, tyrosine, and cholesterol are considered clinically significant

*HPF = high power field
**LPF = low power field

CLINICAL CHEMISTRY REFERENCE VALUES

	REFERENCE RANGES*	
ANALYTE MEASURED	**CONVENTIONAL UNITS**	**SI UNITS**
Alanine aminotransferase (ALT)	3–30 U/L	3–30 U/L
Albumin	3.8–5.0 g/dL	38–50 g/L
Alkaline phosphatase (AP)	20–130 U/L	20–130 U/L
Aspartate aminotransferase (AST)	10–37 U/L	10–37 U/L
Bicarbonate (Total CO_2)	22–28 mEq/L	22–28 mmol/L
Bilirubin (Total)	0.1–1.2 mg/dL	2–21 µmol/L
Bilirubin, Direct	0–0.3 mg/dL	0–6 µmol/L
BNP	100 pg/mL	100 ng/L
BUN	8–18 mg/dL	2.9–6.4 mmol/L
Calcium (ionized)	4.6–5.3 mg/dL	1.15–1.33 mmol/L
Chloride (cl⁻)	98–108 mEq/L	98–108 mmol/L
Cholesterol, Total	140–250 mg/dL (desirable level <200 mg/dL)	3.6–6.5 mmol/L
High-sensitivity C-Reactive Protein (hs-CRP)	Less than 0.5 mg/dL	Less than 5.0 mg/L
Creatine kinase (CK)	30–170 U/L	30–170 U/L
Creatinine kinase (CK-MB)	Less than 14 U/L	Less than 14 U/L
Gamma glutamyltransferase (GGT)	3–40 U/L	3–40 U/L
Glomerular filtration rate (GFR)	Varies with gender and age	
Glucose, serum (fasting)	70–110 mg/dL	3.9-6.1 mol/L
Glucose, plasma (fasting)	66–105 mg/dL	3.7–5.9 mol/L
Glucose, whole blood (fasting)	60–100 mg/dL	3.3-5.6 mol/L
HbA1c (non-diabetic)	4%-5%	
Homocysteine (varies with age)	< 8 µmol/L – < 20 µmol/L	< 8 µmol/L – < 20 µmol/L
Iron	65–165 µg/dL	11.6–29.5 µmol/L
Lactate dehydrogenase (LD)	110–230 U/L	110–230 U/L
Phosphorus (phosphate)	3.0–4.5 mg/dL	0.96–1.44 mmol/L
Potassium (K⁺)	3.8–5.5 mEq/L	3.8–5.5 mmol/L
Sodium (Na⁺)	135–148 mEq/L	135–148 mmol/L
TSH	0.35–5.0 µIU/mL	0.35–5.0 mIU/L
Total Protein	6.0–8.0 g/dL	60–80 g/L
Triglycerides	10–190 mg/dL	0.11–2.15 mmol/L
Uric Acid	3.5–7.5 mg/dL	0.21–0.44 mmol/L

*All reference ranges listed are for serum, unless otherwise indicated. Laboratories must define their own reference intervals.

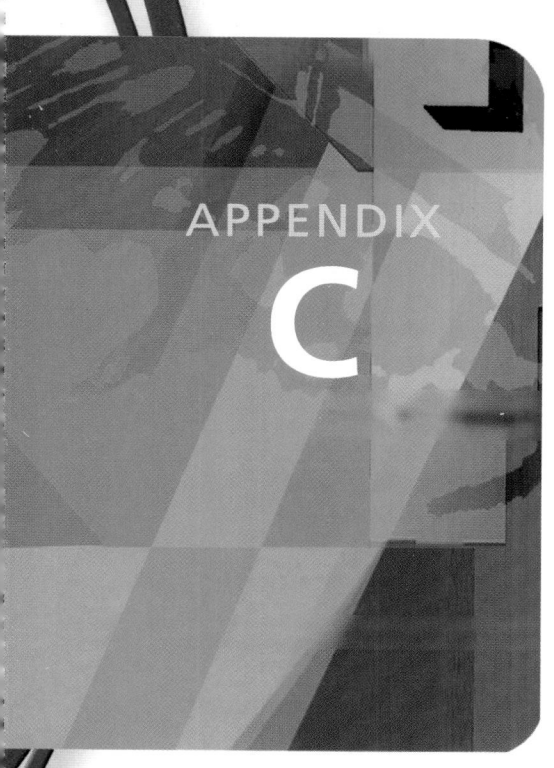

APPENDIX

C

Abbreviations and Acronyms Commonly Used in Medical Laboratories

A	absorbance	CLT	clinical laboratory technician
Ab	antibody	cm	centimeter
ACT	activated clotting time	CNS	central nervous system
AFB	acid-fast bacillus	CO	carbon monoxide
Ag	antigen	CO_2	carbon dioxide
AHG	anti-human globulin	CPD	citrate-phosphate-dextrose
AIDS	acquired immunodeficiency syndrome	CPK	creatine phosphokinase
ALL	acute lymphocytic leukemia	crit	hematocrit
ALP, AP	alkaline phosphatase	CRP	C-reactive protein
ALT	alanine aminotransferase	C & S	culture and sensitivity
AML	acute myelogenous leukemia	CSF	cerebrospinal fluid
ANA	antinuclear antibody	cu mm	cubic millimeter, mm^3
APTT	activated partial thromboplastin time	DAT	direct antiglobulin test
AST	aspartate aminotransferase	dL	deciliter
BA	blood agar	DIC	disseminated intravascular coagulation
bacti	bacteriology	diff	white blood cell differential
BBP	blood-borne pathogen	EBV	Epstein-Barr virus
BP	blood pressure	EDTA	ethylenediaminetetraacetic acid
BSI	body substance isolation	EIA	enzyme immunoassay
BT	bleeding time	EMB	eosin methylene blue
BUN	blood urea nitrogen	ESR	erythrocyte sedimentation rate
C	centigrade, Celsius	E.U.	Ehrlich units
CBC	complete blood count	F	Fahrenheit
cc, ccm	cubic centimeter	FBS	fasting blood sugar
CCU	coronary care unit	FDP	fibrinogen/fibrin degradation products
CFU	colony-forming unit	fL	femtoliter
CGL	chronic granulocytic leukemia	FUO	fever of unknown origin
chol	cholesterol	g	gram
CK	creatine kinase	GC	gonococcus, gonorrhea
Cl	chloride	GFR	glomerular filtration rate
CLL	chronic lymphocytic leukemia	GGT	gamma-glutamyl transferase
CLS	clinical laboratory scientist	GI	gastrointestinal

GTT	glucose tolerance test
GU	genitourinary
HAV	hepatitis A virus
Hb, Hgb	hemoglobin
HBV	hepatitis B virus
hCG	human chorionic gonadotropin
HCl	hydrochloric acid
HCO_3^-	bicarbonate
hs-CRP	high-sensitivity C-reactive protein
Hct	hematocrit
HCV	hepatitis C virus
HDL chol	high-density lipoprotein cholesterol
HDN	hemolytic disease of newborn
H & H	hemoglobin and hematocrit
HIV	human immunodeficiency virus
HLA	human leukocyte antigen
H_2O	water
HPF	high-power field
HSV	herpes simplex virus
ICU	intensive care unit
Ig	immunoglobulin
IgA	immunoglobulin A
IgE	immunoglobulin E
IgG	immunoglobulin G
IgM	immunoglobulin M
IM	infectious mononucleosis
i.m.	intramuscular
ITP	idiopathic thrombocytopenic purpura
IU	international unit
IV, i.v.	intravenous
K	potassium
kg	kilogram
L	liter
LD, LDH	lactate dehydrogenase
LDL chol	low-density lipoprotein cholesterol
LPF	low-power field
µg	microgram
µL, µl	microliter
µmol	micromole
m	meter
M	molar
mcg	microgram
MCH	mean cell hemoglobin
MCHC	mean cell hemoglobin concentration
MCV	mean cell volume
mEq	milliequivalent
mg	milligram
MI	myocardial infarction
MIC	minimum inhibitory concentration
mIU	milli International Unit
mL, ml	milliliter
MLS	medical laboratory scientist
MLT	medical laboratory technician
mm	millimeter
mmol	millimole
mol	mole
MPV	mean platelet volume
MRI	magnetic resonance imaging
MRSA	methicillin-resistant *Staphylococcus aureus*
MSDS	material safety data sheet
MT	medical technologist
N	normal, normality
Na	sodium
NaCl	sodium chloride
nm	nanometer
O.D.	optical density
OGTT	oral glucose tolerance test
O & P	ova and parasites
OPIM	other potentially infectious material
PCV	packed cell volume
pg	picogram
pH	hydrogen ion concentration
PLT	platelet
PMN	polymorphonuclear neutrophil
POC	point of care
POCT	point-of-care test(ing)
POL	physician office laboratory
PP	postprandial
PPE	personal protective equipment
PPM	parts per million
PRC	packed red cells
PSA	prostate specific antigen
PT	prothrombin time, pro-time
QA	quality assessment
QC	quality control
qns	quantity not sufficient
qs	quantity sufficient
RA	rheumatoid arthritis
RBC	red blood cell
RDW	red (cell) distribution width
RF	rheumatoid factors
RhIG	Rh immune globulin
RIA	radioimmunoassay
RNA	ribonucleic acid
rpm	revolutions per minute
RPR	rapid plasma reagin
sed rate	erythrocyte sedimentation rate
SEM	scanning electron microscope
SI	international units (Le Système International d'Unités)
SICU	surgical intensive care unit
sp. gr.	specific gravity
staph	*Staphylococcus*
stat	immediately
STD	sexually transmitted disease
STI	sexually transmitted infection
strep	*Streptococcus*
STS	serological tests for syphilis
TEM	transmission electron microscope
TIA	transient ischemic attack
TIBC	total iron-binding capacity
TSH	thyroid stimulating hormone
UA	urinalysis, uric acid

UP	Universal Precautions
URI	upper respiratory infection
UTI	urinary tract infection
UV	ultraviolet
VD	venereal disease
VDRL	Venereal Disease Research Laboratory
VLDL	very low density lipoproteins
vWF	von Willebrand factor
WBC	white blood cell
XDP	fibrin degradation products

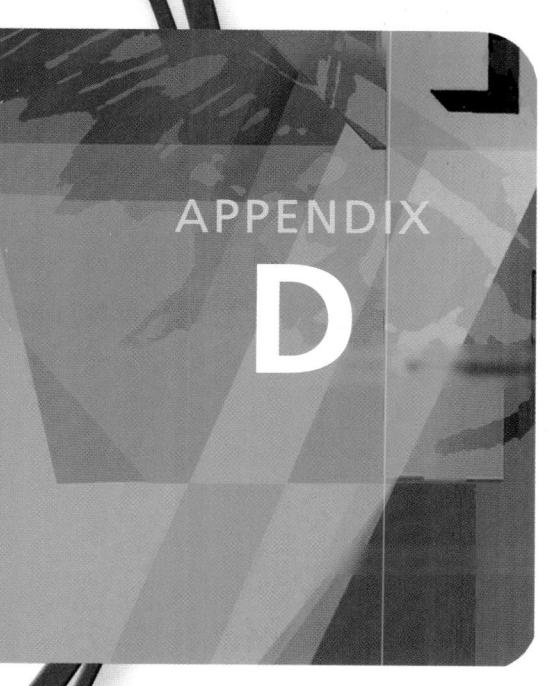

APPENDIX D

Sources of Information: Healthcare Accrediting and Credentialing Agencies, Professional Societies, and Governmental Agencies

Accrediting Agencies

American Association of Blood Banks (AABB)
8101 Glenbrook Road
Bethesda, MD 20814-2749
301.907.6977
www.aabb.org

COLA
9881 Broken Land Parkway, Suite 200
Columbia, MD 21046–1158
800.981.9883
info@COLA.org
www.cola.org

College of American Pathologists, Laboratory Accreditation Program
325 Waukegan Road
Northfield, IL 60093-2750
800.323.4040
www.cap.org

Commission on Accreditation of Allied Health Education Programs (CAAHEP)
1361 Park Street
Clearwater, FL 33756
727.210.2350
mail@caahep.org
www.caahep.org

Council for Higher Education Accreditation (CHEA)
One Dupont Circle Northwest, Suite 510
Washington, DC 20036-1135
202.955.6126
chea@chea.org
www.chea.org

The Joint Commission (JC)
One Renaissance Boulevard
Oakbrook Terrace, IL 60181
630.792.5000
webmaster@jointcommission.org
www.jointcommission.org

National Accrediting Agency for Clinical Laboratory Sciences (NAACLS)
5600 N. River Road, Suite 720
Rosemont, IL 60018
773.714.8880
info@naacls.org
www.naacls.org

Credentialing Agencies, Professional Societies and Other Sources of Information

Advance for Medical Laboratory Professionals
2900 Horizon Drive, Box 61556
King of Prussia, PA 19406-0956
800.355.1088
Publications, laboratorian.advanceweb.com

American Association of Blood Banks (AABB)
8101 Glenbrook Road
Bethesda, MD 20814-2749
301.907.6977
www.aabb.org

American Association for Clinical Chemistry
2101 L Street Northwest, Suite 625
Washington, DC 20037
800.892.1400 or 202.857.0717
www.aacc.org
Journal/Publications: *Clinical Laboratory News, Clinical Chemistry*

899

American Association of Bioanalysts (AAB)
917 Locust Street, Suite 1100
St. Louis, MO 63101-1413
314.241.1445
www.aab.org

American Association of Medical Assistants (AAMA)
20 North Wacker Drive, Suite 1575
Chicago, IL 60606-2903
312.899.1500
www.aama-ntl.org
Journal: *CMA Today*

American Medical Association
515 North State Street
Chicago, IL 60610
800.621.8335
www.ama-assn.org

American Society for Clinical Laboratory Science (ASCLS)
2025 M Street Northwest, Suite 800
Washington DC 20036
202.367.1174
ascls@ascls.org
www.ascls.org

American Society for Clinical Pathology Board of Certification (ASCP BOC)
33 West Monroe Street, Suite 1600
Chicago, IL 60603
800.267.2727
www.ascp.org

American Society for Microbiology (ASM)
1752 N Street Northwest
Washington, DC 20036
202.737.3600
www.asm.org
Journals: *Journal of Clinical Microbiology, Clinical Microbiology Reviews, Clinical and Diagnostic Laboratory Immunology, Journal of Virology*

American Society of Hematology
2021 L Street Northwest, Suite 900
Washington, DC 20036
202.776.0544
www.hematology.org
Journal: *Blood*

American Society of Phlebotomy Technicians (ASPT)
1109 2nd Avenue Southwest
P.O. Box 1831
Hickory, NC 28603
828.294.0078
office@aspt.org
www.aspt.org

Association for Professionals in Infection Control and Epidemiology (APIC)
1275 K Street NW, Suite 1000
Washington, DC 20005-4006
202.789.1890
apicinfo@apic.org
www.apic.org
Journal: *American Journal of Infection Control*

Association of Schools of Allied Health Professions
4400 Jennifer Street Northwest, Suite 333
Washington, DC 20015
202.237.6481
asahp@asahp.org
Journal: *Journal of Allied Health*

Centers for Disease Control and Prevention
1600 Clifton Road
Atlanta, GA 30333
800.311.3435
cdcinfo@cdc.org
www.cdc.gov

Centers for Medicare and Medicaid Services (CMS)
7500 Security Blvd.
Baltimore, MD 21244
www.cms.gov

Clinical and Laboratory Standards Institute (CLSI)
940 West Valley Road, Suite 1400
Wayne, PA 19087-1898
877.447.1888
www.clsi.org

Food and Drug Administration (FDA)
10903 New Hampshire Avenue
Silver Spring, MD 20993
888.INFO.FDA
www.fda.gov

Infection Control Education Institute
3300 North Central Avenue, Suite 300
Phoenix, AZ 85012
800.236.8265
Free online magazine: *Infection Control Today*

National Institute for Occupational Safety and Health (NIOSH)
Centers for Disease Control and Prevention
1600 Clifton Road
Atlanta, GA 30333
800.232.4636
www.cdc.gov/niosh

National Institutes of Health (NIH)
9000 Rockville Pike
Bethesda, MD 20892
e-mail: NIHinfo@od.nih.gov
www.nih.gov

Occupational Safety and Health Administration (OSHA)
U. S. Department of Labor
200 Constitution Avenue
Washington, DC 20210
800.321.OSHA
www.osha.gov

Superintendent of Documents
U. S. Government Printing Office
Washington, DC 20402
866.512.1800
www.gpoaccess.gov

Proficiency Testing
Several private agencies and some state public health laboratories have DHHS approved proficiency testing programs. A listing of approved proficiency testing programs can be obtained through the CDC's Public Health Practice Program Office, Division of Laboratory Systems, www.cdc.gov/dls/

Web sites of interest
American Association for Clinical Chemistry, www.aacc.org (archives of *Clinical Laboratory News*)
American Association of Blood Banks, www.aabb.org
American Cancer Society, www.cancer.org
American Diabetes Association, www.diabetes.org
American Heart Association, www.heart.org
American Red Cross, www.redcross.org
American Society for Microbiology, www.asm.org

Association for Professionals in Infection Control and Epidemiology, www.apic.org
Centers for Disease Control and Prevention, www.cdc.gov
Clinical Laboratory Improvement Amendments, www.cma.gov/clia/
College of American Pathologists, www.cap.org
Digital blood cell morphology software such as CellAtlas iphone application, available free through itunes store at www.apple.com
Federal Drug Administration, www.fda.gov
Lab Tests Online, www.labtestsonline.org
Medscape from WebMD, www.medscape.com
National Cholesterol Education Program, www.nhlbi.nih.gov/about/ncep
National Hemophilia Foundation, www.hemophilia.org
National Institute for Occupational Safety and Health, www.cdc.gov/NIOSH
National Institutes of Health, www.kidney.niddk.nih.gov
National Institutes of Health, www.nih.gov
National Kidney Foundation, www.kidney.org
Occupational Safety and Health Administration, www.osha.gov
World Health Organization, www.who.int

INDEX

Page numbers followed by f and t indicate figures and tables.